BLACKWELL'S
FIVE-MINUTE
VETERINARY
CONSULT

BLACKWELL'S FIVE-MINUTE VETERINARY CONSULT

SMALL MAMMAL

THIRD EDITION

EDITED BY

Barbara L. Oglesbee, DVM, Dipl. ABVP, Dipl. ACEPM
MedVet Avian and Exotics and
The Ohio State University College of Veterinary Medicine
Columbus, Ohio, USA

WILEY Blackwell

Library of Congress Cataloging-in-Publication Data
Names: Oglesbee, Barbara L., editor.
Title: Blackwell's five-minute veterinary consult. Small mammal / edited by
   Barbara L. Oglesbee.
Other titles: Small mammal | Five minute veterinary consult.
Description: Third edition. | Hoboken, New Jersey : Wiley-Blackwell, [2024]
   | Series: Blackwell's five-minute veterinary consult | Includes
   bibliographical references and index.
Identifiers: LCCN 2023023314 (print) | LCCN 2023023315 (ebook) |
   ISBN 9781119456520 (hardback) | ISBN 9781119456506 (adobe pdf) |
   ISBN 9781119456483 (epub)
Subjects: MESH: Animal Diseases | Ferrets | Pets | Rabbits | Rodentia |
   Handbook
Classification: LCC SF997.5.F47 (print) | LCC SF997.5.F47 (ebook) | NLM
   SF 997.5.F47 | DDC 636.976/628–dc23/eng/20231003
LC record available at https://lccn.loc.gov/2023023314
LC ebook record available at https://lccn.loc.gov/2023023315

Cover Design: Wiley
Cover Images: Wiley and Barbara L. Oglesbee

Set in 9/10pt A Garamond Pro by Straive, Pondicherry, India
SKY10068943_030624

I dedicate this book with love to my husband, Michael, and my children, Alexandra and Ian, for their patience and support, and for the sacrifice required to give Mom time to write.

CONTENTS

SECTION III: GUINEA PIGS

SECTION IV: HEDGEHOGS

SECTION V: RABBITS

SECTION VI: RODENTS

SECTION VII: SUGAR GLIDERS

APPENDICES

LIST OF CONTRIBUTORS

NATALIE ANTINOFF, DVM, DIPL.
ABVP–AVIAN PRACTICE
  Medical Director, Texas Avian and
  Exotic Hospital
  Grapevine, TX
  USA

HUGUES BEAUFRERE, DVM, DIPL. ACVM,
DIPL. ABVP–AVIAN PRACTICE, DIPL.
ECZM-AVIAN PRACTICE
  Associate Professor – Medicine and
  Epidemiology
  Companion Zoological Medicine
  School of Veterinary Medicine
  University of California–Davis
  USA

JESSICA COMOLLI, DVM
  Director of Animal Health
  Miami Seaquarium
  Miami, FL
  USA

VITTORIO CAPELLO, DVM, DIPL. ABVP-
EXOTIC COMPANION MAMMAL PRACTICE,
DIPL. ECZM-SMALL MAMMAL PRACTICE
  Clinica Veterinaria S.Siro
  Clinica Veterinaria GranSasso
  Milano
  Italy

CHRISTINE ECKERMANN-ROSS, DVM,
CVA, CVCH,CTPEP
  Avian and Exotic Animal Care, PA
  Raleigh, NC
  USA

MICHELLE G. HAWKINS, VMD, DIPL.
ABVP–AVIAN PRACTICE
  Professor, Department of Medicine and
  Epidemiology
  Companion Avian and Exotic Animal
  Medicine
  School of Veterinary Medicine
  University of California–Davis
  USA

J. JILL HEATLEY, DVM, MS, DIPL.
ABVP–AVIAN PRACTICE, DIPL. ACZM
  Clinical Associate Professor, Zoological
  Medicine
  Department of Small Animal Medicine
  College of Veterinary Medicine
  Texas A&M University
  College Station, TX
  USA

NICHOLAS JEW, DVM
  MedVet Hilliard, Avian and Exotics
  Columbus, OH
  USA

DAN H. JOHNSON, DVM, DIPL.
ABVP–EXOTIC COMPANION MAMMAL
PRACTICE
  Avian and Exotic Animal Care, PA
  Raleigh, NC
  USA

ERIC KLAPHAKE, DVM, DIPL. ABVP, DIPL.
ACZM
  Head Veterinarian, Cheyenne Mountain
  Zoo
  Colorado Springs, CO
  USA

ANGELA M. LENNOX, DVM, DIPL.
ABVP–AVIAN PRACTICE
  Avian & Exotic Animal Clinic of
  Indianapolis
  Indianapolis, IN
  USA

GEORGINA NEWBOLD, DVM DACVO
  Assistant Professor, Clinical
  Ophthalmology
  Department of Veterinary Clinical
  Medicine
  The Ohio State University
  Veterinary Medical Center
  Columbus, OH
  USA

BARBARA L. OGLESBEE, DVM, DIPL.
ABVP–AVIAN PRACTICE
  Specialty Leader-Avian and Exotics,
  MedVet
  Associate Professor, Clinical
  The Ohio State University
  College of Veterinary Medicine
  Columbus, OH
  USA

JOANNE PAUL-MURPHY, DVM, DIPL. ACZM
  Professor Emeritus, Department of
  Medicine and Epidemiology
  Companion Avian and Exotic Pets
  School of Veterinary Medicine
  University of California, Davis
  USA

CHARLY PIGNON, DVM, DIPL.
ECZM-SMALL MAMMAL PRACTICE
  Ecole Nationale Veterinaire d'Alfort
  Department Elevage et Pathologie des
  Equides et des Carnivores
  Maisons-Alfort
  France

CHRISTY L. RETTENMUND, DVM, DIPL.
ACZM
  Senior Staff Veterinarian, Milwaukee
  County Zoo
  Milwaukee, MN
  USA

JEFFREY L. RHODY, DVM, DIPL.
ABVP–EXOTIC COMPANION MAMMAL
  Lakeside Veterinary Center
  Laurel, MD
  USA

RENATA SCHNEIDER, DVM
  Exotic Pet Veterinary Services, Inc.
  Hollywood, FL
  USA

RODNEY SCHNELLBACHER, DVM, DIPL.
ACZM
  Associate Veterinarian, Zoo Miami
  Miami, FL
  USA

AMANDA STEINAGEL, DVM
  Avian & Exotic Services, Mount Laurel
  Animal Hospital
  Mount Laurel, NJ
  USA

THOMAS N. TULLY, JR., DVM, MS, DIPL.
ABVP–AVIAN PRACTICE, DIPL. ECZM
  Professor, Zoological Medicine
  Louisiana State University School of
  Veterinary Medicine
  Baton Rouge, LA
  USA

MICHELLE WILLIS, DVM, DIPL. ACVO
  VCNA City Cats Hospital
  Arlington, MA
  USA

PREFACE

The popularity of Exotic Companion Mammals has increased exponentially in recent years. With this increase, veterinarians in general small animal practice, emergency clinics, and even canine and feline specialty practice are often faced with the difficult challenge of evaluating these often-unfamiliar species. Although excellent in-depth textbooks exist, much of the current information available on these species is scattered in multiple journals, periodicals, conference proceedings, bulletins, and internet resources. For the busy practitioner to keep abreast of all these resources is a daunting task, especially for those simultaneously striving to keep current in canine and feline medicine. Blackwell's *Five-Minute Veterinary Consult: Small Mammals* was designed to bring this information together in a concise, readily accessible format.

Blackwell's *Five-Minute Veterinary Consult* is a quick reference with a unique format that provides consistency and breadth of coverage unparalleled by other texts. Like other editions in the *Five-Minute Veterinary Consult* series, the Small Mammals edition is divided into topics based on presenting problems and diseases. Each topic has an identical format, making finding information easy. Detailed, up-to-date information on the diagnosis and treatment options for all disorders commonly encountered in these species are readily accessible. Individual topics are thoroughly covered within a few pages so that there is little need to cross-reference to other topics within the text.

To make this information quickly available, the book is divided by species into separate sections for chinchillas, guinea pigs, hedgehogs, ferrets, rabbits, rodents, and sugar gliders, with tabs to help quickly identify the section required. Each species section's topics are organized alphabetically so that each can be readily located. A detailed table of contents and index is also provided to help the reader efficiently find the desired topic. The appendix also contains a formulary of commonly used medications.

I am fortunate and pleased to have had the assistance of several outstanding experts in the field of small mammal medicine to serve as contributing authors and as a panel of reviewers for topics presented in this work. Their input has significantly strengthened the text and greatly enhanced each topic's depth and scope of coverage. Unlike that of canine and feline medicine, the amount of information on the disorders of small mammals that have been generated by controlled studies is limited. Much of our cumulative knowledge is based on the shared experience of practicing exotic animal veterinarians. Because of this, many topics in rabbit and ferret medicine are controversial. I have made every attempt to present information with as little bias as possible and having topics reviewed facilitated this. However, the reader is encouraged to utilize the list of suggested readings printed at the end of each topic for additional information and viewpoints.

ABOUT THE COMPANION WEBSITE

This book is accompanied by a companion website:

www.wiley.com/go/mammal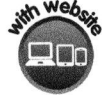

The website includes:

• Handouts

CHINCHILLAS

ALOPECIA

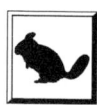

BASICS

DEFINITION
Alopecia is common in chinchillas and is characterized by complete or partial lack of hair in expected areas. It may be multifactorial and can be either a primary or secondary disorder. As many as 60 hairs grow from a single hair follicle in a healthy chinchilla.

PATHOPHYSIOLOGY
• Multifactorial causes
• Disruption in the growth of hair follicles is possible with infection, inflammation, trauma, or blockage of the receptor sites for stimulation of the cycle.

SYSTEMS AFFECTED
• Skin/exocrine
• Behavioral—may cause self-inflicted chewing, biting
• Gastrointestinal—especially dental disease; may cause anorexia, dysphagia, ptyalism
• Hemic/lymphatic/immune
• Ophthalmic—ophthalmic or dental disease may cause epiphora and conjunctivitis resulting in alopecia surrounding one or both eyes.

GENETICS
• Dental disease—avoid breeding affected animals as inheritance of dental disease is suspected.
• Fur chewing—avoid breeding animals that chew fur.

INCIDENCE/PREVALENCE
Common condition in chinchillas

GEOGRAPHIC DISTRIBUTION
N/A

SIGNALMENT
No specific age or sex predilection

SIGNS
• The pattern and degree of hair loss are important for establishing a differential diagnosis.
• Multifocal patches of alopecia—most frequently associated with folliculitis from mycotic or bacterial infection
• Large, diffuse areas of alopecia—indicate follicular dysplasia or metabolic component; not reported in chinchillas but should be considered
• May be acute or slowly progressive in onset

Historical Findings
• Inappropriate diet—fiber deficiency, other nutritional deficiencies
• Inappropriate frequency or complete lack of dust bath; use of inappropriate dust bath materials

• Inappropriate sanitation, ventilation
• Self-inflicted or conspecific barbering
• Drooling, dysphagia
• Ocular or nasal discharge
• History of fur slip, fur chewing

Physical Examination Findings
• Alopecia with or without scaling, crusting—distribution may help differentiate the disease process.
• Broken hair shafts—suggestive of barbering (self-inflicted or conspecific)
• Ptyalism—associated with dental malocclusion; a thorough oral examination is critical for evaluating for premolar/molar malocclusion
• Epiphora—associated with dental malocclusion; a thorough oral examination is critical for evaluating for premolar/molar malocclusion

CAUSES
• Normal shedding pattern—some chinchillas may lose hair in patches when shedding
• Behavioral—barbering; dominant chinchillas may chew or pull out hair of submissive cagemates
• Parasitic—ectoparasites (fleas, lice, and mites)—uncommon in chinchillas because of their dense coat
• Infectious—dermatophytosis, bacterial pyoderma; most often a secondary problem, especially moist dermatitis (e.g., ptyalism, epiphora, and urine scald)
• Trauma—fur slip due to excessive restraint; self- or conspecific-inflicted barbering, bite wounds
• Neoplastic—cutaneous lymphoma, trichofolliculoma, mast cell tumor
• Nutritional—especially protein and fiber deficiencies

RISK FACTORS
Poor husbandry: lack of dust baths, proper ventilation, and sanitation; nutritional deficiencies such as low-fiber diets leading to fur chewing and other deficiencies allowing for immunosuppression; traumatic handling leading to fur slip.

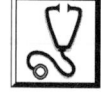

DIAGNOSIS

DIFFERENTIAL DIAGNOSIS

Differentiating Causes
Pattern and degree are important for differential diagnoses.

Symmetrical Alopecia
• Barbering—broken fur shafts identified on close inspection; most commonly on dorsal flanks, around face and ears; can have a "moth-eaten" appearance to the coat. Owners

may or may not observe barbering between animals.
• Fur chewing—very common in chinchillas; may chew on fur constantly or intermittently and fur may regrow in between episodes. Usually chew dorsal flanks and sides, pregnant females may chew temporarily. Coat may have moth-eaten appearance.
• Matted fur associated with high environmental temperature (>80°F/26.7°C), humid environment, or if dust baths are inadequate or not provided.

Multifocal to Focal Alopecia
• Lack of proper dust bath—may cause poor, unkempt coat that becomes matted and sheds abnormally; may cause alopecia and accumulation of scale in matted areas
• Trauma
  ◦ Bite wounds—alopecia, with or without erythema; can abscess; secondary *Staphylococcus* spp. or *Streptococcus* spp. infections may occur
  ◦ Fur slip—alopecia, with or without erythema, no scaling
  ◦ Ear trauma, including frost-bite alopecia with erythema, scaling, necrosis of pinnae
• Fur chewing—may chew on fur constantly or intermittently and fur may regrow in between episodes; usually chew dorsal flanks and sides, pregnant females may chew temporarily
• Dental disease—facial moist dermatitis associated most commonly with ptyalism or epiphora; alopecia, with or without erythema, scale, or ulceration; *Staphylococcus* spp. or *Streptococcus* spp. infections can occur secondary to moist dermatitis.
• Dermatophytosis—*Trichophyton mentagrophytes* are most common, but *Microsporum canis* and *M. gypseum* have been identified; partial or complete alopecia with scaling and pruritis; with or without erythema, not always ring-shaped; may begin as alopecia around eyes, nose, then spread to feet, body, genitals. May be first identified on the "grooming claw" (medial first digit) of hind limbs.
• *Cheyletiella* spp.—reported in chinchillas, lesions are usually located in the intrascapular or tail-base region and are associated with large amounts of white scale. Mites are readily identified on skin scrapes or acetate tape preparations on low power.
• Urinary tract infection—perineal moist dermatitis; alopecia, with or without erythema, scale, or ulceration
• Arthritis of hind limbs—perineal moist dermatitis; alopecia, with or without erythema, scale, or ulceration
• Lumbar spinal spondylosis—perineal moist dermatitis; alopecia, with or without erythema, scale, or ulceration

- Pododermatitis of hind limbs—perineal moist dermatitis; alopecia, with or without erythema, scale, or ulceration
- Abscesses—anywhere on body; alopecia, with or without erythema, scale, ulceration
- Ear mites—alopecia around base of ear; may extend to head, neck, abdomen, perineal region, intense pruritis; brown-beige crusty exudate in ear canal and pinna
- Fleas—patchy alopecia; flea dirt will help differentiate; secondary pyoderma sometimes seen
- Contact dermatitis—alopecia, with or without erythema; scale on ventral abdomen and other contact areas
- Moist dermatitis—alopecia, with or without erythema, scale, or ulceration associated with urinary disease (urine scald), diarrhea, uneaten cecotropes, arthritis, pododermatitis, spinal spondylosis
- Neoplasia—cutaneous lymphoma, cutaneous epitheliotropic lymphoma (mycosis fungoides), trichofolliculoma, mast cell tumors; focal or diffuse alopecia; scaling and erythema; may see crust formation—not reported in chinchillas but should be considered.

CBC/BIOCHEMISTRY/URINALYSIS
To identify evidence of infection, inflammation, and organ function for underlying disease, especially with urine scald, perineal dermatitis, infectious organisms

OTHER LABORATORY TESTS
Fungal cultures—especially DTM for dermatophytes; two negative cultures should be obtained following treatment to ensure clearance of infection.

IMAGING
- Skull radiographs—to identify underlying dental disease in chinchillas with ptyalism, epiphora
- Whole body radiographs—to identify orthopedic, spinal, gastrointestinal, renal, reproductive diseases associated with perineal dermatitis or urine scald
- Abdominal ultrasound—to identify gastrointestinal, renal, reproductive diseases associated with perineal dermatitis or urine scald

DIAGNOSTIC PROCEDURES
- Skin scraping—micro-spatula with flat-ended blade (preferable) or dull edge of scalpel blade
- Acetate tape preparation—evaluate on low-power microscopy for ectoparasites
- Trichogram—cytology of epilated hairs to examine for lice, other ectoparasites, or eggs
- Skin biopsy—especially with suspicion of neoplasia, infectious organisms

- Woods lamp ultraviolet evaluation of *Microsporum canis* lesions; not very useful as a screening tool—many pathogenic dermatophytes, including *T. mentagrophytes,* do not fluoresce; false fluorescence is also common.
- Fungal culture—if dermatophytes are suspected

PATHOLOGIC FINDINGS
Gross and histopathologic findings will differ depending upon the underlying condition.

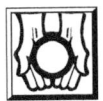

TREATMENT
APPROPRIATE HEALTH CARE
- Patients that appear otherwise normal are typically managed as outpatients; diagnostic evaluation may require brief hospitalization.
- Diseases associated with systemic signs of illness (e.g., pyrexia, depression, anorexia, and dehydration) or laboratory findings of azotemia and or leukocytosis warrant an aggressive diagnostic evaluation and initiation of supportive and symptomatic treatment.

NURSING CARE
- Subcutaneous fluids can be administered (30–50 mL/kg) as needed; IV access is difficult in chinchillas; lateral saphenous vein catheters often kink; consider intraosseous (IO) catheterization if intravascular fluids are needed.
- Base fluid selection on the underlying cause of fluid loss. In most patients, lactated Ringer's solution or Normosol crystalloid fluids are appropriate. Maintenance fluids are estimated at 100 mL/kg/day.

ACTIVITY
Dust baths should be administered at least 2–3 times weekly—minimize during treatment for infectious organisms (especially dermatophytes); do not reuse dust bath. Use only good-quality dust bathing materials.

DIET
- Some chinchillas will develop inappetence. Be certain the chinchilla is eating, or provide assisted syringe feeding of an herbivore critical care diet (e.g., Critical Care for Herbivores, Oxbow Animal Health, Omaha, NE, or Emeraid Herbivore, Lafeber Company, Cornell, IL) if anorectic to prevent the development, or exacerbation of, gastrointestinal dysmotility/GI stasis.
- Increasing water content in foods or via oral or parenteral fluids may increase fluid intake. Provide multiple sources of fresh water, including supplementing fresh water with small amounts of pure fruit juice (no added sugars), high water content vegetables, or soaking or misting fresh vegetables before offering.

CLIENT EDUCATION
- Do not breed animals with malocclusion or that chew their own fur, as both traits are potentially hereditary.
- Disinfect caging and cage materials in cases with infectious organisms; for dermatophytes, use 10% bleach solution.
- Discard wooden cage materials if infectious organisms
- Remove conspecifics if barbering is identified.

SURGICAL CONSIDERATIONS
N/A

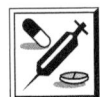

MEDICATIONS
DRUG(S) OF CHOICE
- Varies with specific cause
- Fleas, mites (including *Cheyletiella* spp.), other ectoparasites—ivermectin 1% (0.4 mg/kg SC q10–14d × 3–4 doses); selamectin (Revolution, Zoetis, Parsippany, NJ; 15–30 mg/kg applied topically q21–28d × 3–4 doses); flea shampoos for kittens without permethrins, pyrethrins can be used. Treat all affected animals and clean the environment.
- Dermatophytes—itraconazole (5 mg/kg PO q24h] × 6–8w); terbinafine (20–40 mg/kg PO q24h × 4–6w) or griseofulvin (25 mg/kg PO q24h × 4–6w) for refractory cases; lime sulfur dips q7d has been used successfully—is odiferous and can stain; antifungal shampoos (ketoconazole/chlorhexidine combination) and antifungal sprays (miconazole, enilconazole) are available, but toxicity information not available for chinchillas.
- 0.5%–1% chlorohexidine solution for cleansing of affected areas
- Antihistamines (diphenhydramine, hydroxyzine) for severe pruritis—may cause drowsiness
- Nonsteroidal anti-inflammatory medications (meloxicam 0.5–1 mg/kg SC, PO q24h; carprofen 2–5 mg/kg SC, PO q24h) may be helpful with inflammatory conditions, analgesia for dental disease

CONTRAINDICATIONS
- Oral administration of antibiotics that select against gram-positive bacteria (penicillins, cephalosporins, macrolides, and lincosamides) can cause fatal enteric dysbiosis and enterotoxemia.
- Metronidazole may cause anorexia or reduced appetite in some chinchillas when administered PO; hepatic toxicosis has been anecdotally reported.
- Potentially nephrotoxic drugs (e.g., aminoglycosides, NSAIDs) should be avoided in patients that are febrile, dehydrated, or

CHINCHILLAS

ALOPECIA

azotemic or that are suspected of having pyelonephritis, septicemia, or preexisting renal disease.
• Glucocorticoids or other immunosuppressive agents should be used only when no alternative is available and should be used with caution.
• Do not use fipronil or flea collars as toxicity in chinchillas is not known.
• Do not use organophosphate-containing products in chinchillas.

PRECAUTIONS
• Flea-control products are off-label use in chinchillas; safety and efficacy have not been evaluated in this species.
• Topical flea products such as permethrins and pyrethrins may be toxic in chinchillas.
• Prevent chinchillas and cagemates from licking topical spot-on products until dry.
• Toxicity—if any signs are noted, the animal should be bathed thoroughly to remove any residual products and then treated appropriately.
• Griseofulvin—bone marrow suppression reported in dogs, cats as idiosyncratic reaction or with prolonged therapy; not reported in chinchillas but may occur; consider weekly or bi-weekly CBC. Neurological effects reported in dogs and cats; monitor chinchillas for these signs. Teratogenic in first two trimesters of pregnancy.
• Immunosuppressive agents should be avoided.

POSSIBLE INTERACTIONS
None

ALTERNATIVE DRUGS
Ketoconazole has been utilized for dermatophytes in other species—safety and efficacy are unknown in chinchillas; hepatopathy reported in cats and dogs can be severe.

FOLLOW-UP

PATIENT MONITORING
Varies with cause

PREVENTION/AVOIDANCE
• Provide good-quality dust baths several times weekly to maximize coat quality.
• Feed diets with balanced protein and fiber for chinchillas.
• Separate animals that barber or fur chew from other animals.

POSSIBLE COMPLICATIONS
N/A

EXPECTED COURSE AND PROGNOSIS
Treatment times for dermatophytosis are long (4–8 weeks); treatment diligence necessary to clear infection; continue until two negative cultures are obtained.

MISCELLANEOUS

ASSOCIATED CONDITIONS
• Dental disease
• Musculoskeletal disease

AGE-RELATED FACTORS
N/A

ZOONOTIC POTENTIAL
Dermatophytosis and *Cheyletiella* can cause skin lesions in people.

PREGNANCY/FERTILITY/BREEDING
• Do not breed animals with malocclusion or that chew fur, as both traits are potentially hereditary.
• Griseofulvin contraindicated in pregnant animals during first two trimesters as it can be teratogenic
• Avoid ivermectin in pregnant animals.

SYNONYMS
Ringworm (dermatophytes)
Fur chewing (self-inflicted barbering)

SEE ALSO
Dermatophytosis

ABBREVIATIONS
DTM = dermatophyte test medium
GI = gastrointestinal

INTERNET RESOURCES
N/A

Suggested Reading
Mans C, Donnelly T. Chinchillas. In: Quesenberry KE, Carpenter JW, eds. Ferrets, Rabbits and Rodents 4th ed. Clinical Medicine and Surgery. 2021. St. Louis: Saunders, 2020:298–322.
Martel A, Donnelly T, Mans C. Update on diseases in chinchillas: 2013–2019. Vet Clin Exot Anim 2020;23:321–333.
Mayer J, Mans C. Rodents. In: Carpenter JW, ed. Exotic Animal Formulary, 5th ed. St. Louis: Elsevier, 2018:459–493.
Mitchell MA, Tully TN, eds. Manual of Exotic Pet Practice. St. Louis: Elsevier, 2009:480, 487, 491.
Riggs SM, Mitchell MA. Chinchillas. In: Mitchell MA, Tully TN, eds. Manual of Exotic Pet Practice. St. Louis: Elsevier, 2009:475–486.
Miwa Y, Sladky K. Common surgical procedures of rodents, ferrets, hedgehogs, and sugar gliders. Vet Clin Exot Anim 2016;19:205–244.
Palmerio BS, Roberts H. Clinical approach to dermatologic disease in exotic animals. Vet Clin North Am Exot Anim Pract 2013;16(3):523–577.

Authors Michelle G. Hawkins, VMD DABVP (Avian) and Dan H. Johnson, DVM, DABVP (Exotic Companion Mammal)

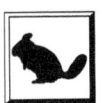

BASICS

DEFINITION
Absence of an appetite for food. The term *pseudoanorexia* is often used to describe the condition in which an animal does not eat because of an inability to prehend, chew, or swallow food rather than because of a lack of interest in food.

PATHOPHYSIOLOGY
• Anorexia is most often associated with systemic disease but can be caused by many different mechanisms, including medications that suppress appetite.
• The control of appetite is a complex interaction between the CNS and the periphery.
• The regulation of food intake also depends on the peripheral control of appetite.
• Inflammatory, infectious, metabolic, or neoplastic diseases can cause inappetence, probably as a result of the release of a variety of chemical mediators.
• Pseudoanorexia is commonly associated with oral pain or inability to chew due to dental disease.

SYSTEMS AFFECTED
Virtually any body system can be affected by anorexia, especially if it persists for more than 24 hours.

INCIDENCE/PREVALENCE
Anorexia and pseudoanorexia are among the most common clinical presentations seen in the chinchilla.

SIGNALMENT
No specific age or sex predisposition to anorexia in general, but signalment predispositions to many of the underlying conditions that cause anorexia

SIGNS
Historical Findings
• Refusal to eat is a common clinical complaint because chinchilla owners often associate a poor appetite with illness.
• Clinical signs associated with anorexia vary and are related to the underlying cause.
• Fecal pellets often become scant and smaller in size.
• Chinchillas with gastrointestinal tract disease (e.g., gastrointestinal stasis or bloat) often initially stop eating pellets or hay but continue to eat treats, followed by complete anorexia.
• Signs of pain, such as teeth grinding, a hunched posture, and reluctance to move, are extremely common in chinchillas with oral disease or problems with gastrointestinal motility.

• Patients with dental disease or disorders causing dysfunction or pain of the face, neck, oropharynx, and esophagus may display an interest in food but be unable to complete prehension and swallowing (pseudoanorexia).
• Pseudoanorectic patients commonly display weight loss, excessive drooling, difficulty in prehension and mastication of food, halitosis, dysphagia, and odynophagia (painful eating); may be preceded by a preference for softer foods such as parsley or romaine lettuce.

Physical Examination Findings
• Reluctance to eat may be the only abnormality identified after an evaluation of the patient history and physical evaluation; this is typical in chinchillas with gastrointestinal tract diseases or pseudoanorexia from oral disease prior to a thorough examination of the oral cavity.
• Most underlying causes of pseudoanorexia can be identified by a thorough examination of the face, mandible, teeth, neck, oropharynx, and esophagus for dental disease, ulceration, traumatic lesions, masses, foreign bodies, and neuromuscular dysfunction.
• A thorough examination of the oral cavity, including the incisors, molars, and buccal and lingual mucosa, is necessary to rule out dental disease. A bivalve nasal speculum (Welch Allyn, Skaneateles Falls, NY) or otoscope may be useful in identifying severe abnormalities; however, many problems will be missed by using this method alone. A thorough examination of the cheek teeth requires heavy sedation or general anesthesia and specialized equipment. Use a focused, directed light source and magnification (or a rigid endoscope, if available) to provide optimal visualization. Use a rodent mouth gag and cheek dilators (Jorgensen Laboratories, Inc., Loveland, CO) to open the mouth and pull buccal tissues away from teeth surfaces to allow adequate exposure. Identify elongation of cheek teeth, irregular crown height, spurs, curved teeth, oral ulcers, or abscesses.
• Significant tooth root abnormalities are commonly present despite normal-appearing crowns. Skull radiographs are especially useful to identify apical disorders in chinchillas; dorsoventral, lateral, and left and right oblique views are necessary for an accurate assessment. CT evaluation may provide even more information.
• Abdominal palpation is an extremely valuable tool in the diagnosis of gastrointestinal hypomotility or stasis disorders. The presence of hair and ingesta is normal and should be palpable in the stomach of a healthy chinchilla. The normal stomach should be easily deformable, feel soft and pliable, and not remain pitted on

compression. A firm, noncompliant stomach or stomach that remains pitted on compression is an abnormal finding.
• Gas distension ("bloat") of the stomach, intestines, or cecum is common in chinchillas with gastrointestinal tract disease.
• Abdominal palpation may also reveal the presence of organomegaly, masses, or gastrointestinal foreign bodies.
• Auscultation of the thorax may reveal cardiac murmurs, arrhythmias, or abnormal breath sounds.
• Auscultation of the abdomen may reveal decreased or absent borborygmus in chinchillas with gastrointestinal hypomotility. Borborygmus may be increased in cases with acute intestinal obstruction.

CAUSES
Anorexia
• Almost any systemic disease process
• Sudden diet change, insufficient water supply, change in husbandry, environmental stress
• Gastrointestinal disease—among the most common causes, especially problems related to gastrointestinal hypomotility or stasis; esophageal foreign body ("choke"); gastric trichobezoar; gas distension ("bloat")
• Pain—acquired dental disease, malocclusion ("slobbers"), apical elongation; orthopedic disorders, urolithiasis
• Metabolic disease—diabetes, hepatic or renal disease, acid–base disorders
• Neoplasia involving any site—uncommon in chinchillas
• Cardiac disease
• Infectious disease—enterotoxemia, enteritis, salmonellosis, listeriosis
• Respiratory disease—bacterial pneumonia
• Reproductive—dystocia, hair ring/paraphimosis, pregnancy toxemia
• Neurologic disease—encephalitis (listeriosis), cerebrospinal nematodiasis
• Psychologic—unpalatable diets, alterations in routine or environment, stress
• Toxicosis/drugs—lead poisoning, metronidazole
• Musculoskeletal disorders—fractures of the long bones of the limbs are relatively common
• Miscellaneous—heat stroke/high environment temperature, inappropriate use of antibiotics, carbohydrate overload, intestinal amyloidosis

Pseudoanorexia
• Any disease process that interferes with chewing or swallowing food
• Diseases causing painful prehension and mastication are extremely common, especially acquired dental disease (e.g., malocclusion, dental abscess, molar impaction, and apical elongation); stomatitis, glossitis, gingivitis

ANOREXIA AND PSEUDOANOREXIA   (CONTINUED)

(e.g., physical agents, caustics, bacterial infections, foreign bodies, and uremia), retrobulbar abscess, oral or glossal neoplasia, musculoskeletal disorders (mandible fracture or subluxation)
• Diseases causing oropharyngeal dysphagia (uncommon); glossal disorders (neurologic, neoplastic), pharyngitis, pharyngeal neoplasia, retropharyngeal disorders (lymphadenopathy, abscess, and hematoma), neuromuscular disorders (CNS lesions, botulism)
• Diseases of the esophagus—foreign body ("choke"), esophagitis, neoplasia, and neuromuscular disorders

RISK FACTORS
• Chinchillas on a diet containing inadequate amounts of long-stem hay are at risk for developing dental disease and gastrointestinal motility disorders.
• Chinchillas with limited exercise or mobility (cage restriction, orthopedic disorders, and obesity) are at a higher risk of developing gastrointestinal problems.
• Anesthesia and surgical procedures commonly cause temporary anorexia.

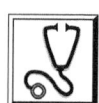

DIAGNOSIS

DIFFERENTIAL DIAGNOSIS
• Pseudoanorexia from dental disease and anorexia due to gastrointestinal disturbance are the two most common causes of inappetence in chinchillas. Decreased gastrointestinal motility can result from improper diet and many disease processes.
• Obtain a minimum database (CBC, biochemistry, and whole-body radiographs) to help delineate underlying medical disorders.
• Questioning about the patient's interest in food and ability to prehend, masticate, and swallow food, along with a thorough examination of the animal's teeth, oropharynx, face, and neck, will help identify pseudoanorexia. If the owners are poor historians, the patient should be observed while eating.
• Obtain a thorough history regarding the animal's environment, diet, other animals, and people in the household. Recent changes involving any of these are suggestive of psychologic anorexia.
• A thorough history regarding the chinchilla's diet, food and water consumption, and physical activity, as well as volume and character of fecal production will aid in the diagnosis of gastrointestinal motility disorders.

• Abnormalities detected in the physical examination or historical evidence of illness indicate the need for a diagnostic workup.

CBC/BIOCHEMISTRY/URINALYSIS
Abnormalities vary with different underlying diseases and causes of anorexia and pseudoanorexia.

OTHER LABORATORY TESTS
Special tests may be necessary to rule out specific diseases suggested by the history, physical examination, or minimum database (see other topics on specific diseases).

IMAGING
• If underlying disease is suspected, but no abnormalities are revealed by the physical examination or minimum database, perform abdominal radiography and abdominal ultrasonography to identify hidden conditions such as gastrointestinal tract disease, hepatic disease, urolithiasis, orthopedic disease, or neoplasia. Consider thoracic radiography to rule out cardiac or pulmonary disease.
• Skull radiographs may identify the presence of and extent of dental disease; dorsoventral, lateral, and left and right oblique views are indicated in most cases.
• The need for advanced diagnostic imaging (e.g., CT, MRI) varies with the underlying condition suspected.

DIAGNOSTIC PROCEDURES/ PATHOLOGIC FINDINGS
Vary with the suspected underlying condition

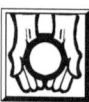

TREATMENT
• Treatment should be directed at the underlying cause.
• Symptomatic therapy includes attention to fluid and electrolyte derangements, reduction in environmental stressors, and modification of the diet.
• Most chinchillas that are anorectic have also refused water and are dehydrated to some degree. Lack of oral intake of fluid also contributes to desiccation of intestinal contents, gastrointestinal hypomotility, and further anorexia. The route of fluid therapy depends on the degree of dehydration, but most anorectic chinchillas will benefit from oral or subcutaneous fluids.
• Subcutaneous fluids can be administered (30–50 mL/kg) as needed; maintenance fluid requirements are estimated at 100 mL/kg/day; in most patients, lactated Ringer's solution or Normosol crystalloid fluids are appropriate.
• Intravenous or intraosseous fluids are required in patients that are severely dehydrated or depressed.

• Direct oral administration of products such as Gatorade (PepsiCo, Purchase, NY) or Pedialyte (Abbott Nutrition, Lake Forest, IL) are indicated if patient is not drinking.
• It is important that patients continue to eat during and following treatment. Continued anorexia will exacerbate gastrointestinal hypomotility and cause further derangement of the gastrointestinal microflora and overgrowth of intestinal bacterial pathogens.
• Chinchillas should be tempted often with parsley, cilantro, dandelion greens, and good-quality grass hay. Many patients will begin to eat these foods, even if they were previously anorectic. Also offer the patient's usual pelleted diet, as the initial goal is to get the chinchilla to eat.
• If the patient refuses these foods, syringe feed a gruel such as Critical Care for Herbivores (Oxbow Animal Health, Omaha, NE) or Emeraid Herbivore (Lafeber Company, Cornell, IL), 15–20 mL/kg PO q6–8h. Larger volumes and more frequent feedings are often accepted; feed as much as the chinchilla will readily accept. Alternatively, pellets can be ground and mixed with fresh greens, vegetable baby foods, water, or juice to form a gruel.
• High-carbohydrate, high-fat nutritional supplements are contraindicated.
• The diet should be permanently modified to include sufficient amounts of roughage and long-stemmed grass hay; foods high in simple carbohydrates should be prohibited or limited to the occasional treat.
• Encourage exercise for 10- to 15-minute intervals every 6–8 hours, unless contraindicated by underlying condition.

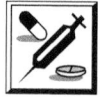

MEDICATIONS
DRUG(S) OF CHOICE
• Depends on the underlying cause
• Anorexia, regardless of the cause, contributes to or causes gastrointestinal tract hypomotility. The use of promotility agents such as metoclopramide (0.2–1.0 mg/kg PO, SC, IM q12h) or cisapride (0.1–0.5 mg/kg PO q8–12h) may be helpful in regaining normal motility; cisapride is available through compounding pharmacies.
• Analgesics such as buprenorphine (0.01–0.05 mg/kg SC, IM, IV q8–12h), meloxicam (0.5–1 mg/kg SC, PO q24h), or carprofen (2–5 mg/kg PO, SC q24h); pain is common in chinchillas with orthopedic disorders, dental disease, and intestinal distention; pain impairs mobility, decreases appetite, and may severely inhibit recovery.

CONTRAINDICATIONS
Avoid promotility agents if gastrointestinal obstruction is present or suspected.

PRECAUTIONS
Meloxicam—use with caution in chinchillas with compromised renal function.

POSSIBLE INTERACTIONS
N/A

ALTERNATIVE DRUGS
N/A

 FOLLOW-UP

PATIENT MONITORING
• Body weight, production of fecal pellets, and hydration can be used to determine if management is effective.

PREVENTION/AVOIDANCE
• Proper diet and husbandry; gradual changes to the diet, environment, or daily regiment when necessary; rapid changes tend to promote gastrointestinal hypomotility.
• Diet should include clean water and sufficient amounts of roughage and long-stemmed hay; inadequate dietary fiber can lead to GI stasis, and other disturbances of gastrointestinal motility. Acquired dental disease in chinchillas appears to have a genetic component; therefore, animals with dental disease should not be allowed to breed.
• A dietary component to acquired dental disease is also considered likely; thus, owners should be advised to increase the amount of long stemmed hay in the diet to increase the grinding motion of the teeth and increase wear.

POSSIBLE COMPLICATIONS
• Dehydration, malnutrition, and cachexia are most likely; these exacerbate the underlying disease.
• Hepatic lipidosis is a possible complication of anorexia, especially in obese chinchillas.
• Breakdown of the intestinal mucosal barrier is a concern in debilitated patients.
• Anorexia may cause enteric dysbiosis and subsequent enterotoxemia.

EXPECTED COURSE AND PROGNOSIS
Varies with different underlying diseases and causes of anorexia and pseudoanorexia.

 MISCELLANEOUS

ASSOCIATED CONDITIONS
See Causes

AGE-RELATED FACTORS
N/A

ZOONOTIC POTENTIAL
N/A

PREGNANCY/FERTILITY/BREEDING
N/A

SYNONYMS
Inappetence
Loss of appetite

SEE ALSO
Acquired dental disease
Gastrointestinal stasis and dilation
Diarrhea
Antibiotic-associated enterotoxemia
Constipation

ABBREVIATIONS
CBC = complete blood count
CNS = central nervous system
CT = computed tomography
MRI = magnetic resonance imaging

INTERNET RESOURCES
N/A

Suggested Reading
Harkness JE, Turner PV, VandeWoude S et al. Harkness and Wagner's Biology and Medicine of Rabbits and Rodents, 5th ed. Ames, IA: Wiley-Blackwell, 2010:210–213, 219, 260–262, 292–302, 321–322, 324–326.
Lennox AM, Gladden JN. Emergency and critical care of small mammals. In: Quesenberry KE, Carpenter JW, eds. Ferrets, Rabbits and Rodents, 4th ed. Clinical Medicine and Surgery. 2021. St. Louis: Saunders, 2020:595–608.
Mans C, Donnelly T. Chinchillas. In: Quesenberry KE, Carpenter JW, eds. Ferrets, Rabbits and Rodents, 4th ed. Clinical Medicine and Surgery. 2021. St. Louis: Saunders, 2020:298–322.
Mans C, Jekl V. Anatomy and disorders of the oral cavity of chinchilla and degus. Vet Clin Exot Anim 2016;19:843–869.
Martel A, Donnelly T, Mans C. Update on diseases in chinchillas: 2013–2019. Vet Clin Exot Anim 2020;23:321–333.
Riggs SM, Mitchell MA. Chinchillas. In: Mitchell MA, Tully TN, eds. Manual of Exotic Pet Practice. St. Louis: Elsevier, 2009:475–486.
Ritzman TK. Diagnosis and clinical management of gastrointestinal conditions in exotic companion mammals (rabbits, guinea pigs, and chinchillas). Vet Clin Exot Anim 2014;17:179–194.
Author Dan H. Johnson, DVM, Dipl. ABVP (Exotic Companion Mammal)

ANTIBIOTIC-ASSOCIATED ENTEROTOXEMIA

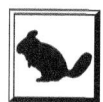

BASICS

OVERVIEW
• The intestinal microflora of the chinchilla is a dynamic mixture of bacteria, protozoa, and fungi.
• The administration of antibiotics to chinchillas can disrupt enteric commensal microflora and lead to bacterial dysbiosis.
• Antibiotics that target gram-positive bacteria and some gram-negative anaerobes—such as lincomycin, clindamycin, erythromycin, ampicillin, amoxicillin, cephalosporins, and penicillins—destroy these beneficial bacteria.
• Because resident enteric microflora competitively inhibits pathogenic bacteria, inappropriate antibiotics permit the growth of pathogenic bacteria such as *Escherichia coli* and *Clostridium* spp. These and other opportunists proliferate, causing enteritis and producing numerous potent enterotoxins.
• Chinchillas are hindgut fermenters; antibiotic-associated disruption in gut flora occurs primarily in the cecum and colon.
• In general, the oral route of antibiotic administration is considered more likely to cause problems than the parenteral route; however, enterotoxemia may also occur with parenteral antibiotic use.
• Pathologic effects are primarily due to toxemia; septicemia is not generally part of the disease.

SIGNALMENT
No specific age or breed predilection

SIGNS
Historical Findings
Antibiotic usage—the use of systemic antibiotics that are primarily gram-positive in spectrum (e.g., penicillins, cephalosporins, and macrolides)

Physical Examination Findings
• Peracute death with no clinical course
• Anorexia, lethargy, depression
• Diarrhea; severe, acute, profuse, often fatal
• Dehydration, hypotension, weakness, hypothermia
• Ileus, bloating, abdominal distension
• Tenesmus, fecal staining of the perineum, rectal prolapse
• Abdominal pain characterized by hunched posture, reluctance to move, stretching out, rolling, bruxism, and/or pain on abdominal palpation
• Respiratory distress, lateral recumbency, fever in end-stage cases

CAUSES
• Systemic (particularly oral) administration of lincomycin, clindamycin, erythromycin, ampicillin, amoxicillin, cephalosporins, and penicillins
• Dysbiosis and enterotoxemia can also occur secondary to stress, poor husbandry, or inappropriate nutrition.

RISK FACTORS
• Improper antibiotic usage
• Stress—improper temperature, poor sanitation, overcrowding, shipping
• Nutrition—sudden diet changes, weaning, insufficient dietary fiber, carbohydrate overload

DIAGNOSIS

DIFFERENTIAL DIAGNOSIS
Consider all causes of enteropathy in chinchillas; more severe illness should prompt a more extensive evaluation:
• Dietary—abrupt change in diet, weaning, excessive fresh green foods or fruit, excessive carbohydrate or sugars, or spoiled food
• Bacterial infection—*Pseudomonas* spp., *Proteus* spp., *Pasteurella* spp., *Salmonella* spp., *Staphylococcus* spp.
• Obstruction—neoplasia, foreign body, intussusception
• Toxic—plant toxins; mycotoxins
• Parasitic—*Giardia* spp., coccidia, nematodes, cestodes, *Cryptosporidium* spp.
• Metabolic disorders—liver disease, renal disease
• Systemic illness may cause diarrhea as a secondary event
• Neoplasia—primary gastrointestinal tumor, or as a sequela to other organ involvement

CBC/BIOCHEMISTRY/URINALYSIS
• Increased PCV and TS seen with dehydration
• TWBC elevation with neutrophilia indicative of a toxic inflammatory response
• Electrolyte abnormalities secondary to anorexia, fluid loss, and dehydration

OTHER LABORATORY TESTS
• Serial antemortem fecal, rectal, or cecal cultures under strict anaerobic conditions
• Demonstration of enterotoxin via fecal assays

IMAGING
Radiographic findings typically demonstrate ileus with significant gas distention of the intestinal tract.

DIAGNOSTIC PROCEDURES
N/A

PATHOLOGIC FINDINGS
• Cecal hemorrhage, ulceration, edema
• Mucosal necrosis, pseudomembrane formation
• Gas and fluid dilation of gut; watery brown, occasionally hemorrhagic, fetid luminal content
• Microscopically, hemorrhages and edema within gut wall, sloughing of enterocytes, and inflammatory infiltrates within the submucosa and mucosa; identifiable bacilli (i.e., *E. coli*) may line the mucosal surface on histologic sections
• Direct smear of mucosa may reveal typical gram-positive, spore-forming clostridial organisms.
• Nonspecific signs—enlarged mesenteric lymph nodes, congested kidneys

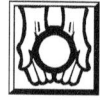

TREATMENT

APPROPRIATE HEALTH CARE
• Chinchillas with mild diarrhea that are otherwise bright and alert usually respond to outpatient treatment.
• Individuals with moderate to severe diarrhea usually require hospitalization and 24-hour care for parenteral medication, fluid therapy, and thermal support.
• Patients exhibiting signs of lethargy, depression, dehydration, and/or shock should be hospitalized even if diarrhea is mild or absent.

NURSING CARE
Fluid Therapy
• Rehydration and correction of electrolyte imbalances are the primary concern.
• Severe volume depletion can occur with acute diarrhea; aggressive shock fluid therapy may be indicated.
• Fluids may be administered by oral, subcutaneous, intravenous, and/or intraosseous routes as indicated by patient condition.
• Mildly affected patients usually respond well to oral and subcutaneous fluids.
• Subcutaneous fluids can be administered (30–50 mL/kg) as needed.
• Intravenous or intraosseous fluids are indicated in patients that are severely dehydrated or depressed.
• Maintenance fluid requirements are estimated at 100 mL/kg/day.
• Rehydration is essential to treatment success in severely ill chinchillas. In most patients, lactated Ringer's solution or Normosol crystalloid fluids are appropriate.
• A warm, quiet environment should be provided.

DIET

• It is imperative that chinchillas continue to eat during treatment and recovery. Prolonged anorexia promotes further derangement of gastrointestinal microflora, encourages overgrowth of intestinal bacterial pathogens, and negatively affects gastrointestinal motility.
• Assisted feeding is typically required until the patient is eating, eliminating, and maintaining body weight.
• Syringe-feeding formulas for rabbits/rodents: Critical Care for Herbivores (Oxbow Animal Health, Omaha, NE), Emeraid Herbivore (Lafeber Co., Cornell, IL), pureed fruit/vegetable baby foods, and blenderized rodent pellets
• Direct oral administration of products such as Gatorade (PepsiCo, Purchase, NY) or Pedialyte (Abbott Nutrition, Lake Forest, IL) indicated if patient not drinking

CLIENT EDUCATION

• Discuss the importance of prevention: appropriate use of antibiotics, proper husbandry, and good nutrition.
• Advise owners to monitor food consumption and fecal output; seek veterinary attention if there is a noticeable decrease in either.

SURGICAL CONSIDERATIONS

• If surgery is indicated (i.e., to correct rectal prolapse), then the patient should first be stabilized.
• Anesthesia, manipulation of the gut, hypothermia, anesthetic agents, and pain all exacerbate gastrointestinal ileus; gastrointestinal stasis is often worse postoperatively. This combination of factors may worsen the prognosis if surgery becomes necessary.

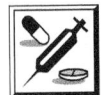

MEDICATIONS
DRUG(S) OF CHOICE
Antibiotic Therapy
• There is little evidence from controlled studies to indicate that antibiotics are efficacious in treating enterotoxemia.
• Antibiotics are indicated in patients with bacterial inflammatory lesions of the gastrointestinal tract, as well as patients with disruption of the intestinal mucosa evidenced by blood in the feces.
• Antibiotic selection should be broad spectrum, based on results of culture and susceptibility testing whenever possible.
• Some choices for empirical use while awaiting culture results include chloramphenicol (30–50 mg/kg PO q12h), trimethoprim sulfa (15–30 mg/kg PO q12h),

or metronidazole (10–20 mg/kg PO, IV q12h)—may cause anorexia or reduced appetite in some chinchillas when administered PO.

Gastrointestinal Agents
• Bismuth subsalicylate (0.3–0.6 mL/kg PO q4–6h PRN; dose cited is extrapolated from rabbit dose)
• Kaolin/pectin (0.2–0.3 mL/kg PO q6–8h PRN; dose cited is extrapolated from guinea pig dose)
• Cholestyramine (2 g/20 mL water PO q24h PRN) has been demonstrated to bind clostridial and other bacterial toxins in humans; anecdotal success in rabbits; may be useful in chinchillas
• Probiotic administration; transfaunation with healthy chinchilla feces may help to reestablish intestinal microflora

CONTRAINDICATIONS

• Anticholinergics (loperamide) in patients with suspected enterotoxin-producing bacteria and invasive bacterial enteritis
• Antibiotics that are primarily gram-positive in spectrum

PRECAUTIONS

• It is important to determine the cause of diarrhea. A general "shotgun" antibiotic approach may be ineffective or detrimental.
• Antibiotic therapy may predispose chinchillas to bacterial dysbiosis and overgrowth pathogenic bacteria. If signs worsen or do not improve, therapy should be adjusted.
• Chloramphenicol may cause aplastic anemia in susceptible people. Clients and staff should use appropriate precautions when handling this drug.
• Metronidazole may cause anorexia or reduced appetite in some chinchillas when administered PO; neurotoxic if overdosed; anecdotal reports of hepatotoxicity
• Isolate affected and exposed animals when infectious disease is suspected.

POSSIBLE INTERACTIONS
N/A

ALTERNATIVE DRUGS
N/A

FOLLOW-UP
PATIENT MONITORING
• Fecal volume and character, appetite, attitude, and body weight
• If diarrhea and other clinical signs do not resolve, consider reevaluation of the diagnosis.

PREVENTION/AVOIDANCE
• Appropriate antibiotic selection

• Providing appropriate diet and husbandry
• Reducing stress and providing sanitary conditions
• When infectious disease is suspected, strict isolation of affected and exposed animals

POSSIBLE COMPLICATIONS

• Antibiotic therapy can promote bacterial dysbiosis and overgrowth of pathogenic bacteria. Use antibiotics with caution, and only use those that are considered safe in chinchillas.
• Dehydration due to fluid loss
• Ileus, bloat, intussusception, tenesmus, rectal prolapse
• Septicemia due to bacterial invasion of enteric mucosa
• Shock, death from enterotoxicosis

EXPECTED COURSE AND PROGNOSIS

• Sudden death without any clinical signs is common.
• Acute, severe diarrhea and lethargy carry a poor prognosis.
• Mild cases where the patient is alert and maintains appetite carry a better prognosis.

MISCELLANEOUS
ASSOCIATED CONDITIONS
• Dehydration
• Malnutrition
• Hypoproteinemia
• Anemia
• Ileus
• Bloat
• Rectal prolapse
• Intussusception, torsion, impaction of cecum/colon
• Hepatic lipidosis

AGE-RELATED FACTORS
• All ages susceptible
• Young and recently weaned animals more commonly affected

ZOONOTIC POTENTIAL
• *E. coli* and *Clostridium* spp. are considered part of the normal gut flora in humans; however, both are also associated with disease.
• Clients should always be advised to follow standard disinfection and hygiene practices when working with affected animals.

PREGNANCY/FERTILITY/BREEDING
Severe diarrhea and associated metabolic disturbance may reduce fertility or cause abortion.

SYNONYMS
Dysbiosis
Clostridial enterotoxicosis

ANTIBIOTIC-ASSOCIATED ENTEROTOXEMIA   (CONTINUED)

SEE ALSO
Diarrhea
Anorexia
Gastrointestinal stasis and dilation

ABBREVIATIONS
PCV = packed cell volume
TS = total solids
TWBC = total white blood cell count

INTERNET RESOURCES
N/A

Suggested Reading
Lennox AM, Gladden JN. Emergency and critical care of small mammals. In: Quesenberry KE, Carpenter JW, eds. Ferrets, Rabbits and Rodents, 4th ed. Clinical Medicine and Surgery. 2021 ed. St. Louis: Saunders, 2020:595–608.
Mans C, Donnelly T. Chinchillas. In: Quesenberry KE, Carpenter JW, eds. Ferrets, Rabbits and Rodents, 4th ed. Clinical Medicine and Surgery. 2021 ed. St. Louis: Saunders, 2020:298–322.
Martel A, Donnelly T, Mans C. Update on diseases in chinchillas: 2013–2019. Vet Clin Exot Anim 2020;23:321–333.
Mayer J, Mans C. Rodents. In: Carpenter JW, ed. Exotic Animal Formulary, 5th ed. St Louis: Elsevier, 2018:459–493.
Mitchell MA, Tully TN, eds. Manual of Exotic Pet Practice. St. Louis: Elsevier, 2009:480, 487, 491.
Riggs SM, Mitchell MA. Chinchillas. In: Mitchell MA, Tully TN, eds. Manual of Exotic Pet Practice. St. Louis: Elsevier, 2009:475–486.
Ritzman TK. Diagnosis and clinical management of gastrointestinal conditions in exotic companion mammals (rabbits, guinea pigs, and chinchillas). Vet Clin Exot Anim 2014;17:179–194.

Author Dan H. Johnson, DVM, Dipl. ABVP (Exotic Companion Mammal)

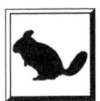

BASICS

DEFINITION
- Left-sided congestive heart failure (L-CHF)—failure of the left side of the heart to advance blood at a sufficient rate to meet the metabolic needs of the patient or to prevent blood from pooling within the pulmonary venous circulation
- Right-sided congestive heart failure (R-CHF)—failure of the right side of the heart to advance blood at a sufficient rate to meet the metabolic needs of the patient or to prevent blood from pooling within the systemic venous circulation

PATHOPHYSIOLOGY
- L-CHF: Low cardiac output causes lethargy, exercise intolerance, syncope, and prerenal azotemia. High hydrostatic pressure causes leakage of fluid from pulmonary venous circulation into pulmonary interstitium and alveoli. When fluid leakage exceeds ability of lymphatics to drain the affected areas, pulmonary edema develops.
- R-CHF: High hydrostatic pressure leads to leakage of fluid from venous circulation into the pleural and peritoneal spaces and interstitium of peripheral tissue. When fluid leakage exceeds ability of lymphatics to drain the affected areas, pleural effusion, ascites, and peripheral edema develop.

SYSTEMS AFFECTED
All organ systems can be affected by either poor delivery of blood or the effects of passive congestion from backup of venous blood.

INCIDENCE/PREVALENCE
- Heart murmurs are extremely common in Chinchillas, with a 23% incidence reported. Most of these are innocent murmurs and typically low grade (I–II/VI).
- Heart murmurs in older animals are more likely to be related to heart disease. These often have higher grade murmurs.

SIGNALMENT
- More common in older animals; no sex differences.

SIGNS
General Comments
Signs vary with underlying cause.

Historical Findings
- Weakness, lethargy, exercise intolerance
- Anorexia or inappetence, weight loss
- Dyspnea or tachypnea
- Syncope
- Abdominal distension with ascites

Physical Examination Findings
L-CHF
- Tachypnea
- Inspiratory and expiratory dyspnea when animal has pulmonary edema
- Prolonged capillary refill time
- Possible murmur
- Possible arrhythmia

R-CHF
- Hepatomegaly
- Ascites
- Cold extremities
- Possible murmur
- Rapid, shallow respiration if animal has pleural effusion

CAUSES
- Hypertrophic cardiomyopathy, mitral valve disease, and congenital abnormalities have been reported.

RISK FACTORS
- Incidence increases with age

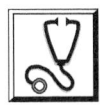

DIAGNOSIS

DIFFERENTIAL DIAGNOSIS
- Innocent heart murmur
- Pleural effusion—neoplasia, trauma resulting in diaphragmatic hernia, pulmonary hemorrhage, pneumothorax
- Dyspnea—rhinitis or sinusitis (rodents are obligate nasal breathers) and primary pulmonary disease (abscess, pneumonia) are most common; neoplasia (heart-based tumors, metastatic neoplasia), pleural effusion
- Ascites, abdominal distension—consider hypoproteinemia, severe liver disease, ruptured bladder, peritonitis, abdominal neoplasia, and abdominal hemorrhage
- Diagnosis is based on history and physical examination findings but is aided with diagnostic imaging, including radiographs and ultrasound.

CBC/BIOCHEMISTRY/URINALYSIS
While nonspecific for cardiac disease, it may help to rule out other underlying disease conditions.

OTHER LABORATORY TESTS
N/A

IMAGING
- Radiography can often identify cardiomegaly and pulmonary effusion and help rule out primary pulmonary disease.
- Echocardiography

DIAGNOSTIC PROCEDURES
- Electrocardiography

PATHOLOGIC FINDINGS
Cardiac findings vary with disease.

TREATMENT

APPROPRIATE HEALTH CARE
- Inpatient—severely debilitated patients or those in respiratory distress
- Discharge stable patients

NURSING CARE
- Oxygen therapy for patients in respiratory distress
- If pleural effusion is present, thoracocentesis has both diagnostic and therapeutic benefits. Sedation can be achieved with midazolam (0.5–2 mg/kg IM) and butorphanol (0.25–1 mg/kg IM).
- Supportive care, including correction of dehydration; administer 5%–10% of body weight in SQ boluses. Fluids should be kept warm to prevent hypothermia; using a 22–25 gauge butterfly needle to administer the fluids can reduce stress on the patient by minimizing restraint. Critical patients may require fluid therapy via an intraosseous catheter.
- Ensure that the patient is kept warm (if hypothermic, an incubator may be required).

ACTIVITY
Restrict activity—remove exercise wheels, ramps from cage

DIET
- Provide adequate nutrition; dyspneic animals may be reluctant to eat and may need assisted feeding with a diet such as Oxbow Critical Care Herbivore (Oxbow Enterprises, Inc., Murdock, NE) or Emeraid Exotic Herbivore (Lafeber's, Cornell, IL).

CLIENT EDUCATION
- CHF is not curable and will progress. Inform the client that cardiac disease is difficult to manage, and prognosis for longer term survival is poor; aim of treatment is palliative as long as quality of life can be maintained.

SURGICAL CONSIDERATIONS
N/A

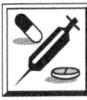

MEDICATIONS

DRUG(S) OF CHOICE
- Drugs for the treatment of cardiac disease in dogs and cats have been extrapolated and are used with variable results in pet rodents.
- Furosemide is recommended at the lowest effective dose to eliminate pulmonary edema and pleural effusion. If fulminate cardiac failure is evident, administer furosemide at 1–4 mg/kg q6–12h IM. Initially, furosemide

CHINCHILLAS

should be administered parenterally. Long-term therapy should be continued orally at 2–10 mg/kg PO q12h.
• Predisposes the patient to dehydration, prerenal azotemia, and electrolyte disturbances.
• Enalapril 0.5 mg/kg PO q24h
• Pimobenden has been used anecdotally at the same doses given to rabbits (0.1–0.3 mg/kg PO q12–24h).

CONTRAINDICATIONS
• Positive inotropic drugs should be avoided in patients with HCM.

PRECAUTIONS
• Treatment regimens for most rodent species are extrapolated from canine or feline doses and should be used with caution and careful patient monitoring.
• ACE inhibitors and digoxin must be used cautiously in patients with renal disease.
• Overzealous diuretic therapy may cause dehydration and hypokalemia.

POSSIBLE INTERACTIONS
• The use of a calcium channel blocker in combination with a beta-blocker should be avoided as clinically significant bradyarrhythmias can develop in other small animals and are likely to also occur in rodents.
• A combination of high-dose diuretics and ACE inhibitors may alter renal perfusion and cause azotemia.

ALTERNATIVE DRUGS
The use of vasodilators, diuretics, and antiarrhythmic drugs in dogs and cats has been extrapolated for use in Chinchillas, but no data exists on their risks vs. benefits.

FOLLOW-UP

PATIENT MONITORING
• Cardiac disease is likely to be progressive; therefore, frequent recheck evaluation is recommended.

• Monitor response to therapy and adjust drug dosages as indicated.
• Radiographs should be repeated 1 week after treatment is started.
• Monitor the patient's weight.
• Monitor the intake of food and water.

PREVENTION/AVOIDANCE
It is unclear at this time how to prevent the development of cardiac disease in chinchillas.

POSSIBLE COMPLICATIONS
• Disease is likely to be progressive.
• Sudden death due to arrhythmias
• Iatrogenic problems associated with medical management

EXPECTED COURSE AND PROGNOSIS
Congestive heart failure is progressive, and the owner should be advised that treatments are palliative to increase patient comfort and control clinical signs.

MISCELLANEOUS

ASSOCIATED CONDITIONS
• Lower respiratory disease
• Renal disease

ZOONOTIC POTENTIAL
N/A

PREGNANCY/FERTILITY/BREEDING
N/A

SYNONYMS
Heart disease
Heart failure

SEE ALSO
Pneumonia

ABBREVIATIONS
ACE = angiotensin-converting enzyme
DCM = dilated cardiomyopathy
HCM = hypertrophic cardiomyopathy
L-CHF = left-sided congestive heart failure
R-CHF = right-sided congestive heart failure

Suggested Reading
Capello V, Lennox AM. Diagnostic imaging of the respiratory system in exotic companion mammals. Vet Clin Exot Anim 2011;14:369–389.
DeCubellis J. Common emergencies in rabbits, guinea pigs, and chinchillas. Vet Clin Exot Anim 2016;19:411–429.
Fitzgerald BC, Dias S, Martorell J. Cardiovascular drugs in avian, small mammal, and reptile medicine. Vet Clin Exot Anim 2018;21:399–442.
Goodman G. Rodents: respiratory and cardiovascular system disorders. In: Keeble E, Meredith A, eds. BSAVA Manual of Rodents and Ferrets. Gloucester: BSAVA, 2009:142–149.
Lennox AM, Gladden JN. Emergency and critical care of small mammals. In: Quesenberry KE, Carpenter JW, eds. Ferrets, Rabbits and Rodents, 4th ed. Clinical Medicine and Surgery. 2021. St. Louis: Saunders, 2020:595–608.
Mans C, Donnelly T. Chinchillas. In: Quesenberry KE, Carpenter JW, eds. Ferrets, Rabbits and Rodents, 4th ed. Clinical Medicine and Surgery. 2021. St. Louis: Saunders, 2020:298–322.
Martel A, Donnelly T, Mans C. Update on diseases in chinchillas: 2013–2019. Vet Clin Exot Anim 2020;23:321–333.
Author Barbara Oglesbee, DVM, Dipl. ABVP (Avian)

CONSTIPATION (LACK OF FECAL PRODUCTION)

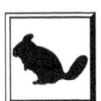

BASICS

DEFINITION
• Constipation—infrequent, incomplete, or difficult defecation with passage of scant, small, hard, or dry fecal pellets

PATHOPHYSIOLOGY
• The most common cause of constipation is feeding too much concentrated diet, which is high in energy and protein, without supplying sufficient roughage or fiber.
• Inadequate dietary fiber can decrease gastrointestinal motility; as motility slows, fecal pellets become smaller, less numerous, and drier than normal.
• Diets low in fiber typically contain high simple carbohydrate concentrations, which provide a ready source of fermentable products that can alter the resident microflora and promote the growth of bacterial pathogens and further suppress gastrointestinal motility.
• Constipation can develop with any disease that impairs passage of feces through the colon. Delayed fecal transit allows removal of additional salt and water, producing drier feces.
• Anorexia due to infectious or metabolic disease, pain, stress, or starvation may cause or exacerbate gastrointestinal hypomotility.

SYSTEMS AFFECTED
Gastrointestinal

SIGNALMENT
• In chinchillas, constipation is more commonly reported than diarrhea.
• No breed or gender predilections are reported.

SIGNS

Historical Findings
• Scant or no production of fecal pellets
• Small, hard, dry feces; occasionally blood stained
• Infrequent defecation
• Inappetence or anorexia
• Signs of pain, hunched posture, stretching out, rolling, reluctance to move
• Inappropriate diet or abrupt diet change
• Recent illness or stressful event
• Weight loss or other evidence of systemic disease
• Confinement, lack of exercise

Physical Examination Findings
• Small, hard fecal pellets; absence of fecal pellets palpable in the colon
• Firm, dry contents may be palpable within the cecum (cecal impaction)
• Gas, fluid, or firm, doughy, or dry gastrointestinal contents may be palpable depending on the underlying cause

• Anorectal prolapse, mass, or other causes of outflow obstruction
• Abnormal function of hind limbs
• Evidence of fur chewing (barbering)
• Obesity
• Other physical examination findings depend on the underlying cause; perform a complete physical examination, including a thorough oral examination.

CAUSES

Dietary and Environmental Causes
• Lack of dietary fiber—indigestible coarse fiber (such as hay) promotes gastrointestinal motility, adds bulk to the ingesta, and holds water, producing plump, moist fecal pellets.
• Excessive carbohydrate—feeding large amounts of simple carbohydrates can promote the growth of *Escherichia coli* and *Clostridium* spp., which can cause enterotoxemia and ileus. Sugary treats and high-carbohydrate, seed-based diets can also promote obesity.
• Obesity—cage confinement, lack of exercise
• Stress—pain, fighting among cagemates, surgery, hospitalization, new environment
• Dehydration—water bottle malfunction, bad tasting water, accidental oversight
• Anorexia—acquired dental disease/malocclusion, excessive fasting, starvation
• Foreign material—ingestion of/impaction with bedding, fibers, or fur

Metabolic and Dental Disease
• Conditions that result in inappetence or anorexia may also promote gastrointestinal hypomotility and constipation. Common causes include dental malocclusion, metabolic disease (renal disease, liver disease), pain (oral, trauma, and postoperative), neoplasia, and toxins.
• Debility—general muscle weakness, dehydration, neoplasia

Drugs
• Anesthetic agents, anticholinergics, opioids
• Barium sulfate, kaolin/pectin, sucralfate
• Diuretics

Painful Defecation
• Anorectal disease—rectal prolapse, anal stricture, abscess, rectal foreign body
• Trauma—fractured pelvis, fractured limb, dislocated hip, perineal bite wound or laceration, perineal abscess

Mechanical Obstruction
• Extraluminal—healed pelvic fracture with narrowed pelvic canal, intrapelvic neoplasia, intestinal compression secondary to large fetuses
• Intraluminal and intramural—intestinal torsion, intussusception, impaction of the cecum or colonic flexure, rectal prolapse, colonic or rectal neoplasia or polyp, rectal

stricture, perineal hernia, congenital defect (atresia ani)

Neuromuscular Disease
• Central nervous system—paraplegia, spinal trauma/disease, intervertebral disk disease, cerebral trauma/disease
• Peripheral nervous system—sacral nerve trauma/disease

RISK FACTORS
• Diets with inadequate indigestible coarse fiber content
• Excessive dietary carbohydrate or sugar
• Inactivity due to pain, obesity, cage confinement
• Anesthesia and surgical procedures
• Metabolic disease resulting in dehydration
• Ingestion of bedding substrate, fibers, fabric
• Barbering, excessive grooming
• Underlying dental, gastrointestinal tract, or metabolic disease
• Spinal, pelvic, or hind-limb trauma

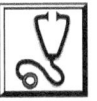

DIAGNOSIS

DIFFERENTIAL DIAGNOSIS
• Dyschezia and tenezmus—may be mistaken for constipation by owners; associated with increased frequency of attempts to defecate and frequent production of small amounts of liquid feces containing blood and/or mucous
• Stranguria—may be mistaken for constipation by owners; can be associated with hematuria and abnormal findings on urinalysis

CBC/BIOCHEMISTRY/URINALYSIS
• Usually normal
• May identify underlying causes of gastrointestinal hypomotility or dehydration
• PCV and TS elevations in dehydrated patients

OTHER LABORATORY TESTS
N/A

IMAGING
• Chinchillas should not be fasted prior to obtaining radiographs.
• A chinchilla's abdomen is normally much larger than its thorax.
• Ileus may be diagnosed radiographically by the presence of severely distended, gas-filled intestinal loops.
• In cases where there is significant gas in the intestines or cecum, radiographic contrast may be poor.
• Contrast radiography may be useful in evaluating gastrointestinal transit time and locating obstructions and displacement of the gastrointestinal tract.

CHINCHILLAS

• Abdominal radiography may reveal colonic or rectal foreign body, colonic or rectal mass, spinal fracture, fractured pelvis, or dislocated hip.

DIAGNOSTIC PROCEDURES
N/A

PATHOLOGIC FINDINGS
N/A

TREATMENT

APPROPRIATE HEALTH CARE
• Remove or ameliorate any underlying cause, if possible.
• Chinchillas that have not produced feces or have been anorectic for over 24 hours should be treated as soon as possible; emergency treatment should be considered in all cases.
• Outpatient care may be appropriate in some cases, but inpatient hospitalization and support should be considered for the majority.

NURSING CARE
• Offer small amounts of fresh food such as apples, carrots, parsley, or cilantro.
• Increase dietary fiber by adding grass or alfalfa hay.
• Omit treats such as grains, dried bananas, or raisins.
• Discontinue any medications that may cause constipation.
• Provide a warm (less than 80°F/26.7°C), quiet environment.

Fluid Therapy
• Fluid support is an essential component of the medical management of all chinchillas with anorexia, gastrointestinal hypomotility, and/or constipation.
• Fluids may be administered by the oral, subcutaneous, intravenous, and/or intraosseous routes as indicated by patient's condition.
• Mildly affected patients usually respond well to oral and subcutaneous fluids. Direct oral administration of products such as Gatorade (PepsiCo, Purchase, NY) or Pedialyte (Abbott Nutrition, Lake Forest, IL) is indicated if the patient is not drinking on its own.
• Subcutaneous fluids can be administered (30–50 mL/kg) as needed; intravenous or intraosseous fluids are indicated in patients that are severely dehydrated or depressed.
• Maintenance fluid requirements are estimated at 100 mL/kg/day. In most patients, lactated Ringer's solution or Normosol crystalloid fluids are appropriate.

ACTIVITY
If the patient is not debilitated, encourage exercise, as activity promotes gastric motility.

DIET
• Patients should be encouraged to eat during and following treatment. Continued anorexia will exacerbate gastrointestinal hypomotility, promote dysbiosis, and encourage the overgrowth of intestinal pathogens.
• To encourage food intake, offer the patient's favorite foods and treats in addition to the usual pelleted diet.
• If the patient refuses these foods, syringe feed a gruel such as Critical Care for Herbivores (Oxbow Animal Health, Omaha, NE) or Emeraid Herbivore (Lafeber Company, Cornell, IL), 15–20 mL/kg PO q6–8h. Larger volumes and more frequent feedings are often accepted. Alternatively, a gruel can be made from ground pellets, fresh greens, vegetable baby foods, water, or juice.
• Assisted or forced feeding is contraindicated in cases of intestinal obstruction (e.g., intussusception, intestinal impaction or torsion, and rectal prolapse).
• High-carbohydrate, high-fat nutritional supplements are contraindicated.
• Encourage oral fluid intake by offering fresh water, fresh foods, or flavoring the water with fruit/vegetable juices.
• Based on history, diet may need to be permanently modified to include sufficient amounts of indigestible, coarse fiber (e.g., long-stemmed grass hay) and limited simple carbohydrates.

CLIENT EDUCATION
• Discuss the importance of dietary modification, if indicated.
• Advise owners to regularly monitor food consumption and fecal output; seek veterinary attention with a noticeable decrease in either.
• Recommend regular follow-up and monitoring for chinchillas with acquired dental disease or malocclusion.

SURGICAL CONSIDERATIONS
• In many cases, constipation and lack of fecal production will resolve with medical treatment alone.
• Surgical manipulation of the intestinal tract, hypothermia, anesthetic agents, and pain all exacerbate gastrointestinal hypomotility; gastrointestinal stasis is often worse postoperatively. The combination of these factors may worsen the prognosis with surgical treatment.
• Surgery may be indicated for torsion, intussusception, intestinal foreign bodies (e.g., bedding, hair), rectal prolapse, extraluminal compression of the gastrointestinal tract, intestinal neoplasia, abscesses, and orthopedic problems.

MEDICATIONS
• Dehydrated patients should be rehydrated with a balanced electrolyte solution.
• Use parenteral medications in animals with severely compromised intestinal motility; oral medications may not be properly absorbed; begin oral medication when intestinal motility begins to return (i.e., fecal production, return of appetite, and radiographic evidence).

DRUG(S) OF CHOICE
• Motility modifiers—cisapride (0.5–1.0 mg/kg PO q8–12h), metoclopramide (0.2–1.0 mg/kg PO, SC, IM q12h); may be indicated in patients with gastrointestinal hypomotility (see contraindications)
• Analgesics—buprenorphine (0.1–0.2 mg/kg SC, IM, IV q8–12h), carprofen (2–5 mg/kg SC, PO q24h), meloxicam (0.5–1 mg/kg PO, SC q24h); intestinal pain, regardless of cause, impairs mobility, decreases appetite, and may severely inhibit recovery
• Petroleum-based laxatives, or lactulose as indicated
• Antibiotics—may be indicated in patients with bacterial overgrowth that sometimes occurs secondary to gastrointestinal hypomotility; indicated in patients with diarrhea, bloat, abnormal fecal cytology, and disruption of the intestinal mucosa (evidenced by blood in the feces); always use broad-spectrum antibiotics, based on culture/sensitivity where possible: chloramphenicol (30–50 mg/kg PO, SC, IM, IV q12h), trimethoprim sulfa (15–30 mg/kg PO, SC, IM q12h), or enrofloxacin (5–15 mg/kg PO, SC, IM q12h); for *Clostridium* spp. overgrowth: metronidazole (10–20 mg/kg PO, IV q12h; use with caution, may cause anorexia or reduced appetite in some chinchillas when administered PO)

CONTRAINDICATIONS
• Anticholinergics
• Assisted or forced feeding is contraindicated in cases of gastrointestinal tract obstruction or rupture.
• Gastrointestinal motility enhancers in patients with suspected mechanical obstruction (e.g., impaction, torsion, intussusception, rectal prolapse, and neoplasia)
• Antibiotics that are primarily gram-positive in spectrum will suppress the growth of commensal flora, allowing overgrowth of enteric pathogens. These include lincomycin, clindamycin, erythromycin, ampicillin, amoxicillin, cephalosporins, and penicillin.

CONSTIPATION (LACK OF FECAL PRODUCTION)

PRECAUTIONS
- Chloramphenicol may cause aplastic anemia in susceptible people. Clients and staff should use appropriate precautions when handling this drug.
- Metronidazole—may cause anorexia or reduced appetite in some chinchillas when administered PO; anecdotal association with liver failure; neurotoxic if overdosed
- Meloxicam—use with caution in cases with suspected renal function

POSSIBLE INTERACTIONS
N/A

ALTERNATIVE DRUGS
N/A

FOLLOW-UP

PATIENT MONITORING
- Monitor appetite and fecal production.
- Chinchillas that are successfully treated will regain a normal appetite; fecal volume and consistency will return to normal.

PREVENTION/AVOIDANCE
- Strict feeding of diets containing adequate indigestible coarse fiber (hay and high-fiber pellets) and low simple carbohydrate content along with access to fresh water likely to prevent episodes
- Obesity prevention; encourage exercise (e.g., provide running wheel) and limit the intake of high-calorie, high-carbohydrate foods.
- Routine fecal examination; treatment of intestinal parasites
- Reduction of stress and prompt treatment of conditions that cause pain
- Be certain that postoperative patients are eating and passing feces prior to release.

POSSIBLE COMPLICATIONS
- Chronic constipation can lead to intestinal torsion, intussusception, impaction of the cecum or colonic flexure, rectal prolapse.

- Death due to gastrointestinal tract rupture, hypovolemic or endotoxic shock
- Postoperative gastrointestinal stasis
- Overgrowth of intestinal bacterial pathogens

EXPECTED COURSE AND PROGNOSIS
- Early medical management of constipation and gastrointestinal hypomotility due to dietary causes, obesity, anesthesia/surgery, or anorexia secondary to pain or other stress usually carries a good to excellent prognosis.
- Surgical removal of foreign material, neoplasia, or surgical correction of intussusception, torsion, impaction, or rectal prolapse carries a guarded to poor prognosis.
- The prognosis for other causes varies.

MISCELLANEOUS

ASSOCIATED CONDITIONS
- Dental disease
- Gastrointestinal hypomotility
- Intestinal torsion
- Intussusception
- Cecal/colonic impaction
- Rectal prolapse
- Hepatic lipidosis
- Renal disease

AGE-RELATED FACTORS
N/A

ZOONOTIC POTENTIAL
N/A

PREGNANCY/FERTILITY/BREEDING
- Pregnancy can produce extraluminal intestinal compression, obstruction.
- If mechanical obstruction is due to narrowed pelvic canal, risk of dystocia is increased.

SYNONYMS
Fecal impaction
Gastrointestinal stasis
Ileus

SEE ALSO
Gastrointestinal stasis and dilation

ABBREVIATIONS
PCV = packed cell volume
TS = total solids

INTERNET RESOURCES
N/A

Suggested Reading
Lennox AM, Gladden JN. Emergency and critical care of small mammals. In: Quesenberry KE, Carpenter JW, eds. Ferrets, Rabbits and Rodents, 4th ed. Clinical Medicine and Surgery. 2021. St. Louis: Saunders, 2020:595–608.
Mans C, Donnelly T. Chinchillas. In: Quesenberry KE, Carpenter JW, eds. Ferrets, Rabbits and Rodents, 4th ed. Clinical Medicine and Surgery. 2021. St. Louis: Saunders, 2020:298–322.
Martel A, Donnelly T, Mans C. Update on diseases in chinchillas: 2013–2019. Vet Clin Exot Anim 2020;23:321–333.
Mayer J, Mans C. Rodents. In: Carpenter JW, ed. Exotic Animal Formulary, 5th ed. St Louis: Elsevier, 2018:459–493.
Mitchell MA, Tully TN, eds. Manual of Exotic Pet Practice. St. Louis: Elsevier, 2009:480, 487, 491.
Riggs SM, Mitchell MA. Chinchillas. In: Mitchell MA, Tully TN, eds. Manual of Exotic Pet Practice. St. Louis: Elsevier, 2009:475–486.
Ritzman TK. Diagnosis and clinical management of gastrointestinal conditions in exotic companion mammals (rabbits, guinea pigs, and chinchillas). Vet Clin Exot Anim 2014;17:179–194.

Author Dan H. Johnson, DVM, Dipl. ABVP (Exotic Companion Mammal)

DENTAL MALOCCLUSION

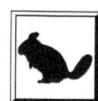 **BASICS**

DEFINITION
- "Malocclusion" is just a single aspect of dental disease of chinchillas, referring to abnormalities of the clinical crowns. Since congenital or developmental abnormalities of the skull have not been documented in this species, "acquired dental disease" is a more accurate terminology.
- Acquired dental disease is a syndrome—a complex of clinical symptoms and signs that may be associated with the syndrome alone or with related diseases (e.g., abscesses).

ANATOMY
- The chinchilla is a rodent species belonging to the suborder Caviomorph or Hystrycomorph ("guinea pig-like" or "porcupine-like" rodent).
- All rodent species are *Simplicidentata*. Unlike rabbits, they have one single maxillary incisor tooth for each quadrant.
- All rodent species have one pair of well-developed maxillary and mandibular incisor teeth, representing the best-known anatomical peculiarity of this order.
- Incisor teeth greatly vary in shape, color, and thickness among rodent species. Incisor teeth of rodents are covered by enamel only over the labial surface. In chinchillas, the enamel is yellow, and incisor teeth have a chisel-shaped occlusal surface.
- Incisor teeth are continually growing throughout life and are open rooted (elodont) in all rodent species.
- Dental formula of chinchilla is $2 \times 1\text{I } 0\text{C } 1\text{P } 3\text{M} = 20$; as with all rodent species and rabbits, chinchillas lack canine teeth, and there is a diastema between the incisor and the premolar tooth.
- Premolar and molar teeth are anatomically indistinguishable and are usually simply called "cheek teeth" for this reason. Each quadrant includes 4 cheek teeth, for a total of 16.
- Cheek teeth of chinchillas are open rooted (elodont); the occlusal surface is rough and uneven due to enamel crests and dentinal grooves.

PATHOPHYSIOLOGY
- Chinchillas have elodont (continuously growing) incisors and cheek teeth (similar to rabbits), which are worn during normal chewing activity.
- The primary cause of dental disease in the chinchillas is insufficient or improper wearing of cheek teeth due to inappropriate diet, in particular, lack of crude fiber.
- Acquired malocclusion and severe deviation of incisor teeth occur most often following acquired dental disease of cheek teeth and uneven chewing. However, it may also be primary following traumatic fractures of the clinical crowns.

SIGNS

Historical Findings
- Chinchillas typically demonstrate clinical signs only when dental disease is advanced. Therefore, routine dental examinations starting at or before 2 years of age (before the onset of clinical signs) are imperative in the diagnosis of early disease to prevent or delay progression.
- When clinical signs develop, a history of reduced activity, decreased food intake, and reduced production of stools are most common.
- Weight loss and emaciation are often present but frequently missed by the owner due to the heavy fur typical of this species.
- Other historical signs are wet fur over the mouth, the chin, and the forelimbs, as dental disease often leads to ptyalism and pawing of the mouth.
- Malocclusion of incisors is common but is rarely a presenting complaint because it is usually missed by the owner.

Physical Examination Findings
- Epiphora and cortical bone deformities of the ventral mandible are common findings in early dental disease. Both are related to elongation of the reserve crowns (roots) and deformation of the apices of maxillary and mandibular cheek teeth.
- The small size and natural chinchilla behaviors make effective oral examination less than optimal or impossible in the awake animal. Complete inspection and proper diagnosis of dental disease should be performed under general anesthesia.
- Intraoral inspection and treatment of dental disease in rodents require specialized equipment. The "table top mouth gag and restrainer" is much easier to use than traditional mouth gags, which are difficult to keep in place due to small patient size and relatively big size of the instruments.
- Smaller, modified "open blade" cheek dilators are available and are much more effective than those used in rabbits as they provide more effective hold on the well-developed buccal folds.
- Inspection by oral endoscopy provides optimal oral visualization for all rodent species. A 14- to 18-cm-long, 2.7-mm-thick, 30-degree rigid endoscope is commonly used. Other magnification devices are helpful but not always sufficient, and many lesions can be missed without the help of stomatoscopy.
- Like rabbits, abnormalities of the occlusal planes can occur in "step mouth" and "wave mouth" patterns.
- Excessive curvature of the reserve crowns leads to apical deformities of the cheek teeth, both maxillary and mandibular.

- Common abnormalities on oral examination include widened interproximal spaces on mandibular cheek teeth and sharp buccal spikes on the maxillary cheek teeth. Coronal elongation of maxillary cheek teeth is frequently accompanied by an increase in height of both the alveolar crest and the gingival margin.

CAUSES AND RISK FACTORS
- Feeding diets insufficient in hay; hay provides an abrasive material to grind coronal surfaces

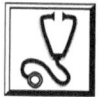 **DIAGNOSIS**

DIFFERENTIAL DIAGNOSIS
For reduced food intake or anorexia—gastrointestinal disease, pain, metabolic disease

CBC/BIOCHEMISTRY/URINALYSIS
Usually normal unless secondary problems or concurrent disease are present.

OTHER LABORATORY TESTS
N/A

IMAGING
- An optimal radiologic study includes five views (lateral; two obliques; ventrodorsal and rostrocaudal). Additional extraoral oblique projections, as well as additional intraoral views, may also be used.
- Modern spiral CT scanning provides excellent detail in small species such as chinchillas. Three-dimensional volume and surface renderings of the head provide tremendous information for diagnosis of dental disease or related problems such as osteomyelitis.

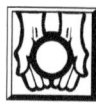 **TREATMENT**

The goal of treatment is restoration of dental anatomy to as close to normal as possible. Extraction of diseased teeth may be part of the dental treatment as well. In most cases, treatment provides only palliation, as effective restoration of dental anatomy to normal is not possible.

APPROPRIATE HEALTH CARE
Unless severely debilitated, treatment of dental disease is performed on an outpatient basis.

DIET
- It is absolutely imperative that the patient continue to eat during and following treatment. Most chinchillas with dental disease present for reduced food intake or anorexia and may be unable to eat solid food for some time following coronal reduction.

Anorexia will cause or exacerbate GI hypomotility, derangement of the gastrointestinal microflora, and overgrowth of intestinal bacterial pathogens.
• Syringe-feed a gruel such as Critical Care for Herbivores (Oxbow Pet Products) or Emerald Herbivore (Lafeber Company, Cornell, IL), 10–15 mL/kg PO q8–12h. Larger volumes and more frequent feedings are often accepted; feed as much as the patient will readily accept.
• Return the patient to a solid food diet as soon as possible to encourage normal occlusion and wear. Increase the amount of tough, fibrous foods and foods containing abrasive silicates such as hay and wild grasses.

CLIENT EDUCATION
• The prognosis is directly related to the stage of dental disease when diagnosis is made. Usually, severe to end-stage dental disease is frequently diagnosed at first presentation.
• Inform the owner that repeated coronal reduction and additional dental treatment will usually be necessary, often life-long, since treatment provides only palliation, and effective restoration of dental anatomy to normal is usually not possible. However, treatment is beneficial to control the progression of dental disease and related clinical signs and symptoms.
• If early dental disease is found on routine examination in a young animal, increasing the amount of coarse fiber in the form of hay may prevent or delay progression of disease.

SURGICAL CONSIDERATIONS
Trimming of the Cheek Teeth (Coronal Reduction)
• Coronal reduction requires general anesthesia.
• Use a focused, directed light source and magnification loops. Adequate visualization and protection of soft tissues require specialized equipment (see "Physical Examination Findings" above).
• A rotating dental unit with a straight handpiece and small metal or silicon burs is used to reduce coronal surfaces.
• Coronal reduction of incisor teeth is usually performed in conjunction with dental treatment of cheek teeth.
• The goal of occlusal adjustment of cheek teeth is to shorten the elongated clinical crowns. This is often difficult to completely accomplish for the maxillary cheek teeth because gingival proliferation limits the depth of reduction.
• Extraction is challenging unless the tooth is loose secondary to periodontal infection; diseased teeth may fracture easily, making complete extraction difficult in selected cases.

MEDICATIONS
DRUGS OF CHOICE
Antibiotics
• Antimicrobial drugs are indicated if bacterial infection is diagnosed.
• Antibiotics should be selected based on the bacterial culture and antimicrobial sensitivity but can be chosen empirically for the initial phase of treatment. A limited number of antibiotics are safe to use in chinchillas, as many cause potentially fatal antibiotic-associated dybiosis and enterotoxemia.
• Use broad-spectrum antibiotics such as enrofloxacin (5–15 mg/kg PO, SC q12h) or trimethoprim-sulfa (15–30 mg/kg PO q12h) for aerobic infections. Anaerobic bacteria may also be causative agent of tooth root abscess; if anaerobes are present, chloramphenicol (30–50 mg/kg PO, SC, IM, IV q12h) has good osseous penetration. Penicillin G (40,000–60,000 IU/kg SC q2–7d) may also be used in severe cases. Monitor closely for loose stool or diarrhea.

Pain Management
• Analgesics such as buprenorphine (0.01–0.05 mg/kg SC, IV q8–12h), meloxicam (0.5–1 mg/kg PO, SC q24h), or carprofen (2–5 mg/kg PO, SC q24h). Pain is common in chinchillas with dental disease; pain impairs mobility, decreases appetite, and may severely inhibit recovery.

CONTRAINDICATIONS
• Oral administration of penicillins, macrolides, lincosamides, and cephalosporins will cause potentially fatal enteric dysbiosis.
• Use of immunosuppressive drugs such as corticosteroids
• Extensive surgery on a debilitated animal, as in case of facial abscesses.

PRECAUTIONS
• Oral administration of antibiotics may cause antibiotic-associated enteritis, dysbiosis, and enterotoxemia.
• Metronidazole may cause anorexia when administered PO in some chinchillas; hepatic toxicity has been anecdotally reported.

FOLLOW-UP
PATIENT MONITORING
• Monitor food intake following treatment. Many patients require assist feeding with hay-based gruel. The duration of assist feeding depends on the severity of disease and on time for improvement.
• Reevaluate and trim as needed. Evaluate the entire oral cavity with each recheck.

PREVENTION/AVOIDANCE
Provide adequate tough, fibrous hay and grasses to encourage normal wear.

POSSIBLE COMPLICATIONS
Periapical infections and abscesses, recurrence, chronic pain, or inability to chew.

EXPECTED COURSE AND PROGNOSIS
In general, the prognosis for dental disease in chinchillas is more guarded than in rabbits since severe to end-stage dental disease is frequently diagnosed at first presentation.
Repeated coronal reduction will usually be necessary, often life-long, since treatment is only palliative, and effective restoration of dental anatomy to normal is usually not possible.

MISCELLANEOUS
AGE-RELATED FACTORS
N/A
ZOONOTIC POTENTIAL
N/A
PREGNANCY/FERTILITY/BREEDING
N/A
SYNONYMS
N/A
SEE ALSO
Anorexia
Nasal discharge and sneezing
ABBREVIATIONS
N/A
INTERNET RESOURCES
N/A

Suggested Reading
Capello V. Diagnostic imaging of dental disease in pet rabbits and rodents. Vet Clin Exot Anim 2016;19(3):757–782.
Capello V, Gracis M. The Chinchilla. In: Lennox AM, ed. Rabbit and Rodent Dentistry Handbook. West Palm Beach, FL: Zoological Education Network, 2005:27–30.
Capello V, Lennox AM. Clinical Radiology of Exotic Companion Mammals. Ames, IA: Wiley Blackwell, 2008.
Capello V, Lennox AM. Small mammal dentistry. In: Quesenberry KE, Carpenter JW, eds. Ferrets, Rabbits and Rodents Clinical Medicine and Surgery, 3rd ed. St Louis: Elsevier Saunders, 2012:452–471.
Crossley DA. Clinical aspects of rodent dental anatomy. J Vet Dent 1995;12(4):131–135.
Mans C, Jekl V. Anatomy and disorders of the oral cavity of chinchillas and degus. Vet Clin Exot Anim 2016;19(3):843–868.
Authors Vittorio Capello, DVM, and Barbara Oglesbee, DVM

DERMATOPHYTOSIS

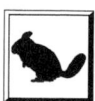

BASICS

DEFINITION
• A cutaneous infection affecting quantified regions of hair, nails, and occasionally the superficial layers of the skin.
• *Trichophyton mentagrophytes* is the organism typically encountered in rodent dermatophytoses.
• *Microsporum canis* and *M. gypseum* are also infrequently isolated and are thought to be acquired from other animals such as dogs and cats.
• Exposure to or contact with dermatophyte does not necessarily result in infection.
• Chinchillas can be asymptomatic carriers.

PATHOPHYSIOLOGY
Dermatophytes are fungal pathogens that use keratin as a nutrient source. Dermatophytes grow in the keratinized layers of hair, nails, and skin; they do not thrive in living tissue or persist in the presence of severe inflammation.

Dermatophytes are readily transmitted by direct contact with spores on fur, in bedding, on grooming equipment, and elsewhere within the environment.

SYSTEMS AFFECTED
Skin/exocrine

GENETICS
Genetics has been implicated as a predisposing factor, but this has not been proven.

INCIDENCE/PREVALENCE
Reported prevalence rates of 5%–30% in rodents; unclear as to specific incidence in chinchillas

GEOGRAPHIC DISTRIBUTION
N/A

SIGNALMENT
More common in young and/or debilitated animals

SIGNS

Historical Findings
• Few or no clinical signs of infection are common
• Lesions often begin as alopecia and dry scaly skin.
• A history of previously confirmed infection or exposure to an infected animal environment is a useful but inconsistent finding.
• Variable pruritis

Physical Examination Findings
• Often begins as focal areas of alopecia
• Classic, well-circumscribed areas of alopecia, crust, scale, and broken hair are often identified first around the eyes, nose, mouth, and feet, but may occur anywhere on the body.
• Scales, crust, erythema are variable, usually in more severe cases.
• Variable pruritis

CAUSES
• Exposure to infected animals, including other chinchillas, other rodents, rabbits, cats, and dogs
• Poor management practices—overcrowding, poor ventilation, dirty environment, poor nutrition
• As in other species, immunocompromised animals or treatment with immunosuppressive medications may predispose to infection, but this has not been clearly demonstrated in chinchillas.

RISK FACTORS
Overcrowding, inappropriate heat and humidity, genetics, age, and pregnancy have been implicated.

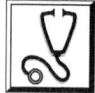

DIAGNOSIS

DIFFERENTIAL DIAGNOSIS
• Fur mites—*Cheyletiella* spp. have been reported in chinchillas and may be concurrent with dermatophytosis. Fur mite lesions are usually located in the intrascapular or tail base region and are associated with large, white scale. Mites are readily identified from skin scrapes or acetate tape reparations under low magnification.
• Ear mites are very rarely reported in chinchillas.
• Fleas—patchy alopecia usually appears in other areas in addition to the head and feet; finding flea dirt will help to differentiate.
• Demodicosis—extremely rare; may occur in association with corticosteroid use; might be identified on deep skin scrape
• Contact dermatitis—usually ventral distribution of lesions; acute onset
• Barbering—by cagemates or self-inflicted; causes hair loss alone without pruritis, scales, or skin lesions
• Lack of grooming due to obesity or underlying dental or musculoskeletal disease may cause an accumulation of scale, especially in the intrascapular region.
• Injection site reactions—especially with irritating substances such as enrofloxacin; may cause alopecia and crusting

CBC/BIOCHEMISTRY/URINALYSIS
Useful for identifying underlying disease.

OTHER LABORATORY TESTS
N/A

IMAGING
N/A

DIAGNOSTIC PROCEDURES
• Skin scraping—micro-spatula with flat-ended blade (preferred) or dull edge of scalpel blade
• Acetate tape preparation—evaluate under low-power microscopy for ectoparasites
• Trichogram—cytology of epilated hairs to examine for lice, other ectoparasites, or eggs
• Skin biopsy—especially helpful in confirming infection and ruling out other causes for lesions

KOH Preparation
A quick diagnosis can sometimes be achieved with a wet mount KOH preparation. Skin scrapings from the periphery of a lesion are placed on a slide with a drop of 10% KOH and gently heated. This dissolves the keratin (hair, keratinocytes), leaving the fungal organisms. A stain such as lactophenol blue may be added, and the slide is examined under the microscope.

Wood's Lamp Examination
Not very useful as a screening tool; many pathogenic dermatophytes do not fluoresce; false fluorescence is common. Lamp should warm up for a minimum of 5 minutes and be exposed to suspicious lesions for up to 5 minutes; a true positive reaction associated with *M. canis* consists of apple-green fluorescence of the hair shaft; keratin associated with epidermal scales and sebum will often produce a false positive fluorescence.

Fungal Culture
• Best means of confirming specific diagnosis
• Hairs that exhibit a positive apple-green fluorescence under a Wood's lamp examination are considered ideal candidates for culture (*M. canis* only).
• Samples for traditional fungal culture should be collected using a sterile brush or spatula to collect skin and hairs from the periphery of an alopecic area; can be inoculated onto a suitable fungal culture medium. Cultures can take 10 days or more for growth to become evident.
• Culture using DTM provides a color change to red when dermatophytes become alkaline; dermatophytes typically produce this color during the early growing phase of their culture; saprophytes, which also produce color, do so in the late growing phase; thus, it is important to examine DTM daily.
• A positive culture indicates existence of a dermatophyte, but this must be differentiated from environmental contamination with a geophilic dermatophyte, which can occur when the feet are cultured.
• Reculture when lesions have disappeared; two negative cultures give best confidence of clearance.

(CONTINUED)

PATHOLOGIC FINDINGS

The diagnosis is usually made on direct microscopic examination of skin scrapings with KOH. Histopathological examination is rarely required to confirm dermatophytic infections. One classic histological pattern is the presence of neutrophils within the stratum corneum. Other common patterns include compact orthokeratosis and a layer of compact orthokeratosis underlying normal orthokeratosis (the so-called "sandwich sign"). Occasionally, the organisms may be seen with routine H and E stain, but commonly a special stain such as GMS or PAS must be used to identify fungal hyphae. Dermatophyte infection of the hair is termed endothrix if it invades the hair shaft and exothrix if it remains on the surface.

TREATMENT

APPROPRIATE HEALTH CARE

• Management of dermatophytosis must be directed at eradication of infectious material from affected animals, in-contact animals, and the environment.
• Environmental treatment is mandatory. Dilute bleach (1:10 solution) is a practical and relatively effective means of environmental decontamination. Concentrated bleach and formalin (1%) combination is more effective at killing spores but is not practical in many situations; chlorhexidine was ineffective in pilot studies. Gloves should be worn during cleaning.
• Patients that appear otherwise normal are typically managed as outpatients; diagnostic evaluation may require brief hospitalization.
• Diseases associated with systemic signs of illness (e.g., pyrexia, depression, anorexia, and dehydration) or laboratory findings of azotemia and/or leukocytosis warrant an aggressive diagnostic evaluation and initiation of supportive and symptomatic treatment.

NURSING CARE

• Gloves should be worn when handling animals with this disease due to the zoonotic nature of the organism.
• Subcutaneous fluids can be administered (30–50 mL/kg) as needed; IV access is difficult in the chinchilla; lateral saphenous vein catheters often kink; consider interosseous (IO) catheterization if intravascular fluids are needed. Base fluid selection on the underlying cause of fluid loss. In most patients, lactated Ringer's solution or Normosol crystalloid fluids are appropriate. Maintenance needs are estimated at 100 mL/kg/day.

ACTIVITY

• Isolate patients and in-contact animals during treatment, as dermatophytosis is very infective and zoonotic.
• Dust baths should be administered less frequently (once weekly); do not reuse dust baths. Use only good-quality dust bathing materials.

DIET

• Some chinchillas will develop inappetence. Be certain the chinchilla is eating, or provide assisted syringe feeding of an herbivore critical care diet (e.g., Critical Care for Herbivores, Oxbow Animal Health, Omaha, NE, or Emeraid Herbivore, Lafeber Company, Cornell, IL) if anorectic to prevent the development, or exacerbation of, gastrointestinal dysmotility/GI stasis.
• Increasing water content in foods or via oral or parenteral fluids may increase fluid intake. Provide multiple sources of fresh water, including supplementing fresh water with small amounts of pure fruit juice (no added sugars), high water content vegetables, or soaking or misting fresh vegetables before offering.

CLIENT EDUCATION

• Dermatophytosis is zoonotic to humans and other household pets.
• Wear gloves when handling affected and in-contact animals and when cleaning the environment.
• Use 10% bleach solution to clean the animal's environment, including all living areas, clothing of the owners, toys, etc. Discard wooden cage materials and toys as they cannot be disinfected adequately.
• Discard previously used dust bath materials.

SURGICAL CONSIDERATIONS

When obtaining biopsy specimens, care should be taken to avoid transfer of organisms to other noninfected sites via contaminated surgical instruments.

MEDICATIONS

DRUG(S) OF CHOICE

Regardless of the therapy chosen, treatment should continue until two negative cultures are obtained 4 weeks apart. In general, a combination of topical therapy and systemic antifungals is required for successful treatment of severe infections.

Topical Therapy

• Prior to topical therapy, affected areas should be gently clipped to expose dermatophyte-infected skin, realizing that

fungal organisms may be transferred to other areas in the process. Thoroughly cleanse clipper blades after use. Always wear gloves when handling the patient.
• Lime sulfur dip (1:16 in water) is safe and efficacious q3–7d. The animal should not be rinsed but should be towel dried. Avoid contact with the eyes and ears as it can be irritating. It is odiferous and can stain. It is the treatment of choice for pregnant chinchillas. Wear gloves when using.
• 2% chlorhexidine/2% miconazole shampoo—shown to have moderate success in cats and dogs; efficacy and toxicity unknown in chinchillas
• 0.2% enilconazole rinse q3–7d—unpredictable toxicity of enilconazole has been reported in cats; recommend caution and advise clients of the concerns, as no information exists on the use of enilconazole in chinchillas and grooming may result in excessive consumption
• Clotrimazole, ketoconazole, or miconazole creams or ointments are not recommended as they are not formulated to penetrate infected hair shafts and follicles; unsuccessful in the dense fur of chinchillas

Systemic Therapy

• Terbinafine 20–40 mg/kg PO q24h × 4–6 weeks; has also been used successfully in other species
• Itraconazole 5 mg/kg PO q24h × 6–8 weeks (or until negative cultures) has been used successfully in chinchillas
• Fluconazole 16 mg/kg PO q24h × 3–4 weeks (or until negative cultures) has been used with success in guinea pigs, no data for chinchillas
• Griseofulvin 25 mg/kg PO q24h × 4–6 weeks (or until negative cultures) for refractory or severe cases; less effective than itraconazole

CONTRAINDICATIONS

The use of corticosteroids (systemic or topical) can severely exacerbate dermatophytosis.

PRECAUTIONS

• Dosages for systemic antifungal medications are extrapolated from dog and cat doses, so caution should always be used and the patient must be closely evaluated for idiosyncratic or toxic reactions.
• Griseofulvin can cause bone marrow suppression and pancytopenia as an idiosyncratic reaction in other species, but this has not been reported in chinchillas; weekly or bi-weekly CBCs are warranted during therapy.
• Ketoconazole and fluconazole can be hepatotoxic; monitor hepatic enzymes during therapy.

DERMATOPHYTOSIS (CONTINUED)

POSSIBLE INTERACTIONS
The imidazole antifungal medications (especially ketoconazole) can induce hepatotoxicity, which could interfere with metabolism of other drugs metabolized by the liver.

ALTERNATIVE DRUGS
• Ketoconazole 5–7 mg/kg PO q12h has been used, but adverse effects (e.g., gastric irritation, hepatotoxicity, and anorexia) are often reported so use with caution.

FOLLOW-UP

PATIENT MONITORING
Repeat fungal cultures toward the end of the treatment regimen and continue treatment until at least one negative culture result is obtained; however, obtaining two negative cultures 4 weeks apart provides greater confidence that dermatophyte infection has been cleared.

PREVENTION/AVOIDANCE
• Quarantine new animals and obtain dermatophyte cultures from all animals entering the household.
• Avoid infected soil to reduce the potential for geophilic dermatophytes.

EXPECTED COURSE AND PROGNOSIS
• Many animals will "self-clear" a dermatophyte infection over a period of a few months; however, recontamination can occur and it is most prudent to treat affected animals.

• Treatment periods can be long (e.g., >30 days); if possible, continue treatment until two negative cultures are obtained.

MISCELLANEOUS

ASSOCIATED CONDITIONS
N/A

AGE-RELATED FACTORS
N/A

ZOONOTIC POTENTIAL
Dermatophytes are zoonotic.

PREGNANCY/FERTILITY/BREEDING
• Lime sulfur dip is the safest treatment for pregnant animals.
• Griseofulvin is teratogenic and should not be used in pregnant chinchillas.
• Ketoconazole can affect steroidal hormone synthesis, especially testosterone, so it should not be used in breeding animals.

SYNONYMS
Ringworm
Fungal infection

SEE ALSO
N/A

ABBREVIATIONS
DTM = dermatophyte test media
KOH = potassium hydroxide
GMS = Gömöri methenamine silver stain
PAS = periodic acid-Schiff
CBC = complete blood count

INTERNET RESOURCES
N/A

Suggested Reading
Donnelly TM, Rush EM, Lackner PA. Ringworm in small exotic pets. Sem Avian Exotic Pet Med 2000;9(2):82–93.
Mans C, Donnelly T. Chinchillas. In: Quesenberry KE, Carpenter JW, eds. Ferrets, Rabbits and Rodents, 4th ed. Clinical Medicine and Surgery. 2021. St. Louis: Saunders, 2020:298–322.
Martel A, Donnelly T, Mans C. Update on diseases in chinchillas: 2013–2019. Vet Clin Exot Anim 2020;23:321–333.
Mayer J, Mans C. Rodents. In: Carpenter JW, ed. Exotic Animal Formulary, 5th ed. St Louis: Elsevier, 2018:459–493.
Mitchell MA, Tully TN, eds. Manual of Exotic Pet Practice. St. Louis: Elsevier, 2009: 480, 487, 491.
Miwa Y, Sladky K. Common surgical procedures of rodents, ferrets, hedgehogs, and sugar gliders. Vet Clin Exot Anim 2016;19:205–244.
Palmerio BS, Roberts H. Clinical approach to dermatologic disease in exotic animals. Vet Clin North Am Exot Anim Pract 2013;16(3):523–577.
Riggs SM, Mitchell MA. Chinchillas. In: Mitchell MA, Tully TN, eds. Manual of Exotic Pet Practice. St. Louis: Elsevier, 2009:475–486.

Authors Michelle G. Hawkins, VMD, DABVP (Avian), Dan H. Johnson, DVM, DABVP (Exotic Companion Mammal)

BASICS

DEFINITION
Abnormal frequency, liquidity, and volume of feces

PATHOPHYSIOLOGY
• Caused by an imbalance in the absorptive, secretory, and motility actions of the intestines.
• Can result from a combination of factors: increased membrane permeability, hypersecretion, and malabsorption.
• Death occurs from loss of electrolytes and water, acidosis, and the manifold effects of toxins.
• A common predisposing cause of diarrhea in chinchillas is disruption of enteric commensal flora by antibiotic usage, stress, or poor nutrition. In a process known as bacterial dysbiosis, resident enteric microflora populations are altered by changes in intestinal motility, carbohydrate fermentation, pH, and substrate production. Beneficial bacteria are destroyed while pathogenic bacteria such as *Escherichia coli* and *Clostridium* spp. are promoted. Bacterial dysbiosis can lead to acute diarrhea, enterotoxemia, ileus, chronic intermittent diarrhea, and/or bloating.
• Antibiotic usage alters normal gut flora, causing severe, acute, often fatal diarrhea. The antibiotics most likely to cause problems are those that are effective against gram-positive bacteria and some gram-negative anaerobes, such as lincomycin, clindamycin, erythromycin, ampicillin, amoxicillin, cephalosporins, and penicillins. These antibiotics are likely to cause problems regardless of the route of administration.

SYSTEMS AFFECTED
• Gastrointestinal
• Endocrine/metabolic—fluid, electrolyte, and acid–base imbalances
• Many of the bacteria responsible for enteritis can also cause septicemia

GENETICS
N/A

INCIDENCE/PREVALENCE
N/A

GEOGRAPHIC DISTRIBUTION
N/A

SIGNALMENT
• Diarrhea is less common in chinchillas than lack of fecal production.
• Breeding females and young chinchillas up to 4 months of age are most susceptible to infectious causes.
• No specific age or gender predilection to noninfectious causes

SIGNS
General Comments
• Diarrhea may occur with or without signs of systemic illness.
• Signs can vary from diarrhea alone in an apparently healthy patient to severe systemic signs. Chinchillas are prey species and instinctively hide illness. Diarrhea is a serious disorder in Chinchillas warranting immediate attention even if no other clinical signs are noted.
• The choice of diagnostic and therapeutic measures depends on the severity of the illness.
• Signs of more severe illness (e.g., anorexia, weight loss, severe dehydration, depression, and shock) should prompt more aggressive diagnostic and therapeutic measures.

Historical Findings
• Stool production ranging from soft, formed to liquid consistency
• Feces smeared on resting board in the cage; fur around the anus matted with feces
• Fecal accidents, changes in fecal consistency and volume, blood or mucous in the feces, or straining to defecate
• Dietary—sudden diet change, weaning, overfeeding fresh green foods or fruit, excessive carbohydrates or sugars; spoiled food; damp, moldy, or immature hay
• Stress—hospitalization, transportation, environmental changes, and concurrent illness all may contribute to alterations in intestinal commensal flora.
• Antibiotic usage—the use of antibiotics that are primarily gram-positive in spectrum, suppressing the growth of commensal flora and allowing overgrowth of enteric pathogens

Physical Examination Findings
• Vary with the severity of disease
• Anorexia, lethargy, depression, lateral recumbency, respiratory distress
• Fever, dehydration, hypotension, weakness, hypothermia
• Rough haircoat, decreased grooming behavior
• Fecal staining of the perineum. An animal may camouflage diarrhea by cleaning itself; therefore, fecal staining of fur may not be apparent.
• Abdominal pain characterized by hunched posture, reluctance to move, stretching out, rolling, bruxism, and/or pain on abdominal palpation
• Tenesmus, hematochezia, intussusception, intestinal impaction, rectal prolapse
• Abdominal distention—due to thickened or fluid-filled bowel loops, impaction, gas accumulation, masses, or organomegaly
• Weight loss in chronically infected animals

• Animals may die acutely without clinical signs.

CAUSES
• Dietary—abrupt change in diet, weaning, excessive fresh green foods or fruit, excessive carbohydrate/sugar, or spoiled food
• Bacterial infection/enterotoxemia—*E. coli*, *Listeria* spp., *Pseudomonas* spp., *Proteus* spp., *Pasteurella* spp., *Salmonella* spp., *Staphylococcus* spp., *Yersinia* spp., and *Clostridium* spp.
• Obstruction—neoplasia, foreign body, intussusception
• Drugs/toxins—administration (particularly PO) of antibiotics lincomycin, clindamycin, erythromycin, ampicillin, amoxicillin, cephalosporins, and penicillins; plant toxins; mycotoxins
• Parasitic—*Giardia* spp., coccidia, nematodes, cestodes, *Cryptosporidium* spp.
• Metabolic disorders—liver disease, renal disease
• Systemic illness may cause diarrhea as a secondary event.
• Neoplasia—primary gastrointestinal tumor, or as a sequela to other organ involvement

RISK FACTORS
• Stress—improper temperature, poor sanitation, overcrowding, shipping
• Sudden diet changes, weaning, insufficient dietary fiber, carbohydrate overload
• Improper antibiotic usage
• Contaminated food
• Immunosuppressors (corticosteroids, concurrent disease), heavy parasite load, and poor nutrition are additional predisposing factors.

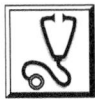

DIAGNOSIS

DIFFERENTIAL DIAGNOSIS
Consider all causes of enteropathy, including diet change, inappropriate antibiotics, enterotoxemia, systemic or metabolic disease, and specific intestinal disorders. A more severe illness should prompt a more extensive evaluation.

CBC/BIOCHEMISTRY/URINALYSIS
• Often normal in mild cases
• Increased PCV and TS are seen with dehydration.
• Hemogram abnormalities consistent with sepsis and/or systemic infection
• TWBC elevation with neutrophilia is indicative of a toxic inflammatory response.
• Anemia is possible with chronic gastrointestinal bleeding.
• Hypoalbuminemia may be seen with protein loss from the intestinal tract.

DIARRHEA (CONTINUED)

• Serum biochemistry abnormalities seen with renal or hepatic disease
• Electrolyte abnormalities secondary to anorexia, fluid loss, and dehydration

OTHER LABORATORY TESTS
Fecal Examination
• Fecal direct examination (with and without Lugol's iodine), fecal floatation, and zinc sulfate centrifugation may demonstrate gastrointestinal parasites or spore-forming bacteria.
• Fecal cytology—may reveal red blood cells or fecal leukocytes, which are associated with inflammation or infection of the intestines
• Fecal gram's stain—may demonstrate large numbers of spore-forming bacteria consistent with *Clostridium* spp. or excessive numbers of gram-negative bacteria
• Fecal culture should be performed if bacterial infection is suspected; however, interpretation may be difficult since *E. coli, Salmonella,* and *Clostridium* spp. may be isolated from clinically healthy chinchillas.
• Fecal occult blood testing—to confirm melena when suspected

IMAGING
• Whole-body radiographs to assess both body cavities
• Varying amounts of gas and ingesta may normally be seen in healthy chinchillas.
• With gastroenteritis, there is usually an increase in gas production and evidence of ingesta in spite of persistent anorexia.
• With ileus, there may be significant gas accumulation ("bloat").
• Contrast radiography may aid in visualization and determination of motility.
• Abdominal ultrasonography may demonstrate intestinal wall thickening, gastrointestinal mass, foreign body, ileus, or mesenteric lymphadenopathy.
• Ultrasound may be difficult to interpret when large amounts of gas are present within the intestinal tract.
• Hyperechogenicity may be seen with hepatic lipidosis or fibrosis; hypoechoic nodules are suggestive of hepatic necrosis, abscess, or neoplasia.

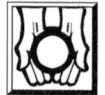

TREATMENT

APPROPRIATE HEALTH CARE
• Treatment must be specific to the underlying cause in order to be successful.
• Chinchillas with mild diarrhea, that are otherwise bright and alert, usually respond to outpatient treatment.
• Individuals with moderate to severe diarrhea usually require hospitalization and 24-hour care for parenteral medication, fluid therapy, and thermal support.
• Patients exhibiting signs of lethargy, depression, dehydration, and/or shock should be hospitalized even if diarrhea is mild or absent.
• When infectious disease is suspected, strict isolation of affected and exposed animals is indicated.

NURSING CARE
Fluid Therapy
• Rehydration and correction of electrolyte imbalances are the mainstays of treatment in most cases.
• Severe volume depletion can occur with acute diarrhea; aggressive shock fluid therapy may be indicated.
• Fluids may be administered by oral, subcutaneous, intravenous, and/or intraosseous routes according to the patient's condition.
• Mildly affected patients usually respond well to oral and subcutaneous fluids. Direct oral administration of products such as Gatorade (PepsiCo, Purchase, NY) or Pedialyte (Abbott Nutrition, Lake Forest, IL) is indicated if the patient is not drinking on its own.
• Subcutaneous fluids can be administered (30–50 mL/kg) as needed; intravenous or intraosseous fluids are indicated in severely dehydrated or depressed animals.
• Maintenance fluid requirements are estimated at 100 mL/kg/day.
• Rehydration is essential to treatment success in severely ill chinchillas. In most patients, lactated Ringer's solution or Normosol crystalloid fluids are appropriate.
• Provide a warm (less than 80°F/26.7°C), quiet environment to reduce stress.

DIET
• Chinchillas must continue to eat during treatment and recovery. Prolonged anorexia promotes further derangement of gastrointestinal microflora, encourages overgrowth of intestinal bacterial pathogens, and negatively affects gastrointestinal motility.
• Assisted feeding is typically required until the patient is eating, eliminating, and maintaining body weight. Use prepared formulations such as Critical Care for Herbivores (Oxbow Animal Health, Omaha, NE) and Emerald Herbivore (Lafeber Company, Cornell, IL). If commercial formula is not available, a gruel may be made by combining blenderized chinchilla pellets with pureed fruit/vegetable baby foods: 15–20 mL/kg PO q6–8h.
• Encourage oral fluid intake: offer fresh water, administer oral fluids via syringe, wet the food, flavor water with fruit or vegetable juices

CLIENT EDUCATION
• Discuss the concept of "prey species"—instinctively hide signs of illness. Any change in fecal consistency or volume should be indicated.
• Discuss the importance of dietary modification, if indicated.
• Advise owners to regularly monitor food consumption and fecal output; seek veterinary attention with noticeable decreases in either.

SURGICAL CONSIDERATIONS
• If surgery is necessary to correct intussusception or impaction, the patient should first be stabilized.
• Surgical manipulation of the intestinal tract, hypothermia, anesthetic agents, and pain may cause or exacerbate gastrointestinal hypomotility. The combination of these factors may worsen the prognosis with surgical treatment.
• Surgery may be indicated for rectal prolapse, intussusception, intestinal foreign bodies (e.g., bedding, hair), extraluminal compression of the gastrointestinal tract, intestinal neoplasia, abscesses, and orthopedic problems.

MEDICATIONS

DRUG(S) OF CHOICE
Antibiotic Therapy
• Indicated in patients with bacterial inflammatory lesions of the gastrointestinal tract; also indicated in patients with disruption of the intestinal mucosa as evidenced by blood in the feces.
• Broad-spectrum antibiotics should be selected, based on the results of culture and susceptibility testing when possible.
• Some choices for empirical use while awaiting culture results include chloramphenicol (30–50 mg/kg PO, SC, IM, IV q12h), trimethoprim sulfa (15–30 mg/kg PO q12h), and enrofloxacin (5–15 mg/kg PO, SC, IM q12h).
• For *Clostridium* spp. overgrowth: metronidazole (10–20 mg/kg PO, IV 12h) caution: may cause anorexia or reduced appetite in some chinchillas when administered PO.

Antiparasitic Agents
• Indicated based upon fecal examination for internal parasites, ova, or cysts
• For nematodes—fenbendazole (20 mg/kg PO q24h × 5 days)
• For cestodes—praziquantal (5–10 mg/kg PO or SQ, repeat in 10 days)
• For coccidia—toltrazuril (10 mg/kg PO q24h × 3 days, skip 3–5 days, repeat for

(CONTINUED)

3 days); sulfadimethoxine (25–50 mg/kg PO q24h × 10 days)
• For *Giardia*—metronidazole (10–50 mg/kg q12h × 5 days; caution may cause anorexia or reduced appetite in some chinchillas when administered PO), fenbendazole (20 mg/kg PO q24h × 5 days), albendazole (25 mg/kg PO q12h × 2 days)

Gastrointestinal Agents
• Bismuth subsalicylate (0.3–0.6 mL/kg PO q4–6h PRN; dose cited is extrapolated from rabbit dose)
• Kaolin/pectin (0.2–0.3 mL/kg PO q6–8h PRN; dose cited is extrapolated from guinea pig dose)
• Loperamide (0.1 mg/kg PO q8h × 3 days, then q24h × 2 days; give in 1 mL water) may be helpful in the treatment of acute diarrhea (see Contraindications)
• Cholestyramine (2 g/20 mL water PO q24h PRN) has been demonstrated to bind clostridial and other bacterial toxins in humans; anecdotal success in rabbits; may be useful in chinchillas
• Transfaunation with healthy chinchilla feces may help to reestablish intestinal microflora.

CONTRAINDICATIONS
• Anticholinergics (loperamide) in patients with suspected intestinal obstruction, glaucoma, intestinal ileus, liver disease, enterotoxin-producing bacteria, and invasive bacterial enteritis
• Antibiotics that are primarily gram-positive in spectrum will suppress the growth of commensal flora, allowing overgrowth of enteric pathogens. These include lincomycin, clindamycin, erythromycin, ampicillin, amoxicillin, cephalosporins, and penicillins.

PRECAUTIONS
• It is important to determine the cause of diarrhea. A general "shotgun" antibiotic approach may be ineffective or detrimental.
• Antibiotic therapy can predispose chinchillas to bacterial dysbiosis and overgrowth of pathogenic bacteria. If signs worsen or do not improve, therapy should be adjusted.
• Chloramphenicol may cause aplastic anemia in susceptible people. Clients and staff should use appropriate precautions when handling this drug.
• Metronidazole may cause anorexia or reduced appetite in some chinchillas when administered PO neurotoxic if overdosed; anecdotal reports of hepatotoxicity
• Isolate affected and exposed animals when infectious disease is suspected.

POSSIBLE INTERACTIONS
N/A

ALTERNATIVE DRUGS
N/A

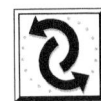

FOLLOW-UP

PATIENT MONITORING
• Fecal volume and character, appetite, attitude, and body weight
• If diarrhea does not resolve, consider reevaluation of the diagnosis.

PREVENTION/AVOIDANCE
• Providing appropriate diet and husbandry
• Reducing stress and providing sanitary conditions
• Appropriate antibiotic selection
• When infectious disease is suspected, strict isolation of affected and exposed animals is indicated.

POSSIBLE COMPLICATIONS
• Antibiotic therapy can promote bacterial dysbiosis and overgrowth of pathogenic bacteria. Use antibiotics with caution, and only use those that are considered safe for chinchillas.
• Dehydration due to fluid loss
• Ileus, bloat, intussusception, tenesmus, rectal prolapse
• Septicemia due to bacterial invasion of enteric mucosa
• Shock, death from enterotoxicosis

EXPECTED COURSE AND PROGNOSIS
Depends on cause and severity of diarrhea

MISCELLANEOUS

ASSOCIATED CONDITIONS
• Dehydration
• Malnutrition
• Hypoproteinemia
• Anemia
• Septicemia
• Peritonitis
• Rectal prolapse
• Intussusception, torsion, impaction of cecum/colon
• Hepatic lipidosis

AGE-RELATED FACTORS
• All ages are susceptible to diarrhea
• Young and recently weaned animals are most severely affected by infectious and parasitic organisms that cause diarrhea.

ZOONOTIC POTENTIAL
• *Cryptosporidium*
• *Salmonella*
• *Giardia*

PREGNANCY/FERTILITY/BREEDING
Severe diarrhea and associated metabolic disturbances may reduce fertility or cause abortion. *Salmonella* spp. infection has been associated with abortion in fur-ranched chinchillas.

SYNONYMS
N/A

SEE ALSO
Anorexia
Antibiotic-associated enterotoxemia
Gastrointestinal stasis and dilation
Giardiasis

ABBREVIATIONS
PCV = packed cell volume
TS = total solids
TWBC = total white blood cell count

INTERNET RESOURCES
N/A

Suggested Reading
Lennox AM, Gladden JN. Emergency and critical care of small mammals. In: Quesenberry KE, Carpenter JW, eds. Ferrets, Rabbits and Rodents, 4th ed. Clinical Medicine and Surgery. 2021. St. Louis: Saunders, 2020:595–608.
Mans C, Donnelly T. Chinchillas. In: Quesenberry KE, Carpenter JW, eds. Ferrets, Rabbits and Rodents, 4th ed. Clinical Medicine and Surgery. 2021. St. Louis: Saunders, 2020:298–322.
Martel A, Donnelly T, Mans C. Update on diseases in chinchillas: 2013–2019. Vet Clin Exot Anim 2020;23:321–333.
Mayer J, Mans C. Rodents. In: Carpenter JW, ed Exotic Animal Formulary, 5th ed. St Louis: Elsevier, 2018:459–493.
Mitchell MA, Tully TN, eds. Manual of Exotic Pet Practice. St. Louis: Elsevier, 2009:480, 487, 491.
Riggs SM, Mitchell MA. Chinchillas. In: Mitchell MA, Tully TN, eds. Manual of Exotic Pet Practice. St. Louis: Elsevier, 2009:475–486.
Ritzman TK. Diagnosis and clinical management of gastrointestinal conditions in exotic companion mammals (rabbits, guinea pigs, and chinchillas). Vet Clin Exot Anim 2014;17:179–194.

Author Dan H. Johnson, DVM, Dipl. ABVP (Exotic Companion Mammal)

DYSPNEA AND TACHYPNEA

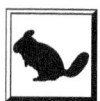 **BASICS**

DEFINITION
Dyspnea is difficulty in breathing or labored breathing; tachypnea is rapid breathing but not necessarily labored. Dyspnea and tachypnea sometimes occur simultaneously.

PATHOPHYSIOLOGY
• Dyspnea and/or tachypnea are common symptoms of respiratory or cardiovascular system disorders.
• Primary respiratory diseases may be divided into upper respiratory tract (URT) and lower respiratory tract (LRT) disorders.
• Nonrespiratory causes of dyspnea may include abnormalities in pulmonary circulation (congestive heart failure), pulmonary vascular tone (CNS disease, shock), oxygenation (anemia), or ventilation (heat stress, obesity, ascites, abdominal organomegaly, and musculoskeletal disease).

SYSTEMS AFFECTED
• Respiratory
• Cardiovascular
• Gastrointestinal
• Nervous system
• Musculoskeletal

GENETICS
Unknown

INCIDENCE/PREVALENCE
• Chinchillas are susceptible to both upper and lower airway disease.
• Esophageal or pharyngeal foreign body obstruction ("choke") is reported to be a common emergency presentation.
• Inflammation of the glottis and pharyngeal tissues is possible following tracheal intubation or attempted intubation.
• Chinchillas are particularly prone to heat stress at temperatures greater than 80°F (26.7°C).
• Cardiac disease is commonly manifested as heart murmur in chinchillas without clinical signs. There is one report of heart failure and acute dyspnea with radiographic evidence of pulmonary edema and cardiomegaly.
• Pulmonary metastatic neoplasia from a primary mammary tumor has been reported.

SIGNALMENT
• All ages and genders affected
• Previous history of dental disease common

SIGNS

General Comments
• Dyspnea and/or tachypnea may be associated with severe pneumonia (usually chronic), cardiovascular disease (acute or chronic), or choke (acute).

• Open-mouthed breathing is a poor prognostic sign because chinchillas are obligate nasal breathers: the rim of the epiglottis is usually situated dorsal to the elongated soft palate to allow air passage from the nose to the trachea during normal respiration; obstruction of nasal passages leads to open mouth breathing.

Historical Findings
• Sneezing, nasal-ocular discharge, facial abscess, dental disease, and ptyalism may be seen with upper respiratory infections.
• Exercise intolerance may occur with URT disease (chinchillas are obligatory nasal breathers), LRT disease, or CHF.
• Anorexia and lethargy are often the only presenting complaints in chinchillas with pneumonia.
• Coughing and frantic pawing at the mouth may occur with choke.
• Prolonged exposure to environmental temperatures greater than 80°F (26.7°C) can result in heat stroke.

Physical Examination Findings
• Stridor, stertor, and open-mouth breathing may occur with upper airway obstruction or pharyngeal/esophageal obstruction, spasm, and tracheal compression.
• Serous or mucopurulent nasal discharge, ocular discharge, facial abscess, dental disease, and ptyalism may occur with upper respiratory disease.
• Patients may indicate pain upon oral examination.
• Harsh inspiratory and expiratory broncho-vesicular sounds are sometimes auscultated with pneumonia.
• Lung sounds may be absent over sites of consolidation (e.g., pulmonary abscesses, neoplasia).
• If lung sounds are absent ventrally and harsh lung sounds are present dorsally, consider pleural effusion
• Fine inspiratory crackles may indicate pulmonary edema.
• Pyrexia is seen with hyperthermia due to heat stress or systemic infectious disease.
• Gastric tympany suggests gastric outflow obstruction.
• Weight loss and poor hair coat are seen in chinchillas with chronic respiratory or dental disease.
• Anorexic chinchillas may show signs of GI hypomotility—scant dry feces, dehydration, firm stomach or cecal contents, and/or gas-filled intestinal loops.
• Cardiac murmur is a common incidental finding in chinchillas but may also be associated with congestive heart failure.

CAUSES

Respiratory causes

Upper Respiratory Tract
• Nasal obstruction—rhinitis/sinusitis most commonly caused by Gram-negative organisms, dental disease (periapical abscess, elongated maxillary tooth roots penetrating into nasal passages, associated with anaerobic bacteria), foreign body, neoplasia (rare), mycotic infection (rare).
• Laryngotracheal obstruction—common to have laryngeal edema following traumatic intubation or attempts at intubation
• Choke—pharyngeal or esophageal spasm, tracheal compression due to food mass or foreign body
• Traumatic airway rupture (rare)

Lower Respiratory Tract
• Pneumonia—most common bacterial agents reported in chinchillas are Gram-negative bacteria (e.g., *Pseudomonas aeruginosa*, *Listeria monocytogenes*, and *Streptococcus pneumoniae*).
• Aspiration pneumonia secondary to force-feeding
• Neoplasia (primary or metastatic, both rare)
• Pulmonary edema (cardiogenic and noncardiac)
• Pneumonitis (allergic)
• Pneumothorax, hemothorax, chylothorax, pleural effusion caused by cardiac or pericardial disease
• Diaphragmatic hernia (rare)

Nonrespiratory causes
• Pain, fever, heat stress, obesity, anxiety
• Cardiac disease—CHF, severe arrhythmias, cardiogenic shock
• Hematologic—anemia
• Metabolic disease—acidosis, uremia
• Abdominal distension—bloat due to gastric obstruction or organomegaly, ascites, or pregnancy

RISK FACTORS
• Dental disease—periapical or tooth root abscess extending into nasal sinuses; low-fiber diets may predispose to dental disease
• Dysphagia, force-feeding—can lead to aspiration
• Elevated environmental temperatures
• Poor husbandry—dirty, urine-soaked bedding (high ammonia concentrations); poor ventilation, prolonged exposure to dust baths
• Bleach, smoke or other inhaled irritants
• Immunosuppression—stress, corticosteroid administration, concurrent disease, and debility increase susceptibility to and extension of bacterial infections.

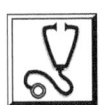

DIAGNOSIS

DIFFERENTIAL DIAGNOSIS

• Tachypnea without dyspnea may be a physiologic response to fear, physical exertion, anxiety, fever, pain, or acidosis.
• Pneumonia usually presents with signs of systemic disease (e.g., emaciation, anorexia, depression, and fever).
• URT dyspnea is often more pronounced on inspiration; nasal discharge, facial abscesses, or signs of dental disease are usually present.
• LRT dyspnea is more often associated with increased expiratory effort but can also present as increased inspiratory effort.
• Pharyngeal mass may cause both inspiratory and expiratory dyspnea, also orthopnea.
• Gastric tympany is an emergency and can be easily palpated, auscultated, and diagnosed radiographically.
• Heat stress is an emergency; typical history includes exposure to elevated environmental temperatures.
• Primary cardiac disease often presents with a constellation of other signs (e.g., heart murmur, arrhythmias, and exercise intolerance).
• Pleural space disease often presents as exaggerated thoracic excursions that generate only minimal airflow at the mouth or nose.
• Neoplasia—uncommon; rule out via imaging.
• Trauma—history and physical examination findings of trauma

CBC/BIOCHEMISTRY/URINALYSIS

• Hemogram—TWBC elevations with neutrophil: lymphocyte ratio shift; toxicity of neutrophils ± bands, monocytosis may suggest chronicity; thrombocytosis associated with active inflammation
• Biochemistry panel—may help to define underlying cause with metabolic diseases; increased liver enzyme activity or bile acids (liver disease), uremia (renal failure), increased CK (muscle wasting, heart disease, or muscle damage if soft tissue abscesses)

OTHER LABORATORY TESTS

• Culture and sensitivity from deep nasal swabs may be useful if URT disease.
• Ultrasound to identify pulmonary abscessation; ultrasound-guided FNA for cytology and culture of abscesses

IMAGING

Radiography

• Skull—nasal obstructions, sinusitis, bone destruction from tooth root abscesses, neoplasia, mycotic, or severe bacterial infections; CT scan or MRI much more useful in diagnosis of URT disease

• Thoracic—pulmonary diseases (small airway disease, pulmonary edema, and pneumonia), pleural space disease (effusion, mediastinal mass, and pneumothorax)
• Cardiac shadow—cardiomegaly, tracheal elevation
• Abdominal—gas-filled stomach due to outflow obstruction (bloat), aerophagia, organomegaly, ascites

Ultrasonography

• Thoracic ultrasound may locate pulmonary abscessation.
• Abdominal ultrasound may be used to evaluate masses, organomegaly, or renal abnormalities.

Echocardiography

Evaluate congenital defects and valvular disease, pericardial effusion, cardiomyopathy

CT Scan

Superior to radiographs for identifying bony changes and severity of dental disease. Can also evaluate the nasal cavity for evidence of fluid or exudates and the soft tissue structures in greater detail to evaluate for signs of abscessation/neoplasia. Contrast CT is useful for evaluating if a tumor is suspected and to detail the extent of a tumor.

DIAGNOSTIC PROCEDURES

• Microbiologic and cytological examinations
• LRT samples—transtracheal washing and bronchoalveolar lavage are difficult procedures in chinchillas and only recommended if able to intubate. Fine-needle aspiration of abscess, fluid, or mass can be performed under ultrasound guidance.
• URT samples—nasal flush rarely yields diagnostic sample; nonspecific inflammation is most commonly found. Deep nasal cultures and cytology showing intracellular bacteria in conjunction with culture results is more meaningful.
• Electrocardiogram—cardiac murmurs and subclinical valvular disorders are common in chinchillas; other cardiac disease is rarely reported but may be underdiagnosed due to lack of clinical investigation.

PATHOLOGIC FINDINGS

Varies with the primary disorder

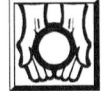

TREATMENT

APPROPRIATE HEALTH CARE

• Severe dyspnea requires hospitalization for supplemental oxygen and stabilization.
• Supply oxygen enrichment (oxygen cage or induction chamber) in a quiet environment.
• Gastric bloat and heat stress require emergency critical care.

• If trauma to the glottis/pharynx has occurred during tracheal intubation attempts, prophylactic NSAID therapy is indicated if/ when animal is well hydrated.
• Nebulization with saline ± antibiotics and/ or mucolytics may be beneficial.
• Systemic antibiotics for bacterial URT or LRT disease. Prolonged course of treatment may be indicated.
• Outpatient—if stable and can be managed at home pending further diagnostics or treatments as necessary

NURSING CARE

• Maintain normal systemic hydration— important to aid mucociliary clearance and secretion mobilization.
• Subcutaneous fluids can be administered (30–50 mL/kg) as needed; IV access can be difficult in the chinchilla; lateral saphenous vein catheters often kink; consider IO catheterization if intravascular fluids are needed. Base fluid selection on the underlying cause of fluid loss. In most patients, isotonic crystalloid fluids (e.g., lactated Ringer's solution, Normosol) are appropriate. Maintenance needs are estimated at 100 mL/ kg/day.
• Fluids by mouth should be avoided in patients with dyspnea or dysphagia.
• Gastric decompression in cases of gastric tympany can be accomplished by passing a large red rubber tube into the stomach through the oral cavity or, alternatively, a needle used as a trocar can be passed percutaneously. Trocarization carries a high risk of gastric or cecal rupture or peritonitis.
• Clinical signs of hyperthermia and shock require reducing the chinchilla's core body temperature to approximately 103°F (39.4°C) with cool crystalloid fluids and cool towels. Treat perfusion deficits with fluid therapy.
• Keep nares clear of nasal discharges in chinchillas with URT disease.
• Thoracocentesis may be both diagnostic and therapeutic in animals with pleural space disease.

ACTIVITY

Restrict activity if severe dyspnea or tachypnea

DIET

• Many chinchillas will develop inappetence. Be certain the chinchilla is eating to prevent the development or exacerbation of gastrointestinal hypomotility/stasis.
• If patient is eating on own, offer a range of normal dietary items including fresh, moist, high-fiber vegetables, chopped hay, and chinchilla pellets.
• If chinchilla is not eating sufficiently on its own, anorexia will often cause GI hypomotility, derangement of the gastrointestinal

microflora, and overgrowth of intestinal bacterial pathogens. Syringe-feeding of a high-fiber diet (e.g., Critical Care for Herbivores, Oxbow Animal Health, Omaha, NE; Emeraid Herbivore, Lafeber Co., Cornell, IL) is critical for the anorexic chinchilla. Administer with caution in cases with dyspnea or dysphagia (aspiration risk). Calculate maintenance caloric requirements using 57 × W0.75 (usually equates to feeding critical care diet at 10–15 mL/kg PO q6–8 hours via syringe) if anorectic. Alternatively, chinchilla pellets can be ground with high-fiber green vegetables to make slurry that can be syringe-fed as above. Ensure appropriate fiber intake to maximize nutrition.
• Rarely, esophagostomy tube is indicated.
• Encourage fluid intake by offering high water content vegetables or by soaking vegetables in water before feeding.
• CAUTION—patients with dyspnea are at risk for aspiration. Ensure patient is in a stable position and is willing to take foods before assisted feeding.

CLIENT EDUCATION
Chinchillas are long-lived and should receive annual physical examinations after reaching adult age. Proper husbandry and appropriate diet can help to reduce many of these problems.

SURGICAL CONSIDERATIONS
• Chinchillas are difficult to intubate due to the palatal ostium in the oropharynx, which complicates providing a secure airway during anesthesia. Chinchillas can be intubated endoscopically.
• Dental disease may be primary cause of URT disorder.

MEDICATIONS
DRUG(S) OF CHOICE
• Systemic antibiotics—based ideally on results from culture and sensitivity testing. Depending on severity of infection, long-term antibiotics (≥6 weeks) are usually indicated. Use broad-spectrum antibiotics such as enrofloxacin (5–15 mg/kg PO, SC q12h) or trimethoprim-sulfa (15–30 mg/kg PO q12h) for aerobic infections; if anaerobes are present as in dental disease, chloramphenicol (30–50 mg/kg PO, SC, IV q12h) has excellent osseous penetration; penicillin G (40,000–60,000 IU/kg SC q2–7d) may also be used in severe cases.
• Topical antibiotics—for treatment of URT infection; use ophthalmic antibiotic preparations without corticosteroids.

• Simethicone has also been suggested to treat gastric bloat to reduce gas in the GI tract; care must be taken to ensure that animal is well hydrated because simethicone can also dehydrate and create mass effect with dehydrated GI contents.
• Cardiac disease in rodents has been treated with similar therapeutics as other companion animals including diuretics, ACE inhibitors, pimobendan, and digoxin.
• NSAIDs such as meloxicam (0.5–1 mg/kg SC, PO q24h), or carprofen (2–5 mg/kg PO, SC q24h), can provide both anti-inflammation and analgesia.
• Analgesia is a critical aspect of therapy if animal is painful such as with osteomyelitis and postsurgical intervention; therefore, the addition of an opioid medication such as buprenorphine (0.1–0.2 mg/kg SC, IM, IV q8–12h) is necessary.

CONTRAINDICATIONS
• Oral antibiotics that select against Gram-positive bacteria (penicillins, macrolides, lincosamides, and cephalosporins) can cause fatal enteric dysbiosis and enterotoxemia.
• Topical and systemic corticosteroids—chinchillas are sensitive to immunosuppressive effects; can exacerbate infectious disease.

PRECAUTIONS
• Metronidazole may cause anorexia or reduced appetite in some chinchillas when administered PO; hepatic toxicity has been anecdotally reported.
• In animals with CHF, blunt chest trauma, or renal disease, iatrogenic fluid overload or pulmonary edema is a potential problem.
• Intravenous administration of crystalloids should be used judiciously. Respiratory rate and effort should be monitored carefully and frequently in these patients.

FOLLOW-UP
PATIENT MONITORING
• Reevaluate the patient at 7–10 days or sooner if the patient's clinical signs are worsening.
• Radiographs—monitor response to therapy in animals with pulmonary disease. Pulmonary edema should be visibly improved within 12 hours if effective therapy is used. Monitor the recurrence of pleural effusion based upon how quickly effusion accumulates. Radiographic evidence of pneumonia improves more slowly than does clinical appearance and may not improve with pulmonary abscesses.

• Cardiac ultrasound may be indicated at intervals of several weeks to months depending on patient condition and treatment.

PREVENTION/AVOIDANCE
Keep in cool, dry environment to prevent respiratory disease. Maintain cool environmental temperatures below 73°F (22.8°C).
Complete oral examination needs to be included in the physical examination of adult chinchillas.

POSSIBLE COMPLICATIONS
• Relapse, progression of disease, and death are common with pneumonia.
• Osteomyelitis is a common sequela to severe, chronic dental infections.
• Surgical intervention for dental disease usually involves repeated occlusal adjustments every 6–12 weeks.

EXPECTED COURSE AND PROGNOSIS
• LRT, URT, and odontogenic infections may take months of multiple therapies to resolve.
• The prognosis for heat stroke and gastric outflow obstruction (bloat) is guarded to grave because most animals are severely affected by the time clinical signs are observed.

MISCELLANEOUS
ASSOCIATED CONDITIONS
• Upper respiratory infection
• Dental disease
• Facial abscesses
• Gastrointestinal hypomotility

ZOONOTIC POTENTIAL
Streptococcus pneumoniae could be considered a potential anthropozoonosis, but it is not known if rodents can acquire the infection from contact with humans.

PREGNANCY/FERTILITY/BREEDING
If dental disease is suspected as the inciting cause, breeders recommend not breeding these animals as inheritance abnormalities are suspected.

SYNONYMS
Choke
Bloat
Snuffles

SEE ALSO
Otitis media and interna
Nasal discharge and sneezing

(CONTINUED)

ABBREVIATIONS

ACE = angiotensin-converting enzyme
CHF = congestive heart failure
CK = creatine kinase
CNS = central nervous system
CT = computed tomography
FNA = fine-needle aspiration
GI = gastrointestinal
LRT = lower respiratory tract
MRI = magnetic resonance imaging
NSAID = nonsteroidal anti-inflammatory
TWBC = total white blood cell count
URT = upper respiratory tract

INTERNET RESOURCES
N/A

Suggested Reading
Capello V, Lennox AM. Diagnostic imaging of the respiratory system in exotic companion mammals. Vet Clin Exot Anim 2011;14: 369–389.
DeCubellis J. Common emergencies in rabbits, guinea pigs, and chinchillas. Vet Clin Exot Anim 2016;19:411–429.
Goodman G. Rodents: respiratory and cardiovascular system disorders. In: Keeble E, Meredith A, eds. BSAVA Manual of Rodents and Ferrets. Gloucester: BSAVA, 2009:142–149.
Lennox AM, Gladden JN. Emergency and critical care of small mammals. In: Quesenberry KE, Carpenter JW, eds. Ferrets, Rabbits and Rodents, 4th ed. Clinical Medicine and Surgery. 2021. St. Louis: Saunders, 2020:595–608.
Mans C, Donnelly T. Chinchillas. In: Quesenberry KE, Carpenter JW, eds. Ferrets, Rabbits and Rodents, 4th ed. Clinical Medicine and Surgery. 2021. St. Louis: Saunders, 2020:298–322.
Mans C, Jekl V. Anatomy and disorders of the oral cavity of chinchilla and degus. Vet Clin Exot Anim 2016;19:843–869.
Martel A, Donnelly T, Mans C. Update on diseases in chinchillas: 2013–2019. Vet Clin Exot Anim 2020;23:321–333.
Riggs SM, Mitchell MA. Chinchillas. In: Mitchell MA, Tully TN, eds. Manual of Exotic Pet Practice. St. Louis: Elsevier, 2009:475–486.

Authors Joanne Paul-Murphy, DVM, Dipl. ACZM, Dan H. Johnson, DVM, Dipl. ABVP (Exotic Companion Mammal)

DYSTOCIA AND DISORDERS OF PREGNANCY

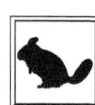

BASICS

DEFINITION
Dystocia is any difficult or abnormal parturition with or without assistance.

Disorders of pregnancy include abortion or retained or mummified fetuses.

PATHOPHYSIOLOGY
• Normal gestation period is 105–115 days.
• Near end of gestation, females that become suddenly startled may spontaneously abort.
• Dystocia is rare in chinchillas but may occur if the fetus is oversized or deformed.
• Female chinchillas are sexually mature at 4–5 months and should be greater than 600 grams body weight prior to breeding. Young females bred too early may experience dystocia.
• Primary uterine inertia may develop if females are poorly conditioned.
• Obesity contributes to dystocia.
• Abortion or mummified fetuses may be caused by improper handling, trauma, inadequate nutrition, septicemia, fever, or interruption of the uterine blood supply.

SYSTEMS AFFECTED
Reproductive system

GENETICS
N/A

INCIDENCE/PREVALENCE
• Dystocia is uncommon.
• Abortion or mummified fetuses are more common.

GEOGRAPHIC DISTRIBUTION
N/A

SIGNALMENT
Female chinchillas with a history of being with one or more male chinchillas. Breeding may not have been observed because it generally occurs at night.

Historical Findings
• Mating occurred 105–115 days prior to presentation.
• Mammary gland development occurs at 60 days gestation.
• It is normal for chinchillas nearing parturition to become less active, anorectic, and aggressive toward previously compatible cage mates.
• In late gestation, the gravid female may become constipated.
• It is normal for female to writhe, stretch, and vocalize during delivery, but these behaviors terminate after all fetuses are delivered.
• Abnormal behaviors include intermittently straining for over 2 hours or biting at the lateral body wall.
• If fetuses get stuck in the birth canal, the female may injure or cannibalize them.

• Vaginal discharge or perineal staining—serosanguinous or hemorrhagic
• Female may lick and bite at her vulva.
• Anorexia
• Lethargy
• Abortion may take place unnoticed because the female will immediately ingest the aborted kits. Abortion should be suspected if a female chinchilla suddenly loses weight.
• Female may ignore the newborn kits if dead or mummified fetuses remaining in the uterus.

Physical Examination Findings
• Palpation of fetal masses in caudal abdomen
• Painful abdomen
• Gentle abdominal palpation to determine if uterine contractions present
• Female may have an inappropriate body score, either underconditioned or overconditioned.
• Female may be restless, anxious, and irritable.
• Hunched posture, straining, or lethargy and weakness if labor has been prolonged
• Vaginal discharge may be bloody or green colored.

CAUSES AND RISK FACTORS
• Oversized fetuses—often associated with breeding young females
• Fetal malposition in birth canal
• Uterine inertia, ineffective uterine contractions
• Abnormality of vaginal vault such as stricture, hyperplasia, aplasia, intraluminal, or extraluminal mass in vagina

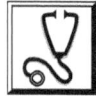

DIAGNOSIS

DIFFERENTIAL DIAGNOSIS
Differentiate from normal pregnancy by palpation as early as 60 days, radiographic evidence 6 weeks after mating, or abdominal ultrasound.

CBC/BIOCHEMISTRY/URINALYSIS
• Hemogram—depends on length and cause of dystocia. If fetal death has occurred, may see toxic heterophils. Anemia presents with prolonged abortion or dystocia where blood loss is significant. Thrombocytosis with acute inflammation.
• Biochemistry panel—prolonged dystocia may result in hypoglycemia, dehydration, and hypocalcemia. Hypocalcemia can present with uterine inertia.

OTHER LABORATORY TESTS
N/A

IMAGING
• Radiography of the abdomen and pelvic area will determine number, size, and position of fetuses. Fetal skeletons are visualized beyond 6 weeks of gestation.

• Ultrasonography is useful for determining if fetuses are viable in addition to the number of fetuses present.
• Ultrasonography can determine if uterine inertia present.

DIAGNOSTIC PROCEDURES
N/A

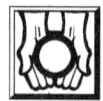

TREATMENT

APPROPRIATE HEALTH CARE
• Oxytocin can be administered to promote delivery within 30 minutes of administration.
• Glucose and calcium supplementation can be delivered orally if indicated by biochemistry values. Glucose can be added if intravenous fluids being administered. Do not administer calcium intravenously.
• Post-abortion females can be treated with flushing the reproductive tract gently with an antiseptic solution and administration of appropriate parenteral antibiotics.

SURGICAL TREATMENT
• Cesarean section indicated if fetuses are viable and chinchilla does not respond to oxytocin, or with fetal oversize or malposition.
• Cesarean section has a good prognosis if performed within the first 2–3 hours, but less successful if dystocia has been ongoing for several hours.

NURSING CARE
• Fluid therapy with balanced electrolyte solutions (e.g., lactated Ringer's solution, Normosol) should be initiated as soon as possible. Subcutaneous fluids can be administered (30–50 mL/kg) as needed.
• IV access is challenging in the chinchilla; use cephalic or lateral saphenous vein catheters or consider IO catheterization if intravascular fluids are needed and for venous access during surgery. Maintenance needs are estimated at 100 mL/kg/day.
• Postoperative management includes assisted feeding, fluids, analgesics, and broad-spectrum antibiotics.
• Bandage the abdomen if incision site in contact with the cage floor.

ACTIVITY
Reduced activity in the 2-week postoperative period.

CLIENT EDUCATION
• Owners should be educated about proper nutrition and cautioned about the detrimental effects of overfeeding chinchillas.
• Owners should know the sex of their pet and only breed if homes for offspring are previously established.
• A few days before expected parturition, the dust bath should no longer be offered to

avoid dust entering the vagina and causing irritation.

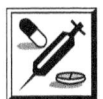

MEDICATIONS

DRUG(S) OF CHOICE
• Administer oxytocin (0.2–3.0 IU/kg IM or SC) to induce uterine contractions. Can be repeated once within 15–20 minutes. If kits not delivered within 45–60 minutes, surgical intervention is indicated.
• Pain management is essential during and following surgery. Multimodal therapy is recommended for perioperative analgesia with an anxiolytic, opioid, and NSAID: Midazolam (0.3–0.7 mg/kg IM), butorphanol (0.2–2.0 mg/kg SC, IM, IV q4h), or buprenorphine (0.01–0.05 mg/kg SC, IM, IV q6–8h) plus meloxicam (0.5–1 mg/kg SC, PO q24h) and carprofen (2–5 mg/kg PO, SC q24h).
• Antibiotic therapy may be indicated if vaginitis present or surgical intervention occurred and incision is difficult to maintain in a clean environment. Antimicrobial choice should be broad spectrum or based upon results of culture and sensitivity if surgical tissues are cultured.

CONTRAINDICATIONS
• Oxytocin is contraindicated with obstructive dystocia (fetus too large for pelvic delivery), malposition, or if long-standing fetal death.
• Oral administration of antibiotics that select against gram-positive bacteria (penicillins, cephalosporins, macrolides, and lincosamides) can cause fatal enteric dysbiosis and enterotoxemia.
• Avoid potentially nephrotoxic drugs (e.g., aminoglycosides, NSAIDs) in patients that are febrile or dehydrated, or have preexisting renal disease.

PRECAUTIONS
• Avoid drugs that reduce blood pressure or induce cardiac dysrhythmia until dehydration is resolved.
• During surgery, avoid excessive handling of gastrointestinal tissues to reduce postoperative ileus or fibrous adhesions.

• Obese chinchillas are at greater risk of anesthetic complications.

POSSIBLE INTERACTIONS
None

ALTERNATIVE DRUGS
N/A

FOLLOW-UP

PATIENT MONITORING
• Ensure gastrointestinal motility by making sure the patient is eating, well hydrated, and passing normal feces prior to release.
• If vaginal delivery, use ultrasonography to insure all fetuses have been delivered.

PREVENTION/AVOIDANCE
• Breed chinchillas when mature and in good body condition after 6 months of age.
• Avoid overfeeding the breeding female.
• Chinchilla females do not typically build nests at parturition; however, a nesting box may decrease neonatal mortality caused by drafts or cold stress.
• OVH to prevent future pregnancies.

POSSIBLE COMPLICATIONS
• Loss of neonates if treatment is not provided promptly
• Postoperative gastrointestinal ileus may take days to weeks to resolve.

EXPECTED COURSE AND PROGNOSIS
• The prognosis is fair to good if neonates can be vaginally delivered.
• The chinchilla is generally tolerant of Cesarean section if undertaken early in the course of dystocia and the patient is in good body condition.

MISCELLANEOUS

ASSOCIATED CONDITIONS
Following delivery of kits, vaginitis, metritis, or pyometra can occur from ascending bacterial infection.

AGE-RELATED FACTORS
Breeding young females may lead to dystocia if fetuses are oversized.

ZOONOTIC POTENTIAL
N/A

PREGNANCY/FERTILITY/BREEDING
N/A

SYNONYMS
N/A

SEE ALSO
N/A

ABBREVIATIONS
NSAIDs = nonsteroidal anti-inflammatory drugs
OVH = ovariohysterectomy

INTERNET RESOURCES
N/A

Suggested Reading
Hoefer H, Latney L. Rodents: urogenital and reproductive disorders. In: Keeble E, Meredith A, eds. BSAVA Manual of Rodents and Ferrets. Gloucester: BSAVA, 2009:216–218.
Kondert L, Mayer J. Reproductive medicine in guinea pigs, chinchillas and degus. Vet Clin Exot Anim 2017;20:609–628.
Lennox AM, Gladden JN. Emergency and critical care of small mammals. In: Quesenberry KE, Carpenter JW, eds. Ferrets, Rabbits and Rodents, 4th ed. Clinical Medicine and Surgery. 2021. St. Louis: Saunders, 2020:595–608.
Mans C, Donnelly T. Chinchillas. In: Quesenberry KE, Carpenter JW, eds. Ferrets, Rabbits and Rodents, 4th ed. Clinical Medicine and Surgery. 2021. St. Louis: Saunders, 2020:298–322.
Martel A, Donnelly T, Mans C. Update on diseases in chinchillas: 2013–2019. Vet Clin Exot Anim 2020;23:321–333.
Riggs SM, Mitchell MA. Chinchillas. In: Mitchell MA, Tully TN, eds. Manual of Exotic Pet Practice. St. Louis: Elsevier, 2009:475–486.

Authors Joanne Paul-Murphy, DVM, Dipl. ACZM Dan H. Johnson, DVM, Dipl. ABVP (Exotic Companion Mammal)

DYSURIA, HEMATURIA, AND POLLAKIURIA

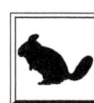

BASICS

DEFINITION
• Dysuria—difficult or painful urination
• Hematuria—the presence of blood in the urine. It is important to differentiate true hematuria from blood originating from the reproductive tract in females and from orange, red, or red-brown colored urine caused by the excretion of dietary pigments (porphyrins) via the urine.
• Pollakiuria—voiding small quantities of urine with increased frequency

PATHOPHYSIOLOGY
• Inflammatory and noninflammatory disorders of the lower urinary tract may decrease bladder compliance and storage capacity by damaging compliance of the bladder wall or by stimulating sensory nerve endings located in the bladder or urethra. Sensations of bladder fullness, urgency, and pain stimulate premature micturition and reduce functional bladder capacity. Dysuria and pollakiuria are generally caused by lesions of the urinary bladder and/or urethra, but these clinical signs do not exclude concurrent involvement of the upper urinary tract or disorders of other body systems.
• The most common causes of dysuria, pollakiuria, and hematuria in the chinchilla are cystitis, pyometra, dystocia, and in males, fur rings causing paraphimosis. Urolithiasis is less common in the chinchilla than in other small mammalian pets.
• Inadequate water intake leading to a more concentrated urine and factors that impair complete evacuation of the bladder, such as lack of exercise, obesity, cystitis, neoplasia, or neuromuscular diseases may be associated with these signs.
• "Fur rings," a circumferential ring of hair around the distal penis, commonly occurs in males and can cause paraphimosis and urethral obstruction, which can be very painful.

SYSTEMS AFFECTED
• Renal/urologic—bladder, urethra; fur rings
• Reproductive—pyometra, dystocia
• Integument—fur rings

GENETICS
N/A

INCIDENCE/PREVALENCE
Fur rings are very common in males, especially if dust baths are not provided on a routine basis.

GEOGRAPHIC DISTRIBUTION
N/A

SIGNALMENT
• Depending on the cause can occur in any age and either gender

SIGNS

Historical Findings
• Straining to urinate; small, frequent urinations; and/or urinating when picked up by the owners
• Hematuria, or thick, white- or tan-appearing urine
• Urine staining in the perineal area, urine scald, moist pyoderma
• Anorexia, weight loss, lethargy, bruxism, and a hunched posture in chinchillas with chronic or obstructive lower urinary tract disease
• Gross hematuria—In males: most often found with fur rings, In females: most often due to expulsion of blood from the reproductive tract during micturition due to uterine disorders or with dystocia. Hematuria is rare with urolithiasis or UTI
• Pollakiuria or stranguria; evidence of urine retention
• Hunched posture, vocalizing during urination may be associated with pain
• Hunched posture, ataxia, or difficulty ambulating in chinchillas with musculoskeletal or neurological disease
• Signs of uremia with partial or complete urinary tract obstruction—anorexia, weight loss, lethargy, bruxism, tenesmus, hunched posture

Physical Examination Findings
• If significant blood loss via hematuria has occurred, the patient may have pale mucous membranes or generalized paleness of the skin, face, and legs.
• A circumferential ring of hair around the distal penis is consistent with fur rings.
• Large, turgid bladder (or inappropriate size remains after voiding efforts) upon palpation of the urinary bladder—can occur with pollakiuria or with uroliths
• Manual expression of the bladder may reveal hematuria or sometimes "sludgy," thick, white-tan material, even in animals that have normal-appearing voided urine—this is less common in chinchillas than in rabbits/guinea pigs, but occasionally occurs.
• Hematuria, stranguria, pollakiuria
• Enlarged kidney—may be palpable if nephritis or nephrolithiasis
• Signs of uremia—dehydration, anorexia, lethargy, weakness, hypothermia, bradycardia, high rate or shallow respirations; stupor, coma, and/or seizures occur rarely, often in terminal cases; tachycardia resulting from ventricular dysrhythmias induced by hyperkalemia

• Thick, palpable uterus may be found with endometritis or pyometra; pups may be palpable if dystocia is the cause.
• Bladder palpation may demonstrate cystoliths; failure to palpate calculi does not exclude them from consideration.
• Organomegaly may suggest other organ system involvement or neoplasia.

CAUSES

Urinary System
• Urinary tract infection—bacterial urethritis, cystitis, pyelonephritis, nephritis
• Urethral plugs, fur rings—in males
• Urolithiasis—urinary bladder or urethra
• Trauma—especially bite wounds
• Iatrogenic—catheterization, overdistention of the bladder during contrast radiography, surgery
• Neoplasia (uncommon in chinchillas)

Reproductive System
• Endometrial hyperplasia
• Pyometra, endometritis, vaginitis, dystocia
• Neoplasia (rare)

Other Organ Systems
• Neurological/musculoskeletal—any disease that inhibits normal posturing for urination (e.g., pododermatitis, arthritis) may predispose
• Urine scald—can cause ascending inflammation, leading to urethral spasm
• Other abdominal organomegaly may put undue pressure on the urinary system and cause straining to urinate.

RISK FACTORS
• Inadequate water intake—dirty water bowls, unpalatable water, inadequate water provision, changing water sources
• Urine retention—underlying bladder pathology, neuromuscular disease, painful conditions causing a reluctance to ambulate (e.g., pododermatitis, arthritis)
• Inadequate cage cleaning may cause some chinchillas to avoid urinating.
• Obesity has been suggested but not a proven cause in chinchillas.
• Lack of exercise
• Diseases, diagnostic procedures, or treatments that (1) alter normal host urinary tract offenses and predispose to infection, (2) predispose to formation of uroliths, or (3) damage urothelium or other tissues of the lower urinary tract
• Mural or extramural diseases that compress the bladder or urethral lumen
• Unlike rabbits and guinea pigs, excess dietary calcium does not appear to predispose chinchillas to crystalluria or urolithiasis.

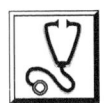

DIAGNOSIS

DIFFERENTIAL DIAGNOSIS

Differentiating from Other Abnormal Patterns of Micturition
• Rule out polyuria—increased frequency and volume of urine
• Rule out urethral obstruction—stranguria, anuria, overdistended urinary bladder, signs of postrenal uremia

Differentiating Causes of Dysuria, Pollakiuria, Hematuria
• Cystitis—bacteriuria; painful, thickened bladder
• Uterine disease—chinchillas with uterine disease often strain and expel blood when urinating, blood may mix with urine and be mistaken for hematuria
• Fur rings or urethral plugs—should be identified on physical examination
• Neoplasia—hematuria; palpable masses in the urethra or bladder possible; radiographs ultrasound may differentiate; considered rare in chinchillas
• Neurogenic disorders—flaccid bladder wall; residual urine in the bladder lumen after micturition; neurologic deficits to hind legs, tail, perineum, and anal sphincter
• Iatrogenic disorders—history of catheterization, reverse flushing, contrast radiography, or surgery
• Hypercalciuria (bladder sludge)—considered rare in chinchillas; thick, white-to-beige urine, sometimes streaked with fresh blood; radiopaque bladder
• Urolithiasis—palpable uroliths in the bladder, radio-opacities within the bladder; less common in chinchillas than in other small exotic mammals

CBC/BIOCHEMISTRY/ URINALYSIS
• CBC—TWBC elevations with neutrophil: lymphocyte ratio shift; toxicity of neutrophils ± bands, monocytosis suggest inflammation/ infection; thrombocytosis associated with active inflammation; may be anemic if hematuria is severe
• Biochemistry panel—lower urinary tract disease complicated by urethral obstruction may be associated with azotemia. With complete (or nearly complete) obstruction, changes in electrolytes such as hyperkalemia, hypochloremia, hyponatremia may occur.
• Patients with concurrent pyelonephritis have impaired urine concentrating capacity, leukocytosis, and azotemia.
• Disorders of the urinary bladder are best evaluated with urine specimen collected by cystocentesis.

• Urinalysis including both a standard dipstick and microscopic examination of the sediment. Reported urine specific gravity for chinchillas is >1.045 and urine pH is 8.5. Identification of neoplastic cells in urine sediment indicates urinary tract neoplasia (rare). Bacteriuria, pyuria (>0–1 WBC/hpf), and hematuria (>0–3 RBC/hpf) may indicate urinary or reproductive tract inflammation.
• A trace amount of protein is considered normal in the urine of chinchillas. In a recent study of 41 clinically normal chinchillas, the majority (40/41 [98%]) had more than a trace amount of protein as determined by a urine dipstick.
• Crystalluria is common in chinchillas, but calcium carbonate crystalluria is uncommon and not considered normal. Hypercrystalluria should increase suspicion for causing disease.

OTHER LABORATORY TESTS
• Prior to antibiotic use, culture the urine or bladder wall if high numbers of red or white blood cells, bacteria, or a combination of these are present on sediment examination. Collecting urine via cystocentesis is preferable as free-catch samples are commonly contaminated.
• Aerobic/anaerobic bacterial urine culture and sensitivity—the most definitive means of identifying and characterizing bacterial urinary tract infection; negative urine culture results suggest a noninfectious cause, unless the patient was on concurrent antibiotics or has an anaerobic infection. There are anecdotal reports of anaerobic urinary infections in chinchillas, so choose this culture technique if anaerobic infection suspected.
• If surgery is necessary to relieve obstruction from urolithiasis, collect and submit the calculi for analysis and culture and sensitivity, and submit the bladder wall for culture and sensitivity.
• Calculi-containing calcium carbonate requires specific methodologies to differentiate from calcium oxalate monohydrate crystals; the laboratory chosen for analysis must be able to perform these methods. Confirm the lab's ability to perform these techniques in advance, since human and some veterinary laboratories unfamiliar with exotic animal samples do not differentiate calcium oxalate from calcium carbonate.

IMAGING
• Survey abdominal radiography and abdominal ultrasound are important means of identifying and localizing causes of dysuria, pollakiuria, and hematuria.
• Urinary calculi in chinchillas are generally radiopaque, allowing for ease of identification using survey radiography. However, if

multiple calculi or significant GI gas are present, the anatomic locations of the calculi using survey radiography alone may be obscured.
• In a recent review of 15 cases, calculi were only found within the bladder and/or urethra. Obstructive calculi are most likely to be found in the urethra (males and females) but could also be found in the kidneys or ureters.
• Contrast (negative or positive) cystography can be employed to evaluate filling defects in the bladder or bladder masses.
• Ultrasound is useful for anatomic location of urinary calculi and for evaluating anatomic changes in the kidneys, ureters, or bladder such as hydronephrosis or hydroureter, ureteral or cystic mucosal thickening, or perforation, and for evaluating other organ systems.
• Excretory intravenous pyelograms (IVPs) are useful to further elucidate relative functional abnormalities in the kidneys or ureters.
• CT images are obtained more rapidly than IVP, using significantly less contrast material but at a greater cost.

DIAGNOSTIC PROCEDURES
Bacterial culture/sensitivity—of urine, bladder wall, or if exudates present; recommended if high numbers of RBC or WBC, bacteria, or a combination are present on urine sediment examination. If surgical urolithiasis patient, recommend bladder wall culture as generally more rewarding.

PATHOLOGIC FINDINGS
Gross lesions associated with hematuria or dysuria depend on the underlying disease.
　　Refer to specific causes.

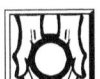

TREATMENT

APPROPRIATE HEALTH CARE
• Patients with nonobstructive urinary tract diseases are typically managed as outpatients; diagnostic evaluation may require brief hospitalization.
• Dysuria, pollakiuria, or hematuria associated with systemic signs of illness (e.g., pyrexia, depression, anorexia, and dehydration) or laboratory findings of azotemia and or leukocytosis warrant an aggressive diagnostic evaluation and initiation of supportive and symptomatic treatment.
• Chinchillas with urinary obstruction should be hospitalized, emergency supportive and symptomatic therapy should be provided until surgical intervention to relieve the obstruction can be performed. Medical treatment of urolithiasis has been

DYSURIA, HEMATURIA, AND POLLAKIURIA   (CONTINUED)

unrewarding to date, and surgical removal of calculi is most often required. Postoperative management includes supportive and symptomatic treatment and pain management therapies.

NURSING CARE

• Subcutaneous fluids can be administered (30–50 mL/kg) as needed; IV access is difficult in the chinchilla; lateral saphenous vein catheters often kink; consider intraosseous (IO) catheterization if intravascular fluids are needed. Base fluid selection on evidence of dehydration, azotemia, and electrolyte imbalances. In most patients, lactated Ringer's solution or Normosol crystalloid fluids are appropriate. Maintenance fluid needs are estimated to be 100 mL/kg/day. In obstructed patients, fluid therapy should be based on treatment modalities used in cats with obstructive urinary disease; normal saline should be administered until patient electrolyte status is determined.

• Fur rings can be gently removed using lubricating products. The distal penis may need to be lubricated prior to removal attempts, to loosen the hair. The chinchilla may require sedation or anesthesia to remove if painful.

• In females, gently flush the bladder using a 3.5-Fr red rubber catheter under deep sedation and analgesia to attempt to remove the calculi. Catheterizing males is much more complicated due to the small size and curvature of the urethra; attempts at retropulsion into the bladder have been unrewarding.

ACTIVITY

• Long-term—increased activity level by providing large exercise areas to encourage voiding and prevent recurrence. Activity should be reduced during the immediate postoperative period if surgery is required for urinary obstruction.

• Dust baths should be offered every 3 days or twice weekly to reduce the potential for fur rings.

DIET

• Many affected chinchillas are anorectic or have a decreased appetite. It is an absolute requirement that the patient continues to eat during and following treatments. Anorexia may cause or exacerbate gastrointestinal hypomotility and cause derangement of the gastrointestinal microflora and overgrowth of intestinal bacterial pathogens.

• Offer a large selection of fresh, moist greens such as cilantro, lettuces, parsley, carrots tops, dark leafy greens, and good-quality grass hay.

• If the patient refuses these foods, syringe-feed Critical Care for Herbivores (Oxbow Animal Health, Omaha, NE) or Emeraid

Herbivore (Lafeber Company, Cornell, IL), 15–20 mL/kg PO q6–8h. Larger volumes and more frequent feedings are often accepted; feed as much as the patient will readily accept. Alternatively, pellets can be ground and mixed with fresh greens, vegetable baby foods, water, or sugar-free juice to form a gruel.

CLIENT EDUCATION

• Limiting risk factors such as obesity, sedentary life, and inappropriate diet combined with increasing water consumption is necessary to minimize or delay recurrence of lower urinary tract disease. Even with these changes, however, recurrence may occur.

• Surgical removal of urinary tract obstructions does not alter the causes responsible for their formation. Unfortunately, the causes of urolithiasis in chinchillas are not known, limiting dietary calcium intake does not appear to be a factor, and recurrence is likely.

• Fur rings are very common in males; owners should inspect the penis and prepuce frequently to reduce the potential for severe conditions. Dust baths at least twice weekly are recommended and reduce the potential for fur rings.

SURGICAL CONSIDERATIONS

• Surgery is necessary to relieve obstructions if medical attempts are unsuccessful. Urolithiasis is reported mostly in males, and most uroliths are located either in the urinary bladder or urethra. Surgical removal of bladder stones has been rewarding, while attempts at dislodging urethral stones and flushing them retrograde into the bladder have not.

• Surgery may be required if the distal penis of males becomes necrotic.

• Surgery may be required for patients with cystic hypercrystalluria or "sludge" that do not respond to medical therapy.

• Postoperative management includes assisted feeding, fluids, analgesics, and antibiotics based on culture and sensitivity results. However, recurrence of the disease is common.

MEDICATIONS

DRUG(S) OF CHOICE

• Antibiotic choice should be based upon the results of culture and sensitivity (see Contraindications). Until results are obtained, use broad-spectrum antibiotics such as enrofloxacin (5–15 mg/kg PO, SC q12h) or trimethoprim-sulfa (15–30 mg/kg PO q12h).

• Reduction of inflammation and analgesia should be provided, especially if pain is

causing reduced frequency of voiding, and pain management is essential during and following surgery. Perioperative analgesic choices include butorphanol (0.2–2.0 mg/kg SC, IM, IV q4h) or buprenorphine (0.01–0.05 mg/kg SC, IM, IV q8–12h). Meloxicam (0.5–1 mg/kg SC, PO q24h) and carprofen (2–5 mg/kg PO, SC q24h) provide anti-inflammatory relief as well as analgesia.

• Procedures for relief of obstruction generally require administering sedatives and/or anesthetics. When substantial physiological and/or biochemistry derangements exist, begin with fluid administration and other supportive measures first. Calculate the dosage of sedative or anesthetic drug using the low end of the recommended range or give only to effect.

CONTRAINDICATIONS

• Oral administration of antibiotics that select against gram-positive bacteria (penicillins, cephalosporins, macrolides, and lincosamides) can cause fatal enteric dysbiosis and enterotoxemia.

• Potentially nephrotoxic drugs (e.g., aminoglycosides, NSAIDs) should be avoided in patients that are febrile, dehydrated, or azotemic or that are suspected of having pyelonephritis, septicemia, or preexisting renal disease.

• Glucocorticoids or other immunosuppressive agents

PRECAUTIONS

• Metronidazole may cause anorexia or reduced appetite in some chinchillas when administered PO; hepatic toxicity has been anecdotally reported.

• Avoid drugs that reduce blood pressure or induce cardiac dysrhythmia until any dehydration is resolved.

• If obstructed or significant renal insufficiency is evident, modify dosages of all drugs that require renal metabolism or elimination.

• If obstructed or significant renal insufficiency is evident, avoid nephrotoxic drugs (NSAIDs, aminoglycosides).

POSSIBLE INTERACTIONS
None

ALTERNATIVE DRUGS
N/A

FOLLOW-UP

PATIENT MONITORING

• Response to treatment by clinical signs, serial physical examinations, laboratory testing, and radiographic and ultrasonic evaluations appropriate for each specific cause.

• Monitor for reduction and cessation of clinical signs. Generally, a positive response occurs within a few days after instituting appropriate antibiotic therapy for lower urinary tract infections and supportive therapy.
• Ensure gastrointestinal motility by making sure the patient is eating, well hydrated, and passing normal feces.
• Assess urine production and hydration status frequently while hospitalized, or have owners monitor daily at home, adjusting fluid administration accordingly.
• Verify the ability to urinate adequately; failure to do so may require urinary catheterization or cystocentesis to alleviate urine retention.
• Follow-up examination should be performed within 7–10 days of discharge from hospital, or sooner if the clinical signs are not reduced.
• Ideally, recheck of urine culture and sensitivity should be performed 3–5 days after the cessation of antibiotics when lower urinary tract infections are present.
• Since calcium carbonate crystalluria is not considered normal in chinchillas, clinicians should consider close monitoring for future development of urolithiasis in chinchillas diagnosed with calcium carbonate crystalluria.

PREVENTION/AVOIDANCE
• Prevention is based on the specific underlying cause. Limiting risk factors such as obesity, sedentary life, and inappropriate diet combined with increasing water consumption are necessary to minimize or delay recurrence of urinary tract diseases. Even with these changes, however, recurrence may occur.
• For chinchillas with urolithiasis, increased water intake is the primary means of preventing recurrence; unlike rabbits and guinea pigs, reduction of dietary calcium intake is not a major concern.
• Frequent dust baths should be provided to reduce the potential for fur rings.

POSSIBLE COMPLICATIONS
• Anemia
• Urine scald; myiasis; pododermatitis

• Distal penile necrosis if fur ring is chronic
• Urinary tract obstruction with urolithiasis or hypercrystalluria

EXPECTED COURSE AND PROGNOSIS
• Depends on the underlying disease. Generally, the prognosis for animals with uncomplicated lower urinary tract infection is good to excellent. The prognosis for patients with complicated infection is determined by the prognosis for the other urine abnormalities.
• Outcome for urolithiasis in chinchillas appears to be associated with urolith location. Chinchillas with calculi in the urinary bladder alone have a fair to good prognosis following surgical removal. However, recurrence rate is approximately 50% with mean recurrence interval of 68 days. Chinchillas with uroliths in the urethra have poor prognosis, as flushing calculi into the bladder for removal is rarely successful. Recurrence of urolithiasis is reported in about 50% of cases.
• If dust baths are not provided on a consistent basis, fur rings may be seen with more frequency.

MISCELLANEOUS
ASSOCIATED CONDITIONS
• Urolithiasis
• Pyometra, other uterine disorders
• Gastrointestinal hypomotility or dysbiosis
• Pyoderma (urine scald)

AGE-RELATED FACTORS
N/A

ZOONOTIC POTENTIAL
N/A

PREGNANCY/FERTILITY/BREEDING
• Lower urinary tract infections may ascend into the reproductive tract via the vagina. If untreated, the potential for development of vaginal or uterine infections increases.
• Dystocia may cause irreparable damage to the uterus, potentially precluding breeding in the future.

SYNONYMS
None

SEE ALSO
Urolithiasis

ABBREVIATIONS
CT = computed tomography
IVP = intravenous pyelogram
RBC = red blood cell
TWBC = total white blood cell count
WBC = white blood cell

INTERNET RESOURCES
N/A

Suggested Reading
Doss GA, Mans C, Houseright RA et al. Urinalysis in chinchillas (*Chinchilla lanigera*). J Am Vet Med Assoc 2016;248(8):901–907.
Hallman RM, Brandão J. Diagnostic imaging of the renal system in exotic companion mammals. Vet Clin Exot Anim 2020;23:195–214.
Lennox AM, Gladden JN. Emergency and critical care of small mammals. In: Quesenberry KE, Carpenter JW, eds. Ferrets, Rabbits and Rodents, 4th ed. Clinical Medicine and Surgery. 2021. St. Louis: Saunders, 2020:595–608.
Mans C, Donnelly T. Chinchillas. In: Quesenberry KE, Carpenter JW, eds. Ferrets, Rabbits and Rodents, 4th ed. Clinical Medicine and Surgery. 2021. St. Louis: Saunders, 2020:298–322.
Martel-Arquette A, Mans C. Urolithiasis in chinchillas: 15 cases (2007 to 2011). J Small Anim Pract 2016;57:260–264.
Martel-Arquette A, Donnelly T, Mans C. Update on diseases in chinchillas: 2013–2019. Vet Clin Exot Anim 2020;23:321–333.
Riggs SM, Mitchell MA. Chinchillas. In: Mitchell MA, Tully TN, eds. Manual of Exotic Pet Practice. St. Louis: Elsevier, 2009:475–486.

Authors Michelle G. Hawkins, VMD, Dipl. ABVP (Avian Practice) Dan H. Johnson, DVM, Dipl. ABVP (Exotic Companion Mammal)

GASTROINTESTINAL STASIS AND DILATION

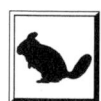

BASICS

DEFINITION
• Gastrointestinal stasis—severe ileus of the digestive tract with little or no caudal movement of ingesta
• Gastrointestinal dilation—accumulation of ingesta (food, fluid, and fur) and gas in the stomach, intestines, and cecum

PATHOPHYSIOLOGY
• Chinchillas, like rabbits and guinea pigs, are monogastric, hind-gut fermenters; they have a functional cecum and require a high-fiber diet. Chinchillas produce two types of fecal pellets: nitrogen-rich cecotropes and nitrogen-poor fecal pellets.
• Fiber is broken down in the cecum by a variety of microorganisms that are nourished by a constant supply of water and nutrients from the stomach and small intestine.
• These same microorganisms produce volatile fatty acids which, in turn, affect appetite and gut motility.
• Any disturbance in this mutually beneficial relationship can result in gastrointestinal hypomotility—increased gastrointestinal transit time—characterized by decreased frequency of cecocolonic segmental contractions; in severe cases, this leads to ileus with little to no caudal movement of ingesta ("gastrointestinal stasis"), and accumulation of ingesta and gas within the digestive tract ("gastrointestinal dilation").
• Proper hind-gut fermentation and gastrointestinal tract motility are dependent on the ingestion of large amounts of roughage, long-stemmed hay, and water.
• Diets that contain inadequate amounts of long-stemmed, coarse fiber predispose the patient to gastrointestinal stasis. However, unlike rabbits and guinea pigs, gastrointestinal transit time in chinchillas is not directly affected by a reduction in dietary fiber; instead, decreased fiber intake alters large bowel ecology in a way that threatens favorable microorganisms and promotes bacterial pathogens (e.g., *E coli* and *Clostridium*) and toxin production.
• Diets that are low in coarse fiber typically contain high simple carbohydrate concentrations, which provide a ready source of fermentable products. These can alter cecal fermentation, pH, and substrate production such that enteric microflora populations are altered ("bacterial dysbiosis") and result in diarrhea, enterotoxemia, ileus, or gas accumulation.
• As nausea and gastrointestinal discomfort lead to anorexia, fiber and water intake are further reduced and the process becomes self-perpetuating.
• Anorexia due to infectious or metabolic disease, pain, stress, or starvation may cause or exacerbate gastrointestinal hypomotility.
• If prolonged, gastrointestinal stasis often leads to hepatic lipidosis, dehydration, and other secondary complications.
• Like rabbits and guinea pigs, chinchillas cannot vomit. In the healthy digestive tract, a moderate amount of gas is normally produced by the fermentation process and eliminated by peristalsis. With gastrointestinal stasis, however, there can be excessive gas production, and, without normal motility, the stomach and intestines can overfill with gas and become distended ("bloat").
• Gastrointestinal stasis and dilation are not diseases but are symptoms that one or more of the factors governing gastrointestinal motility and commensal microorganisms are out of order.

SYSTEMS AFFECTED
• Gastrointestinal
• Musculoskeletal—loss of muscle mass may occur as a result of inappetence

INCIDENCE/PREVALENCE
Gastrointestinal stasis and dilation are among the most common clinical presentations seen in the chinchilla.

SIGNALMENT
No age or gender predilections for gastrointestinal stasis and gastrointestinal dilation, but signalment predispositions to many of the underlying conditions that cause gastrointestinal stasis and dilation

SIGNS

Historical Findings
• Decreased appetite—patients often initially stop eating pellets or hay but continue to eat treats, followed later by complete anorexia.
• Decreased fecal production—fecal pellets become small, hard, dry, scant to nonexistent; occasionally blood-stained
• Signs of abdominal pain—bruxism, hunched posture, reluctance to move, and failure to groom; affected animals may stretch out or roll in an attempt to relieve pain.
• Abdominal distension—animals affected by bloat are often swollen, lie on their sides, hesitate to stir, and may be dyspneic.
• Diarrhea in cases of dysbiosis
• Systemic (particularly oral) administration of antibiotics
• Inappropriate diet (e.g., cereals, grains, commercial pellets only, and lack of long-stemmed hay) or abrupt changes in the diet
• Excessive fasting, inability to consume a normal quantity of food (e.g., dental disease)
• Recent illness, pain, or stressful event
• Fur chewing in cases of gastric trichobezoar
• Gastric tympany—recent parturition/lactating female, hay rich in clover, overeating

Physical Examination Findings
• Small, hard fecal pellets or absence of fecal pellets palpable in the colon
• Abdominal palpation may reveal gas, fluid, or firm, doughy gastrointestinal contents, depending on the underlying cause; a firm, noncompliant stomach or stomach that remains pitted on compression is an abnormal finding. The presence of firm ingesta in the stomach of a patient that has been anorectic for 1–3 days is compatible with the diagnosis of gastrointestinal stasis.
• Abdominal distention—due to ileus, fluid-filled bowel loops, gas accumulation
• Pain on abdominal palpation
• Decreased or absent borborygmus
• Soft stools, diarrhea, or perineal staining in some cases
• Initially patients are bright and alert, but with severe or prolonged stasis or dilation may present depressed, lethargic, or in shock.
• Rough hair coat, failure to groom
• Signs of pain including bruxism, hunched posture, and reluctance to move
• Lateral recumbency, respiratory distress, dehydration, hypotension, weakness, and hypothermia in severe cases
• Weight loss in chronically affected chinchillas
• Palpable gastric foreign body and evidence of fur chewing in cases of trichobezoar
• Other physical examination findings depend on the underlying cause; perform a complete physical examination, including a thorough oral examination.

CAUSES AND RISK FACTORS

Dietary and Environmental Causes
• Gastrointestinal stasis and dilation in chinchillas is most commonly associated with insufficient dietary fiber and/or excessive stress.
• Chinchillas that do not receive enough fiber are more susceptible to gastrointestinal hypomotility and dysbiosis, whereas those that have adequate fiber intake are more resistant. A diet high in roughage such as grasses and long-stemmed hay is ideal.
• Gastrointestinal disorders are promoted by a diet consisting primarily of commercial pellets, especially those containing seeds, oats, or other high-carbohydrate treats. Feeding cereal products (e.g., bread, crackers, and breakfast cereals) and foods high in sugar (e.g., fruits, yogurt drops, other treats) results in carbohydrate overload and further increases the risk.
• Stressful conditions such as improper temperature, poor sanitation, and overcrowding have a negative effect on gut

motility. Gastrointestinal motility is regulated in part by the autonomic nervous system; stress increases the adrenal output of epinephrine and inhibits peristalsis.
• Common causes of stress include dental disease (e.g., malocclusion, molar elongation, and odontogenic abscesses), metabolic disease (e.g., renal disease, liver disease), pain (e.g., oral, trauma, postoperative, and urolithiasis), anxiety (e.g., dyspnea, fear, fighting, and lack of hide box), neoplasia, infection, parasitism, and environmental changes (e.g., boarding, new pets, and unfamiliar noises).
• Gastric trichobezoars in the chinchilla are associated with fur chewing rather than insufficient dietary fiber.
• Gastric dilation (bloat) is associated with overeating, consuming hay that has not matured or is rich in clover, sudden changes in diet (especially the addition of fresh greens and fruits), and gastrointestinal inflammation.

Anorexia or Inappetence
• Because intestinal microflora depends on a steady flow of water and nutrients, any event leading to inappetence or anorexia (e.g., presurgical fasting, sudden changes in the diet) or dehydration (e.g., sipper malfunction, bad-tasting water, and careless mistake) can trigger gastrointestinal dysbiosis, stasis, and/or dilation.
• Common causes of anorexia include dental disease (malocclusion, molar elongation, and tooth root abscesses), metabolic disease (renal disease, liver disease), pain (oral, trauma, and postoperative pain), neoplasia, toxins, changes in the environment, or accidental starvation.

Other Factors
• Other factors that can contribute to gastrointestinal stasis and dilation include toxin ingestion, foreign material (e.g., scoopable cat litter, fur, and carpet fiber), obesity, inactivity, confinement, and certain drugs (e.g., anesthetics, anticholinergics, opioids, and antibiotics).
• Inappropriate antibiotics can damage enteric microflora, promote the growth of pathogens associated with gastrointestinal stasis, and lead to antibiotic-associated enterotoxemia.
• Gastric tympany can result from overeating and sudden dietary changes. It has been reported in lactating females 2–3 weeks postpartum and may be related to hypocalcemia.

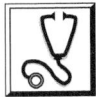

DIAGNOSIS
DIFFERENTIAL DIAGNOSIS
• Gastrointestinal stasis and dilation must be differentiated from acute pyloric or small

intestinal obstruction, as acute obstruction represents a life-threatening emergency. With acute gastrointestinal obstruction, acute onset of anorexia, abdominal pain, and reluctance to move often progress to lateral recumbency and signs of hypovolemic shock (e.g., pale mucous membranes, decreased capillary refill time, weak pulses, hypothermia). Stomach is severely distended, tympanic, and full of gas and/or fluid. Patients are often in shock and require emergency decompression. Monitor rectal temperature; hypothermic patients are critically ill.
• For palpable mass in the cranial abdomen—neoplasia, abscess, hepatomegaly, trichobezoar, normal gastric contents
• For gastric tympany—volvulus, esophageal foreign body ("choke"), acute pyloric or intestinal obstruction (e.g., hair, other foreign body), sudden dietary change, overeating, hypocalcemia-related condition of lactating females
• For anorexia—acquired dental disease, metabolic disease, pain, stress, neoplasia, cardiac disease, toxin, sudden diet change, infection
• For decreased fecal output—anorexia, constipation, intestinal foreign body, intussusception, intestinal neoplasia
• For diarrhea—bacterial or parasitic infections; dysbiosis secondary to stress, improper diet, or antibiotic use; partial obstruction by gastrointestinal foreign body, trichobezoar, or neoplasia; infiltrative bowel disease

CBC/BIOCHEMISTRY/URINALYSIS
• These tests are often normal.
• May identify underlying causes of gastrointestinal hypomotility and/or dilation
• PCV and TS may be elevated with dehydration.
• Serum liver enzymes may be elevated with liver disease, especially with secondary hepatic lipidosis.
• If the intestinal tract has been perforated, an inflammatory leukogram may be seen.

OTHER LABORATORY TESTS
N/A

IMAGING
• Chinchillas should not be fasted prior to obtaining radiographs.
• Gastric contents are normally present and visible on radiographs.
• Moderate to severe distension of the stomach with ingesta (food, fluid, and hair) is usually visible with gastrointestinal hypomotility; a distended stomach in spite of anorexia implies gastrointestinal stasis.
• A halo of gas can be observed around the inspissated stomach contents in some cases of gastrointestinal stasis, and there can be

moderate to severe gas distension throughout the digestive tract, including the cecum.
• Small fecal balls or the absence of fecal balls in the colon is highly suggestive of hypomotility.
• Severe distention of the stomach with fluid and/or gas is radiographic evidence of acute small intestinal obstruction, which constitutes a surgical emergency.

OTHER DIAGNOSTIC PROCEDURES
N/A

PATHOLOGIC FINDINGS
N/A

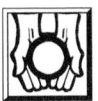

TREATMENT
APPROPRIATE HEALTH CARE
• Outpatient care may be appropriate for chinchillas exhibiting mild decreases in appetite and fecal production, but inpatient hospitalization and support are recommended in the majority of cases.
• Chinchillas exhibiting anorexia and lack of fecal production should be treated as soon as possible; those that have been showing signs for over 24 hours should be seen on an emergency basis.
• Therapy should also be directed at the underlying cause (e.g., dietary, stress, pain, etc.), when known.

NURSING CARE
General
• Medical management of gastrointestinal stasis and dilation centers on basic supportive care.
• Warmth, stress reduction, pain relief, fluid replacement, and nutritional support are important first-aid measures.
• The clinician should consider hospitalization in a quiet environment so that the patient can be observed, its progress monitored, and additional nursing care provided as needed.
• Chinchillas should be housed in a dark, quiet space away from natural predators' noise and odors.
• Provide thermal support using incubators, heating pads, or radiant heat emitters; to avoid causing heat stress, ambient temperature should not exceed 80°F (26.7°C).

Fluid Therapy
• Fluid therapy—both oral and parenteral administration—is an essential component of the medical management of all patients with gastrointestinal hypomotility.
• Oral fluid administration will aid in the rehydration of inspissated gastric contents. Direct oral administration of products such

CHINCHILLAS

GASTROINTESTINAL STASIS AND DILATION (CONTINUED)

as Gatorade (PepsiCo, Purchase, NY) or Pedialyte (Abbott Nutrition, Lake Forest, IL) is indicated for patients not drinking on their own.
• Mildly affected chinchillas usually respond well to oral and subcutaneous fluids, intestinal motility modifiers, analgesics, and dietary modification described below.
• Subcutaneous fluids can be administered (30–50 mL/kg) as needed. In most patients, lactated Ringer's solution or Normosol crystalloid fluids are appropriate.
• Intravenous or intraosseous fluids are required in patients that are severely dehydrated or depressed and to replace fluid losses from acute diarrhea. Maintenance fluid requirements are estimated at 100 mL/kg/day.
• Warm parental fluids to body temperature prior to administration.
• Supplemental fluids are gradually tapered once drinking and urine output return to normal.

ACTIVITY
• If the patient is not debilitated, encourage activity for at least 10–15 minutes every 6–8 hours since activity promotes gastric motility.
• Supervised time out of the cage and access to a safe grazing area provides additional enrichment and fiber intake.
• Gentle massage of the abdomen may assist in moving gas and ingesta through the digestive tract.

DIET
• It is important that patients continue to eat during and following treatment. Continued anorexia will exacerbate gastrointestinal hypomotility and cause further derangement of the gastrointestinal microflora and overgrowth of intestinal bacterial pathogens.
• Chinchillas may be tempted with parsley, cilantro, dandelion greens, and good-quality grass hay. Many patients will begin to eat these foods, even if they were previously anorectic. Also offer the patient's usual pelleted diet.
• If the patient refuses these foods, syringe-feed a gruel such as Critical Care for Herbivores (Oxbow Animal Health, Omaha, NE) or Emeraid Herbivore (Lafeber Company, Cornell, IL), 15–20 mL/kg PO q6–8h. Larger volumes and more frequent feedings are often accepted; feed as much as the chinchilla will readily accept. Alternatively, pellets can be ground and mixed with fresh greens, vegetable baby foods, water, or juice to form a gruel.
• High-carbohydrate, high-fat nutritional supplements are contraindicated.
• Encourage oral fluid intake: offer fresh water, administer oral fluids via syringe, wet the food, or flavor water with fruit or vegetable juices. (see fluid therapy)

• The diet should be permanently modified to include sufficient amounts of roughage and long-stemmed grass hay; foods high in simple carbohydrates should be prohibited or limited to the occasional treat.

CLIENT EDUCATION
• Discuss the importance of dietary modification, making diet changes gradually, and reducing/preventing stress.
• Advise owners to regularly monitor food consumption and fecal output; seek veterinary attention with a noticeable decrease in either.

SURGICAL CONSIDERATIONS
• Gastrointestinal stasis and dilation are usually treated medically; surgery is generally contraindicated. Surgical manipulation of the intestinal tract, hypothermia, anesthetic agents, and pain all exacerbate gastrointestinal hypomotility; gastrointestinal stasis is often worse postoperatively. The combination of these factors results in significantly worsened prognosis with surgical treatment.
• Gastric trichobezoars are often associated with fur chewing. As with hairballs in rabbits, medical treatment usually resolves the problem; however, surgery may be indicated in rare cases.
• Chinchillas affected by bloat should be treated by decompression by passing a stomach tube (orgastric decompression).

MEDICATIONS
Use parenteral medications in animals with severely compromised intestinal motility; oral medications may not be properly absorbed. Begin oral medication when intestinal motility begins to return (fecal production, return of appetite, radiographic evidence).

DRUG(S) OF CHOICE
• Motility modifiers such as metoclopramide (0.2–1.0 mg/kg PO, SC, IM q12h) or cisapride (0.1–0.5 mg/kg PO q8–12h) may be helpful in regaining normal motility; these may be used in alone or in conjunction; cisapride is available through compounding pharmacies. Promotility agents are contraindicated if intestinal obstruction or perforation is suspected.
• Analgesics such as buprenorphine (0.1–02 mg/kg SC, IM, IV q8–12h), meloxicam (0.5–1 mg/kg SC, PO q24h), and carprofen (2–5 mg/kg PO, SC q24h) are indicated in most cases. Intestinal pain, either postoperative or from gas distention and ileus, impairs mobility, decreases appetite, and may severely inhibit recovery.

• Anxiety can be safely reduced in chinchillas with injectable midazolam (0.25–0.5 mg/kg IM).
• Antibiotic therapy—recommended in cases where gastrointestinal stasis leads to secondary bacterial overgrowth, as indicated by diarrhea, abnormal fecal cytology, or bloody stool. Broad-spectrum antibiotics such as chloramphenicol (30–50 mg/kg PO q12h), trimethoprim sulfa (15–30 mg/kg PO q12h), or enrofloxacin (5–15 mg/kg PO q12h) should be selected.
• If *Clostridium* spp. overgrowth and enterotoxemia are suspected—metronidazole (10–20 mg/kg PO, IV q12h; may cause anorexia or reduced appetite in some chinchillas when administered PO) and cholestyramine (2 g/20 cc water, divided q24h PO or by gavage; binds bacterial toxins; dose cited is for a typical rabbit)
• Simethicone (20 mg/kg PO q8–12h) may be indicated in cases of gas distention.
• Lactating females with gastric tympany may respond favorably to calcium gluconate (100 mg/kg IV) administered slowly to effect.
• Probiotics (lactobacillus, yogurt) are of questionable efficacy; however, transfaunation with feces from a healthy individual may be indicated in cases of dysbiosis.

CONTRAINDICATIONS
• Avoid promotility agents if gastrointestinal obstruction or perforation is present or suspected.
• Anticholinergics (loperamide, atropine, and glycopyrrolate) in patients with suspected intestinal obstruction, glaucoma, intestinal ileus, liver disease, enterotoxin-producing bacteria, and invasive bacterial enteritis.
• Antibiotics that are primarily gram-positive in spectrum will suppress the growth of commensal flora, allowing overgrowth of enteric pathogens. These include lincomycin, clindamycin, erythromycin, ampicillin, amoxicillin, cephalosporins, and penicillins.

PRECAUTIONS
• NSAIDs (meloxicam, carprofen)—use with caution in chinchillas with compromised renal function.
• Chloramphenicol—may cause aplastic anemia in susceptible people. Clients and staff should use appropriate precautions when handling this drug.
• Metronidazolemay cause anorexia or reduced appetite in some chinchillas when administered PO: neurotoxic if overdosed; anecdotal reports of hepatotoxicity.

POSSIBLE INTERACTIONS
N/A

ALTERNATIVE DRUGS
N/A

FOLLOW-UP

PATIENT MONITORING
• Monitor hydration, appetite, and production of fecal pellets.
• Chinchillas that are successfully treated will regain a normal appetite and begin to produce normal volumes of feces.

PREVENTION/AVOIDANCE
• Gastrointestinal hypomotility (and the myriad problems related to it) can be avoided through strict feeding of diets containing adequate amounts of indigestible coarse fiber (long-stemmed hay) and low simple carbohydrate content, along with access to fresh water.
• Allow sufficient daily exercise.
• Prevent obesity.
• Minimize changes in the daily routine that might cause stress in small herbivores and avoid sudden changes the diet.
• Be certain that clean water is available and presented in a familiar manner (sipper vs. bowl).
• Avoid over-fasting patients prior to surgery, control perioperative pain and stress, and encourage patients to eat as soon as possible following surgery.
• Be certain that all postoperative patients are eating and passing feces prior to release.

POSSIBLE COMPLICATIONS
• Continued ileus leading to metabolic derangements and death
• Death due to gastric rupture
• Overgrowth of bacterial pathogens; clostridial enterotoxicosis

EXPECTED COURSE AND PROGNOSIS
• Depends on severity and underlying cause
• If caught early, mild cases usually respond to outpatient medical management and diet correction; the prognosis is generally excellent to good.
• Moderately severe cases generally respond to several days of hospitalization and intensive supportive care. These cases carry a good to fair prognosis; the patient usually improves and is discharged for additional care at home.
• In advanced cases—those that went unnoticed for several days prior to presentation—the prognosis is usually guarded to poor; hepatic lipidosis, shock, and other complications frequently make treatment unrewarding.
• The prognosis following gastrotomy or enterotomy is guarded to poor. Surgical correction of gastric trichobezoar, if indicated, carries a better prognosis than for surgical treatment of acute intestinal blockage by hair.

MISCELLANEOUS

ASSOCIATED CONDITIONS
• Anorexia
• Acquired dental disease
• Diarrhea
• Dehydration
• Antibiotic-associated enterotoxemia
• Constipation
• Hepatic lipidosis

AGE-RELATED FACTORS
N/A

ZOONOTIC POTENTIAL
N/A

PREGNANCY/FERTILITY/BREEDING
N/A

SYNONYMS
Ileus
Bloat

SEE ALSO
Anorexia
Diarrhea
Constipation (lack of fecal production)
Antibiotic-associated enterotoxemia

ABBREVIATIONS
PCV = packed cell volume
TS = total solids

INTERNET RESOURCES
N/A

Suggested Reading
Lennox AM, Gladden JN. Emergency and critical care of small mammals. In: Quesenberry KE, Carpenter JW, eds. Ferrets, Rabbits and Rodents, 4th ed. Clinical Medicine and Surgery. 2021. St. Louis: Saunders, 2020:595–608.
Mans C, Donnelly T. Chinchillas. In: Quesenberry KE, Carpenter JW, eds. Ferrets, Rabbits and Rodents, 4th ed. Clinical Medicine and Surgery. 2021. St. Louis: Saunders, 2020:298–322.
Martel A, Donnelly T, Mans C. Update on diseases in chinchillas: 2013–2019. Vet Clin Exot Anim 2020;23:321–333.
Mayer J, Mans C. Rodents. In: Carpenter JW, ed. Exotic Animal Formulary, 5th ed. St Louis: Elsevier, 2018:459–493.
Mitchell MA, Tully TN, eds. Manual of Exotic Pet Practice. St. Louis: Elsevier, 2009:480, 487, 491.
Riggs SM, Mitchell MA. Chinchillas. In: Mitchell MA, Tully TN, eds. Manual of Exotic Pet Practice. St. Louis: Elsevier, 2009:475–486.
Ritzman TK. Diagnosis and clinical management of gastrointestinal conditions in exotic companion mammals (rabbits, guinea pigs, and chinchillas). Vet Clin Exot Anim 2014;17:179–194.
Author Dan H. Johnson, DVM, Dipl. ABVP (Exotic Companion Mammal)

GIARDIASIS

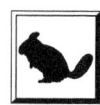

BASICS

OVERVIEW
• Enteric infection with the protozoan parasite *Giardia* spp.
• Often found in low numbers in normal chinchillas
• Numbers increase and active infection develops with stress and poor husbandry.
• Motile (flagellated) organisms attach to surface of enterocytes in small intestine, especially duodenum through jejunum.
• Malabsorption syndrome, severe diarrhea, and even death may result.
• Severe *Giardia* infection can predispose animals to other opportunistic infections.
• Its importance as a reservoir for human infection is not known.

SIGNALMENT
• No breed, age, or sex predilections have been described.
• Most reports have been in group-housed chinchillas, in fur ranches, and research colonies.
• Incidence in pet chinchillas is relatively low.

SIGNS
• Infection may be asymptomatic.
• Illness is typically chronic or intermittent.
• Appetite loss
• Sticky black feces, diarrhea
• Weight loss, debilitation
• Poor condition of fur

CAUSES AND RISK FACTORS
• *Giardia* is transmitted by oral ingestion of cysts, usually from contaminated water.
• Animals housed indoors and bred in captivity are less likely to acquire infection.
• Stress and poor husbandry facilitate *Giardia* infection and make it worse.
• Infection is often innocuous until a high parasite load develops.

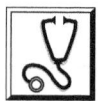

DIAGNOSIS

DIFFERENTIAL DIAGNOSIS
Consider all causes of enteropathy, including diet change, inappropriate antibiotics, enterotoxemia, systemic or metabolic disease, and specific intestinal disorders. More severe illnesses should prompt a more extensive evaluation.

CBC/BIOCHEMISTRY/URINALYSIS
• Usually normal with mild illness
• Increased PCV and TS are possible with dehydration

OTHER LABORATORY TESTS
• Often visible in fresh fecal wet mount with saline: motile organisms, tear-drop-shaped, $10–18 \times 7–15$ μm; "falling leaf" swimming pattern with two nuclei and four pairs of flagella. Specimen should be <10 minutes old. Addition of Lugol's iodine enhances appearance and kills organism, enabling inspection.
• Cysts—seen as crescent shapes with zinc sulfate fecal floatation; $8–13 \times 7–10$ μm
• Fecal ELISA is not superior to zinc sulfate floatation; its usefulness in chinchillas is unknown
• Fecal PCR assays—inconsistent results; should not be used as sole means of confirming *Giardia* infection.
• Organisms are shed intermittently—lack of visualization does not rule out infection. Collect samples over several days to increase probability of detection.

IMAGING
N/A

DIAGNOSTIC PROCEDURES
N/A

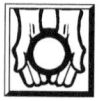

TREATMENT
Treat as outpatients unless debilitated or dehydrated

MEDICATIONS

DRUG(S) OF CHOICE
• Metronidazole 10–20 mg/kg q12h × 5 days
• Fenbendazole 20 mg/kg PO q24h × 5 days
• Albendazole 25 mg/kg PO q12h × 2 days
• Fluid therapy if dehydrated

CONTRAINDICATIONS AND PRECAUTIONS
• Metronidazole—may cause anorexia or reduced appetite in some chinchillas when administered PO; neurotoxic if overdosed; anecdotal reports of hepatotoxicity
• Albendazole—teratogenicity reported in mammals

FOLLOW-UP
Serial fecal examinations to confirm efficacy of treatment

MISCELLANEOUS

ZOONOTIC POTENTIAL
• *Giardia* is the most common intestinal parasite in humans residing in North America.
• *Giardia* spp. may not be highly host specific; no conclusive evidence that cysts shed by chinchillas are infective for humans

PREGNANCY/FERTILITY/BREEDING
Albendazole reported to be teratogenic in mammals

SEE ALSO
Diarrhea

ABBREVIATIONS
ELISA = enzyme-linked immunosorbent assay
PCV = packed cell volume
TS = total solids
PCR = polymerase chain reaction

Suggested Reading
Lennox AM, Gladden JN. Emergency and critical care of small mammals. In: Quesenberry KE, Carpenter JW, eds. Ferrets, Rabbits and Rodents, 4th ed. Clinical Medicine and Surgery. 2021. St. Louis: Saunders, 2020:595–608.
Mans C, Donnelly T. Chinchillas. In: Quesenberry KE, Carpenter JW, eds. Ferrets, Rabbits and Rodents, 4th ed. Clinical Medicine and Surgery. 2021. St. Louis: Saunders, 2020:298–322.
Martel A, Donnelly T, Mans C. Update on diseases in chinchillas: 2013–2019. Vet Clin Exot Anim 2020;23:321–333.
Mayer J, Mans C. Rodents. In: Carpenter JW, ed. Exotic Animal Formulary, 5th ed. St Louis: Elsevier, 2018:459–493.
Mitchell MA, Tully TN, eds. Manual of Exotic Pet Practice. St. Louis: Elsevier, 2009:480, 487, 491.
Riggs SM, Mitchell MA. Chinchillas. In: Mitchell MA, Tully TN, eds. Manual of Exotic Pet Practice. St. Louis: Elsevier, 2009:475–486.
Ritzman TK. Diagnosis and clinical management of gastrointestinal conditions in exotic companion mammals (rabbits, guinea pigs, and chinchillas). Vet Clin Exot Anim 2014;17:179–194.

Author Dan H. Johnson, DVM, DABVP (Exotic Companion Mammal)

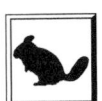

BASICS

DEFINITION
• Nasal discharge may be unilateral or bilateral, serous, mucoid, mucopurulent, purulent, hemorrhagic (epistaxis), or contain food material.
• Sneezing is the reflexive expulsion of air through the nasal cavity and is commonly caused by irritation of the nasal passages and associated with nasal discharge.

PATHOPHYSIOLOGY
• Mucous cells and glands of the nasal epithelium produce secretions. Irritation of the nasal mucosa (by mechanical, chemical, or inflammatory stimulation) increases nasal secretion production.
• Mucosal irritation and accumulated secretions are a potent stimulus of the sneeze reflex; sneezing may be the first sign of nasal discharge. Sneezing frequency often decreases with chronic disease.
• Dental disease is very common in chinchillas and is often associated with mucopurulent oculonasal discharge.
• Bacterial rhinitis can begin in the nasal cavity and may spread via the eustachian tubes to the inner or middle ears, into the sinuses, via the nasolacrimal duct to the eye, via the trachea to the lower respiratory tract.
• Allergic rhinitis has been proposed in the chinchilla but is very difficult to confirm.

Types of Nasal Discharge and Common Associations
• Serous—mild irritation, allergies, acute phase of inflammation, early bacterial infection
• Mucoid—allergies or contact irritation, acute inflammation or infection, early neoplastic conditions
• Purulent or mucopurulent—dental disease involving sinuses, bacterial infections, nasal foreign bodies, rarely mycotic in chinchillas
• Serosanguinous—destructive processes (bacterial pathogens, primary nasal tumors [rare])

SYSTEMS AFFECTED
• Respiratory—mucosa of the upper respiratory tract, including the nasal cavities, sinuses, and nasopharynx
• Ophthalmic—extension via nasolacrimal ducts causing ocular discharge
• Musculoskeletal—primary dental disease with extension of infection into sinuses
• Neurologic—extension of infection via eustachian tube causing vestibular signs from otitis interna/media
• Gastrointestinal—secondary GI stasis due to anorexia or pain; difficulty eating with upper respiratory obstruction (chinchilla is obligate nasal breather)
• Hemic/Lymphatic/Immune—may develop leukocytosis due to infection and inflammation
• Hepatobiliary—may develop hepatic lipidosis if anorectic due to pain or head tilt

GENETICS
Unknown

INCIDENCE/PREVALENCE
Primary bacterial rhinitis is less frequent than in rabbits; however, dental disease is very common in chinchillas with concurrent nasal discharge, which can progress to otitis interna.

GEOGRAPHIC DISTRIBUTION
N/A

SIGNALMENT
• Young animals—bacterial infections
• Middle-aged to older animals—nasal tumors, dental disease, bacterial infections
• Chinchillas with previous history of dental disease

SIGNS

General Comments
Related to the severity and extent of infection; may range from none to severe mucopurulent or serosanguinous nasal discharge

Historical Findings
• Nasal discharge and sneezing may be reported as concurrent problems. Information concerning both the initial and present character of the discharge and whether it was originally unilateral or bilateral are important historical findings.
• The response to previous antibiotic therapy may be helpful in determining bacterial involvement. Bacterial infections, dental disease, or foreign body will often respond initially to antibiotic therapy but commonly relapse after treatment. Nasal tumors typically show little response.
• History of ocular discharge; ptyalism with tooth involvement; head tilt, vestibular signs, scratching at ears with extension into the ears
• History of feeding diets consisting of commercial pelleted foods without the addition of long-stemmed hay or grasses common with dental disease

Physical Examination Findings
• Secretions or dried discharges on the hair around the nose and front limbs
• Concurrent dental disease, especially tooth root impaction. Findings may include ptyalism, anorexia, nasal discharge, ocular discharge, and exophthalmia. Always perform a thorough oral exam (which requires sedation or anesthesia).
• Ocular discharge—may be serous with nasolacrimal duct occlusion or mucopurulent; conjunctivitis secondary to nasolacrimal duct obstruction or extension of upper respiratory infection; exophthalmos with retrobulbar abscess
• Head tilt if rhinitis or dental disease has progressed along eustachian tube(s) to middle or inner ear.
• Bony involvement (tooth root abscess, tumor, and bacterial) may cause facial swelling and pain.
• Lethargy, anorexia, or depression with pain, extension of infection to lower respiratory tract or hematogenous spread
• Dyspnea, stridor—especially when exertion is combined with complete nasal occlusion (chinchillas are obligate nasal breathers) or extension of infection to lower respiratory tract

CAUSES
• Bacterial—most common agents identified in chinchillas are *Pseudomonas aeruginosa* and *Listeria monocytogenes*.
• Odontogenic infections—common isolates from these sites include anaerobic bacteria
• Dental disease—periapical or tooth root abscesses, elongated maxillary premolar or molar tooth roots penetrating into nasal passages
• Foreign objects, especially hay, straw, or other bedding material
• Allergies or irritants—dust, bedding, plant material
• Neoplasia—rare
• Unilateral discharge often is associated with nonsystemic processes—dental-related disease, nasal tumors, or foreign bodies
• Discharge may be unilateral or bilateral with bacterial respiratory tract infections, allergies, nasal tumors, dental disease, or foreign bodies.

RISK FACTORS
• Dental disease—extending infection
• Poor husbandry—inappropriate diet; ammonia build up in urine-soaked bedding
• Immunosuppression—stress, corticosteroid administration, concurrent disease, debility increases susceptibility to and extension of bacterial infections

DIAGNOSIS

DIFFERENTIAL DIAGNOSIS
Allergic, irritant, neoplastic, infectious, inflammatory, and traumatic disorders

CBC/BIOCHEMISTRY/URINALYSIS
• Hemogram—TWBC elevations with neutrophil: lymphocyte ratio shift; toxicity of neutrophils, bands; monocytosis may suggest

chronicity; thrombocytosis associated with active inflammation
• Biochemistry panel—usually normal unless concurrent disease, elevations in CK with muscle damage if soft tissue abscesses are present. Hepatic enzymes elevated if concurrent anorexia and hepatic lipidosis.

OTHER LABORATORY TESTS
• Culture and sensitivity from deep nasal swabs may be useful; best to obtain during sedation
• Further evaluation of liver function can be obtained with bile acid concentrations.

IMAGING
• Skull radiography—radiography of the nasal cavities can be helpful in cases of chronic nasal discharge, especially to rule out bacterial rhinitis/sinusitis, neoplasia, foreign body, or associated dental disease. It is difficult to evaluate the nasal cavity of the chinchilla on skull radiographs; therefore, the patient should be anesthetized and carefully positioned. A full skull series is warranted to evaluate the entire skull. Radiographs should be evaluated for dental disease, as this is a common precursor to rhinitis. All other bones of the skull should be evaluated for signs of sclerosis or lysis, as damage to the nasal, temporal, and mandibular bones may be present with rhinitis or neoplasia. Examine bullae for evidence of concurrent otitis; sclerosis of the bullae and surrounding bones may indicate chronicity.
• CT or MRI—superior to radiographs for identifying dental disease and associated changes affecting the nasal cavity. Can evaluate the nasal cavity for evidence of fluid or exudates. Can examine soft tissue structures in greater detail to evaluate for signs of abscessation/neoplasia. Contrast is useful for evaluating vascular changes associated with neoplasia, whereas abscesses do not take up contrast.

DIAGNOSTIC PROCEDURES
• Bacterial culture and sensitivity testing
• Deep nasal cultures may be useful in chinchillas with rhinitis. A heavy growth of a single organism is usually significant. A lack of growth does not rule out bacterial disease, since the infection may be in an inaccessible, deep area of the nasal cavity or sinuses.
• Deep nasal cytology showing intracellular bacteria in conjunction with a positive culture is strongly suggestive of bacterial infection; cytology showing nonspecific inflammatory response is most commonly found, often difficult to interpret, and may indicate allergic rhinitis.
• Rhinoscopy requires a narrow endoscope but can be extremely valuable to visualize nasal abnormalities, retrieve foreign bodies,

or obtain biopsy samples; sometimes the only method of identifying foreign bodies
• Biopsy—when tumor is suspected

PATHOLOGIC FINDINGS
Purulent exudates within the nasal cavity, microscopic evidence of degenerative neutrophils with or without intracellular bacteria; variable degrees of osteomyelitis

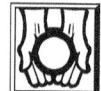

TREATMENT
APPROPRIATE HEALTH CARE
• Inpatient—severe debilitating infection, anorexia, or concurrent hepatic lipidosis; indicated if neurological signs present due to concurrent otitis
• Outpatient—if stable and can be managed at home pending further diagnostics or treatments as necessary
• Treat associated dental disease—extractions, complete debridement of abscesses
• Remove environmental allergens/irritants (dust bath provided for limited time, moldy hay, or bedding; provide good ventilation)

NURSING CARE
• Provide oxygen supplementation if the patient appears to be dyspneic. Chinchillas are obligate nasal breathers; thus, nasal discharge can cause severe dyspnea. Keep nostrils clear of discharge.
• Symptomatic treatment and nursing care are important in the treatment of chinchillas with sneezing and nasal discharge. Patient hydration, nutrition, warmth, and hygiene (keeping nostrils clean) are important.
• Subcutaneous fluids can be administered (30–50 mL/kg) as needed; IV access is difficult in the chinchilla; lateral saphenous vein catheters often fail; crystalloid fluids (e.g., lactated Ringer's solution or Normosol) are appropriate in most patients. Maintenance fluid needs are estimated at 100 mL/kg/day. CAUTION: risk of aspiration with open-mouth breathing and/or vestibular signs; fluids by mouth should be avoided.
• Housing support—for chinchillas that are falling and rolling due to vestibular disorders; provide housing such that the chinchilla is propped up by towels or other bedding materials to minimize these signs.

ACTIVITY
Return to normal activity as soon as possible. Restrict activity if severe vestibular signs to avoid injury.

DIET
• Affected chinchillas often develop inappetence. Be certain the chinchilla is eating to prevent the development or

exacerbation of gastrointestinal dysmotility/ GI stasis or hepatic lipidosis.
• If patient is eating on own, offer range of normal diet at home, including fresh, moist, high-fiber vegetables, chopped hay, and pellets.
• If chinchilla is not eating sufficiently on own, syringe-feeding a high-fiber critical diet is indicated: Critical Care for Herbivores (Oxbow Animal Health, Omaha, NE) or Emeraid Herbivore (Lafeber Company, Cornell, IL), 15–20 mL/kg PO q6–8h. Calculate caloric needs based on metabolic needs. Alternatively, chinchilla pellets can be ground with high-fiber green vegetables to make slurry that can be syringe-fed as above. Ensure high fiber intake to maximize dietary needs. High-carbohydrate, high-fat nutritional supplements are contraindicated.
• Encourage fluid intake with high-water vegetables, or by soaking vegetables in water before feeding.
• CAUTION—risk of aspiration with open-mouth breathing and/or vestibular signs. Ensure patient is in a stable position and willing to take foods by mouth before assisted feeding.

CLIENT EDUCATION
• Discuss the need to correct or prevent risk factors.
• Rhinitis due to bacterial infection may require long course of treatment.
• If dental disease is the underlying cause, this is a lifelong condition requiring consistent and repeated treatments for occlusal adjustments. By the time root elongations can be readily detected, they are irreversible; therefore, timely treatment of crown elongation is highly recommended.

SURGICAL CONSIDERATIONS
• If dental disease is the primary problem, may require extractions followed by periodic (every 6–8 weeks) occlusal adjustments.
• Chinchillas are difficult to intubate due to the palatal ostium in the oropharynx, which complicates providing a secure airway during anesthesia. Chinchillas can be intubated endoscopically. Normal chinchillas can be maintained under gas anesthesia via nasal mask; URT congestion and open-mouth breathing complicate inhalant anesthesia.

MEDICATIONS
DRUG(S) OF CHOICE
• Systemic antibiotics—based ideally on results from culture and sensitivity testing.
• Depending on severity of infection, long-term antibiotics: 6 weeks minimally, up to months or even lifelong treatment in

(CONTINUED)

NASAL DISCHARGE AND SNEEZING

chronic, recurrent, bacterial rhinitis/sinusitis. Use broad-spectrum antibiotics such as enrofloxacin (5–15 mg/kg PO, SC q12h) or trimethoprim-sulfa (15–30 mg/kg PO q12h) for aerobic infections. Anaerobic bacteria are usually causative agent of tooth root abscess; if anaerobes are present, chloramphenicol (30–50 mg/kg PO, SC, IV q12h) has good osseous penetration; penicillin G (40,000–60,000 IU/kg SC q2–7d) may also be used in severe cases. Monitor closely for loose stool or diarrhea.
• Intranasal antibiotics—use ophthalmic preparations of antibiotics without corticosteroids.
• Nasal secretions clear more easily if the patient is well hydrated; fluid therapy should be considered if hydration is marginal.
• Antihistamines have been used for chinchillas with allergic rhinitis, and symptomatically for infectious rhinitis; use is anecdotal, dosages extrapolated from other species (e.g., diphenhydramine 2.0 mg/kg PO, SC q8–12h).
• Nebulization with saline ± antibiotics and/or mucolytics may help to clear airways and treat infection.
• Topical ophthalmic preparations, such as those containing quinolones, to treat associated conjunctivitis
• Topical otic preparations if indicated for concurrent otitis
• Analgesia—pain relief is a critical aspect of therapy if concurrent dental disease, osteomyelitis, or neoplasia is present. Nonsteroidal anti-inflammatory such as meloxicam (0.5–1 mg/kg PO, SC q24h) and carprofen (2–5 mg/kg PO q24h) can provide both anti-inflammation and analgesia. However, with osteomyelitis or neoplasia addition of an opioid medication such as buprenorphine (0.01–0.05 mg/kg SC, IM, IV q8–12h) is recommended.

CONTRAINDICATIONS
• Oral antibiotics that select against Gram-positive bacteria (penicillins, macrolides, lincosamides, and cephalosporins) can cause fatal enteric dysbiosis and enterotoxemia.
• Topical and systemic corticosteroids—chinchillas are also sensitive to their immunosuppressive effects; can exacerbate bacterial infections
• Nasal decongestants containing phenylephrine can exacerbate nasal inflammation and cause nasal ulceration and purulent rhinitis.

PRECAUTIONS
• Metronidazole may cause anorexia or reduced appetite in some chinchillas when administered PO; hepatic toxicity has been anecdotally reported.

• The bones of the skull are relatively thin in this species; potential for fractures of maxillary bones or nasal fistulas if dental extractions required

POSSIBLE INTERACTIONS
Some topical otic medications may induce contact irritation; reevaluate all worsening cases.

ALTERNATIVE DRUGS
N/A

FOLLOW-UP

PATIENT MONITORING
• Reevaluate patient at 7–10 days or sooner if patient is worsening.
• Regular 6-month clinical assessment and monitoring for relapse of clinical signs
• Dental disease requires routine occlusal adjustments.

PREVENTION/AVOIDANCE
Treating otitis or upper respiratory infections in the early stages may prevent otitis media/interna.

POSSIBLE COMPLICATIONS
• Dyspnea as a result of nasal obstruction; chinchillas are obligate nasal breathers
• Osteomyelitis is a possible sequela to severe, chronic infection
• Surgical intervention (for otitis)—because of the extensive compartmentalization of the chinchilla bullae, this procedure is not commonly performed.
• Loss of appetite, gastrointestinal stasis, hepatic lipidosis

EXPECTED COURSE AND PROGNOSIS
Rhinitis/sinusitis may resolve after one course of therapy or may take months of multiple therapies to resolve.

MISCELLANEOUS

ASSOCIATED CONDITIONS
• Lower respiratory infection
• Dental disease
• Gastrointestinal hypomotility

AGE-RELATED FACTORS
N/A

ZOONOTIC POTENTIAL
N/A

PREGNANCY/FERTILITY/BREEDING
If dental disease is suspected as the inciting cause, breeders recommend not breeding these animals as inheritance abnormalities are suspected.

SYNONYMS
Snuffles

SEE ALSO
Dyspnea and tachypnea
Otitis media and interna

ABBREVIATIONS
CT = computed tomography
GI = gastrointestinal
MRI = magnetic resonance imaging
TWBC = total white blood cell count
URT = upper respiratory tract

Suggested Reading
Capello V, Cauduro A. Clinical technique: application of computed tomography for diagnosis of dental disease in the rabbit, guinea pig, and chinchilla. J Exot Pet Med 2008;17(2):93–101.
Capello V, Lennox AM. Diagnostic imaging of the respiratory system in exotic companion mammals. Vet Clin Exot Anim 2011;14:369–389.
DeCubellis J. Common emergencies in rabbits, guinea pigs, and chinchillas. Vet Clin Exot Anim 2016;19:411–429.
Goodman G. Rodents: respiratory and cardiovascular system disorders. In: Keeble E, Meredith A, eds. BSAVA Manual of Rodents and Ferrets. Gloucester: BSAVA, 2009:142–149.
Lennox AM, Gladden JN. Emergency and critical care of small mammals. In: Quesenberry KE, Carpenter JW, eds. Ferrets, Rabbits and Rodents, 4th ed. Clinical Medicine and Surgery. 2021. St. Louis: Saunders, 2020:595–608.
Mans C, Donnelly T. Chinchillas. In: Quesenberry KE, Carpenter JW, eds. Ferrets, Rabbits and Rodents, 4th ed. Clinical Medicine and Surgery. 2021. St. Louis: Saunders, 2020:298–322.
Mans C, Jekl V. Anatomy and disorders of the oral cavity of chinchilla and degus. Vet Clin Exot Anim 2016;19:843–869.
Martel A, Donnelly T, Mans C. Update on diseases in chinchillas: 2013–2019. Vet Clin Exot Anim 2020;23:321–333.
Riggs SM, Mitchell MA. Chinchillas. In: Mitchell MA, Tully TN, eds. Manual of Exotic Pet Practice. St. Louis: Elsevier, 2009:475–486.

Authors Joanne Paul–Murphy, DVM, Dipl. ACZM Dan H. Johnson, DVM, Dipl. ABVP (Exotic Companion Mammal)

OTITIS MEDIA AND INTERNA

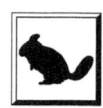

BASICS

DEFINITION
Inflammation of the middle ear (otitis media) and inner ear (otitis interna) characterized by the accumulation of purulent material or fluid in the middle ear, pain associated with the ear, bulging of the tympanum, and if the tympanum is perforated, drainage of purulent material into the ear canal. The chinchilla is a model for otitis media in humans, and much literature is available as to the anatomy, physiology, diagnosis, and treatment of this disease because of this.

PATHOPHYSIOLOGY
Most commonly arises from the eustachian tubes from infection in the oropharynx and upper respiratory system. Extension of external ear disease is less common.

SYSTEMS AFFECTED
• Respiratory—most infections begin in the upper respiratory tract or oropharynx and spread via the Eustachian tubes.
• Behavioral—lethargy, anorexia, and abnormal neurological signs
• Gastrointestinal—secondary GI stasis due to pain
• Hemic/Lymphatic/Immune—may develop leukocytosis due to infection and inflammation
• Hepatobiliary—may develop hepatic lipidosis if overconditioned and anorectic due to pain or head tilt
• Musculoskeletal—abscesses may extend into soft tissues surrounding infected ear
• Nervous—may develop abnormalities associated with cranial nerve VII (facial nerve paresis/paralysis) or cranial nerve VIII (head tilt, torticollis, and nystagmus)
• Ophthalmic—extension via nasolacrimal ducts from upper respiratory infections

GENETICS
Unknown

INCIDENCE/PREVALENCE
Subclinical disease is a common a sequella to upper respiratory tract disorders and can easily be missed; clinical disease is less common, but generally chronic and difficult to eliminate infection.

GEOGRAPHIC DISTRIBUTION
N/A

SIGNALMENT
N/A

SIGNS

General Comments
Signs are related to the severity and extent of infection; may range from none to nervous system involvement and bullae discomfort

Historical Findings
• Most common—acute onset of vestibular signs; often severe
• Torticollis can be severe; affected chinchillas often unable or unwilling to lift head
• May lean, veer, circle, or roll toward affected side
• Head tilt toward affected side
• Anorexia or bruxism due to nausea
• Pain manifested as reluctance to chew, shaking head, pawing affected ear, holding affected ear down, inappetence, reluctance to move
• Facial nerve abnormalities: facial symmetry; whisker movement and ability to blink reduced or absent on affected side; ocular discharge, decreased tear production
• Often history of past or current upper respiratory infection

Physical Examination Findings
Neurological Examination Findings
• Damage to neurological structures depends upon severity and location of disease
• Vestibular component of cranial nerve VIII—ipsilateral head tilt
• Nystagmus—resting or positional (most common); rotatory or horizontal; doesn't appear to aid in differentiation of central from peripheral
• Strabismus—ipsilateral ventral deviation of globe with extension of neck
• Ipsilateral leaning, falling, rolling
• Cranial nerve VII—facial nerve signs include ipsilateral paresis/paralysis of the affected ear, eyelids, lips, and nares; reduced tear production, with chronic cranial nerve VII damage, the affected side of the face may be contracted caused by fibrosis of denervated muscles; deficits can be bilateral
Otoscopic Examination
• Aural erythema, white or tan creamy discharge from ear; Otitis externa is usually the result of extension of infection from otitis media via a ruptured tympanic membrane. The external canal should be clean in a normal chinchilla; any exudate warrants further examination of the middle ear
• The external ear canal is short and wide allow easy visualization of the tympanum. The tympanic membrane should be uniform in appearance and semitransparent. Hyperemia, increased vascularization, increases in opacity, or bulging tympanic membrane on otoscopic examination indicates middle ear disease.
Other Findings
• Nasal or ocular discharge
• Facial abscesses, or abscesses at base of the ear
• Pain—upon oral or aural examination or palpation
• Corneal ulceration—inability to blink and dry eye resulting from cranial nerve VII damage, eyelid paralysis

CAUSES
• Bacterial—most common cause; usually extension of infection from URI. Agents identified in chinchillas are *Pseudomonas aeruginosa*, *Listeria monocytogenes*, and oral bacteria including various anaerobes
• Fungal—yeast (*Malassezia* spp., *Candida* spp.) are possible but not common
• Trauma—cagemate aggression causing external infections
• Polyps—at tympanum causing external ear disease
• Foreign bodies—uncommon
• Neoplasia—uncommon

RISK FACTORS
• Past or current upper respiratory tract infection. Immunosuppression—stress, corticosteroid administration, concurrent disease, debility; increases susceptibility to and extension of bacterial infections
• Dental disease—infection extending via eustachian tubes
• Overexuberant external ear canal flushing
• Ear cleansing solutions—may be irritating to middle or inner ear; avoid if tympanum is ruptured
• Ototoxic or immunosuppressive ear medications—many otic medications contain corticosteroids which reduce inflammation but may permit growth of bacteria if antibiotics are not effective. Based on research in chinchillas for human diseases, certain medications may be ototoxic.

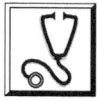

DIAGNOSIS

DIFFERENTIAL DIAGNOSIS
• Dental disease
• Pain from otitis externa causing chinchilla to hold ear abnormally can be confused with otitis media signs; chinchillas with otitis media commonly demonstrate neurologic abnormalities associated with vestibular disease such as nystagmus, torticollis, ataxia, circling, and head tilt.
• Central vestibular disease—bacterial infection/abscesses most common; parasites (e.g., *Baylisascaris* spp. aberrant larval migrans and *Sarcocystis neurona* [if housed outdoors], *Toxoplasma gondii* [if housed with cats]); may see severe lethargy, stupor, and other CNS signs
• History of use of ototoxic drugs
• Neoplasia—uncommon; rule out via imaging of the skull
• Trauma—history and physical examination findings of trauma

CBC/BIOCHEMISTRY/URINALYSIS
• Hemogram—TWBC elevations with neutrophil: lymphocyte ratio shift; toxicity of neutrophils ± bands, monocytosis may

suggest chronicity; thrombocytosis associated with active inflammation
• Biochemistry panel—usually normal unless concurrent disease, elevations in CK with muscle damage if soft tissue abscesses are present

OTHER LABORATORY TESTS
N/A

IMAGING
• Skull radiography—a full skull series is warranted to evaluate the entire skull: bullae may appear cloudy if exudates are present, sclerosis of the bullae and surrounding bones may indicate chronicity; bony lysis indicates osteomyelitis; even with severe cases, bullae sometimes appear normal on radiographs.
• Radiographs should be evaluated for dental disease, as this is a common precursor to ear disease. All other bones of the skull should be evaluated for signs of sclerosis or lysis as damage to the nasal, temporal, and mandibular bones may be present. It is difficult to evaluate the nasal cavity of the chinchilla on skull radiographs.
• CT—superior to radiographs for identifying bony changes associated with bullae disease and severity of dental disease. Can evaluate nasal cavity for evidence of fluid/exudate and soft tissue structures for signs of abscessation/neoplasia. Contrast is not very useful for evaluating bullae and nasal disease, as abscesses do not take up contrast; however, if a tumor is suspected, contrast CT is warranted to determine the extent of neoplasia.

DIAGNOSTIC PROCEDURES
• Cytolologic examination and bacterial culture. Samples can be obtained from the bullae using a transbular approach using a 18–20g needle punctured through the bone on dorsal aspect of the bulla. General anesthesia and sterile technique are required. Once entered, a 20–22g catheter can be used to flush the bulla with warm sterile saline.
• Samples obtained from deep within the external ear canal are less accurate but can be helpful. Culture and sensitivity from deep nasal swabs generally not useful
• Microscopic examination of ear swab if otitis externa is present
• Biopsy—when deep tissue infection, tumor or osteomyelitis is suspected.

PATHOLOGIC FINDINGS
Purulent exudates within the middle ear cavity surrounded by a thickened bulla, microscopic evidence of degenerative neutrophils with or without intracellular bacteria; variable degrees of osteomyelitis

TREATMENT
APPROPRIATE HEALTH CARE
• Inpatient—severe debilitating infection, neurological signs
• Outpatient—if stable and can be managed at home pending further diagnostics or treatments as necessary

NURSING CARE
• Flushing of the bullae using a transbulbar approach as described above (diagnostic procedures). Most infections are chronic by the time clinical signs are noted and the bullae contain thick exudate. Complete cure is unlikely, and the goal is to manage disease and prevent progression.
• Concurrent otitis externa—clean ears with warm saline flush; dry ear with cotton swabs ± low vacuum suction; general anesthesia is necessary to provide thorough cleaning.
• Subcutaneous fluids can be administered (30–50 mL/kg) as needed; IV access is difficult in the chinchilla; lateral saphenous vein catheters often kink; consider intraosseous (IO) catheterization if intravascular fluids are needed. Base fluid selection on the underlying cause of fluid loss. In most patients, lactated Ringer's solution or Normosol crystalloid fluids are appropriate. Maintenance fluids estimated to be 100 mL/kg/day. Fluids by mouth should be avoided in patients with extreme head tilt. Housing support—for chinchillas that are falling and rolling, provide housing such that the chinchilla is propped up by towels or other bedding materials to minimize these signs.

ACTIVITY
Restrict activity if severe vestibular signs to avoid injury; encourage return to normal activity as soon as possible

DIET
Many chinchillas will develop inappetence. Be certain the chinchilla is eating to prevent the development, or exacerbation of, gastrointestinal dysmotility/GI stasis.
• If patient is eating on own, offer range of normal diet at home, including fresh, moist, high-fiber vegetables, chopped hay, and pellets. May need to offer in more than one place in the cage so that the patient can get to food if vestibular signs prevent normal activity.
• If chinchilla is not eating sufficiently on own, syringe feed a high-fiber diet. The chinchilla usually accepts Critical Care for Herbivores (Oxbow Animal Health, Omaha, NE) or Emerald Herbivore (Lafeber Company, Cornell, IL), 15–20 mL/kg PO

q6–8h. Alternatively, chinchilla pellets can be ground with high-fiber green vegetables to make slurry that can be syringe-fed as above. Ensure appropriate fiber intake to maximize nutrition.
• Rarely, esophagostomy tube indicated
• Encourage fluid intake with high-water vegetables, or by soaking vegetables in water before feeding.
• CAUTION—patients with vestibular signs are at risk for aspiration due to abnormal body posture. Ensure the patient is in a stable position and is willing to take food before assisted feeding.

CLIENT EDUCATION
• Warn the client that otitis media/interna can be extremely frustrating to treat, especially in chronic cases. Successful outcomes require long-term therapies, client compliance, and in severe cases, surgical intervention.
• Warn clients that neurological signs, especially head tilt and facial nerve damage, may be permanent. Some chinchillas improve minimally due to the extensive compartmentalization of the bullae in chinchillas; however, many will maintain a good quality of life.

SURGICAL CONSIDERATIONS
• Indicated when ear canal is severely stenotic, when infection is refractory to medical management, or when neoplasia is diagnosed
• Chinchillas are difficult to intubate due to the palatal ostium in the oropharynx, which complicates providing a secure airway during anesthesia. Chinchillas can be intubated endoscopically.
• Total ear canal ablation is not usually necessary in chinchillas but may be indicated if otitis media is associated with recurrent otitis externa or neoplasia, especially when aural pain reduces quality of life.
• Bullae osteotomy—to date, there is little information regarding surgical approaches due to the extensive compartmentalization of the chinchilla bullae. Several research studies using the chinchilla as a model for human otitis media have reported successful bullae osteotomy, but the surgical procedures have not been clearly outlined.

MEDICATIONS
DRUG(S) OF CHOICE
• Systemic antibiotics—based ideally on results from culture and sensitivity testing. Depending on severity of infection, long-term antibiotics (6 weeks minimally, up to months or even lifelong treatment in some severe cases). Use broad-spectrum antibiotics

OTITIS MEDIA AND INTERNA

such as enrofloxacin (5–15 mg/kg PO, SC q12h) or trimethoprim-sulfa (15–30 mg/kg PO q12h) for aerobic infections; if anaerobes are present, chloramphenicol (30–50 mg/kg PO, SC, IV q12h) has excellent bony penetration; penicillin G (40,000–60,000 IU/kg SC q2–7d) may also be used in severe cases.

• Topical antibiotics—for treatment of concurrent otitis externa; use otic preparations of antibiotics without corticosteroids.

• Analgesia—pain relief is a critical aspect of therapy. Nonsteroidal anti-inflammatory medications such as meloxicam (0.5–1 mg/kg PO, SC q24h) and carprofen (2–5 mg/kg PO, SC q24h) can provide both anti-inflammation and analgesia. However, with osteomyelitis and postsurgical intervention, addition of an opioid medication such as buprenorphine (0.01–0.05 mg/kg SC, IV q8–12h) is necessary.

• Severe vestibular signs or seizures—midazolam (1–2 mg/kg IM) during acute phase

• Meclizine (2–12 mg/kg PO q24h) may reduce clinical vestibular signs, control nausea, and induce mild sedation.

CONTRAINDICATIONS

• Oral antibiotics that select against gram-positive bacteria (penicillins, macrolides, lincosamides, and cephalosporins) can cause fatal enteric dysbiosis and enterotoxemia.

• Topical and systemic corticosteroids—chinchillas are also sensitive to their immunosuppressive effects; can exacerbate otitis externa.

• Ruptured tympanum or associated neurological deficits—avoid the use of oil-based or irritating external ear preparations (chlorhexidine) and aminoglycosides, which can be ototoxic.

PRECAUTIONS

• Metronidazole may cause anorexia or reduced appetite in some chinchillas when administered PO; hepatic toxicity has been anecdotally reported.

• Avoid overexuberant flushing of external ear as this can exacerbate signs of otitis media/interna.

• The bones of the skull are relatively thin in this species; potential for fractures of surrounding bones if pinhole or other surgical incision is made into the bullae

POSSIBLE INTERACTIONS

Some topical otic medications may induce contact irritation; reevaluate all worsening cases.

ALTERNATIVE DRUGS

Azithromycin and Clarithromycin have been experimentally used to eliminate bacterial otitis media in chinchillas. These should be used with caution as they may cause intestinal dysbiosis.

FOLLOW-UP

PATIENT MONITORING

• Monitor for corneal ulceration—secondary to facial nerve paresis/paralysis or abrasion during vestibular episodes.

• Reevaluate patient at 7–10 days or sooner if patient is worsening.

PREVENTION/AVOIDANCE

Treating otitis or upper respiratory infections in the early stages may prevent otitis media/interna.

POSSIBLE COMPLICATIONS

• Corneal ulceration

• Persistence of vestibular and facial nerve damage

• Severe infections may spread to the CNS.

• Osteomyelitis is a common sequela to severe, chronic infections.

• Surgical intervention—because of the extensive compartmentalization of the chinchilla bullae, this procedure is not commonly performed.

EXPECTED COURSE AND PROGNOSIS

• Otitis media/interna—may take months of multiple therapies to resolve; recurrence is common

• When medical management is ineffective, surgical considerations should be explored.

• Vestibular signs often resolve, but recurrence does occur in many patients.

• Residual deficits cannot be predicted until a long course of therapy has been attempted; long-term quality of life is good for chinchillas with mild-moderate residual head tilt or facial nerve damage.

MISCELLANEOUS

ASSOCIATED CONDITIONS

• Upper respiratory infection

• Dental disease

• Facial abscesses

AGE-RELATED FACTORS
N/A

ZOONOTIC POTENTIAL
N/A

PREGNANCY/FERTILITY/BREEDING

If dental disease is suspected as the inciting cause, breeders recommend not breeding these animals as inheritance abnormalities are suspected.

SYNONYMS

Middle ear, inner ear disease

SEE ALSO

Nasal discharge and sneezing

ABBREVIATIONS

CNS = central nervous system
CK = creatine kinase
C/S = culture and sensitivity
CT = computed tomography
TWBC = total white blood cell count

INTERNET RESOURCES
N/A

Suggested Reading

Capello V, Lennox AM. Diagnostic imaging of the respiratory system in exotic companion mammals. Vet Clin Exot Anim 2011;14:369–389.

Mancinelli E. Neurologic examination and diagnostic testing in rabbits, ferrets and rodents. J Exot Pet Med 2015;24:52–64.

Mans C, Donnelly T. Chinchillas. In: Quesenberry KE, Carpenter JW, eds. Ferrets, Rabbits and Rodents, 4th ed. Clinical Medicine and Surgery. 2021. St. Louis: Saunders, 2020:298–322.

Martel A, Donnelly T, Mans C. Update on diseases in chinchillas: 2013–2019. Vet Clin Exot Anim 2020;23:321–333.

Mayer J, Mans C. Rodents. In: Carpenter JW, ed. Exotic Animal Formulary, 5th ed. St Louis: Elsevier, 2018:459–493.

Meredith AL, Richardson J. Neurologic disease of rabbits and rodents. J Exot Pet Med 2015;24:21–33.

Mitchell MA, Tully TN, eds. Manual of Exotic Pet Practice. St. Louis: Elsevier, 2009:480, 487, 491.

Miwa Y, Sladky K. Common surgical procedures of rodents, ferrets, hedgehogs, and sugar gliders. Vet Clin Exot Anim 2016;19:205–244.

Palmerio BS, Roberts H. Clinical approach to dermatologic disease in exotic animals. Vet Clin North Am Exot Anim Pract 2013;16(3):523–577.

Riggs SM, Mitchell MA. Chinchillas. In: Mitchell MA, Tully TN, eds. Manual of Exotic Pet Practice. St. Louis: Elsevier, 2009:475–486.

Authors Michelle G. Hawkins, VMD, Dipl. ABVP (Avian) Dan H. Johnson, DVM, Dipl. ABVP (Exotic Companion Mammal)

PENILE DISORDERS: PHIMOSIS, PARAPHIMOSIS, AND BALANOPOSTHITIS

BASICS

DEFINITION
- Phimosis—the inability to protrude or extend the glans penis from the prepuce
- Paraphymosis—the inability to reduce or fully reduce the glans penis into the prepuce
- Balanoposthitis—inflammation of the prepuce and glans penis, usually secondary to infection, fur rings, or accumulation of smegma

PATHOPHYSIOLOGY
- Phimosis—may be congenital, most often acquired secondary to trauma, infection or inflammation (e.g., fur rings) with scar tissue formation
- Paraphimosis—the penis is sigmoid shaped and long, contains a 1 cm long os penis, with the glans penis retracted fully into the prepuce when flaccid. Fur often accumulates at the base of the glans penis, deep within the prepuce, and can form a constricting ring. These are generally referred to as "Fur Rings" and predispose to paraphimosis. Accumulations of smegma or balanoposthitis can also lead to paraphimosis.
- Balanoposthitis—Fur rings and accumulation of smegma can serve as a nidus for bacterial infection, resulting in infection or abscess formation

SYSTEMS AFFECTED
- Renal/urologic—bladder, urethra with urethral constriction
- Reproductive—breeding failure
- Integument—fur rings, urine scald
- Systemic—sepsis with infection, abscess; anorexia and weight loss with pain, urine retention, or infection

INCIDENCE/PREVALENCE
Penile and preputial disorders are one of the most common problems seen in pet chinchillas

SIGNALMENT
Usually middle-aged to older chinchillas; young chinchillas if phimosis is congenital

SIGNS

Historical Findings
- Can be asymptomatic until infection is severe—it is important to fully extrude and examine the penis as part of routine examination in all male chinchillas
- Excessive grooming around penis
- Breeding failure
- Dysuria, stranguria
- Hyporexia, anorexia, depression with pain, or secondary infection

Physical Examination Findings
- It is important to fully extrude and examine the penis as part of routine examination in all male chinchillas
- Phimosis—the glans penis cannot be extruded; may see urine retention within the prepuce, swelling, inflammation or abscess formation under the prepuce, excessive grooming in region
- Paraphymosis—the glans penis is extended from the prepuce; the glans may appear inflamed, edematous, or dry and firm. With prolonged exposure, can become necrotic. Full extrusion from the prepuce may demonstrate fur rings, accumulation of smegma and other debris, exudate, or abscess
- Balanoposthitis—excessive smegma accumulation, inflammation, swelling, exudate, or abscess formation; fur rings often contribute
- Alopecia, moist dermatitis around penis with urine scald or excessive grooming
- If infection becomes generalized or urinary outflow is constricted—anorexia, lethargy, fever, dehydration

CAUSES

Phimosis
- Most often due to inflammation and scar formation from fur rings, accumulation of smega, infection, or abscess
- Trauma
- Congenital
- Neoplasia—possible, but not yet reported

Paraphimosis
- Fur rings are the most common cause; excessive smegma accumulation, or balanoposthitis/abscesses. With chronic exposure, the glans penis may become dried out or even necrotic
- Trauma, self-mutilation of exposed glans penis

Balanopostitis
- Infection can be secondary to or the cause of paaraphimosis; fur rings and excessive smegma accumulation serve as nidus of infection. Underlying systemic *Pseudomonas aeruginosa* infection has been a reported cause in the absence of fur rings.
- May lead to large abscess formation in the penis or prepuce

RISK FACTORS
- Lack of routine cleaning of the prepuce
- Unsanitary conditions
- Lack of dust baths may predispose to fur rings

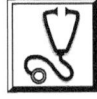

DIAGNOSIS

DIFFERENTIAL DIAGNOSIS
For stranguira, dysuria:

- Cystitis—bacteriuria; painful, thickened bladder
- Urolithiasis—palpable uroliths in the bladder, radio-opacities within the bladder; less common in chinchillas than in other small exotic mammals

CBC/BIOCHEMISTRY/URINALYSIS
- CBC—usually normal unless infection is severe or becomes systemic
- Biochemistry panel—if urethral obstruction occurs—may see azotemia, changes in electrolytes such as hyperkalemia, hypochloremia, hyponatremia
- Urinalysis—to rule out bacterial cystitis

OTHER LABORATORY TESTS
- Cytology of purulent discharge—Diff-Quick and Gram's stain to direct therapy
- Bacterial culture and sensitivity testing of exudate

IMAGING
- Radiographs to rule out urinary calculi as a cause of dysuria

TREATMENT

APPROPRIATE HEALTH CARE
- Patients with nonobstructive penile disorders are typically managed as outpatients
- Chinchillas with urinary obstruction should be hospitalized, emergency supportive and symptomatic therapy should be provided until the obstruction is resolved.

NURSING CARE
- Fur rings can be gently removed using lubricating products. The distal penis may need to be lubricated or soaked in warm saline solution prior to removal attempts to loosen the hair. The chinchilla may require sedation or anesthesia to remove if painful. Fur rings may need to be carefully cut to remove.
- Clean all accumulation smegma and preputial discharge with dilute (0.125%) chlorohexidine solution
- Paraphimosis
  - If chronic, the exposed glans penis may be coated with a hard, dry coating of desquamated cells and debris. Soak in warm saline solution until coating softens and gently remove; may require sedation. Fully replace the glans penis back into the prepuce
  - If exposed glans penis is swollen, edematous—clean with dilute chlorhexidine solution—coat with sugar to reduce swelling, coat with lubricant such as petroleum jelly to replace into prepuce.

PENILE DISORDERS: PHIMOSIS, PARAPHIMOSIS, AND BALANOPOSTHITIS (CONTINUED)

◦ If edema and swelling are severe—do not attempt to force into prepuce. Apply ointments or hydrocolloid gel topically 3–4 times daily until swelling resolves. An E collar is needed to prevent grooming or mutilation.

ACTIVITY
• No restriction required.

DIET
• If anorectic or have a decreased appetite assist feed Critical Care for Herbivores (Oxbow Animal Health, Omaha, NE) or Emeraid Herbivore (Lafeber Company, Cornell, IL), 15–20 mL/kg PO q6–8h. Larger volumes and more frequent feedings are often accepted; feed as much as the patient will readily accept.

CLIENT EDUCATION
• Instruct and encourage clients to extrude and clean the glans penis regularly
• Dust baths at least twice weekly are recommended and reduce the potential for fur rings.

SURGICAL CONSIDERATIONS
• Phimosis—gently break down adhesions using sharp/blunt dissection under general anesthesia. Postoperative management entails daily extrusion of the penis, cleaning with dilute chlorhexidine solution, and application of antibiotic/steroid combination ointment to the penis until healing occurs, then reduce to once weekly
• Surgery may be required if the distal penis of males becomes necrotic.
• Abscesses may require surgical drainage

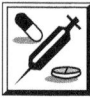

MEDICATIONS

DRUG(S) OF CHOICE
• Antibiotics if bacterial infection is present—ideally based on culture and sensitivity testing. Broad-spectrum antibiotics commonly used in chinchillas include enrofloxacin (5–15 mg/kg PO, SC, IM q12h), trimethoprim sulfa (15–30 mg/kg PO q12h), and chloramphenicol (30–50 mg/kg PO, SC, IM, IV q8–12h).
• Analgesics meloxicam (0.5–1 mg/kg SC, PO q24h) or carprofen (2–5 mg/kg PO, SC q24).

CONTRAINDICATIONS
If the exposed glans penis is severely edematous, do not force it back into the prepuce

PRECAUTIONS
Meloxicam—use with caution in chinchillas with compromised renal function.

POSSIBLE INTERACTIONS
N/A

ALTERNATIVE DRUGS
N/A

FOLLOW-UP

PATIENT MONITORING
• Owners should be instructed to extrude and clean the glans penis regularly

PREVENTION/AVOIDANCE
• Regular inspection of the glans penis
• Regular fur baths
• Clean environment

POSSIBLE COMPLICATIONS
• Constriction of the penis causing urinary outflow obstruction and subsequent uremia
• Extension of infection, formation of abscesses, or bacterial sepsis with balanoposthitis
• Necrosis of the exposed glans penis with chronicity
• Self-mutilation

EXPECTED COURSE AND PROGNOSIS
• Phimosis—adhesions may recur
• Paraphymosis—good prognosis if fur rings, smegma, and other accumulations are removed and exposed tissues are kept moist
• Balanopostosis—depends on severity

MISCELLANEOUS

ASSOCIATED CONDITIONS
See Causes

AGE-RELATED FACTORS
N/A

ZOONOTIC POTENTIAL
N/A

PREGNANCY/FERTILITY/BREEDING
Can prevent successful breeding until treatment

SYNONYMS
Fur rings

SEE ALSO
Dysuria and hematuria

ABBREVIATIONS
N/A

INTERNET RESOURCES
N/A

Suggested Reading
Kondert L, Mayer J. Reproductive medicine in guinea pigs, chinchillas and degus. Vet Clin Exot Anim 2017;20:609–628.
Lennox AM, Gladden JN. Emergency and critical care of small mammals. In: Quesenberry KE, Carpenter JW, eds. Ferrets, Rabbits and Rodents, 4th ed. Clinical Medicine and Surgery. 2021. St. Louis: Saunders, 2020:595–608.
Mans C, Donnelly TM. Update on diseases of chinchillas. Vet Clin Exot Anim 2013;16:383–406.
Mans C, Donnelly T. Chinchillas. In: Quesenberry KE, Carpenter JW, Orcutt C, eds. Ferrets, Rabbits and Rodents: Clinical Medicine and Surgery, 4th ed. St. Louis, MO: Elsevier, 2020:298–323.
Martel-Arquette A, Donnelly T, Mans C. Update on diseases in chinchillas: 2013–2019. Vet Clin Exot Anim 2020;23: 321–333.
Martel-Arquette A, Mans C. Management of Phimosis and Balanoposthitis in a pet chinchilla (*Chinchilla lanigera*). J Exot Pet Med 2016;25:60–64.
Riggs SM, Mitchell MA. Chinchillas. In: Mitchell MA, Tully TN, eds. Manual of Exotic Pet Practice. St. Louis: Elsevier, 2009:475–486.
Author Barbara Oglesbee, DVM, Dipl. ABVP (Avian)

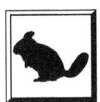

BASICS

DEFINITION
Polyuria is greater than normal urine production, and polydipsia is greater than normal water consumption. The average water intake of the chinchilla is approximately 10 mL/100 g BW/day. Chinchillas fed large amounts of high-moisture leafy vegetables will drink less water than those on a diet primarily of hay and/or pellets. Chinchillas offered water from an open dish drink more than those offered water from a nipple water bottle. Urine production reported for rodents is approximately 3.3–4.2 mL/100 g BW/day; values are not available specifically for chinchillas.

PATHOPHYSIOLOGY
• Urine production and water consumption are controlled by interactions between the hypothalamus, the pituitary gland, and the kidneys.
• Polydipsia generally occurs as a response to polyuria to maintain circulating fluid volume.
• The patient's plasma becomes hypertonic, activating thirst mechanisms.
• Occasionally, polyuria may occur as a response to polydipsia. The patient's plasma becomes relatively hypotonic because of excessive water intake and ADH secretion, resulting in polyuria.

SYSTEMS AFFECTED
• Renal/Urologic
• Reproductive
• Hepatic
• Endocrine/Metabolic
• Cardiovascular—alterations in circulating fluid volume

CAUSES
Primary Polyuria
• Upper urinary tract disease—renal failure, pyelonephritis
• Lower urinary tract disease—infection, urolithiasis, neoplasia, anatomic, or neurologic problem
• Pyometra
• Osmotic diuresis—diabetes mellitus (only reported in one chinchilla to date), post-obstructive diuresis, ingestion, or administration of large quantities of solute (sodium chloride, glucose)
• Ingestion of nephrotoxic plants (lilies)
• Iatrogenic—administration of nephrotoxic drugs (aminoglycosides), diuretics (furosemide and mannitol), corticosteroids, anticonvulsants (phenytoin), alcohol

• Hyperthyroidism (not reported in chinchillas)
• Diabetes insipidus—central, renal
• Hepatic failure
• Hypokalemia
• Traumatic, neoplastic

Primary Polydipsia
• Behavioral problems (especially boredom), pyrexia, pain
• Organic disease of the anterior hypothalamic thirst center of neoplastic, traumatic, or inflammatory origin (not reported in chinchillas)
• Psychogenic drinking

RISK FACTORS
• Renal or hepatic disease
• Selected electrolyte disorders
• Administration of diuretics, anticonvulsants, nephrotoxic drugs
• Exposure to nephrotoxic plants (lilies)

DIAGNOSIS

DIFFERENTIAL DIAGNOSIS
Differentiating Similar Signs
• Differentiate polyuria from an abnormal increase in frequency of urination (pollakiuria). Pollakiuria is often associated with dysuria, stranguria, or hematuria. Patients with polyuria void large quantities of urine and patients with pollakiuria generally void small quantities of urine.
• Measuring urine-specific gravity may provide evidence of adequate urine concentrating capacity (>1.045).

Differentiating Causes
• If associated with progressive weight loss—consider renal failure, hepatic failure, pyometra, neoplasia, pyelonephritis, and possibly diabetes mellitus (one report in chinchillas)
• If associated with polyphagia or cataracts—consider diabetes mellitus.
• If associated with recent estrus in an intact female chinchilla—consider pyometra
• If associated with fever in an intact female chinchilla—consider pyometra
• If associated with abdominal distension—consider hepatic failure and neoplasia
• If associated with hypercrystalluria—consider nephrolithiasis or renal failure
• If post-obstructive, diuresis can cause polyuria.
• Diabetes insipidus—central vs. renal
• Hypokalemia
• Iatrogenic—corticosteroids, anticonvulsants, nephrotoxic drugs

CBC/BIOCHEMISTRY/URINALYSIS
• CBC—elevated TWBC, neutrophilia suggests inflammation, infection; elevated platelet counts suggests inflammation
• Relative hypernatremia suggests primary polyuria; hyponatremia suggests primary polydipsia.
• Elevated BUN (>25 mg/dL) and creatinine (>1.0 mg/dL) are consistent with renal causes, but also consider prerenal causes such as dehydration resulting from inadequate compensatory polydipsia.
• Elevated hepatic enzymes suggest hepatic insufficiency.
• Hyperglycemia suggests diabetes mellitus and stress.
• Hypoalbuminemia suggests renal or hepatic disease.
• WBC casts and/or bacteriuria: should consider pyelonephritis
• Urinalysis, including both a standard dipstick and microscopic examination of the sediment, should be performed, preferably from a cystocentesis sample. If voided, assume sample contamination.
• Urine sediment evaluation may reveal calcium carbonate, calcium oxalate, or struvite crystals; if excessive consider urolithiasis, cystitis.
• Glucosuria and ketonuria may be identified with diabetes mellitus. Ketonuria can also be associated with starvation or prolonged anorexia, especially during pregnancy.
• Bacteriuria, pyuria (>0–1 WBC/hpf), hematuria (>0–3 RBC/hpf), and proteinuria indicate urinary or reproductive tract inflammation but are not specific to differentiate infectious and noninfectious causes of lower urinary tract disease; trace protein is considered normal in the urine of chinchillas as determined by urine dipstick.
• Identification of neoplastic cells in urine sediment indicates urinary tract neoplasia (rare).

OTHER LABORATORY TESTS
• Prior to antibiotic use, culture the urine or bladder wall if pyuria, hematuria, bacteriuria, or a combination of these are present on sediment examination.
• Aerobic/anaerobic bacterial urine culture and sensitivity—the most definitive means of identifying and characterizing bacterial urinary tract infection; negative urine culture results suggest a noninfectious cause unless the patient was on concurrent antibiotics or has an anaerobic infection. Chronic pyelonephritis cannot be completely ruled out by negative pyuria, bacteriuria.
• If surgery is necessary to relieve obstruction from urolithiasis, collect and submit the calculi for analysis and culture and sensitivity and submit the bladder wall for culture and sensitivity.

CHINCHILLAS

IMAGING
Abdominal radiography and ultrasonography may provide additional evidence for renal disease (e.g., primary renal disease, urolithiasis), hepatic disease, pancreatic disease, reproductive disease (e.g., pyometra).

PATHOLOGIC FINDINGS
Depend upon the underlying cause

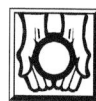

TREATMENT

APPROPRIATE HEALTH CARE
• Patients with uncomplicated PU/PD that appear otherwise normal are typically managed as outpatients; diagnostic evaluation may require brief hospitalization.
• Diseases associated with systemic signs of illness (e.g., pyrexia, depression, anorexia, and dehydration) or laboratory findings of azotemia and or leukocytosis warrant an aggressive diagnostic evaluation and initiation of supportive and symptomatic treatment.
• Chinchillas with urinary obstruction should be hospitalized; emergency supportive and symptomatic therapy should be provided until surgical intervention to relieve the obstruction is performed. Medical treatment of calcium-based urolithiasis has been unrewarding to date, and surgical removal of calculi is most often required. Postoperative management including supportive and symptomatic treatment as well as pain management therapies.

NURSING CARE
• Ensure that patient has adequate water available at all times until the causes for the PU/PD are understood and that the patient has adequate water intake.
• Subcutaneous fluids can be administered (30–50 mL/kg) as needed; IV access is difficult in the chinchilla; lateral saphenous vein catheters often kink; consider intraosseous (IO) catheterization if intravascular fluids are needed. Base fluid selection on the underlying cause of fluid loss. In most patients, lactated Ringer's solution or Normosol crystalloid fluids are appropriate. Maintenance fluids are estimated at 100 mL/kg/day.

ACTIVITY
• Activity should be reduced during the time of tissue repair if surgery is required for any disease.
• Dust baths should be administered daily, or at least 2–3 times weekly—minimize during treatment for infectious organisms; do not reuse dust bath.

DIET
• Many chinchillas with PU/PD develop inappetence. Be certain the chinchilla is eating; if anorectic, provide assisted syringe-feeding of an herbivore critical care diet to prevent the development or exacerbation of gastrointestinal dysmotility/GI stasis.
• Increasing water content in foods or via oral or parenteral fluids may increase fluid intake. Provide multiple sources of fresh water, including supplementing fresh water with small amounts of pure fruit juice (no added sugars), high-water-content vegetables, or soaking or misting fresh vegetables before offering.
• Provide a high-fiber, low-calcium hay sources such as timothy, oat, or grass hays and timothy-based pellets, and offer a variety of fresh vegetables. Because chinchillas do not excrete excess calcium in the urine, dietary calcium restriction is not considered a factor in urolith prevention.

CLIENT EDUCATION
• Limit risk factors and increase water consumption until the cause of the PU/PD is identified.
• Surgical removal of urinary tract obstructions does not alter the causes responsible for their formation; limiting risk factors such as described above are necessary to minimize or delay recurrence.

SURGICAL CONSIDERATIONS
If calcium-based urolithiasis is present, surgery is considered the treatment of choice as medical dissolution is unrewarding.

MEDICATIONS

DRUG(S) OF CHOICE
Based upon cause of underlying disease

CONTRAINDICATIONS
• Oral administration of antibiotics that select against Gram-positive bacteria (penicillins, cephalosporins, macrolides, and lincosamides) can cause fatal enteric dysbiosis and enterotoxemia.
• Potentially nephrotoxic drugs (e.g., aminoglycosides, NSAIDs) should be avoided in patients that are febrile, dehydrated, or azotemic or who are suspected of having pyelonephritis, septicemia, or preexisting renal disease.
• Glucocorticoids, or other immunosuppressive agents

PRECAUTIONS
• Metronidazole may cause anorexia or reduced appetite in some chinchillas when administered PO; hepatic toxicosis has been anecdotally reported.

• Until underlying renal or hepatic disease has been excluded, use caution in administering any drug eliminated by these pathways.

FOLLOW-UP

PATIENT MONITORING
• Hydration status by clinical assessment of dehydration and serial evaluation of body weight
• Fluid intake and urine output—provide a useful baseline for assessing adequacy of hydration therapy

PREVENTION/AVOIDANCE
Will depend upon the underlying cause of these signs

POSSIBLE COMPLICATIONS
• Dehydration
• Gastrointestinal hypomotility/GI stasis
• Urine scald
• Pododermatitis, myiasis if sedentary

EXPECTED COURSE AND PROGNOSIS
Will depend upon the underlying cause of these signs

MISCELLANEOUS

ASSOCIATED CONDITIONS
• Bacterial urinary tract infections
• Hypercrystalluria, urolithiasis
• Diabetes mellitus

PREGNANCY/FERTILITY/BREEDING
Pyometra can affect fertility or decisions regarding suitability of this patient for future breeding.

SEE ALSO
Dysuria, hematuria, and pollakiuria
Gastrointestinal stasis and dilation

ABBREVIATIONS
ADH = antidiuretic hormone
BUN = blood urea nitrogen
RBC = red blood cell
TWBC = total white blood cells
WBC = white blood cell

Suggested Reading
Doss GA, Mans C, Houseright RA et al. Urinalysis in chinchillas (*Chinchilla lanigera*). J Am Vet Med Assoc 2016; 248(8):901–907.
Hallman RM, Brandão J. Diagnostic imaging of the renal system in exotic companion mammals. Vet Clin Exot Anim 2020;23:195–214.

(CONTINUED)

Lennox AM, Gladden JN. Emergency and critical care of small mammals. In: Quesenberry KE, Carpenter JW, eds. Ferrets, Rabbits and Rodents, 4th ed. Clinical Medicine and Surgery. 2021. St. Louis: Saunders, 2020:595–608.

Mans C, Donnelly T. Chinchillas. In: Quesenberry KE, Carpenter JW, eds. Ferrets, Rabbits and Rodents, 4th ed. Clinical Medicine and Surgery. 2021. St. Louis: Saunders, 2020:298–322.

Martel-Arquette A, Donnelly T, Mans C. Update on diseases in chinchillas: 2013–2019. Vet Clin Exot Anim 2020;23:321–333.

Martel-Arquette A, Mans C. Urolithiasis in chinchillas: 15 cases (2007 to 2011). J Small Anim Pract 2016;57:260–264.

Reavill D, Lennox A. Disease overview of the urinary tract in exotic companion mammals and tips on clinical management. Vet Clin Exot Anim 2020;23:169–193.

Riggs SM, Mitchell MA. Chinchillas. In: Mitchell MA, Tully TN, eds. Manual of Exotic Pet Practice. St. Louis: Elsevier, 2009:475–486.

Author Michelle G. Hawkins, VMD, Dipl. ABVP (Avian)

Dan H. Johnson, DVM, Dipl. ABVP (Exotic Companion Mammal)

UROLITHIASIS

CHINCHILLAS

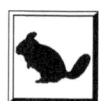

BASICS

DEFINITION
The formation of concretions (calculi, stones) composed of various salts and minerals anywhere along the urinary tract (kidneys, ureters, bladder, and/or urethra).

PATHOPHYSIOLOGY
• Urolithiasis is relatively uncommon and poorly described in chinchillas.
• Chinchillas excrete calcium primarily through the feces and do not rely on urinary excretion of calcium to maintain calcium homeostasis, while crystalluria is common in chinchillas, calcium carbonate crystalluria is rare and considered abnormal.
• Calcium carbonate uroliths are the predominant calculi identified in chinchillas.
• Factors leading to urolithiasis in chinchillas are unclear, although the alkaline pH of normal chinchilla urine may favor mineral precipitation and the formation of calculi.
• Whereas rabbits and guinea pigs excrete excess dietary calcium via the urine, chinchillas do not. Even chinchillas fed high levels of dietary calcium excrete only a small amount (between 1% and 3% of dietary intake) in the urine. No correlation between dietary calcium and stone formation has been established in chinchillas.
• Inadequate water intake leads to a more concentrated urine and factors that impair complete evacuation of the bladder, such as lack of exercise, obesity, cystitis, neoplasia, or neuromuscular diseases may be associated with urolith production.

SYSTEMS AFFECTED
• Renal/Urologic
• Gastrointestinal, neuromuscular, and cardiovascular systems may all be affected in patients with uremia.

GENETICS
N/A

INCIDENCE/PREVALENCE
• Except for penile fur rings, urinary tract or urogenital diseases are uncommon in chinchillas.
• Urolithiasis is less common in chinchillas than in other small herbivores.

GEOGRAPHIC DISTRIBUTION
N/A

SIGNALMENT
Urolithiasis is predominantly diagnosed in male chinchillas; mean age is 3.4 years, and the range is 11 months to 11 years; most chinchillas diagnosed with urolithiasis are less than 4 years of age.

SIGNS

Historical Findings
• Reduced appetite, activity; hematuria, pollakiuria, stranguria, anuria; nibbling at prepuce, dribbling urine; occasionally asymptomatic
• Hunched posture, vocalizing during urination may be associated with pain.
• Signs of uremia that develop when urinary tract obstruction is complete (or nearly complete)—anorexia, weight loss, lethargy, bruxism, tenesmus, hunched posture.
• Postural problems, ataxia, or difficulty ambulating in chinchillas with musculoskeletal or neurological disease that impair complete evacuation of the bladder
• Urine scald, moist pyoderma possible with urinary incontinence

Physical Examination Findings
• Hematuria, stranguria, or pollakiuria
• Dehydration, unkempt appearance, fur chewing, penile fur ring, perianal staining
• Discomfort during palpation of the bladder or caudal abdomen
• Large, turgid bladder (or inappropriate size remains after voiding efforts) upon palpation of the urinary bladder; ruptured bladder
• May detect cystoliths on palpation, but not always palpable
• Signs of uremia—dehydration, anorexia, lethargy, weakness, hypothermia, bradycardia, high rate or shallow respirations, stupor or coma; seizures occur rarely, often in terminal cases; tachycardia resulting from ventricular dysrhythmias induced by hyperkalemia
• No abnormal findings reported in some

CAUSES
Unknown for chinchillas; however, based upon causative factors for urolithiasis in rabbits and rodents, consider the following:
• Inadequate water intake—dirty water bowls, unpalatable water, inadequate water provision, changing water sources
• Urine retention—underlying bladder pathology, neuromuscular disease; painful conditions causing a reluctance to ambulate, such as musculoskeletal disease (pododermatitis, arthritis) or dental disease; inadequate cage cleaning
• Decreased activity, lack of exercise; obesity
• Renal disease
• Unlike rabbits and guinea pigs, excess dietary calcium does not appear to cause urolithiasis in chinchillas.

RISK FACTORS
Unknown, but gender appears to be important as the overwhelming majority of uroliths are diagnosed in males; the larger diameter and straighter nature of the female chinchilla urethra may more easily allow stone passage without intervention than the male.

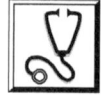

DIAGNOSIS

DIFFERENTIAL DIAGNOSIS
• Cystitis
• Constipation
• Fur rings
• Uterine disease
• Neurogenic disorders
• Neoplasia (uncommon in chinchillas)
• Almost any systemic disease process that results in anorexia, weight loss, lethargy, bruxism, and/or hunched posture (e.g., gastrointestinal stasis, dental disease, renal failure, etc.)

CBC/BIOCHEMISTRY/URINALYSIS
• Hemogram is usually normal.
• Biochemistry panel—urolithiasis with complete (or nearly complete) obstruction can cause postrenal azotemia and/or electrolyte abnormalities (e.g., hyperkalemia, hypochloremia, and hyponatremia).
• Urinalysis including both a standard dipstick and microscopic examination of the sediment
• Crystalluria is common in chinchillas, but calcium carbonate crystalluria is uncommon and not considered normal. Hypercrystalluria should increase suspicion for causing disease.
• In a recent study of 41 clinically normal chinchillas, crystals were observed in 28 of 41 (68%) samples; 27 of those samples contained amorphous crystals (amorphous phosphates), three contained calcium phosphate crystals, and only one contained calcium carbonate crystals.
• A trace amount of protein is considered normal in the urine of chinchillas. In the same study mentioned above, the majority (40/41 [98%]) of clinically normal chinchillas had more than a trace amount of protein as determined by a urine dipstick.

OTHER LABORATORY TESTS
• If surgery is necessary to relieve obstruction from urolithiasis, collect and submit the calculi for analysis and culture and sensitivity, and submit the bladder wall for culture and sensitivity.
• Calculi-containing calcium carbonate requires specific methodologies to differentiate from calcium oxalate monohydrate crystals; the laboratory chosen for analysis must be able to perform these methods. Confirm the lab's ability to perform these techniques in advance, since human and some veterinary laboratories unfamiliar with exotic animal samples do not differentiate calcium oxalate from calcium carbonate.

IMAGING
• The overwhelming majority of urinary calculi in chinchillas are radiopaque (calcium carbonate) allowing for ease of identification using survey radiography. However, if multiple calculi or significant GI gas are present, the anatomic locations of the calculi using survey radiography alone may be obscured.
• In one review of 15 cases, calculi were only found within the bladder and/or urethra. Obstructive calculi are most likely to be found in the urethra (males and females) but could also be found in the kidneys or ureters.
• Ultrasound is useful for anatomic location of the calculi and for evaluating anatomic changes in the kidneys or ureters, such as hydronephrosis or hydroureter, ureteral mucosal inflammation, or perforation.
• Excretory intravenous pyelograms (IVPs) are useful to further elucidate relative functional abnormalities in the kidneys or ureters. The time to image collection is longer than for computed tomography (CT), but the excretory IVP can be performed at a lower cost and is practical for most veterinary practices.
• CT images are obtained more rapidly than IVP, using significantly less contrast material.

DIAGNOSTIC PROCEDURES
• Urethral endoscopy can be performed to identify the location of the calculi if present in this region. Endoscopy can also be performed through a surgical incision into the bladder to attempt to identify the location of calculi within the proximal neck of the bladder.

PATHOLOGIC FINDINGS
On gross examination, urinary calculi may vary in size from sand-like to large concentric stones. Pathologic findings have not been described in chinchillas; however, in rabbits and guinea pigs, these vary from thickening of the urethra, bladder, or ureteral mucosa with congestion in more chronic cases to intramural and/or intraluminal hemorrhage. Perforations of the ureter may be identified with chronic, complete obstructions. Microscopic changes seen in acute cases may include ulceration, hemorrhage, and infiltration with heterophils. Chronic cases are characterized by infiltration of leukocytes and mononuclear cells in the lamina propria, and occasionally fibroblast proliferation.

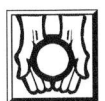

TREATMENT
APPROPRIATE HEALTH CARE
• Complete obstruction is a medical emergency that can be life threatening. Chinchillas with urinary obstruction should be hospitalized, and emergency supportive therapy should be provided until surgical intervention to relieve the obstruction can be performed. Medical treatment of urolithiasis is unrewarding, and surgical removal of calculi is usually required.
• Partial obstruction may or may not be an emergency, but these patients may be at greater risk for complete obstruction; may cause irreversible urinary tract damage if not treated promptly.
• Treat as inpatient until chinchilla's ability to urinate has been restored.
• Treatment has three major components: combating metabolic derangements associated with postrenal uremia; restoring and maintaining a patent pathway for urine outflow; and implementing a specific treatment for the underlying cause of urine retention, if present.

NURSING CARE
• Fluid therapy should be initiated in patients with evidence of dehydration, azotemia, and electrolyte imbalances. Fluid therapy should be based on treatment modalities used in cats with obstructive urinary disease. Normal saline is recommended until electrolyte status of patient is known.
• Subcutaneous fluids can be administered (30–50 mL/kg) as needed. IV access is difficult in chinchillas; lateral saphenous vein catheters often kink; consider IO catheterization if intravascular fluids are needed. Maintenance fluid needs are estimated at 100 mL/kg/day.
• In females, gentle flushing of urethral calculi back into the bladder can be attempted. Gently flush the bladder using a 3.5 Fr red rubber catheter under deep sedation and analgesia to attempt to remove the calculi. Catheterizing males is much more difficult due to the small size and curved nature of the male urethra; calculi often adhere tightly to the urethral mucosa, making successful retropulsion of a urolith back into the bladder unlikely.

ACTIVITY
• Reduced during the time of tissue repair after surgery
• Long term—increase activity level by providing large exercise areas to encourage voiding and prevent recurrence (unproven but based on experience in other small herbivores).

DIET
• Many chinchillas with urinary tract obstruction are anorectic or have decreased appetite. It is an absolute requirement that the patient continue to eat during and following treatments. Anorexia may cause or exacerbate gastrointestinal hypomotility and cause derangement of the gastrointestinal microflora with overgrowth of intestinal bacterial pathogens.
• Chinchillas may be tempted with parsley, cilantro, dandelion greens, and good-quality grass hay. Many patients will begin to eat these foods, even if they were previously anorectic. Also offer the patient's usual pelleted diet.
• If the patient refuses these foods, syringe-feed a gruel such as Critical Care for Herbivores (Oxbow Animal Health, Omaha, NE) or Emeraid Herbivore (Lafeber Company, Cornell, IL), 15–20 mL/kg PO q6–8h. Larger volumes and more frequent feedings are often accepted; feed as much as the chinchilla will readily accept. Alternatively, pellets can be ground and mixed with fresh greens, vegetable baby foods, water, or juice to form a gruel.
• High-carbohydrate, high-fat nutritional supplements are contraindicated (promote dysbiosis).

CLIENT EDUCATION
• Urethral calculi are often tightly adhered to the urethral mucosa and can be difficult to impossible to retropulse during catheterization, especially in males. Prepare clients for this possibility and the option of humane euthanasia if unsuccessful.
• Surgical removal of calclui does not alter the causes responsible for their formation; recurrence rate after surgery can be as high as 50% with mean time to recurrence of 68 day (range 19–1440 days).
• Limiting risk factors in other small herbivores such as obesity, sedentary life, and inappropriate diet combined with increasing water consumption may minimize or delay recurrence; unfortunately, even with these changes, recurrence is possible.

SURGICAL CONSIDERATIONS
• Cytotomy to remove cystic calculi; advise owners of high recurrence rates. Submit calculi for analysis and culture; submit the bladder wall for culture and sensitivity.
• Postoperative management includes assisted feeding, fluids, analgesics, and antibiotics based on culture and sensitivity results. Rate of recurrence of urolithiasis is high.

MEDICATIONS
DRUG(S) OF CHOICE
• Medical dissolution of calcium-based uroliths is considered ineffective small herbivores.
• Pain management is essential during and following surgery or if pain is causing reduced frequency of voiding. Perioperative analgesic

UROLITHIASIS   (CONTINUED)

CHINCHILLAS

choices include buprenorphine (0.01–0.05 mg/kg SC, IM, IV q8–12h), meloxicam (0.5–1 mg/kg SC, PO q24h), and carprofen (2–5 mg/kg PO, SC q24h). Use NSAIDs with caution in case of renal compromise.

• Procedures for relief of obstruction generally require administering sedatives and/or anesthetics. When substantial derangements exist, begin with fluid administration and other supportive measures. Calculate the dosage of sedative or anesthetic drug using the low end of the recommended range or give only to effect.

• Antibiotics, if indicated, should be selected based upon results of culture and sensitivity (see Contraindications). Broad-spectrum antibiotics commonly used in chinchillas include enrofloxacin (5–15 mg/kg PO, SC, IM q12h), trimethoprim sulfa (15–30 mg/kg PO q12h), and chloramphenicol (30–50 mg/kg PO, SC, IM, IV q8–12h).

CONTRAINDICATIONS

• Oral administration of antibiotics that select against gram-positive bacteria (penicillins, cephalosporins, macrolides, and lincosamides) can cause fatal enteric dysbiosis and enterotoxemia.

• Potentially nephrotoxic drugs (e.g., aminoglycosides, NSAIDs) in patients that are febrile, dehydrated, or azotemic or that are suspected of having pyelonephritis, septicemia, or preexisting renal disease

• Glucocorticoids or other immunosuppressive agents

PRECAUTIONS

• Avoid drugs that reduce blood pressure or induce cardiac dysrhythmia until dehydration is resolved.

• Modify dosages of all drugs that require renal metabolism or elimination.

• Avoid nephrotoxic drugs (NSAIDs, aminoglycosides).

POSSIBLE INTERACTIONS

None

ALTERNATIVE DRUGS

N/A

FOLLOW-UP

PATIENT MONITORING

• Ensure gastrointestinal motility by making sure the patient is eating, well hydrated, and passing normal feces prior to release.

• Assess urine production and hydration status frequently, adjusting fluid administration rate accordingly.

• Verify the ability to urinate adequately; inability may require urinary catheterization to combat urine retention, or cystocentesis.

• Since calcium carbonate crystalluria is not considered normal in chinchillas, clinicians should consider close monitoring for future development of urolithiasis in chinchillas diagnosed with calcium carbonate crystalluria.

PREVENTION/AVOIDANCE

• Fluid therapy and encouraging water intake in chinchillas have been recommended to prevent urolithiasis. Chinchillas prefer open dish drinkers vs. nipple water bottles, and this can be used as a method to increase water consumption. While increasing water intake is intended to reduce the risk of hypercalciuria and supersaturation of urine, it remains unclear whether this is a risk factor in chinchillas and whether increased water intake would be aid in prevention of development or recurrence of uroliths in chinchillas.

• In most other species, reduction in dietary calcium is recommended to prevent urinary calculi; however, no correlation between dietary calcium and stone formation has been established for chinchillas; therefore, it remains questionable whether reducing dietary calcium content in chinchillas will aid in urolith prevention.

POSSIBLE COMPLICATIONS

• Severe electrolyte imbalances, uremia with complete obstruction

• Urine scald

• Failure to detect or treat effectively may lead to pyelonephritis

• Pododermatitis

EXPECTED COURSE AND PROGNOSIS

• Outcome in chinchillas appears to be associated with urolith location. In one study, 4 out of 6 chinchillas diagnosed with urethral calculi were euthanized because of the inability to dislodge urethral calculi and flush them into the urinary bladder for removal. In contrast, chinchillas with uroliths located in the urinary bladder alone appeared to have a good short-term outcome.

• In the same study, recurrence of urolithiasis was reported in 50% (5/10) of chinchillas that underwent cystotomy for successful urolith removal. The time to recurrence was less than 68 days in 3/5 animals, and the survival time was shorter in animals with recurrence than in animals without recurrence.

MISCELLANEOUS

ASSOCIATED CONDITIONS

• Urinary tract infections

• Vaginitis, pyometra from ascending bacterial infection of the lower urinary tract

AGE-RELATED FACTORS

Most affected chinchillas are less than 4 years of age.

ZOONOTIC POTENTIAL

N/A

PREGNANCY/FERTILITY/BREEDING

While there is no documented evidence that urolithiasis has a hereditary component, it is generally recommended to avoid breeding these animals in the future.

SYNONYMS

Urinary tract stones

SEE ALSO

Dysuria, hematuria, and pollakiuria

ABBREVIATIONS

CT = computed tomography
IVP = intravenous pyelogram
NSAID = nonsteroidal anti-inflammatory drug

INTERNET RESOURCES

N/A

Suggested Reading

Doss GA, Mans C, Houseright RA et al. Urinalysis in chinchillas (*Chinchilla lanigera*). J Am Vet Med Assoc 2016;248(8):901–907.

Hallman RM, Brandão J. Diagnostic imaging of the renal system in exotic companion mammals. Vet Clin Exot Anim 2020;23:195–214.

Lennox AM, Gladden JN. Emergency and critical care of small mammals. In: Quesenberry KE, Carpenter JW, eds. Ferrets, Rabbits and Rodents, 4th ed. Clinical Medicine and Surgery. 2021. St. Louis: Saunders, 2020:595–608.

Mans C, Donnelly T. Chinchillas. In: Quesenberry KE, Carpenter JW, eds. Ferrets, Rabbits and Rodents, 4th ed. Clinical Medicine and Surgery. 2021. St. Louis: Saunders, 2020:298–322.

Martel-Arquette A, Donnelly T, Mans C. Update on diseases in chinchillas: 2013–2019. Vet Clin Exot Anim 2020;23:321–333.

Martel-Arquette A, Mans C. Urolithiasis in chinchillas: 15 cases (2007 to 2011). J Small Anim Pract 2016;57:260–264.

Reavill D, Lennox A. Disease overview of the urinary tract in exotic companion mammals and tips on clinical management. Vet Clin Exot Anim 2020;23:169–193.

Riggs SM, Mitchell MA. Chinchillas. In: Mitchell MA, Tully TN, eds. Manual of Exotic Pet Practice. St. Louis: Elsevier, 2009:475–486.

Authors Michelle G. Hawkins, VMD, Dipl. ABVP (Avian Practice)
Dan H. Johnson, DVM, Dipl. ABVP (Exotic Companion Mammal)

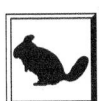

BASICS

DEFINITION
• Weight loss is considered clinically important when it exceeds 10% of the normal body weight and is not associated with fluid loss.
• Cachexia is defined as a state of extremely poor health associated with anorexia, weight loss, weakness, and mental depression and is often the result of chronic disease.

PATHOPHYSIOLOGY
• Weight loss can result from many different pathophysiological mechanisms that share a common feature—insufficient caloric intake or availability to meet metabolic needs.
• Insufficient caloric intake or availability can be caused by (1) a high-energy need (e.g., the characteristic of a hypermetabolic state); (2) inadequate energy intake, including insufficient quantity or quality of food, or inadequate nutrient assimilation (e.g., with anorexia dysphagia or malabsorption disorders); or (3) excessive loss of nutrients or fluid, which can occur in patients with gastrointestinal losses, glucosuria, or proteinuria.
• There is little published regarding caloric requirements for chinchillas. In general, growing, pregnant, lactating chinchillas will require higher caloric density than that necessary for adult maintenance.

SYSTEMS AFFECTED
Any body system can be affected by weight loss, especially if severe or the result of systemic disease.

SIGNALMENT
No sex or breed predilection

SIGNS

Historical Findings
• It is diagnostically important to know whether the patient's appetite is normal, increased, decreased, or absent.
• Important historical information includes the type of diet, environment (chewing habits and access to potential gastrointestinal foreign bodies), signs of dental disease, chronic respiratory disease, abscesses, signs of gastrointestinal disease (including lack of fecal production or scant feces), diarrhea, or any signs of a specific disease.
• Signs of pain, such as bruxism, a hunched posture, or reluctance to move are extremely common in chinchillas with dental disease or gastrointestinal hypomotility.
• Pseudo-anorectic patients commonly display excessive drooling, difficulty in pretension and mastication of food, halitosis, dysphagia, bruxism, and odynophagia (painful eating).

Physical Examination Findings
• Most underlying causes of pseudo-anorexia can be identified by a thorough examination of the face, mandible, teeth, neck, oropharynx, and esophagus for dental disease, ulceration, traumatic lesions, foreign bodies, masses, and neuromuscular dysfunction.
• A thorough examination of the oral cavity, including the incisors, molars, and mucosa is essential to rule out dental disease. Use of an otoscope, nasal speculum, or endoscope is required to adequately perform a thorough examination of the cheek teeth. A complete examination requires heavy sedation or general anesthesia.
• Examine the face for evidence of chronic upper respiratory disease, such as secretions or dried discharge around the nose and front limbs, ocular discharge, exophthalmos, facial swelling, or pain.
• Abdominal palpation is a valuable tool in the diagnosis of gastrointestinal stasis/hypomotility. The normal stomach should be easily deformable and feel soft and pliable; palpation may also reveal organomegaly, masses, or gastrointestinal foreign bodies.
• Gas distention of the stomach, intestines, or cecum can cause severe bloating in the chinchilla, which can be life threatening. With bloating, the abdomen may be taut or tympanic.
• Auscultation of the intestines and cecum may reveal decreased borborygmi in patients with GI stasis.
• Auscultation of the thorax may reveal cardiac murmurs, arrhythmias, or abnormal breath sounds.

CAUSES

Increased Use of Calories
• Catabolism—fever, inflammation, cancer; very common, especially chronic upper respiratory disease, abscesses (subcutaneous, joint, facial, intrathoracic, and intra-abdominal)
• Increased physical activity
• Pregnancy, lactation, growth

Pseudoanorexia
Dental disease is extremely common and can cause dysphagia—inability to prehend or chew food

Maldigestive/Malabsorptive Disorders
• Gastrointestinal hypomotility/gastrointestinal stasis—very common
• Intestinal dysbiosis, chronic intermittent diarrhea—common
• Coccidiosis—young or debilitated animals

Metabolic Disorders
• Organ failure—cardiac, hepatic, and renal failure are common
• Secondary hepatic lipidosis can develop in an overconditioned chinchilla with significant weight loss.
• Cancer cachexia—many neoplastic conditions can cause weight loss

Dietary Causes
• Insufficient particle size of hay, or excessive simple carbohydrates—very common, leads to secondary gastrointestinal disorders and dental disease
• Insufficient or poor-quality diet

Neuromuscular Disease and Pain
• Dental disease—very common
• Degenerative joint disease (arthritis)
• Facial abscesses—often associated with dental disease or trauma
• Ulcerative pododermatitis—very common
• CNS disease—brain abscesses or other infections (*Listeria monocytogenes*, LCMV) can be associated with anorexia or pseudoanorexia
• Fur rings of the penis in male chinchillas are common; if left undetected, can cause pain, paraphimosis, and necrosis in severe cases.

Excessive Nutrient Loss
• Protein-losing enteropathy (secondary to infectious or infiltrative disease)
• Protein-losing nephropathy—may be seen in older chinchillas with chronic renal failure

RISK FACTORS
Any disease process in the chinchilla can cause weight loss; cachexia can occur if the disease process is chronic.

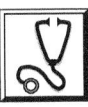

DIAGNOSIS

• If a previous body weight is not available, subjectively assess the patient for thin body condition, emaciation, cachexia by using a body condition scoring system (e.g., BCS 1–9). Assess the patient for dehydration by evaluating skin/eyelid turgor, evidence of sunken eyes, and the mucous membranes.
• Once weight loss is confirmed, seek the underlying cause.

DIFFERENTIAL DIAGNOSIS
• Categorize the weight loss as occurring within normal, increased, or decreased appetite.
• Differential diagnosis for a chinchilla with weight loss despite a normal or increased appetite is much different and shorter than for one with decreased appetite or anorexia.
• Determine what the patient's appetite was at the onset of the weight loss; any condition can lead to anorexia if it persists long enough for the patient to become debilitated.

WEIGHT LOSS AND CACHEXIA   (CONTINUED)

• Dental disease is one of the most common causes of pseudoanorexia and weight loss in chinchillas.
• Some loss of muscle mass occurs in chinchillas as a normal aging change.

CBC/BIOCHEMISTRY/URINALYSIS
• Used to identify infectious, inflammatory, and metabolic diseases, including organ failure and secondary hepatic lipidosis
• A minimum database is always important, but especially when history and physical examination provide little information.

OTHER LABORATORY TESTS
• Based upon the most likely differential diagnoses and the specific findings of the history and physical examination
• Fecal direct examination, fecal flotation to rule out coccidiosis

IMAGING
• Abdominal radiography and ultrasonography should be utilized to evaluate gastrointestinal disorders, hepatic, renal, and urogenital diseases, or internal abscesses. Secondary hepatic lipidosis is best evaluated through imaging using ultrasonography.
• Skull radiography may help rule out dental disease, but CT provides a broader evaluation of the relationship of the teeth to one another, the nasal cavity, and the bones of the skull.
• Thoracic radiography is used initially to evaluate for cardiac and respiratory diseases. Because of the small thorax, ultrasonography can sometimes be used to localize and guide aspiration of respiratory masses/abscesses. Echocardiography is used to evaluate for specific cardiac diseases.

DIAGNOSTIC PROCEDURES
Will vary depending upon the suspected underlying cause of the weight loss

PATHOLOGIC FINDINGS
Will vary depending upon the suspected underlying cause of the weight loss

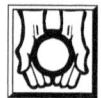

TREATMENT
APPROPRIATE HEALTH CARE
• Inpatient—severe debilitating disease with anorexia that requires hospitalization and support
• Especially if patient was previously obese, secondary hepatic lipidosis may develop and must be aggressively treated in the hospital if identified.
• Outpatient—if stable and can be managed at home pending further diagnostics or treatments

NURSING CARE
• Subcutaneous fluids can be administered (50–100 mL/kg) as needed; IV access is difficult in the chinchilla; lateral saphenous vein catheters often kink; consider intraosseous (IO) catheterization if intravascular fluids are needed.
• Base fluid selection on the underlying cause of fluid loss. In most patients, lactated Ringer's solution or Normosol crystalloid fluids are appropriate. Fluids can be administered by mouth in some stable patients. Maintenance fluid needs are estimated at 100 mL/kg/day.

ACTIVITY
• Dust baths should be administered daily, or at least 2–3 times weekly—minimize during treatment for infectious organisms; do not reuse dust bath.
• Activity should be reduced during the time of tissue repair if surgery is required for any disease.

DIET
• Be certain the chinchilla is eating, as it is imperative that the chinchilla began eating as soon as possible, regardless of the underlying cause. Continued anorexia exacerbates gastrointestinal hypomotility and can cause further derangements in intestinal bacterial pathogens.
• Offer a large selection of fresh, moist greens such as romaine lettuce, carrot tops, spinach, collard greens, and parsley and a good-quality grass hay, as well as the chinchilla's usual pelleted diet, as the initial goal is to get the chinchilla to eat.
• If the patient refuses these foods, syringe-feed Critical Care for Herbivores (Oxbow Animal Health, Omaha, NE) or Emeraid Herbivore (Lafeber Company, Cornell, IL), 15–20 mL/kg PO q6–8h. Larger volumes and more frequent feedings are often accepted; feed as much as the patient will readily accept. Alternatively, pellets can be ground and mixed with fresh greens, vegetable baby foods, water, or sugar-free juice to form a gruel.
• High-carbohydrate, high-fat nutritional supplements are contraindicated in these hind-gut fermenters.

CLIENT EDUCATION
• Virtually any disease in the chinchilla can cause weight loss, and in a previously obese patient may lead to hepatic lipidosis, which requires hospitalization, aggressive supportive care, and can still carry a guarded prognosis.
• Evaluate the environment and husbandry and ensure appropriate general care; modify as necessary depending on the disease process identified.

SURGICAL CONSIDERATIONS
Heavy sedation is usually necessary for complete oral examination; benzodiazepines are relatively safe even in the very ill animal. General anesthesia evaluation should be used with caution until the underlying disease processes are identified.

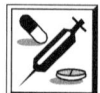

MEDICATIONS
DRUG(S) OF CHOICE
Depends on the underlying cause of a weight loss.

FOLLOW-UP
PATIENT MONITORING
The level of patient monitoring depends upon the underlying cause of the weight loss. Regardless, the patient should be weighed 1–2 times daily until weight is stabilized. Inexpensive gram scales can be purchased by the owner for home monitoring.

PREVENTION/AVOIDANCE
Breeders and owners should weigh their chinchillas routinely, to identify potential problems before they become chronic. In general, if the chinchilla steadily decreases body weight without any untoward clinical signs, a veterinarian should be consulted.

POSSIBLE COMPLICATIONS
• Cachexia can lead to irreversible organ failure and even sudden death if not identified and treated as quickly as possible.
• Significant weight loss in a previously obese chinchilla can lead to a negative energy and hepatic lipidosis.

EXPECTED COURSE AND PROGNOSIS
• Will depend upon the underlying cause of the disease
• Hepatic lipidosis carries a guarded prognosis, even with aggressive supportive care.

MISCELLANEOUS
PREGNANCY/FERTILITY/BREEDING
Pregnancy and lactation can be associated with weight loss due to increased caloric expenditure.

SEE ALSO
Dental malocclusion
Anorexia

Gastrointestinal hypomotility and gastrointestinal stasis

ABBREVIATIONS

CNS = central nervous system
CT = computed tomography
LCMV = lymphocytic choriomeningitis virus

INTERNET RESOURCES

N/A

Suggested Reading
Capello V. Diagnosis and treatment of dental disease in pet rodents. J Exot Pet Med 2008;17:114–123.
Harkness JE, Turner PV, VandeWoude S et al. Harkness and Wagner's Biology and Medicine of Rabbits and Rodents, 5th ed. Ames, IA: Wiley-Blackwell, 2010:210–213, 219, 260–262, 292–302, 321–322, 324–326.
Lennox AM, Gladden JN. Emergency and critical care of small mammals. In: Quesenberry KE, Carpenter JW, eds. Ferrets, Rabbits and Rodents, 4th ed. Clinical Medicine and Surgery. 2021. St. Louis: Saunders, 2020:595–608.
Mans C, Donnelly T. Chinchillas. In: Quesenberry KE, Carpenter JW, eds. Ferrets, Rabbits and Rodents, 4th ed. Clinical Medicine and Surgery. 2021. St. Louis: Saunders, 2020:298–322.
Mans C, Jekl V. Anatomy and disorders of the oral cavity of chinchilla and degus. Vet Clin Exot Anim 2016;19:843–869.
Martel A, Donnelly T, Mans C. Update on diseases in chinchillas: 2013–2019. Vet Clin Exot Anim 2020;23:321–333.
Riggs SM, Mitchell MA. Chinchillas. In: Mitchell MA, Tully TN, eds. Manual of Exotic Pet Practice. St. Louis: Elsevier, 2009:475–486.
Ritzman TK. Diagnosis and clinical management of gastrointestinal conditions in exotic companion mammals (rabbits, guinea pigs, and chinchillas). Vet Clin Exot Anim 2014;17:179–194.

Authors Michelle G. Hawkins, VMD, Dipl. ABVP (Avian)
Dan H. Johnson, DVM, Dipl. ABVP (Exotic Companion Mammal)

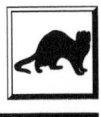

FERRETS

FERRET ADRENAL DISEASE (HYPERADRENOCORTICISM)

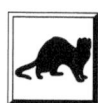

BASICS

DEFINITION
• Spontaneous hyperadrenocorticism is a disorder resulting in the excessive production of estrogens, androgens, and estrogen-related compounds by the adrenal cortex.
• Clinical signs are due to the deleterious effects of the elevated circulating estrogen and androgen concentrations on multiple organ systems. Clinical signs caused by the space-occupying effects of the tumor may also be seen.
• Cortisol concentrations are not significantly elevated in ferrets with adrenal disease.

PATHOPHYSIOLOGY
• Ferret adrenal disease is caused by excessive secretion of sex steroids from adrenocortical hyperplasia, adrenal adenomas, or carcinoma.
• Unilateral disease is somewhat more common than bilateral adrenal disease.
• Hyperadrenocorticism resulting from pituitary corticotroph tumors or hyperplasia oversecreting ACTH has not been documented in the ferret.
• Iatrogenic hyperadrenocorticism resulting from excessive exogenous administration of glucocorticoids has not been reported in ferrets.

SYSTEMS AFFECTED
• Ferret adrenal disease is a multisystemic disorder.
• Signs referable to the skin or reproductive tract predominate.
• Bone marrow suppression may also occur.
  The degree to which each system is involved varies; in some patients, signs referable to one system may predominate; others have several systems involved to a comparable degree.

GENETICS
Unknown: A genetic predisposition has been suspected since many of the ferrets in North America come from similar breeding stock; however, reports in other countries are continuously increasing, possibly due to changing husbandry practices with more frequent early neutering and indoor housing.

INCIDENCE/PREVALENCE
Considered one of the most common disorders in ferrets, affecting up to 70% of pet ferrets in the United States. More than 95% of ferrets with bilaterally symmetric progressive alopecia have ferret adrenal disease.

GEOGRAPHIC DISTRIBUTION
Ferret adrenal disease is seen more commonly in ferrets in North America as compared with Europe. This may be due to genetics, early neutering practices, or differing husbandry practices.

SIGNALMENT
Breed Predilections
N/A

Predominant Sex
Seen primarily in neutered animals—equal incidence in male and female animals. Females may be presented for evaluation more frequently than males because of the prominent appearance of vulvar swelling.

Mean Age and Range
Generally, a disorder of middle-aged animals, 3–4 years old. The reported age range is 1–7 years.

SIGNS
General Comments
• Severity may vary greatly, depending on the duration and magnitude of sex steroid excess.
• In some cases, the space-occupying and catabolic effects of the neoplastic process contribute.

Historical and Physical Examination Findings
• Alopecia is the most common clinical sign. Hair loss may be sudden and progressive or may begin in spring and regrow later in the year, followed by progressive alopecia the following spring. In most cases, bilaterally symmetric alopecia begins in the tail region and progresses cranially. Other patterns, such as diffuse thinning of the hair coat or alopecia over the shoulder region, can also be seen. In severe cases, the ferret will become completely bald. The skin usually has a normal appearance but can appear thickened.
• About 30% of affected ferrets are pruritic; secondary pyoderma is sometimes seen.
• Swollen vulva in spayed females is extremely common.
• Stranguria due to paraurethral/urogenital cysts, abscesses, or prostatic hyperplasia in both males and females—common, often life-threatening consequence; large cysts can be palpable
• Sexual aggression or return of sexual behavior in neutered animals
• Thinning of the skin, muscle atrophy, and pot-bellied appearance in chronic disease
• Occasionally, mammary gland hypertrophy
• Rarely—anemia, polydipsia, and polyuria
• Occasionally, the affected adrenal gland is palpably enlarged.

CAUSES
Functional adrenal hyperplasia, adenoma, or adenocarcinomas most common

RISK FACTORS
Evidence suggests that adrenal disease may be related to neutering. The gonads and adrenals arise embryonically from the urogenital ridge; some gonadal cells are likely present in the adrenals. Stimulation of these cells by pituitary gonadotropin may cause hypertrophy of these steroid-secreting cells.

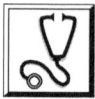

DIAGNOSIS

DIFFERENTIAL DIAGNOSIS
• For alopecia and pruritus: seasonal alopecia, pyoderma, flea allergy dermatitis, dermatophytes, mast cell tumor, and cutaneous lymphoma
• For swollen vulva in spayed females: ovarian remnant, intact female
• For stranguria: cystitis, urolithiasis

CBC/BIOCHEMISTRY/URINALYSIS
• Usually normal
• Rarely, in chronic cases, the hemogram may show nonregenerative anemia, leucopenia, or thrombocytopenia due to estrogen excess.
• Hypoglycemia may be present—due to concurrent insulinoma since many ferrets in this age range will also have pancreatic tumors

OTHER LABORATORY TESTS
• Elevations in plasma estradiol, androstenedione, and 17-hydroxyprogesterone combined (available through the Clinical Endocrinology Laboratory, Department of Comparative Medicine, University of Tennessee) are supportive of the diagnosis. However, this does not differentiate FAD from ovarian remnant; does not distinguish between hyperplasia, adenoma, or carcinoma as all 3 will cause an elevation in these hormones.
• Elevations in serum cortisol are rarely seen.
• Unlike the diagnosis in dogs, ACTH response test and low-dose dexamethasone suppression tests are not diagnostic and are not pertinent to the diagnosis.
• Urinary cortisol:creatinine ratio may be elevated in ferrets with hypercortisolism, although this is rare.

IMAGING
• Ultrasonography is the most useful diagnostic test. Normal adrenal glands average 2–3.7 mm in width and 4–8 mm in length. Diseased glands often have an enlarged pole (>3.9 mm wide), appear rounded, have abnormal echogenicity, or may be mineralized. Keep in mind that some ferrets with functional adrenal disease may initially have normal-appearing glands on ultrasound.
• CT scan will also identify an enlarged adrenal gland.
• Radiographs may occasionally demonstrate an enlarged adrenal gland in ferrets with large tumors.

(CONTINUED) FERRET ADRENAL DISEASE (HYPERADRENOCORTICISM)

• In ferrets with prostatomegaly or urogenital cysts, single or multiple cystic structures may be visible around the urinary bladder.
• Examine the prostate and paraurethral tissues, spleen, pancreas, mesenteric lymph nodes, and liver for concurrent disease, especially in older ferrets.

PATHOLOGIC FINDINGS
• Gross examination reveals enlargement of the adrenal gland, irregular surface or discoloration of the affected gland, or cysts or differences in texture within the affected gland.
• Occasionally, bilateral tumors are found.
• Invasion into the liver, kidney, vena cava, or other abdominal organs in some patients with adrenal adenocarcinoma
• Metastasis rarely occurs.
• Microscopically—may see adrenocortical hyperplasia, adrenocortical adenoma, carcinoma, or leiomyosarcoma

TREATMENT
APPROPRIATE HEALTH CARE
• Ferret adrenal disease may be treated with adrenalectomy or managed medically. The decision as to which form of treatment is appropriate is multifactorial; which gland is affected (left vs. right), the surgeon's experience and expertise, the severity of clinical signs, age of the animal, concurrent diseases, and financial issues should be considered.
• Surgical removal of the affected adrenal gland(s) is often curative. This procedure may require special surgical expertise, especially if the right adrenal gland is diseased (see Surgical Considerations, below).
• Medical treatment (see Medications, below) may cause a sufficient reduction in clinical signs. Depending on the circumstances, medical treatment may be preferred. However, medical treatment is not curative, must be administered lifelong and is not known to affect adrenal tumor size or potential metastasis.
• Hospitalization is usually required for patients with urethral obstruction due to prostate disease, severely depressed patients, and during the postsurgical recovery period for those undergoing adrenalectomy.

NURSING CARE
N/A

DIET
Normal diet is returned 2–6 hours postsurgery.

CLIENT EDUCATION
• If surgical treatment is elected, the affected adrenal can usually be identified and removed during exploratory laparotomy, even if the affected gland could not be identified by preoperative imaging techniques.
• If the right or both adrenal glands are affected, surgical treatment is more difficult and referral may be required, depending on the surgeon's experience.
• If medical treatment is opted, owners should be advised that medical treatment is lifelong; that metastasis, although rare, may occur; the space-occupying and catabolic effects of neoplasia may become significant.

SURGICAL CONSIDERATIONS
• Adrenalectomy is often curative for unilateral adrenocortical hyperplasia, adenomas, and adenocarcinomas.
• Both adrenals should be observed and palpated. Normal glands are light pink with homogenous color and density, 2–3.7 mm in width, and 4–8 mm in length. Indications for removal include gross enlargement of the adrenal gland, irregular surface or discoloration, and cysts or differences in texture within the affected gland.
• Several techniques for adrenalectomy have been advocated, and problems may be associated with each surgical option, depending on the surgeon's expertise. Refer to the suggested reading list for a more detailed description of surgical procedures.
• Left adrenalectomy is generally a relatively uncomplicated procedure.
• Right adrenalectomy requires special surgical expertise. The proximity of the right adrenal to the vena cava and the potential for vena cava invasion by malignant tumors make complete excision a high-risk procedure. Referral to a surgeon or clinician with experience is recommended when possible.
• Many surgeons advocate debulking, rather than complete removal of the right adrenal, as this procedure carries less risk of life-threatening complications. If this method is chosen, signs of clinical disease will return, necessitating repeat surgery or medical therapy alone.
• If both adrenals are affected, removal of the left adrenal gland and a subtotal adrenalectomy of the right gland is often recommended. Eventually, however, the ferret is likely to become symptomatic, requiring complete removal of the remaining gland or medical management.
• Removal of both adrenals may cause iatrogenic adrenal insufficiency (Addison's disease), requiring close monitoring and medical management.
• Always explore the entire abdominal cavity during surgery since concurrent liver disease,

gastrointestinal tract disease, insulinoma, lymphoma, or other neoplastic diseases are extremely common. Biopsy the liver and any enlarged lymph nodes to check for metastases.

MEDICATIONS
DRUG(S) OF CHOICE
Medical Treatment of Adrenal Disease

GnRH Analogs
• Treatment with a GnRH agonist is indicated even if adrenalectomy is performed to prevent the recurrence of disease in the remaining adrenal gland.
• The GnRH agonist deslorelin acetate (Suprelorin-F®, Virbac Animal Health) is labeled for the treatment of adrenal disease in domestic ferrets in the United States. It is a 4.7-mg slow-release deslorelin implant reported to provide alleviation of clinical signs lasting from 8 to 20 months. Alleviation of clinical signs may be more likely in patients with adrenal hyperplasia or adenoma; adenocarcinomas may be less likely to respond. Deslorelin has no demonstrated effect on adrenal tumor growth or metastasis. In Europe, 9.4-mg deslorelin implants are available and may be effective for up to 2–4 years.
• Leuprolide acetate, a GnRH analog, is a potent gonadotropin secretion inhibitor and suppresses LH and FSH, downregulating their receptor sites. It is available as a 1- or 4-month depot injection and may alleviate the dermal and reproductive organ signs of adrenal disease in ferrets. Reported dosages: Lupron® 30-day depot, 100–250 µg/kg IM q4w until signs resolve, then q4–8w PRN, lifelong. Larger ferrets often require the higher end of the dose range. This drug has no effect on adrenal tumor growth or metastasis. This drug has become challenging to acquire and often prohibitively expensive in the United States.

Other Treatments
• Melatonin implants are available commercially (Ferretonin® 2.7-mg— ferrets < 600 g) and 5.4-mg implants—most ferrets (Melatek, LLC) and have been used in ferrets with adrenal disease to alleviate alopecia and, possibly, aggressive behavior, prostatomegaly, or vulvar swelling. Implants are repeated every 4 months as needed, lifelong. Alleviation of clinical signs may be more likely in patients with adrenal hyperplasia or adenoma; adenocarcinomas may be less likely to respond. Melatonin has

FERRET ADRENAL DISEASE (HYPERADRENOCORTICISM)   (CONTINUED)

FERRETS

no demonstrated effect on adrenal tumor growth or metastasis.

If Surgical Treatment Is Opted
• Continued, life-long treatment with a GnRH analog is recommended following unilateral adrenalectomy to prevent disease in the remaining gland.
• In ferrets with concurrent insulinoma, or if a combination of left and subtotal right adrenalectomy is performed, administer prednisone 0.25–1 mg/kg PO q12h for 1 week, then gradually tapering the dose over 1–2 weeks.
• If subtotal or total bilateral adrenalectomy is performed, long-term treatment with glucocorticoids is often necessary. The dosage is titrated to the individual patient and tapered to the lowest dosage interval necessary to prevent clinical signs of hypoadrenocorticism. Many ferrets have accessory adrenal tissue, and some may be weaned from exogenous steroids completely if carefully monitored. However, some ferrets do become critically ill due to hypoadrenocorticism even with prednisone supplementation, and treatment with mineralocorticoid may also be required. Treatment is initiated based on clinical signs and electrolyte status (signs typically occur within days to weeks postoperatively). Fludrocortisone (0.05–0.1 mg/kg PO q24h or divided q12h) or deoxycorticosterone pivalate (DOCP) (2 mg/kg IM q21d). Carefully monitor electrolyte status.

CONTRAINDICATIONS
N/A

ALTERNATIVE DRUGS
N/A

PRECAUTIONS
N/A

FOLLOW-UP

PATIENT MONITORING
• Most ferrets can be successfully managed with GnRH analog treatment alone.
• Response to therapy is evident by the remission of clinical signs, particularly hair regrowth, regression of vulvar swelling, and reduction in the size of urogenital cysts or prostatic tissue. Urogenital signs usually resolve within days of surgery.
• Monitor serum glucose concentrations before, during, and following surgery since many ferrets have concurrent insulinomas and develop postoperative hypoglycemia.
• Following unilateral adrenalectomy or subtotal adrenalectomy, monitor for return of clinical signs since tumor recurrence is common. Ideally, continued lifelong treatment with a GnRH analog is recommended.
• In ferrets with bilateral adrenalectomy, monitor for the development of Addison's disease (lethargy, weakness, anorexia, and periodic evaluation of serum electrolytes).

PREVENTION/AVOIDANCE
Anecdotal reports suggest that annual treatment with Deslorelin may prevent disease. These can be used to prevent the onset of estrus or sexual development in intact animals, precluding the need for surgical alteration.

POSSIBLE COMPLICATIONS
• Recurrence of tumor or development of tumor in the remaining gland in patients with unilateral or subtotal bilateral adrenalectomy
• Rarely, metastasis in patients with carcinomas
• Invasion of right adrenal tumors into the vena cava or liver
• Cachexia due to the catabolic effects of neoplasia
• Development of postoperative hypoglycemia in patients with concurrent undiagnosed insulinoma
• Addison's disease or death in ferrets with bilateral adrenalectomy

EXPECTED COURSE/PROGNOSIS
• Following surgical removal of the affected gland(s), a reduction in vulvar swelling is seen within 2 days to 2 weeks, and the haircoat returns to normal within 2–4 months. A reduction in the size of paraurethral cysts or prostatomegaly may occur as soon as 1–2 days postoperatively.
• Response to medical therapy may vary with tumor type; on average, clinical signs are controlled for 2 or more years.
• Prognosis is variable and depends on tumor type, age of the animal, presence of concurrent disease, and mode of treatment.
• Dermal and/or urogenital signs will worsen without treatment.
• Carcinomas rarely metastasize. If metastasis occurs, the prognosis is fair to poor.

MISCELLANEOUS

ASSOCIATED CONDITIONS
Insulinomas, lymphoma, cardiomyopathy, and/or nonspecific splenomegaly are often concurrently found in ferrets with adrenal disease.

AGE-RELATED FACTORS
Older animals are more likely to have concurrent heart disease, renal disease, or other neoplasia.

ZOONOTIC POTENTIAL
N/A

PREGNANCY/FERTILITY/BREEDING
N/A

SYNONYMS
Hyperadrenocorticism

SEE ALSO
Insulinoma
Lower urinary tract infection
Prostatomegaly
Urogenital cystic disease

ABBREVIATIONS
FSH = follicular-stimulating hormone
GnRH = gonadotropic-releasing hormone
LH = luteinizing hormone

Suggested Reading
Di Girolamo N, Huyun M. Disorders of the urinary and reproductive systems in ferrets. In: Quesenberry KE, Carpenter JW, eds. Ferrets, Rabbits and Rodents, 4th ed. Clinical Medicine and Surgery. St. Louis: Saunders, 2020:39–54.
Di Girolamo N, Selleri P. Medical and surgical emergencies in ferrets. Vet Clin Exot Anim Pract. 2016;19:431–464.
Jekl V, Hauptman K. Reproductive medicine in ferrets. Vet Clin Exot Anim Pract 2017;20:629–663.
Lennox AM, Wagner RA. Comparison of 4.7-mg deslorelin implants and surgery for the treatment of adrenocortical disease in ferrets. J Exot Pet Med. 2012;21:332–335.
Schoemaker NJ, Van Zealand YRA. Endocrine diseases of ferrets. In: Quesenberry KE, Carpenter JW, eds. Ferrets, Rabbits and Rodents, 4th ed. Clinical Medicine and Surgery. St. Louis: Saunders, 2020:77–91.
Schoemaker NJ, van Deijk R, Muijlaert B et al. Use of a gonadotropin releasing hormone agonist implant as an alternative for surgical castration in male ferrets (*Mustela putorius furo*). Theriogenology 2008;70:161–167.
Swiderski JK, Seim HB, MacPhail CM et al. Long-term outcome of domestic ferrets treated surgically for hyperadrenocorticism: 130 cases (1995–2004). J Am Vet Med Assoc 2008;232:1338–1343.
Wagner RA, Piché CA, Jöchle W et al. Clinical and endocrine responses to treatment with deslorelin acetate implants in ferrets with adrenocortical disease. Am J Vet Res 2005;66:910–914.

Author Barbara Oglesbee, DVM, DABVP (Avian)

ALEUTIAN DISEASE VIRUS (PARVOVIRUS)

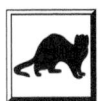

BASICS

DEFINITION
• Aleutian mink disease virus (ADV) are parvoviruses that can infect mink and ferrets. Both mink and ferret strains exist. Both can affect either species, but virulence is greater in species-specific strains.
• ADV is an immune-mediated, chronic systemic illness characterized by wasting and nervous system signs.
• Not all ferrets infected with ADV will become clinically ill.
• Ferrets may be persistently infected but remain asymptomatic; may be persistently infected and develop clinical disease (sometimes months to years after infection); or may eliminate the virus, with or without showing clinical signs.

PATHOPHYSIOLOGY
• Transmission occurs via both aerosol and oral routes. Direct contact with urine, saliva, blood, and feces is most common, but transmission may also occur through fomites.
• Unlike parvoviral infections in dogs and cats, disease is caused by the long-term effects of immune-complex deposition, not by the cytotoxic effect of the virus.
• Exposure to the virus causes an antibody response and subsequent plasma cell proliferation; however, the antibody response is not protective.
• Virus–antibody complex deposition results in glomerulonephritis, arteritis, and lymphoplasmacytic infiltrates in the liver, kidneys, spleen, lymph nodes, gastrointestinal tract, and nervous tissues.
• The course of the disease is usually protracted, extending over 18–24 months.
• It is presumed that ferrets with antibody titers to ADV are shedding virus; however, the mode or duration of viral shedding is currently unknown.

SYSTEMS AFFECTED
• Hemic/Lymphatic/Immune—hypergammaglobulinemia; thymus, lymph nodes, spleen: plasmacytic infiltration
• Renal—membranoproliferative glomerulonephritis, lymphoplasmacytic nephritis
• Hepatobiliary—bile duct hyperplasia, portal lymphoplasmacytic hepatitis
• Nervous—nonsuppurative encephalomyelitis, nonsuppurative meningitis
• Gastrointestinal—lymphoplasmacytic enteritis
• Cardiovascular—lymphoplasmacytic arteritis
• Respiratory—interstitial pneumonia, pleural effusion
• Ophthalmic—anterior uveitis

GENETICS
Unknown

INCIDENCE/PREVALENCE
• Most common in breeding facilities, animal shelters, and pet stores
• Although rates within individual colonies of ferrets from 42% to 60% have been reported, the overall incidence in the pet ferret population appears to be low (8.5%–10%).

GEOGRAPHIC DISTRIBUTION
Worldwide

SIGNALMENT
No age or sex predilection

SIGNS

General Comments
Suspect ADV infection in ferrets with chronic wasting, other nonspecific signs (lethargy, intermittent anorexia), or neurologic signs combined with hypergammaglobulinemia.

Historical Findings
• Chronic, progressive weight loss
• Nonspecific signs: lethargy, anorexia, poor hair coat, and collapse
• Neurologic signs include rear limb paresis, which may progress cranially, fecal and/or urinary incontinence, and head tremors
• Melena or frank hemorrhage from the GI tract
• Coughing, dyspnea

Physical Examination Findings
• Emaciation and muscle wasting are consistent features.
• Rear limb paresis, muscle atrophy in the rear limbs
• Head tremors
• Splenomegaly may be palpated.
• Occasionally, enlarged mesenteric lymph nodes are palpable.
• Pale mucous membranes with anemic animals
• Signs of dehydration

RISK FACTORS
• Exposure to mink
• Exposure to ADV-positive ferrets
• Crowding and poor sanitation increase the risk of infection.
• Copathogens such as parasites, viruses, and certain bacterial species are hypothesized to exacerbate illness; ferrets with ADV are presumed to be immunosuppressed and therefore more susceptible to other pathogens.

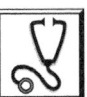

DIAGNOSIS

GENERAL COMMENTS
Definitive diagnosis of ADV requires viral isolation or detection in tissue samples. A presumptive diagnosis can be made based on the presence of supportive clinical signs, hypergammaglobulinemia, and positive serologic or PCR testing.

DIFFERENTIAL DIAGNOSIS
• For chronic wasting: gastrointestinal foreign bodies, *Helicobacter mustelae*, infiltrative bowel disease (eosinophilic gastroenteritis, lymphoplasmacytic enteritis, and lymphosarcoma), neoplasia, and estrogen-induced anemia
• For rear limb paresis and tremors: spinal cord disease, insulinoma, heavy metal toxicosis, CDV, and rabies

CBC/BIOCHEMISTRY/URINALYSIS
• Serum protein electrophoresis: The hallmark of ADV is hypergammaglobulinemia. Gammaglobulins usually represent >20% of total protein; hypoalbuminemia may also be seen.
• Leukopenia and/or anemia—occasionally seen
• Increased BUN and creatinine with severe renal disease
• Increased liver enzymes in ferrets with hepatic involvement

OTHER LABORATORY TESTS
Serologic Testing
• Both ELISA and PCR testing are available. Positive serologic testing indicates current or previous infection; however, a correlation between positive titer and shedding has not been established.

IMAGING
• Abdominal radiographs are usually normal but may reveal splenomegaly and either an increase or decrease in the size of the kidneys. Thoracic radiographs may demonstrate pleural effusion or an interstitial pattern in animals with pneumonia (rare).
• Radiographs may be helpful to rule out other causes of rear limb paresis, such as vertebral disorders.

PATHOLOGIC FINDINGS
• Gross changes are often absent, other than emaciation and muscle wasting. Other reported changes include an enlarged spleen, enlarged mesenteric lymph nodes, small kidneys, pleural effusion, hemorrhagic pneumonia, lung lobe consolidation, cardiomegaly, and frank hemorrhage into the small intestinal lumen.

FERRETS

• Histopathology demonstrates immune complex deposition and lymphoplasmacytic infiltration, including portal and periportal lymphoplasmacytic hepatitis, membranoproliferative glomerulonephritis, interstitial lymphoplasmacytic nephritis, nonsuppurative encephalomyelitis, perivascular accumulations of plasmacytes and astrocytic hypertrophy in spinal cord, hemorrhagic interstitial pneumonia, and multifocal arteritis (may include cardiac muscle).

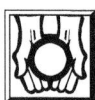

TREATMENT

APPROPRIATE HEALTH CARE
• Symptomatic and supportive only—there is no specific treatment for ADV
• Intensity depends on the severity of signs on examination.
• Proper, strict isolation procedures are essential. Exercise care to prevent the spread of ADV, a very stable virus.

NURSING CARE
Symptomatic therapy includes attention to fluid and electrolyte derangements, reduction in environmental stressors, and modification of the diet to improve palatability.

ACTIVITY
N/A

DIET
• If anorexic, assist feed an easily digestible high-protein/high-fat diet such as Lafeber Carnivore Critical Care Diet (Lafeber Company, Cornell, IL) or Oxbow Carnivore Critical Care Diet (Oxbow Animal Health, Omaha, NE); if these are unavailable, offer chicken baby foods; may also add dietary supplement such as Nutri-Cal (EVSCO Pharmaceuticals) to increase caloric content to these foods.
• Sick ferrets should receive a minimum of 400 kcal/kg BW per day

CLIENT EDUCATION
• Inform about the need for thorough disinfection, especially if other ferrets are on the premises. See prevention/avoidance.
• Inform owners that most ferrets never develop clinical signs. However, when clinical signs do appear, the prognosis is guarded to grave.

SURGICAL CONSIDERATIONS
N/A

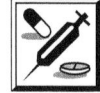

MEDICATIONS

DRUG(S) OF CHOICE
Treat secondary or opportunistic infections with the appropriate antibiotic or antiparasitic agent.

CONTRAINDICATIONS
N/A

PRECAUTIONS
N/A

POSSIBLE INTERACTIONS
N/A

ALTERNATIVE DRUGS
N/A

FOLLOW-UP

PATIENT MONITORING
N/A

PREVENTION/AVOIDANCE
• Vaccines are not available and would be contraindicated due to the immune-mediated effects of this disease.
• The virus can survive for months, especially in the presence of gross debris. Thoroughly clean all organic debris and apply a 1:30 dilution of bleach (5% sodium hypochlorite).
• It is assumed that all serologically positive ferrets are capable of shedding virus. Serologically positive animals should not be housed in the same home as serologically negative animals.

POSSIBLE COMPLICATIONS
Secondary bacterial, parasitic, or viral infections

EXPECTED COURSE AND PROGNOSIS
• Prognosis is good in asymptomatic ferrets testing positive on serology. Most of these ferrets will never develop clinical disease. If clinical disease eventually develops, the prognosis depends on the strain of virus and the organ system affected

• Prognosis is guarded in severely affected ferrets and ferrets demonstrating neurologic signs. Signs may or may not progress, and there are no predictive diagnostic tests available.

MISCELLANEOUS

ASSOCIATED CONDITIONS
N/A

AGE-RELATED FACTORS
N/A

ZOONOTIC POTENTIAL
N/A

PREGNANCY/FERTILITY/BREEDING
No in-utero infections have been reported in ferrets.

SYNONYMS
Mink parvovirus

SEE ALSO
Paresis and paralysis
Weight loss and cachexia

ABBREVIATIONS
ADV = Aleutian disease virus
CDV = canine distemper virus
ELISA = enzyme-linked immunosorbent assay
GI = gastrointestinal
PCR = polymerase chain reaction

Suggested Reading
Huynh M, Piazza S. Musculoskeletal and neurologic diseases. In: Quesenberry KE, Carpenter JW, eds. Ferrets, Rabbits and Rodents, 4th ed. Clinical Medicine and Surgery. 2021. St. Louis: Saunders, 2020:117–130.
Morrisey JK, Malakoff RJ. Cardiovascular and other diseases of ferrets. In: Quesenberry KE, Carpenter JW, eds. Ferrets, Rabbits and Rodents, 4th ed. Clinical Medicine and Surgery. 2021. St. Louis: Saunders, 2020:5–70.
Virtanen J, Zalewski A, Kołodziej-Sobocińska M et al. Diversity and transmission of Aleutian mink disease virus in feral and farmed American mink and native mustelids. Virus Evol 2021;7(2). veab075.
Author Barbara Oglesbee, DVM, DABVP (Avian)

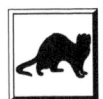

BASICS

DEFINITION
• Extremely common disorder in ferrets
• May be associated with a multifactorial cause
• May be the primary problem or only a secondary phenomenon

PATHOPHYSIOLOGY
• Multifactorial causes
• All the disorders represent a disruption in the growth of the hair follicle from endocrine abnormalities, infection, or trauma.

SYSTEMS AFFECTED
• Skin/Exocrine
• Endocrine/Metabolic

SIGNALMENT
• No specific age or sex predilection
• Ferret adrenal disease, the most common cause of alopecia, is seen primarily in middle-aged (3–7 years old) neutered animals—equal incidence in male and female animals

SIGNS
• The pattern and degree of hair loss are important for establishing a differential diagnosis.
• Large diffuse areas of alopecia—indicate a follicular dysplasia or metabolic component
• Multifocal patches of alopecia—most frequently associated with folliculitis from bacterial, mycotic, or parasitic infection
• May be acute in onset or slowly progressive

CAUSES
• Endocrine—ferret adrenal disease is the most common cause of alopecia in pet ferrets; seasonal alopecia is common in intact animals
• Infectious—bacterial pyoderma, dermatophytosis; most often a secondary problem
• Parasitic—ear mites, fleas, and sarcoptic mange
• Neoplastic—cutaneous lymphoma, mast cell tumor
• Immunologic—contact dermatitis has been anecdotally reported in ferrets. Cutaneous lesions resembling urticaria or histologic lesions characteristic of allergic reactions in other species have also been anecdotally reported; however, there are no confirmed cases of atopy, food allergy, or other allergic dermatitis in ferrets.

RISK FACTORS
N/A

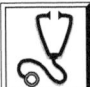

DIAGNOSIS

DIFFERENTIAL DIAGNOSIS
Differentiating Causes
Pattern and degree—important features for formulating a differential diagnosis

Symmetrical
• Ferret adrenal disease—over 95% of neutered ferrets with bilaterally symmetric alopecia have adrenal disease. Hair loss may be sudden and progressive, or may begin in spring, initially regrow later in the year, and be followed by progressive alopecia the following spring. Alopecia frequently begins in the tail region and progresses cranially. Other patterns, such as diffuse thinning of the hair coat or alopecia over the shoulder region, can also be seen. In severe cases, the ferret will become completely bald. In most cases, the skin has a normal appearance, although skin thickening may be seen. Many ferrets are pruritic, and secondary pyoderma is occasionally seen. Other signs related to adrenal disease, such as a swollen vulva in spayed females, are common.
• Seasonal flank alopecia—in intact animals (or females with ovarian remnant), bilaterally symmetric alopecia begins at the tail base and progresses throughout the breeding season (March–August for females, December–July for males). Alopecia is not as extensive as in ferrets with adrenal disease.
• Hyperestrogenism (females)—symmetrical alopecia of the flanks and perineal and inguinal regions with enlarged vulva and mammary glands

Multifocal to focal
• Ear mites—partial to complete alopecia caudal to the ears; waxy brown aural discharge; excoriations around pinna
• Fleas—patchy alopecia at tail base and in cervical and dorsal thoracic region; excoriations; secondary pyoderma
• Sarcoptic mange—two forms reported—generalized with diffuse alopecia and intense pruritus and local form affecting the feet with secondary pododermatitis
• Bacterial folliculitis—multifocal area of circular alopecia to coalescing large areas of hair loss; epidermal collarettes
• Dermatophytosis—partial to complete alopecia with scaling; with or without erythema; not always ringlike; may begin as small papules
• Neoplasia—cutaneous lymphoma, cutaneous epitheliotropic lymphoma—diffuse, generalized truncal alopecia with scaling and erythema, later nodule, and plaque formation; mast cell tumor—focal alopecia with pruritus, scaling, and often covered with black crusts

CBC/BIOCHEMISTRY/URINALYSIS
• Inflammatory leukocytosis with neutrophilia may be seen with pyoderma.
• Lymphocytosis may be seen with cutaneous lymphoma.
• Nonregenerative anemia, leucopenia, or thrombocytopenia with estrogen excess

OTHER LABORATORY TESTS
• Elevations in plasma estradiol, androstenedione, and 17-hydroxyprogesterone combined (available through the Clinical Endocrinology Laboratory, Department of Comparative Medicine, University of Tennessee) are supportive of the diagnosis.

IMAGING
Ultrasonography—evaluate adrenal glands for evidence of ferret adrenal disease; generally requires an ultrasonographer experienced in evaluating ferret adrenal glands.

DIAGNOSTIC PROCEDURES
• Response to therapy as a trial
• Fungal culture
• Skin scraping
• Cytology
• Skin biopsy

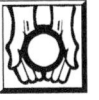

TREATMENT
• Treatment must be specific to the underlying cause to be successful.
• Ferret adrenal disease may be treated with adrenalectomy or managed medically. The decision as to which form of treatment is appropriate is multifactorial; which gland is affected (left vs. right), the surgeon's experience and expertise, the severity of clinical signs, age of the animal, concurrent diseases, and financial issues should be considered.
• Hyperestrogenism—ovariohysterectomy or surgical removal of ovarian remnant
• Mast cell tumor—surgical excision

MEDICATIONS
DRUG(S) OF CHOICE
Varies with the specific cause
• Ferret Adrenal Disease—the GnRH agonist deslorelin acetate (Suprelorin-F®, Virbac Animal Health) is labeled for the treatment of adrenal disease in domestic ferrets in the United States. It is a 4.7-mg slow-release deslorelin implant reported to provide alleviation of clinical signs lasting from 8 to

FERRETS

ALOPECIA

20 months. Alleviation of clinical signs may be more likely in patients with adrenal hyperplasia or adenoma; adenocarcinomas may be less likely to respond. Deslorelin has no demonstrated effect on adrenal tumor growth or metastasis. In Europe, 9.4-mg deslorelin implants are available and may be effective for up to 2–4 years.
• Ear mites—ivermectin (0.4 mg/kg PO, SC q14-28d); selamectin (Revolution, Pfizer) 15 mg/kg topically q30d
• Fleas—fipronil (Frontline, Boehringer Ingelheim) 0.2–0.4 mL/animal applied topically q30d; imidacloprid (Advantage, Bayer) 10 mg/kg topically q30d; imidacloprid and moxidectin (Advantage Multi for Cats, Bayer) 0.4 mL/animal topically q30d; selamectin (Revolution, Pfizer) 15 mg/kg topically q30d
• Sarcoptic mange—ivermectin 0.2–0.4 mg/kg SC q14d for 3 to 4 doses; selamectin (Revolution, Pfizer) 15 mg/kg topically q30d
• Bacterial folliculitis—shampoos and antibiotic therapy, preferably based on culture and susceptibility testing; good initial choices include amoxicillin/clavulanate (13–25 mg/kg PO q12h), cephalexin (15–30 mg/kg PO q12h), or trimethoprim/sulfa (15–30 mg/kg PO q12h)
• Dermatophytosis—topical therapy—miconazole shampoo (with or without chlorhexidine) plus fluconazole (10 mg/kg PO q12h) or ketoconazole (10–15 mg/kg PO q24h) or itraconazole (10–20 mg/kg PO q24h) for 4–8 weeks
• Neoplasia—various chemotherapy protocols

CONTRAINDICATIONS
Do not administer topical and systemic ivermectin simultaneously.

PRECAUTIONS
Ivermectin
Anecdotally associated with birth defects when used in pregnant jills

Topical Antiparasitic Agents
• Flea shampoos, sprays, or powders—use cautiously and sparingly to minimize ingestion during grooming
• Antibacterial shampoos—use cautiously as may cause excessive dryness and pruritus

POSSIBLE INTERACTIONS
None

ALTERNATIVE DRUGS
For Adrenal Disease:
• Leuprolide acetate, a GnRH analog, is a potent gonadotropin secretion inhibitor and suppresses LH and FSH, downregulating their receptor sites. It is available as a 1- or 4-month depot injection and may alleviate the dermal and reproductive organ signs of adrenal disease in ferrets. Reported dosages: Lupron® 30-day depot, 100–250 µg/kg IM q4w until signs resolve, then q4–8w PRN, lifelong. Larger ferrets often require the higher end of the dose range. This drug has no effect on adrenal tumor growth or metastasis. This drug has become challenging to acquire and often prohibitively expensive in the United States.
• Melatonin implants are available commercially (Ferretonin® 2.7-mg—ferrets < 600-g) and 5.4-mg implants—most ferrets (Melatek, LLC) and have been used in ferrets with adrenal disease to alleviate alopecia and, possibly, aggressive behavior, prostatomegaly, or vulvar swelling. Implants are repeated every 4 months as needed, lifelong. Alleviation of clinical signs may be more likely in patients with adrenal hyperplasia or adenoma; adenocarcinomas may be less likely to respond. Melatonin has no demonstrated effect on adrenal tumor growth or metastasis.

FOLLOW-UP

PATIENT MONITORING
Varies with cause

POSSIBLE COMPLICATIONS
N/A

MISCELLANEOUS

ASSOCIATED CONDITIONS
Other types of neoplasia, especially insulinoma and lymphoma, are often found in ferrets with adrenal disease.

AGE-RELATED FACTORS
N/A

ZOONOTIC POTENTIAL
Dermatophytosis can cause skin lesions in people.

PREGNANCY/FERTILITY/BREEDING
Avoid griseofulvin and ivermectin in pregnant animals.

SYNONYMS
None

SEE ALSO
Adrenal disease (hyperadrenocorticism)
Dermatophytosis
Ear mites
Fleas
Hyperestrogenism
Lymphoma
Mast cell tumor

ABBREVIATIONS
FSH = follicular-stimulating hormone
LH = luteinizing hormone
LHRH = luteinizing hormone-releasing hormone

Suggested Reading
d'Ovidio D, Santoro D. Dermatologic diseases of ferrets. In: Quesenberry KE, Carpenter JW, eds. Ferrets, Rabbits and Rodents, 4th ed. Clinical Medicine and Surgery. 2021. St. Louis: Saunders, 2020:109–116.
Hoppmann E, Wilson Barron H. Ferret and rabbit dermatology. J Exot Pet Med 2007;16:225–237.
Schoemaker NJ, Van Zealand YRA. Endocrine diseases of ferrets. In: Quesenberry KE, Carpenter JW, eds. Ferrets, Rabbits and Rodents, 4th ed. Clinical Medicine and Surgery. St. Louis: Saunders, 2020:77–91.
Schoemaker NJ, van Deijk R, Muijlaert B et al. Use of a gonadotropin releasing hormone agonist implant as an alternative for surgical castration in male ferrets (*Mustela putorius furo*). Theriogenology 2008;70:161–167.
Swiderski JK, Seim HB, MacPhail CM et al. Long-term outcome of domestic ferrets treated surgically for hyperadrenocorticism: 130 cases (1995–2004). J Am Vet Med Assoc 2008;232:1338–1343.
Wagner RA, Piché CA, Jöchle W et al. Clinical and endocrine responses to treatment with deslorelin acetate implants in ferrets with adrenocortical disease. Am J Vet Res 2005;66:910–914.
Author Barbara Oglesbee, DVM, DABVP (Avian)

BASICS

DEFINITION
- The lack or loss of appetite for food; appetite is psychologic and depends on memory and associations, compared with hunger, which is physiologically aroused by the body's need for food; the existence of appetite in animals is assumed.
- The term *pseudoanorexia* is used to describe animals that have a desire for food but are unable to eat because they cannot prehend, chew, or swallow food.

PATHOPHYSIOLOGY
- Anorexia is most often associated with systemic disease but can be caused by many different mechanisms.
- The control of appetite is a complex interaction between the CNS and the periphery.
- Inflammatory, infectious, metabolic, or neoplastic diseases can cause inappetence, probably as a result of the release of a variety of chemical mediators.

SYSTEMS AFFECTED
All body systems are affected; breakdown of the intestinal mucosal barrier is particularly important in sick patients.

SIGNALMENT
Depends on the underlying cause

SIGNS
- Refusal to eat is a common complaint presented by ferret owners, because a poor appetite is strongly associated with illness.
- Reluctance to eat may be the only abnormality identified after an evaluation of the patient history and physical examination; this is typical in ferrets with many types of gastrointestinal tract diseases or psychologic causes of anorexia.
- Patients with disorders causing dysfunction or pain of the face, neck, oropharynx, and esophagus may display an interest in food but be unable to complete prehension and swallowing (pseudoanorexia).
- Pseudoanorectic patients commonly display weight loss, halitosis, excessive drooling, difficulty in prehension and mastication of food, dysphagia, and odynophagia (painful eating).
- Most underlying causes of pseudoanorexia can be identified by a thorough examination of the face, neck, oropharynx, and esophagus for traumatic lesions, masses, foreign bodies, dental disease, ulceration, and neuromuscular dysfunction.
- Clinical signs in true anorexia vary and are related to the underlying cause.

CAUSES
Anorexia
- Almost any systemic disease process
- Gastrointestinal disease is one of the most common causes—especially GI foreign body, gastric ulceration, epizootic catarrhal enteritis (ECE), or infiltrative bowel diseases
- Endocrine disease—especially insulinoma
- Metabolic disease—especially hepatic or renal disease
- Neoplasia involving any site—especially lymphoma
- Cardiac failure
- Pain
- Infectious disease
- Respiratory disease
- Neurologic disease
- Psychologic—unpalatable diets, alterations in routine or environment, stress
- Toxicosis and drugs
- Musculoskeletal disorders
- Acid–base disorders
- Miscellaneous—motion sickness, high environmental temperature, etc.

Pseudoanorexia
- Any disease process that interferes with the swallowing reflex
- Diseases causing painful prehension and mastication; stomatitis, glossitis, gingivitis (e.g., physical agents, caustics, bacterial infections, viral infections, foreign bodies, uremia), oral or glossal neoplasia (especially squamous cell carcinoma), neurologic disorders (rabies, tetanus, and CNS lesions), musculoskeletal disorders (mandible fracture or subluxation) dental disease, salivary gland disorders, and retrobulbar abscess
- Diseases causing oropharyngeal dysphagia (much less common in ferrets); glossal disorders (neurologic, neoplastic), pharyngitis, pharyngeal neoplasia, retropharyngeal disorders (lymphadenopathy, abscess, hematoma, and sialocele), neuromuscular disorders (CNS lesions, botulism)
- Diseases of the esophagus—esophagitis, neoplasia, and neuromuscular disorders (unusual in ferrets)

RISK FACTORS
N/A

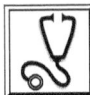

DIAGNOSIS

DIFFERENTIAL DIAGNOSIS
- Gastrointestinal disease is the most common cause of anorexia in ferrets, followed by systemic disease.
- Obtain a minimum database (CBC, biochemistry, and radiographs) to help eliminate the possibility of underlying medical disorders.
- Questioning about the patient's interest in food and its ability to prehend, masticate, and swallow food, along with a thorough examination of the animal's oropharynx, face, and neck, will help identify pseudoanorexia; if the owners are poor historians the patient should be observed while eating.
- A thorough history regarding the animal's environment, diet, other animals and people in the household, and any recent changes involving any of these helps identify psychologic anorexia.
- Any abnormalities detected in the physical examination or historical evidence of illness mandates a diagnostic workup for the identified problem.

CBC/BIOCHEMISTRY/URINALYSIS
Abnormalities vary with different underlying diseases and causes of pseudoanorexia and anorexia.

OTHER LABORATORY TESTS
Special tests may be necessary to rule out specific diseases suggested by the history, physical examination, or minimum database (see other topics on specific diseases).

IMAGING
- If underlying disease is suspected but no abnormalities are revealed by the physical examination or minimum database, perform abdominal radiography and abdominal ultrasonography to identify hidden conditions such as GI tract disease, hepatic disease, or neoplasia. Consider thoracic radiography to rule out cardiac or pulmonary disease.
- The need for further diagnostic imaging varies with the underlying condition suspected (see other topics on specific diseases).

DIAGNOSTIC PROCEDURES
Vary with underlying condition suspected (see other topics regarding specific diseases)

TREATMENT
- Treat underlying cause.
- Ferrets often become hypoglycemic within 1–4 hours of the onset of anorexia. Insulinomas are very common in middle-aged to older ferrets and may be subclinical. Monitor blood glucose concentrations and begin IV fluid therapy with 2.5%–5% dextrose as indicated to correct hypoglycemia.
- Symptomatic therapy includes attention to fluid and electrolyte derangements, reduction in environmental stressors, and modification of the diet to improve palatability.
- Symptomatic therapy includes attention to fluid and electrolyte derangements, reduction in environmental stressors, and modification of the diet to improve palatability.

ANOREXIA

FERRETS

• If refusing solid food, most ferrets will accept assist feeding with an easily digestible high-protein/high-fat diet such as Lafeber Carnivore Critical Care Diet (Lafeber Company, Cornell, IL) or Oxbow Carnivore Critical Care Diet (Oxbow Animal Health, Omaha, NE); may also add dietary supplement such as Nutri-Cal (EVSCO Pharmaceuticals) to increase caloric content to these foods.

• Easily digestible, high-protein diets such as chicken baby food are often helpful in ferrets recovering from ECE or inflammatory bowel disease.

• The caloric recommendation for sick ferrets is approximately 400 kcal/kg BW per day (although this may be a high estimate).

• Techniques for providing enteral nutrition include assisted syringe-feeding or placement of nasogastric, esophagostomy, gastrostomy, or jejunostomy tubes.

• Parenteral nutrition may be provided via infusion through a polyurethane jugular catheter using a syringe pump.

MEDICATIONS

DRUG(S) OF CHOICE

• Depends on the underlying cause

• Gastrointestinal antisecretory agents are helpful to treat, and possibly prevent gastritis in anorectic ferrets. Ferrets continually secrete a baseline level of gastric hydrochloric acid and, as such, anorexia itself may predispose to gastric ulceration. Those successfully used in ferrets include omeprazole (4 mg/kg PO q24h) famotidine (0.25–0.5 mg/kg PO, SC, IV q24h), and cimetidine (10 mg/kg PO, SC, IM, IV q8h)

• Anti-emetics—metoclopramide (0.2–1.0 mg/kg PO, SC, IM q6–8h), Ondansetron (1mg/kg PO q12–24h), or maropitant citrate (1 mg/kg SC q24h).

• Analgesics may promote appetite in painful conditions—butorphanol (0.1–0.5 mg/kg SC, IM, IV q4–6h), hydromorphone (0.1–0.2 mg/kg SC, IM, IV q6–8h), tramadol (10 mg/kg PO q12–24h), gabapentin (3–5 mg/kg PO q8–12h), and meloxicam (0.2 mg/kg SC, PO q24h, reduce to 0.1 mg/kg q24h)

CONTRAINDICATIONS

Avoid antiemetics or promotility agents if gastrointestinal obstruction is present or suspected.

PRECAUTIONS

Use nonsteroidal anti-inflammatory agents with caution in ferrets with gastrointestinal or renal disease.

POSSIBLE INTERACTIONS

N/A

ALTERNATIVE DRUGS

• Capromorelin (Entyce) has been anecdotally used at canine doses

FOLLOW-UP

PATIENT MONITORING

Body weight and hydration to determine if management is effective

POSSIBLE COMPLICATIONS

• Dehydration, malnutrition, and cachexia are most likely; these exacerbate the underlying disease.

• Ferrets secrete a baseline level of gastric hydrochloric acid and may develop gastric ulcerations when anorexic.

• Hepatic lipidosis is a possible complication of anorexia, especially in obese ferrets.

• Breakdown of the intestinal mucosal barrier is a concern in debilitated patients.

MISCELLANEOUS

ASSOCIATED CONDITIONS

Hypoglycemia may occur in anorectic ferrets with insulinoma, kits, and cachectic patients and in some medical conditions (e.g., advanced liver disease).

AGE-RELATED FACTORS

Nutritional support and/or glucose-containing fluids may be necessary to treat or prevent hypoglycemia in anorectic kits, ferrets with insulinoma, or emaciated ferrets.

ZOONOTIC POTENTIAL

N/A

PREGNANCY/FERTILITY/BREEDING

N/A

SYNONYMS

Inappetence

SEE ALSO

Epizootic catarrhal enteritis
Gastritis
Gastroduodenal ulcers
Gastrointestinal foreign bodies
Inflammatory bowel disease
Insulinoma
Lymphoma

ABBREVIATIONS

CNS = central nervous system
ECE = epizootic catarrhal enteritis
IBD = infiltrative bowel disease

Suggested Reading
Di Girolamo N, Selleri P. Medical and surgical emergencies in ferrets. Vet Clin Exot Anim 2016;19:431–464.
Hoefer HL. Gastrointestinal diseases of ferrets. In: Quesenberry KE, Carpenter JW, eds. Ferrets, Rabbits, and Rodents, 4th ed. Clinical Medicine and Surgery. 2021. St. Louis: Saunders, 2020:27–38.
Huynh M, Pignon C. Gastrointestinal disease in exotic small mammals. J Exot Pet Med 2013;22(2):118–131.
Johnson-Delaney CA. Geriatric ferrets. Vet Clin Exot Anim Pract 2020;23(3): 549–565.
Johnson-Delaney CA. Ferret nutrition. Vet Clin Exot Anim Pract 2014;17(3): 449–470.
Lennox AM, Gladden JN. Emergency and critical care of small mammals. In: Quesenberry KE, Carpenter JW, eds. Ferrets, Rabbits and Rodents, 4th ed. Clinical Medicine and Surgery. 2021. St. Louis: Saunders, 2020:595–608.
Powers LV, Perpiñán D. Basic anatomy, physiology, and husbandry of ferrets. In: Quesenberry KE, Orcutt CJ, Mans C, Carpenter JW, eds. Ferrets, Rabbits, and Rodents, 4th ed. St. Louis, MO, USA: Elsevier, 2020:1–2.
Schoemaker NJ, van Zeeland YRA. Endocrine diseases of ferrets. In: Quesenberry KE, Carpenter JW, eds. Ferrets, Rabbits and Rodents, 4th ed. Clinical Medicine and Surgery. 2021. St. Louis: Saunders, 2020:77–91.

Author Barbara Oglesbee, DVM, DABVP (Avian)

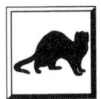

BASICS

DEFINITION
The escape of fluid, either transudate or exudate, into the abdominal cavity between the parietal and visceral peritoneum

PATHOPHYSIOLOGY
Ascites can be caused by the following:
• CHF and associated interference in venous return
• Depletion of plasma proteins associated with inappropriate loss of protein from renal or gastrointestinal disease—protein-losing nephropathy or enteropathy, respectively
• Obstruction of the vena cava or portal vein, or lymphatic drainage due to neoplastic occlusion
• Overt neoplastic effusion
• Peritonitis—infective or inflammatory
• Liver cirrhosis

SYSTEMS AFFECTED
• Cardiovascular
• Gastrointestinal
• Renal/Urologic
• Hemic/Lymph/Immune

SIGNALMENT
No age or sex predisposition

SIGNS
• Episodic weakness, rear limb paresis, or ataxia
• Lethargy
• Abdominal distension
• Abdominal discomfort when palpated
• Dyspnea from abdominal distension or associated pleural effusion
• Anorexia
• Weight gain

CAUSES
• CHF—most common
• Abdominal neoplasia
• Abdominal hemorrhage
• Hypoproteinemia
• Renal disease
• Cirrhosis of liver
• Ruptured bladder
• Peritonitis

RISK FACTORS
N/A

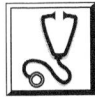

DIAGNOSIS

DIFFERENTIAL DIAGNOSIS
Differentiating Abdominal Distension
Without Effusion
• Organomegaly—splenomegaly (most common), renomegaly (renal cysts), and hepatomegaly
• Obesity—extremely common
• Abdominal neoplasia
• Pregnancy
• Gastric dilatation (rare)

Differentiating Diseases
• Transudate—right-sided CHF, hypoproteinemia, cirrhosis of liver, renal disease, and ruptured bladder
• Exudate—peritonitis, abdominal neoplasia, and hemorrhage

CBC/BIOCHEMISTRY/URINALYSIS
• Neutrophilic leukocytosis occurs in patients with systemic infection.
• Albumin is low in patients with impaired liver synthesis, gastrointestinal loss, or renal loss.
• Liver enzymes are low to normal in patients with impaired liver synthesis; high in patients with liver inflammation and chronic passive congestion
• BUN and creatinine are high in patients with renal failure; BUN may be low in patients with impaired liver synthesis.
• Glucose is low in patients with concurrent insulinoma or impaired liver synthesis.

OTHER LABORATORY TESTS
To detect hypoproteinemia—protein electrophoresis

IMAGING
• Thoracic and abdominal radiography to evaluate cardiac size and rule out organomegaly
• Ultrasonography of the heart, liver, spleen, pancreas, kidney, bladder, and abdomen can often determine cause.

DIAGNOSTIC PROCEDURES
• Abdominocentesis—remove approximately 1–3 mL of abdominal fluid via aseptic technique; a portion of the sample for bacterial culture and antibiotic sensitivity
• Allows characterization of the fluid type and determination of potential underlying cause (following parameters extrapolated from canine and feline data):

Transudate
• Clear and colorless
• Protein <2.5 g/dL
• Specific gravity <1.018
• Cells <1000/mm³—neutrophils and mesothelial cells

Modified Transudate
• Red or pink; may be slightly cloudy
• Protein 2.5–5.0 g/dL
• Specific gravity >1.018
• Cells <5000/mm³—neutrophils, mesothelial cells, erythrocytes, and lymphocytes

Exudate (Nonseptic)
• Pink or white; cloudy
• Protein 2.5–5.0 g/dL
• Specific gravity >1.018
• Cells 5,000–50,000/mm³—neutrophils, mesothelial cells, macrophages, erythrocytes, and lymphocytes

Exudate (Septic)
• Red, white, or yellow; cloudy
• Protein. >4.0 g/dL
• Specific gravity >1.018
• Cells 5,000–100,000/mm³—neutrophils, mesothelial cells, macrophages, erythrocytes, lymphocytes, and bacteria

Hemorrhage
• Red; spun supernatant clear and sediment red
• Protein >5.5 g/dL
• Specific gravity 1.007–1.027
• Cells consistent with peripheral blood
• Does not clot

Urine
• Clear to pale yellow
• Protein >2.5 g/dL
• Specific gravity 1.000–1.040
• Cells 5,000–50,000/mm³—neutrophils, erythrocytes, lymphocytes, and macrophages

TREATMENT
• Can design treatment on an outpatient basis, with follow-up or inpatient care, depending on physical condition and underlying cause
• If patients are markedly uncomfortable when lying down or become more dyspneic with stress, consider removing enough ascites to reverse these signs.
• For exudate ascites control, address the underlying cause; corrective surgery may be indicated, followed by specific therapeutic management (e.g., tumor removed, abdominal bleeding controlled, and blood transfusion administered).

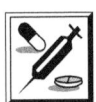

MEDICATIONS

DRUG(S) OF CHOICE
• Patients with liver insufficiency or CHF—diuretics such as furosemide (1–4 mg/kg PO, SC, IV, IM q8–12h); sodium restriction possibly helpful, but difficult to achieve in ferrets
• Patients with hypoproteinemia and associated ascitic fluid accumulation—can treat as above with the addition of hetastarch; administer an IV bolus (10 mL/kg) slowly over 2–3 hours; then as a constant rate infusion of 1–2 mL/kg/hr for 24 hours with a maximum infusion of 20 mL/kg/day; hetastarch increases plasma oncotic pressure and pulls fluid into the intravascular space.

ASCITES (CONTINUED)

FERRETS

• Systemic antibiotic therapy is dictated by bacterial identification and sensitivity testing in patients with septic exudate ascites.

CONTRAINDICATIONS
N/A

PRECAUTIONS
N/A

POSSIBLE INTERACTIONS
N/A

ALTERNATIVE DRUGS
N/A

FOLLOW-UP

PATIENT MONITORING
• Varies with the underlying cause
• Check sodium, potassium, BUN, creatinine, and weight fluctuations periodically if the patient is maintained on a diuretic.

POSSIBLE COMPLICATIONS
Aggressive diuretic administration may cause hypokalemia.

MISCELLANEOUS

ASSOCIATED CONDITIONS
N/A

AGE-RELATED FACTORS
N/A

ZOONOTIC POTENTIAL
N/A

PREGNANCY/FERTILITY/BREEDING
N/A

SYNONYMS
Abdominal effusion

SEE ALSO
Lymphoma
Hepatomegaly
Congestive heart failure

ABBREVIATIONS
BUN = blood urea nitrogen
CHF = congestive heart failure

Suggested Reading
Di Girolamo N, Selleri P. Medical and surgical emergencies in ferrets. Vet Clin North Am Exot Anim Pract 2016;19: 431–464.
Johnson-Delaney CA. Geriatric ferrets. Vet Clin Exot Anim Pract 2020;23(3): 549–650.
Lennox AM, Gladden JN. Emergency and critical care of small mammals. In: Quesenberry KE, Carpenter JW, eds. Ferrets, Rabbits and Rodents, 4th ed. Clinical Medicine and Surgery. 2021. St. Louis: Saunders, 2020:595–608.
Morrisey JK, Malakoff RJ. Cardiovascular and other diseases of ferrets. In: Quesenberry KE, Carpenter JW, eds. Ferrets, Rabbits and Rodents, 4th ed. Clinical Medicine and Surgery. 2021. St. Louis: Saunders, 2020:5–70.
Van Zeeland YA, Schoemaker N. Ferret cardiology. Vet Clin Exot Anim 2022;25:541–562.
Williams BH, Wyre NR. Neoplasia in ferrets. In: Quesenberry KE, Carpenter JW, eds. Ferrets, Rabbits and Rodents, 4th ed. Clinical Medicine and Surgery. 2021. St. Louis: Saunders, 2020:92–108.
Author Barbara Oglesbee, DVM, DABVP (Avian)

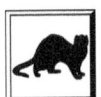

BASICS

DEFINITION
• A sign of sensory dysfunction that produces incoordination of the limbs, head, and/or trunk
• Three clinical types—sensory (proprioceptive), vestibular, and cerebellar; all produce changes in limb coordination, but vestibular and cerebellar ataxia also produce changes in head and neck movement.

PATHOPHYSIOLOGY

Sensory
• Proprioceptive pathways in the spinal cord relay limb and trunk position to the brain.
• When the spinal cord is slowly compressed, proprioceptive deficits are usually the first signs observed, because these pathways are located more superficially in the white matter and their larger sized axons are more susceptible to compression than are other tracts.
• Generally accompanied by weakness owing to early concomitant upper motor neuron involvement

Cerebellar
• The cerebellum regulates, coordinates, and smoothes motor activity.
• Proprioception is normal because the ascending proprioceptive pathways to the cortex are intact; weakness does not occur because the upper motor neurons are intact.
• Inadequacy in the performance of motor activity; strength preservation; no proprioceptive deficits

Vestibular (unusual in ferrets)
• Diseases that affect the vestibular receptors, the nerve in the inner ear, or the nuclei in the brainstem cause various degrees of disequilibrium with ensuing vestibular ataxia.
• Affected animal leans, tips, falls, or even rolls toward the side of the lesion; may be accompanied by head tilt

SYSTEMS AFFECTED
Nervous—spinal cord (and brainstem); cerebellum; vestibular system

SIGNALMENT
Any age or sex

SIGNS
• Important to define the type of ataxia to localize the problem
• Only hind limbs affected—likely weakness due to systemic or metabolic disease (most common cause of ataxia in ferrets), or a spinal cord disorder
• Only one limb involved—consider a lameness problem
• All or both ipsilateral limbs affected—cerebellar
• Head tilt—vestibular (rare)

CAUSES

Metabolic (most common cause of rear limb ataxia)
• Hypoglycemia from insulinomas—extremely common cause
• Electrolyte disturbances—especially with GI foreign bodies, severe hepatic disease, or sepsis
• Anemia—seen with hyperestrogenism, leukemia, and CRF

Neurologic
Spinal Cord (most common neurologic cause)
• Neoplastic—primary bone tumors (esp. chondroma, chondrosarcoma); multiple myeloma and metastatic tumors that infiltrate the vertebral body (especially lymphoma)
• Traumatic—intervertebral disc herniation; fracture or luxation
• Infectious—discospondylitis (rare)

Cerebellar
• Neoplastic—any tumor of the CNS (primary or secondary) localized to the cerebellum
• Infectious—canine distemper virus; rabies (rear limb ataxia may be the only clinical sign in ferrets with rabies) and any other CNS infection affecting the cerebellum
• Inflammatory, idiopathic, immune-mediated—ADV-induced encephalomyelitis
• Toxic—metronidazole

Vestibular
• Infectious—canine distemper virus; otitis media or interna (rare)
• Neoplastic
• Traumatic
• Inflammatory, immune-mediated—ADV-induced meningoencephalomyelitis
• Toxic—metronidazole

Miscellaneous
• Respiratory compromise
• Cardiac compromise
• Drugs—acepromazine; antihistamines; antiepileptic

RISK FACTORS
N/A

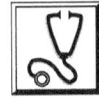

DIAGNOSIS

DIFFERENTIAL DIAGNOSIS
• Differentiate the types of ataxia
• Differentiate from other disease processes that can affect gait—musculoskeletal; metabolic; cardiovascular; respiratory
• Musculoskeletal disorders—typically produce lameness and a reluctance to move

• Systemic illness and endocrine, cardiovascular, and metabolic disorders—can cause ataxia, especially of the pelvic limbs; usually other signs present such as weight loss, inappetence, ptyalism, hair loss, murmurs, arrhythmias, or collapse with exercise suspect a non-neurologic cause; obtain minimum data from hemogram, biochemistry analysis, and urinalysis.
• Head tilt or nystagmus—likely vestibular
• Intention tremors of the head or hypermetria—likely cerebellar; sometimes metabolic disease
• Only limbs affected—likely spinal cord dysfunction if all four limbs affected: lesion is in the cervical area or is multifocal to diffuse. Only pelvic limbs affected: may be metabolic disease or spinal cord dysfunction; spinal lesion is anywhere below the second thoracic vertebra

CBC/BIOCHEMISTRY/URINALYSIS
Normal unless metabolic cause (e.g., hypoglycemia, electrolyte imbalance, and anemia)

OTHER LABORATORY TESTS
• Hypoglycemia—simultaneous fasting glucose and insulin determination—may be supportive of a diagnosis of insulinoma if the insulin assay used has been validated for use in ferrets. Do not fast the ferret for longer than 4–6 hours. Monitor blood glucose concentrations every 30–60 minutes and discontinue testing when glucose concentration falls below 70 mg/dL.
• Anemia—differentiates as nonregenerative or regenerative on the basis of the reticulocyte count or bone marrow aspirate.
• Electrolyte imbalance—correct the problem; see if ataxia resolves.
• Serum electrophoresis—hypergammaglobulinemia (gammaglobulins >20% of total protein) seen in ferrets with ADV.
   Fluorescent antibody test (IFA)—to rule out CDV; can be performed on peripheral blood or buffy coat smears, conjunctival or mucous membrane scrapings. False negatives may occur. Vaccination will not affect the results.

IMAGING
• Spinal radiographs—if spinal cord dysfunction suspected
• Bullae radiographs—if peripheral vestibular disease is suspected (rare in ferrets); CT or MRI scans superior
• Thoracic radiographs—identify neoplasia, cardiopulmonary disease
• CT or MRI—if cerebellar disease suspected; evaluate potential brain disease
• Abdominal ultrasonography—if neoplasia, hepatic, renal, adrenal, or pancreatic dysfunction suspected
• Echocardiography—if cardiac disease is suspected

ATAXIA

FERRETS

DIAGNOSTIC PROCEDURES
- CSF—may confirm nervous system causes
- Myelography—may establish evidence of spinal cord compression. Use 22-g spinal needle; infuse iohexol (0.25–0.50 mL/kg)
- Location for CSF tap or myelography—atlanto-occipital region or L5-L6 region.

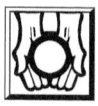

TREATMENT
- Usually outpatient, depending on the severity and acuteness of clinical signs
- Exercise—restrict if spinal cord disease suspected
- Client should monitor gait for increasing dysfunction or weakness; if paresis worsens or paralysis develops, other testing is warranted.

MEDICATIONS
DRUG(S) OF CHOICE
Not recommended until the source or cause of the problem is identified

CONTRAINDICATIONS
N/A

PRECAUTIONS
N/A

POSSIBLE INTERACTIONS
N/A

ALTERNATIVE DRUGS
N/A

FOLLOW-UP
PATIENT MONITORING
Periodic neurologic examinations to assess condition

POSSIBLE COMPLICATIONS
- Depend on the underlying cause
- Spinal cord or neuromuscular disease—progression to weakness and possibly paralysis
- Hypoglycemia—seizures, stupor, and coma

MISCELLANEOUS
ASSOCIATED CONDITIONS
N/A

AGE-RELATED FACTORS
N/A

ZOONOTIC POTENTIAL
Rabies—rare cause of ataxia in ferrets, but when present has extreme zoonotic potential. Rabies cases must be strictly quarantined and confined to prevent exposure to humans and other animals. Local and state regulations must be adhered to carefully and completely.

PREGNANCY/FERTILITY/BREEDING
N/A

SYNONYMS
N/A

SEE ALSO
See specific diseases
Aleutian disease virus (parvovirus)
Gastrointestinal foreign bodies
Insulinoma
Paresis and paralysis

ABBREVIATIONS
ADV = Aleutian disease virus
CDV = canine distemper virus
CNS = central nervous system
CSF = cerebrospinal fluid
CT = computed tomography
IFA = immunofluorescent antibody test
MRI = magnetic resonance imaging

Suggested Reading
Di Girolamo N, Selleri P. Medical and surgical emergencies in ferrets. Vet Clin Exot Anim 2016;19:431–464.
Huynh M, Piazza S. Musculoskeletal and neurologic diseases. In: Quesenberry KE, Carpenter JW, eds. Ferrets, Rabbits and Rodents, 4th ed. Clinical Medicine and Surgery. 2021. St. Louis: Saunders, 2020:117–130.
Johnson-Delaney CA. Geriatric ferrets. Vet Clin Exot Anim 2020;23:549–565.
Kiupel M, Perpiñán D. Viral diseases of ferrets. In: Fox JG, Marini RP, eds. Biology and Diseases of the Ferret, 3rd ed. John Wiley & Sons, 2014:439–517.
Lennox AM, Gladden JN. Emergency and critical care of small mammals. In: Quesenberry KE, Carpenter JW, eds. Ferrets, Rabbits and Rodents, 4th ed. Clinical Medicine and Surgery. 2021. St. Louis: Saunders, 2020:595–608.
Mancinelli E. Neurologic examination and diagnostic testing in rabbits, ferrets and rodents. J Exot Pet Med 2015;24:52–64.
Schoemaker NJ, van Zeeland YRA. Endocrine diseases of ferrets. In: Quesenberry KE, Carpenter JW, editors. Ferrets, Rabbits and Rodents, 4th ed. Clinical Medicine and Surgery. 2021, St. Louis: Saunders; 2020. p. 77-91
Author Barbara Oglesbee, DVM, DABVP (Avian)

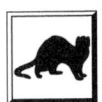

BASICS

DEFINITION
Bradyarrhythmias are defined as bradycardia (<140 bpm in a ferret) associated with arrhythmia. These include sinus bradycardia, sinoatrial block, atrial standstill, and atrioventricular heart block. In humans, there are three types: respiratory sinus arrhythmia associated with vagal tone response, benign sinus arrhythmia associated with well-conditioned athletes, and sick sinus syndrome associated with pathological conditions.

PATHOPHYSIOLOGY
Rhythm disturbances result from abnormalities of impulse formation, impulse conduction, or both. Bradyarrhythmias result from decreased intrinsic pacemaker function or from conduction blockage within the AV node or the His-Purkinje system.

SYSTEMS AFFECTED
Cardiac

GENETICS
N/A

INCIDENCE/PREVALENCE
• A pronounced benign sinus arrhythmia is common and considered to be normal in a healthy ferret.
• Sinus bradycardias can be seen as sequela to insulinomas (hypoglycemia), a common neoplasia of older ferrets.
• Second-degree AV blocks have been reported as normal in some ferrets. More severe AV blocks and other forms of bradyarrhythmias are considered rare or underreported.

GEOGRAPHIC DISTRIBUTION
Worldwide

SIGNALMENT
Species
All ferrets are susceptible.

Breed Predilections
None reported at this time

Mean Age and Range
Benign sinus bradyarrhythmias can be seen at any age. Insulinoma-induced bradycardia would be more typical in ferrets over 2.5 years of age.

Predominant Sex
None

SIGNS
Historical Findings
• Often incidental during examination or anesthetic episode; most animals are asymptomatic
• History of insulinoma

Physical Examination Findings
• Heart rate less than 140 bpm
• Pronounced change in heart rhythm in association with respiration—sinus arrhythmia
• Pronounced change in heart rhythm overall—other bradyarrhythmias

CAUSES
Decreased intrinsic pacemaker function or blocks in conduction within the AV node or the His-Purkinje system.

RISK FACTORS
Concurrent insulinoma, primary cardiac disease, severe systemic disease

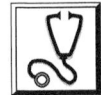

DIAGNOSIS

DIFFERENTIAL DIAGONSIS
• Insulinoma
• Primary cardiac disease
• Other severe systemic disease
• Occlusion of caudal vena cava, such as for surgery of right adrenalectomy in advanced cases

CBC/BIOCHEMISTRY/URINALYSIS
May be useful in identifying underlying disease if present

OTHER LABORATORY TESTS
N/A

IMAGING
Radiographs and echocardiography may reveal underlying structural heart disease if present. Insulinomas are rarely diagnosed by these modalities.

DIAGNOSTIC PROCEDURES
Consultation with an ACVIM specialist or cardiologist is highly recommended.

ECG
• Bradyarrhythmia with no relationship between P waves and QRS complexes indicates AV dissociation.
• Regular QRS rhythm with 1:1 relationship between P waves and QRS complexes indicates no AV block.
• P waves preceding QRS complexes indicate sinus bradycardia (if P waves normal) or sinus arrest with escape atrial bradycardia (if P waves abnormal).
• P waves after QRS complexes indicate sinus arrest with junctional or ventricular escape rhythm and retrograde atrial activation; ventricular escape rhythm results in wide QRS complex while junctional escape rhythm usually has narrow QRS
• When QRS rhythm irregular, P waves usually outnumber QRS complexes; some P waves produce QRS complexes, but some do not (second-degree AV block).

• Irregular QRS rhythm with 1:1 relationship between P waves and following QRS complexes usually indicates sinus arrhythmia with gradual acceleration and deceleration of sinus rate (if P waves normal).
• Pauses in otherwise regular QRS rhythm may be caused by blocked P waves, sinus arrest, or sinus exit block, as well as by second-degree AV block.

Atropine Response Test
Administer 0.04 mg/kg atropine IM and repeat ECG in 20–30 minutes to determine whether AV block is due to high vagal tone.

PATHOLOGIC FINDINGS
• Variable, depending on underlying cause
• Often heart appears grossly normal

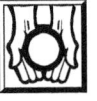

TREATMENT

APPROPRIATE HEALTH CARE
• Treat underlying primary insulinoma, primary cardiac disease, or systemic disease as appropriate.
• If an arrhythmia of concern, treat as if a feline; no ferret-specific recommendations

NURSING CARE
Treat symptomatically and for underlying etiology when appropriate

ACTIVITY
Dependent on severity and cause, best to allow ferret to self-regulate

DIET
N/A

CLIENT EDUCATION
Similar to feline guidance for clinically relevant arrhythmias

SURGICAL CONSIDERATIONS
Placement of a pacemaker may be considered, but decision should be deferred to cardiologist

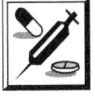

MEDICATIONS

DRUG(S) OF CHOICE
• Atropine (0.02–0.04 mg/kg SC, IM) may be helpful in diagnosis and control of bradyarrhythmias.
• Third-degree heart block: isoproterenol (40–50 µg/kg PO q12h or 20–25 µg/kg SC, IM q4–6h) or metaproterenol (0.25–1.0 mg/kg PO q12h). Generally, parenteral administration has best success in treating block, but often not practical.
• Corticosteroids may be helpful if managing patient with bradyarrhythmias secondary to insulinoma

BRADYARRHYTHMIAS   (CONTINUED)

FERRETS

CONTRINDICATIONS
N/A

PRECAUTIONS
N/A

ALTERNATIVE DRUGS
N/A

 FOLLOW-UP

PATIENT MONITORING
Recheck auscultation and ECG recommended weekly to monthly if addressing underlying causes

PREVENTION/AVOIDANCE
None known

POSSIBLE COMPLICATIONS
- Death
- Pulmonary edema
- Ascites
- Weakness
- Seizures

EXPECTED COURSE AND PROGNOSIS
Variable from incidental finding to death

 MISCELLANEOUS

ASSOCIATED CONDITIONS
- Insulinoma
- Primary cardiac disease
- Severe generalized systemic disease

AGE-RELATED FACTORS
Older ferrets more prone to insulinomas and primary cardiac disease, so bradyarrhythmia can occur secondarily

ZOONOTIC POTENTIAL
N/A

PREGNACY/FERTILITY/BREEDING
None

ABBREVIATIONS
ECG = electrocardiography
AV = atrioventricular

SYNONYMS
None

INTERNET RESOURCES
http://www.merck.com/mmpe/sec07/ch075/ch075a.html

Suggested Reading
Calicchio K, Bennett R, Laraio L et al. Collateral circulation in ferrets (*Mustela putorius*) during temporary occlusion of the caudal vena cava. Am J Vet Res 2016;77(5):540–547.

Di Girolamo N, Selleri P. Medical and surgical emergencies in ferrets. Vet Clin North Am Exot Anim Pract 2016;19: 431–464.

Dudás-Györki Z, Szabó Z, Manczur F et al. Echocardiographic and electrocardiographic examination of clinically healthy, conscious ferrets. J Small Anim Pract 2011;52(1): 18–25.

Fitzgerald B, Dias S, Martorell J. Cardiovascular drugs in avian, small mammal, and reptile medicine. Vet Clin North Am Exot Anim Pract 2018;21(2): 399–442.

Malakoff RL, Laste NJ, Orcutt CJ. Echocardiographic and electrocardiographic findings in client-owned ferrets: 95 cases (1994–2009). J Am Vet Med Assoc 2012;241(11):1484–1489.

Morrisey JK, Kraus MS. Cardiovascular and other diseases of ferrets. In: Quesenberry KE, Carpenter JW, eds. Ferrets, Rabbits and Rodents, 4th ed. Clinical Medicine and Surgery. St. Louis: Saunders, 2020:55–71.

Van Zeeland YA, Schoemaker N. Ferret cardiology. Vet Clin Exot Anim 2022;25: 541–562.

Author Eric Klaphake, DVM, DABVP, DACZM

BASICS

DEFINITION
• An acute contagious disease with respiratory, cutaneous, gastrointestinal, and CNS manifestations
• Caused by CDV, a Morbillivirus in the Paramyxoviridae family
• Distemper is uniformly fatal in ferrets.

PATHOPHYSIOLOGY
• Natural route of infection—airborne and droplet exposure through contact with affected animals or fomites
• From the nasal cavity, pharynx, and lungs, macrophages carry the virus to local lymph nodes, where virus replication occurs; spreads via viremia to the surface epithelium of respiratory, gastrointestinal, and urogenital tracts and to the CNS
• Viremia occurs within 2 days of exposure, and virus can be detected in nasal exudates within 5–13 days postexposure.
• Incubation period is 7–10 days
• Shedding from all bodily fluids begins 7 days post exposure
• In unvaccinated ferrets—death occurs from 12 to 35 days postexposure, depending on the strain of virus

SYSTEMS AFFECTED
• Multisystemic—all lymphatic tissues; surface epithelium in the respiratory, alimentary, and urogenital tracts; endocrine and exocrine glands
• Nervous—skin; gray and white matter in the CNS

GENETICS
N/A

INCIDENCE/PREVALENCE
• Ferrets—sporadic outbreaks in unvaccinated colonies and animal shelters
• Wildlife (raccoons, skunks, and fox)—common

GEOGRAPHIC DISTRIBUTION
Worldwide

SIGNALMENT
Species
• Most species of the order Carnivora— Canidae, Hyaenidae, Mustelidae, Procyonidae, Viverridae
• Infection in large cats, marine mammals, and javelinas has also been reported

Breed Predilection
N/A

Mean Age and Range
Young animals are more susceptible than are adults.

Predominant Sex
N/A

SIGNS
• Catarrhal phase occurs 7–10 days postexposure—fever, serous nasal and ocular discharge, sneezing, depression, and anorexia
• 10–15 days following exposure, a characteristic, erythematous, pruritic rash appears on the chin and lips and spreads caudally to the inguinal area.
• Mucopurulent nasocular discharge occurs with secondary bacterial infections, and crusts appear on the eyes, nose, and chin
• Hardening of the footpads (hyperkeratosis) and nose is common.
• Coughing is common, since the primary site of virus replication is the lungs; secondary bacterial pneumonia is common in ferrets not treated with antibiotics.
• Vomiting, diarrhea, and melena occur in some ferrets
• CNS signs are seen in many infected ferrets; signs often (but not always) occur following systemic disease; depends on the virus strain; either acute gray matter disease (seizures and myoclonus with depression) or subacute white matter disease (incoordination ataxia, paresis, paralysis, and muscle tremors); meningeal signs of hyperesthesia and cervical rigidity may be seen in both.

CAUSES
• CDV, a Morbillivirus within the Paramyxoviridae family, same virus that infects dogs; closely related to measles virus, rinderpest virus of cattle, and phocine (seal) and dolphin distemper viruses
• Secondary bacterial infections frequently involve the respiratory and gastrointestinal systems.

RISK FACTORS
Contact of nonimmunized animals with CDV-infected animals (ferrets, dogs, or wild carnivores)

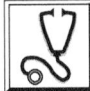

DIAGNOSIS
A presumptive diagnosis of CDV may be made in any unvaccinated ferret with fever as well as characteristic respiratory and cutaneous signs.

DIFFERENTIAL DIAGNOSIS
• Influenza virus—CDV can be difficult to differentiate from influenza virus during the early, catarrhal phase. Influenza is self-limiting, whereas CDV will progress, and dermatologic signs will follow.
• Enteric signs—differentiate from helicobacter, ECE, GI foreign body, inflammatory bowel disease. Respiratory or

dermatologic signs seen with CDV do not occur with these diseases.
• CNS signs—rabies

CBC/BIOCHEMISTRY/URINALYSIS
Lymphopenia during early infection

OTHER LABORATORY TESTS
Immunoflorescent antibody test (IFA)—can be performed on peripheral blood or buffy coat smears, conjunctival or mucous membrane scrapings. False negatives may occur. Vaccination will not affect the results.

IMAGING
Radiographs—determine the extent of pneumonia; lung lobe consolidation is common

DIAGNOSTIC PROCEDURES
Postmortem diagnosis—histopathology, immunofluorescence, and/or immunocytochemistry, virus isolation, and/or PCR; preferred tissues from lungs, stomach, urinary bladder, lymphs, and brain

PATHOLOGIC FINDINGS
Gross
• Mucopurulent discharges—from eyes and nose, bronchopneumonia, catarrhal enteritis, and skin pustules; probably caused by secondary bacterial infections; commonly seen
• Generalized dermatitis
• Footpads and nose—hyperkeratosis
• Lungs—patchy consolidation due to interstitial pneumonia

Histologic
• Intracytoplasmic eosinophilic inclusion bodies—frequently found in the epithelium of the bronchi, liver, and urinary bladder; also seen in reticulum cells and leukocytes in lymphatic tissues
• Inclusion bodies in the CNS—glial cells and neurons; frequently intranuclear; can also be found in the cytoplasm
• Staining by fluorescent antibody or immunoperoxidase may detect viral antigens where inclusion bodies are not seen.

TREATMENT
APPROPRIATE HEALTH CARE
Inpatients and in isolation, to prevent infection of other ferrets and dogs

NURSING CARE
• Symptomatic supportive care may prolong the life of the animal by days to weeks; however, CDV is uniformly fatal in ferrets.
• Intravenous fluids—with anorexia and diarrhea

ACTIVITY
Limited

CANINE DISTEMPER VIRUS   (CONTINUED)

FERRETS

DIET
Depends on the extent of gastrointestinal involvement; offer meat baby foods if anorexic

CLIENT EDUCATION
Inform client that mortality rate is 100%.

SURGICAL CONSIDERATIONS
N/A

MEDICATIONS

DRUGS OF CHOICE
• Antiviral drugs—none known to be effective
• Antibiotics—to reduce secondary bacterial infection because CDV is highly immunosuppressive

CONTRAINDICATIONS
Corticosteroids—do not use because they augment the immunosuppression and may enhance viral dissemination

PRECAUTIONS
N/A

POSSIBLE INTERACTIONS
N/A

ALTERNATIVE DRUGS
N/A

FOLLOW-UP

PATIENT MONITORING
• Monitor for signs of pneumonia or dehydration from diarrhea in the acute phase of the disease.
• Monitor for development of rash or hyperkeratosis
• Monitor for CNS signs.

PREVENTION/AVOIDANCE
• Avoid infection of kits by isolation to prevent infection from wildlife (e.g., raccoons, fox, and skunks) or from CDV-infected dogs or ferrets.
• Recovered dogs are not carriers.

Vaccines
• MLV-CD—prevents infection and disease. Only chick embryo-adapted vaccines should be used in ferrets. The approved vaccines

available in the US are Fervac-D (United Vaccines, Inc., Madison WI) and PureVax (Merial, Athens, GA).
• Canine or ferret tissue culture-adapted vaccines can induce disease and should never be used.
• Begin vaccination at 6–8 weeks of age and vaccinate every 3–4 weeks until the ferret is 14 weeks old, followed by annual boosters.
• Killed vaccines do not offer reliable, consistent protection.

Maternal Antibody
Most kits lose protection from maternal antibody at 6–12 weeks of age.

POSSIBLE COMPLICATIONS
• Hypersensitivity reactions to CDV vaccination are common and may be fatal.
• Signs may vary from pruritus and lethargy to severe reactions characterized by acute, hemorrhagic diarrhea, vomiting, collapse, and rarely, death. Premedication with diphenhydramine (2 mg/kg IM) 20 minutes prior to vaccination is recommended. Monitor ferrets for 30 minutes following vaccination for adverse reaction.

EXPECTED COURSE AND PROGNOSIS
• Death—12–35 days after infection; mortality rate approximately 100%
• Euthanasia—owner may elect once definitive diagnosis is made.

MISCELLANEOUS

ASSOCIATED CONDITIONS
Secondary bacterial rhinitis and pneumonia

AGE-RELATED FACTORS
Unvaccinated ferrets of any age are extremely susceptible to infection followed by death due to CDV

ZOONOTIC POTENTIAL
Possible that humans may become subclinically infected with CDV; immunization against measles virus also protects against CDV infection

PREGNANCY/FERTILITY/BREEDING
In utero infection of fetuses—occurs in dogs, but has not been documented in ferrets

SYNONYMS
Paramyxovirus
Hard pad disease

ABBREVIATIONS
CDV = canine distemper virus
ECE = epizootic catarrhal enteritis
IFA = immunofluorescent antibody test

Suggested Reading
Greenacre CB. Incidence of adverse events in ferrets vaccinated with distemper or rabies vaccine: 143 cases (1995–2001). J Am Vet Med Assoc 2003;223:663–665.
Huynh M, Piazza S. Musculoskeletal and neurologic diseases. In: Quesenberry KE, Carpenter JW, eds. Ferrets, Rabbits and Rodents, 4th ed. Clinical Medicine and Surgery. 2021. St. Louis: Saunders, 2020: 117–130.
Kiupel M, Perpiñán D. Viral diseases of ferrets. In: Fox JG, Marini RP, eds. Biology and Diseases of the Ferret, 3rd ed. John Wiley & Sons, 2014:439–517.
Mancinelli E. Neurologic examination and diagnostic testing in rabbits, ferrets and rodents. J Exot Pet Med 2015;24:52–64.
Moore GE, Glickman NW, Ward MP et al. Incidence of and risk factors for adverse events associated with distemper and rabies vaccine administration in ferrets. J Am Vet Med Assoc 2005;226(6):909–912.
Munday JS, Stedman NL, Richey LJ. Histology and immunohistochemistry of seven ferret vaccination-site fibrosarcomas. Vet Pathol 2003;40(3):288–293.
Perpinan D, Ramis A, Tomás A et al. Outbreak of canine distemper in domestic ferrets (*Mustela putorius furo*). Vet Rec 2008;163:246–250.
Zehnder AM, Hawkins MG, Koski MA et al. An unusual presentation of canine distemper virus infection in a domestic ferret (*Mustela putorius furo*). Vet Dermatol 2008;19:232–238.

Author Barbara Oglesbee, DVM, DABVP (Avian)

BASICS

OVERVIEW
- A slow-growing, low-grade malignant neoplasia thought to arise from cellular remnants of the notochord
- Grows in areas where remnants of notochord remain associated with the spinal cord. In ferrets, this most commonly occurs on the tail tip.

SIGNALMENT
- All ferrets are susceptible.
- Often first noted in young kits (as young as 3 months), slow-growing nature can present as concern at any age.

SIGNS
Historical Findings
Slow growing lump on tail tip, few reports of cervical form with slow growing regional mass

Physical Examination Findings
Irregular, round, white-gray, firm, clublike swelling of tail tip, though can occur at other tail locations

CAUSES AND RISK FACTORS
Neoplastic growth of notochord cell remnants

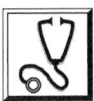

DIAGNOSIS

DIFFERENTIAL DIAGONSIS
- Other bone, soft tissue, or dermatological neoplasia
- Cyst
- Abscess/granuloma

CBC/BIOCHEMISTRY/URINALYSIS
N/A

IMAGING
Radiographs—focally extensive lytic and proliferative vertebral lesion

DIAGNOSTIC PROCEDURES
Histopathology of affected tissue to confirm diagnosis

TREATMENT
Outpatient after surgical removal

CLIENT EDUCATION
Inform that tumors rarely metastasize; progress locally in most cases but should be removed. Non-tail chordomas have a poor prognosis.

SURGICAL CONSIDERATIONS
- Amputation of affected tail region with wide margins
- Submit tissues for histologic diagnosis.

MEDICATIONS

DRUG(S) OF CHOICE
- Pain Management—butorphanol (0.1–0.5 mg/kg SC, IM, IV q4-6h), hydromorphone (0.1–0.2 mg/kg SC, IM, IV q6-8h), tramadol (10 mg/kg PO q12-24h), Gabapentin (3–5 mg/kg PO q8-12h), and meloxicam (0.2 mg/kg SC, PO q24h, reduce to 0.1 mg/kg q24h)

CONTRINDICATIONS/POSSIBLE INTERACTIONS
N/A

FOLLOW-UP

PATIENT MONITORING
Monitor amputation site.

PREVENTION/AVOIDANCE
None known

POSSIBLE COMPLICATIONS
- Death
- Metastasis
- Pathological fracture at site

EXPECTED COURSE AND PROGNOSIS
- Considered malignant, though slow to develop; metastasis can occur but is rare
- Removal is generally curative if on tail tip

Suggested Reading

Camus M, Rech R, Choy F, Fiorello C, Howerth E. Pathology in practice. Chordoma on the tip of the tail of a ferret. J Am Vet Med Assoc 2009;235(8): 949–951.

Frohlich J, Donovan T. Cervical chordoma in a domestic ferret (*Mustela putorius furo*) with pulmonary metastasis. J Vet Diagn Invest 2015;27(5):656–659.

MacPhail C. Ferret soft tissue surgery. In: Bennett A, Pye GW, eds. Surgery of Exotic Animals. Wiley-Blackwell, 2021:277–296.

Munday J, Brown C, Richey L. Suspected metastatic coccygeal chordoma in a ferret (*Mustela putorius furo*). J Vet Diagn Invest 2004;16(5):454–458.

Williams BH, Wyre NR. Neoplasia in ferrets. In: Quesenberry KE, Carpenter JW, eds. Ferrets, Rabbits and Rodents, 4th ed. Clinical Medicine and Surgery. 2021. St. Louis: Saunders, 2020:92–108.

Author Eric Klaphake, DVM, DABVP, DACZM

FERRETS

CLOSTRIDIAL ENTEROTOXICOSIS

BASICS

OVERVIEW
- Clostridial enterotoxicosis is a relatively uncommon disease in ferrets. Two clinical syndromes may be seen with clostridial enterotoxicosis. One is a syndrome characterized by diarrhea due to enterotoxin production by certain strains of enteric *Clostridium perfringens* (CP). The second, more serious syndrome is characterized by acute gastrointestinal bloating due to gas production by CP organisms.
- CP is a common enteric inhabitant generally found in the vegetative form living in a symbiotic relationship with the host.
- Certain strains of CP (type A) are genetically capable of producing enterotoxin that binds to the enteric mucosa, alters cell permeability, and results in cell damage and/or subsequent cell death. Depending on the strain of organism and host defenses, CP may cause mild disease with anorexia and diarrhea, or life-threatening disease characterized by severe abdominal distention, GI bloating, and in some cases, peracute death.
- Enterotoxin production is associated with enteric sporulation of CP.
- A number of intrinsic host-related factors appear to influence enterotoxin production and pathogenicity of CP.

SIGNALMENT
- A relatively uncommon disease in ferrets; often a co-pathogen
- No age or sex predilections

SIGNS
General Comments
Clinical syndromes are associated with either diarrhea or serious, life-threatening disease associated with severe gastrointestinal bloating.

Historical Findings
- Most common—large or small bowel diarrhea, often green in color with mucus, small amounts of fresh blood, small scant stools, and tenesmus with an increased frequency of stools; other signs include anorexia, abdominal discomfort, or generalized unthriftiness
- Occasionally, acute severe bloating of the stomach and/or small intestines with gas occurs (bloat syndrome). Severity of signs depend on the degree of gastric/intestinal distension, which may vary from moderate to severe. Signs include acute depression, ptyalism, anorexia, weakness, collapse, or

acute death. Owners may note progressive abdominal distension.
- May be a history of prolonged antibiotic use
- Severe acute bloat syndrome has been associated with eating rancid whole prey (ferrets often hide food then eat days later) or household garbage
- May be a nosocomial (hospital acquired) disease with signs precipitated during or shortly following hospitalization or boarding

Physical Examination Findings
Mild to moderate diarrhea
- Abdominal discomfort and gas- or fluid-filled intestines may be detected on palpation.
- May be evidence of blood or mucus in the feces

Bloat syndrome
- Abdominal distension
- Tympanic cranial abdomen
- Tachycardia
- Tachypnea
- Signs of hypovolemic shock (e.g., pale mucous membranes, decreased capillary refill time, and weak pulses)

CAUSES AND RISK FACTORS
- Not known if enterotoxigenic CP is a true acquired infection or an opportunistic pathogen.
- Only certain strains of CP can produce enterotoxin, and certain animals are affected clinically.
- Disease may be associated with small intestinal bacterial overgrowth.
- Clostridia overgrowth may occur secondary to prolonged antibiotic use.
- Stress factors to the gastrointestinal tract, dietary change, concurrent disease, or hospitalization may initiate disease.
- Bloat syndrome has been reported following overeating of meat, or unsanitary feeding conditions, but has also been seen following hospitalization and/or surgical procedures.
- Overgrowth of CP may occur secondary to GI foreign bodies or other concurrent gastrointestinal disease.

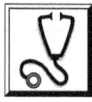

DIAGNOSIS
Patients with chronic intermittent clinical signs—always evaluate during the onset of episodes.

DIFFERENTIAL DIAGNOSIS
- More common causes of diarrhea in ferrets include epizootic catarrhal enteritis (ECE), infiltrative GI tract diseases (lymphoma, inflammatory bowel diseases)

- Consider all causes of diarrhea, including systemic or metabolic disease, as well as specific intestinal disorders.
- For bloat syndrome, consider GI foreign body, aerophagia, gastrointestinal outflow obstruction

CBC/BIOCHEMISTRY/URINALYSIS
- With mild/moderate diarrhea—usually normal
- With bloat syndrome, expect hemogram abnormalities consistent with acute inflammation and hemoconcentration/shock; electrolyte abnormalities and acid–base alterations may be seen.

OTHER LABORATORY TESTS
Fecal direct examination, fecal flotation, zinc sulfate centrifugation to rule out gastrointestinal parasites in patients with diarrhea

Microbiology
Anaerobic fecal cultures may demonstrate high concentrations of CP organisms but occasionally are negative due to the fastidious nature of the organism.

Fecal Cytology
- Large numbers of CP spores in the feces in a patient with evidence of clinical disease
- Cytology—make a thin fecal smear on a microscope slide, air dry or heat fix, and stain with Diff-Quick or Wright's stain or use malachite green, a specific spore stain.
- CP spores have a "safety-pin" appearance—an oval structure with a dense body at one end of the spore wall; bacteria with terminal spores may also be seen.
- Examine for spores shortly after onset of clinical signs.

IMAGING
- Radiographs may be normal in ferrets with mild to moderate disease; occasionally, excessive amount of gas is visible in the large and/or small bowel.
- With bloat syndrome, moderate to severe gastric, small, and/or large bowel gas distension.

DIAGNOSTIC PROCEDURES
- Exploratory laparotomy may be needed to evaluate the extent of gastric pathology and to rule out GI foreign bodies, neoplasia, and intestinal inflammatory diseases.
- Abdominocentesis and cytology may help determine if perforation has occurred in ferrets with gastric bloat.

PATHOLOGIC FINDINGS
With bloat syndrome, grossly dilated, thin-walled stomach and intestines, diffuse necrosis of mucosa on histologic examination

TREATMENT

APPROPRIATE HEALTH CARE
• Most patients with mild to moderate diarrhea can be treated as outpatients.
• Hospitalize when diarrhea is severe, resulting in dehydration and electrolyte imbalance; administer supportive fluids based on hydration status.
• Bloat syndrome requires inpatient management.
• Patients require immediate medical therapy with special attention to establishing improved cardiovascular function and gastric decompression.
• Shock/fluid therapy should accompany gastric decompression; give isotonic fluids at the rate of 90 mL/kg within the first 30–60 minutes, the general treatment of choice for hypovolemic (shock) patients.
• Supportive fluids based on hydration status are recommended for animals not in shock.
• Gastric decompression by orogastric intubation with an appropriate-sized rubber catheter may be necessary
• Orogastric intubation may need to be repeated to maintain gastric decompression.

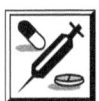

MEDICATIONS

DRUG(S) OF CHOICE

Antibiotics
• Most patients respond well to appropriate antibiotic therapy (e.g., amoxicillin 20–30 mg/kg PO, SC q8–12h), clindamycin (5.5–10 mg/kg PO q12h), or metronidazole (20 mg/kg PO q12h).
• Patients with chronic disease may require prolonged antibiotic therapy.
• For pain relief with mild to moderate GI distention—buprenorphine (0.01–0.05 mg/kg SC, IM, IVq6–12h), butorphanol (0.2–0.5 mg/kg SC, IM, IV q8–12h)

CONTRAINDICATIONS
N/A

PRECAUTIONS
N/A

POSSIBLE INTERACTIONS
N/A

ALTERNATIVE DRUGS
N/A

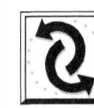

FOLLOW-UP

PATIENT MONITORING
• Monitor patients closely for recurrence of dilation or cardiorespiratory decompensation.
• Response to therapy supports the diagnosis; repeat diagnostics are rarely necessary.

PREVENTION/AVOIDANCE
Infection is associated with environmental contamination; disinfection is difficult.

POSSIBLE COMPLICATIONS
• Gastrointestinal necrosis or rupture may occur after treatment.
• Gastric dilation may recur.

EXPECTED COURSE AND PROGNOSIS
• Most animals with mild to moderate diarrhea respond well to therapy; chronic patients may require long-term therapy; failure to respond suggests concurrent disease; further diagnostic evaluation is indicated.
• The prognosis is fair to grave following gastrointestinal bloat, depending on the degree of distension and time elapsed to treatment.

MISCELLANEOUS

ASSOCIATED CONDITIONS
Frequently other enteric disease

AGE-RELATED FACTORS
N/A

ZOONOTIC POTENTIAL
Unknown

PREGNANCY/FERTILITY/BREEDING
N/A

SYNONYMS
Bloat syndrome

SEE ALSO
Diarrhea
Gastrointestinal foreign bodies
Inflammatory bowel disease

ABBREVIATIONS
CP = *Clostridium perfringens*
ECE = epizootic catarrhal enteritis
GI = gastrointestinal

Suggested Reading
Di Girolamo N, Selleri P. Medical and surgical emergencies in ferrets. Vet Clin Exot Anim 2016;19:431–464.
Hoefer HL. Gastrointestinal diseases of ferrets. In: Quesenberry KE, Carpenter JW, eds. Ferrets, Rabbits, and Rodents, 4th ed. Clinical Medicine and Surgery. 2021. St. Louis: Saunders, 2020:27–38.
Huynh M, Pignon C. Gastrointestinal disease in exotic small mammals. J Exot Pet Med 2013;22(2):118–131.
Johnson-Delaney CA. Geriatric ferrets. Vet Clin Exot Anim Pract 2020;23(3):549–565.
Livingstone M. Dealing with gastrointestinal disease in ferrets. In Practice 2022;44:169–179.
Murray J, Kiupel M, Maes RK. Ferret coronavirus-associated diseases. Vet Clin North Am Exot Anim Pract 2010;13(3):543–560.
Powers LV. Bacterial and parasitic diseases of ferrets. Vet Clin North Am Exot Anim Pract 2009;12:531–561.

Author Barbara Oglesbee, DVM, DABVP-Avian

FERRETS

COCCIDIOSIS

FERRETS

BASICS

OVERVIEW
- An enteric infection, associated with *Isospora* spp. in pet ferrets; *Eimeria* spp. has been reported to cause disease in laboratory and free-ranging ferrets.
- Strictly host specific (i.e., no cross transmission)
- Usually asymptomatic infection in adults; may cause moderate to severe clinical disease in young ferrets
- Asexual multiplication occurs in intestinal epithelial cells, causes cellular damage and disease
- Following asexual multiplication, sexual reproduction results in shedding of oocysts in the feces.
- Oocysts become infective 1–4 days after shedding in the feces.
- May be a co-pathogen with *Desulfovibrio* spp. (proliferative bowel disease)
- Occasionally, hepatic infection in young ferrets

SIGNALMENT
Young ferrets, usually 6–16 weeks of age

SIGNS
- Often asymptomatic
- Rectal prolapse
- Watery-to-mucoid, sometimes blood-tinged, diarrhea
- Tenesmus
- Weakness, lethargy, dehydration, and weight loss with severe infection or hepatic infection
- Thickened, ropy intestines and enlarged mesenteric lymph nodes may be palpable.
- With hepatic involvement, may see jaundice

CAUSES AND RISK FACTORS
- Infected ferrets contaminating environment with oocysts of *Isospora* spp. or *Eimeria* spp.
- Stress
- Enteric infection with *Desulfovibrio* spp. or other co-pathogens

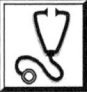

DIAGNOSIS

DIFFERENTIAL DIAGNOSIS
- Consider all causes of diarrhea, including systemic or metabolic disease, as well as specific intestinal disorders.
- Blood and mucus in stool is also seen with *Desulfovibrio* spp., *Clostridia*, *Campylobacter*, and *Salmonella*. These organisms all can cause disease alone or be co-pathogens with coccidia.
- Wasting, thickened GI tract and palpable mesenteric lymph nodes—consider ECE, *Desulfovibrio*, *Clostridia*, *Campylobacter*, and lymphoma

CBC/BIOCHEMISTRY/URINALYSIS
- Usually normal; may see hemoconcentration if dehydrated
- Increased liver enzymes, and bile acids with hepatic involvement

OTHER LABORATORY TESTS
N/A

IMAGING
N/A

DIAGNOSTIC PROCEDURES
- Fecal examination for oocysts using routine fecal floatation
- Oocysts range in size from 10 to 45 μm.

TREATMENT
- Usually treated as an outpatient
- Inpatient if debilitated
- Fluid therapy if dehydrated

MEDICATIONS

DRUG(S) OF CHOICE
- Sulfadimethoxine—(50 mg/kg PO on the first day, then 30 mg/kg q24h or 9 days)
- Sulfadiazine-trimethoprim (30 mg/kg q24h PO for 14d)
- Amprolium (19 mg/kg PO q24h) for at least 2 weeks

CONTRAINDICATIONS/POSSIBLE INTERACTIONS
N/A

FOLLOW-UP
Fecal examination for oocysts 1–2 weeks following treatment

MISCELLANEOUS

AGE-RELATED FACTORS
Disease in young patients 6–16 weeks old

SEE ALSO
Proliferative bowel disease
Epizootic catarrhal enteritis
Dyschezia and hematochezia

ABBREVIATIONS
ECE = epizootic catarrhal enteritis
PBD = proliferative bowel disease

Suggested Reading
Di Girolamo N, Selleri P. Medical and surgical emergencies in ferrets. Vet Clin Exot Anim 2016;19:431–464.
Hoefer HL. Gastrointestinal diseases of ferrets. In: Quesenberry KE, Carpenter JW, eds. Ferrets, Rabbits, and Rodents, 4th ed. Clinical Medicine and Surgery. 2021. St. Louis: Saunders, 2020:27–38.
Huynh M, Pignon C. Gastrointestinal disease in exotic small mammals. J Exot Pet Med 2013;22(2):118–131.
Johnson-Delaney CA. Geriatric ferrets. Vet Clin Exot Anim Pract 2020;23(3):549–565.
Livingstone M. Dealing with gastrointestinal disease in ferrets. In Practice 2022;44: 169–179.
Murray J, Kiupel M, Maes RK. Ferret coronavirus-associated diseases. Vet Clin North Am Exot Anim Pract 2010;13(3): 543–560.
Powers LV. Bacterial and parasitic diseases of ferrets. Vet Clin North Am Exot Anim Pract 2009;12:531–561.

Author Barbara Oglesbee, DVM, DABVP-Avian

CONGESTIVE HEART FAILURE

BASICS

DEFINITION
• Left-sided congestive heart failure (L-CHF)—failure of the left side of the heart to advance blood at a sufficient rate to meet the metabolic needs of the patient or to prevent blood from pooling within the pulmonary venous circulation
• Right-sided congestive heart failure (R-CHF)—failure of the right side of the heart to advance blood at a sufficient rate to meet the metabolic needs of the patient or to prevent blood from pooling within the systemic venous circulation

PATHOPHYSIOLOGY
• The most common causes of CHF in the ferret are dilated cardiomyopathy (DCM) and acquired valvular disease.
• L-CHF: Low cardiac output causes lethargy, exercise intolerance, syncope, and prerenal azotemia. High hydrostatic pressure causes leakage of fluid from the pulmonary venous circulation into the pulmonary interstitium and alveoli. When fluid leakage exceeds the ability of lymphatics to drain the affected areas, pulmonary edema develops.
• R-CHF: High hydrostatic pressure leads to leakage of fluid from venous circulation into the pleural and peritoneal space and interstitium of peripheral tissue. When fluid leakage exceeds the ability of lymphatics to drain the affected areas, pleural effusion, ascites, and peripheral edema develop.

SYSTEMS AFFECTED
All organ systems can be affected by either poor delivery of blood or the effects of passive congestion from backup of venous blood.

INCIDENCE/PREVALENCE
Very common syndrome in clinical practice, especially DCM

SIGNALMENT
Most commonly seen in middle-aged to older ferrets (>4 years of age)

SIGNS
General Comments
Signs vary with the underlying cause and are often vague.

Historical Findings
• Weakness, lethargy, exercise intolerance—usually manifested as rear limb paresis or paralysis in ferrets
• Anorexia
• Coughing and dyspnea
• Abdominal distension

Physical Examination Findings
L-CHF
• Tachypnea
• Inspiratory and expiratory dyspnea when the animal has pulmonary edema
• Pulmonary crackles and wheezes
• Prolonged capillary refill time
• Possible murmur or gallop
• Weak femoral pulses

R-CHF
• Rapid, shallow respiration if the animal has pleural effusion
• Jugular venous distention or jugular pulse in some animals
• Hepatomegaly
• Splenomegaly (may be due to congestion or incidental finding in older ferrets)
• Ascites is usually a finding later in the course of disease
• Possible murmur or gallop
• Muffled heart sounds if the ferret has a pleural or pericardial effusion
• Weak femoral pulses
• Peripheral edema (very rare)

CAUSES
Pump (Muscle) Failure of Left or Right Ventricle
Idiopathic DCM is one of the most common causes of congestive heart failure in the ferret.

Volume Overload of the Left Heart
• Degenerative valvular disease is the most common echocardiographic finding in ferrets. The aortic valve is the most commonly affected, followed by the mitral valve. Minor insufficiency of the aortic valve is very common and typically does not cause disease. More severe regurgitation can cause LSHF, especially if combined with mitral insufficiency.
• Valvular endocardiosis has also been reported
• Ventricular septal defect anecdotally reported; other congenital defects have not been reported but should be considered

Pressure Overload to Left Heart
Causes reported in other mammals, such as systemic hypertension, subaortic stenosis, or left ventricular tumors have not yet been reported in ferrets. However, these causes should be considered since there is nothing that would preclude these diseases in ferrets, and they may be underreported.

Pressure Overload to Right Heart
• Heartworm disease is the most common cause of R-CHF in the ferret.
• Causes reported in other mammals, such as chronic obstructive pulmonary disease, pulmonary thromboembolism, pulmonic stenosis, right ventricular tumors, or primary

pulmonary hypertension, have not yet been reported in ferrets. However, these causes should be considered since there is nothing that would preclude these diseases in ferrets, and they may be underreported.

Impediment to Filling of Left Heart
• Hypertrophic cardiomyopathy (rare)
• Pericardial effusion with tamponade
• Restrictive pericarditis
• Left atrial masses (e.g., tumors and thrombus), pulmonary thromboembolism, and mitral stenosis have not been reported in ferrets. However, these causes should be considered since there is nothing that would preclude these diseases in ferrets, and they may be underreported.

Impediment to Right Ventricular Filling
• Pericardial effusion
• Restrictive pericarditis
• Right atrial or caval masses and tricuspid stenosis have not yet been reported in ferrets. However, these causes should be considered since there is nothing that would preclude these diseases in ferrets, and they may be underreported.

Rhythm Disturbances
• Bradycardia (AV block)
• Tachycardia (e.g., atrial fibrillation, atrial tachycardia, and ventricular tachycardia)

RISK FACTORS
• No heartworm prophylaxis
• Risk factors for other diseases have not been evaluated

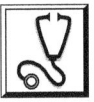

DIAGNOSIS

DIFFERENTIAL DIAGNOSIS
• Rear limb weakness—consider metabolic diseases, including hypoglycemia (especially insulinoma), anemia (hyperestrogenism, blood loss from GI tract, leukemia, and CRF), gastrointestinal foreign body; neurologic disease, including CNS or spinal cord disease, CDV or rabies
• Pleural effusion—mediastinal lymphoma, other neoplasia, abscess, chylothorax
• Cough—infection (influenza virus, CDV, bacterial tracheitis, bronchitis, and pneumonia); neoplasia; heartworm disease
• Dyspnea—intrathoracic fat accumulation, neoplasm (mediastinal lymphoma), primary pulmonary disease, pleural effusion, trauma resulting in diaphragmatic hernia, pulmonary hemorrhage, pneumothorax; airway obstruction due to foreign body
• Ascites, abdominal distension—consider hypoproteinemia, severe liver disease,

CONGESTIVE HEART FAILURE   (CONTINUED)

FERRETS

ruptured bladder, peritonitis, abdominal neoplasia, and abdominal hemorrhage

CBC/BIOCHEMISTRY/URINALYSIS
• CBC is usually normal; may be a stress leukogram
• Mild to moderately high alanine transaminase, aspartate transaminase, and serum alkaline phosphatase with R-CHF
• Prerenal azotemia in some animals

OTHER LABORATORY TESTS
Heartworm serologic testing—ELISA (snap heartworm antigen test, Idexx Laboratories)—may have a false negative if low worm burdens are present or in early infections

IMAGING
Radiographic Findings
• Generalized cardiomegaly—increased sternal or diaphragmatic contact; tracheal elevation. In normal ferrets, minimal or no contact occurs between the heart and the sternum or the heart and the diaphragm.
• In obese ferrets, pericardial fat can mimic cardiomegaly.
• Pulmonary edema (L-CHF) or pleural effusion or both are extremely common findings.
• Hepatomegaly and splenomegaly may be seen (R-CHF); ascites is a common finding
• The different forms of cardiomyopathy cannot be differentiated by radiography.
• Important tool for ruling out mediastinal lymphoma in dyspneic ferrets

Echocardiography
• Echocardiography is the diagnostic modality of choice to differentiate forms of cardiomyopathy, cardiac masses, heartworm disease, and pericardial effusion.
• Findings vary markedly with cause.

DIAGNOSTIC PROCEDURES
Electrocardiographic Findings
• Ferrets resist attachment of alligator clips; use padded clips, soft clips, or sedation to perform ECG; some ferrets may be distracted when fed treats such as Nutri-Cal while performing the ECG
• Pronounced respiratory sinus arrhythmias are common in normal ferrets and should not be over-interpreted.
• First- or second-degree heart block are common findings both in normal ferrets and in ferrets with CHF.
• The ECG of normal ferrets differs from the feline ECG in that R waves are taller, and a short QT interval and/or elevated ST segment are commonly seen.
• Both ventricular and supraventricular arrhythmias can be seen.
• May show atrial or ventricular enlargement patterns.
• Sinus tachycardia (HR >280) is common.

Abdominocentesis
Analysis of ascitic fluid in patients with R-CHF generally reveals modified transudate.

Pleural Effusion Analysis
Pleural effusion typically is a modified transudate with a total protein of less than 4.0 g/dL and nucleated cell counts of less than 2500/mL (these values have been extrapolated from other mammalian species to be used as a guideline). Analysis of the pleural effusion is important to rule out other causes of pleural effusion such as pyothorax, lymphosarcoma, or chylothorax.

PATHOLOGIC FINDINGS
Cardiac findings vary with disease

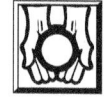

TREATMENT
APPROPRIATE HEALTH CARE
• Severely dyspneic, weak, or anorectic ferrets with congestive heart failure should be treated as inpatients.
• Mildly affected animals can be treated as outpatients.

NURSING CARE
• Supplemental oxygen therapy for dyspneic animals
• Minimize handling of critically dyspneic animals.
• Thoracocentesis is both therapeutic and diagnostic. If there is significant pleural effusion, drain each hemithorax with a 20-gauge butterfly catheter after the ferret is stable enough to be handled. When performing thoracocentesis, be aware that the heart is located much more caudally within the thorax in the ferret as compared to dogs and cats. Sedation—butorphanol (0.2–0.5 mg/kg IM) or midazolam (0.25–1.0 mg/kg IM, SC)
• If hypothermic, external heat (incubator or heating pad) is recommended.

ACTIVITY
Restrict activity

CLIENT EDUCATION
CHF is not curable. Symptoms can be managed but will progress.

SURGICAL CONSIDERATIONS
N/A

MEDICATIONS
DRUG(S) OF CHOICE
Diuretics
• Furosemide is recommended at the lowest effective dose to eliminate pulmonary edema

and pleural effusion. If the ferret is in fulminant cardiac failure, administer furosemide at 2–4 mg/kg q8–12h IM or IV. Initially, furosemide should be administered parenterally. Long-term therapy should be continued at a dose of 1–4 mg/kg q8–12h PO. The pediatric elixir is generally well accepted.
• Predisposes the patient to dehydration, prerenal azotemia, and electrolyte disturbances

Venodilators
• Nitroglycerin (2% ointment) 1/16–1/8 inch applied topically can be used in conjunction with diuretics in the acute management of CHF to further reduce preload. Nitroglycerin will lower the dose of furosemide and is particularly useful in patients with hypothermia or dehydration.
• May be useful in animals with chronic L-CHF when used intermittently

ACE Inhibitors
• Enalapril is recommended for long-term maintenance to reduce afterload and preload. Begin with a dose of 0.25–0.5 mg/kg PO q48h and increase to 0.5 mg/kg PO q24h if well tolerated (see Precautions). Enalapril can be compounded into a suspension by a compounding pharmacy for ease of administration.
• Captopril has also been used (1/8 of a 12.5 mg tablet q48h)

Positive Inotropes
• Pimobendan—(0.5–1.25 mg/kg PO q12h) is a calcium channel sensitizer that dilates arteries and increases myocardial contractility. Used as a first-line agent in treating ferrets with DCM and those with refractory CHF due to valvular disease.

Beta-Blockers
• Propranolol (0.2–1.0 mg/kg q8–12h), atenolol (3.125–6.25 mg/ferret PO q24h), or benazepril (0.25–0.5 mg/kg PO q24h)
• Beneficial effects may include slowing of sinus rate and correcting atrial and ventricular arrhythmias.
• Role in asymptomatic patients unresolved

Calcium Channel Blockers
• Used to treat tachyarrhythmia and/or hypertrophic cardiomyopathy at 1.5–7.5 mg/ferret PO q12h
• Diltiazem (2.5–7.5 mg/ferret q12h)
• Beneficial effects may include slower sinus rate, resolution of supraventricular arrhythmias, improved diastolic relaxation, and peripheral vasodilation, but has not been documented in ferrets

Digoxin
• Digoxin is used in animals with DCM at a dose of 0.005–0.01 mg/kg PO

(CONTINUED)

• Digoxin is also indicated to treat supraventricular arrhythmias (e.g., sinus tachycardia, atrial fibrillation, and atrial or junctional tachycardia) in patients with CHF.

CONTRAINDICATIONS

Positive inotropic drugs should be avoided in patients with HCM

PRECAUTIONS

• Ferrets are very sensitive to the hypotensive effects of ACE inhibitors and may become weak and lethargic. The dosage should be reduced if this side effect is observed or hypotension is documented.
• ACE inhibitors and digoxin must be used cautiously in patients with renal disease.
• Atenolol, enalapril, propranolol, and diltiazem may all cause lethargy, anorexia, and hypotension.
• Overzealous diuretic therapy may cause dehydration and hypokalemia.

POSSIBLE INTERACTIONS

• The use of a calcium channel blocker in combination with a beta-blocker should be avoided as clinically significant bradyarrhythmias can develop in other small animals and are likely to also occur in ferrets.
• Combination of high-dose diuretics and ACE inhibitors may alter renal perfusion and cause azotemia

ALTERNATIVE DRUGS

• Potassium supplementation for hypokalemia; use potassium supplements cautiously in animals receiving ACE inhibitor or spironolactone

FOLLOW-UP

PATIENT MONITORING

• Monitor renal status, electrolytes, hydration, respiratory rate and effort, heart rate, body weight, and abdominal girth.
• If azotemia develops, reduce the dosage of diuretics. If azotemia persists and the animal

is also on an ACE inhibitor, reduce or discontinue the ACE inhibitor. Use digoxin with caution if azotemia develops.
• Monitor ECG if arrhythmias are suspected.
• Check digoxin concentration periodically. Therapeutic range (as extrapolated from dogs and cats) is between 1 and 2 ng/dL 8–12 hours post-pill.

PREVENTION/AVOIDANCE

• Minimize stress and exercise in patients with heart disease.
• Prescribing an ACE inhibitor early in the course of heart disease in patients with mitral valve disease and DCM may slow the progression of heart disease and delay the onset of CHF. Consider this in asymptomatic animals if they have DCM or if they have mitral valve disease and radiographic or echocardiographic evidence of left heart enlargement.

POSSIBLE COMPLICATIONS

• Sudden death due to arrhythmias
• Iatrogenic problems associated with medical management (see above)

EXPECTED COURSE AND PROGNOSIS

Prognosis varies with the underlying cause

MISCELLANEOUS

ASSOCIATED CONDITIONS
N/A

AGE-RELATED FACTORS
• DCM seen in young animals
• Degenerative heart conditions and HCM are generally seen in middle-aged to old animals

ZOONOTIC POTENTIAL
N/A

PREGNANCY/FERTILITY/BREEDING
N/A

SYNONYMS
N/A

SEE ALSO
Dyspnea
Heartworm disease

ABBREVIATIONS
ACE = angiotensin-converting enzyme
CDV = canine distemper virus
CRF = chronic renal failure
DCM = dilated cardiomyopathy
HCM = hypertrophic cardiomyopathy
L-CHF = left-sided congestive heart failure
R-CHF = right-sided congestive heart failure

Suggested Reading
Di Girolamo N, Selleri P. Medical and surgical emergencies in ferrets. Vet Clin North Am Exot Anim Pract 2016;19: 431–464.
Dudás-Györki Z, Szabó Z, Manczur F et al. Echocardiographic and electrocardiographic examination of clinically healthy, conscious ferrets. J Small Anim Pract 2011;52(1): 18–25.
Fitzgerald B, Dias S, Martorell J. Cardiovascular drugs in avian, small mammal, and reptile medicine. Vet Clin North Am Exot Anim Pract 2018;21(2): 399–442.
Malakoff RL, Laste NJ, Orcutt CJ. Echocardiographic and electrocardiographic findings in client-owned ferrets: 95 cases (1994–2009). J Am Vet Med Assoc 2012;241(11):1484–1489.
Morrisey JK, Kraus MS. Cardiovascular and other diseases of ferrets. In: Quesenberry KE, Carpenter JW, eds. Ferrets, Rabbits and Rodents, 4th ed. Clinical Medicine and Surgery. St. Louis: Saunders, 2020:55–71.
Van Zeeland YA, Schoemaker N. Ferret cardiology. Vet Clin Exot Anim 2022;25: 541–562.

Author Barbara Oglesbee, DVM, DABVP-Avian

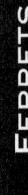

FERRETS

COUGHING

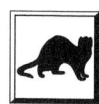

BASICS

DEFINITION
A sudden forceful expiration of air through the glottis, usually accompanied by an audible sound, which is preceded by an exaggerated inspiratory effort

PATHOPHYSIOLOGY
• One of the most powerful reflexes in the body
• Induced by stimulation of either afferent fibers of the pharyngeal distribution of the glossopharyngeal nerves or sensory endings of the vagus nerves located in the larynx, trachea and larger bronchi
• Begins with an inspiratory phase followed in sequence by an inspiratory pause, glottis closure, increased intrathoracic pressure, and glottis opening
• Serves as an early warning system for the pharynx and respiratory system and as a protective mechanism

SYSTEMS AFFECTED
• Respiratory
• Musculoskeletal—because of the role played in the reflex by inspiratory and expiratory muscles of respiration
• Cardiovascular

SIGNALMENT
No age or sex predilection

SIGNS
N/A

CAUSES
Upper Respiratory Tract Diseases
• Nasopharyngeal—rhinitis or sinusitis (influenza virus, bacterial, and CDV); nasopharyngeal foreign body or tumor
• Laryngeal—inflammation; foreign body; injuries; tumors
• Tracheal—inflammation (inhalation of irritating substances and heat); infections (viral and bacterial); foreign body; tumor

Lower Respiratory Tract Diseases
• Bronchial—inflammation; infection (influenza, CDV, and bacterial); foreign body
• Pulmonary/vascular—pulmonary edema; heartworm disease, tumor (esp. lymphoma); infection; aspiration pneumonia

Other Diseases
• Pleural—tumor (mediastinal lymphoma), infection (bacterial and fungal); inflammation
• Esophageal—inflammation; foreign body; tumor

RISK FACTORS
• Esophageal, gastroesophageal, and upper gastrointestinal disorders—predispose the patient to aspiration pneumonia
• Environmental factors—exposure to viral, bacterial diseases; exposure of ferrets to mosquitoes without effective heartworm prophylaxis

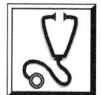

DIAGNOSIS

DIFFERENTIAL DIAGNOSIS
Similar Signs
• Sneezing and coughing—expiratory events that may occur together in certain conditions (e.g., rhinitis, sinusitis, and regurgitation); may confuse both the owner and the history; forceful expiration of a sneeze: mouth usually closed; cough: mouth usually open

Causes
• Patterns and characteristics—may suggest an underlying cause
• Nocturnal—may be associated with early stages of left-sided CHF
• Precipitated by exercise or excitement—frequently the result of inflammation or irritation involving the larynx, trachea, and bronchi
• Harsh and prolonged—suggests the involvement of the major airways
• Productive—suggests fluid or mucus in the expectorated material
• Dry—indicates lack of mucus or fluid production

CBC/BIOCHEMISTRY/URINALYSIS
• CBC—may suggest possible causes: e.g., neutrophilia with infection
• Mild to moderate elevations in ALT—suggest liver congestion secondary to pulmonary disease or right heart failure

OTHER LABORATORY TESTS
• Filaria serologic test—evaluate for heartworm disease; false negatives common as ferrets are rarely microfilaremic
• Serologic tests that identify adult *D. immitis* antigen are of some use; however, false-negative results are common with low worm burdens or early infection—ELISA (snap heartworm antigen test, Idexx Laboratories)

IMAGING
• Radiographs—particularly useful for evaluating patients with nasal, sinus, tracheal, cardiac, and lower respiratory tract disorders
• Thoracic ultrasound—useful for patients with primary cardiac disease and pleural effusion

DIAGNOSTIC PROCEDURES
• Thoracocentesis—with pleural effusion
• CT scan—better evaluate nasal and sinus disorders
• Transtracheal wash with cytologic examination and culture—evaluate lower respiratory tract disorders

TREATMENT
• Outpatient—unless CHF is diagnosed or marked alteration in pulmonary function or hemoptysis noted
• Exercise restriction—best enforced until a cause is established and corrected, especially when activity aggravates the condition
• Inform the client that a wide variety of conditions can be responsible for the cough, and a fairly extensive workup may be required to define and treat the underlying cause.
• Surgical intervention—may be indicated for tumors involving the respiratory system

MEDICATIONS
DRUG(S) OF CHOICE
• Symptomatic treatment without other abnormalities—broad-spectrum antibiotics; bronchodilator-expectorant; appropriate follow-up evaluations
• Collect airway specimens for bacterial culture and sensitivity testing before administering antibiotics.
• Broad-spectrum antibiotics—for suspected infection when results of bacterial culture and sensitivity testing are pending (e.g., trimethoprim/sulfonamide at 15–30 mg/kg PO, SC q12h; enrofloxacin at 5–10 mg/kg PO, SC, IM q12h; or a cephalosporin (Cephalexin 15–25 mg/kg PO q8–12h).
• Bronchodilator—theophylline (4.25–10 mg/kg q8–12h) or terbutaline (0.01 mg/kg SC, IM) with or without the use of expectorants—may be beneficial for a variety of diseases affecting the trachea and lower respiratory airways
• Cough suppressants are rarely indicated in ferrets; avoid in patients with coughs secondary to bacterial respiratory infection and CHF.
• Therapeutic thoracocentesis—perform for any patient with a marked pleural effusion.

FERRETS

(CONTINUED)

CONTRAINDICATIONS
• Corticosteroids—do not use in animals with infectious causes of cough
• Cough suppressants—do not use in any patient in which either a respiratory infection or clinically important heart disease is suspected.

PRECAUTIONS
• Cough suppressants—indiscriminate use may obscure the warning signs of serious cardiac and pulmonary disorders and predispose the patient to serious complications or even death.
• Bronchodilator therapy—may cause tachyarrhythmias
• Diuretics—do not use in patients with primary airway disease; drying of secretions decreases the clearance of mucus and exudate

POSSIBLE INTERACTIONS
Theophylline bronchodilators—clearance may be inhibited by other drugs (e.g., enrofloxacin and chloramphenicol); signs of toxicity may develop with the addition of such drugs

ALTERNATIVE DRUGS
N/A

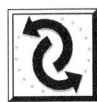 FOLLOW-UP

PATIENT MONITORING
• Follow-up thoracic radiographs—in 10–14 days with bronchopulmonary disease; in 3–4 weeks to monitor potential tumors

POSSIBLE COMPLICATIONS
• Complete control does not guarantee the resolution of the inciting cause.
• Serious respiratory dysfunction and even death may be caused by underlying disease.

 MISCELLANEOUS

ASSOCIATED CONDITIONS
• Heavy breathing
• Dyspnea

AGE-RELATED FACTORS
N/A

ZOONOTIC POTENTIAL
Influenza virus

PREGNANCY/FERTILITY/BREEDING
N/A

SEE ALSO
Canine distemper virus
Congestive heart failure
Influenza virus
Nasal discharge and sneezing
Pneumonia

ABBREVIATIONS
ALT = alanine aminotransferase
CDV = canine distemper virus
CHF = congestive heart failure
CT = computed tomography
ELISA = enzyme-linked immunosorbent assay

Suggested Reading
Capello V, Lennox AM. Diagnostic imaging of the respiratory system in exotic companion mammals. Vet Clin Exot Anim 2011;14:369–389.
Di Girolamo N, Selleri P. Medical and surgical emergencies in ferrets. Vet Clin North Am Exot Anim Pract 2016;19: 431–464.
Fitzgerald B, Dias S, Martorell J. Cardiovascular drugs in avian, small mammal, and reptile medicine. Vet Clin North Am Exot Anim Pract 2018;21(2): 399–442.

Johnson-Delaney CA. Ferret respiratory system: clinical anatomy, physiology, and disease. Vet Clin Exot Anim 2011;14:357–367.
Kiupel M, Perpiñán D. Viral diseases of ferrets. In: Fox JG, Marini RP, eds. Biology and Diseases of the Ferret, 3rd ed. John Wiley & Sons, 2014:439–517.
Lennox A. Respiratory disorders in ferrets. Vet Clin Exot Anim 2021;24:483–493.
Morrisey JK, Malakoff RJ. Cardiovascular and other diseases of ferrets. In: Quesenberry KE, Carpenter JW, eds. Ferrets, Rabbits and Rodents, 4th ed. Clinical Medicine and Surgery. 2021. St. Louis: Saunders, 2020:5–70.
Perpiñán D. Respiratory diseases of ferrets. In: Quesenberry KE, Carpenter JW, eds. Ferrets, Rabbits and Rodents, 4th ed. Clinical Medicine and Surgery. 2021. St. Louis: Saunders, 2020:71–76.
Swenson SL, Koster LG, Jenkins-Moore M et al. Natural cases of 2009 pandemic H1N1 Influenza A virus in pet ferrets. J Vet Diagn Invest 2010;22:784–788.

Author Barbara Oglesbee DVM, DABVP (Avian)

FERRETS

CRYPTOSPORIDIOSIS

FERRETS

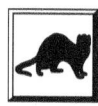

BASICS

OVERVIEW
• *Cryptosporidium* spp.—coccidian protozoan; causes gastrointestinal disease in ferrets, dogs, cats, humans, calves, and rodents; ubiquitous in nature; worldwide distribution; enteric life cycle
• Infection and clinical disease may occur in immunosuppressed ferrets, or as a co-pathogen with other primary gastrointestinal pathogens.
• Infection—when sporulated oocysts are ingested, sporozoites are released and penetrate intestinal epithelial cells; after asexual reproduction, merozoites are released to infect other cells
• Immunocompetent animals—asymptomatic
• Immunocompromised animals—intestinal disease

SIGNALMENT
No sex or breed predilection

SIGNS
• Most infections subclinical
• Intractable diarrhea that may last for weeks; yellow/beige diarrhea, anorexia, and depression

CAUSES AND RISK FACTORS
• Ingestion of contaminated water or feces; feeding raw meat
• Immunosuppression, corticosteroid therapy
• May be co-pathogen or secondary to ECE

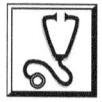

DIAGNOSIS

DIFFERENTIAL DIAGNOSIS
• Dietary indiscretion or intolerance
• Other parasites—giardiasis, coccidiosis
• Infectious agents—ECE, Aleutian disease virus, salmonella, campylobacter, clostridium
• Organ disease—renal, hepatic
• Neoplasia—intestinal lymphoma, insulinoma
• Infiltrative diseases—inflammatory bowel disease

CBC/BIOCHEMISTRY/URINALYSIS
Usually normal, unless an underlying immunosuppressive disease

OTHER LABORATORY TESTS
N/A

IMAGING
N/A

DIAGNOSTIC PROCEDURES
• Sugar and zinc sulfate flotation—specific gravity 5 1.18; concentrate fecal oocysts (oocysts are 3–6 μm so routine salt flotation often fails); oocysts best visualized after staining with modified acid-fast stain
• Submitting feces to a laboratory—mix one part 100% formalin with nine parts feces to inactivate oocysts and decrease health risk to laboratory personal
• Intestinal biopsy—cytologic and histopathologic identification of intracellular organisms; diagnostic but impractical; can produce false-negative results

PATHOLOGIC FINDINGS
• Gross lesions—not well described in ferrets, possibly enlarged mesenteric lymph nodes; hyperemic intestinal mucosa; fix specimens in Bouin or formalin solution within hours of death because autolysis causes rapid loss of the intestinal surface containing the organisms
• Microscopic lesions—parasites may be found on the tips of the brush border of intestinal villi, eosinophilic infiltration of the small intestinal lamina propria

TREATMENT
• Disease is usually self-limiting. Treat underlying disease or co-pathogens. Most recover within 2–3 weeks.
• Mild diarrhea—oral glucose–electrolyte solution
• Severe diarrhea with dehydration—parenteral fluids

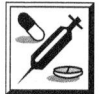

MEDICATIONS

DRUG(S) OF CHOICE
• No reported efficacious treatment in ferrets

CONTRAINDICATIONS/POSSIBLE INTERACTIONS
• Paromycin has been used in other mammalian species; use caution if attempting to use this medication in ferrets, may cause renal failure.

FOLLOW-UP
• Monitor oocyst shedding in the feces 2–3 weeks in immunocompetent animals, longer shedding possible in immunocompromised ferrets.
• Prognosis excellent; if cause of immunosuppression can be overcome, most animals recover within 2–3 weeks

MISCELLANEOUS

ZOONOTIC POTENTIAL
Not reported in humans, but warn clients of potential zoonotic transmission from organisms in feces and that immunocompromised people (HIV infection, chemotherapy, and systemic corticosteroids) may be at risk

ABBREVIATIONS
ECE = epizootic catarrhal enteritis

Suggested Reading
Di Girolamo N, Selleri P. Medical and surgical emergencies in ferrets. Vet Clin Exot Anim 2016;19:431–464.
Hoefer HL. Gastrointestinal diseases of ferrets. In: Quesenberry KE, Carpenter JW, eds. Ferrets, Rabbits, and Rodents, 4th ed. Clinical Medicine and Surgery. 2021. St. Louis: Saunders, 2020:27–38.
Huynh M, Pignon C. Gastrointestinal disease in exotic small mammals. J Exot Pet Med 2013;22(2):118–131.
Johnson-Delaney CA. Geriatric ferrets. Vet Clin Exot Anim Pract 2020;23(3): 549–565.
Livingstone M. Dealing with gastrointestinal disease in ferrets. In Practice 2022;44: 169–179.
Murray J, Kiupel M, Maes RK. Ferret coronavirus-associated diseases. Vet Clin North Am Exot Anim Pract 2010;13(3): 543–560.
Powers LV. Bacterial and parasitic diseases of ferrets. Vet Clin North Am Exot Anim Pract 2009;12:531–561.
Author Barbara Oglesbee, DVM, DABVP-Avian

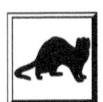

BASICS

OVERVIEW
- A cutaneous fungal infection affecting the cornified regions of hair, nails, and occasionally the superficial layers of the skin
- Isolated organisms include *Microsporum canis, Trichophyton mentagrophytes*
- Exposure to or contact with a dermatophyte does not necessarily result in an infection.
- Dermatophytic pseudomycetoma (DPM) has been reported in ferrets. DPM lesions extend beyond the epidermis and hair follicle to involve the dermis and subcutaneous adipose tissue, resulting in nodular, draining tracts.

SIGNALMENT
- Uncommon disease of ferrets
- Usually occurs in young or immunosuppressed animals

SIGNS
Historical Findings
- Lesions may begin as alopecia, papules, or a poor hair coat.
- A history of previously confirmed infection or exposure to an infected animal or environment is a useful but not consistent finding.

Physical Examination Findings
- Often begins as papules and areas of alopecia
- Scales, crust, erythema—variable, usually in more advanced cases
- Thickening of the skin, hyperkeratosis seen in chronic disease
- With DPM—single or multiple raised, firm draining cutaneous nodules
- Lesions may occur anywhere on the body.

CAUSES AND RISK FACTORS
- Exposure to affected animals, including other ferrets and cats
- Poor management practices
- Immunocompromising diseases or immunosuppressive medications predispose to infection.

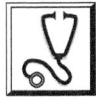

DIAGNOSIS

DIFFERENTIAL DIAGNOSIS
Differentiating Causes
- Ferret adrenal disease—rule out adrenal disease, since this is the most common cause of alopecia and may occur in conjunction with dermatophytosis. Adrenal disease causes bilaterally symmetric alopecia. Alopecia begins in the tail region and progresses

cranially. In severe cases, the ferret will become completely bald. In most cases, the skin has a normal appearance, although some ferrets are pruritic and secondary pyoderma is occasionally seen. Other signs related to adrenal disease, such as a swollen vulva in spayed females, may be seen.
- Seasonal flank alopecia—in intact animals (or females with ovarian remnant), bilaterally symmetric alopecia begins at the tail base and progresses throughout the breeding season (March–August for females, December–July for males)
- CDV—characteristic rash usually follows a catarrhal phase characterized by naso-ocular discharge depression and anorexia. Pruritic, erythematous rash appears on the chin and lips and spreads caudally to the inguinal area; pododermatitis is characterized by hyperkeratinization of the footpads, erythema, and swelling. CDV is uniformly fatal, and signs other than pododermatitis alone will be seen.
- Neoplasia—can be nodular, inflamed, swollen, or ulcerative, depending on tumor type. Mast cell tumors are most common; appear as raised alopecic nodules; may become ulcerated or covered with a thick black crust; may be single or multiple, usually pruritic, and found on the neck and trunk
- Ear mites—partial to complete alopecia caudal to the ears; waxy brown aural discharge; excoriations around pinna; may be pruritic; differentiate by otic examination and skin scrape
- Fleas—patchy alopecia at the tail base and in cervical and dorsal thoracic region; pruritic; excoriations; secondary pyoderma sometimes seen
- Bacterial dermatitis—usually secondary infection—localized or multifocal areas alopecia depending on the primary cause, lesions may appear ulcerated, pruritus sometimes seen
- Sarcoptic mange—two forms reported—local form affecting the feet with intense pruritus and secondary pododermatitis and generalized form with diffuse or focal alopecia and pruritus
- Demodicosis—extremely rare, has been reported in association with corticosteroid use; mites will be present on skin scrape
- Hypersensitivity/contact irritant—uncommon cause; dermatitis localized to the area of contact with an irritant

CBC/BIOCHEMISTRY/URINALYSIS
Not useful for diagnosis

OTHER LABORATORY TESTS
To rule out ferret adrenal disease: Elevations of serum estradiol, androstenedione, and 17-hydroxyprogesterone combined are most diagnostic (available through the University

of Tennessee Clinical Endocrinology Laboratory, Department of Comparative Medicine).

IMAGING
Ultrasonography—evaluate adrenal glands for evidence of ferret adrenal disease

DIAGNOSTIC PROCEDURES
Fungal Culture
- Best means of confirming the diagnosis
- Pluck hairs from the periphery of an alopecic area; do not use a random pattern.

Skin Biopsy
- Necessary for the diagnosis of DPM

Wood's Lamp Examination
Not a very useful screening tool; many pathogenic dermatophytes do not fluoresce; false fluorescence is common; a true positive reaction associated with *M. canis* consists of apple-green fluorescence of the hair shaft; keratin associated with epidermal scales and sebum will often produce a false-positive fluorescence.

TREATMENT

APPROPRIATE HEALTH CARE
- Mild cases may resolve spontaneously with no treatment
- Consider quarantine owing to the infective and zoonotic nature of the disease.
- Environmental treatment, including fomites, is important, especially in recurrent cases; dilute bleach (1:10) is a practical and relatively effective means of providing environmental decontamination; concentrated bleach and formalin (1%) are more effective at killing spores, but their use is not as practical in many situations; chlorhexidine was ineffective in pilot studies.
- DPM—surgical excision of lesions, combined with both topical and systemic treatment may control infection

MEDICATIONS

DRUG(S) OF CHOICE
- Topical therapy—alone or in combination with systemic treatment; miconazole shampoo (with or without chlorhexidine)
- Fluconazole (10 mg/kg PO q12h)
- Ketoconazole (10–15 mg/kg PO q24h) for 4–8 weeks. Anorexia and vomiting have been anecdotally reported.
- Itraconazole (5–10 mg/kg PO q24h) for 4–8 weeks. Available as an oral syrup; fewer side effects anecdotally reported

• Griseofulvin—for treatment of refractory cases or severely affected animals; 25 mg/kg PO q12h for 4–6 weeks; administer with a high-fat meal; gastrointestinal upset is a possible common side effect; alleviate by reducing the dose or dividing the dose for more frequent administration

CONTRAINDICATIONS
N/A

PRECAUTIONS
Griseofulvin
• Bone marrow suppression (anemia, pancytopenia, and neutropenia) reported in dogs/cats as an idiosyncratic reaction or with prolonged therapy; not yet reported in ferrets but may occur; weekly or biweekly CBC is recommended
• Neurologic side effects reported in dogs and cats—monitor for this possibility in ferrets
• Do not use during the first two trimesters of pregnancy; it is teratogenic.

Ketoconazole
• Hepatopathy has been reported in dogs and cats; unknown in ferrets

Itraconazole
• Vasculitis and necroulcerative skin lesions and hepatotoxicity reported in dogs; unknown in ferrets

POSSIBLE INTERACTIONS
N/A

ALTERNATIVE DRUGS
N/A

FOLLOW-UP

PATIENT MONITORING
Repeat fungal cultures toward the end of the treatment regimen and continue treatment until at least one culture result is negative.

PREVENTION/AVOIDANCE
• Initiate a quarantine period and obtain dermatophyte cultures of all animals entering the household to prevent reinfection from other animals.
• Avoid infective soil, if a geophilic dermatophyte is involved.

POSSIBLE COMPLICATIONS
False-negative dermatophyte cultures

EXPECTED COURSE AND PROGNOSIS
• Some animals will "self-clear" a dermatophyte infection over a period of a few months.
• Treatment for the disease hastens clinical cure and helps reduce environmental contamination.
• For DPM—the prognosis is guarded, infection may recur or progress despite aggressive treatment.

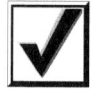

MISCELLANEOUS

ASSOCIATED CONDITIONS
N/A

AGE-RELATED FACTORS
N/A

ZOONOTIC POTENTIAL
Dermatophytosis is zoonotic.

PREGNANCY/FERTILITY/BREEDING
• Griseofulvin is teratogenic.
• Ketoconazole can affect steroidal hormone synthesis, especially testosterone.

SYNONYM
Ringworm

Suggested Reading
d'Ovidio D, Santoro D. Dermatologic diseases of ferrets. In: Quesenberry KE, Carpenter JW, eds. Ferrets, Rabbits and Rodents (4th ed.). Clinical Medicine and Surgery. 2021. St. Louis: Saunders, 2020:109–116.
Fox JG. Mycotic diseases. In: Fox JG, Marini RP, eds. Biology and Diseases of the Ferret, 3rd ed. Ames, IA: Wiley Blackwell, 2014: 573–585.
Giner J, Bailey J, Juan-Sallés C, Joiner K, Martínez-Romero EG, Oster S. Dermatophytic pseudomycetomas in two ferrets (*Mustela putorius furo*). Vet Dermatol 2018;29(5):452–454.
Hoppmann E, Wilson Barron H. Ferret and rabbit dermatology. J Exot Pet Med 2007; 16:225–237.

Author Barbara Oglesbee, DVM, DABVP (Avian)

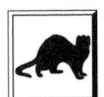

BASICS

DEFINITION
Abnormal frequency, liquidity, and volume of feces.

PATHOPHYSIOLOGY
• Caused by an imbalance in the absorptive, secretory, and motility actions of the intestines
• May or may not be associated with inflammation of the intestinal tract (enteritis)
• Ingestion of osmotically active foodstuffs that are poorly digestible. Fiber content contributes to the osmotic force exerted by a diet. Ferrets should not be fed a high-fiber or high-carbohydrate diet.
• Many of the infectious causes of diarrhea are related to increased secretion. Normally, the intestinal epithelium secretes fluid and electrolytes to aid in the digestion, absorption, and propulsion of foodstuffs. In disease states, this secretion can overwhelm the absorptive activity and produce a secretory diarrhea.
• Inflammatory and infectious diarrhea—often produced by changes in secretion, motility, and absorptive ability; inflammation can also cause changes in intestinal wall permeability, causing loss of fluid and electrolytes and decreased absorptive ability.

SYSTEMS AFFECTED
• Gastrointestinal
• Endocrine/Metabolic—fluid, electrolyte, and acid–base imbalances

SIGNALMENT
No specific age or gender predilection

SIGNS

General Comments
• Patients can be placed into categories according to the severity of their illness. The extent of diagnostic workup and treatment is determined by the category.
• Mild illness—patients are alert, active, and have no other clinical signs.
• Moderate illness—patients remain alert and active but have other clinical signs such as anorexia, vomiting, or weight loss.
• Severe illness—patients are depressed, dehydrated, or listless and may also show signs listed under moderate illness.

Historical Findings
• Chewing habits—young ferrets (usually <1 year old) commonly ingest toys, foam rubber, or cloth
• History of diet change or ingestion of garbage, spoiled food
• History of recent exposure to other ferrets

• History of stress or other causes of immunosuppression
• Past history of acute, infectious diarrhea (e.g., ECE) or clinical *Helicobacter mustelae*
• There may be no history of changes in environment or husbandry in ferrets with IBD

Small Bowel
• Larger volume of feces than normal
• Weight loss and polyphagia with malabsorption and maldigestion
• Melena
• Voluminous stools or "bird seed" consistency to feces may be seen with malabsorptive disorders.
• With many infectious diseases, especially epizootic catarrhal enteritis (ECE; aka "green slime disease"), feces are often mucoid and green.
• Diarrhea can be profuse and recurrent with severe weight loss.

Large Bowel
• Dark, liquid feces; fresh blood; green mucus or mucoid feces
• Frequency of defecation increased, and volume often decreased
• Hematochezia, tenesmus, and/or mucus
• Dyschezia in ferrets with rectal or distal colonic disease
• Rectal prolapse, either intermittent or continuous, may be present
• Weight loss and polyphagia

Physical Examination Findings
• Dehydration
• Emaciation
• Fecal staining of the perineum
• Poor haircoat—seen with chronic disease (infiltrative intestinal disease, hepatic disease, and metabolic disorders)
• Abdominal distention may be due to thickened or fluid-filled intestinal loops, masses, ascites, or organomegaly (especially splenomegaly)
• Mesenteric lymph nodes are often palpably enlarged.

CAUSES
• Bacterial infection—*Helicobacter mustelae* (most common bacterial infection); *Campylobacter* spp., *Clostridium* spp., and *Salmonella* spp. can be co-pathogens or primary pathogens in debilitated or stressed ferrets; *Mycobacterium avium-intracellulare*
• Viral infection—Epizootic Catarrhal Enteritis (very common cause of diarrhea), Rotavirus (rare)
• Infiltrative—lymphoplasmacytic gastroenteritis (very common cause); eosinophilic gastroenteritis (common); proliferative bowel disease common in young ferrets (*Desulfovibrio* spp.)
• Parasitic causes—coccidia, giardia (both are unusual and may be primary pathogens, or

secondary to ECE), *Cryptosporidium* spp. (rare)
• Neoplasia—lymphoma (common cause of diarrhea), adenocarcinoma (unusual)
• Obstruction—foreign body (common cause), neoplasia, intussusception
• Metabolic disorders—common; liver disease, renal disease
• Dietary—very common; diet changes, eating spoiled food, dietary intolerance
• Drugs and toxins—vaccine reaction (hemorrhagic diarrhea with CDV vaccination), plant toxins
• Maldigestion—hepatobiliary disease and pancreatitis (both are rare)

RISK FACTORS
• Exposure to other ferrets
• Dietary changes or inappropriate diet
• Unsupervised chewing
• Feeding raw meat products
• Past history of clinical ECE or *H. mustelae* infection
• Vaccine reaction

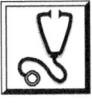

DIAGNOSIS

DIFFERENTIAL DIAGNOSIS

Differentiating Causes
• Melena and anorexia most common with *H. mustelae* or gastrointestinal foreign body
• Thickened intestinal loops and palpably enlarged mesenteric lymph nodes are common with lymphoplasmacytic enteritis, eosinophilic enterocolitis, ECE, or lymphoma.
• Bile-stained (green) mucous-covered diarrhea is seen most commonly with ECE.
• Granular, birdseed-like feces seen with maldigestive/malabsorptive disorders and ECE
• Tenesmus, dyschezia, and rectal prolapse in young ferrets with coccidia or proliferative bowel disease
• A large amount of fresh blood in the feces is more common with salmonellosis.

CBC/BIOCHEMISTRY/URINALYSIS
• Increased hematocrit and serum protein concentration are seen with dehydration
• Anemia may be seen with chronic gastrointestinal bleeding
• TWBC elevation with neutrophilia may be seen with bacterial enteritis.
• TWBC elevation with lymphocytosis or normal TWBC with relative lymphocytosis can be suggestive of lymphoma.
• Eosinophilia (as high as 35%) in ferrets with eosinophilic enterocolitis
• Hypoalbuminemia may be seen with protein loss from the intestinal tract, especially with proliferative bowel disease.

FERRETS

• Serum biochemistry abnormalities may suggest renal or hepatic disease; ALT elevations are usually seen with ECE

OTHER LABORATORY TESTS
• Fecal direct examination, fecal flotation, and zinc sulfate centrifugation may demonstrate gastrointestinal parasites
• Fecal cytology—may reveal RBC or fecal leukocytes, which are associated with inflammatory bowel disease or invasive bacterial strains.
• Fecal culture should be performed if abnormal bacteria are observed on the fecal Gram stain, or if salmonella is suspected.

IMAGING
Radiographic Findings
• Survey abdominal radiography may indicate intestinal obstruction, organomegaly, mass, foreign body, or ascites.
• Contrast radiography may indicate mucosal irregularities, mass, severe ileus, foreign body, stricture, or rarely, thickening of the intestinal wall.
• Abdominal ultrasonography may demonstrate intestinal wall thickening, gastrointestinal mass, foreign body, ileus, or mesenteric lymphadenopathy. Hyperechogenicity may be seen with hepatic lipidosis or fibrosis; hypoechoic nodules are suggestive of hepatic necrosis, abscess, or neoplasia.

DIAGNOSTIC PROCEDURES
Surgical Considerations
Exploratory laparotomy and surgical biopsy should be pursued if there is evidence of obstruction or intestinal mass, and or for a definitive diagnosis of gastrointestinal inflammatory or infiltrative diseases or *H. mustelae*.

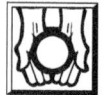

TREATMENT
• Treatment must be specific to the underlying cause to be successful.
• Patients with mild disease usually respond to outpatient treatment.
• Patients with moderate to severe disease usually require hospitalization and 24-hour care for parenteral medication and fluid therapy.

NURSING CARE
Fluid Therapy
• Essential in the treatment of patients with diarrhea. The route and type of fluids will depend on the severity of the disease.
• Subcutaneous and/or oral fluids may be sufficient in patients with mild disease.
• An intravenous route is most effective in severely dehydrated patients. Initially, a

balanced fluid (e.g., lactated Ringer's solution) may be used.
• Correct electrolyte and acid–base disturbances in patients with moderate to severe disease
• Patients with hypoproteinemia may benefit from treatment with hetastarch; administer an IV bolus (10 mL/kg) slowly over 2–3 hours; then as a constant rate infusion of 1 mL/kg/hr for 24 hours, not to exceed 20 mL/kg/day; hetastarch increases plasma oncotic pressure and pulls fluid into the intravascular space.

DIET
• If the patient has been anorectic, assist feed an easily digestible high-protein/high-fat diet such as Lafeber Carnivore Critical Care Diet (Lafeber Company, Cornell, IL) or Oxbow Carnivore Critical Care Diet (Oxbow Animal Health, Omaha, NE); may also add dietary supplement such as Nutri-Cal (EVSCO Pharmaceuticals) to increase caloric content to these foods.
• Easily digestible, high-protein diets such as chicken baby food are often helpful in ferrets recovering from ECE or inflammatory bowel disease.
• The caloric recommendation for sick ferrets is approximately 400 kcal/kg BW per day (although this may be a high estimate).

SURGICAL CONSIDERATIONS
Exploratory laparotomy to remove foreign bodies or tumors

MEDICATIONS
DRUG(S) OF CHOICE
Antibiotic Therapy
• Indicated in patients with bacterial inflammatory lesions in the gastrointestinal tract. Also indicated in patients with disruption of the intestinal mucosa evidenced by blood in the feces. Selection should be based on the results of culture and susceptibility testing when possible.
• Some choices for empirical use while waiting for culture results include trimethoprim sulfa (15–30 mg/kg PO, SC q12h), amoxicillin (20 mg/kg PO, SC q12h), or enrofloxacin (5–10 mg/kg PO, SQ, IM q12h)
• Proliferative bowel disease— chloramphenicol (50 mg/kg, IM, SQ, PO q12h)
• Giardiasis, anaerobic bacterial infections— metronidazole (20 mg/kg PO q12h)
• *H. mustelae*— the combination of amoxicillin (30 mg/kg PO q8–12h) plus metronidazole (20 mg/kg PO q 8–12h) and bismuth subsalicylate (17.5 mg/kg PO q12h

or 1 mL/kg of regular strength preparation [262 mg/15 mL] PO q8–12h) is a common, inexpensive treatment regimen; however, many ferrets find this unpalatable. Dosing every 8 hours may be necessary to eliminate infection. Combine this treatment with an antisecretory agent (see below). Treat for at least 2 (often 3–4) weeks. The combination of clarithromycin (12.5 mg/kg PO q8–12h) and ranitidine bismuth citrate or ranitidine HCl (24 mg/kg PO q8–12h) for 2 weeks has also been reported to be effective in the eradication of *Helicobacter* spp. Ranitidine is no longer approved for human use in the US and can be difficult to find. The combination of clarithromycin (50 mg/kg PO q24h or divided q12h); omeprazole (4 mg/kg PO q24h); metronidazole (20 mg/kg PO q12h) for 14 days has also been used for eradication

Gastrointestinal Antisecretory Agents
• Are helpful to treat, and possibly preventing gastritis in anorectic ferrets. Ferrets continually secrete a baseline level of gastric hydrochloric acid and, as such, anorexia itself may predispose to gastric ulceration. Those successfully used in ferrets include omeprazole (4 mg/kg PO q24h) famotidine (0.25–0.5 mg/kg PO, SC, IV q24h), and cimetidine (10 mg/kg PO, SC, IM, IV q8h)

Corticosteroids
• Often helpful in the treatment of inflammatory bowel diseases (treat underlying disease whenever possible)— prednisone (1.25–2.5 mg/kg PO q24h); when signs resolve, gradually taper the corticosteroid dose to (0.5–1.25 PO mg/kg) every other day

Anticholinergics
• Loperamide (0.2 mg/kg PO q12h) may be helpful in the symptomatic treatment of acute diarrhea (see Contraindications, Precautions).
• Cobalamin—ferrets with chronic diarrhea: 250 µg/kg SC weekly for 6 weeks, followed by 250 µg/kg q2w for 6 weeks, then monthly. Check cobalamin concentrations one month after administration to determine if continued therapy is warranted.

CONTRAINDICATIONS
• Anticholinergics in patients with suspected intestinal obstruction, glaucoma, intestinal ileus, liver disease, enterotoxin-producing bacteria, and invasive bacterial enteritis
• Anticholinergics exacerbate most types of chronic diarrhea and should not be used for empirical treatment.

PRECAUTIONS
• Loperamide may cause hyperactivity in ferrets.

• It is important to determine the cause of diarrhea. A general shotgun antibiotic approach may be ineffective or detrimental.
• Some ferrets will become anorectic when administered high doses of amoxicillin.

POSSIBLE INTERACTIONS
N/A

ALTERNATE DRUGS
See specific diseases for a more complete discussion of treatment.

FOLLOW-UP

PATIENT MONITORING
• Fecal volume and character, appetite, attitude, and body weight
• In patients with ECE, stool may not return to a normal consistency for several weeks. Occasionally, diarrhea will recur months after the initial resolution of clinical signs.
• If diarrhea does not resolve, consider reevaluation of the diagnosis.

POSSIBLE COMPLICATIONS
• Septicemia due to bacterial invasion of enteric mucosal
• Dehydration due to fluid loss

MISCELLANEOUS

ASSOCIATED CONDITIONS
• Septicemia
• Rectal prolapse

AGE-RELATED FACTORS
• Kits 4–6 weeks of age more susceptible to rotavirus
• Inflammatory bowel disease more common in middle-aged to older ferrets
• Older ferrets demonstrate more severe clinical signs with ECE.
• Intestinal foreign bodies, proliferative bowel disease, and coccidia are seen more commonly in ferrets <1 year of age

ZOONOTIC POTENTIAL
• Cryptosporidiosis
• Giardia

PREGNANCY/FERTILITY/BREEDING
N/A

SEE ALSO
Eosinophilic gastroenteritis
Epizootic catarrhal enteritis
Giardiasis
Helicobacter mustelae
Lymphoplasmacytic enteritis and gastroenteritis
Proliferative bowel disease

ABBREVIATIONS
ALT = alanine aminotransferase
CDV = canine distemper virus
ECE = epizootic catarrhal enteritis
IBD = inflammatory bowel disease
TWBC = total white blood cell count

Suggested Reading
Cazzini P, Watson MK, Gottdenker N et al. Proposed grading scheme for inflammatory bowel disease in ferrets and correlation with clinical signs. J Vet Diagn Invest 2020;32(1):17–24.

Di Girolamo N, Selleri P. Medical and surgical emergencies in ferrets. Vet Clin Exot Anim 2016;19:431–464.
Hoefer HL. Gastrointestinal diseases of ferrets. In: Quesenberry KE, Carpenter JW, eds. Ferrets, Rabbits, and Rodents (4th ed.). Clinical Medicine and Surgery. 2021. St. Louis: Saunders, 2020:27–38.
Johnson-Delaney CA. Geriatric ferrets. Vet Clin Exot Anim Pract 2020;23(3): 549–565.
Livingstone M. Dealing with gastrointestinal disease in ferrets. In Practice 2022;44: 169–179.
Murray J, Kiupel M, Maes RK. Ferret coronavirus-associated diseases. Vet Clin North Am Exot Anim Pract 2010;13(3): 543–560.
Watson MK, Cazzini P, Mayer J et al. Histology and immunohistochemistry of severe inflammatory bowel disease versus lymphoma in the ferret (*Mustela putorius furo*). J Vet Diagn Invest 2016;28(3): 198–206.

Author Barbara Oglesbee, DVM, DABVP-Avian

DISSEMINATED IDIOPATHIC MYOFASCIITIS (DIM)

FERRETS

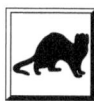 **BASICS**

DEFINITION
• A severe, suppurative inflammatory myopathy of young, domestic ferrets affecting primarily muscle but also surrounding connective tissue
• Characterized by an acute onset of weakness, ataxia, posterior paresis, pain, depression, pyrexia, inappetence, and dehydration, with rapid deterioration
• Also known as DIM, myositis, and polymositis

PATHOPHYSIOLOGY
• Inflammation of mostly skeletal but some smooth/cardiac muscle—results in muscle weakness, myalgia, and atrophy
• The etiology is unknown at this time but believed to be autoimmune or immune-mediated based on similarities to conditions seen in humans and canines.

SYSTEMS AFFECTED
• Neuromuscular—inflammation in muscles and connective tissue, some atrophy
• Gastrointestinal—difficulty swallowing, sometimes diarrhea
• Lymphatic/splenic—enlarged lymph nodes common
• Respiratory—nasal discharge or dyspnea sometimes seen
• Cardiac—heart muscle can be affected

GENETICS
Unknown

INCIDENCE/PREVALENCE
Relatively newly diagnosed condition, so true incidence is unknown; prevalence spiked in 2004–2005 and has since significantly decreased

GEOGRAPHIC DISTRIBUTION
Seen primarily in North American populations at this time

SIGNALMENT
Species
All ferrets are susceptible

Breed Predilections
None reported at this time

Mean Age and Range
Most are less than 18 months of age (5–48 months reported range)

Predominant Sex
None

SIGNS
Historical Findings
• Acute to subacute onset, with rapid deterioration (usually within 12–36 hours)

• May have history of recent vaccination. Early cases were all seen in ferrets vaccinated with a distemper vaccine that is no longer on the market. Since then, no definite correlation with vaccination in confirmed cases.

Physical Examination Findings
Affected ferrets have multiple symptoms, including (in order of frequency):
• Fever (104–108°F)
• Lethargy
• Paresis (especially posterior)
• Depression
• Inappetence
• Dehydration
• Caudal pain (rear legs and lumbosacral region; hyperesthesia)—may vocalize or try to bite
• Abnormal stools (e.g., green stools, diarrhea, and mucoid stools)
• Lymphadenopathy
• SQ masses
• Weight loss
• Tachycardia/heart murmur
• Serous nasal discharge
• Pinpoint, orange dermal lesions
• Ocular discharge
• Labored or congested breathing; coughing; panting
• Bruxism
• Pale gums
• Edema
• Seizures

CAUSES
Unknown at this time, likely autoimmune or immune mediated

RISK FACTORS
Unknown

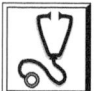 **DIAGNOSIS**

Definitive diagnosis is based on histopathology of affected skeletal muscle

DIFFERENTIAL DIAGNOSIS
• Neoplasia
• Aleutian disease
• Canine distemper
• Coronavirus
• Sarcocystis
• Toxoplasmosis
• Myesthenia gravis
• Toxin
• Trauma
• Intervertebral disc prolapse
• Ferret systemic coronavirus
• Bacterial infection
• Other viral infection

CBC/BIOCHEMISTRY/URINALYSIS
• Eventually develop a moderate to marked mature neutrophilia (occasional left shift) with slight to moderate toxicity of neutrophils
• Mild to moderate anemia (initially nonregenerative but can become regenerative)
• Mild hyperglycemia and hypoalbuminemia
• Mild elevation of ALT
• Paradoxically, there is no elevation of creatine kinase or AST.

OTHER LABORATORY TESTS
• Testing for other infectious diseases, such as Aleutian disease, canine distemper virus, and sarcocystis are all negative.
• Bacterial cultures are negative.

IMAGING
Splenomegaly and enlarged mesenteric lymph nodes are common, nonspecific findings.

DIAGNOSTIC PROCEDURES
Histopathology of skeletal muscle via biopsy for ante-mortem diagnosis. Biopsies from a minimum of three sites are recommended. Suggested sites include lumbar region, hind limbs, shoulder, or temporal muscles. CT, MRI, CSF tap and cytology, EMG, Nerve Conduction Velocity Studies, Tensilon (edrophonium HCL)/physostigmine testing may help rule out other etiologies while awaiting histopathology.

PATHOLOGIC FINDINGS
• Inapparent or subtle gross lesions in acute cases
• Red and white mottling of esophagus
• White streaks in diaphragm, lumbar, and leg muscles
• Marked atrophy of diaphragm and skeletal muscle in advanced cases
• Lymphadenopathy and splenomegaly
• Occasional bronchopneumonia likely secondary to esophageal disease
• Multifocal mild to severe suppurative to pyogranulomatous inflammation in the fascia between skeletal and cardiac muscle bundles, rarely causing necrosis of muscle fibers
• Inflammation can extend into adipose tissue, and muscle atrophy and fibrosis seen in chronic cases

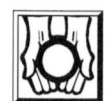 **TREATMENT**

APPROPRIATE HEALTH CARE
Inpatient—provide supportive care while awaiting response to medical therapy, although the prognosis is usually poor, and treatment may be prolonged.

NURSING CARE
Provide general supportive care

ACTIVITY
Often self-limiting due to disease

DIET
Minimize potential esophageal reflux

CLIENT EDUCATION
Prognosis is generally poor; may respond initially to treatment, then relapse; prolonged treatment regimen

SURGICAL CONSIDERATIONS
None

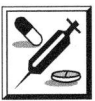

MEDICATIONS

DRUG(S) OF CHOICE
Some ferrets have improved or recovered completely with a combination of three drugs:
• Prednisolone 1 mg/kg PO q12h × 3 months, then q24h until recovered, then wean off
• Cyclophosphamide SQ 10 mg/kg q2w × 2 treatments, then q4w × 3 treatments or until recovered
• Chloramphenicol 50 mg/kg PO q12h × 6–8 weeks

CONTRAINDICATIONS
If disease confirmed, likely mortality outweighs side effects of treatments, but make owner aware of risks of each drug

PRECAUTIONS
Cyclophosphamide—may see GI toxicity or neutropenia; administer subcutaneous fluids to reduce risk of hemorrhagic cystitis

ALTERNATIVE DRUG(S)
Acupuncture may be of benefit.

FOLLOW UP

PATIENT MONITORING
Perform CBC before each cyclophosphamide treatment.

PREVENTION/AVOIDANCE
None known at this time

POSSIBLE COMPLICATIONS
• Death
• Aspiration pneumonia
• Paresis

EXPECTED COURSE AND PROGNOSIS
• Death likely, poor prognosis in most cases; sporadic improvement or recovery has been reported with combination treatment listed above
• Relapse common

MISCELLANEOUS

ASSOCIATED CONDITIONS
Splenomegaly

AGE-RELATED FACTORS
Usually seen in ferrets less than 18 months old

ZOONOTIC POTENTIAL
N/A

PREGNACY/FERTILITY/BREEDING
Unknown

ABBREVIATIONS
None

SYNONYMS
Polymyositis
Suppurative myositis
Myofasciitis

INTERNET RESOURCES
None

Suggested Reading
Antinoff A, Giovonella C. Musculoskeletal and neurologic diseases. In: Quesenberry K, Carpenter J, eds. Ferrets, Rabbits, and Rodents: Clinical Medicine and Surgery, 3rd ed. Elsevier Saunders: St Louis, MO, 2012:132–140.
Garner M, Ramsell K, Schoemaker NJ et al. Myofasciitis in the domestic ferret. Vet Pathol 2007;44(1):25–38.
Müller K, Dietert K, Kershaw O. The first report of a disseminated idiopathic myofasciitis in a ferret (*Mustela putorius furo*) from Germany. Berl Munch Tierarztl Wochenschr 2015;128(1–2):70–75.
Papageorgiou S, Krikonis K, Quinton J-F, Gnirs K. Motor and sensory nerve conduction study in the ferret. J Exot Pet Med 2018;27(4):38–47.
Ramsell K, Garner M. Disseminated idiopathic myofasciitis in ferrets. Vet Clin Exot Anim 2010;13(3):561–575.

Author Eric Klaphake, DVM, DABVP, DACZM

FERRETS

DYSCHEZIA AND HEMATOCHEZIA

BASICS

DEFINITION
- Dyschezia—painful or difficult defecation
- Hematochezia—bright red blood in the feces

PATHOPHYSIOLOGY
- Result from various causes of inflammation or irritation of the rectum or anus
- Hematochezia may also occur with diseases of the colon.

SYSTEMS AFFECTED
Gastrointestinal

SIGNALMENT
- Coccidiosis and proliferative bowel disease (PBD) and seen primarily in ferrets <6 months of age
- No sex or age predilection in ferrets with other types of inflammatory bowel disease

SIGNS

Historical Findings
- Crying out during defecation
- Tenesmus common
- Mucoid, bloody diarrhea in patients with colonic disease
- Severe weight loss, ataxia, weakness, muscle tremors, abdominal discomfort, or generalized unthriftiness in ferrets with severe PBD
- Anorexia, weight loss, muscle wasting, vomiting, ptyalism, and/or pawing at the mouth seen with other types of inflammatory bowel disease and epizootic catarrhal enteritis (ECE)

Physical Examination Findings
- Inflammatory bowel diseases—cachexia; thickened, ropy intestines, enlarged mesenteric lymph nodes and splenomegaly often palpable
- Proliferative bowel disease—distal colon may be palpably thickened, mesenteric lymph nodes may be enlarged; fecal and urine staining of perineum; partial to complete rectal prolapse

CAUSES

Colonic Disease
- Proliferative bowel disease (*Desulfovibrio* spp.)—very common in young ferrets
- Coccidiosis—common cause in young ferrets
- Inflammation—inflammatory bowel disease (lymphoplasmacytic gastroenteritis, eosinophilic gastroenteritis)
- Epizootic catarrhal enteritis (ECE)
- Neoplasia—lymphoma most common, adenocarcinoma

Rectal/Anal Disease (rare)
- Rectal or anal foreign body
- Trauma—bite wounds, etc.
- Neoplasia—adenocarcinoma, lymphoma

Extraintestinal Disease
- Prostatic disease—Prostatic cysts, abscesses, or hyperplasia can occur in middle-aged ferrets with adrenal disease
- Fractured pelvis or hind limb
- Intrapelvic neoplasia

RISK FACTORS
Stress, poor hygiene, concurrent disease

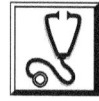

DIAGNOSIS

DIFFERENTIAL DIAGNOSIS
- Dysuria, stranguria, or hematuria—abnormal findings on urinalysis, such as pyuria, crystalluria, bacteriuria with UTI or urolithiasis; hair loss, palpable caudal abdominal mass with paraurethral cystic disease or prostatic hyperplasia

CBC/BIOCHEMISTRY/URINALYSIS
- Usually normal
- May reflect underlying cause (e.g., inflammatory leukogram with infectious disease, eosinophilia with EGE, increased ALT with ECE)
- Hypoproteinemia with chronic diarrhea
- Dehydration—elevated PCV, TP, and azotemia; reflecting fluid loss from the GI tract

OTHER LABORATORY TESTS
Fecal direct examination, fecal flotation, or zinc sulfate centrifugation may demonstrate gastrointestinal parasites.

Microbiology
- Aerobic and anaerobic fecal cultures rule out clostridia or salmonella
- PCR *Desulfovibrio* spp. in ferrets with proliferative bowel disease.
- Fecal cytology may demonstrate *Clostridia* or other organisms, increased WBC or RBC numbers

IMAGING
- Pelvic radiographs may reveal urogenital cysts or prostatic disease, foreign body, or fracture.
- Ultrasonography may demonstrate prostatic disease or caudal abdominal masses.

DIAGNOSTIC PROCEDURES
Definitive diagnosis of inflammatory bowel disease requires biopsy and histopathology, usually obtained via exploratory laparotomy.

TREATMENT
- Most patients with mild to moderate diarrhea can be treated as outpatients.
- Hospitalize when diarrhea is severe, resulting in dehydration and electrolyte imbalance; administer supportive fluids based on hydration status.
- Rehydration is essential to treatment success in severely ill ferrets. Initially, a balanced fluid (e.g., lactated Ringer's solution) may be used.
- Supplementation with 5% dextrose is beneficial in anorectic, hypoglycemic patients
- Proper, strict isolation procedures are essential in patients with suspected infectious diseases.

DIET
- If anorexic, assist feed an easily digestible high-protein/high-fat diet such as Lafeber Carnivore Critical Care Diet (Lafeber Company, Cornell, IL) or Oxbow Carnivore Critical Care Diet (Oxbow Animal Health, Omaha, NE); if these are unavailable, offer chicken baby foods; may also add dietary supplement such as Nutri-Cal (EVSCO Pharmaceuticals) to increase caloric content to these foods.

MEDICATIONS

DRUG(S) OF CHOICE
- Depends on the underlying cause; see discussion under specific diseases.
- For coccidia—sulfadimethoxine—(50 mg/kg PO on the first day, then 30 mg/kg q24h or 9 days) or sulfadiazine-trimethoprim (30 mg/kg q24h PO for 14d) or amprolium (19 mg/kg PO q24h) for at least 2 weeks
- For PBD—chloramphenicol palmitate (50 mg/kg PO q12h × 14d) or chloramphenicol sodium succinate (50 mg/kg PO, IM q12h × 14d) or metronidazole (20 mg/kg PO q12h × 10–14d)
- Antibiotics are indicated in most patients with hematochezia due to disruption of the intestinal mucosa. Selection should be based on results of culture and susceptibility testing when possible. Some choices for empirical use while waiting for culture results include trimethoprim sulfa (15–30 mg/kg PO, SC q12h), amoxicillin (20–30 mg/kg PO, SC q12h), or enrofloxacin (5–10 mg/kg PO q12h)

CONTRAINDICATIONS
N/A

PRECAUTIONS
N/A

POSSIBLE INTERACTIONS
N/A

ALTERNATIVE DRUGS
N/A

 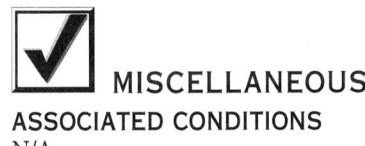

FOLLOW-UP

PATIENT MONITORING
Monitor patients for recurrence of diarrhea or concurrent diseases such as GI ulceration or enteric co-pathogens.

POSSIBLE COMPLICATIONS
• Rectal prolapse
• Dehydration, malnutrition, hypoproteinemia, anemia, and diseases secondary to therapy or resulting from the above-mentioned problems
• May see fecal incontinence with rectal disease

MISCELLANEOUS

ASSOCIATED CONDITIONS
N/A

AGE-RELATED FACTORS
• Coccidia and PBD more common in young ferrets
• Infiltrative (inflammatory, neoplastic) diseases more common in older ferrets

ZOONOTIC POTENTIAL
N/A

PREGNANCY/FERTILITY/BREEDING
N/A

SYNONYMS
N/A

SEE ALSO
Diarrhea
Lymphoplasmacytic enteritis and gastroenteritis
Proliferative bowel disease
Rectal and anal prolapse

ABBREVIATIONS
ALT = alanine aminotransferase
ECE = epizootic catarrhal enteritis
EGE = eosinophillic gastroenteritis
GI = gastrointestinal
IBD = inflammatory bowel disease
PBD = proliferative bowel disease
PCV = packed cell volume
TP = total protein

Suggested Reading
Di Girolamo N, Selleri P. Medical and surgical emergencies in ferrets. Vet Clin Exot Anim 2016;19:431–464.
Hoefer HL. Gastrointestinal diseases of ferrets. In: Quesenberry KE, Carpenter JW, eds. Ferrets, Rabbits, and Rodents, 4th ed. Clinical Medicine and Surgery. 2021. St. Louis: Saunders, 2020:27–38.
Huynh M, Pignon C. Gastrointestinal disease in exotic small mammals. J Exot Pet Med 2013;22(2):118–131.
Lennox AM, Gladden JN. Emergency and critical care of small mammals. In: Quesenberry KE, Carpenter JW, eds. Ferrets, Rabbits and Rodents, 4th ed. Clinical Medicine and Surgery. 2021. St. Louis: Saunders, 2020:595–608.
MacPhail C. Ferret soft tissue surgery. In: Bennett A, Pye GW, eds. Surgery of Exotic Animals. Wiley-Blackwell, 2021:277–296.
Miwa Y, Sladky K. Common surgical procedures of rodents, ferrets, hedgehogs, and sugar gliders. Vet Clin Exot Anim 2016;19:205–244.
Mullen HS, Scavelli TD, Quesenberry KE et al. Gastrointestinal foreign body in ferrets: 25 cases (1986–1990). J Am Anim Hosp Assoc 1992;28:13–19.
Author Barbara Oglesbee, DVM, DABVP-Avian

DYSPHAGIA

FERRETS

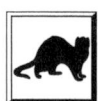

BASICS

OVERVIEW
• Dysphagia may be defined as difficulty swallowing, resulting from the inability to prehend, form, and move a bolus of food through the oropharynx into the esophagus.
• Swallowing difficulties can be caused by mechanical obstruction of the oral cavity or pharynx, neuromuscular dysfunction resulting in weak or uncoordinated swallowing movements, or pain associated with prehension, mastication, or swallowing.

SYSTEMS AFFECTED
• Neuromuscular
• Nervous
• Gastrointestinal
• Respiratory

SIGNALMENT
No breed, sex, or age predilections have been described.

SIGNS
Historical Findings
• Drooling, gagging, weight loss, ravenous appetite, repeated attempts at swallowing, swallowing with the head in an abnormal position, coughing (due to aspiration), regurgitation, painful swallowing, and occasionally anorexia are all possible.
• Ascertain onset and progression.
• Foreign bodies cause acute dysphagia; oropharyngeal disease may cause chronic or intermittent signs.

Physical Examination Findings
• A thorough oral examination, with the patient sedated or anesthetized is most important.
• Observe for asymmetry, foreign body, inflammation, tumor, edema, abscessed teeth, and loose teeth.
• Observe the patient eating; this may localize the abnormal phase of swallowing.
• Perform a complete neurologic examination, with emphasis on the cranial nerves.

CAUSES
• Pain because of dental disease (e.g., tooth fractures and abscesses), mandibular trauma, stomatitis, glossitis, and pharyngeal inflammation may also disrupt normal prehension, bolus formation, and swallowing.
• Anatomic or mechanical lesions—consider pharyngeal inflammation (e.g., abscess, inflammation), pharyngeal or retropharyngeal foreign body, retropharyngeal lymphadenomegaly, neoplasia, temporomandibular joint disorders (e.g.,

luxation, fracture), mandibular fracture, and pharyngeal trauma.
• Neuromuscular disorders—megaesophagus has rarely been reported in the ferret. Cranial nerve deficits that impair prehension and bolus formation and masticatory muscle myositis have not been reported in ferrets but should be considered.
• Rabies may cause dysphagia by affecting both the brainstem and peripheral nerves.
• Other CNS disorders, especially those involving the brainstem, should be considered if an anatomic, mechanical lesion or pain is not found.

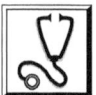

DIAGNOSIS

DIFFERENTIAL DIAGNOSIS
• Must be differentiated from vomiting and regurgitation from esophageal disease
• Exaggerated or repeated efforts to swallow—characteristic of dysphagia; most useful means of distinguishing it from vomiting or regurgitation
• Vomiting is associated with abdominal contractions; dysphagia is not.

CBC/BIOCHEMISTRY/URINALYSIS
• Inflammatory conditions may cause leukocytosis.
• High serum creatine phosphokinase activity may indicate a muscular disorder.

OTHER LABORATORY TESTS
N/A

IMAGING
• Obtain survey radiographs of the skull and neck; give particular attention to the mandibles, temporomandibular joint, teeth, and pharyngeal and retropharyngeal area.
• Ultrasonography of the pharynx may be useful in patients with mass lesions and for obtaining ultrasound-guided biopsy specimens.
• Fluoroscopy, with or without positive contrast, is useful in evaluating pharyngeal movement in other mammals with suspected pharyngeal dysphagia and may have similar value in ferrets.
• Computed tomography and/or magnetic resonance imaging may be useful to identify suspected intracranial mass.

DIAGNOSTIC PROCEDURES
• Excisional or incisional biopsies of a mass lesion
• Pharyngoscopy
• Electromyography of the pharyngeal musculature has been used in other small animals to confirm the presence of a neuromuscular disorder, usefulness in ferrets is unknown.

TREATMENT
• Determine the underlying cause to develop a treatment plan and accurate prognosis.
• Direct primary treatment at the underlying cause.
• Nutritional support is important for all dysphagic patients.
• Patients with oral disease may be able to swallow a gruel or liquid diet; take care to avoid aspiration when feeding orally. Make gruel from chicken baby foods or an easily digestible high-protein/high-fat diet such as Lafeber Carnivore Critical Care Diet (Lafeber Company, Cornell, IL) or Oxbow Carnivore Critical Care Diet (Oxbow Animal Health, Omaha, NE); may also add dietary supplement such as Nutri-Cal (EVSCO Pharmaceuticals) to increase caloric content to these foods
• Surgical excision of a mass lesion and foreign body may be curative or temporarily improve the signs of dysphagia.

MEDICATIONS
DRUG(S) OF CHOICE
• Dysphagia is not immediately life-threatening, direct drug therapy at the underlying cause.

CONTRAINDICATIONS
N/A

PRECAUTIONS
• Use barium sulfate with caution in patients with evidence of aspiration.
• Use corticosteroids with caution or not at all in patients with evidence of, or at risk for, aspiration.

POSSIBLE INTERACTIONS
N/A

ALTERNATIVE DRUGS
N/A

FOLLOW-UP
PATIENT MONITORING
• Daily for signs of aspiration pneumonia (e.g., depression, fever, mucopurulent nasal discharge, coughing, and dyspnea)
• Body condition and hydration status daily; if oral nutrition does not meet requirements, gastrostomy tube feeding may be necessary.

POSSIBLE COMPLICATIONS
• Aspiration pneumonia is a common complication with swallowing disorders.
• Feeding multiple small meals with the patient in an upright position and maintaining this position for 10–15 minutes after feeding may help prevent aspiration of food.

MISCELLANEOUS
ASSOCIATED CONDITIONS
Aspiration pneumonia
AGE-RELATED FACTORS
• Young ferrets are more likely to ingest foreign objects and suffer facial trauma.
• Older ferrets are more likely to have oral pain from dental disease.
ZOONOTIC POTENTIAL
• Consider rabies in any patient with dysphagia, especially if the animal's rabies vaccination status is unknown or questionable or it has been exposed to a potentially rabid animal.
• If a dysphagic animal dies of rapidly progressive neurologic disease, submit the head to a qualified laboratory designated by the local or state health department for rabies examination.

PREGNANCY/FERTILITY/BREEDING
N/A

SYNONYMS
N/A

SEE ALSO
Pneumonia, aspiration
Vomiting
Weight loss and cachexia

Suggested Reading
Blanco MC, Fox JG, Rosenthal K et al. Megaesophagus in nine ferrets. J Am Vet Med Assoc 1994;205:444–447.
Couturier J, Huynh M, Boussarie D et al. Autoimmune myasthenia gravis in a ferret. J Am Vet Med Assoc 2009;235:1462–1466.
Garner MM, Ramsell K, Schoemaker NJ et al. Myofasciitis in the domestic ferret. Vet Pathol 2007;44:25–38.
Hoefer HL. Gastrointestinal diseases of ferrets. In: Quesenberry KE, Carpenter JW, eds. Ferrets, Rabbits, and Rodents, 4th ed. Clinical Medicine and Surgery. 2021. St. Louis: Saunders, 2020:27–38.
Huynh M, Pignon C. Gastrointestinal disease in exotic small mammals. J Exot Pet Med 2013;22(2):118–131.
Johnson-Delaney CA. Geriatric ferrets. Vet Clin Exot Anim Pract 2020;23(3): 549–565.
Schwarz LA, Solano M, Manning A et al. The normal upper gastrointestinal examination in the ferret. Vet Radiol Ultrasound 2003;44(2):165–172.
Webb J, Graham J, Fordham M, DeCubellis J, Buckley F, Hobbs J, Berent A, Weisse C. Diagnosis and treatment of esophageal foreign body or stricture in three ferrets (*Mustela putorius furo*). J Am Vet Med Assoc 2017;251(4):451–457.
Author Barbara Oglesbee, DVM, DABVP-Avian

DYSURIA AND POLLAKIURIA

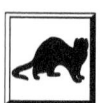

FERRETS

BASICS

DEFINITION
- Dysuria—difficult or painful urination
- Pollakiuria—voiding small quantities of urine with increased frequency

PATHOPHYSIOLOGY
- Inflammatory and noninflammatory disorders of the lower urinary tract may decrease bladder compliance and storage capacity by damaging structural components of the bladder wall or by stimulating sensory nerve endings located in the bladder or urethra. Sensations of bladder fullness, urgency, and pain stimulate premature micturition and reduce functional bladder capacity. Dysuria and pollakiuria are caused by lesions of the urinary bladder and/or urethra; these clinical signs do not exclude concurrent involvement of the upper urinary tract or disorders of other body systems.
- In ferrets, the most common cause of urinary tract obstruction are urethral calculi followed by extraluminal compression of the urethra by periurethral (prostastic or prostatic remnants) swelling, abcesses, or cysts that occur secondary to ferret adrenal disease.

SYSTEMS AFFECTED
Renal/Urologic—bladder, urethra, and prostate gland

SIGNALMENT
More common in males than females

SIGNS

Historical Findings
- Frequent trips to the litterbox
- Loss of housebreaking
- Tenesmus
- Feeding "grain free" diets containing plant proteins especially legumes and soy products
- Alopecia, increased sexual aggression, or vulvar swelling seen in ferrets with adrenal disease-associated parurethral cystic disease
- Anorexia, weight loss, weakness in ferrets with chronic disease, or urethral blockage

Physical Examination Findings
- May be normal
- Caudal abdominal mass associated with the bladder (prostatic tissue or paraurethral cysts)
- Turgid, painful bladder on abdominal palpation with obstruction or cystitis
- Thickened bladder wall on abdominal palpation possible

CAUSES

Urinary Bladder
- Urinary tract infection—bacterial; can be primary or secondary to urogenital cystic disease

- Urolithiasis—especially cysteine and struvite
- Neoplasia (unusual)
- Trauma
- Iatrogenic—e.g., catheterization, palpation, reverse flushing, overdistension of the bladder during contrast radiography, and surgery

URETHRA
- Urinary tract infection
- Urethrolithiasis—especially cysteine and struvite
- Extraluminal compression by paraurethral cysts
- Urethral plugs—in ferrets with abscessed paraurethral cysts—thick, tenacious exudate from cysts enters urine in the bladder and may plug urethra
- Neoplasia—local invasion by malignant neoplasms of adjacent structures
- Trauma
- Iatrogenic—see previous section

Prostate Gland and Paraurethral Tissues
- Paraurethral cystic disease—caused by excessive androgen production associated with ferret adrenal disease (paraurethral cysts, prostatic cysts, or hyperplasia); most common cause of stranguria; equally likely to occur in both male and female ferrets
- Neoplasia—rare

RISK FACTORS
- Feeding ferret, cat, or dog foods that contain plant-based proteins may lead to the development of struvite urolithiasis.
- Feeding ferret, cat, or dog foods that contain soy products, grain, or legumes may lead to the development of cysteine urolithiasis.
- A genetic basis for the formation of cysteine uroliths is suspected; research is ongoing.
- Urogenital cysts, prostatic hyperplasia, or prostatic cysts are caused by excess hormone formation due to Ferret adrenal disease.

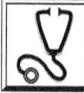

DIAGNOSIS

DIFFERENTIAL DIAGNOSIS

Differentiating from Other Abnormal Patterns of Micturition
- Rule out polyuria—increased frequency and volume of urine
- Rule out urethral obstruction—stranguria, anuria, overdistended urinary bladder, and signs of postrenal uremia

Differentiate Causes of Dysuria and Pollakiuria
- Rule out urinary tract infection—hematuria; malodorous or cloudy urine; small, painful, and thickened bladder

- Rule out urolithiasis—may see hematuria; palpable uroliths in urethra or bladder
- Rule out prostatic or paraurethral cystic diseases—alopecia, swollen vulva, increased sexual aggression, palpable caudal abdominal mass, depression, weakness, malodorous, or cloudy urine
- Rule out neoplasia—may see hematuria; palpable masses in urethra or bladder
- Rule out neurogenic disorders—rare finding; flaccid bladder wall; residual urine in bladder lumen after micturition; other neurologic deficits to hind legs, tail, perineum, and anal sphincter
- Rule out iatrogenic disorders—history of catheterization, reverse flushing, contrast radiography, or surgery

CBC/BIOCHEMISTRY/URINALYSIS
- Results often normal. Lower urinary tract disease complicated by urethral obstruction may be associated with azotemia, hyperphosphatemia, acidosis, and hyperkalemia. Patients with concurrent pyelonephritis may have impaired urine-concentrating capacity, leukocytosis, and azotemia. Dehydrated patients may have elevated total plasma protein.
- Hemogram may rarely show nonregenerative anemia, leucopenia, or thrombocytopenia due to estrogen excess in ferrets with adrenal disease
- Hypoglycemia may be present—usually due to concurrent insulinoma
- Disorders of the urinary bladder are best evaluated with a urine specimen collected by cystocentesis. Urethral disorders are best evaluated with a voided urine sample or by comparison of results of analysis of voided and cystocentesis samples (Caution: cystocentesis may induce hematuria).
- Pyuria (normal value 0–5 WBC/hpf), hematuria (normal value 0–10 RBC/hpf), and proteinuria (normal value 0–33 mg/dL) may indicate abscessed paraurethral cysts or urinary tract inflammation, but these are nonspecific findings that may result from infectious and noninfectious causes of lower urinary tract disease.
- Identification of bacteria in urine sediment suggests that urinary tract infection or abscessed paraurethral cysts are causing or complicating lower urinary tract disease. Consider contamination of urine during collection and storage when interpreting urinalysis results.
- Identification of neoplastic cells in urine sediment indicates urinary tract neoplasia. Use caution in establishing a diagnosis of neoplasia based on urine sediment examination.
- Crystalluria occurs in some normal patients, patients with urolithiasis, or patients with lower urinary tract disease unassociated with uroliths.

OTHER LABORATORY TESTS
• Quantitative urine culture—the most definitive means of identifying and characterizing bacterial urinary tract infection; negative urine culture results suggest a noninfectious cause
• Cytologic evaluation of urine sediment, urethral discharges, or vaginal discharges may help in evaluating patients with localized urinary tract disease.
• Elevations serum estradiol, androstenedione, and 17-hydroxyprogesterone combined are most diagnostic for adrenal disease. (Available through the University of Tennessee Clinical Endocrinology Laboratory, Department of Comparative Medicine)

IMAGING
Survey abdominal radiography, contrast urethrocystography and cystography, urinary tract ultrasonography, and excretory urography are important means of identifying and localizing causes of dysuria and pollakiuria.

DIAGNOSTIC PROCEDURES
N/A

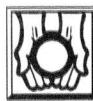

TREATMENT
• Patients with nonobstructive lower urinary tract diseases are typically managed as outpatients; diagnostic evaluation may require brief hospitalization.
• Dysuria and pollakiuria associated with systemic signs of illness (e.g., pyrexia, depression, anorexia, vomiting, and dehydration) or laboratory findings of azotemia or leukocytosis warrant more aggressive diagnostic evaluation and initiation of supportive and symptomatic treatment.
• Treatment depends on the underlying cause and specific sites involved. See specific chapters describing diseases listed in section on causes.
• Clinical signs of dysuria and pollakiuria often resolve rapidly following specific treatment of the underlying cause(s).

MEDICATIONS
DRUGS OF CHOICE
• Depend on the underlying cause
• If bacterial cystitis is demonstrated, begin treatment with a broad-spectrum antibiotic. Some choices for empirical use while waiting for culture results include trimethoprim sulfa (15–30 PO, SC mg/kg q12h), amoxicillin (10–30 mg/kg PO, SC q12h), or enrofloxacin (5–10 mg/kg PO, SQ, IM q12h). Modify antibacterial treatment based on results of urine culture and susceptibility testing.

CONTRAINDTICATIONS
Potentially nephrotoxic drugs (e.g., gentamicin) in patients that are febrile, dehydrated, or azotemic or that are suspected of having pyelonephritis, septicemia, or preexisting renal disease

PRECAUTIONS
N/A

POSSIBLE INTERACTIONS
N/A

ALTERNATIVE DRUGS
N/A

FOLLOW-UP
PATIENT MONITORING
• Response to treatment by clinical signs, serial physical examinations, laboratory testing, and radiographic and ultrasonic evaluations appropriate for each specific cause
• Refer to specific chapters describing diseases listed in section on causes.

POSSIBLE COMPLICATIONS
• Refer to specific chapters describing diseases listed in section on causes.

MISCELLANEOUS
ASSOCIATED CONDITIONS
• Ferret adrenal disease
• Insulinomas are commonly seen in ferrets with adrenal disease.

• Ferrets on poor-quality diets are more prone to dental diseases.

AGE-RELATED FACTORS
N/A

ZOONOTIC POTENTIAL
N/A

PREGNANCY/FERTILITY/BREEDING
N/A

SYNONYMS
N/A

SEE ALSO
Adrenal disease
Lower urinary tract infection
Paraurethral cysts
Urinary tract obstruction
Urolithiasis

ABBREVIATIONS
N/A

Suggested Reading
Di Girolamo N, Huyun M. Disorders of the urinary and reproductive systems in ferrets. In: Quesenberry KE, Carpenter JW, eds. Ferrets, Rabbits and Rodents, 4th ed. Clinical Medicine and Surgery. St. Louis: Saunders, 2020:39–54.
Di Girolamo N, Selleri P. Medical and surgical emergencies in ferrets. Vet Clin Exot Anim Pract 2016;19:431–464.
Hallman RM, Brandão J. Diagnostic imaging of the renal system in exotic companion mammals. Vet Clin Exot Anim 2020;23:195–214.
Hanak EB, Di Girolamo N, DeSilva U, Marschang RE, Brandao JL et al. Variation in mineral types of uroliths from ferrets (*Mustela putorius furo*) submitted for analysis in North America, Europe, or Asia over an 8-year period. J Am Vet Med Assoc 2021;259:757–763.
Reavill DR, Lennox AM. Disease overview of the urinary tract in exotic companion mammals and tips on clinical management. Vet Clin Exot Anim 2020;23(1):169–193.
Author Barbara Oglesbee, DVM, DABVP (Avian)

FERRETS

DYSPNEA AND TACHYPNEA

FERRETS

BASICS

DEFINITION
Dyspnea is difficult or labored breathing, tachypnea is rapid breathing (not necessarily labored), and hyperpnea is deep breathing. In animals, the term *dyspnea* often is applied to labored breathing that appears to be uncomfortable.

PATHOPHYSIOLOGY
• Nonrespiratory causes of dyspnea may include abnormalities in pulmonary vascular tone (CNS disease, shock), pulmonary circulation (congestive heart failure), oxygenation (anemia), or ventilation (obesity, ascites, abdominal organomegaly, and musculoskeletal disease).
• Primary respiratory diseases may be divided into upper and lower respiratory tract; the latter can be subdivided into obstructive and restrictive causes.

Systems Affected
• Respiratory
• Cardiovascular
• Nervous (secondary to hypoxia)

SIGNALMENT
Any

SIGNS

Historical Findings
• Orthopnea (recumbent dyspnea), restlessness, and poor sleeping may occur in ferrets with pleural space disease (mediastinal mass, effusions, abscesses, and diaphragmatic hernias) or CHF.
• Exercise intolerance may occur with lower respiratory tract disease or CHF.
• Sneezing or naso-ocular discharge may be seen with upper respiratory infections.
• Coughing is less common in ferrets but may occur with dyspnea in ferrets with tracheal or LRT disease.
• History of obesity or chronic use of corticosteroids

Physical Examination Findings
• Upper airway obstruction—stridor, stertor
• Pulmonary edema—fine inspiratory crackles
• Pneumonia—harsh inspiratory and expiratory bronchovesicular sounds
• Pleural effusion, intrathoracic fat accumulation, or diaphragmatic hernia—dull percussion and absent lung sounds ventrally, harsh lung sounds dorsally
• Mediastinal mass—noncompressible thorax
• Pyrexia (CDV, influenza, and bacterial infections)
• Weight loss and poor hair coat in ferrets with chronic respiratory disease
• Obesity in ferrets with intrathoracic fat accumulation

CAUSES

Nonrespiratory Causes
• Cardiac disease (very common)—congestive heart failure, heartworm disease, severe arrhythmias, and cardiogenic shock
• Intrathoracic fat accumulation (very common)—fat pads surrounding the heart, in the mediastinum, and within lung parenchyma can cause significant dyspnea in obese ferrets and/or those on chronic corticosteroid treatment.
• Mediastinal mass (lymphoma most common)
• Neuromuscular disease—severe CNS disease (trauma, inflammation, neoplasia), rib fractures, spinal disease (trauma, disc extrusion), megaesophagus
• Metabolic disease—acidosis, uremia
• Hematologic—anemia (estrogen toxicity, blood loss)
• Other—anxiety, pain, obesity, ascites, organomegaly, fever, heat stroke

Respiratory Causes

Upper Respiratory Tract (URT)
• Nasal obstruction—rhinitis/sinusitis (viral, bacterial, and mycotic) granuloma, foreign body, neoplasia
• Laryngotracheal obstruction—foreign body, neoplasia
• Traumatic airway rupture
• Extraluminal tracheal compression—hilar lymphadenopathy (lymphoma)

Lower Respiratory Tract (LRT)
• Obstructive—pulmonary edema (cardiogenic and noncardiac); pneumonia—viral (CDV, influenza), bacterial and neoplasia (primary, metastatic) most common; mycotic, pulmonary contusion (trauma); consolidated lung lobe; pneumonitis (allergic, parasitic, not documented in ferrets); intrathoracic tracheal disease (foreign body, neoplasia)
• Restrictive—pleural effusion caused by cardiac or pericardial disease, mediastinal masses (lymphoma); diaphragmatic hernias; hemothorax; pneumothorax; chylothorax

RISK FACTORS
• Exposure to other ferrets
• Obesity, chronic corticosteroid use
• Trauma, bite wounds
• CDV in poorly vaccinated animals
• Poor ventilation
• Immunosuppression

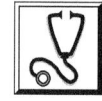

DIAGNOSIS

DIFFERENTIATING CAUSES
• Gagging and retching associated with nausea or vomiting may be mistaken for dyspnea.

• Tachypnea without dyspnea may be a physiologic response to fear, physical exertion, anxiety, fever, pain, or acidosis.
• Infectious causes (pneumonia, sinusitis/rhinitis) usually present with signs of systemic disease (emaciation, anorexia, and depression)
• Primary cardiac disease often presents with a constellation of other signs (e.g., heart murmur, arrhythmias, and ascites).
• URT dyspnea is often more pronounced on inspiration.
• LRT dyspnea is more often associated with expiratory effort.
• Tracheal mass or foreign body may cause both inspiratory and expiratory dyspnea.
• Pleural space disease often presents as exaggerated thoracic excursions that generate only minimal airflow at the mouth or nose.

CBC/BIOCHEMISTRY/URINALYSIS
• Hemogram—inflammatory leukocytosis (pneumonia, sinusitis), anemia with chronic disease
• Biochemistry panel—increased liver enzyme activity or bile acids (liver disease), increased CK (muscle wasting, heart disease)

OTHER LABORATORY TESTS
• Cytologic examination, bacterial and mycotic culture—on samples from tracheal wash, deep nasal swabs, pleural fluid, or fine needle aspirates of masses
• Serologic tests that identify adult *D. immitis* antigen are of some use; however, false-negative results are common with low worm burdens or early infections—ELISA (snap heartworm antigen test, Idexx Laboratories)
• The fluorescent antibody test for CDV—on blood or mucous membrane scrapings

IMAGING

Radiography
• Skull—may demonstrate nasal obstruction, sinusitis, boney destruction from neoplasia, or mycotic infections
• Thoracic—may reveal pulmonary diseases (small airway disease, pulmonary edema, and pneumonia), pleural space disease (effusions, mediastinal mass, fat accumulation), pneumothorax, and hernias
• Cardiac shadow—cardiomegaly with heart disease
• Abdominal—organomegaly, ascites

Ultrasonography
• Echocardiography to evaluate pericardial effusion, cardiomyopathy, heartworm disease, congenital defects, and valvular disease
• Thoracic ultrasound may be beneficial in some animals with mediastinal mass lesions, but the beam is often greatly attenuated by any air in surrounding lung lobes.

- Abdominal ultrasound may be used to evaluate masses or organomegaly.

DIAGNOSTIC PROCEDURES
- Tracheal wash—cytology and culture
- Thoracocentesis—fluid analysis and culture

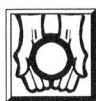

TREATMENT
- Airway—if URT is obstructed, intubation (if possible) or tracheostomy may be required.
- Breathing—supply O_2 enrichment (O_2 cage or induction chamber) in a quiet environment. Ventilate only if the animal has bradypnea, pulmonary arrest, or is hypoventilating from exhaustion. If the hypoventilation is from pleural space disease, artificial ventilation and O_2 supplementation do little until the chest is evacuated.
- Thoracocentesis—may be both diagnostic and therapeutic in animals with pleural space disease. In acutely dyspneic animals, perform tap prior to radiography. A negative tap for air or fluid suggests solid pleural space (fat, mass, abscess, or hernia), primary pulmonary, or cardiac disease. If there is significant pleural effusion, drain each hemithorax with a 20-gauge butterfly catheter after the ferret is stable enough to be handled. When performing thoracocentesis be aware that the heart is located much more caudally within the thorax in the ferret compared with dogs and cats. Sedation or anesthesia is necessary.
- Surgery may be necessary to remove foreign bodies, obtain samples for biopsy, or to debulk tumors, abscesses, or granulomas.

MEDICATIONS
DRUG(S) OF CHOICE
- Oxygen is the single most useful drug in the treatment of acute severe dyspnea.
- See primary disorder for definitive therapy.

CONTRAINDICATIONS
- In animals with CHF and blunt chest trauma, iatrogenic fluid overload and pulmonary edema is a potential problem.

Intravenous administration of crystalloids should be used judiciously.
- Respiratory rate and effort should be monitored carefully and frequently in these patients.

PRECAUTIONS
Corticosteroids should be used with caution in patients with suspected infectious diseases.

POSSIBLE INTERACTIONS
N/A

ALTERNATIVE DRUGS
N/A

FOLLOW-UP
PATIENT MONITORING
- Repeat any abnormal tests
- Radiographs—monitor response to therapy in animals with pulmonary disease. If effective therapy is used, pulmonary edema should be visibly improved within 12 hours of therapy. Monitor the recurrence of pleural effusion, based on how quickly effusion accumulates.
- Cardiac ultrasound—3–12 weeks, depending on the condition

POSSIBLE COMPLICATIONS
- Depends on the underlying disease
- Relapse, progression of disease, and death are common.

MISCELLANEOUS
ASSOCIATED CONDITIONS
- Obesity
- Lymphoma
- Splenomegaly

ZOONOTIC POTENTIAL
Influenza virus

PREGNANCY/FERTILITY/BREEDING
N/A

SYNONYMS
N/A

SEE ALSO
See Causes

ABBREVIATIONS
CHF = congestive heart failure
CDV = canine distemper virus
CK = creatine kinase
CNS = central nervous system
ELISA = enzyme-linked immunosorbent assay
URT = upper respiratory tract
LRT = lower respiratory tract

Suggested Reading
Capello V, Lennox AM. Diagnostic imaging of the respiratory system in exotic companion mammals. Vet Clin Exot Anim 2011;14:369–389.
Di Girolamo N, Selleri P. Medical and surgical emergencies in ferrets. Vet Clin North Am Exot Anim Pract 2016;19: 431–464.
Fitzgerald B, Dias S, Martorell J. Cardiovascular drugs in avian, small mammal, and reptile medicine. Vet Clin North Am Exot Anim Pract 2018;21(2): 399–442.
Johnson-Delaney CA. Ferret respiratory system: clinical anatomy, physiology, and disease. Vet Clin Exot Anim 2011;14: 357–367.
Kiupel M, Perpiñán D. Viral diseases of ferrets. In: Fox JG, Marini RP, eds. Biology and Diseases of the Ferret, 3rd ed. John Wiley & Sons, 2014:439–517.
Lennox A. Respiratory disorders in ferrets. Vet Clin Exot Anim 2021;24:483–493.
Morrisey JK, Malakoff RJ. Cardiovascular and other diseases of ferrets. In: Quesenberry KE, Carpenter JW, eds. Ferrets, Rabbits and Rodents, 4th ed. Clinical Medicine and Surgery. 2021. St. Louis: Saunders, 2020:5–70.
Perpiñán D. Respiratory diseases of ferrets. In: Quesenberry KE, Carpenter JW, eds. Ferrets, Rabbits and Rodents, 4th ed. Clinical Medicine and Surgery. 2021. St. Louis: Saunders, 2020:71–76.
Swenson SL, Koster LG, Jenkins-Moore M et al. Natural cases of 2009 pandemic H1N1 Influenza A virus in pet ferrets. J Vet Diagn Invest 2010;22:784–788.

Author Barbara Oglesbee DVM, DABVP (Avian)

FERRETS

EAR MITES

BASICS

OVERVIEW
• Otodectes cynotis mite infestation is common in ferrets. Many ferrets are asymptomatic, but intense irritation of the external ear can also be seen.
• Sequelae to infestation is rare in ferrets; however, secondary bacterial or mycotic infections or otitis interna/media have been anecdotally reported. These sequelae are usually a consequence of overzealous cleaning of the ear canal.

SIGNALMENT
No breed or sex predilection

SIGNS
• Thick, red-brown or black crusts in the outer ear—may or may not be associated with mite infestation; this type of exudate is usually a normal finding in ferrets
• Pruritus primarily located around the ears, head, and neck; occasionally generalized
• Alopecia and excoriations around the pinnae may occur, owing to the intense pruritus.
• Signs of otitis interna/media such as head tilt and vestibular signs have been anecdotally reported in ferrets with ear mites.

CAUSES AND RISK FACTORS
Otodectes cynotis

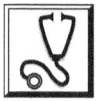

DIAGNOSIS

DIFFERENTIAL DIAGNOSIS

Exudate in the Ear Canal
• Normal finding—most ferrets normally have a black to brown crumbly exudate in the ear canal
• Bacterial or mycotic otitis externa—rare in ferrets; may occur secondary to mite infestation; differentiate by microscopic examination of exudate

Pruritus/Alopecia
• Fleas—patchy alopecia usually appears in other areas in addition to head, especially tail region; finding flea dirt will help to differentiate
• Sarcoptic mange—intense pruritus; can be generalized or localized to feet
• Contact dermatitis—usually ventral distribution

• Ferret adrenal disease—usually bilaterally symmetric alopecia, with or without pruritus, beginning at the tail region and extending dorsally; however, it is possible to see unusual distributions of alopecia (such as the head alone) in ferrets with adrenal disease.

CBC/BIOCHEMISTRY/URINALYSIS
Normal

OTHER LABORATORY TESTS
N/A

IMAGING
N/A

DIAGNOSTIC PROCEDURES
• Ear swabs placed in mineral oil—usually a very effective means of identification
• Skin scrapings—identify mites, occurrence outside of the ear canal is extremely rare in ferrets

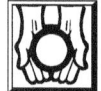

TREATMENT
• Contagious; important to treat all in-contact animals
• Thoroughly clean and treat the environment.
• Cleaning of the ear canal may not enhance treatment in the ferret. Overzealous cleaning of the ear canal may cause irritation, secondary bacterial or mycotic infections, or rupture of the tympanum.

MEDICATIONS

DRUG(S) OF CHOICE
• Topical ivermectin: 1% ivermectin diluted 1:10 in propylene glycol, administered in ears at 400 mcg/kg q2w × 2 treatments
• Ivermectin (0.4 mg/kg PO, SC q14-28d)
• Selamectin (Revolution, Pfizer) 15 mg/kg topically q30d or Imidacloprid (10%) and moxidectin (1%) (Advantage-Multi, Bayer)—0.4 mL/animal topically q30d
• It is not necessary to clean the ears thoroughly to remove debris prior to topical administration of ivermectin since debris may aid in the retention of medication in the canal.

CONTRAINDICATIONS
• Avoid overzealous cleaning of the ear canal
• Ivermectin—do not use pregnant jills
• Do not use topical and parenteral or oral ivermectin concurrently

PRECAUTIONS
N/A

ALTERNATIVE DRUGS
• Topical Ivermectin—0.5–1 mg/kg in ears, repeat in 14 days; do not use concurrently with oral or parenteral ivermectine

FOLLOW-UP
• An ear swab and physical examination should be done 1 month after therapy commences.
• For most patients, the prognosis is good.
• Infestation is more likely to recur or fail to respond to treatment with parenteral ivermectin or topical thiabendazole.

MISCELLANEOUS

ZOONOTIC POTENTIAL
The mites will also bite humans (rare).

SEE ALSO
Adrenal disease (hyperadrenocorticism)
Dermatophytosis
Fleas and flea infestation
Pruritus

Suggested Reading
d'Ovidio D, Santoro D. Dermatologic diseases of ferrets. In: Quesenberry KE, Carpenter JW, eds. Ferrets, Rabbits and Rodents, 4th ed. Clinical Medicine and Surgery. 2021. St. Louis: Saunders, 2020:109–116.
Fehr M, Koestlinger S. Ectoparasites in small exotic mammals. Vet Clin Exot Anim 2013;16:611–657.
Fisher M, Beck W, Hutchinson MJ. Efficacy and safety of selamectin (Stronghold*/Revolution™) used off-label in exotic pets. Int J Appl Res Vet Med 2007;5:87–96.
Hoppmann E, Wilson Barron H. Ferret and rabbit dermatology. J Exot Pet Med 2007;16:225–237.
Patterson MM, Kirchain SM. Comparison of three treatments for control of ear mites in ferrets. Lab Anim Sci 1999;49:655–657.
Author Barbara Oglesbee, DVM, DABVP (Avian)

EOSINOPHILLIC GASTROENTERITIS

BASICS

DEFINITION
An inflammatory disease of the stomach and intestine characterized by a transmucosal infiltration of eosinophils with resultant inflammation and thickening of the affected areas. Eosinophilic granulomas are often found in the mesenteric lymph nodes, and a peripheral eosinophilia is occasionally present.

PATHOPHYSIOLOGY
• The underlying cause of the tissue and circulating eosinophilia is unknown. Although a parasitic or allergic cause has been suspected, parasites are usually not found, and allergies have not been well documented in ferrets.
• Eosinophils contain granules with substances that directly damage the surrounding tissues.

SYSTEMS AFFECTED
Gastrointestinal—usually affects the stomach and small intestine; large intestine and mesenteric nodes commonly affected, and occasionally liver

GENETICS
N/A

INCIDENCE/PREVALENCE
• True incidence is unknown
• Less common in ferrets than lymphoplasmacytic gastroenteritis

GEOGRAPHIC DISTRIBUTION
N/A

SIGNALMENT
Mean Age and Range
Young to middle age, range—6 months to 4 years

Predominant Sex
None reported

SIGNS
Historical Findings
Chronic diarrhea with or without mucus or blood, anorexia, weight loss, and vomiting are the most common client complaints.

Physical Examination Findings
• Dehydration and emaciation
• Thickened intestinal loops and enlarged mesenteric lymph nodes may be palpated.
• Splenomegaly usually present—most often due to nonspecific, age-related change; rarely, eosinophilic infiltration may occur
• Hepatomegaly may be noted in a few cases where infiltrates occur in the liver, or due to other, concurrent hepatic disease.

CAUSES
• The cause is unknown, although food allergies are strongly suspected. Other theories include parasitic or idiopathic.
• Idiopathic eosinophilic gastroenteritis; hypereosinophilic syndrome has been suggested, since some affected ferrets have a peripheral eosinophilia and occasionally, eosinophilic infiltration into liver, spleen, lymph nodes, and skin.
• Immune-mediated—food allergy suspected; often associated with other forms of inflammatory bowel disease. Some ferrets respond very well to conversion to a novel protein source diet, or respond to anti-inflammatory or immunosuppressive doses of corticosteroids, suggesting a hypersensitivity reaction.
• Parasitic—parasites not usually found

RISK FACTORS
N/A

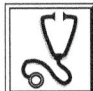

DIAGNOSIS

DIFFERENTIAL DIAGNOSIS
• Common causes of weight loss, anorexia, diarrhea, and vomiting include GI foreign body, lymphosarcoma, gastric ulcers, viral or bacterial enteritis, and other types of inflammatory bowel disease.
• Intestinal biopsy differentiates the other causes of inflammatory bowel disease from eosinophilic gastroenteritis.

CBC/BIOCHEMISTRY/URINALYSIS
• Hemogram occasionally reveals a peripheral eosinophilia (up to 35% eosinophils); however, not seen in every ferret with EGE
• Panhypoproteinemia or hypoalbuminemia may be present due to protein-losing enteropathy.

OTHER LABORATORY TESTS
• Multiple fecal flotations and direct smears are needed to rule in or out intestinal parasitism; however, GI parasites are rare in ferrets.

IMAGING
• Plain abdominal radiographs provide little information.
• Barium contrast radiography may occasionally demonstrate thick intestinal walls and mucosal irregularities but does not provide any information about etiology or the nature of the thickening.
• Ultrasonography—to rule out other diseases; can be used to examine the liver, spleen, and mesenteric lymph nodes

DIAGNOSTIC PROCEDURES
Definitive diagnosis requires biopsy and histopathology, usually obtained via exploratory laparotomy.

PATHOLOGIC FINDINGS
• Stomach and intestinal tract may appear grossly normal or diffusely thickened, or may contain patchy, multifocal areas of thickening
• Ulcerations and erosions may also be seen.
• Eosinophilic infiltrates can be patchy in the intestine; multiple biopsies may be necessary to obtain a diagnostic sample.
• Mesenteric lymph nodes are often grossly enlarged.
• Histopathology—affected areas of the GI tract reveal a diffuse infiltrate of eosinophils into the lamina propria, submucosa, and occasionally the serosa; villous atrophy may be apparent; other inflammatory cell populations may be found along with eosinophils; focal eosinophilic granulomas may be seen in affected lymph nodes.

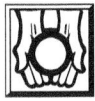

TREATMENT

APPROPRIATE HEALTH CARE
• Most can be treated on an outpatient basis.
• Patients that are dehydrated, emaciated, or have other concurrent illnesses may require hospitalization until they are stabilized.

NURSING CARE
If the patient is dehydrated, any balanced fluid such as lactated Ringer's solution is adequate (for a patient without other concurrent disease); otherwise, select fluids on the basis of secondary diseases. If held NPO due to vomiting, provide a dextrose-containing fluid, and monitor blood glucose concentration.

ACTIVITY
No need to restrict unless severely debilitated

DIET
• Highly digestible diets with novel protein sources may be useful for eliciting remission, although an allergic cause has not been documented, and little information is available regarding the efficacy of these diets. If attempted, choose feline diets since ferrets have high nutritional protein and fat requirements. Foods that have anecdotally reported to elicit remission include feline lamb and rice diets, diets consisting exclusively of one type of meat (lamb, duck, and turkey), or a "natural prey diet" consisting of whole rodents. Avoid diets that contain plant-based proteins (peas, soy, and grains), since these have been associated with

EOSINOPHILLIC GASTROENTERITIS

the development of urinary calculi. If remission is elicited, continue the diet for at least 8–13 weeks; this diet may need to be fed lifelong.
• Anorexic ferrets may refuse dry foods but are often willing to eat canned cat foods or pureed meats.

CLIENT EDUCATION
• This can be a very frustrating disease to treat. Novel protein source trial diets are only occasionally effective, and client compliance is essential. Often clients have more than one ferret, or give their ferrets treats, and have difficulty feeding one exclusive type of food.
• In many cases, trial diets are ineffective. Some ferrets may never respond, or respond initially to medical therapy and diet manipulation but become refractory to treatment with time.
• Explain the potential for long-term therapy.

SURGICAL CONSIDERATIONS
N/A

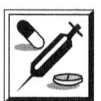

MEDICATIONS

DRUG(S) OF CHOICE
• Corticosteroids—mainstay of treatment; prednisone (1.25–2.5 mg/kg PO q24h) for at least 1–2 weeks
• Gradually taper corticosteroids to 0.25–1 mg/kg qod; some ferrets will relapse when dosage is lowered and may require long-term therapy with higher doses of prednisone.
• Many ferrets fail to respond to prednisone therapy or initially respond but become refractory to treatment with time.
• Other immunosuppressive drugs such as azathioprine (0.9 mg/kg PO q24–72h) have been used in ferrets that become refractory to prednisone treatment.

CONTRAINDICATIONS
N/A

PRECAUTIONS
• In ferrets with concurrent infectious diseases, use corticosteroids with caution.

POSSIBLE INTERACTIONS
N/A

ALTERNATIVE DRUGS
• Empirical use of antiparasitic agents has been advocated, although no parasitic causes have been documented, and intestinal parasites are rare in ferrets. These drugs are generally safe to use, and a trial is unlikely to cause harm. Those used anecdotally include ivermectin (0.4 mg/kg SC once, repeat in 2 weeks) and metronidazole (10–15 mg/kg PO q12h)

FOLLOW-UP

PATIENT MONITORING
• Initially frequent for some more severely affected patients; monitor severity of diarrhea and peripheral eosinophil counts.
• Patients with less severe disease—may be checked 2–5 weeks after the initial evaluation; monthly to bimonthly thereafter

PREVENTION/AVOIDANCE
If a food intolerance or allergy is suspected or documented, avoid that particular item and adhere strictly to dietary changes.

POSSIBLE COMPLICATIONS
• Weight loss, debilitation, and death in refractory cases
• Adverse effects of prednisone therapy (rare)

EXPECTED COURSE AND PROGNOSIS
The prognosis is good to fair in those animals that respond clinically to corticosteroid and or dietary therapy; poor to grave if clinical response is not observed.

MISCELLANEOUS

ASSOCIATED CONDITIONS
Many affected ferrets also have splenomegaly (nonspecific in aged ferrets).

AGE-RELATED FACTORS
N/A

ZOONOTIC POTENTIAL
N/A

PREGNANCY/FERTILITY/BREEDING
N/A

SYNONYMS
N/A

SEE ALSO
Anorexia
Diarrhea
Inflammatory Bowel Disease
Lymphoplasmacytic enteritis and gastroenteritis

ABBREVIATIONS
GI = gastrointestinal

Suggested Reading
Cazzini P, Watson MK, Gottdenker N et al. Proposed grading scheme for inflammatory bowel disease in ferrets and correlation with clinical signs. J Vet Diagn Invest 2020; 32(1):17–24.
Di Girolamo N, Selleri P. Medical and surgical emergencies in ferrets. Vet Clin Exot Anim 2016;19:431–464.
Hoefer HL. Gastrointestinal diseases of ferrets. In: Quesenberry KE, Carpenter JW, eds. Ferrets, Rabbits, and Rodents, 4th ed. Clinical Medicine and Surgery. 2021. St. Louis: Saunders, 2020:27–38.
Johnson-Delaney CA. Geriatric ferrets. Vet Clin Exot Anim Pract 2020;23(3): 549–565.
Livingstone M. Dealing with gastrointestinal disease in ferrets. In Practice 2022;44: 169–179.
Murray J, Kiupel M, Maes RK. Ferret coronavirus-associated diseases. Vet Clin North Am Exot Anim Pract 2010; 13(3):543–560.
Watson MK, Cazzini P, Mayer J et al. Histology and immunohistochemistry of severe inflammatory bowel disease versus lymphoma in the ferret (*Mustela putorius furo*). J Vet Diagn Invest 2016;28(3): 198–206.

Author Barbara Oglesbee, DVM, DABVP-Avian

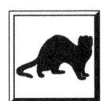

BASICS

DEFINITION
• An enteric viral disease caused by a novel coronavirus, ferret group A coronavirus (FECV). Disease is characterized initially by anorexia, vomiting, and lethargy, followed by profuse green, mucous-covered diarrhea. Due to characteristic diarrhea, pet owners refer to this disease as "green slime disease."
• Following the hypersecretory phase, chronic, intermittent, malabsorptive diarrhea is commonly seen.
• Typically, high morbidity and low mortality rates are seen.
• Clinical signs are usually seen within 48–72 hours following exposure to clinically affected ferrets or asymptomatic carriers.

PATHOPHYSIOLOGY
• Initial lesions of ECE are caused by an enteric coronavirus, although secondary bacterial and/or parasitic infections may contribute.
• Coronavirus infection causes lymphocytic infiltration, villous atrophy, and blunting of intestinal villi, as well as vacuolar degeneration and necrosis of apical (villous tip) epithelium.
• Initial intestinal lesions cause a hypersecretory, mucoid diarrhea, and vomiting.
• Following the hypersecretory phase, some ferrets recover with no further clinical signs; other ferrets develop chronic or intermittent disease due to villous atrophy and/or secondary infections
• Hepatic degeneration and necrosis are often seen in ferrets with ECE; the mechanism for this has not been described.

SYSTEMS AFFECTED
• Gastrointestinal—small intestinal villi and adjacent mucosal epithelium
• Hepatobiliary—hepatic degeneration and necrosis common
• Hemic/Lymphatic/Immune—mesenteric lymphoid hyperplasia
• Musculoskeletal—muscle wasting due to intestinal malabsorption
• Endocrine/Metabolic—fluid, electrolyte, and acid–base imbalances

INCIDENCE/PREVALENCE
• Seen most commonly in breeding facilities, animal shelters, pet stores, or wherever kits are reared

GEOGRAPHIC DISTRIBUTION
Seen most commonly in North America

SIGNALMENT
Mean Age and Range
• Older ferrets are more severely affected
• Young kits, 6–16 weeks of age, usually have mild to moderate disease or are asymptomatic carriers.

Predominant Sex
N/A

SIGNS
Historical Findings
• Recent exposure to or acquisition of a new ferret, either symptomatic or asymptomatic carriers (usually kits from a pet store or shelter), is key to the diagnosis. Contact may be either direct or through fomites.
• Within 48–72 hours of exposure, sudden onset of anorexia, lethargy, and often, repeated episodes of vomiting
• Diarrhea usually (but not always) seen—profuse, bright-green-colored, large mucous component; lasts several days and may recur
• Sudden profound weight loss common, especially in older animals with diarrhea
• In breeding facilities, pet stores, or multi-ferret households, all animals show varying degrees of clinical signs within a short period of time; younger animals are often less seriously affected
• Following the acute phase, chronic or intermittent diarrhea (often lasting months) is seen due to villous atrophy and subsequent malabsorption. Diarrhea is often granular ("bird seed" or "millet seed") in appearance; pale brown to green in color; mucus or fresh blood is sometimes seen
• Some ferrets will appear to completely recover, then relapse weeks to months later
• Lethargy, chronic wasting, inappetence may be seen for weeks to months

Physical Examination Findings
• Dehydration, weight loss, and abdominal discomfort are consistent features.
• Thickened, ropy intestinal loops may be palpated.
• Occasionally, enlarged mesenteric lymph nodes are palpable.
• Splenomegaly is a common, nonspecific finding.

RISK FACTORS
• Ferrets from kennels, animal shelters, pet shops, or elsewhere where ferrets have congregated are at greatest risk.
• Older ferrets are at higher risk of severe infection, especially with concurrent insulinoma, and gastrointestinal, cardiac, or adrenal disease.
• Co-pathogens such as parasites, viruses, and certain bacterial species (e.g., *Helicobacter*

mustelae, *Campylobacter* spp., *Clostridium* spp.) and *Cryptosporidium* spp. hypothesized to exacerbate illness
• Crowding and poor sanitation increases the risk of infection, especially in kennels or animal shelters.

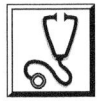

DIAGNOSIS

DIFFERENTIAL DIAGNOSIS
• Gastrointestinal foreign bodies—common cause of similar signs, especially in young ferrets; often may differentiate by history
• *Helicobacter mustelae*—disease induced by *H. mustelae* often occurs secondary to ECE; likely related to stress and anorexia or general debility
• *Clostridium* spp., *Campylobacter* spp., *Salmonella* spp., or other enteric bacterial infections—should be considered as differential diagnoses. Enteritis caused by bacteria alone is uncommon. Generally, these agents are co-pathogens or secondary invaders.
• Gastrointestinal parasites—*Giardia*, *Coccidia*, *Cryptosporidium* spp. (may be primary pathogens or secondary to ECE)
• Lymphoma—may cause identical clinical signs; differentiate by characteristic ECE history and on plasma biochemistry—ALT often extremely elevated with ECE; elevated in lymphoma if hepatic involvement
• Metabolic disorders—liver disease, renal disease, pancreatic disease
• Dietary—diet changes, eating spoiled food, dietary intolerance
• Infiltrative—proliferative bowel disease (*Desulfovibrio* spp.), lymphoplasmacytic gastroenteritis, eosinophilic gastroenteritis
• Intussusception
• Toxin ingestion

CBC/BIOCHEMISTRY/URINALYSIS
• Increased PCV due to dehydration
• Increased ALT (often >700 U/L) and ALP are commonly seen in acute disease due to liver necrosis or mobilization of fat stores.
• Persistent lymphocytosis in ferrets with chronic disease
• Hypoalbuminemia and mild increases in globulins are commonly seen in patients with chronic disease due to inflammatory bowel disease.

OTHER LABORATORY TESTS
• PCR on intestinal biopsy or fecal sample. The virus is shed intermittently, so false negatives can occur with fecal testing.

FERRETS

IMAGING
- If done as part of the diagnostic workup, abdominal radiographs may reveal a generalized small intestinal ileus.
- Useful to rule out GI foreign body
- Useful to rule in or out other causes of diarrhea

DIAGNOSTIC PROCEDURES
- Definitive diagnosis requires biopsy and histopathology, usually obtained via exploratory laparotomy.
- Immunohistochemistry is used to detect coronaviral antigen in intestinal biopsy
- Fecal direct examination, fecal flotation, and zinc sulfate centrifugation may demonstrate gastrointestinal parasites (often co-pathogens).
- Fecal cytology—may reveal RBC or fecal leukocytes, which can be associated with inflammatory bowel disease or invasive bacterial strains.
- Fecal culture should be performed if abnormal bacteria are observed on the fecal Gram's stain, or if salmonella is suspected (may be co-pathogens)

PATHOLOGIC FINDINGS
- Gross changes include hyperemia of the small intestine with green, mucoid diarrhea in the lumen in the acute phase. With chronic disease, see thinning of the intestinal wall with loss of villi.
- Mesenteric lymph nodes are often enlarged.
- Multifocal hepatic degeneration and necrosis are common.
- Histopathology reveals intestinal lymphocytic or lymphoplasmacytic inflammation and necrosis of apical epithelium, often with severe villus atrophy.

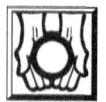

TREATMENT

APPROPRIATE HEALTH CARE
- Symptomatic and supportive
- Intensity depends on the severity of signs on examination
- Prompt, intensive inpatient care favors treatment success.
- Proper, strict isolation procedures are essential.

NURSING CARE
- Hospitalize patients that are dehydrated, anorectic, or severely debilitated.
- Rehydration is essential to treatment success in severely ill ferrets. Initially, a balanced fluid (e.g., lactated Ringer's solution) may be used.

- Correct electrolyte and acid-base disturbances in patients with moderate to severe disease
- Supplementation with 5% dextrose is beneficial in anorectic, hypoglycemic patients.
- Patients with hypoproteinemia may benefit from treatment with hetastarch; administer an IV bolus (10 mL/kg) slowly over 2–3 hours; then as a constant rate infusion of 1 mL/kg/h for 24 hours, with a maximum of 20 mL/kg/day; hetastarch increases plasma oncotic pressure and pulls fluid into the intravascular space.

ACTIVITY
Restrict until symptoms abate.

DIET
- If anorexic, assist feed an easily digestible high-protein/high-fat diet such as Lafeber Carnivore Critical Care Diet (Lafeber Company, Cornell, IL) or Oxbow Carnivore Critical Care Diet (Oxbow Animal Health, Omaha, NE); if these are unavailable, offer chicken baby foods; may also add dietary supplement such as Nutri-Cal (EVSCO Pharmaceuticals) to increase caloric content to these foods.
- Warming the food to body temperature or offering via syringe may increase acceptance.
- Ferrets exhibiting malabsorptive diarrhea (characterized by grainy feces, and weight loss) often respond well to a diet consisting of chicken-based human baby foods and high-calorie dietary supplements until the diarrhea resolves.

CLIENT EDUCATION
- Inform owners about the need for thorough disinfection, especially if other ferrets are on the premises.
- Warn owners that malabsorptive diarrhea may persist for weeks to months, requiring long-term treatment.
- Warn owners that Inflammatory Bowel disease (IBD) may develop, requiring life-long treatment.

SURGICAL CONSIDERATIONS
Exploratory laparotomy and biopsy to confirm diagnosis

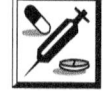

MEDICATIONS

DRUG(S) OF CHOICE
- Treat secondary/concurrent infections (especially *H. mustelae*)
- Antibiotic therapy—indicated in patients with hypersecretory diarrhea, bloody diarrhea, or when secondary infections are

identified. For empirical treatment, use broad-spectrum antibiotics such as cephalexin (15–30 mg/kg PO q12), trimethoprim sulfa (15–30 mg/kg PO, SC q12h), amoxicillin/clavulanate (13–25 mg/kg PO q12h), or Enrofloxacin (10–20 mg/kg PO, IM, IV q12h)
- Antiemetics—metoclopramide (0.2–1.0 mg/kg PO, SC, IM q6–8h), Ondansetron (1 mg/kg PO q12–24h) or maropitant citrate (1 mg/kg SC q24h)
- Gastrointestinal antisecretory agents are helpful to treat, and possibly preventing gastritis in anorectic ferrets. Ferrets continually secrete a baseline level of gastric hydrochloric acid, and as such, anorexia itself may predispose to gastric ulceration. Those successfully used in ferrets include omeprazole (0.7 mg/kg PO q24h), famotidine (0.25–0.5 mg/kg PO, SC, IV q24h), and cimetidine (5–10 mg/kg PO, SC, IM q8h)
- For chronic, malabsorptive disease—administration of prednisone (0.25–0.5 mg/kg PO q12h) may be helpful until signs abate

CONTRAINDICATIONS
N/A

PRECAUTIONS
- Ensure all secondary/concurrent bacterial or parasitic infections have been successfully treated before administering corticosteroid therapy.

POSSIBLE INTERACTIONS
N/A

ALTERNATIVE DRUGS
N/A

FOLLOW-UP

PATIENT MONITORING
N/A

PREVENTION/AVOIDANCE
- No vaccine is currently available
- Isolate all ferrets with suspected ECE

POSSIBLE COMPLICATIONS
- Septicemia/endotoxemia
- Chronic malabsorptive diarrhea
- Dehydration, death
- Intussusception

EXPECTED COURSE AND PROGNOSIS
- Prognosis is guarded in severely affected ferrets.
- Prognosis is good for ferrets that receive prompt initial treatment and survive the initial crisis of illness.
- Many ferrets will develop chronic IBD.

MISCELLANEOUS

ASSOCIATED CONDITIONS
- Helicobacter mustelae
- Lymphoplasmacytic enteritis
- Giardiasis
- Inflammatory Bowel Disease

AGE-RELATED FACTORS
- Older ferrets suffer a higher rate of severe illness.
- Young kits often have mild disease or are asymptomatic.

ZOONOTIC POTENTIAL
N/A

PREGNANCY/FERTILITY/BREEDING
N/A

SYNONYMS
Green slime disease
Infectious hepatitis and enteritis of ferrets
Ferret coronavirus

SEE ALSO
Anorexia
Diarrhea
Gastroduodenal ulcers
Lymphoplasmacytic enteritis and gastroenteritis
Vomiting

ABBREVIATION
ALPE = alkaline phosphatase
ALT = alanine aminotransferase
ECE = epizootic catarrhal enteritis
IBD = inflammatory bowel disease
PCV = packed cell volume

Suggested Reading
Doria-Torra G, Vidaña B, Ramis A, Amarilla S, Martínez J. Coronavirus infection in ferrets: antigen distribution and inflammatory response. Vet Pathol 2016;53(6): 1180–1186.
Hoefer HL. Gastrointestinal diseases of ferrets. In: Quesenberry KE, Carpenter JW, eds. Ferrets, Rabbits and Rodents, (4th ed.). Clinical Medicine and Surgery. 2021. St. Louis: Saunders, 2020:27–38.
Huynh M, Pignon C. Gastrointestinal disease in exotic small mammals. J Exot Pet Med 2013;22(2):118–131.
Li T, Yoshizaki S, Kataoka M et al. Determination of ferret enteric coronavirus genome in laboratory ferrets. *Emerg Infect Dis* 2017;*23*(9):1568–1570.
Murray J, Kiupel M, Maes RK. Ferret coronavirus-associated diseases. Vet Clin North Am Exot Anim Pract 2010;13(3):543–560.
Terada Y, Minami S, Noguchi K et al. Genetic characterization of coronaviruses from domestic ferrets, Japan. Emerg Infect Dis 2014;20(2):284–287.

Author Barbara Oglesbee, DVM, DABVP-Avian

FERRET SYSTEMIC CORONAVIRUS (FRSCV)

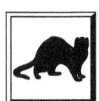

BASICS

DEFINITION
• An emerging systemic disease associated with a novel coronavirus in the genus *Alphacoronavirus*
• Characterized by pyogranulomatous perivasculitis and peritonitis that resembles FIP in cats and has a high mortality rate

PATHOPHYSIOLOGY
• Unknown at this time, but theorized to be similar to the dry form of FIP in cats—a mutated form of virus may become more virulent in certain individuals that lack a proper antibody response, causing a hypersensitivity response, resulting in clinical disease
• Local perivascular viral replication and subsequent pyogranulomatous tissue reaction produce the observed lesions, usually in multiple organs

SYSTEMS AFFECTED
• Multisystemic—pyogranulomatous or granulomatous lesions on the serosal surface of abdominal organs (most often the intestinal serosa or mesentery)
• Gastrointestinal
• Central nervous system—lesions can occur throughout the CNS
• Respiratory
• Cardiac
• Renal
• Hepatic
• Lymphatic
• Ocular

GENETICS
Unknown

INCIDENCE/PREVALENCE
Unknown

GEOGRAPHIC DISTRIBUTION
Seen in North American, European and Japanese populations at this time

SIGNALMENT

Species
All domestic ferrets are susceptible.

Breed Predilections
None reported at this time

Mean Age and Range
Mean of 11 months of age and range of 2–36 months.

Predominant Sex
None

SIGNS

Historical Findings
Nonspecific, as with "dry" form of FIP in cats

Physical Examination Findings
• Diarrhea ("birdseed-like" in late stages)
• Weight loss
• Lethargy
• Hyporexia to anorexia
• Vomiting
• Chronic wasting
• Hind limb paresis/paraparesis
• Ataxia/head tilt
• Tremors/seizures
• Sneezing/labored, congested breathing/coughing/panting
• Bruxism
• Nasal discharge
• Dehydration
• Systolic heart murmur
• Jaundice
• Focal skin erythema
• Green urine
• Reddened rectal mucosa/rectal prolapse
• Splenomegaly
• Renomegaly
• Abdominal masses—polyadenomegaly
• Peripheral lymphadenopathy
• Fever
• Corneal stromal opacity

CAUSES
Mutation of and/or hypersensitivity response to a novel *Alphacoronavirus*

RISK FACTORS
Age (younger more susceptible)

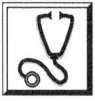

DIAGNOSIS

Diagnosis is based on a combination of clinical signs, histopathology, exclusion of other diseases causing similar signs, and specific immunohistochemistry assays along with PCR testing.

DIFFERENTIAL DIAGNOSIS
Rule out other disease that may cause similar signs, such as
• Ferret enteric coronavirus (FRECV)
• Lymphoma
• Other neoplasia
• Aleutian disease
• Toxin
• Gastrointestinal foreign body
• Trauma
• Bacterial infection
• Mycobacteriosis
• Other viral infection
• Disseminated idiopathic myofasciitis

CBC/BIOCHEMISTRY/URINALYSIS
• CBC: Typical findings include nonregenerative anemia and thrombocytopenia
• Biochemistry: Hyperglobulinemia (hypergammaglobulinemia), hypoalbuminemia, and increased globulin:albumin ratio; increases in BUN, ALT, ALP, GGT—depending on organ system affected
• Urinalysis—Bilverdinuria common

OTHER LABORATORY TESTS
• Protein electrophoresis—polyclonal gammopathy is suggestive of the diagnosis
• Serology for ferret coronavirus—to confirm exposure only; positive test is not diagnostic; tests for feline coronavirus serology are NOT cross-reactive
• Ferret enteric coronavirus PCR test on feces, swab, or tissue indicates presence of virus, not FRSCV or FRECV
• Negative Aleutian disease antibody test or Ferret Aleutian Disease PCR on feces or swab

IMAGING
Radiography and ultrasound may demonstrate abdominal masses, splenomegaly, renomegaly, polyadenomegaly. Micro-CT for neurologic signs suggesting head granulomas or better elucidation of abdominal masses

DIAGNOSTIC PROCEDURES
Immunohistochemistry staining of coronavirus antigen in macrophages within areas of granulomatous inflammation, followed by genotype specific reverse transcription PCR to differentiate from FRECV

PATHOLOGIC FINDINGS
• Gross lesions resemble dry form of FIP
• Multifocal to coalescing white-tan, irregular, 0.5–2.0 cm nodules or plaques on intestinal serosa and/or mesentery; lesions are usually oriented along vascular pathways
• Similar nodules sometimes seen on serosa of liver, kidneys, spleen, or lung
• Mesenteric lymphadenopathy
• Splenomegaly, renomegaly, and/or hepatomegaly
• Severe pyogranulomatous inflammation seen histologically

TREATMENT

APPROPRIATE HEALTH CARE
• Hospitalize for general supportive care
• Most die or are euthanized

NURSING CARE
Supportive care, including fluid therapy, gastroprotectants, antiemetics, antidiarrheal therapy, broad-spectrum antibiotics, and cobalamin supplementation

ACTIVITY
Often self-limiting due to disease

DIET

If anorexic, assist feed an easily digestible high-protein/high-fat diet such as Lafeber Carnivore Critical Care Diet (Lafeber Company, Cornell, IL) or Oxbow Carnivore Critical Care Diet (Oxbow Animal Health, Omaha, NE); if these are unavailable, offer chicken baby foods; may also add dietary supplement such as Nutri-Cal (EVSCO Pharmaceuticals) to increase caloric content to these foods.

CLIENT EDUCATION

Poor prognosis; most die or are euthanized. Some may respond initially to treatment, then relapse; long treatment regimen; may be contagious to other ferrets

SURGICAL CONSIDERATIONS

Antemortem biopsy of granulomas

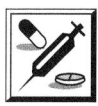

MEDICATIONS

DRUG(S) OF CHOICE

Disease is Immune Mediated; Therapy is Directed at Immune Modulation
• Prednisolone 1–2 mg/kg PO q12h until clinical improvement, then slowly wean off
• Doxycycline has been used as both an antibiotic and for its anti-inflammatory properties (10 mg/kg PO q12h)
• Amoxicillin/clavulanic acid (13–25 mg/kg PO q8–12h) as general antibiotic for secondary bacterial infection

Gastric Protectants
• Sucralfate (Carafate)—75–100 mg/kg PO 10–15 minutes before feeding or prednisone administration
• Cimetidine—10 mg/kg PO q8h—may be preferred; others include omeprazole (0.7 mg/kg PO q24h); famotidine (0.25–0.5 mg/kg PO, IV, SQ q24h)

Antiemetics
• Metoclopramide (0.2–1.0 mg/kg PO, SC, IM q6–8h)
• Maropitant citrate (Cerenia) has been used at dog dosage (1 mg/kg SC q24h)

CONTRAINDICATIONS

N/A

PRECAUTIONS

• If disease is confirmed, the likelihood of mortality without treatment outweighs the side effects of experimental drugs used for treatment, but make owner aware of the risks of each drug

ALTERNATIVE DRUGS

S-Adenosylmethionine (SAMe) and Silybin have been used along with immune-modulating therapy and supportive care.

FOLLOW-UP

PATIENT MONITORING

Recheck CBC, protein electrophoresis

PREVENTION/AVOIDANCE

Be careful with mixing new older and younger ferrets; FRECV is ubiquitous, so preventing exposure to virus is difficult; practice good sanitation and hygiene to avoid spread of the virus.

POSSIBLE COMPLICATIONS

Death

EXPECTED COURSE AND PROGNOSIS

• The prognosis is poor to grave in most cases; death due to progression of disease or euthanasia is likely.
• Some survive with immune modulation and supportive care therapy; supportive care may be required long term, and relapse is common in those that survive the initial course of disease.

MISCELLANEOUS

ASSOCIATED CONDITIONS

Splenomegaly

AGE-RELATED FACTORS

Usually less than 18 months old

ZOONOTIC POTENTIAL

N/A

PREGNANCY/FERTILITY/BREEDING

Unknown

SYNONYMS

Ferret infectious peritonitis
FIP-like disease

ABBREVIATIONS

ALP = alkaline phosphatase
ALT = alanine aminotransferase
BUN = blood urea nitrogen
FIP = ferret infectious peritonitis
FRECV = ferret enteric coronavirus
FRSCV = ferret systemic coronavirus
GGT = gamma glutamyl transferase
PCR = polymerase chain reaction

INTERNET RESOURCES

None

Suggested Reading
Autieri C, Miller C, Scott K, Kilgore A, Papscoe V, Garner M, Fox J. Systemic coronaviral disease in 5 ferrets. Comp Med 2015;65(6):508–516.
Doria-Torra G, Vidaña B, Ramis A, Amarilla S, Martínez J. Coronavirus infection in ferrets: antigen distribution and inflammatory response. Vet Pathol 2016;53(6):1180–1186.
Gnirs K, Quinton J, Dally C, Nicolier A, Ruel Y. Cerebral pyogranuloma associated with systemic coronavirus infection in a ferret. J Small Anim Pract. 2016;57:36–39.
Hoefer HL. Gastrointestinal diseases of ferrets. In: Quesenberry KE, Carpenter JW, eds. Ferrets, Rabbits and Rodents (4th ed.). Clinical Medicine and Surgery. 2021. St. Louis: Saunders, 2020:27–38.
Huynh M, Pignon C. Gastrointestinal disease in exotic small mammals. J Exot Pet Med 2013;22(2):118–131.
Li T, Yoshizaki S, Kataoka M, Doan Y, Ami Y, Suzaki Y, Wakita T. Determination of ferret enteric coronavirus genome in laboratory ferrets. *Emerg Infect Dis* 2017; *23*(9):1568–1570.
Lindemann D, Eshar D, Schumacher L, Almes K, Rankin A. Pyogranulomatous panophthalmitis with systemic coronavirus disease in a domestic ferret (*Mustela putorius furo*). Vet Ophthalmol 2016;19: 167–171.
Murray J, Kiupel M, Maes RK. Ferret coronavirus-associated diseases. Vet Clin North Am Exot Anim Pract 2010;13(3): 543–560.
Terada Y, Minami S, Noguchi K, Mahmoud H, Shimoda H, Mochizuki M, Maeda K. Genetic characterization of coronaviruses from domestic ferrets, Japan. Emerg Infect Dis 2014;20(2):284–287.

Author Eric Klaphake, DVM, DABVP, DACZM

FLEAS AND FLEA INFESTATION

BASICS

OVERVIEW
- Flea infestation—large number of fleas and flea dirt
- Heavy infestations may cause anemia, especially in young ferrets
- Fleabite hypersensitivity has not been documented in ferrets; however, some ferrets appear to be significantly more pruritic than others, suggesting that a hypersensitivity reaction may exist in these animals.

SIGNALMENT
- Incidence varies with climatic conditions and flea population
- No age or sex predilection
- Clinical signs vary with individual animals
- Young animals more likely to develop anemia

SIGNS

Historical Findings
- History of flea infestation in other pets, including dogs and cats
- Some animals asymptomatic
- Biting, chewing, scratching, or excessive licking
- Signs of fleas and flea dirt

Physical Examination Findings
- Depends on the severity of the reaction and the degree of exposure to fleas (i.e., seasonal vs. year-round)
- Finding fleas and flea dirt
- Papules, alopecia, excoriations, and scaling, often in the tail region, but may appear anywhere
- Secondary bacterial infections sometimes seen
- Pale mucous membranes, tachycardia in anemic animals

CAUSES AND RISK FACTORS
Exposure to other flea-infested animals within the household; keeping animals outdoors

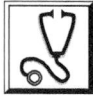

DIAGNOSIS

DIFFERENTIAL DIAGNOSIS
- Ferret adrenal disease—rule out ferret adrenal disease, since this is the most common cause of alopecia and may occur in conjunction with fleas. Ferrets with adrenal disease may be extremely pruritic; secondary pyoderma may be present. Alopecia generally is symmetric, gradual in onset, begins at the tail base, and progresses cranially. Other signs, such as vulvar swelling in females, often seen. May be concurrent with flea infestation.

- Otodectes (ear mites)—usually not pruritic; lesions typically localized to areas surrounding ears; black/brown waxy exudate present
- Sarcoptic mange—unusual mite; sometimes may differentiate based on skin scraping, but mites not always present; therapeutic trial with ivermectin may differentiate; however, concurrent flea and sarcoptes infestation may occur.
- Contact dermatitis—usually ventral distribution of lesions; acute onset

CBC/BIOCHEMISTRY/URINALYSIS
Usually normal; hypereosinophilia inconsistently detected and not well documented

OTHER LABORATORY TESTS
- Skin scrapings—negative
- Flea combings—fleas or flea dirt usually found in affected ferrets
- Cytology of ear exudate—no mites seen

IMAGING
Abdominal ultrasound to rule out adrenal disease

DIAGNOSTIC PROCEDURES
- Diagnosis is usually based on historical information, the distribution of lesions and finding fleas or flea dirt

PATHOLOGIC FINDINGS
- Superficial dermatitis is occasionally seen

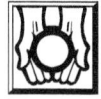

TREATMENT

CLIENT EDUCATION
Inform owners that controlling exposure to fleas is currently the only means of therapy.

MEDICATIONS

DRUG(S) OF CHOICE
- Corticosteroids—anti-inflammatory dosages for symptomatic relief while the fleas are being controlled; prednisone 0.25–1.0 mg/kg q 24h PO divided
- Antihistamines—hydroxyzine (2 mg/kg PO q8h); diphenhydramine (0.5–2.0 mg/kg PO, IM, IV q8–12h); chlorpheniramine (1–2 mg/kg PO q8–12h)
- Fipronil (Frontline, Boehringer Ingelheim) 0.2–0.4 mL/animal applied topically q30d
- Imidacloprid (Advantage, Bayer) 10 mg/kg topically q30d; Imidacloprid and moxidectin (Advantage Multi for Cats, Bayer) 0.4 mL/ animal topically q30d
- Selamectin (Revolution, Pfizer) 15 mg/kg topically q30d

- Systemic treatments—limited benefit because they require a flea bite to be effective; may help animals with flea infestation; lufenuron (Program, Novartis) for cats has been used anecdotally in ferrets at 30–45 mg/kg PO q30d
- Sprays and powders—usually contain pyrethrins and pyrethroids (synthetic pyrethrins) or carbaryl with an insect growth regulator or synergist; products labeled for use in kittens and puppies are anecdotally considered safe and generally effective, advantages are low toxicity and repellent activity; disadvantages are frequent applications and expense
- Indoor treatment—fogs and premises sprays; usually contain organophosphates, pyrethrins, and/or insect growth regulators; apply according to manufacturer's directions; treat all areas of the house; can be applied by the owner; advantages are weak chemicals and generally inexpensive; disadvantage is labor intensity; premises sprays concentrate the chemicals in areas that most need treatment. Safety of product usage in a ferret's environment is unknown.
- Professional exterminators—advantages are less labor intensive; relatively few applications; sometimes guaranteed; disadvantages are strength of chemicals and cost; specific recommendations and guidelines must be followed. Safety of product usage in a ferret's environment is unknown.
- Inert substances—boric acid, diatomaceous earth, and silica aerogel; treat every 6–12 months; follow manufacturer's recommendations; very safe and effective if applied properly
- Outdoor treatment—concentrated in shaded areas; sprays usually contain pyrethroids or organophosphates and an insect growth regulator; powders are usually organophosphates; product containing nematodes (Steinerma carpocapsae) is very safe and chemical free.
- Antibiotics—may be necessary to treat secondary pyoderma, if severe

CONTRAINDICATIONS
- Do not use flea collars on ferrets.
- Do not use organophosphate-containing products on ferrets.
- Do not use straight permethrin sprays or spot-ons on ferrets.

PRECAUTIONS
- Prevent ferrets or their cagemates from licking topical spot-on products before they are dry.
- Pyrethrin/pyrethroid-type flea products— adverse reactions include depression, hypersalivation, muscle tremors, vomiting, ataxia, dyspnea, and anorexia.

• Toxicity—if any signs are noted, the animal should be bathed thoroughly to remove any remaining chemicals and treated appropriately.

POSSIBLE INTERACTIONS
With the exception of lufenuron used concurrently with fipronil or imidacloprid, do not use more than one flea treatment at a time.

ALTERNATIVE DRUGS
N/A

FOLLOW-UP
PATIENT MONITORING
• Pruritus and alopecia—should decrease with effective flea control; if signs persist evaluate for other causes or concurrent disease (e.g., ferret adrenal gland disease)
• Fleas and flea dirt—should decrease with effective flea control; however, absence is not always a reliable indicator of successful treatment in very sensitive animals

PREVENTION/AVOIDANCE
• Year-round warm climates—may require year-round flea control
• Seasonally warm climates—usually begin flea control in May or June

POSSIBLE COMPLICATIONS
• Secondary bacterial infections
• Adverse reaction to flea control products

EXPECTED COURSE AND PROGNOSIS
Prognosis is good, if strict flea control is instituted.

MISCELLANEOUS
ASSOCIATED CONDITIONS
N/A

AGE-RELATED FACTORS
Use caution with flea control products in young animals

ZOONOTIC POTENTIAL
In areas of moderate to severe flea infestation, people can be bitten by fleas; usually, papular lesions are located on the wrists and ankles.

PREGNANCY/FERTILITY/BREEDING
Carefully follow the label directions of each individual product to estimate its safety; however, bear in mind that these products have not been used extensively in pregnant ferrets, and safety is unknown.

SYNONYMS
N/A

SEE ALSO
Adrenal disease (Hyperadrenocorticism)
Dermatophytosis
Ear mites
Sarcoptic mange

ABBREVIATIONS
N/A

Suggested Reading
d'Ovidio D, Santoro D. Dermatologic diseases of ferrets. In: Quesenberry KE, Carpenter JW, eds. Ferrets, Rabbits and Rodents, 4th ed. Clinical Medicine and Surgery. 2021. St. Louis: Saunders, 2020:109–116.
Fehr M, Koestlinger S. Ectoparasites in small exotic mammals. Vet Clin Exot Anim 2013;16:611–657.
Fisher M, Beck W, Hutchinson MJ et al. Efficacy and safety of selamectin (Stronghold®/Revolution™) used off-label in exotic pets. Int J Appl Res Vet Med 2007; 5:87–96.
Hoppmann E, Wilson Barron H. Ferret and rabbit dermatology. J Exot Pet Med 2007; 16:225–237.
Patterson MM, Kirchain SM. Comparison of three treatments for control of ear mites in ferrets. Lab Anim Sci 1999;49:655–657.
Author Barbara Oglesbee DVM, DABVP (Avian)

FERRETS

GASTRITIS

BASICS

DEFINITION
• Inflammation of the gastric mucosa
• The presence of gastric erosions and ulcers depends on the inciting cause and duration

PATHOPHYSIOLOGY
• Irritation of the gastric mucosa by chemical irritants, drugs, or infectious agents, resulting in an inflammatory response in the mucosal surface that may extend to involve submucosal layers
• Ferrets secrete a baseline level of gastric hydrochloric acid and may develop gastric ulcerations when anorexic.
• Immune-mediated disease may also produce chronic inflammation.

SYSTEMS AFFECTED
• Gastrointestinal
• Respiratory—aspiration pneumonia is infrequently seen secondary to vomiting; it is more likely if concurrent esophageal disease exists or the patient is debilitated.

INCIDENCE/PREVALENCE
Relatively common, especially when due to *Helicobacter mustelae* or gastric foreign bodies

SIGNALMENT
• Gastritis due to helicobacter or gastric foreign bodies is seen most commonly in ferrets 3 months to 3 years of age, and in older ferrets, or ferrets with other, underlying disorders
• Gastric foreign bodies are more common in young (<2 years old) ferrets

SIGNS

Historical Findings
• Vomiting is a relatively uncommon sign of GI tract disease in ferrets as compared with dogs or cats. When present, vomitus may be bile stained and may contain undigested food, flecks of blood, or digested blood ("coffee grounds").
• Weight loss and muscle wasting due to chronic anorexia are the most common signs of gastritis in ferrets.
• Decreased appetite, will only accept certain foods, such as the popular "duck soups" or homemade foods
• Ptyalism, pawing at the mouth, bruxism
• Diarrhea, sometimes with blood or mucus
• May see melena with ulceration
• Abdominal pain
• Lethargy, poor haircoat

Physical Examination Findings
• Often normal
• May be thin with persistent anorexia

• May have pale mucous membranes with anemia from chronic blood loss
• Abdominal palpation may elicit cranial abdominal pain, splenomegaly, and/or enlarged mesenteric lymph nodes.

CAUSES
• Infectious—*Helicobacter mustelae*, viral (ECE, CDV)
• Dietary indiscretion—foreign objects, trichobezoar, chemical irritants, spoiled foods
• Inflammatory—eosinophilic gastroenteritis, lymphoplasmacytic gastroenteritis
• Metabolic/endocrine disease—chronic liver disease, uremia
• Toxins—cleaning agents, heavy metals
• Drugs—NSAIDs, possibly glucocorticoids
• Miscellaneous—anorexia, stress

RISK FACTORS
• Environmental—unsupervised/free-roaming pets are more likely to ingest inappropriate foods or materials, intentionally or unintentionally.
• Anorexia due to starvation or GI or metabolic disease may cause gastric ulcers.
• Potentially poor sanitary conditions and overcrowding may facilitate the spread of infection.
• Medications—NSAIDs, glucocorticoids

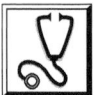

DIAGNOSIS

DIFFERENTIAL DIAGNOSIS
• All the causes listed above are included in the differential diagnosis of gastritis; sometimes no identifiable cause is found for observed gastric inflammation.
• For ptyalism, pawing at the mouth—insulinoma or other causes of hypoglycemia; any condition causing nausea (GI lymphoma, hepatic or renal disease, and lower intestinal tract disease), mouth pain, dental disease
• Idiopathic gastritis—diagnosis of exclusion; often characterized by a predominantly lymphoplasmacytic infiltrate (superficial or diffuse)

CBC/BIOCHEMISTRY/URINALYSIS
• Hemogram is usually unremarkable unless systemic disease present
• Hemoconcentration if severe dehydration
• Regenerative anemia with ulceration
• May see eosinophilia with eosinophilic gastroenteritis
• May see leukocytosis with neutrophilia and lymphocytosis with helicobacter-induced disease
• Azotemia with low urine specific gravity in uremic gastritis

• Increased serum hepatic enzyme activities or hypoalbuminemia with ECE or chronic hepatic disease

OTHER LABORATORY TESTS
• Fecal flotation—to screen for gastrointestinal parasitism

IMAGING
• Survey abdominal radiographs—usually normal, but may reveal radiodense foreign objects, a thickened gastric wall, or gastric outlet obstruction with persistent gastric distension
• Contrast radiography—may detect foreign objects, outlet obstruction, delayed gastric emptying, or gastric wall defects
• Ultrasonography—may be used to evaluate stomach and intestinal wall thickness and gastric foreign objects; can be used to examine the liver, spleen, and mesenteric lymph nodes

DIAGNOSTIC PROCEDURES
• Laparotomy for gastric biopsy and histopathology may be required for definitive diagnosis; if laparotomy is performed, should biopsy, even if gastric mucosa appears normal
• Many patients may be unsuitable candidates for surgery (severely debilitated, concurrent disease, or owner financial constraints). Alternatively, a presumptive diagnosis of helicobacter-induced disease may be made based on the identification of suggestive clinical signs, exclusion of other diagnoses, and a favorable response to empirical treatment.
• Foreign objects can occasionally be identified and retrieved via endoscopy. However, the small size of the patient and subsequent limitations on instrument size often limit the use of endoscopy.

PATHOLOGIC FINDINGS
• Helicobacter gastritis—gastric mucosal ulceration and granular-appearing mucosa due to inflammatory reaction. Lesions appear most commonly in the pyloric antrum. On histopathologic examination, gastric spiral organisms seen on silver-stained sections; lymphoplasmacytic gastritis and lymphoid follicle hyperplasia
• Idiopathic gastritis—inflammatory infiltrates vary; most often lymphocytes and plasma cells; can see eosinophils, and/or histiocytes
• Eosinophilic gastroenteritis—diffuse infiltrate of eosinophils into the lamina propria, submucosa, and occasionally the serosa; focal eosinophilic granulomas may be seen in affected lymph nodes
• The distribution of lesions may be patchy, so take several biopsy specimens.

TREATMENT

APPROPRIATE HEALTH CARE

• Most patients are stable at presentation unless vomiting is severe enough to cause dehydration.
• Can typically manage as outpatient, pending diagnostic testing or undergoing clinical trials of special diets or medications
• If the patient is dehydrated or vomiting becomes severe, hospitalize and institute appropriate intravenous fluid therapy. If held NPO due to vomiting, provide a dextrose-containing fluid, and monitor blood glucose concentration.

DIET

• Ferrets rarely have intractable vomiting such that holding NPO for long periods is necessary. If holding NPO, monitor ferrets carefully for hypoglycemia. A fast of greater than 4 hours can be dangerous. Insulinomas are extremely common in middle-aged ferrets and may be the cause of signs of gastritis, or may occur simultaneously with other causes of gastritis.
• Can use novel protein sources if a dietary allergy is suspected. Feed diets for a minimum of 3 weeks to assess adequacy of response.

Anorexia

• If anorexic, assist feed an easily digestible high-protein/high-fat diet such as Lafeber Carnivore Critical Care Diet (Lafeber Company, Cornell, IL) or Oxbow Carnivore Critical Care Diet (Oxbow Animal Health, Omaha, NE); if these are unavailable, offer chicken baby foods; may also add dietary supplement such as Nutri-Cal (EVSCO Pharmaceuticals) to increase caloric content to these foods.
• Warming the food to body temperature or offering it via syringe may increase acceptance.
• Ferrets exhibiting malabsorptive diarrhea (characterized by grainy feces, and weight loss) often respond well to a diet consisting of chicken-based human baby foods and high-calorie dietary supplements until the diarrhea resolves.

Client Education

• Gastritis has numerous causes.
• Diagnostic work-up—may be extensive; usually requires a biopsy for a definitive diagnosis

SURGICAL CONSIDERATIONS

• Gastrotomy for removal of foreign objects
• Surgical management if a mass is causing a gastric outflow obstruction

MEDICATIONS

DRUG(S) OF CHOICE

• If helicobacter infection is confirmed or suspected—specific treatment for helicobacter—the combination of amoxicillin (30 mg/kg PO q8–12h) plus metronidazole (20 mg/kg PO q 8–12h) and bismuth subsalicylate (17.5 mg/kg PO q12h or 1 mL/kg of regular strength preparation [262 mg/15 mL] PO q8–12h) is a common, inexpensive treatment regimen; however, many ferrets find this unpalatable. Dosing every 8 hours may be necessary to eliminate infection. Combine this treatment with an antisecretory agent (see below). Treat for at least 2 (often 3–4) weeks. The combination of clarithromycin (12.5 mg/kg PO q8–12h) and ranitidine bismuth citrate or ranitidine HCl (24 mg/kg PO q8–12h) for 2 weeks has also been reported to be effective in the eradication of *Helicobacter* spp. Ranitidine is no longer approved for human use in the US and can be difficult to find. The combination of clarithromycin (50 mg/kg PO q24h or divided q12h); omeprazole (4 mg/kg PO q24h); and metronidazole (20 mg/kg PO q12h) for 14 days has also been used for eradication.
• Gastrointestinal antisecretory agents are helpful to treat and possibly prevent gastritis in anorectic ferrets. Ferrets continually secrete a baseline level of gastric hydrochloric acid and, as such, anorexia itself may predispose to gastric ulceration. Those successfully used in ferrets include omeprazole (4 mg/kg PO q24h), famotidine (0.25–0.5 mg/kg PO, SC, IV q24h), and cimetidine (10 mg/kg PO, SC, IM, IV q8h)
• Sucralfate suspension (25 mg/kg PO q8h) protects ulcerated tissue (cytoprotection) by binding to ulcer sites.
• Administer antibiotic(s) with activity against enteric gram-negatives and anaerobes parenterally if a suspected break in the gastrointestinal mucosal barrier or aspiration pneumonia
• Glucocorticoids (prednisone 1.25–2.5 mg/kg PO q24h, gradually taper to 0.25–1 mg/kg QOD) may decrease inflammation in patients with chronic gastritis secondary to suspected immune-mediated mechanisms (eosinophilic or lymphoplasmacytic gastroenteritis)
• Antiemetics should be reserved for patients with refractory vomiting that have not responded to treatment of the underlying disease. Options include metoclopramide (0.2–1.0 mg/kg PO, SC, IM q6–8h), ondansetron (1mg/kg PO q12-24h), or maropitant citrate (1 mg/kg SC q24h).

• Metoclopramide (0.2–1.0 mg/kg PO, SC, IM q6–8h) or cisapride (0.5 mg/kg PO q8–12h) to increase gastric emptying and normalize intestinal motility gastric emptying is delayed or duodenogastric reflux is present

CONTRAINDICATIONS

• Do not use prokinetics (metoclopramide or cisapride) if gastric outlet obstruction is present.
• Alpha-adrenergic blockers such as chlorpromazine should not be used in dehydrated patients since they can cause hypotension.

FOLLOW-UP

PATIENT MONITORING

• Resolution of clinical signs indicates a positive response.
• Monitor blood glucose concentration in animals held NPO for hypoglycemia, do not fast for >4 hours
• Repeat biopsy if signs decrease but do not resolve.

PREVENTION/AVOIDANCE

• Avoid medications (e.g., NSAIDs) and foods that cause gastric irritation in the patient.
• Use antisecretory agents in anorexic ferrets.
• Prevent unsupervised roaming and the potential for dietary indiscretion.
• Avoid overcrowding and unsanitary conditions.

POSSIBLE COMPLICATIONS

• Gastric erosions and ulcers with progressive mucosal damage, hemorrhage, and anemia from ulcers; perforation
• Aspiration pneumonia

EXPECTED COURSE AND PROGNOSIS

Varies with the underlying cause

MISCELLANEOUS

ASSOCIATED CONDITIONS

• Gastrointestinal foreign bodies
• Insulinoma, adrenal disease, lymphoma, and cardiac disease are common in middle-aged to older ferrets and may predispose to the development of gastric ulceration.

AGE-RELATED FACTORS

Young animals are more likely to ingest foreign objects and have helicobacter-induced gastritis.

SEE ALSO

Eosinophilic gastroenteritis
Gastroduodenal ulcers

GASTRITIS

FERRETS

Helicobacter mustelae
Lymphoplasmacytic enteritis and gastroenteritis
Vomiting

ABBREVIATIONS
CDV = canine distemper virus
ECE = epizootic catarrhal enteritis
GI = gastrointestinal
NSAIDs = nonsteroidal anti-inflammatory drugs

Suggested Reading
Doria-Torra G, Vidaña B, Ramis A, Amarilla S, Martínez J. Coronavirus infection in ferrets: antigen distribution and inflammatory response. Vet Pathol 2016;53(6):1180–1186.
Hoefer HL. Gastrointestinal diseases of ferrets. In: Quesenberry KE, Carpenter JW, eds. Ferrets, Rabbits, and Rodents, 4th ed. Clinical Medicine and Surgery. 2021 ed. St. Louis: Saunders, 2020:27–38.
Huynh M, Pignon C. Gastrointestinal disease in exotic small mammals. J Exot Pet Med 2013;22(2):118–131.
Johnson-Delaney CA. Geriatric ferrets. Vet Clin Exot Anim Pract 2020;23(3):549–565.
Li T, Yoshizaki S, Kataoka M et al. Determination of ferret enteric coronavirus genome in laboratory ferrets. *Emerg Infect Dis* 2017;*23*(9):1568–1570.
Murray J, Kiupel M, Maes RK. Ferret coronavirus-associated diseases. Vet Clin North Am Exot Anim Pract 2010;13(3):543–560.
Terada Y, Minami S, Noguchi K et al. Genetic characterization of coronaviruses from domestic ferrets, Japan. Emerg Infect Dis 2014;20(2):284–287.

Author Barbara Oglesbee, DVM, DABVP-Avian

GASTRODUODENAL ULCERS

BASICS

DEFINITION
Erosive lesions that extend through the mucosa and into the muscularis mucosa

PATHOPHYSIOLOGY
• Gastroduodenal ulcers result from single or multiple factors altering, damaging, or overwhelming the normal defense and repair mechanisms of the gastric mucosal barrier.
• The most common cause of gastric ulceration is *Helicobacter mustelae*-induced disease.
• Ferrets secrete a baseline level of gastric hydrochloric acid and may develop gastric ulcerations when anorexic.

SYSTEMS AFFECTED
• Gastrointestinal—gastric fundus and antrum are the most common sites of ulceration.
• Cardiovascular/hemic—acute hemorrhage may result in anemia with subsequent tachycardia, systolic heart murmur, and/or hypotension.
• Respiratory—tachypnea may be present with anemia; aspiration pneumonia possible secondary to vomiting

INCIDENCE/PREVALENCE
• True incidence unknown; probably more common than clinically recognized
• *Helicobacter*-induced gastric ulceration is one of the most common causes of anorexia, melena, and vomiting in ferrets in North America; the incidence in other countries has not been reported.

SIGNALMENT
Mean Age and Range
Most common in ferrets 3 months to 3 years of age; also seen in older ferrets with underlying disease conditions, stress, or immunosuppression

SIGNS
General Comments
Some animals may be asymptomatic with significant gastroduodenal ulcer disease.

SIGNS
Historical Findings
Anorexia, ptyalism, bruxism, diarrhea, melena, vomiting, abdominal pain, weight loss, and weakness are the most common clinical signs. Many affected ferrets will paw at the mouth when nauseated.

Physical Examination Findings
• May have signs of dehydration from fluid and electrolyte loss due to vomiting or diarrhea

• Pallor of the mucous membranes with chronic blood loss
• Weight loss—indicates chronic disease
• Poor hair coat or alopecia
• Fecal staining of the perineum
• Mesenteric lymph nodes are often palpably enlarged.
• Splenomegaly is a common, usually nonspecific, finding.
• Signs related to underlying disorders
• Can be normal in patients with early or mild disease

CAUSES
• *Helicobacter mustelae* is the most common cause of GI ulcer disease in North American ferrets
• Gastric foreign bodies
• Anorexia from any origin may cause gastric ulcers.
• Gastric neoplasia
• Metabolic disease—hepatic disease, renal failure
• Drugs—NSAIDs
• Gastritis—lymphocytic/plasmacytic gastroenteritis, eosinophilic gastroenteritis
• Stress/major medical illness—shock, severe illness, hypotension, trauma, major surgery, burns, heat stroke, sepsis
• Lead poisoning
• Neurologic disease—head trauma, intervertebral disk disease

RISK FACTORS
• Stress, concurrent illness (e.g., epizootic catarrhal enteritis [ECE], other intestinal pathogens, insulinoma, lymphoma)
• Administration of ulcerogenic drugs (NSAIDs)
• Concurrent administration of NSAIDs and glucocorticoids
• Hypovolemic or septic shock

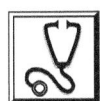

DIAGNOSIS

DIFFERENTIAL DIAGNOSIS
• For melena: esophageal disease (neoplasia, esophagitis, foreign body)—differentiate by contrast radiography and/or endoscopy; coagulopathies (DIC, anticoagulant rodenticide poisoning; nasal or oropharyngeal disease (neoplasia, fungal infection)—blood may be swallowed, and hematemesis and melena can occur; may differentiate on clinical signs and physical examination findings; Pepto-Bismol may cause black, tarry stools.
• For ptyalism, pawing at the mouth—insulinoma or other causes of hypoglycemia; any condition causing nausea (GI lymphoma, hepatic or renal disease, and lower intestinal tract disease)

• In young ferrets, GI foreign bodies (in older ferrets, trichobezoars) can cause identical clinical signs and may contribute to gastric ulceration.
• Similar clinical signs may be seen with GI neoplasia, ECE, bacterial enteritis, or inflammatory bowel disease.

CBC/BIOCHEMISTRY/URINALYSIS
• Regenerative anemia is seen with chronic blood loss and may be severe
• Hypoproteinemia—may be present due to alimentary hemorrhage
• Leukocytosis with neutrophilia and lymphocytosis can be seen with helicobacter infection; may see mature neutrophilia, left-shift neutrophilia with sepsis, and gastroduodenal ulcer perforation
• May see elevated BUN, creatinine, and isosthenuria—if ulcers are due to renal disease
• May see elevated liver enzymes, hyperbilirubinemia, and/or hypoalbuminemia—if ulcers are due to liver disease

OTHER LABORATORY TESTS
• Fecal flotation—to screen for gastrointestinal parasitism
• For helicobacter—culture usually requires gastric biopsy and specialized isolation techniques and media; success rates are low

IMAGING
• Radiography—usually normal with ulceration alone; helpful to rule out underlying disease (e.g., gastric foreign body, neoplasia) or other causes of GI tract disease
• GI contrast studies rarely demonstrate mucosal irregularities or filling defects.
• Abdominal ultrasonography usually will not detect a gastroduodenal ulcer; it may identify a gastric or duodenal mass, gastric or duodenal wall thickening, and/or abdominal lymphadenopathy.

DIAGNOSTIC PROCEDURES
• To establish a causal relationship between infection with helicobacter and clinical signs, a gastric biopsy is needed. Exploratory laparotomy is often useful to evaluate the extent of gastric pathology and to rule out GI foreign bodies, neoplasia, and intestinal inflammatory diseases, but is not indicated in every case. Biopsy is performed via laparotomy. Evidence of characteristic histologic lesions combined with documentation of the organism is needed to support helicobacter infection as the cause of clinical disease.
• Alternatively, a presumptive diagnosis may be made based on the identification of suggestive clinical signs, exclusion of other diagnoses, and a favorable response to empirical treatment. Many patients may be unsuitable candidates for surgery

FERRETS

(severely debilitated, concurrent disease, or owner financial constraints).

PATHOLOGIC FINDINGS
• Stomach—gastric mucosal ulceration and granular-appearing mucosa due to the inflammatory reaction. Lesions appear most commonly in the pyloric antrum. On histopathologic examination, lymphocytic plasmacytic gastritis and lymphoid follicle hyperplasia are commonly seen, especially with helicobacter infection
• May identify *Helicobacter* spp. in gastric biopsy specimens (silver stains help identify *Helicobacter*)

TREATMENT

APPROPRIATE HEALTH CARE
• Treat any underlying causes.
• Can treat on an outpatient basis if the cause is identified and removed, vomiting is not excessive, and gastroduodenal bleeding is minimal
• Ferrets that are anorexic, vomiting, or dehydrated require hospitalization; treat as inpatients—those with severe gastroduodenal bleeding and/or ulcer perforation
• May need emergency management of hemorrhage or septic peritonitis

NURSING CARE
• Intravenous fluids to maintain hydration
• May need transfusions in patients with severe gastroduodenal hemorrhage

ACTIVITY
Restricted

DIET
• If anorexic, assist feed an easily digestible high-protein/high-fat diet such as Lafeber Carnivore Critical Care Diet (Lafeber Company, Cornell, IL) or Oxbow Carnivore Critical Care Diet (Oxbow Animal Health, Omaha, NE); if these are unavailable, offer chicken baby foods; may also add dietary supplement such as Nutri-Cal (EVSCO Pharmaceuticals) to increase caloric content to these foods.
• Warming the food to body temperature or offering it via syringe may increase acceptance.

CLIENT EDUCATION
Explain the difficulty of establishing a diagnosis without invasive techniques such as gastric biopsy.

SURGICAL CONSIDERATIONS
Surgical treatment is indicated if hemorrhage is uncontrolled and severe, gastroduodenal ulcer perforates, and/or a potentially resectable tumor is identified.

MEDICATIONS

DRUG(S) OF CHOICE
• If helicobacter infection is confirmed or suspected–specific treatment for helicobacter—the combination of amoxicillin (30 mg/kg PO q8–12h) plus metronidazole (20 mg/kg PO q 8–12h) and bismuth subsalicylate (17.5 mg/kg PO q12h or 1 mL/kg of regular strength preparation [262 mg/15 mL] PO q8–12h) is a common, inexpensive treatment regimen; however, many ferrets find this unpalatable. Dosing every 8 hours may be necessary to eliminate the infection. Combine this treatment with an antisecretory agent (see below). Treat for at least 2 (often 3–4) weeks. The combination of clarithromycin (12.5 mg/kg PO q8–12h) and ranitidine bismuth citrate or ranitidine HCl (24 mg/kg PO q8–12h) for 2 weeks has also been reported to be effective in the eradication of *Helicobacter* spp. Ranitidine is no longer approved for human use in the US and can be difficult to find. The combination of clarithromycin (50 mg/kg PO q24h or divided q12h); omeprazole (4 mg/kg PO q24h); metronidazole (20 mg/kg PO q12h) for 14 days has also been used for eradication
• Gastrointestinal antisecretory agents are helpful to treat and possibly prevent gastritis in anorectic ferrets. Ferrets continually secrete a baseline level of gastric hydrochloric acid and, as such, anorexia itself may predispose to gastric ulceration. Those successfully used in ferrets include omeprazole (4 mg/kg PO q24h), famotidine (0.25–0.5 mg/kg PO, SC, IV q24h), and cimetidine (10 mg/kg PO, SC, IM, IV q8h)
• Sucralfate suspension (25 mg/kg PO q8h) protects ulcerated tissue (cytoprotection) by binding to ulcer sites.
• Administer antibiotic(s) with activity against enteric gram-negatives and anaerobes parenterally if a suspected break in the gastrointestinal mucosal barrier or aspiration pneumonia
• Glucocorticoids (prednisone 1.25–2.5 mg/kg PO q24h, gradually taper to 0.25–1 mg/kg QOD) may decrease inflammation in patients with chronic gastritis secondary to suspected immune-mediated mechanisms (eosinophilic or lymphoplasmacytic gastroenteritis)
• Antiemetics should be reserved for patients with refractory vomiting that have not responded to treatment of the underlying disease. Options include metoclopramide (0.2–1.0 mg/kg PO, SC, IM q6–8h), Ondansetron (1mg/kg PO q12-24h), or maropitant citrate (1 mg/kg SC q24h).

• Metoclopramide (0.2–1.0 mg/kg PO, SC, IM q6–8h) or cisapride (0.5 mg/kg PO q8–12h) to increase gastric emptying and normalize intestinal motility gastric emptying is delayed or duodenogastric reflux is present

CONTRAINDICATIONS
• Do not use prokinetics (metoclopramide or cisapride) if gastric outlet obstruction is present.
• Alpha-adrenergic blockers such as chlorpromazine should not be used in dehydrated patients since they can cause hypotension.

POSSIBLE INTERACTIONS
• Cimetidine may interfere with the metabolism of other drugs.
• H_2 blockers prevent the uptake of omeprazole by oxyntic cells.
• Sucralfate may alter the absorption of other drugs.

FOLLOW-UP

PATIENT MONITORING
• Assess improvement in clinical signs
• Can check PCV, TP, and BUN until they return to normal
• If vomiting persists or recurs after cessation of *Helicobacter* therapy, a biopsy may be needed to determine whether the infection has been eradicated.

PREVENTION/AVOIDANCE
• Avoid gastric irritants (e.g., NSAIDs) and stress
• Administer antisecretory agents to anorexic ferrets.

POSSIBLE COMPLICATIONS
• Gastroduodenal ulcer perforation and possible sepsis
• Severe blood loss requiring transfusion
• Aspiration pneumonia
• Death—sepsis, hemorrhage

EXPECTED COURSE AND PROGNOSIS
• Varies with the underlying cause
• Patients with malignant gastric neoplasia, renal failure, liver failure, sepsis, and gastric perforation—poor
• Gastroduodenal ulcers secondary to helicobacter infection, inflammatory bowel disease, or NSAID administration—may be good to excellent, depending on the severity

MISCELLANEOUS

AGE-RELATED FACTORS
Neoplasia more common in older animals

ZOONOTIC POTENTIAL
Further investigation is needed to determine/evaluate a possible zoonotic potential for *Helicobacter* spp.

PREGNANCY/FERTILITY/BREEDING
Avoid metronidazole in pregnant animals.

ASSOCIATED CONDITIONS
• Gastrointestinal foreign bodies
• Insulinoma, adrenal disease, lymphoma, and cardiac disease are common in middle-aged to older ferrets and may predispose to the development of gastric ulceration.

SEE ALSO
Gastrointestinal and esophageal foreign bodies
Helicobacter mustelae
Inflammatory bowel disease

Melena
Vomiting

ABBREVIATIONS
BUN = blood urea nitrogen
DIC = disseminated intravascular coagulation
ECE = epizootic catarrhal enteritis
GI = gastrointestinal
NSAIDs = nonsteroidal anti-inflammatory drugs
PCV = packed cell volume
TP = total protein

Suggested Reading

Di Girolamo N, Selleri P. Medical and surgical emergencies in ferrets. Vet Clin Exot Anim 2016;19:431–464.
Hoefer HL. Gastrointestinal diseases of ferrets. In: Quesenberry KE, Carpenter JW, eds. Ferrets, Rabbits, and Rodents, 4th ed. Clinical Medicine and Surgery. 2021 ed. St. Louis: Saunders, 2020:27–38.
Huynh M, Pignon C. Gastrointestinal disease in exotic small mammals. J Exot Pet Med 2013;22(2):118–131.
Johnson-Delaney CA. Geriatric ferrets. Vet Clin Exot Anim Pract 2020;23(3):549–565.
Livingstone M. Dealing with gastrointestinal disease in ferrets. In Practice 2022;44:169–179.
Murray J, Kiupel M, Maes RK. Ferret coronavirus-associated diseases. Vet Clin North Am Exot Anim Pract 2010;13(3):543–560.

Author Barbara Oglesbee, DVM, DABVP-Avian

GASTROINTESTINAL AND ESOPHAGEAL FOREIGN BODIES

BASICS

DEFINITION
A non-food item located in the esophagus, stomach, or intestine

PATHOPHYSIOLOGY
• Ferrets are extremely fond of chewing, especially on rubber or foam rubber objects, plastic, and cloth. Therefore, gastrointestinal foreign bodies (GI FBs) are a common occurrence, especially in young ferrets <2 years of age. Trichobezoars acquired through grooming may also form GI FBs, especially in older ferrets.
• Some small or easily deformed foreign bodies will pass through the gastrointestinal tract with the ingesta and will subsequently be eliminated from the body in the feces. Larger, nondeformable material may cause a partial or complete outflow obstruction, most commonly of the stomach or intestines.
• Underlying disorders causing abnormal or delayed GI transit may contribute to GI FB rendition (e.g., lymphoma, IBD, gastric ulcers, and *Helicobacter gastroenteritis*).
• Retained objects of insufficient size to cause an outflow obstruction may cause mechanical irritation to the mucosa.

SYSTEMS AFFECTED
• Gastrointestinal—if an obstruction has occurred, the patient may become dehydrated from fluid loss via vomiting or regurgitation. If a perforation has occurred, mediastinitis or peritonitis may develop.
• Musculoskeletal—loss of muscle mass may occur due to inappetence.
• Multisystemic—heavy metal toxicosis can cause multisystemic changes.

INCIDENCE/PREVALENCE
Exact incidence not reported; however, GI FBs are anecdotally one of the most common causes of clinical disease in pet ferrets.

SIGNALMENT
• Younger ferrets (<2 years) are more likely to ingest toys or other objects.
• Trichobezoars are more commonly seen in older ferrets.

SIGNS

Historical Findings
Gastric
• Pronounced weakness and reluctance to move are commonly seen in acute obstructions.
• Inappetence, anorexia, weight loss, chronic wasting, and lethargy are the most common signs, especially with chronic disease.

• Anorexia may wax and wane.
• Signs of nausea such as ptyalism, bruxism, and pawing at the mouth are also common.
• Vomiting may also occur but is seen less frequently than the signs listed above.
• Hematemesis and/or melena may be present if the FB has caused a gastric erosion or ulcer.

Intestinal
• Acute onset of severe weakness, depression, and anorexia, often with no other clinical signs, is the most common presentation in young ferrets with GI FB.
• Anorexia, lethargy, diarrhea, and bruxism are the most common signs in older ferrets.
• Diarrhea is common.
• Vomiting occasionally occurs but is unusual in ferrets with GI FB.
• Melena may be present if the foreign body has caused intestinal erosion or ulcer.
• Depression and signs of pain such as reluctance to move occur in acute obstructions.

Physical Examination Findings
• Intestinal foreign bodies are often palpable; gastric foreign bodies often are not.
• Pain may be elicited on abdominal palpation.
• Gas- or fluid-filled stomach or intestines sometimes are palpable.
• Emaciation is seen in chronic cases.
• May have signs of dehydration from fluid and electrolyte loss due to vomiting or diarrhea
• Pallor of the mucous membranes with chronic blood loss

Esophagus
• Esophageal foreign bodies are rare in ferrets.
• Regurgitation, ptyalism, anorexia, and persistent attempts at swallowing may be seen.

CAUSES
• Most retained foreign bodies are simply too large to pass through the intestinal tract.
• Gastrointestinal lymphoma, gastritis, or metabolic disease resulting in severe ileus may cause retention of a foreign object that would normally pass.
• Young ferrets are particularly fond of chewing or swallowing rubber toys and foam rubber.

RISK FACTORS
• Unsupervised access to toys or other objects to chew
• Underlying gastrointestinal tract disease

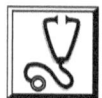

DIAGNOSIS

DIFFERENTIAL DIAGNOSIS
• Any disease that may cause ptyalism, bruxism, regurgitation, vomiting, anorexia, or weight loss should be considered in the differential diagnosis. The most common causes of these signs include GI FB, *Helicobacter mustelae* gastritis, epizootic catarrhal enteritis (ECE), lymphoma, and inflammatory bowel diseases.
• *Helicobacter mustelae*-induced gastritis may cause similar clinical signs. *Helicobacter*-induced disease may be a primary pathogen and mimic GI FB or may occur as a consequence of GI FB (mechanical irritation of the gastric mucosa caused by the FB, or stress)
• Differential diagnoses for ptyalism, pawing at the mouth—insulinoma or other causes of hypoglycemia; any condition causing nausea (GI lymphoma, *Helicobacter*, ECE, hepatic or renal disease, and lower intestinal tract disease)
• Melena and anorexia most common with *H. mustelae* or GI FB
• Abdominal palpation may be helpful when differentiating causes of anorexia, weight loss, and gastrointestinal signs—thickened intestinal loops and palpably enlarged mesenteric lymph nodes are more common with eosinophilic enterocolitis, lymphoplasmacytic enteritis, ECE, or lymphoma, and less likely with GI FB
• In patients with diarrhea, the character of diarrhea may be helpful in differentiating causes—bile-stained (green), mucous-covered diarrhea is seen most commonly with ECE; granular, "bird seed"—like feces seen with maldigestion/malabsorptive disorders; tenesmus, dyschezia, and rectal is associated with colonic disease.

CBC/BIOCHEMISTRY/URINALYSIS
• These tests are often normal.
• Inflammatory leukogram may be seen with FB-induced gastritis
• PCV and TS elevation in dehydrated patients
• Anemia from gastric bleeding is rare.
• If the intestinal tract has been perforated, an inflammatory leukogram may be seen.

IMAGING

Radiography
• Radiographs are valuable to delineate the type and location of some radiopaque foreign bodies, especially metallic substances. If gas is visualized in the mediastinum or pleural space, perforation of the esophagus should be

(CONTINUED) GASTROINTESTINAL AND ESOPHAGEAL FOREIGN BODIES

considered. Gas distension of the stomach is sometimes observed with gastric foreign bodies. This gas occasionally may provide enough contrast to make the ingested object also visible.

• A sudden change in the diameter of intestinal loops is highly suggestive of a foreign body. A mechanical ileus or displacement of bowel loops can sometimes (but not always) be seen. In many cases, however, radiographs can appear normal, especially in patients with soft or foam rubber toy FB.

• Localized free gas in the peritoneal cavity is seen with peritonitis resulting from gastrointestinal perforation.

• Plication of the intestines as observed with a linear foreign body is extremely rare in ferrets.

Positive Contrast Radiography

• A positive contrast study may reveal a delay in intestinal transit time and will sometimes document the presence of radiolucent objects. Barium is the contrast agent of choice to delineate a foreign body or ulceration. It is, however, contraindicated in ferrets with suspected perforation or intractable vomiting/regurgitation. In these instances, Iohexidol should be used.

Ultrasonography

Abdominal ultrasound can be useful in documenting a gastric or intestinal FB.

DIAGNOSTIC PROCEDURES

Upper GI endoscopy may be used to diagnose esophageal and gastric FBs. However, the small size of the patient and subsequent limitations on instrument size often limits the use of endoscopy. Endoscopy, when feasible, is superior to radiography in evaluating inflammation, punctures, lacerations, erosions, and ulcers.

TREATMENT

APPROPRIATE HEALTH CARE

• Esophageal FBs are considered an emergency since the incidence of complications increases with the length of time the foreign body is present.

• Gastric FBs are considered an urgency rather than an emergency unless the patient has evidence of gastric erosion or signs of toxicosis.

• Intestinal FBs are usually an emergency since the incidence of complications increases with the length of time the FB is present.

NURSING CARE

• Patients are usually anorectic or dehydrated. Fluid therapy using a balanced electrolyte solution should be administered before and during surgery.

• Older ferrets often have clinical or subclinical insulinomas and will become hypoglycemic if anorexic. Administer dextrose-containing fluid and monitor blood glucose concentration.

ACTIVITY

Restrict activity for 5–7 days postoperatively.

DIET

• If the ferret has been eating, the diet does not require modification. Most ferrets will resume eating soft food within 12–24 hours post-surgery.

• If anorexic, assist feed an easily digestible high-protein/high-fat diet such as Lafeber Carnivore Critical Care Diet (Lafeber Company, Cornell, IL) or Oxbow Carnivore Critical Care Diet (Oxbow Animal Health, Omaha, NE); if these are unavailable, offer chicken baby foods; may also add dietary supplement such as Nutri-Cal (EVSCO Pharmaceuticals) to increase caloric content to these foods.

CLIENT EDUCATION

• Discuss possible complications prior to treatment, especially if surgery is required.

• Remove objects commonly ingested from the environment, especially rubber toys.

SURGICAL CONSIDERATIONS

• Esophageal FBs are rare and may be removed via endoscopy.

• Gastric and intestinal FBs are usually removed by surgery. This allows for assessment of the intestinal tract, liver, and spleen, along with biopsy specimen collection when indicated.

• Carefully observe the adrenals and pancreas, since concurrent disease is often present, especially in middle-aged to older animals

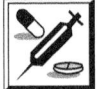

MEDICATIONS

DRUG(S) OF CHOICE

• If gastric ulceration is evident, treatment for *Helicobacter mustelae* is indicated. The combination of amoxicillin (30 mg/kg PO q8–12h) plus metronidazole (20 mg/kg PO q 8–12h) and bismuth subsalicylate (17.5 mg/kg PO q12h or 1 mL/kg of regular strength preparation [262 mg/15 mL] PO q8–12h) is a common, inexpensive treatment regimen; however, many ferrets find this unpalatable. Dosing every 8 hours may be necessary to eliminate infection. Combine this treatment with an antisecretory agent (see below). Treat for at least 2 (often 3–4) weeks. The combination of clarithromycin (12.5 mg/kg PO q8–12h) and ranitidine bismuth citrate

or ranitidine HCl (24 mg/kg PO q8–12h) for 2 weeks has also been reported to be effective in the eradication of *Helicobacter* spp. Ranitidine is no longer approved for human use in the US and can be difficult to find. The combination of clarithromycin (50 mg/kg PO q24h or divided q12h); omeprazole (4 mg/kg PO q24h); metronidazole (20 mg/kg PO q12h) for 14 days has also been used for eradication.

• Gastrointestinal antisecretory agents are helpful to treat and possibly prevent gastritis in anorectic ferrets. Ferrets continually secrete a baseline level of gastric hydrochloric acid and, as such, anorexia itself may predispose to gastric ulceration. Those successfully used in ferrets include omeprazole (4 mg/kg PO q24h), famotidine (0.25–0.5 mg/kg PO, SC, IV q24h), and cimetidine (10 mg/kg PO, SC, IM, IV q8h).

• Sucralfate suspension (25 mg/kg PO q8h) protects ulcerated tissue (cytoprotection) by binding to ulcer sites.

• Postoperative analgesics.

FOLLOW-UP

PATIENT MONITORING

• After the FB has been removed, assess the mucosa for damage. Mucosal ulceration may occur due to infection with *Helicobacter mustelae* or mucosal injury. Usually, the degree of mucosal injury is proportional to the length of time the object is within the gastrointestinal tract and the texture of the object.

• Monitor the patient for at least 2 months after the FB removal for evidence of stricture formation at the site of the FB.

PREVENTION/AVOIDANCE

• The ferret should be closely supervised during times of access to potential foreign bodies.

• Avoid giving rubber toys to young ferrets.

• To prevent trichobezoars, administer a cat laxative regularly, especially during periods of heavy shedding.

POSSIBLE COMPLICATIONS

Other than the possibility of stricture formation at the site of removal, complications following the removal of gastric foreign bodies are rare.

EXPECTED COURSE AND PROGNOSIS

The prognosis following the removal of an intestinal foreign body is usually good to excellent. Patients can usually be released within 36–48 hours.

GASTROINTESTINAL AND ESOPHAGEAL FOREIGN BODIES (CONTINUED)

FERRETS

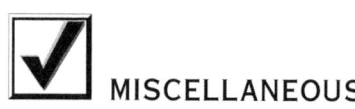

MISCELLANEOUS

ASSOCIATED CONDITIONS
- Gastritis due to Helicobacter mustelae
- GI lymphoma
- Inflammatory bowel diseases (eosinophilic or lymphoplasmacytic)
- Insulinoma

AGE-RELATED FACTORS
- There is a higher incidence of foreign bodies in younger ferrets.
- Older ferrets are more likely to have concurrent diseases such as insulinoma or adrenal disease.
- Lymphoma may be seen in any age ferret.

SEE ALSO
Anorexia
Gastritis
Helicobacter mustelae

Insulinoma
Lymphoma
Lymphoplasmacytic enteritis and gastroenteritis

ABBREVIATIONS
ALT = alanine aminotransferase
ECE = epizootic catarrhal enteritis
FB = foreign body
GI = gastrointestinal
IBD = inflammatory bowel disease
PCV = packed cell volume
TS = total solids

Suggested Reading
Di Girolamo N, Selleri P. Medical and surgical emergencies in ferrets. Vet Clin Exot Anim 2016;19:431–464.
Hoefer HL. Gastrointestinal diseases of ferrets. In: Quesenberry KE, Carpenter JW, eds. Ferrets, Rabbits, and Rodents, 4th ed. Clinical Medicine and Surgery. 2021. St. Louis: Saunders, 2020:27–38.
Huynh M, Pignon C. Gastrointestinal disease in exotic small mammals. J Exot Pet Med 2013;22(2):118–131.
Lennox AM, Gladden JN. Emergency and critical care of small mammals. In: Quesenberry KE, Carpenter JW, eds. Ferrets, Rabbits and Rodents, 4th ed. Clinical Medicine and Surgery. 2021. St. Louis: Saunders, 2020:595–608.
MacPhail C. Ferret soft tissue surgery. In: Bennett A, Pye GW, eds. Surgery of Exotic Animals. Wiley-Blackwell, 2021:277–296.
Miwa Y, Sladky K. Common surgical procedures of rodents, ferrets, hedgehogs, and sugar gliders. Vet Clin Exot Anim 2016;19:205–244.
Mullen HS, Scavelli TD, Quesenberry KE et al. Gastrointestinal foreign body in ferrets: 25 cases (1986–1990). J Am Anim Hosp Assoc 1992;28:13–19.

Author Barbara Oglesbee, DVM, DABVP-Avian

BASICS

OVERVIEW
• Enteric infection with the protozoan parasite, *Giardia* spp.
• Usually a co-pathogen with other enteric infectious agents, primary infection is rare
• Waterborne transmission of cysts; dogs or cats in household may serve as reservoir
• Motile (flagellated) organisms attach to surface of enterocytes in small intestine, especially duodenum through jejunum
• Malabsorption syndrome with soft, voluminous, or grainy "bird seed"-appearing stools
• Importance as a reservoir for human infections not known

SIGNALMENT
• Uncommon cause of gastrointestinal disease
• No breed, sex, or age predilections have been described.

SIGNS
• May be asymptomatic
• Intermittent diarrhea, or may be acute with co-pathogens
• Soft, mucoid, or grainy "millet seed" or "bird seed"-appearing feces
• Weight loss, poor hair coat
• Persistence may lead to chronic debilitation.

CAUSES AND RISK FACTORS
• Giardia transmitted by oral ingestion of cysts, usually from water supplies. Ferrets are usually housed indoors and do not have access to most water sources; dogs or cats may serve as a reservoir within a household.
• Infection is often innocuous until a high parasite load develops.
• Debilitated ferrets, especially those with enteric disease (e.g., ECE, helicobacter, and GI lymphoma) are more likely to shed *Giardia*. Treatment of both primary disease and giardiasis is usually necessary for resolution of clinical signs.

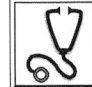 **DIAGNOSIS**

DIFFERENTIAL DIAGNOSIS
Other causes of maldigestion and malabsorption (e.g., ECE, GI lymphoma, and inflammatory bowel disease) are much more common.

CBC/BIOCHEMISTRY/URINALYSIS
Usually normal, peripheral eosinophilia not documented, but may be suggestive.

OTHER LABORATORY TESTS
N/A

IMAGING
N/A

DIAGNOSTIC PROCEDURES
• Motile organisms, tear drop-shaped, 10–18 × 7–15 μm; "falling leaf" appearance with two nuclei and flagella. Sometimes visible in fresh fecal wet mount with saline. Specimen should be <10 minutes old. Addition of iodine may enhance appearance.
• Cysts—seen as crescent shapes with zinc sulfate fecal flotation; 8–13 × 7–10 μm.
• Fecal ELISA not superior to zinc sulfate flotation, its usefulness in ferrets is unknown.
• Organisms are shed intermittently—lack of visualization does not rule out infection. Collect samples over several days to increase the probability of identification.

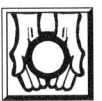 **TREATMENT**

Treat as outpatients unless debilitated or dehydrated.

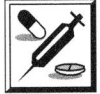 **MEDICATIONS**

DRUG(S) OF CHOICE
• Metronidazole 50 mg/kg q24h for 5 days
• Treat all identified copathogens

CONTRAINDICATIONS/POSSIBLE INTERACTIONS
Metronidazole bitter taste; anorexia; vomiting; neurotoxic if overdosed

 FOLLOW-UP

Serial fecal examinations to confirm the efficacy of treatment.

 MISCELLANEOUS

ZOONOTIC POTENTIAL
• *Giardia* is the most common intestinal parasite in humans residing in North America.
• *Giardia* spp. may not be highly host specific; no conclusive evidence indicates that cysts shed by ferrets are infective for humans.

ABBREVIATIONS
ECE = epizootic catarrhal enteritis
ELISA = enzyme-linked immunosorbent assay
GI = gastrointestinal

Suggested Reading
Di Girolamo N, Selleri P. Medical and surgical emergencies in ferrets. Vet Clin Exot Anim 2016;19:431–464.
Hoefer HL. Gastrointestinal diseases of ferrets. In: Quesenberry KE, Carpenter JW, eds. Ferrets, Rabbits, and Rodents, 4th ed. Clinical Medicine and Surgery. 2021. St. Louis: Saunders, 2020:27–38.
Huynh M, Pignon C. Gastrointestinal disease in exotic small mammals. J Exot Pet Med 2013;22(2):118–131.
Johnson-Delaney CA. Geriatric ferrets. Vet Clin Exot Anim Pract 2020;23(3):549–565.
Livingstone M. Dealing with gastrointestinal disease in ferrets. In Practice 2022;44:169–179.
Murray J, Kiupel M, Maes RK. Ferret coronavirus-associated diseases. Vet Clin North Am Exot Anim Pract 2010;13(3):543–560.
Powers LV. Bacterial and parasitic diseases of ferrets. Vet Clin North Am Exot Anim Pract 2009;12:531–561.
Author Barbara Oglesbee, DVM, DABVP-Avian

FERRETS

GINGIVITIS AND PERIODONTAL DISEASE

FERRETS

BASICS

OVERVIEW
- Gingivitis—a reversible inflammatory response of the marginal gumline; the earliest phase of periodontal disease
- Periodontal disease—inflammation of some or all of the tooth's support structures (gingiva, cementum, periodontal ligament, and alveolar bone)
- Caused by bacteria located in the gingival crevice; initially, a pellicle forms on the enamel surface of a clean tooth; the pellicle is composed of proteins and glycoproteins deposited from saliva and gingival crevicular fluid; the pellicle attracts bacteria that soon adhere, forming plaque; the plaque thickens, eventually becomes mineralized and transforms into calculus, which is rough and irritating to the gingiva.
- Calculus formation is a common finding in ferrets; this occasionally lead to gingivitis; periodontal disease with bone loss and abscess formation is rare in ferrets.
- The severity of gingivitis is likely determined by the host's immunocompetency and local oral factors.

SIGNALMENT
- Middle-aged to older ferrets
- Calculus formation is a common finding; gingivitis is occasionally seen; severe periodontal disease is rare.

SIGNS
- Usually detected during routine wellness examinations
- Variable degrees of plaque and calculus formation
- Halitosis
- Erythremic or edematous gingiva
- Gingival surfaces may bleed easily on contact
- Pustular discharge and bone loss uncommon finding
- Fractured canine teeth are a common finding in ferrets; pain is uncommon unless dental pulp is exposed.

CAUSES AND RISK FACTORS
- Plaque accumulation
- Feeding homemade or whole prey diets. Soft diet promotes gingivitis through accumulation of plaque
- Chewing habits
- Lack of oral health care
- Metabolic diseases such as uremia may predispose
- Specific bacterial pathogens and the role of aerobic vs. anaerobic bacteria and bacterial endotoxin formation have not been described in ferrets.

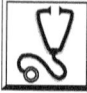

DIAGNOSIS

DIFFERENTIAL DIAGNOSIS
- For ptylaism, pawing at mouth—consider nausea secondary to GI disease or hypoglycemia/insulinoma. These are much more common causes than dental disease.
- Oral neoplasia
- Stomatitis

CBC/BIOCHEMISTRY/URINALYSIS
May help identify risk factors

OTHER LABORATORY TESTS
N/A

IMAGING
- No radiographic changes are usually evident, since severe periodontal disease is uncommon in ferrets.
- Radiographs are indicated if abscess or severe periodontal disease is suspected.

DIAGNOSTIC PROCEDURES
- Anesthetized oral examination allows more thorough visual examination of all dental surfaces; use of a periodontal probe may help distinguish between gingivitis and periodontitis (normal sulcal depths not described in ferrets; 1 mm in cats)
- Biopsy and histopathology to rule out oral neoplasia

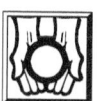

TREATMENT
- Modify behavior to avoid chewing hard objects and eliminate repetitive trauma, if possible.
- Regular dental prophylaxis can be performed before lesions develop.
- Hard food leaves less substrate on the teeth than soft food; chewing also helps to clean teeth mechanically.
- Professional periodontal therapy may reverse gingivitis.
- Dental cleaning—complete oral examination; supragingival removal of plaque and calculus; subgingival scaling; polishing; subgingival irrigation; extractions are rarely necessary.
- A gentle technique is necessary when cleaning; ferret teeth are more fragile than canine or feline teeth.

MEDICATIONS

DRUG(S) OF CHOICE
- Lactoperoxidase- and chlorhexidine-containing dentifrices are effective in retarding plaque but are difficult to use in ferrets.
- Topically applied chlorhexidine, 0.4% stannous fluoride gel also reduce the inciting plaque formation.
- Antibiotics are generally not necessary in patients with mild gingivitis; for severe disease—clindamycin (5.5–10 mg/kg PO q12h) or clavulanic acid/amoxicillin (13–25 mg/kg PO q12h).

POSSIBLE INTERACTIONS
N/A

ALTERNATIVE DRUGS
N/A

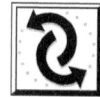

FOLLOW-UP

PATIENT MONITORING
Regular oral reexaminations are necessary to determine the proper interval between periodontal therapies and assess the effectiveness of oral home care; these steps can cure gingivitis and help to avoid the progression to periodontitis.

POSSIBLE COMPLICATIONS
Uncontrolled periodontitis invariably leads to tooth loss.

MISCELLANEOUS

ASSOCIATED CONDITIONS
N/A

AGE-RELATED FACTORS
N/A

ZOONOTIC POTENTIAL
None

Suggested Reading
Hoefer HL. Gastrointestinal diseases of ferrets. In: Quesenberry KE, Carpenter JW, eds. Ferrets, Rabbits, and Rodents, 4th ed. Clinical Medicine and Surgery. 2021. St. Louis: Saunders, 2020:27–38.

Johnson-Delaney CA. Ferret nutrition. Vet Clin Exot Anim Pract 2014;17(3): 449–470.

Johnson-Delaney CA. Geriatric ferrets. Vet Clin Exot Anim Pract 2020;23(3): 549–565.

Nemec A, Zadravec M, Račnik J. Oral and dental diseases in a population of domestic ferrets (*Mustela putorius furo*). J Small Anim Pract 2016;57(10):553–560.

Author Barbara Oglesbee, DVM, DABVP (Avian)

HEARTWORM DISEASE

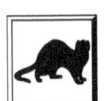

BASICS

OVERVIEW
- Disease caused by infection with *Dirofilaria immitis*
- Worms may lodge in the right ventricle, cranial vena cava, or main pulmonary artery
- Usually very low worm burden (range 1–21 adult worms, 1–2 more common); microfilaremia is less common (50%–60% of infected ferrets)
- Severe cardiac disease may be seen in ferrets with very low worm burdens (1–2 adults)
- High right ventricular afterload causes myocardial hypertrophy and, in some animals, congestive heart failure (CHF).
- Pulmonary hypertension and embolization occur, especially following adulticide therapy

SIGNALMENT
- May be seen in any age ferret
- Common disease in tropical and semitropical zones, especially along the Atlantic and Gulf coasts in the United States
- All unprotected ferrets are at risk in endemic regions.

SIGNS
General Comments
Clinical signs may vary from absent, to mild-moderate signs (lethargy, anorexia), to signs of fulminant heart failure. Most ferrets, however, present with severe signs of CHF. Signs of CHF occur with very low adult worm burdens due to the small size of the ferret heart.

Historical Findings
- Animals may be asymptomatic
- Sudden onset, often over a course of days to weeks of weakness, loss of appetite with rapid progression to profound weakness and respiratory distress or sudden death.

Physical Examination Findings
- Labored breathing, rales, or crackles—ferrets with severe pulmonary hypertension or pleural effusion
- Systolic murmur
- Pale mucus membranes or cyanosis
- Muffled heart sounds, lack of chest compliance, and dyspnea characterized by rapid shallow respirations may be associated with pleural effusion
- Tachycardia, ascites, and hepatomegaly indicate RSHF

CAUSES AND RISK FACTORS
- Infection with *D. immitis*
- Residence in endemic regions
- Lack of prophylaxis

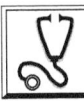

DIAGNOSIS

DIFFERENTIAL DIAGNOSIS
- Other causes of CHF (e.g., dilated cardiomyopathy)
- Mediastinal lymphoma

CBC/BIOCHEMISTRY/URINALYSIS
- Usually normal
- Mild to moderate anemia, monocytosis, and mild hyperchloremia sometimes seen
- Eosinophilia and basophilia—not usually seen in ferrets with HW disease
- Bilirubinuria and trace hematuria common

OTHER LABORATORY TESTS
- Modified Knott's test—limited usefulness; microfilaria are present in <50% of affected ferrets
- Low worm burdens (fewer than five worms) and single-sex infections commonly result in false-negative results; negative result does not rule out heartworm disease
- Serologic tests that identify adult *D. immitis* antigen are of some use; however, false-negative results are common in ferrets with low worm burdens or early infections. ELISA (SNAP heartworm antigen test, Idexx Laboratories) appears to be most useful—60%–80% of experimentally infected ferrets were antigen positive 4 months after infection.

IMAGING
Radiographic Findings
- Pleural effusion is a very common finding.
- Cardiomegaly, right atrial enlargement, and enlarged vena cava are common; main pulmonary artery segment enlargement and arterial enlargement and tortuosity vary but are usually absent
- Parenchymal lung infiltrates of variable severity—surround lobar arteries; may extend into most or all of one or multiple lung lobes when thromboembolism occurs
- Diffuse, symmetrical, alveolar, and interstitial infiltrates occasionally occur.

Echocardiographic Findings
- May be extremely helpful in the diagnosis when performed by an experienced practitioner
- Parallel, linear echodensities produced by heartworms may be detected in the right ventricle, right atrium, and pulmonary arteries.
- Dilation of pulmonary arteries.

DIAGNOSTIC PROCEDURES
Electrocardiographic Findings
- Usually normal
- Heart rhythm disturbances—occasionally seen (atrial fibrillation most common) in severe infection

Pathologic Findings
- Large right heart
- Pulmonary arterial myointimal proliferation
- Pulmonary thromboembolism
- Hepatomegaly and congestion in animals with R-CHF

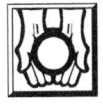

TREATMENT

APPROPRIATE HEALTH CARE
General Comments
- Treatment options include adulticide therapy followed by long-term treatment with prednisone and ivermectin (symptomatic animals), or treatment with prednisone and ivermectin alone (asymptomatic animals). Both have high mortality rates.
- Treatment with adulticide therapy carries the risk of complications from worm emboli and toxicity of the adulticide drug itself. Emboli can occur up to 3 months following adulticide treatment. Mortality rate is 40%–60%.
- Treatment with long-term ivermectin and prednisone allows a slower kill of adult heartworms, and perhaps less risk of worm emboli. However, most ferrets do not survive more than 3 months.

NURSING CARE
- Symptomatic ferrets are often in fulminant heart failure and should be hospitalized and stabilized.
- Thoracocentesis is indicated in ferrets with pleural effusion. When performing thoracocentesis be aware that the heart is located much more caudally within the thorax of the ferret compared with dogs and cats.
- It may be necessary to repeat thoracocentesis frequently to relieve dyspnea over a several-month period.

ACTIVITY
Severe restriction of activity required for at least 4–6 weeks after adulticide administration

CLIENT EDUCATION
- Survival rates in symptomatic ferrets with either treatment protocol is poor. Reported treatment survival rates vary between 33% and 40%.
- Reinfection can occur unless appropriate prophylaxis administered.

FERRETS

HEARTWORM DISEASE (CONTINUED)

FERRETS

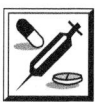

MEDICATIONS

DRUG(S) OF CHOICE

Symptomatic Ferrets—Stabilize Animals with R-CHF Before Adulticide Treatment
• Supplemental oxygen; thoracocentesis if indicated
• If the ferret is in fulminant cardiac failure, administer furosemide at 2–4 mg/kg q8–12h IM or IV. Initially, furosemide should be administered parenterally. Long-term therapy should be continued at a dose of 1–2 mg/kg PO q12h.
• Enalapril may be needed for long-term maintenance in ferrets with CHF to reduce afterload and preload. Begin with a dose of 0.25–0.5 mg/kg PO q48h and increase to q24h dosing if well tolerated.
• Prednisone is administered at a dose of 1 mg/kg PO q24h or divided q12h
• Theophylline (4.25 mg/kg PO q8–12h) may be useful in severely dyspneic ferrets.

Adulticide Treatment
• Melarsomine dihydrochloride—2.5 mg/kg IM, followed by two injections 24 hours apart 30 days later. About 40% mortality rate is due to the high risk of post-treatment embolus formation.
• Thiacetarsamide sodium 0.22 mL/kg IV q12h × 2 days also has high (60%) mortality risk.
• Ivermectin (0.05–0.1 mg/kg SC q30d) until microfilaremia resolves and clinical signs improve may be a safer treatment, but many ferrets symptomatic for CHF do not survive.
• Concurrent treatment with prednisone is indicated to protect against pulmonary emboli. Begin administration of prednisone 1 mg/kg PO q24h or divided q12h concurrently with adulticide treatment. Continue treatment for at least 4 months.

CONTRAINDICATIONS
Adulticide treatment in patients with renal failure or hepatic failure.

PRECAUTIONS
• Melarsomine dihydrochloride may cause local muscle necrosis; sudden death with 12 hours postinjection has been anecdotally reported.
• Standard adulticide therapy in ferrets with severe infection is associated with high mortality due to subsequent pulmonary thromboembolism; may occur up to 3 months following adulticide therapy; concurrent prednisone therapy will reduce this risk.

POSSIBLE INTERACTIONS
None

ALTERNATIVE DRUGS
Moxidectin (Pro-Heart Injectable) has been anecdotally used as a safe and effective adulticide at 0.17–2.0 mg/ferret SC followed by monthly preventative ivermectin treatment and prednisone

FOLLOW-UP

PATIENT MONITORING
• Perform an antigen test 3–4 weeks after microfilaricide administration
• Repeat thoracic radiographs periodically to determine efficacy of therapy

PREVENTION/AVOIDANCE

Heartworm Prophylaxis Should Be Provided for All Ferrets at Risk
• Imidacloprid with moxidectin (Advantage Multi, Bayer)—20 mg imidacloprid/2 mg moxidectin/kg applied topically once a month appears to be 100% effective in preventing heartworm disease.
• Selamectin (Revolution, Pfizer)—18 mg/kg applied topically once a month appears to be 95%–100% effective in preventing heartworm disease.
• Ivermectin—0.05 mg/kg PO q30d; dilute injectable formula in propylene glycol to a concentration of 0.5 mg/mL and dispense in a light-protected bottle.

POSSIBLE COMPLICATIONS
• Sudden death
• Post-adulticide pulmonary thromboembolic complications—may occur up to 3–4 months after treatment
• Thrombocytopenia, disseminated intravascular coagulation
• Melarsomine adverse effects—sudden death within 12–24 hours of injection; pulmonary thromboembolism; injection site reaction (myositis); lethargy or depression; causes elevations of hepatic enzymes in dogs and possibly in ferrets

EXPECTED COURSE AND PROGNOSIS
• Fair to guarded prognosis for animals with asymptomatic infection
• Guarded to poor prognosis in ferrets with signs of CHF

MISCELLANEOUS

ASSOCIATED CONDITIONS
N/A

AGE-RELATED FACTORS
N/A

ZOONOTIC POTENTIAL
N/A

PREGNANCY/FERTILITY/BREEDING
Adulticide treatment should be delayed if possible.

SYNONYMS
N/A

SEE ALSO
Congestive heart failure

ABBREVIATIONS
CHF = congestive heart failure
ELISA = enzyme-linked immunosorbent assay
RCHF = right-sided congestive heart failure

Suggested Reading
Di Girolamo N, Selleri P. Medical and surgical emergencies in ferrets. Vet Clin North Am Exot Anim Pract 2016;19:431–464.
Dudás-Györki Z, Szabó Z, Manczur F et al. Echocardiographic and electrocardiographic examination of clinically healthy, conscious ferrets. J Small Anim Pract 2011;52(1):18–25.
Fitzgerald B, Dias S, Martorell J. Cardiovascular drugs in avian, small mammal, and reptile medicine. Vet Clin North Am Exot Anim Pract 2018;21(2):399–442.
Malakoff RL, Laste NJ, Orcutt CJ. Echocardiographic and electrocardiographic findings in client-owned ferrets: 95 cases (1994–2009). J Am Vet Med Assoc 2012;241(11):1484–1489.
Morrisey JK, Kraus MS. Cardiovascular and other diseases of ferrets. In: Quesenberry KE, Carpenter JW, eds. Ferrets, Rabbits and Rodents, 4th ed. Clinical Medicine and Surgery. St. Louis: Saunders, 2020:55–71.
Van Zeeland YA, Schoemaker N. Ferret cardiology. Vet Clin Exot Anim 2022;25:541–562.

Author Barbara Oglesbee, DVM, DABVP-Avian

BASICS

DEFINITION
Helicobacter mustelae are microaerophilic gram-negative urease-positive, spiral bacteria. *H. mustelae* infection in ferrets is associated with gastritis and peptic ulcerative disease.

PATHOPHYSIOLOGY
• Nearly 100% of ferrets acquired from commercial breeders in the United States are colonized with *Helicobacter* by weaning. However, only a small percentage of these ferrets will develop clinically significant helicobacter-associated disease. Disease is seen most commonly in ferrets that have been stressed or have other concurrent diseases.
• Gastric colonization by *H. mustelae* can cause hypergastrinemia-induced peptic ulcer disease in ferrets; colonization usually results in diffuse antral gastritis, focal glandular atrophy, and often superficial gastritis in the remainder of the stomach. Mucosal damage is the result of direct toxic effects of the bacteria and severe lymphoplasmacytic inflammatory reaction.
• *H. mustelae* has also been associated with gastric adenocarcinomas in ferrets; chronically diseased ferrets are at increased risk for developing gastric mucosa-associated lymphoid tissue (MALT) lymphoma.

SYSTEMS AFFECTED
• Gastrointestinal
• Hemic/Lymphatic/ Immune—mesenteric lymphoid hyperplasia
• Musculoskeletal—muscle wasting with severe disease
• Endocrine/Metabolic—fluid, electrolyte, and acid–base imbalances

GENETICS
N/A

INCIDENCE/PREVALENCE
• *H. mustelae* is highly prevalent in ferrets—nearly 100% of ferrets acquired from commercial breeders in the United States are colonized by weaning. *H. mustelae* can be isolated from the feces of ferrets shortly after weaning but shedding ceases by 20 weeks of age. Although helicobacter can be found in a large percentage of ferrets, not all will become ill.
• Ferrets that are stressed are more likely to develop clinically significant disease.
• Helicobacter-induced disease is one of the most common causes of anorexia, melena, and vomiting in young ferrets.

GEOGRAPHIC DISTRIBUTION
Seen more commonly in North America as compared to Europe, but prevalence in other countries has not been reported.

SIGNALMENT
Species/Breed Predilections
N/A

Mean Age and Range
Helicobacter-induced disease can be seen in any aged ferret.

Predominant Sex
N/A

SIGNS
Historical Findings
Anorexia, ptyalism, bruxism, diarrhea, melena, vomiting, abdominal pain, weight loss, and weakness are the most common clinical signs. Many affected ferrets will paw at the mouth when nauseated.

Physical Examination Findings
• May be normal in patients with early or mild disease
• Pallor of the mucous membranes due to chronic blood loss possible
• May have signs of dehydration from fluid and electrolyte loss due to vomiting or diarrhea
• Weight loss—indicates chronic disease
• Poor hair coat or alopecia
• Fecal staining of the perineum
• Mesenteric lymph nodes are often palpably enlarged.
• Splenomegaly is commonly detected; usually is a nonspecific finding

CAUSES
Helicobacter mustelae

RISK FACTORS
Stress, concurrent illness (e.g., epizootic catarrhal enteritis [ECE], other intestinal pathogens, insulinoma, lymphoma, or other neoplasia)

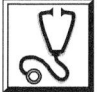

DIAGNOSIS

GENERAL COMMENTS
• High *H. mustelae* prevalence rates exist in ferrets in the United States. A combination of organism identification and demonstration of characteristic histologic lesions, or identification of organism and exclusion of other diagnoses, is necessary to support a causal relationship between helicobacter infection and clinical disease
• A presumptive diagnosis may be made on the identification of suggestive clinical signs, exclusion of other diagnoses, and a favorable response to empirical treatment.

DIFFERENTIAL DIAGNOSIS
• In young ferrets, GI foreign bodies will cause identical clinical signs and may contribute to gastric ulceration; in

middle-aged to older ferrets, trichobezoars are common GI foreign bodies.
• Gastric ulceration may result from stress or anorexia.
• Gastric ulcers may also be seen secondary to renal disease or the use of nonsteroidal anti-inflammatory agents.
• Similar clinical signs may be seen with GI neoplasia, ECE, *Salmonella* spp., or inflammatory bowel disease.

CBC/BIOCHEMISTRY/URINALYSIS
• Regenerative anemia seen with chronic blood loss and may be severe
• May reflect fluid and electrolyte abnormalities secondary to vomiting and/or diarrhea
• Leukocytosis with neutrophilia and lymphocytosis is common

OTHER LABORATORY TESTS
Culture—usually requires gastric biopsy and specialized isolation techniques and media; success rates are low.

IMAGING
• Radiography and ultrasonography—usually normal
• GI contrast studies occasionally demonstrate mucosal irregularities or filling defects.

DIAGNOSTIC PROCEDURES
• In order to establish a causal relationship between infection with helicobacter and clinical signs, a gastric biopsy is needed. Exploratory laparotomy is often useful to evaluate the extent of gastric pathology and to rule out GI foreign bodies, neoplasia, and intestinal inflammatory diseases, but is not indicated in every case. Biopsy is performed via laparotomy. Evidence of characteristic histologic lesions combined with documentation of the organism is needed to support helicobacter infection as the cause of clinical disease.
• Alternatively, a presumptive diagnosis may be made based on identification of suggestive clinical signs, exclusion of other diagnoses, and a favorable response to empirical treatment. Many patients may be unsuitable candidates for surgery (severely debilitated, concurrent disease, or owner financial constraints).

PATHOLOGICAL FINDINGS
Stomach—gastric mucosal ulceration and granular-appearing mucosa due to the inflammatory reaction. Lesions appear most commonly in the pyloric antrum. On histopathologic examination, gastric spiral organisms can be seen on silver-stained sections; lymphoplasmacytic gastritis and lymphoid follicle hyperplasia

FERRETS

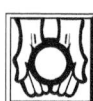

TREATMENT

APPROPRIATE HEALTH CARE
- Ferrets that are anorexic, vomiting, or dehydrated require hospitalization.
- Ferrets that will still eat and are not vomiting may be treated on an outpatient basis.
- There is no indication at present for treating asymptomatic animals with helicobacter infection.

NURSING CARE
- Fluid therapy using a balanced electrolyte solution should be administered to anorectic or dehydrated patients.
- A warm, quiet environment should be provided for recovery.

ACTIVITY
N/A

DIET
- If anorexic, assist feed an easily digestible high-protein/high-fat diet such as Lafeber Carnivore Critical Care Diet (Lafeber Company, Cornell, IL) or Oxbow Carnivore Critical Care Diet (Oxbow Animal Health, Omaha, NE); if these are unavailable, offer chicken baby foods; may also add dietary supplement such as Nutri-Cal (EVSCO Pharmaceuticals) to increase caloric content to these foods.
- Warming the food to body temperature or offering via syringe may increase acceptance.
- Administer these supplements several times a day.

CLIENT EDUCATION
Explain the difficulty of establishing a definitive diagnosis without invasive techniques such as gastric biopsy.

SURGICAL CONSIDERATIONS
N/A

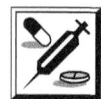

MEDICATIONS

DRUG(S) OF CHOICE
- When possible, identify and treat all underlying diseases.
- Specific treatment for helicobacter—the combination of amoxicillin (30 mg/kg PO q8–12h) plus metronidazole (20 mg/kg PO q 8–12h) and bismuth subsalicylate (17.5 mg/kg PO q12h or 1 mL/kg of regular strength preparation [262 mg/15 mL] PO q8–12h) is a common, inexpensive treatment regimen; however, many ferrets find this unpalatable. Dosing every 8 hours may be necessary to eliminate infection. Combine this treatment with an antisecretory agent (see below). Treat for at least 2 (often 3–4) weeks.

- The combination of clarithromycin (12.5 mg/kg PO q8–12h) and ranitidine bismuth citrate or ranitidine HCl (24 mg/kg PO q8–12h) for 2 weeks has also been reported to be effective in the eradication of *Helicobacter* spp. Ranitidine is no longer approved for human use in the US and can be difficult to find. The combination of clarithromycin (50 mg/kg PO q24h or divided q12h); omeprazole (4 mg/kg PO q24h); metronidazole (20 mg/kg PO q12h) for 14 days has also been used for eradication
- Other antisecretory agents successfully used in ferrets include omeprazole (4 mg/kg PO q24h), famotidine (0.25–0.5 mg/kg PO, SC, IV q24h), and cimetidine (5–10 mg/kg PO, SC, IM, IV q6–8h)
- Sucralfate suspension (25 mg/kg PO q8h) protects ulcerated tissue (cytoprotection) by binding to ulcer sites.

CONTRAINDICATIONS
Avoid nonsteroidal anti-inflammatory medications in ferrets with gastric ulcers.

PRECAUTIONS
N/A

POSSIBLE INTERACTIONS
- Cimetidine may interfere with metabolism of other drugs.
- Sucralfate may alter absorption of other drugs.

FOLLOW-UP

PATIENT MONITORING
- No noninvasive tests are currently available to confirm the eradication of gastric helicobacter
- If vomiting persists or recurs after cessation of combination therapy, pursue other diseases as the cause of clinical signs.

PREVENTION/AVOIDANCE
- Identify and treat any underlying disease.
- Gastrointestinal antisecretory agents are helpful to treat and possibly prevent gastritis in anorectic ferrets. Ferrets continually secrete a baseline level of gastric hydrochloric acid and, as such, anorexia itself may predispose to gastric ulceration.
- Avoid overcrowding and unsanitary conditions.

POSSIBLE COMPLICATIONS
- Hemorrhage and anemia from ulcers
- Perforation
- Recurrence

EXPECTED COURSE AND PROGNOSIS
- Most infections are eradicated by using the treatment regimen described above.

- Some ferrets with chronic infections are severely debilitated and will not respond to treatment.
- Recurrence is common, especially under stressful conditions. Repeat therapy may be necessary.

MISCELLANEOUS

ASSOCIATED CONDITIONS
- Metabolic disease
- Gastrointestinal foreign bodies
- ECE

AGE-RELATED FACTORS
Gastric *Helicobacter* organisms appear to be acquired at a young age.

ZOONOTIC POTENTIAL
The high prevalence of *Helicobacter* spp. in ferrets raises the possibility that household pets may serve as a reservoir for the transmission of *Helicobacter* spp. to people; however, no cases have been documented.

PREGNANCY/FERTILITY/BREEDING
Avoid metronidazole in pregnant animals.

SYNONYMS
Helicobacter-associated gastric disease

SEE ALSO
Gastrointestinal and esophageal foreign bodies
Lymphoplasmacytic enteritis and gastroenteritis
Melena
Vomiting

ABBREVIATIONS
ECE = epizootic catarrhal enteritis
GI = gastrointestinal

Suggested Reading
Di Girolamo N, Selleri P. Medical and surgical emergencies in ferrets. Vet Clin Exot Anim 2016;19:431–464.
Hoefer HL. Gastrointestinal diseases of ferrets. In: Quesenberry KE, Carpenter JW, eds. Ferrets, Rabbits, and Rodents, 4th ed. Clinical Medicine and Surgery. 2021. St. Louis: Saunders, 2020:27–38.
Huynh M, Pignon C. Gastrointestinal disease in exotic small mammals. J Exot Pet Med 2013;22(2):118–131.
Johnson-Delaney CA. Geriatric ferrets. Vet Clin Exot Anim Pract 2020;23(3):549–565.
Livingstone M. Dealing with gastrointestinal disease in ferrets. In Practice 2022;44: 169–179.
Murray J, Kiupel M, Maes RK. Ferret coronavirus-associated diseases. Vet Clin North Am Exot Anim Pract 2010;13(3): 543–560.

Author Barbara Oglesbee, DVM, DABVP-Avian

BASICS

DEFINITION
High absolute or relative concentrations of feminizing sex hormones such as estradiol, estriol, and estrone. Severe aplastic anemia and blood loss due to abnormal clotting from estrogen-induced bone marrow suppression is the most common and severe effect of hyperestrogenism.

PATHOPHYSIOLOGY
• Severe hyperestrogenism is seen in intact females (Jills). Ferrets are induced ovulators. Ovulation is induced by stimulation of the cervix by mating or artificial means and is followed by pregnancy or pseudopregnancy lasting 41–43 days. If not bred, most Jills will remain in estrus. Serum estrogen concentration will remain elevated for the remainder of the breeding season (March–August in the Northern hemisphere and from August–January in the Southern hemisphere).
• Following 41–43 days of pregnancy or pseudopregnancy, estrus will return during the breeding season.
• Estrogen causes severe bone marrow suppression of erythroid, myeloid, and megakaryocytic cell lines. Jills are at risk of developing life-threatening anemia and blood loss due to thrombocytopenia if allowed to remain in estrus for more than 1 month. Death usually occurs after 2 months of estrus.
• Hyperestrogenism is also occasionally seen in neutered ferrets of either gender with ferret adrenal disease. Adrenal cortical hyperplasia or neoplasia causes increased production of sex steroids and is one of the most common diseases of ferrets. The bone marrow suppressive effects of hyperestrogenism in ferrets with adrenal disease is usually mild.
• Other organs affected include the skin and urogenital tract.

SYSTEMS AFFECTED
• Hemic/Lymphatic/Immune—aplastic anemia
• Urogenital—feminization, swollen vulva, pyometra, and urogenital cysts
• Skin/Exocrine—alopecia
• Neuromuscular—weakness, ataxia, or paresis from anemia; paresis or paralysis due to subdural hematoma formation (rare)

INCIDENCE/PREVALENCE
• Hyperestrogenism due to prolonged estrus is less common in the United States, since most ferrets are neutered before arriving at pet store, approximately 5–6 weeks of age.
• 50% or more of unbred jills will develop bone marrow toxicity.

• Hyperestrogenism is a less common manifestation of ferret adrenal disease.

SIGNALMENT
• Sexually mature females (>8–12 months of age)
• Endogenous hyperestrogenism is most common in young, intact, female ferrets. It is occasionally seen in spayed females if an ovarian remnant is present.

SIGNS
Historical Findings
• Prolonged estrus characterized by prominent, swollen vulva
• Bilaterally symmetric alopecia, usually beginning at the tail base and progressing cranially.
• Hematuria
• Melena
• Anorexia, depression, and lethargy
• Rear limb weakness, ataxia, paresis, or paralysis

Physical Examination Findings
• Large, turgid vulva
• Pale mucous membranes are manifestations of anemia and bone marrow suppression.
• Petechiation, ecchymosis, or other signs of hemorrhage
• Systolic murmur associated with anemia
• Serous or purulent vaginal discharge
• Bilateral, symmetrical alopecia beginning at the tail base
• Paraurethral cyst or abscess
• Cutaneous hyperpigmentation
• Fever and depression, due to pneumonia, septicemia, or pyometra may be caused by neutropenia associated with bone marrow suppression
• Splenomegaly
• Gynecomastia (rare)
• Galactorrhea (rare)

CAUSES AND RISK FACTORS
• Failure to breed intact females
• Ovarian remnant in neutered females
• Ferret adrenal disease—estrogen-secreting adrenal tumors—may cause mild anemia

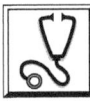

DIAGNOSIS

DIFFERENTIAL DIAGNOSIS
• Rule out adrenal disease—(usually seen in ferrets >2 years of age) signs not as severe and slower in onset
• For anemia—blood loss (trauma, gastric ulceration, and fleas), rodenticide toxicity, immune-mediated hemolytic anemia, severe hepatic disease, neoplasia, anemia of chronic disease, renal failure

• For alopecia—adrenal disease, seasonal alopecia, ectoparasites, mast cell tumor, and dermatophytosis

CBC/BIOCHEMISTRY/URINALYSIS
• Nonregenerative anemia (clinical signs usually apparent when PCV falls to <20%), thrombocytopenia (hemorrhage occurs when platelet counts fall below 20,000/μL), and leukocytosis initially, followed by leukopenia
• Normal PCV (46%–61%), erythrocyte count (17.0×10^6 cells/μL), and reticulocyte count (10%) are higher in ferrets than in other mammals.
• Hematuria

OTHER LABORATORY TESTS
• High serum estrogen (estradiol) concentration to help confirm a suspected diagnosis
• Examination of vaginal cytology may reveal numerous cornified cells or purulent exudate in ferrets with pyometra.

IMAGING
Radiography and ultrasonography to diagnose pyometra or to detect enlarged adrenals in ferrets with adrenal disease

DIAGNOSTIC PROCEDURES
• Examination of bone marrow aspirate reveals hypoplasia of the myeloid, erythroid, and megakaryocytic lines.
• In spayed females with swollen vulva—hCG challenge test. 100 IU of hCG IM once at least 2 weeks following onset of vulvar swelling. If swelling subsides 3–4 days postinjection, an ovarian remnant is likely. Some ovarian remnants do not respond to a single injection of hCG, requiring a second injection 2 weeks later. If the vulva remains swollen, HAC is most likely the cause.

PATHOLOGIC FINDINGS
• Gross examination—swollen vulva; pale mucous membranes; petechia and ecchymosis; tan-pink bone marrow; hemorrhage in GI tract, uterus, or urinary bladder; hydrometra or pyometra; pneumonia; subdural hemorrhage in brain or spinal cord; enlargement of the adrenal gland(s) seen with adrenal disease
• Histopathologic examination— hypocellular bone marrow, hemosiderosis in liver, spleen, and lymph nodes, suppurative pneumonia or metritis may be seen.

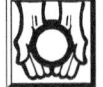

TREATMENT

APPROPRIATE HEALTH CARE
Hospitalization is required in ferrets exhibiting clinical signs related to anemia or hemorrhage. Asymptomatic ferrets in estrus

FERRETS

less than 1 month may be treated on an outpatient basis.

NURSING CARE
• Indications for whole blood transfusion are the same as those for dogs or cats. In general, most ferrets will benefit from a transfusion when the PCV falls below 15%, depending on clinical signs. Identifiable blood groups have not been demonstrated in ferrets, and transfusion reactions are unlikely, even after multiple transfusions. However, administration of dexamethasone sodium phosphate 4–6 mg/kg by slow IV injection once prior to transfusion has been recommended as a precaution. Healthy, large males with a normal PCV are the most appropriate blood donors. Up to 0.6% of donor's body weight can be safely collected (usually, 6–12 mL, depending on the size of the ferret and volume required). Collect blood from anesthetized donor ferret via the anterior vena cava or jugular vein into a syringe with 1 mL acid-citrate-dextrose anticoagulant per 7 mL of blood, or 5 units of heparin per mL of blood. (Volume of blood to be transfused is estimated in the same manner as for cats.) Administer blood within 4 hours of collection. Blood should be filtered during administration to the recipient. Administer blood slowly initially, at a rate of 0.5 mL/kg for the first 20 minutes, while monitoring for transfusion reaction. Follow transfusion with IV administration of 0.9% NaCl to meet maintenance and dehydration needs.
• Supportive care, such as fluid therapy, warmth, and adequate nutrition, are required for recovery.

ACTIVITY
Limited if anemic

DIET
If normal diet is refused, most ferrets will accept high-calorie diets such as Eukanuba Maximum Calorie diet (Iams Co., Dayton, OH), Feline a/d (Hills Products, Topeka, KS), chicken-based baby foods, or Clinicare Feline liquid diet (Abbott Laboratories, North Chicago, IL); may also add dietary supplement such as Nutri-Cal (EVSCO Pharmaceuticals) to increase caloric content to these foods. Warming the food to body temperature or offering via syringe may increase acceptance.

CLIENT EDUCATION
• Seek medical attention for any ferret remaining in estrus for over 2 weeks.
• Ferrets with complications such as thrombocytopenia, pyometra, and pneumonia are poor surgical risks and often do not respond well to medical treatment.
• Nonbreeding females should be neutered.

SURGICAL CONSIDERATIONS
• Ovariohysterectomy is the treatment of choice. This is usually a relatively safe procedure in ferrets with PCV >30. Ferrets with PCV <30 will usually require a blood transfusion prior to surgery. Ferrets that are extremely anemic, thrombocytopenic, and with secondary infections such as pneumonia or pyometra are poor surgical risks and should be stabilized if possible prior to surgery (transfusion as needed and medical treatment with hCG—see below).
• Perform celiotomy in ferrets with ovarian remnant. Ovarian tissue may be small and is located at the caudolateral pole of the kidney. These ferrets are usually not severely anemic presurgery, but a blood transfusion may be required if intraoperative hemorrhage is extensive.
• Ferret adrenal disease may be treated with adrenalectomy or managed medically. The decision as to which form of treatment is appropriate is multifactorial: which gland is affected (left vs. right), surgeon's experience and expertise, severity of clinical signs, age of the animal, concurrent diseases, and financial issues should be considered.

MEDICATIONS
DRUG(S) OF CHOICE
To induce ovulation and terminate estrus:
• Human chorionic gonadotropin (hCG)—administer 100 IU per ferret IM to stimulate ovulation and end estrus. Signs of estrus (particularly vulvar swelling) should diminish within 3–4 days. If signs are still apparent 1 week posttreatment, repeat the injection. Treatment is only effective after day 10 of estrus.
• Leuprolide acetate (100–250 ug/kg IM)
Other treatments:
• Administer antibiotics to treat secondary infections.
• Other supportive care measures include the administration of iron dextran (10 mg/kg IM once); anabolic and corticosteroids have also been used.

CONTRAINDICATIONS
N/A

ALTERNATIVE DRUGS
• GnRH—20 μg per ferret IM or SC may also be used to stimulate ovulation. Injection may be repeated q1–2w as needed. Treatment is only effective after day 10 of estrus.
• Erythropoietin may be considered to stimulate erythroid and granulocytic production at the level of the bone marrow.

FOLLOW-UP
PATIENT MONITORING
Monitor response to treatment by remission of clinical signs—reduction in vulvar swelling is good initial indicator of response to treatment. Repeat CBC 1–2 weeks posttreatment to monitor bone marrow response.

PREVENTION/AVOIDANCE
• Perform OHE on all females not used for breeding.
• For intact, breeding Jills:
  ○ Sham breeding using vasectomized males ("V-Hobs") to induce pseudopregnancy
  ○ If not breeding, administer deslorelin acetate 4.7 mg implant. Suppresses ovulation for 2 years. If the owner desires to breed the Jill post-deslorelin treatment, the first breeding typically results in pseudopregnancy. A normal pregnancy typically occurs with the second breeding.
  ○ Do not allow intact females to remain in heat for longer than 2 weeks—induce ovulation by breeding or administration of hCG

POSSIBLE COMPLICATIONS
• Death due to blood loss and anemia during of following surgery. This is particularly a risk in severely anemic and thrombocytopenic patients that do not respond immediately to treatment with hCG.
• Death due to bronchopneumonia or septicemia
• Hemolysis following transfusion
• Permanent suppression of bone marrow (rare).

EXPECTED COURSE AND PROGNOSIS
• Estrus will be terminated within 1 week post administration of hCG in 95% of ferrets
• Signs of estrus will usually resolve within 1 week of surgery for removal of ovarian remnant, OHE, or adrenalectomy.
• Ferrets with a PCV >25% usually carry a good prognosis and respond to treatment with hCG. Perform OHE following termination of estrus to prevent future episodes.
• Ferrets with a PCV of 15%–25% or below carry a fair to guarded prognosis, depending on the severity of clinical signs and other factors such as age and concurrent diseases. Intensive medical treatment and, in some cases, multiple transfusions are required prior to or following OHE.

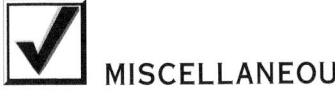

MISCELLANEOUS

ASSOCIATED CONDITIONS
- Pyometra
- Paraurethral cysts
- Insulinoma or lymphoma are commonly seen in ferrets with adrenal disease.
- Splenomegaly is a common, nonspecific finding.

AGE-RELATED FACTORS
Female <2 years of age are most likely to develop hyperestrogenism due to ovarian remnant or prolonged estrus. Females >2 years of age are more likely to develop a milder degree of hyperestrogenism due to adrenal disease.

SEE ALSO
Adrenal disease (hyperadrenocorticism)
Pyometra and stump pyometra

ABBREVIATIONS
GnRH = gonadotropin-releasing hormone
HAC = hyperadrenocorticism
Hb = hemoglobin
hCG = human chorionic gonadotropin
OHE = ovariohysterectomy
PCV = packed cell volume

Suggested Reading
Di Girolamo N, Huyun M. Disorders of the urinary and reproductive systems in ferrets. In: Quesenberry KE, Carpenter JW, eds. Ferrets, Rabbits and Rodents, 4th ed. Clinical Medicine and Surgery. St. Louis: Saunders, 2020:39–54.

Di Girolamo N, Selleri P. Medical and surgical emergencies in ferrets. Vet Clin Exot Anim Pract 2016;19:431–464.

Jekl V, Hauptman K. Reproductive medicine in ferrets. Vet Clin Exot Anim Pract 2017;20:629–663.

Lennox AM, Wagner RA. Comparison of 4.7-mg deslorelin implants and surgery for the treatment of adrenocortical disease in ferrets. J Exot Pet Med 2012;21:332–335.

Schoemaker NJ, Van Zealand YRA. Endocrine diseases of ferrets. In: Quesenberry KE, Carpenter JW, eds. Ferrets, Rabbits and Rodents, 4th ed. Clinical Medicine and Surgery. St. Louis: Saunders, 2020:77–91.

Wagner RA, Piché CA, Jöchle W, Oliver JW. Clinical and endocrine responses to treatment with deslorelin acetate implants in ferrets with adrenocortical disease. Am J Vet Res 2005;66:910–914.

Author Barbara Oglesbee, DVM, DABVP (Avian)

FERRETS

HYPOGLYCEMIA

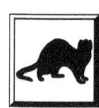

BASICS

DEFINITION
Abnormally low blood glucose concentration

PATHOPHYSIOLOGY
Mechanisms Responsible for Hypoglycemia
- Excess insulin or insulin-like factors; insulinoma (pancreatic islet b-cell neoplasia) most common cause in ferrets
- Reduction of hormones needed to maintain normal serum glucose (e.g., iatrogenic hypoadrenocorticism)
- Reduced hepatic gluconeogenesis (e.g., hepatic disease, sepsis)
- Overuse (sepsis, neoplasia)
- Reduced intake or underproduction (e.g., kits, severe malnutrition, or starvation)

SYSTEMS AFFECTED
- Nervous
- Musculoskeletal

SIGNALMENT
Variable, depending on the underlying cause

SIGNS
- Most animals have episodic signs
- Weakness
- Nausea—often manifested as ptyalism and pawing at the mouth
- Ataxia
- Lethargy and depression
- Muscle fasciculation
- Posterior paresis
- Abnormal mentation (stargazing)
- Exercise intolerance
- Abnormal behavior—irritability, aggressiveness
- Stupor
- Collapse
- Seizures (rare)
- Some animals appear normal aside from findings associated with underlying disease.

CAUSES
Endocrine
- Insulinoma—most frequent cause of hypoglycemia; one of the most common diseases seen in pet ferrets
- Iatrogenic insulin overdose
- Iatrogenic hypoadrenocorticism

Hepatic Disease
- Severe hepatitis (e.g., toxic and inflammatory)
- Cirrhosis

Overuse
- Neoplasia
- Sepsis

Reduced Intake/Underproduction
- Young kits
- Severe malnutrition or starvation

RISK FACTORS
- Low energy intake predisposes hypoglycemia in patients with conditions causing overuse and underproduction.
- Fasting, excitement, exercise, and eating foods that contain simple sugars may increase the risk of hypoglycemic episodes in patients with insulinoma.

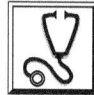

DIAGNOSIS

DIFFERENTIAL DIAGNOSIS
- Patients with hyperinsulinism—usually present with signs of hypoglycemia or have a normal physical examination
- Patients with cirrhosis and severe hepatitis—usually have other signs of their disease (e.g., gastrointestinal signs, icterus, and ascites or edema)
- Patients with sepsis—critical; usually in shock; pyrexia or hypothermia revealed by examination; may have gastrointestinal signs
- Patients with iatrogenic hypoadrenocorticism—waxing, waning, nonspecific signs (e.g., vomiting, diarrhea, melena, and weakness); history of surgery for adrenal disease; Addisonian patients that present in a crisis usually display hypovolemia and hyperkalemia rather than hypoglycemia (e.g., shock, bradycardia, and dehydration).

Laboratory Findings

Drugs that may alter laboratory results
N/A

Disorders that may alter laboratory results
- Lipemia, hemolysis, and icterus may interfere with spectrophotometric assays.
- Delayed serum separation artificially lowers glucose concentration; must separate serum after collection to prevent cellular glucose use
- Refrigerate or freeze serum sample not analyzed within 12 hours.
- Blood glucose reagent strips require whole blood.
- Measure glucose concentration in whole blood immediately following collection.

CBC/BIOCHEMISTRY/URINALYSIS
- Hypoglycemia—BG <60 mg/dL is found during symptomatic hypoglycemic episodes in patients with insulinoma (normal value 90–100 mg/dL)
- Normoglycemia is seen in some patients, due to counterregulatory hormone production (epinephrine, glucocorticoids, glucagon, etc.). If insulinoma is suspected but

the patient is normoglycemic, perform a carefully monitored fast for no longer than 4 hours. Serum glucose concentrations of <60 mg/dL is suggestive.
- Patients with chronic insulinomas often become tolerant of hypoglycemia and often appear asymptomatic even with BG <60 mg/dL. Treatment is directed at controlling the frequency and severity of hypoglycemic events, not at tightly controlling BG concentration.
- Patients with cirrhosis, severe hepatitis, and hepatic neoplasia may have anemia associated with chronic disease, high liver enzyme activities, hyperbilirubinemia, hypoalbuminemia, and low urinary specific gravity.

OTHER LABORATORY TESTS
- Simultaneous fasting glucose/insulin determination—may be helpful (but usually not necessary) when insulinoma is suspected; high plasma insulin in the face of hypoglycemia suggests insulinoma
- Fasting and postprandial serum bile acids—indicated when functional hepatic disease is suspected; however, normal values in ferrets have not been reported
- Bacterial culture of blood—indicated when sepsis is suspected

IMAGING
- CT scan, abdominal radiography, and ultrasonography—useful in patients with neoplastic processes (may see organomegaly or masses) as well as cirrhosis (microhepatica, hyperechogenicity) and severe hepatitis (hepatomegaly); pancreatic insulinomas are rarely detectable radiographically but may be seen on ultrasonic examination if sufficiently large
- Thoracic radiography—to detect metastasis if neoplasia is suspected

DIAGNOSTIC PROCEDURES
Ultrasound-guided or surgical biopsy—useful to evaluate for cirrhosis, hepatitis, and neoplasia

TREATMENT
- Treat as inpatients animals with clinical hypoglycemia; treat underlying disease.
- If able to eat (i.e., responsive, no vomiting), feeding is the most important component of initial treatment.
- If unable to eat, start continuous fluid therapy with 2.5% dextrose; if clinical signs persist, use a 5% dextrose solution.
- Surgery may be indicated if insulinoma is the cause of hypoglycemia.

(CONTINUED)

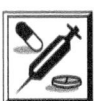

MEDICATIONS

DRUG(S) OF CHOICE

Emergency/Acute Treatment
In hospital
• Most signs of hypoglycemia will respond to oral dextrose or glucose. Begin by administering 0.5–1.0 ml of dextrose or corn syrup. When signs abate, follow this with a small, high-protein meal such as chicken baby food, Lafeber Carnivore Critical Care Diet (Lafeber Company, Cornell, IL) or Oxbow Carnivore Critical Care Diet (Oxbow Animal Health, Omaha, NE). Do not continue to administer oral dextrose or supplements that contain sugars as this will cause a release of insulin and rebound hypoglycemia.
• If no response to oral treatment, administer 50% dextrose, 0.25–2.0 mL IV slow bolus (1–3 minutes) to effect to control seizures/severe hypoglycemic signs. Do not continue to administer once clinical signs begin to abate, or dextrose will cause a release of insulin and rebound hypoglycemia. Follow with a small meal, as described above.
• If symptoms abate after oral treatment or IV bolus of dextrose, manage on an inpatient or outpatient basis with frequent feeding of high-protein foods. Depending on the severity, food should be offered or assist-fed every 1–4 hours. Normal GI transit time is 4 hours, so do not allow the ferret to go without eating for more than 3–4 hours.
• If the ferret is hospitalized and IV fluids are indicated, begin with a balanced electrolyte solution. Empirical treatment with IV dextrose solutions will cause a continuous release of insulin and rebound hypoglycemia.
• If food is refused, NPO is necessary during hospitalization, or signs are not controlled with oral or IV dextrose boluses, begin IV fluid therapy with 2.5% dextrose and 0.45% saline. This may be increased to 5% dextrose solution if needed to control clinical signs. Do not attempt to tightly control blood glucose concentrations. Treatment is aimed at controlling clinical signs of hypoglycemia.

Long-Term Treatment
• See chapter on insulinoma for treatment of insulinoma.
• Young kits with hypoglycemia—increase the frequency of feeding (nursing or hand feeding)

• Other causes of hypoglycemia require treating the underlying disease and do not usually need long-term treatment.

CONTRAINDICATIONS
Insulin

PRECAUTIONS
• 50% dextrose causes tissue necrosis and sloughing if given extravascularly; never administer dextrose in concentrations over 5% without confirmed vascular access.
• Dextrose bolus—suitable for an acute hypoglycemic crisis to effect only. Continued administration will cause insulin release and rebound hypoglycemia. Administering a dextrose bolus without following with frequent feedings can predispose to subsequent hypoglycemic episodes.
• Barbiturates and diazepam in patients with hypoglycemic seizures—they do not treat the cause of the seizure and they may worsen hepatoencephalopathy.

POSSIBLE INTERACTIONS
N/A

ALTERNATIVE DRUGS
N/A

FOLLOW-UP

PATIENT MONITORING
• At home—for return or progression of clinical signs of hypoglycemia; assess serum glucose if signs recur
• Single, intermittent serum glucose determinations may not truly reflect the glycemic status of the patient because of the normal production of counterregulatory hormones.
• Other monitoring is based on the underlying disease.

POSSIBLE COMPLICATIONS
Recurrent, progressive episodes of hypoglycemia

MISCELLANEOUS

ASSOCIATED CONDITIONS
Prolonged hypoglycemia can cause transient (hours to days) to permanent blindness from laminar necrosis of the occipital cerebral cortex.

AGE-RELATED FACTORS
Neonatal animals have poor glycogen storage capacity and a reduced ability to perform gluconeogenesis; thus, short periods of fasting can cause hypoglycemia.

ZOONOTIC POTENTIAL
N/A

PREGNANCY/FERTILITY/BREEDING
• Hypoglycemia can lead to weakness and dystocia.
• Pregnancy coupled with fasting causes hypoglycemia in rare instances.

SYNONYMS
N/A

SEE ALSO
See specific causes
Insulinoma

Suggested Reading
Schoemaker NJ. Ferret oncology: diseases, diagnostics, and therapeutics. Vet Clin Exot Anim Pract 2017;20(1):183–208.
Schoemaker NJ, van Zeeland YRA. Endocrine diseases of ferrets. In: Quesenberry KE, Carpenter JW, eds. Ferrets, Rabbits and Rodents, 4th ed. Clinical Medicine and Surgery. 2021. St. Louis: Saunders, 2020:77–91.
Schoemaker NJ, van Zeeland YR. Ferrets. In: Graham JE, Doss GA, Beaufrère H, eds. Exotic Animal Emergency and Critical Care Medicine, 2021:201–237.
Williams BH, Wyre NR. Neoplasia in ferrets. In: Quesenberry KE, Carpenter JW, eds. Ferrets, Rabbits and Rodents, 4th ed. Clinical Medicine and Surgery. 2021. St. Louis: Saunders, 2020:92–108.
Wu RS, Liu YJ, Chu CC, Heng HG, Chia MY, Wang HC, Chen KS. Ultrasonographic features of insulinoma in six ferrets. Vet Radiol Ultrasound 2017;58(5):607–612.
Author Barbara Oglesbee, DVM, DABVP (Avian)

FERRETS

IBUPROFEN AND ACETAMINOPHEN TOXICITY

BASICS

DEFINITION
Ingestion of and clinical manifestations of toxic effects of the NSAID ibuprofen and the non-NSAID acetaminophen (aka paracetamol/APAP).

PATHOPHYSIOLOGY
Pathophysiology is not known specifically in ferrets for either drug. Ibuprofen nonselectively blocks the conversion of arachidonic acid into various prostaglandins that mediate pain and inflammation, regulating mucus and bicarbonate synthesis, maintaining water homeostasis, stimulating repair of gastrointestinal epithelia cells, and controlling blood flow to the stomach and kidneys. The principal toxic metabolite of acetaminophen is produced by the hepatic cytochrome P-450 enzyme system. An acute overdose depletes glutathione stores in the liver, which normally detoxify this metabolite. The toxin accumulates, causing hepatocellular necrosis and possibly damages other organs. Like cats, ferrets seem more acutely sensitive to this toxicity.

SYSTEMS AFFECTED
- Circulatory—impaired platelet aggregation and clot formation (ibuprofen); methemoglobinemia (acetaminophen)
- GI—direct cytotoxic effects on gastric mucosa leading to GI upset, ulceration, and hemorrhage (ibuprofen)
- Renal—disruption of vasodilatory prostaglandins that maintain blood flow to the kidneys, decrease GFR, inhibit tubular ion transport; worsened by preexisting disease or dehydration (ibuprofen)
- Hepatic—inhibit hepatic function (ibuprofen), hepatocellular necrosis (acetaminophen)
- CNS—most commonly affected system—ataxia, tremors, drowsiness to coma, seizures, episodes of apnea associated with metabolic acidosis (ibuprofen)

SIGNALMENT
All ages, though perhaps younger ferrets are more intrinsically inquisitive to getting into and ingesting nonfood items.

SIGNS
Historical Findings
- Chewed pill vials/pills
- Owner self-treating

Physical Examination Findings
- Ibuprofen: CNS depression, seizures, anorexia, vomiting, diarrhea, and melena
- Acetominophen: progressive depression, ptalism, vomiting, abdominal pain, tachypnea, cyanosis, and possible dark-colored urine

CAUSES
Ingestion of ibuprofen or acetominophen

RISK FACTORS
- Free roaming
- Easy medication access (in purse, on tables)

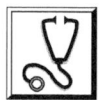

DIAGNOSIS

DIFFERENTIAL DIAGNOSIS
- Circulatory—rodenticide toxicity, metastatic adrenal/pancreatic neoplasia affecting liver, and other toxins
- GI—other ingested toxins, foreign body ingestion, adrenal/pancreatic disease, IBD, and infection
- Renal—Chronic renal failure, renal cysts, other ingested toxins (ethylene glycol), and infection
- Hepatic—other ingested toxins, neoplasia, and infection
- CNS—other toxins, neoplasia, trauma, and infection

CBC/BIOCHEMISTRY/URINALYSIS
CBC
- Ibuprofen—may identify anemia and/or thrombocytopenia
- Acetaminophen—methemoglobinemia

Biochemistry
- Ibuprofen—increased BUN, creatinine, phosphorus, sometimes liver enzymes, and elevated CPK if seizures
- Acetaminophen—increased ALT and ALP
- Bilirubin is infrequently elevated in ferrets with liver disease.

OTHER LABORATORY TESTS
- Urinalysis: isosthenuria (ibuprofen), hematuria/hemoglobinuria (acetaminophen)
- Ibuprofen analysis on serum, urine, and hepatic tissue
- Acetaminophen analysis on serum (must be within 1–3 hours of ingestion), blood glutathione decreased

IMAGING
Radiography
- Possible pulmonary edema in advanced cases of acetaminophen toxicity

DIAGNOSTIC PROCEDURES
- Hepatic biopsy—via ultrasound-guided needle, laparoscopy, or laparotomy
- Coagulation profile—before hepatic biopsy

TREATMENT

APPROPRIATE HEALTH CARE
- Acute ibuprofen exposure—induce vomiting/gastric lavage if <2 hours from ingestion, otherwise gavage activated charcoal (watch for aspiration); IV/IO fluids to prevent renal failure, famotidine, omeprazole, sucralfate, or other GI protectants; maropitant for vomiting, midazolam, or diazepam for seizures.
- Acute acetaminophen exposure—same as ibuprofen, consider blood transfusion if anemia severe; *N*-acetylcysteine.
- Chronic exposure—GI protectants for at least a week post-exposure; nutritional support

ACTIVITY
Restricted cage rest while undergoing primary therapy

DIET
- If normal diet is refused, most ferrets will accept high-calorie carnivore critical care diets (Oxbow Animal Health, Omaha, NE; Lafeber, Cornell, IL). Warming the food to body temperature or offering via syringe may increase acceptance.
- Administer these supplements several times a day.
- Sick ferrets should receive 300–400 kcal/kg BW per day.

CLIENT EDUCATION
- Inform client that treatment depends on exposure dose and concurrent health issues.
- Acetaminophen toxicity severity usually tapers after 12–48 hours.

SURGICAL CONSIDERATIONS
NA

MEDICATIONS

DRUG(S) OF CHOICE
- GI protectants—famotidine, omeprazole, sucralfate
- Antiemetics—maropitant
- Acetaminophen—N-acetylcysteine

CONTRAINDICATIONS
- Simultaneous administration of corticosteroids

POSSIBLE INTERACTIONS
- Avoid corticosteroids, anticoagulants, other NSAIDs

ALTERNATIVE DRUGS
N/A

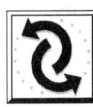

FOLLOW-UP

PATIENT MONITORING
- Physical assessment
- CBC, biochemistry, urinalysis—assess progression
- Repeat ibuprofen and acetaminophen/glutathione testing if case relevant

POSSIBLE COMPLICATIONS
Can lead to renal and/or hepatic failure or death

MISCELLANEOUS

ASSOCIATED CONDITIONS
N/A

AGE-RELATED FACTORS
N/A

ZOONOTIC POTENTIAL
N/A

PREGNANCY/FERTILITY/BREEDING
N/A

ABBREVIATIONS
ALP = alkaline phosphatase
ALT = alanine aminotransferase
APAP = acetyl-*para*-aminophenol
BUN = blood urea nitrogen
CNS = central nervous system
CPK = creatine phosphokinase
GFR = glomerular filtration rate
GI = gastrointestinal
IBD = inflammatory bowel disease
NSAID = nonsteroidal anti-inflammatory drug

Suggested Reading
Court M. Acetaminophen UDP-glucuronosyltransferase in ferrets: species and gender differences, and sequence analysis of ferret UGT1A6. J Vet Pharmacol Ther 2001;24:415–422.
Graham J. Ibuprofen and acetaminophen toxicity. In: Mayer J, Donnelly T, eds. Clinical Veterinary Advisor: Birds and Exotic Pets. St. Louis, MO: Elsevier, 2013:464–465.
Overman M. A review of ferret toxicoses. J Exot Pet Med 2015;24(4):398–402.
Petritz O, Chen S. Therapeutic contraindications in exotic pets. Vet Clin Exot Anim Pract 2018;21(2):327–340.
Richardson J, Balabuszko R. Ibuprofen ingestion in ferrets: 43 cases. J Vet Emerg Crit Care 2001;11(1):53–59.
Author Eric Klaphake, DVM, DACZM, DABVP

FERRETS

INFLAMMATORY BOWEL DISEASE

FERRETS

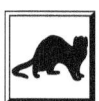

BASICS

OVERVIEW
• A group of gastrointestinal diseases characterized by inflammatory cellular infiltrates in the lamina propria of the small or large intestine, with associated clinical signs
• An abnormal mucosal immune response to certain causative factors resulting in the recruitment of inflammatory cells to the intestine and cellular damage
• Inflammatory response is usually lymphocytic, lymphoplasmacytic, or eosinophilic
• Lymphocytic infiltration into the lamina propria of the intestines is a common inflammatory response to many infectious agents or environmental stimuli.
• Plasmacytic infiltration indicates chronicity or a more severe inflammatory reaction.
• The cause of tissue eosinophilia is unknown, although a parasitic or allergic cause has been suspected, parasites are usually not found, and allergies have not been well documented in ferrets.
• The exact mechanisms, antigens, and patient factors involved in initiation and progression remain unknown.

SIGNALMENT
No sex or age predilection

SIGNS
• Anorexia
• Weight loss, muscle wasting
• "Bird seed" consistency to feces
• Diarrhea, sometimes with blood or mucus
• Melena
• Vomiting
• Ptyalism, pawing at the mouth (due to nausea)
• Physical examination—cachexia; thickened, ropy intestines; enlarged mesenteric lymph nodes; and splenomegaly often palpable

CAUSES AND RISK FACTORS
• Pathogenesis is most likely multifactorial.
• Lymphocytic or lymphoplasmacytic infiltrates may be associated with *Helicobacter mustelae*, epizootic catarrhal enteritis (ECE), Aleutian disease virus (ADV), giardia, salmonella, campylobacter, cryptosporidiosis, or other infectious agents.
• Foreign body ingestion
• Meat proteins, food additives, artificial coloring, preservatives, and milk proteins may play a role.

DIAGNOSIS

DIFFERENTIAL DIAGNOSIS
• Intestinal lymphosarcoma resembles IBD in both clinical presentation and physical exam findings
• Gastrointestinal foreign body
• Infectious diseases (e.g., *Helicobacter mustelae*, ECE, giardiasis, salmonellosis, campylobacter enteritis, cryptosporidiosis, and mycobacteriosis)

CBC/BIOCHEMISTRY/URINALYSIS
• Lymphocytic or lymphocytic/plasmacytic—results often normal; these tests help rule in or out some other differential diagnoses
• Eosinophilic—hemogram may reveal a peripheral eosinophilia (up to 35% eosinophils)
• Panhypoproteinemia or hypoalbuminemia may be present due to protein-losing enteropathy.

OTHER LABORATORY TESTS
• Fecal direct examination, fecal flotation, and zinc sulfate centrifugation may demonstrate gastrointestinal parasites
• Fecal cytology—may reveal RBC or fecal leukocytes, which are associated with inflammatory bowel disease or invasive bacterial strains
• Fecal culture should be performed if abnormal bacteria are observed on the fecal gram's stain, or if salmonella is suspected.

IMAGING
• Plain abdominal radiographs provide little information.
• Barium contrast radiography may demonstrate thick intestinal walls and mucosal irregularities but does not provide any information about etiology or the nature of the thickening.
• Ultrasonography—may be used to measure stomach and intestinal wall thickness, and to rule out other diseases; can be used to examine the liver, spleen, and mesenteric lymph nodes

DIAGNOSTIC PROCEDURES
Definitive diagnosis requires biopsy and histopathology, usually obtained via exploratory laparotomy

PATHOLOGIC FINDINGS
Infiltration of intestines with inflammatory cells

TREATMENT

APPROPRIATE HEALTH CARE
Outpatient, unless the patient is debilitated from dehydration, hypoproteinemia, or cachexia

NURSING CARE
If the patient is dehydrated, any balanced fluid such as lactated Ringer's solution is adequate (for a patient without other concurrent disease); otherwise, select fluids on the basis of secondary diseases. If held NPO due to vomiting, provide a dextrose-containing fluid and monitor blood glucose concentration.

ACTIVITY
No need to restrict unless severely debilitated.

DIET
• Highly digestible diets with novel protein sources may be useful for eliciting remission, although an allergic cause has not be documented, and little information is available regarding the efficacy of these diets. If attempted, choose feline diets since ferrets have high nutritional protein and fat requirements. Foods that have anecdotally reported to elicit remission include feline lamb and rice diets, diets consisting exclusively of one type of meat (lamb, duck, and turkey), or a "natural prey diet" consisting of whole rodents. Avoid diets that contain plant-based proteins (peas, soy, and grains), since these have been associated with the development of urinary calculi. If remission is elicited, continue the diet for at least 8–13 weeks; this diet may need to be fed lifelong.
• Anorexic ferrets may refuse dry foods but are often willing to eat canned cat foods or pureed meats.

CLIENT EDUCATION
• Emphasize to the client that IBD is not necessarily cured as much as controlled.
• Relapses are common; the client must be prepared to be patient during the various food and medication trials that are often necessary to get the disease under control.
• A severely debilitated patient may need hospitalization and parenteral nutrition.

(CONTINUED)

MEDICATIONS

DRUG(S) OF CHOICE
• Treat the underlying cause (e.g., helicobacter, salmonella, giardia, etc.) if found; if gastric lesions are present, empirical treatment for helicobacter is indicated.
• Immunosuppressive agents: Prednisone (2 mg/kg PO q24h or divided q12h); when signs resolve, gradually taper the corticosteroid dose by 1/2 every other week to effect (usually 0.5–1 mg/kg every other day) or Azathioprine (0.9 mg/kg PO q24–72h)
• Antibiotics used for immune modulating effect or to modify intestinal include metronidazole (10–15 mg/kg PO q12–24h); tylosin (25 mg/kg PO q12–24h); tetracycline 2 (0–25 mg q8–12h)
• Cobalamin for ferrets with chronic diarrhea—250 μg/kg SC weekly for 6 weeks, followed by 250 μg/kg q2w for 6 weeks, then monthly. Check cobalamin concentrations 1 month after administration to determine if continued therapy is warranted.
• See specific diseases for more detailed discussion of treatment.

CONTRAINDICATIONS
If secondary problems are present, avoid therapeutic agents that might be contraindicated for those conditions.

PRECAUTIONS
See discussion under specific diseases.

POSSIBLE INTERACTIONS
See discussion under specific diseases.

ALTERNATIVE DRUGS
See discussion under specific diseases.

FOLLOW-UP

PATIENT MONITORING
• Periodic reevaluation may be necessary until the patient's condition stabilizes.
• No other follow-up may be required except yearly physical examinations and assessment during relapse.

PREVENTION/AVOIDANCE
N/A

POSSIBLE COMPLICATIONS
Dehydration, malnutrition, adverse drug reactions, hypoproteinemia, anemia, and diseases secondary to therapy or resulting from the above-mentioned problems

EXPECTED COURSE AND PROGNOSIS
• Varies with specific type of IBD
• See discussion under specific diseases.

MISCELLANEOUS

ASSOCIATED CONDITIONS
See discussion under specific diseases.

AGE-RELATED FACTORS
N/A

ZOONOTIC POTENTIAL
N/A

PREGNANCY/FERTILITY/BREEDING
N/A

SYNONYMS
N/A

SEE ALSO
Anorexia
Diarrhea
Lymphoplasmacytic gastroenteritis
Eosinophilic enteritis and gastroenteritis

ABBREVIATIONS
ADV = Aleutian disease virus
ECE = epizootic catarrhal enteritis
IBD = inflammatory bowel disease

Suggested Reading
Cazzini P, Watson MK, Gottdenker N et al. Proposed grading scheme for inflammatory bowel disease in ferrets and correlation with clinical signs. J Vet Diagn Invest 2020;32(1):17–24.
Di Girolamo N, Selleri P. Medical and surgical emergencies in ferrets. Vet Clin Exot Anim 2016;19:431–464.
Hoefer HL. Gastrointestinal diseases of ferrets. In: Quesenberry KE, Carpenter JW, eds. Ferrets, Rabbits, and Rodents, 4th ed. Clinical Medicine and Surgery. 2021. St. Louis: Saunders, 2020:27–38.
Johnson-Delaney CA. Geriatric ferrets. Vet Clin Exot Anim Pract 2020;23(3): 549–565.
Livingstone M. Dealing with gastrointestinal disease in ferrets. In Practice 2022;44: 169–179.
Murray J, Kiupel M, Maes RK. Ferret coronavirus-associated diseases. Vet Clin North Am Exot Anim Pract 2010;13(3): 543–560.
Watson MK, Cazzini P, Mayer J et al. Histology and immunohistochemistry of severe inflammatory bowel disease versus lymphoma in the ferret (*Mustela putorius furo*). J Vet Diagn Invest 2016;28(3): 198–206.
Author Barbara Oglesbee, DVM, DABVP-Avian

FERRETS

INFLUENZA VIRUS

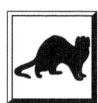

BASICS

DEFINITION
A common, self-limiting viral respiratory disease of ferrets characterized by sneezing, rhinitis, fever, conjunctivitis, and occasionally pneumonia.

PATHOPHYSIOLOGY
Human influenza types A and B (class Orthomyxoviridae), including H1N1, are pathogenic in ferrets. Transmission occurs from human to ferret or ferret to human. Virus replication occurs in the nasal mucosa, causing rhinitis and conjunctivitis within 48 hours following exposure. Occasionally, infection spreads to the lungs, causing pneumonia.

SYSTEMS AFFECTED
• Respiratory—rhinitis; interstitial pneumonia
• Ophthalmic—acute serous conjunctivitis without keratitis or corneal ulcers
• Gastrointestinal—anorexia, occasionally vomiting

GENETICS
None

INCIDENCE/PREVALENCE
Common, especially in multiferret households or facilities, or during influenza epizootics in humans

GEOGRAPHIC DISTRIBUTION
Worldwide

SIGNALMENT
No age or sex predilection

SIGNS
Historical Findings
• Sudden onset
• Anorexia
• Serous nasal or ocular discharge
• Sneezing
• Dyspnea or coughing if pneumonia occurs
• Lethargy
• Occasionally otitis
• Occasionally vomiting

Physical Examination Findings
• Generally alert and in good condition
• Fever
• Conjunctivitis
• Serous naso-ocular discharge, becoming purulent with secondary bacterial infections

CAUSES
• Human influenza types A and B, belonging to the class Orthomyxoviridae
• Secondary bacterial infections frequently occur

RISK FACTORS
• Exposure to affected humans or ferrets
• Multiferret facilities

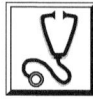

DIAGNOSIS

DIFFERENTIAL DIAGNOSIS
General Comments
Diagnosis is usually presumptive, based on a history of exposure to affected humans or other ferrets and the presence of suggestive clinical signs.

Differentiating Similar Causes
• Canine distemper virus (CDV)—the presence of other clinical signs will help to differentiate CDV from influenza virus infection. In ferrets with CDV, facial dermatitis (rash, crusts) and hyperkeratotic foot pads are seen following the onset of nasal discharge. These signs are followed by severe respiratory signs, neurologic signs, and death. Fluorescent antibody testing on conjunctival smears, mucous membrane scrapings, or blood smears can be used to diagnose CDV.
• Nasal foreign bodies—usually unilateral with purulent, mucopurulent, and blood-tinged discharge
• Dental related disease—abscess, oronasal fistula—rare in ferrets; differentiate based on oral exam
• Fungal infections—cryptococcosis, blastomycosis—also rare; chronic infection, whereas influenza is self-limiting
• Nasal tumors—usually associated with serosanguinous or blood-tinged discharges; may cause unilateral discharge initially then progress to bilateral discharge as the disease extends through the nasal septum.

CBC/BIOCHEMISTRY/URINALYSIS
• No characteristic or consistent findings. Leukopenia may be seen in early infection; leukocytosis in ferrets with secondary bacterial infections.
• Increases in BUN, creatinine, ALT depending on the level of dehydration, and severity of disease.

OTHER LABORATORY TESTS
• Serologic testing—not readily available; rarely necessary. A rising titer indicates active infection; however, clinical signs generally resolve prior to receiving test results.
• Immunofluorescence assays, ELISA, or AGID—available from many veterinary diagnostic laboratories for type A influenza viruses, including H1N1. Antibodies can usually be detected by 3 days post-infection
• Fluorescent antibody test to rule out CDV—on conjunctival or mucous

membrane scrapings, or peripheral blood smears

IMAGING
• Skull radiographs—to differentiate Influenza from nasal tumors, fungal rhinitis, or dental disease
• Radiographs of the lungs—for evidence of pneumonia

DIAGNOSTIC PROCEDURES
• Cell cultures to isolate the virus—oral pharynx; lung tissue; secretions from the nose and conjunctiva may be used if obtaining a definitive diagnosis is necessary

PATHOLOGIC FINDINGS
• Gross—reddened, swollen mucosa in the upper respiratory tract; serous to mucoid nasal or discharge
• Histopathologic—vacuolar degeneration of epithelial cells, progressing to epithelial necrosis, with sloughing of epithelial cells and infiltration of inflammatory cells (chiefly neutrophils in the early phase, then mononuclear cells) followed by epithelial cell regeneration and hyperplasia

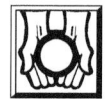

TREATMENT

APPROPRIATE HEALTH CARE
Outpatient, unless severe pneumonia occurs

NURSING CARE
• Clean eyes and nose as indicated
• Provide palatable foods (see Diet, below)
• Fluid therapy using a balanced electrolyte solution should be administered to anorectic or dehydrated patients. Subcutaneous route is sufficient in most patients unless severe secondary bacterial pneumonia is present.
• Oxygen—with severe, secondary bacterial pneumonia

ACTIVITY
Patients should be restricted from contact with humans and other ferrets to prevent transmission of the disease.

DIET
• No restrictions
• If normal diet is refused, most ferrets will accept high-calorie diets such as Eukanuba Maximum Calorie diet (Iams Co., Dayton, OH), Feline a/d (Hills Products, Topeka, KS), chicken-based baby foods, or Clinicare Feline liquid diet (Abbott Laboratories, North Chicago, IL); may also add dietary supplement such as Nutri-Cal (EVSCO Pharmaceuticals) to increase caloric content to these foods.
• Warming the food or offering via syringe may increase acceptance.

CLIENT EDUCATION
• Discuss the potential for zoonosis—can be transmitted from human to ferret, ferret to ferret, or ferret to human.
• Most infections are self-limiting, unless patient is immunosuppressed or develops severe, secondary bacterial infections.

SURGICAL CONSIDERATIONS
None

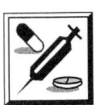

MEDICATIONS

DRUG(S) OF CHOICE
• Broad-spectrum antibiotics—indicated for secondary bacterial infections (e.g., trimethoprim/sulfonamide (15–30 mg/kg PO, SC q12h); enrofloxacin (10–30 mg/kg PO, SC, IM q12h); or amoxicillin/clavulanate (13–25 mg/kg PO q12h)
• Antihistamines such as chlorpheniramine (1.0–2.0 mg/kg PO q8–12h) or diphenhydramine (0.5–2.0 mg/kg PO, IM, IV q8–12h) may help to alleviate nasal discharge.
• Antibiotic eye ointments—to reduce secondary bacterial infections of the conjunctiva

CONTRAINDICATIONS
None

PRECAUTIONS
N/A

POSSIBLE INTERACTIONS
None

ALTERNATIVE DRUGS
None

FOLLOW-UP

PATIENT MONITORING
• Monitor for development of dyspnea associated with pneumonia
• Monitor for development of secondary bacterial rhinitis, conjunctivitis, or sinusitis
• No specific laboratory tests needed for monitoring

PREVENTION/AVOIDANCE
Avoid exposure to humans or ferrets exhibiting clinical signs of influenza.

POSSIBLE COMPLICATIONS
• Interstitial pneumonia—most serious complication
• Secondary bacterial infections of the lungs or upper airways

EXPECTED COURSE AND PROGNOSIS
• Clinical disease—usually appears within 48 hours after exposure
• Recovery is usually rapid, occurring within 7 days of the onset of clinical signs
• Prognosis is excellent unless severe secondary bacterial infections develop

MISCELLANEOUS

ASSOCIATED CONDITIONS
N/A

AGE-RELATED FACTORS
N/A

ZOONOTIC POTENTIAL
High

PREGNANCY/FERTILITY/BREEDING
N/A

SYNONYMS
N/A

SEE ALSO
Canine distemper virus
Cough
Nasal discharge (sneezing, gagging)

ABBREVIATIONS
AGID = agar gel immunodiffusion
CDV = canine distemper virus
ELISA = enzyme-linked immunosorbent assay

Suggested Reading
Capello V, Lennox AM. Diagnostic imaging of the respiratory system in exotic companion mammals. Vet Clin Exot Anim 2011;14:369–389.
Johnson-Delaney CA. Ferret respiratory system: clinical anatomy, physiology, and disease. Vet Clin Exot Anim 2011;14: 357–367.
Kiupel M, Perpiñán D. Viral diseases of ferrets. In: Fox JG, Marini RP, eds. Biology and Diseases of the Ferret, 3rd ed. John Wiley & Sons, 2014:439–517.
Lennox A. Respiratory disorders in ferrets. Vet Clin Exot Anim 2021;24:483–493.
Perpiñán D. Respiratory diseases of ferrets. In: Quesenberry KE, Carpenter JW, eds. Ferrets, Rabbits and Rodents, 4th ed. Clinical Medicine and Surgery. 2021. St. Louis: Saunders, 2020:71–76.
Swenson SL, Koster LG, Jenkins-Moore M et al. Natural cases of 2009 pandemic H1N1 Influenza A virus in pet ferrets. J Vet Diagn Invest 2010;22(5):784–788.
Author Barbara Oglesbee DVM, DABVP (Avian)

INSULINOMA

BASICS

DEFINITION
Pancreatic islet b-cell neoplasm that secretes an excess quantity of insulin leading to clinical signs of hypoglycemia.

Insulinomas are extremely common in ferrets. Disease is due to the effects of hypoglycemia rather than space-occupying effects or metastasis, and the disease is managed, not cured. Multiple tumors are present in the pancreas and the number of tumors will progress with time. The therapeutic goal is to regulate blood glucose concentrations, thereby limiting clinical signs of hypoglycemia.

PATHOPHYSIOLOGY
Excessive insulin secretion leads to excessive glucose uptake and use by insulin-sensitive tissues and reduced hepatic production of glucose; this causes hypoglycemia and its associated clinical signs.

SYSTEMS AFFECTED
• Nervous—stargazing, ataxia, seizures, disorientation, abnormal behavior, collapse, and posterior paresis
• Musculoskeletal—weakness and muscle fasciculations
• Gastrointestinal—nausea, vomiting

SIGNALMENT
• Insulinoma is one of the most common diseases seen in pet ferrets; incidence reported as 25% of all neoplasms diagnosed in ferrets
• Usually seen in ferrets over 2 years old, mean 4 years of age
• No sex predilection reported

SIGNS

General Comments
• Signs are typically episodic.
• The rate of decline of serum glucose concentration affects the type and severity of clinical signs.
• Signs may or may not be related to fasting, excitement, exercise, and eating.
• Ferrets usually demonstrate more than one clinical sign, and they progress with time.

Historical Findings
• Abnormal mentation, dullness, irritability, stargazing, nausea (characterized by ptyalism and pawing at the mouth), weakness (usually hind limb paresis), depression, ataxia, tremors, and stupor are most common; also, seizures (generalized and focal), vomiting, collapse, muscle fasciculations, abnormal behavior, polyuria and polydipsia, and exercise intolerance
• Many of the hypoglycemic episodes may go unwitnessed, giving owners the impression of acute onset.

Physical Examination Findings
• Often within normal limits unless examined during a hypoglycemic episode, then clinical signs as noted above
• Pancreatic tumors are usually not palpable
• Emaciation and muscle wasting are seen in ferrets with chronic disease
• Splenomegaly is often an incidental finding on abdominal palpation
• Signs of concurrent ferret adrenal disease (especially alopecia) are commonly seen

CAUSES
Insulin-producing adenoma or carcinoma of the pancreas

RISK FACTORS
• Fasting, excitement, exercise, and eating may increase the risk of hypoglycemic episodes.
• Excessive carbohydrate intake may predispose to the development of clinical disease
• Concurrent gastrointestinal disease, especially GI foreign body or IBD, may increase the risk and complicate the management of hypoglycemic episodes.

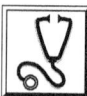

DIAGNOSIS

DIFFERENTIAL DIAGNOSIS
• For hypoglycemia—fasting, starvation, gastrointestinal foreign body, intractable vomiting, severe hepatic disease, and sepsis
• Seizures and collapse—must consider cardiovascular (e.g., syncope), metabolic (e.g., anemia most common), hepatoencephalopathy, hypocalcemia, iatrogenic (hypoadrenocorticism rare cause following adrenalectomy), and neurologic (e.g., epilepsy, neoplasia, toxin, and inflammatory disease) causes
• Posterior paresis and weakness—consider cardiovascular (e.g., arrhythmias, heart failure, and pericardial effusion), metabolic (e.g., anemia, hypokalemia, and hypocalcemia), neurologic and neuromuscular (e.g., spinal cord disease), and toxic (e.g., botulism, chronic organophosphate exposure, and lead poisoning) causes
• Muscle fasciculations—consider metabolic (e.g., electrolyte imbalances) and toxic (e.g., tetanus and strychnine poisoning) causes

CBC/BIOCHEMISTRY/URINALYSIS
• Hypoglycemia—BG <60 mg/dL is found during symptomatic hypoglycemic episodes in patients with insulinoma (normal value 90–100 mg/dL).
• Normoglycemia is seen in some patients, due to counterregulatory hormone production (epinephrine, glucocorticoids, glucagon, etc.). If insulinoma is suspected but the patient is normoglycemic, perform a

carefully monitored fast for no longer than 4 hours. Serum glucose concentration of <60 mg/dL is suggestive.
• Patients with chronic insulinomas often become tolerant of hypoglycemia and often appear asymptomatic even with BG <60 mg/dL. Treatment is directed at controlling the frequency and severity of hypoglycemic events, not at tightly controlling BG concentration.
• Be certain to perform serum glucose concentration testing immediately following venipuncture, since storage of serum not separated from red cells will cause a falsely lowered value.
• The practice of feeding flavored nutritional supplements or peanut butter to aid in restraint or venipuncture should be strictly avoided prior to or during collection of blood for serum glucose concentration, as this will cause a falsely elevated value.

OTHER LABORATORY TESTS
• Simultaneous fasting glucose and insulin determination—results are not consistently reliable, and insulin assay not readily available. If measuring insulin is elected, it should be measured along with serum glucose; a single insulin measurement alone is not meaningful. After initiating fast, collect blood samples hourly or bi-hourly for serum glucose determination and serum storage; when the serum glucose drops below 60 mg/dL (usually within 2–4 hours), submit that sample for serum insulin determination. Be certain that the insulin assay used has been validated for use in ferrets. Normal insulin concentrations reported to be between 5 and 40 μU/ml
• Interpretation: high insulin in the face of hypoglycemia, insulinoma likely; normal insulin in the face of hypoglycemia, insulinoma possible; low insulin with hypoglycemia, insulinoma less likely
• Determination of serum insulin concentration is not usually necessary. In most cases, the finding of hypoglycemia with suggestive clinical signs justifies a presumptive diagnosis.

IMAGING
Abdominal radiography is often normal, except for splenomegaly (usually an incidental finding). Pancreatic nodules or metastatic nodules in regional lymph nodes, spleen, or liver can sometimes be seen on abdominal ultrasonography. Concurrent adrenal tumor(s) are commonly found.

DIAGNOSTIC PROCEDURES
N/A

PATHOLOGIC FINDINGS
• Multiple nodules of variable size within the pancreas are usually seen.

- Most insulinomas can be identified grossly at surgery; often gentle palpation is required for detection. Occasionally, no tumor can be identified grossly, but multiple small tumors are present within the pancreas; a biopsy is necessary to identify these.
- Metastasis is relatively uncommon; when it occurs, areas include the regional lymph nodes, spleen, liver, and local adipose tissue.
- Micrometastasis within the pancreas is common.
- Histopathologically, they appear as either carcinoma or adenoma, but both behave malignantly.

TREATMENT

APPROPRIATE HEALTH CARE
- Treatment is directed toward managing the clinical signs of hypoglycemia. Most ferrets will be asymptomatic if BG is maintained above 60 mg/dL. However, many ferrets with chronic disease will be asymptomatic at this or even lower BG concentrations. The goal of management is to resolve symptoms during acute hypoglycemic episodes, mitigate the severity of signs in future episodes, and limit, for as long as possible, the frequency of episodes. It is neither possible nor beneficial to attempt tight regulation of BG. The number of pancreatic tumors will increase over time, and the disease will progress. Fortunately, severe, uncontrollable hypoglycemia usually only occurs in older ferrets with long-term disease.
- Most can be treated on an outpatient basis after medical management of a hypoglycemic crisis.
- If signs of hypoglycemia cannot be managed and hospitalization is necessary, look for concurrent disorders, especially gastrointestinal disease. GI disorders can exacerbate hypoglycemic episodes.

NURSING CARE
- Most signs of hypoglycemia will respond to oral dextrose or glucose. Begin by administering 0.5–1.0 ml of dextrose or corn syrup. When signs abate, follow this with a small, high-protein meal such as chicken baby food, Lafeber Carnivore Critical Care Diet (Lafeber Company, Cornell, IL) or Oxbow Carnivore Critical Care Diet (Oxbow Animal Health, Omaha, NE). Do not continue to administer oral dextrose or supplements that contain sugars as this will cause a release of insulin and rebound hypoglycemia.
- If no response to oral treatment, administer 50% dextrose, 0.25–2.0 mL IV slow bolus (1–3 minutes) to effect to control seizures/severe hypoglycemic signs. Do not continue

to administer once clinical signs begin to abate, or dextrose will cause a release of insulin and rebound hypoglycemia. Follow with a small meal, as described above.
- If symptoms abate after oral treatment or IV bolus of dextrose, manage on an inpatient or outpatient basis with frequent feeding of high-protein foods. Depending on the severity, food should be offered or assist-fed every 1–4 hours. Normal GI transit time is 4 hours, so do not allow the ferret to go without eating for more than 3–4 hours.
- If the ferret is hospitalized and IV fluids are indicated, begin with a balanced electrolyte solution. Empirical treatment with IV dextrose solutions will cause a continuous release of insulin and rebound hypoglycemia.
- If food is refused, NPO is necessary during hospitalization, or signs are not controlled with oral or IV dextrose boluses, begin IV fluid therapy with 2.5% dextrose and 0.45% saline. This may be increased to 5% dextrose solution if needed to control clinical signs. Do not attempt to tightly control blood glucose concentrations. Treatment is aimed at controlling clinical signs of hypoglycemia.

ACTIVITY
Restricted

DIET
- The first and most important aspect of management (with or without medical or surgical treatment). With early disease, feeding frequent meals alone is often sufficient. Eventually, as the disease progresses, medical treatment is added.
- Depending on the severity, food should be offered or assist-fed every 1–4 hours. Normal GI transit time is 4 hours, so do not allow the ferret to go without eating for more than 3–4 hours.
- The diets should consist of high-quality ferret or cat foods that are high in animal proteins and low in carbohydrates and simple sugars.
- Do not feed sugary treats, as these will cause an increase in blood glucose concentration and a rebound release of insulin.

CLIENT EDUCATION
- Advise the owner that the disease is managed, not cured, and will eventually progress. It is not possible to remove all of the tumors, and more will develop over time. Treatment is aimed at maintaining normal blood glucose concentrations and minimizing the number and severity of hypoglycemic events.
- The owner should be aware of signs of hypoglycemia. Mild signs may be alleviated by administering a small amount (1/4 to 1/2 teaspoon) of corn syrup (preferred), honey, or other syrups (taking care to avoid being

bitten). Follow this with a small, high-protein meal such as your ferret's normal food, "duck soup," or chicken baby food. DO NOT continue to feed sugary foods. This will only cause the insulin to spike, causing another hypoglycemic event. Emphasize the importance of avoiding sugary or carbohydrate-based treats; many commercial treats and supplements contain simple sugars. If collapse or seizures occur, they should be instructed to seek immediate medical attention.
- Make sure that high-quality, high-protein foods are always available. Feed at least four to six small meals a day, during waking hours. Be sure to feed the ferret immediately upon awakening and just before going to sleep at night. Ferrets with advanced disease will require food available 24 hours a day.
- Insulinomas are progressive, even with surgical treatment, since complete excision of all nodules is rare.

SURGICAL CONSIDERATIONS
- Surgery confirms the diagnosis, can provide temporary remission, and can sometimes improve response to medical treatment.
- In most cases multiple nodules are present. Nodules appear as white to pink raised areas on the surface of the pancreas; however, nodules may be buried within the parenchyma—careful palpation is required for detection. Debulk large nodules or perform a partial pancreatectomy if multiple small nodules are present. Small, nonpalpable nodules remain, and clinical signs will eventually return.
- Surgical excision of nodules does not guarantee remission. In some cases, no benefit is seen.
- Occasionally, nodules are too small to detect by gross examination. If no nodules are detected, biopsy the pancreas and submit for histopathological examination.
- Always explore the entire abdominal cavity—concurrent adrenal disease is extremely common.
- Administer 2.5% dextrose in 0.45% saline or 5% dextrose solutions pre-, inter-, and postoperatively. Withhold food for up to 6 hours postoperatively (monitor blood glucose concentrations), then offer a high-protein diet. Continue fluid therapy SQ or IV until the ferret is eating normally and released.
- Measure serum glucose concentration after surgery and every 6–12 hours until concentration reaches >70 mg/dL.
- If serum glucose concentration does not increase postoperatively, begin medical treatment.

INSULINOMA (CONTINUED)

FERRETS

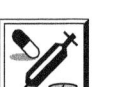

MEDICATIONS

DRUG(S) OF CHOICE

Emergency/Acute Therapy
See Nursing Care above

Long-Term Therapy
• Medical therapy is indicated when clinical signs return in patients that had previous surgical therapy.
• Initially, dietary management alone is usually effective, especially in younger ferrets. Feed frequent high-quality protein meals, no longer than 2–4 hours between feedings.
• When frequent feeding is no longer effective, begin treatment with glucocorticoids. Prednisolone—initial dosage of 0.25–0.5 mg/kg PO q12h; can gradually increase up to 2.2 mg/kg PO q12h if needed. Begin at the low end of the dosage range and increase as needed to control signs of hypoglycemia. Serum glucose concentration will usually maintain in the range of 70–90 mg/dL and signs will abate initially with prednisolone and diet modification. With time and the progression of tumors, more insulin will be released, and clinical signs will recur. Gradually increase the dose of prednisone as signs of hypoglycemia recur.
• Diazoxide (benzothiadiazine)—added after dietary modification and prednisone treatment are no longer effective. Diazoxide acts by directly inhibiting pancreatic insulin secretion and stimulating hepatic gluconeogenesis. Reduce prednisone dose to back to 1–1.25 mg/kg PO q12h and begin diazoxide at a dose of 5–10 mg/kg PO per day, divided q8–12h. If needed, the dose can be gradually increased to 30 mg/kg PO per day (divided into 2–3 doses). Administer with food.

CONTRAINDICATIONS
Insulin

PRECAUTIONS
• Dextrose bolus—suitable for an acute hypoglycemic crisis to effect only. Continued administration will cause insulin release and rebound hypoglycemia. Administering a dextrose bolus without following with frequent feedings can predispose to subsequent hypoglycemic episodes.
• Diazoxide—can cause vomiting, diarrhea, or anorexia; these effects can be mitigated if administered with a meal. In humans, causes bone marrow suppression, cataract formation, aplastic anemia, tachycardia, and thrombocytopenia; it is unknown if these occur in ferrets.
• Prednisolone and diazoxide may each cause fluid retention and increase preload in ferrets with congestive heart failure.

• Chronic use of prednisolone can cause severe, sometimes life-threatening obesity in ferrets. Fat accumulation in the thorax, including around the heart and within the lung parenchyma, can cause progressive, severe dyspnea. Fat accumulation within the abdomen can cause lethargy, exercise intolerance, and general malaise.

POSSIBLE INTERACTIONS
N/A

ALTERNATIVE DRUGS
Octreotide (1–2 µg/kg q8–12h SC), a synthetic somatostatin analogue, has been anecdotally used in some ferrets with mixed efficacy.

FOLLOW-UP

PATIENT MONITORING
• Postoperative in-hospital serum glucose determinations—monitor every 6–12 hours for the first 2–3 days or until euglycemic. Most ferrets will be euglycemic within 1–2 days after surgery. If hypoglycemia persists, treatment with prednisone is necessary.
• Some ferrets will develop transient hyperglycemia after debulking the pancreas. At home, the urine may be monitored for glucose 2–3 times daily for the next week. In most cases, hyperglycemia is transient (resolving in 1–2 weeks) and does not require treatment.
• Following medical treatment—monitor at home for return or progression of clinical signs of hypoglycemia and adjust medication based on clinical signs. Do not attempt tight regulation of serum glucose concentration (treat the symptoms, not the numbers).

PREVENTION/AVOIDANCE
N/A

POSSIBLE COMPLICATIONS
• Rarely, iatrogenic pancreatitis occurs due to handling of the pancreas during surgery. Clinical signs include nausea, anorexia, and vomiting. Withhold food and continue fluid therapy with 2.5%–5% dextrose until euglycemic and appetite returns.
• Postoperative hyperglycemia occasionally occurs and usually resolves without treatment. Rarely, hyperglycemia will persist, resulting in clinical signs of diabetes mellitus (in one case, postoperative diabetes was seen in a ferret with a mixed insulinoma/glucagonoma). See Diabetes mellitus chapter for treatment.

EXPECTED COURSE AND PROGNOSIS
• With surgical treatment, relatively few ferrets will remain euglycemic long term. Most ferrets will require medical treatment within 6 months.

• With medical treatment alone, clinical signs will be controlled for periods of 6 months to 2 years, depending on the age of onset, number and type of tumor.

MISCELLANEOUS

ASSOCIATED CONDITIONS
• Ferret adrenal disease and splenomegaly are commonly found in ferrets with insulinomas.
• Gastrointestinal disorders often exacerbate hypoglycemic episodes.

AGE-RELATED FACTORS
Older ferrets may not benefit from surgery, since mean survival times are relatively equivalent with medical therapy alone in older animals.

ZOONOTIC POTENTIAL
N/A

PREGNANCY/FERTILITY/BREEDING
N/A

SYNONYMS
B-cell tumor
Hyperinsulinism
Insulin-producing pancreatic tumor
Insulin-secreting tumor
Islet cell adenocarcinoma
Islet cell tumor

SEE ALSO
Hypoglycemia

Suggested Reading
Schoemaker NJ. Ferret oncology: diseases, diagnostics, and therapeutics. Vet Clin Exot Anim Pract 2017;20(1):183–208.
Schoemaker NJ, van Zeeland YRA. Endocrine diseases of ferrets. In: Quesenberry KE, Carpenter JW, eds. Ferrets, Rabbits and Rodents, 4th ed. Clinical Medicine and Surgery. 2021. St. Louis: Saunders, 2020:77–91.
Schoemaker NJ, van Zeeland YR. Ferrets. In: Graham JE, Doss GA, Beaufrère H, eds. Exotic Animal Emergency and Critical Care Medicine, 2021:201–237.
Williams BH, Wyre NR. Neoplasia in ferrets. In: Quesenberry KE, Carpenter JW, eds. Ferrets, Rabbits and Rodents, 4th ed. Clinical Medicine and Surgery. 2021. St. Louis: Saunders, 2020:92–108.
Wu RS, Liu YJ, Chu CC, Heng HG, Chia MY, Wang HC, Chen KS. Ultrasonographic features of insulinoma in six ferrets. Vet Radiol Ultrasound 2017; 58(5):607–612.

Author Barbara Oglesbee, DVM, DABVP (Avian)

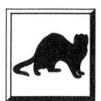

BASICS

GENERAL
• Can be infectious, inflammatory, toxic, or neoplastic.
• In ferrets, infectious and hepatic lipidosis is most common, followed by biliary disease and neoplasia

SYSTEMS AFFECTED
• Hepatobiliary—inflammation, cholestasis
• Gastrointestinal—vomiting, diarrhea
• Pulmonary—compromised ventilatory space with hepatomegaly or ascites

SIGNALMENT
Middle-aged to older animals more commonly affected

SIGNS
Historical Findings
• Often subclinical disease
• Anorexia or decreased appetite
• Non-specific findings such as weight loss, weakness, general malaise, and unkempt haircoat
• Diarrhea
• Exposure to other ferrets with infectious causes—most commonly ECE
• Icterus with cholestatic disorders
• Abdominal distention or palpable mass with neoplasia or ascites

Physical Examination Findings
• Depend on underlying cause
• Fluid wave with ascites
• Hepatomegaly or mass in region of liver
• Jaundice—with cholestatic disorders; most noticeable on nose, foot pads
• Dehydration, thin body condition
• Abdominal pain

CAUSES
• Hepatic lipidosis—especially in obese ferrets or with chronic corticosteroid use
• Infectious hepatitis—inflammation secondary to chronic inflammatory bowel disease (e.g., eosinophilic gastroenteritis, lymphoplasmacytic gastroenteritis), ADV, ECE
• Cholestatic disorders—blockage of bile ducts with inspissated bile plugs and gall bladder mucoceles are the most common cause. May be secondary to chronic lymphocytic hepatitis from ascending inflammatory process from the intestinal tract (IBD, helicobacter, ECE). Other, less common causes include Pancreatic islet cell neoplasia; other neoplasms arising near or involving the bile duct, abscess, proximal duodenitis or duodenal foreign body
• Neoplasia—lymphoma; bile duct cystadenoma are most common, hepatoma;

hepatocellular carcinoma; bilary carcinoma, hemangioma.hemangiosarcoma; various metastatic tumors
• Acute hepatic necrosis—toxins; drugs; ischemia
• High central venous pressure—right-sided congestive heart failure; cardiomyopathy; neoplasia; pericardial disease; heartworm disease; pulmonary hypertension; severe arrhythmia
• Hepatic abscesses
• Extramedullary hematopoiesis

RISK FACTORS
• Chronic gastrointestinal tract disease—ECE, IBD, foreign body
• Cardiac disease
• Obesity, chronic corticosteroid use—hepatic lipidosis

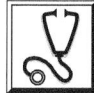

DIAGNOSIS

DIFFERENTIAL DIAGNOSIS
Differentiating Similar Causes
• History of chronic gastrointestinal disease. Hepatic inflammation (lymphocytic hepatitis) can occur secondary to chronic IBD, *Helicobacter gastroenteritis*, ECE, chronic gastrointestinal foreign bodies
• Signs of acute gastrointestinal disease—infiltration into the liver of infectious agents (e.g., coronavirus, parvovirus, and bacterial hepatitis)
• Signs of cardiac disorders (e.g., heart murmur, jugular distention, and muffled heart sounds)—hepatic congestion
• Obesity, history of chronic corticosteroid use—hepatic lipidosis
• Jaundice—cholelithiasis, cholestasis
• Palpable or radiographic evidence of hepatomegaly—neoplasia, congestion

CBC/BIOCHEMISTRY/URINALYSIS
CBC
• Leukogram—to identify underlying conditions (leukocytosis with neutrophilia with bacterial disease; may see lymphocytosis in young ferrets or lymphopenia in older ferrets with lymphoma; peripheral eosinophilia with eosinophilic gastroenteritis)
• Panhypoproteinemia or hypoalbuminemia is seen with protein-losing enteropathy

Biochemistry
• Moderate to high ALT and ALP with inflammatory disorders, primary hepatic neoplasia, hepatic lipidosis, or vacuolar hepatopathy
• Mild to moderately high liver enzymes with metastatic neoplasia, venous outflow obstruction, or infiltrative disorders

• Elevated Bilirubin, ALT in ferrets with cholestatic disorders

Urinalysis
Bilirubinuria in ferrets with cholestatic disorders

IMAGING
Abdominal Radiography
• Hepatomegaly—extension of a rounded liver margin caudal to the costal arch; caudal-dorsal displacement of stomach; mass effect with neoplasia

Thoracic Radiography
• Right and left lateral views—screen for metastasis and underlying disorders
• Cardiac, pulmonary, pericardial disorders

Abdominal Ultrasonography
• To identify choleliths, gall bladder mucocele, and bile duct distension
• Abdominal effusions—distribution and echogenic patterns
• Diffuse enlargement with normal echogenicity—congestion; cellular infiltration; inflammation; extramedullary hematopoiesis
• Diffuse enlargement with hyperechoic parenchyma (minor nodularity)—lipidosis; glycogen accumulation; inflammation; diffuse early fibrosis

DIAGNOSTIC PROCEDURES
• Fine-needle aspiration—23- or 25-gauge 2.5–3.75-cm (1–1.5-in) needle; aspirated with ultrasound guidance
• Cytology—may reveal infectious agents, neoplasia, inflammation, or extramedullary hematopoiesis
• Hepatic biopsy—if findings suggest primary hepatic disease and imaging rules out other obvious diagnoses; via ultrasound-guided needle, laparoscopy, or laparotomy
• Microbial culture—aerobic and anaerobic bacterial
• Coagulation profile—before liver biopsy (limited information on normal ferrets available)
• Abdominal effusion paracentesis—cytology; protein content; cultures

TREATMENT

APPROPRIATE HEALTH CARE
• General supportive goals—eliminate inciting cause; optimize conditions for hepatic regeneration; prevent complications; reverse derangements associated with hepatic failure
• Important derangements—dehydration and hypovolemia; hepatic encephalopathy; hypoglycemia; acid–base and electrolyte abnormalities; coagulopathies;

LIVER DISEASE   (CONTINUED)

FERRETS

gastrointestinal ulcerations; sepsis; endotoxemia

NURSING CARE

- Hospitalize patients that are anorectic, dehydrated, or in heart or liver failure
- Rehydration is essential to treatment success in severely ill ferrets.
- Fluids are usually supplemented with potassium chloride, 5% dextrose if anorexic or concurrent insulinoma
- Heart failure or ascites—avoid sodium-rich fluids

ACTIVITY

Restricted cage rest while undergoing primary therapy

DIET

- If refusing solid food, most ferrets will accept assist feeding with an easily digestible high-protein/high-fat diet such as Lafeber Carnivore Critical Care Diet (Lafeber Company, Cornell, IL) or Oxbow Carnivore Critical Care Diet (Oxbow Animal Health, Omaha, NE); may also add dietary supplement such as Nutri-Cal (EVSCO Pharmaceuticals) to increase caloric content to these foods.
- Easily digestible, high-protein diets such as chicken baby food are often helpful in ferrets recovering from ECE or inflammatory bowel disease.
- Sick ferrets should receive 300–400 kcal/kg BW per day.

CLIENT EDUCATION

- Warn client that many causes are life threatening, although others are less serious and may be amenable to treatment.
- Inform client that a thorough workup is essential for attaining a definitive diagnosis.

SURGICAL CONSIDERATIONS

- May be indicated for resection of primary or focal hepatic mass lesions (neoplasia, abscess)
- Choledochotomy to remove inspissated bile and/or cholelith, or cholecystectomy may be indicated

MEDICATIONS

DRUG(S) OF CHOICE

- Treat underlying intestinal tract disease when indicated (see specific disorders)
- Infectious (e.g., bacterial) diseases—appropriate antimicrobial agents
- Ursodiol (10–15 mg/kg PO q24h) has been very successful in treatment of bile duct obstruction, and gall bladder mucoceles in ferrets.
- Cardiac causes—diuretics (e.g., furosemide) ACE inhibitors, Pimobenden

CONTRAINDICATIONS

Avoid hepatotoxic medications

POSSIBLE INTERACTIONS

N/A

ALTERNATIVE DRUGS

N/A

FOLLOW-UP

PATIENT MONITORING

- Physical assessment and hepatic imaging—reassess liver size, resolution of cholestasis
- CBC, biochemistry—assess the progression of hepatic dysfunction
- Thoracic radiographs, ECG, and echocardiography—assess previous abnormalities

POSSIBLE COMPLICATIONS

Many causes are life threatening.

MISCELLANEOUS

ASSOCIATED CONDITIONS

ECE
Helicobacter
IBD
Cardiac disease
Lymphoma

AGE-RELATED FACTORS

More common in middle-aged to older ferrets

ZOONOTIC POTENTIAL

N/A

PREGNANCY/FERTILITY/BREEDING

N/A

ABBREVIATIONS

ADV = Aleutian disease virus
ALT = alanine aminotransferase
ALP = alkaline phosphatase
ECE = epizootic catarrhal enteritis
IBD = inflammatory bowel disease

Suggested Reading
Hall BA, Ketz-Riley CJ. Cholestasis and cholelithiasis in a domestic ferret (*Mustela putorius furo*). J Vet Diagn Invest 2011;23(4):836–839.
Hauptman K, Jekl V, Knotek Z. Extrahepatic biliary tract obstruction in two ferrets (*Mustela putorius furo*). J Small Anim Pract 2011;52(7):371–375.
Hauptman K, Sívková A, Jekl V. Cholestasis with obstruction of the biliary tract in a ferret (*Mustela putorius furo*). Veterinářství 2019;69(2):69–72.
Hoefer HL. Gastrointestinal diseases of ferrets. In: Quesenberry KE, Carpenter JW, eds. Ferrets, Rabbits, and Rodents, 4th ed. Clinical Medicine and Surgery. 2021. St. Louis: Saunders, 2020:27–38.
Huynh M, Guillaumot P, Hernandez J, Ragetly G. Gall bladder rupture associated with cholecystitis in a domestic ferret (*Mustela putorius*). J Small Anim Pract 2014;55(9):479–482.
Huynh M, Laloi F. Diagnosis of liver disease in domestic ferrets (*Mustela putorius*). Vet Clin Exot Anim Pract 2013;16(1):121–144.
Huynh M, Pignon C. Gastrointestinal disease in exotic small mammals. J Exot Pet Med 2013;22(2):118–131.
Rhody JL, Williams BH. Exocrine pancreatic adenocarcinoma and associated extrahepatic biliary obstruction in a ferret. J Exot Pet Med 2013;22(2):206–211.

Author Barbara Oglesbee, DVM, DABVP (Avian)

LOWER URINARY TRACT INFECTION

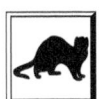

BASICS

OVERVIEW
- Result of microbial colonization of the urinary bladder and/or proximal portion of the urethra
- Microbes, usually aerobic bacteria, ascend the urinary tract under conditions that permit them to persist in the urine or adhere to the epithelium and subsequently multiply. Urinary tract colonization requires at least transient impairment of the mechanisms that normally defend against infection. Inflammation of infected tissues results in the clinical signs and laboratory test abnormalities exhibited by patients.
- Some ferrets with adrenal disease develop paraurethral or prostatic cysts. Cysts may become secondarily infected, leading to abscess formation. Exudate from these cysts/abscesses may drain into the urinary bladder or urethra resulting in thick purulent exudate mixed with urine in the bladder. In some cases, this exudate can be thick enough to cause urethral blockage.

SYSTEMS AFFECTED
Renal/Urologic—lower urinary tract

INCIDENCE/PREVALENCE
Uncommon in ferrets as compared with cats and dogs

SIGNALMENT
- More common in female ferrets than in males
- All ages affected, but occurrence increases with age because of a greater frequency of other urinary lesions (e.g., uroliths, prostate or paraurethral cystic disease, and tumors) that predispose to secondary urinary tract infection.

SIGNS

Historical Findings
- None in some patients
- Pollakiuria—frequent voiding of small volumes
- Dysuria
- Urinating in places that are not customary
- Hematuria and cloudy or malodorous urine in some patients
- Signs of adrenal disease, especially alopecia in many patients

Physical Examination Findings
- No abnormalities in some animals
- Acute infection—bladder or urethra may seem tender on palpation
- Palpation of the bladder may stimulate urination, even in normal ferrets.
- Chronic infection—wall of the bladder or urethra may be palpably thickened or abnormally firm.

- Paraurethral cysts palpable in some ferrets with ferret adrenal disease

CAUSES AND RISK FACTORS
- Most common—Escherichia, Staphylococcus, and Proteus spp.
- Conditions that cause urine stasis or incomplete emptying of the bladder, such as paraurethral cystic disease or urolithiasis, predispose to LUTI.

DIAGNOSIS

DIFFERENTIAL DIAGNOSIS
- LUTI may mimic other causes of pollakiuria, dysuria, hematuria, and/or outflow obstruction, the most common of which is urolithiasis and urogenital cystic disease.
- Ferrets with urogenital cysts usually have other signs of adrenal disease, especially bilaterally symmetric alopecia.
- Differentiate from other causes by urinalysis, urine culture, radiography, and ultrasonography.

CBC/BIOCHEMISTRY/URINALYSIS
- Results of CBC and serum biochemistry normal
- Pyuria (normal value 0–1 WBC/hpf) is most commonly associated with urinary tract infection, but noninfectious urinary lesions can also cause pyuria. Hematuria (normal value 0–3 RBC/hpf) and proteinuria (normal value 0–33 mg/dL) indicate urinary tract inflammation, but these are nonspecific findings that may result from infectious and noninfectious causes of lower urinary tract disease.
- Some paraurethral or prostatic cysts may become secondarily infected, forming abscesses that drain into the urinary bladder or urethra. Thick, purulent exudate from these abscesses may mix with urine in the bladder, resulting in significant pyuria and bacteriuria. In some cases, this exudate can be thick enough to cause urethral blockage.
- Identification of bacteria in urine sediment suggests that urinary tract infection is causing or complicating lower urinary tract disease or may be seen in ferrets with abscessed urogenital cysts. If small numbers of bacteria are seen, consider contamination of urine during collection and storage when interpreting urinalysis results.

OTHER LABORATORY TESTS

Urine Culture and Sensitivity Testing
- Urine culture is necessary for definitive diagnosis.
- Correct interpretation of urine culture results requires obtaining the specimen in a manner that minimizes contamination,

handling, and storing the specimen so that numbers of viable bacteria do not change in vitro and using a quantitative culture method. Keep the specimen in a sealed sterile container; if the culture is not started right away, the urine can be refrigerated up to 8 hours without important changes in the results.
- Cystocentesis—the preferred technique for obtaining urine for culture. Sedation is usually required.

IMAGING
Survey and contrast radiographic studies as well as ultrasound of the bladder or urethra may detect an underlying urinary tract lesion (i.e., paraurethral cystic disease or urolithiasis).

DIAGNOSTIC PROCEDURES
N/A

PATHOLOGIC FINDINGS
N/A

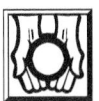

TREATMENT

APPROPRIATE HEALTH CARE
Treat as outpatient unless another urinary abnormality (e.g., obstruction) requires inpatient treatment

CLIENT EDUCATION
Prognosis for cure of simple urinary tract infection is excellent; prognosis for complicated urinary tract infection depends on the underlying abnormality. Compliance with recommendations for treatment and follow-up evaluations is crucial for optimum results.

SURGICAL CONSIDERATIONS
Except when a concomitant disorder requires surgical intervention, management does not involve surgery.

MEDICATIONS

DRUG(S) OF CHOICE
- Base choice of drug on results of sensitivity test.
- Antibiotics that concentrate in the urine are most appropriate. Initial choices include trimethoprim-sulfadiazine (15–30 mg/kg PO, SC q12h), amoxicillin/clavulanate (13–25 mg/kg PO q12h), cephalexin (15–30 mg/kg PO q8–12h), or enrofloxacin (5–10 mg/kg PO, SC, IM q12h).
- For acute, uncomplicated infection, treat with antimicrobial drugs for at least 2 weeks. Appropriate duration of treatment for

FERRETS

complicated lower urinary tract infection depends on the underlying problem.

PRECAUTIONS
Because of potential nephrotoxicity with long-term administration, use aminoglycosides only when there are no alternatives.

 FOLLOW-UP

PATIENT MONITORING
• When antibacterial drug efficacy is in doubt, culture the urine 2–3 days after starting treatment. If the drug is effective, the culture will be negative.
• Continue treating at least 1 week after resolution of hematuria, pyuria, and proteinuria. Failure of urinalysis findings to return to normal while an episode of urinary tract infection is being treated with an effective antibiotic (i.e., as indicated by negative urine culture) generally indicates some other urinary tract abnormality (e.g., urogenital cysts, urolith, tumor). Rapid recrudescence of signs when treatment is stopped generally indicates either a concurrent urinary tract abnormality or that the infection extends into some deep-seated site (e.g., prostatic or renal parenchyma).
• Successful cure of an episode of urinary tract infection is best demonstrated by performing a urine culture 7–10 days after completing antimicrobial therapy.

PREVENTION/AVOIDANCE
• Treat underlying adrenal disease in ferrets with urogenital cystic disease.
• Feed high-quality ferret or cat foods to avoid urolithiasis.

POSSIBLE COMPLICATIONS
Failure to detect or treat effectively may lead to pyelonephritis

EXPECTED COURSE AND PROGNOSIS
• If not treated, expect infection to persist indefinitely. Associated health risks include development of extension of infection to other portions of the urinary tract (e.g., the kidneys) or beyond (e.g., septicemia and bacterial endocarditis).
• Generally, the prognosis for animals with uncomplicated lower urinary tract infection is good to excellent. The prognosis for animals with complicated infection is determined by the prognosis for the other urinary abnormality.

 MISCELLANEOUS

ASSOCIATED CONDITIONS
• Struvite urolithiasis
• Ferret adrenal disease

AGE-RELATED FACTORS
Complicated infection is more common in middle-aged to old than young animals.

SYNONYMS
Bacterial cystitis

Urethritis
Urethrocystitis

SEE ALSO
Adrenal disease (hyperadrenocorticism)
Dysuria and pollakiuria
Parurethral cysts
Urolithiasis

ABBREVIATION
LUTI = lower urinary tract infection

Suggested Reading
Di Girolamo N, Huyun M. Disorders of the urinary and reproductive systems in ferrets. In: Quesenberry KE, Carpenter JW, eds. Ferrets, Rabbits and Rodents, 4th ed. Clinical Medicine and Surgery. St. Louis: Saunders, 2020:39–54.
Di Girolamo N, Selleri P. Medical and surgical emergencies in ferrets. Vet Clin Exot Anim Pract 2016;19:431–464.
Hallman RM, Brandão J. Diagnostic imaging of the renal system in exotic companion mammals. Vet Clin Exot Anim 2020; 23:195–214.
Reavill DR, Lennox AM. Disease overview of the urinary tract in exotic companion mammals and tips on clinical management. Vet Clin Exot Anim 2020; 23(1):169–193.
Wagner RA, Piché CA, Jöchle W et al. Clinical and endocrine responses to treatment with deslorelin acetate implants in ferrets with adrenocortical disease. Am J Vet Res 2005;66:910–915.
Author Barbara Oglesbee, DVM, DABVP (Avian)

LYMPHADENOPATHY (LYMPHADENOMEGALY)

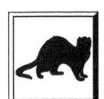

BASICS

DEFINITION
Abnormally large lymph nodes, generalized or localized to a single node or group of regional nodes

PATHOPHYSIOLOGY
• Can result from hyperplasia of lymphoid elements, inflammatory infiltration, or neoplastic proliferation within the lymph node
• Because of their filtration function, lymph nodes often act as sentinels of disease in the tissues they drain; inflammation of any tissue is often accompanied by enlargement of the draining nodes, which most likely results from reactive lymphoid hyperplasia but may also be caused by extension of the inflammatory process into the nodes (lymphadenitis).
• Neoplastic proliferation may be either primary (malignant lymphoma) or metastatic. Malignant lymphoma is the most common cause of lymphadenomegaly in ferrets.

SYSTEMS AFFECTED
Hemic/Lymph/Immune

SIGNALMENT
No breed, sex, or age predilection

SIGNS
• Peripheral lymphadenomegaly or mild enlargement of mediastinal or mesenteric nodes typically do not directly cause clinical signs.
• Severe—may cause mechanical obstruction and interference with the function of adjacent organs, signs of which depend on the affected lymph node, and may include dysphagia, regurgitation, respiratory distress, dyschezia, and limb swelling.
• May be systemically ill from the underlying disease process

CAUSES
Neoplasia
• Lymphoma—most common cause of lymphadenomegaly
• Metastatic neoplasia

Lymphoid Hyperplasia
• Localized or systemic infection caused by infectious agents of all categories (i.e., bacteria, viruses, and protozoa) when infection does not directly involve the node—common cause of mesenteric lymphadenomegaly
• Aleutian disease virus (ADV) infection—generalized hyperplasia
• Antigenic stimulation by factors other than infectious agents (e.g., inflammatory bowel disease)

Lymphadenitis
• Bacteria—capable of causing purulent lymphadenitis, which may progress to abscessation; a few (e.g., *Mycobacterium* spp.) induce granulomatous lymphadenitis (unusual in ferrets)
• Fungi—systemic infections cryptococcosis most commonly reported
• Eosinophilic—may be associated with allergic inflammation of the organ being drained by the affected lymph node; may be encountered in a patient with gastrointestinal eosinophilic disease, or in a lymph node draining a mast cell tumor

RISK FACTORS
• Malignant lymphoma—possibly close association with other ferrets with lymphoma
• Lymphadenomegaly caused by metastatic neoplasms—vary with the type of primary neoplasm
• Impaired immune function predisposes to infection and, therefore, to lymphadenitis.

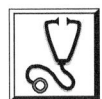

DIAGNOSIS

DIFFERENTIAL DIAGNOSIS
• For peripheral lymphadenomegaly—subcutaneous fat can surround the peripheral lymph nodes and have a firm consistency mimicking lymphadenomegaly. This is extremely common in obese ferrets and can sometimes be found in ferrets with normal body weight. Fine-needle aspiration is often nondiagnostic since the node is hidden deep within the fat deposits; a lymph node biopsy is usually necessary to differentiate lymphoma from a normal node surrounded by fat deposits.
• For mesenteric lymphadenomegaly—reactive nodes due to chronic gastrointestinal inflammatory or infiltrative disease such as *Helicobacter mustelae* gastritis, lymphoplasmacytic gastroenteritis, eosinophilic gastroenteritis, or ECE. Hyperplastic lymph nodes can resemble lymphosarcoma on both gross and histologic examination and may be difficult to distinguish. If the mesenteric lymph nodes are the only area of lymphocyte proliferation observed, hyperplasia is more likely than neoplasia.
• Palpable lymph nodes in normal ferrets—mandibular, prescapular, axillary, superficial inguinal, and popliteal nodes
• Severe lymph node enlargement—most likely to develop in patients with lymphoma
• Lesser degrees of enlargement—attributable to reactive hyperplasia, lymphadenitis, or neoplasia
• Extent of enlargement in patients with metastatic disease varies widely

• Multiple lymph nodes affected throughout the body—likely the result of lymphoma or systemic infection that causes either lymphadenitis or lymphoid hyperplasia
• Abscessation and metastatic neoplasms usually affect a single lymph node.

CBC/BIOCHEMISTRY/URINALYSIS
• Cytopenias—seen with lymphoma, anemia of chronic disease, stress, splenic disease, or neoplastic infiltration of the bone marrow; also seen with viral disease
• Lymphocytosis—may suggest lymphoid neoplasia; atypical lymphocytes in the blood help establish a diagnosis of lymphoid neoplasia
• Eosinophilia—may occur in animals with lymphadenopathy owing to eosinophilic gastroenteritis; relation to parasitic disease has not been established
• Neutrophilia, with or without a left shift—may develop in patients with lymphoid hyperplasia, or neoplasia
• Hyperglobulinemia—may develop in patients with ADV, chronic inflammatory disease, or lymphoid neoplasia

OTHER LABORATORY TESTS
N/A

IMAGING
• Radiography and ultrasonography—involvement of lymph nodes within the body cavity
• Lesions associated with lymph node enlargement may be detected in other organs, for example, pneumonia, gastroenteritis, or primary tumor in animals with lymphadenomegaly caused by metastatic neoplasia.

DIAGNOSTIC PROCEDURES
Cytologic Examination
• Aspirates from affected lymph nodes may help determine the major category of lymphadenomegaly (i.e., hyperplasia, inflammation, or neoplasia). Successful fine-needle aspiration of peripheral nodes is more difficult to perform in ferrets—the nodes are frequently surrounded by firm fat deposits.
• It is often difficult to distinguish severe lymphoid hyperplasia from malignant lymphoma based on fine-needle aspirate alone; thus, a biopsy is usually necessary for diagnosis.
• Lymphoid hyperplasia and lymphoma may be difficult to distinguish on gross or histologic examination. If the peripheral or mesenteric lymph nodes are the only area of lymphocyte proliferation observed and the ferret is otherwise asymptomatic, sampling of more than one node and submitting to a pathology lab familiar with ferrets may be needed for an accurate diagnosis.

LYMPHADENOPATHY (LYMPHADENOMEGALY)   (CONTINUED)

FERRETS

• Rarely, aspirates from lymph nodes affected by lymphadenitis contain high proportions of neutrophils, macrophages, and/or eosinophils, depending on the cause of the inflammation; specific infectious agents, such as bacteria and systemic fungi, may be evident.
• Aspirates from lymph nodes containing metastatic neoplasia contain populations of cells that are not seen in normal nodes; the appearance of such cells varies widely, depending on the type of neoplasm.

Other
• Since a diagnosis often cannot be made by cytologic examination, excisional biopsy is preferable to needle biopsy.
• The cytologic diagnosis of lymphoma should be confirmed by histopathologic examination of an excised lymph node, and sampling of more than one node may be needed for accurate diagnosis.

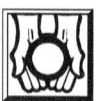

TREATMENT
• Because of the many disease processes and specific agents that can cause lymphadenomegaly, treatment depends on establishing the underlying cause.
• In animals with lymphoma, treatment includes combination chemotherapy or corticosteroids alone.

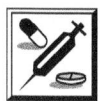

MEDICATIONS
DRUG(S) OF CHOICE
Appropriate medications vary with the cause of lymph node enlargement.

CONTRAINDICATIONS
N/A

PRECAUTIONS
N/A

POSSIBLE INTERACTIONS
N/A

ALTERNATIVE DRUGS
N/A

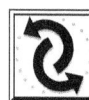

FOLLOW-UP
PATIENT MONITORING
Lymph node size to assess efficacy of treatment

POSSIBLE COMPLICATIONS
N/A

MISCELLANEOUS
ASSOCIATED CONDITIONS
• Lymph node hyperplasia is often components or manifestations of systemic disease
• Lymphoma may involve other organs (e.g., liver, spleen, intestines, kidneys, and skin) with a variety of clinical consequences.
• Many middle-aged to older ferrets with lymphoma have concurrent insulinoma or ferret adrenal disease.

AGE-RELATED FACTORS
None

ZOONOTIC POTENTIAL
Caution should be exercised when performing fine-needle aspiration in animals that may have systemic fungal disease.

PREGNANCY/FERTILITY/BREEDING
N/A

SEE ALSO
Epizootic catarrhal enteritis
Helicobacter mustelae
Inflammatory bowel disease
Lymphoma

ABBREVIATIONS
ADV = Aleutian disease virus
ECE = epizootic catarrhal enteritis

Suggested Reading
Dias S. Guide to diagnosing and treating neoplasia in ferrets. In Practice 2022;44(6): 340–347.
Dulli R, Clark SD. Digital cytology in exotic practice. Vet Clin Exot Anim 2022;25: 663–678.
Hoefer HL. Gastrointestinal diseases of ferrets. In: Quesenberry KE, Carpenter JW, eds. Ferrets, Rabbits and Rodents. Clinical Medicine and Surgery, 4th ed. St. Louis: Saunders, 2014:27–38.
Johnson-Delaney CA. Geriatric ferrets. Vet Clin Exot Anim Pract 2020;23(3): 549–650.
Kiupel M, Perpiñán D. Viral diseases of ferrets. In: Fox JG, Marini RP, eds. Biology and Diseases of the Ferret, 4th ed. Wiley, 2020:27–38.
Suran JN, Latney LV, Wyre NR. Radiographic and ultrasonographic findings of the spleen and abdominal lymph nodes in healthy domestic ferrets. J Small Anim Pract 2017;58(8):444–453.
Williams BH, Wyre NR. Neoplasia in ferrets. In: Quesenberry KE, Carpenter JW, eds. Ferrets, Rabbits and Rodents, 4th ed. Clinical Medicine and Surgery. 2021. St. Louis: Saunders, 2020:92–108.

Author Barbara Oglesbee, DVM, DABVP (Avian)

BASICS

DEFINITION
Proliferation of neoplastic lymphocytes in solid tissues, lymph nodes, bone marrow, and visceral organs

PATHOPHYSIOLOGY
• Lymphocytic or lymphoblastic lymphoma is seen most commonly in ferrets.
• Less often, a polymorphic lymphoma resembling lymphoma associated with a viral etiology in other species is seen. A retroviral etiology has been proposed but not conclusively demonstrated in ferret lymphosarcoma. Clusters of disease seen in cohabiting ferrets are suggestive of a viral etiology. Proposed viral agents include FeLV, Aleutian disease virus (parvo virus), and Ferret retrovirus.
• Gastric or MALT (mucosal-associated lymphoid tissue) lymphosarcoma has been associated with chronic *Helicobacter mustelae* gastritis; a causative effect has not been established.
• T-cell lymphosarcoma can be seen in epitheliotropic (cutaneous), periorbital, or mediastinal lymphoma.

SYSTEMS AFFECTED
• Hemic/Lymphatic/Immune—peripheral and/or mesenteric lymphadenomegaly with or without splenic, hepatic, and/or bone marrow involvement and circulating malignant lymphocytes (multicentric)
• Gastrointestinal—infiltration of stomach, intestines, and associated lymph nodes
• Respiratory—proliferation of neoplastic lymphocytes in mediastinal lymph nodes or thymus may lead to respiratory signs. Lungs are less commonly infiltrated.
• Miscellaneous (extranodal)—proliferation of or invasion by neoplastic lymphocytes in the bone marrow and ocular, cutaneous, mucocutaneous, neural, renal, cardiac, and other tissues

GENETICS
No documentation of genetic basis

INCIDENCE/PREVALENCE
Although the exact incidence is not well documented, it is one of the most common diseases seen in pet ferrets; third most common neoplasm (following insulinoma and adrenal neoplasia).

GEOGRAPHIC DISTRIBUTION
N/A

SIGNALMENT

Mean Age and Range
• Ferrets under 2 years of age are more likely to develop an aggressive, lymphoblastic form. Most often, the mediastinal form is seen

• Older ferrets are more likely to develop a less aggressive, lymphocytic form. Most often multicentric or intestinal.

Predominant Sex
None

SIGNS

General Comments
Depend on anatomic form, organ systems affected, and stage of disease

Historical Findings
• All forms of malignant lymphoma—nonspecific; anorexia; lethargy; weight loss; occurrence of clinical signs may be cyclical
• Multicentric—possibly no signs in early stages; generalized, painless lymphadenomegaly; may note distended abdomen secondary to hepatomegaly, splenomegaly, or ascites; anorexia, weight loss, and depression with progression of disease
• Gastrointestinal—anorexia; weight loss; lethargy; vomiting; diarrhea; abdominal discomfort; melena; tenesmus with mesenteric or sublumbar lymphadenomegaly
• Mediastinal—labored breathing; exercise intolerance secondary to mass(es) and/or effusion; coughing; difficulty swallowing; regurgitation; anorexia; weight loss
• Cutaneous—solitary or multiple masses, most often affecting feet and extremities; swollen, hyperemic extremities; cutaneous epitheliotropic lymphoma (mycosis fungoides) may be pruritic with dermal thickening and crusting or ulcerated
• Solitary form—depends on location; splenic form: abdominal distention, discomfort; periorbital lymphosarcoma: facial deformity, protrusion of the globe; spinal cord lymphosarcoma: quickly progressing posterior paresis may be seen; kidney: signs of renal failure

Physical Examination Findings
• Multicentric—generalized, painless, irregular, movable, large lymph node(s), and/or hepatosplenomegaly; pale mucous membranes secondary to anemia if bone marrow involvement is present
• Gastrointestinal—weight loss, possibly palpable abdominal mass or thickened bowel loops
• Mediastinal—noncompressible cranial thorax; dyspnea, cyanosis—often induced by physical examination; tachypnea; muffled heart sounds secondary to pleural effusion
• Extranodal—splenic: splenomegaly due to EMH or splenic lymphoma; cutaneous: raised plaques, thickened and crusted dermis; neural: dementia, seizures, and paralysis; renal: renomegaly and renal failure; cardiac: arrhythmias

CAUSES
No proven cause—a viral etiology has been proposed

RISK FACTORS
Possibly exposure to other ferrets with lymphosarcoma within the household. There is some speculation that FeLV may be involved; ferrets should not be housed with FeLV-positive cats.

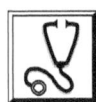

DIAGNOSIS

DIFFERENTIAL DIAGNOSIS
• For peripheral lymphadenomegaly—subcutaneous fat can surround the peripheral lymph nodes and have a firm consistency mimicking lymphadenomegaly. This is common in obese ferrets. Fine-needle aspiration is often nondiagnostic since the node is hidden deep within the fat deposits; a lymph node biopsy is usually necessary to differentiate lymphoma from a normal node surrounded by fat deposits.
• For mesenteric lymphadenomegaly—reactive nodes due to chronic gastrointestinal inflammatory or infiltrative disease such as *Helicobacter mustelae* gastritis, lymphoplasmacytic gastroenteritis, eosinophilic gastroenteritis, ferret coronavirus, or ECE. Hyperplastic lymph nodes can resemble lymphosarcoma on both gross and histologic examination and may be difficult to distinguish. If the mesenteric lymph nodes are the only area of lymphocyte proliferation observed, hyperplasia is more likely than neoplasia.
• For mediastinal form—congestive heart failure; chylothorax; hemothorax; thymoma
• Alimentary form—foreign body ingestion; intestinal ulceration; ECE; inflammatory bowel disease; intussusception; other gastrointestinal tumor
• Cutaneous form—mast cell tumor, other cutaneous neoplasm, chronic inflammatory disease

CBC/BIOCHEMISTRY/URINALYSIS
• Anemia (PCV <45%; nonregenerative) is the most common laboratory abnormality and may be severe in ferrets with leukemia.
• Both lymphocytosis and lymphopenia are reported in ferrets with lymphoma; however, overall lymphocytosis is rare in ferrets with lymphoma.
• Hepatic or renal values may be elevated if these organs are affected
• Hypercalcemia can be seen with T-cell lymphoma

FERRETS

OTHER LABORATORY TESTS
• Hyperproteinemia and hyperglobulinemia are rare findings associated with T-cell lymphoma.
• Immunohistochemistry can be performed to determine T-cell or B-cell origin.

IMAGING
• Thoracic radiography—may reveal sternal or tracheobronchial lymphadenomegaly, widened mediastinum, mediastinal masses, and pleural effusion
• Abdominal radiography—may reveal sublumbar or mesenteric lymphadenomegaly, intestinal mass, abdominal effusions, or hepatomegaly; splenomegaly is common due to EMH or splenic lymphoma
• Ultrasonography—often necessary to detect mesenteric or sublumbar lymphadenomegaly, nodules, or infiltrates in visceral organs, and sometimes even intestinal wall thickening or masses

DIAGNOSTIC PROCEDURES
• Examine bone marrow aspirate when nonregenerative anemia, other cytopenia, or abnormal circulating lymphocytes are observed.
• Lymph node biopsy—may be diagnostic when peripheral lymphadenomegaly is present. The popliteal lymph nodes are most readily accessible. Hyperplastic lymph nodes can resemble lymphosarcoma on both gross and histologic examination and may be difficult to distinguish. If the peripheral lymph nodes are the only area of lymphocyte proliferation observed and the ferret is otherwise asymptomatic, sampling of more than one node and submitting to a pathology lab familiar with ferrets may be needed for an accurate diagnosis.
• FNA of mediastinal or mesenteric lymph nodes may be performed using ultrasound guidance. However, it is often difficult to differential hyperplasia from lymphoma based on an aspirate alone; exploratory laparotomy and biopsy may be necessary for definitive diagnosis

PATHOLOGIC FINDINGS
• Cut section—homogenous, white masses, and sometimes with areas of necrosis
• Monomorphic or polymorphic population of discrete round neoplastic cells that efface and replace parenchyma of lymph nodes and visceral organs or bone marrow

TREATMENT
GENERAL COMMENTS
• Many ferrets with lymphoma are asymptomatic, and the diagnosis is often incidental. It can be difficult to predict whether or not treatment is helpful in these cases. Some ferrets may remain asymptomatic for years with no treatment at all. In others, signs of disease may be cyclic and may wane with or without treatment, making the evaluation of treatment success difficult.
• Treatment is indicated in any ferret with aggressive lymphosarcoma or in ferrets with clinical signs attributable to lymphoma.

APPROPRIATE HEALTH CARE
• Inpatient—intravenous chemotherapy and supportive care for debilitated, anorexic, or dehydrated patients
• Outpatient—once stable, most patients can be treated on an outpatient basis after remission; some protocols allow owner to administer drugs orally at home; instruct owner to wear latex gloves when administering these drugs.

NURSING CARE
• Fluid therapy—for animals with advanced disease and dehydrated patients
• Thoracocentesis or abdominocentesis—recommended with marked pleural or abdominal effusion

ACTIVITY
Restrict in patients with low WBC or platelet count

DIET
• If the patient has been anorectic, assist feed an easily digestible high-protein/high-fat diet such as Lafeber Carnivore Critical Care Diet (Lafeber Company, Cornell, IL) or Oxbow Carnivore Critical Care Diet (Oxbow Animal Health, Omaha, NE); may also add dietary supplement such as Nutri-Cal (EVSCO Pharmaceuticals) to increase caloric content to these foods.
• The caloric recommendation for sick ferrets is approximately 400 kcal/kg BW per day (although this may be a high estimate).

CLIENT EDUCATION
• Warn the client that chemotherapy is rarely curative and relapse often occurs.
• Inform the client that the side effects of chemotherapy drugs depend on the type used but are usually associated with the gastrointestinal tract and bone marrow.
• Note that the quality of life is good while the patient is receiving chemotherapy, and while it is in remission, add that some protocols are associated with serious morbidity, whereas others have little morbidity.

SURGICAL CONSIDERATIONS
• To relieve intestinal obstructions and remove solitary masses
• To obtain specimens for histopathologic examination
• Splenectomy to reduce tumor load in ferrets with splenic lymphoma

MEDICATIONS
DRUG(S) OF CHOICE
• Combination chemotherapy—many protocols exist with similar remission and survival times. Most are based on feline protocols. An oncologist should be consulted for recommendations.
• Corticosteroids alone—(prednisolone 1–2 mg/kg PO q12–24h) is often an effective short-term palliative therapy (1–2 months). Do not begin treatment with prednisone alone if the owner is willing to undertake combination therapy; the response to combination therapy will be significantly diminished.
• Retinoids (isotretinoin 2 mg/kg PO q24h) have been used as a palliative treatment in ferrets with cutaneous epitheliotropic lymphoma with some success.

CONTRAINDICATIONS
Close monitoring of CBC is necessary when using most chemotherapeutics; if neutrophil count is <1000, any myelosuppressive chemotherapy should be postponed.

PRECAUTIONS
• Use extreme caution when handling chemotherapeutic agents.

POSSIBLE INTERACTIONS
All chemotherapy drugs must be given according to published protocols as many have overlapping side effects.

ALTERNATIVE TREATMENTS
• Many alternative treatment protocols exist; consultation with an oncologist is recommended.
• Radiation is an excellent adjunct or primary therapy, especially with large solitary masses.

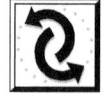

FOLLOW-UP
PATIENT MONITORING
• Signs of toxicity in ferrets receiving chemotherapy for lymphoma include anorexia, lethargy, weakness, vomiting, and hair loss.
• CBC and platelet count—24 hours prior to administration of cytotoxic agents, if severe leukopenia or neutropenia (neutrophils < 1000 cells/mm^3; PCV < 30%) is noted, discontinue therapy
• Physical examination and cytologic or histologic evaluation on all nonresponsive lymph nodes

PREVENTION/AVOIDANCE
N/A

POSSIBLE COMPLICATIONS

• With prednisolone treatment—severe obesity with accumulation of fat within the thorax causing dyspnea and large intrabdominal fat deposits
• With chemotherapy—leukopenia, neutropenia, anemia, thrombocytopenia, vomiting, diarrhea, anorexia, cardiotoxicity (doxorubicin), alopecia, sepsis, and tissue sloughing—with extravasated dose

EXPECTED COURSE AND PROGNOSIS

• Ferrets with mediastinal, splenic, cutaneous lymphoma or those with peripheral node involvement alone tend to respond well to chemotherapy. Many ferrets will live up to 2–3 years.
• Ferrets with polymorphic lymphoma respond poorly to chemotherapy, often present moribund, and do not survive long.
• Primary CNS, diffuse gastrointestinal, and multiorgan involvement—associated with poor response to treatment

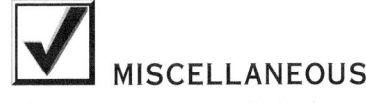 **MISCELLANEOUS**

ASSOCIATED CONDITIONS

Insulinoma and adrenal disease are commonly found in ferrets with lymphoma.

AGE-RELATED FACTORS

See above

ZOONOTIC POTENTIAL

None

PREGNANCY/FERTILITY/BREEDING

Treatment of pregnant ferrets is contraindicated.

SYNONYMS

Lymphosarcoma
Malignant lymphoma

ABBREVIATIONS

CBC = complete blood count
CNS = central nervous system
ECE = epizootic catarrhal enteritis
EMH = extrameduallary hematopoiesis
FNA = fine-needle aspiration
PCV = packed cell volume
WBC = white blood cell count

Suggested Reading
Bean AD, Fisher PG, Reavill DR, Kiupel M. Hypercalcemia associated with lymphomas in the ferret (*Mustela putorius furo*): four cases. J Exot Pet Med 2019;1(29):147–153.
Bernhard C, Flenghi L, Nicolier A, Mentré V. Cutaneous epitheliotropic T-cell lymphoma in ferrets (*Mustela putorius furo*): 3 cases (2014–2021). J Exot Pet Med 2023;1(44):30–34.
Dias S. Guide to diagnosing and treating neoplasia in ferrets. In Practice 2022;44(6):340–347.
Dulli R, Clark SD. Digital cytology in exotic practice. Vet Clin Exot Anim 2022;25:663–678.
Johnson-Delaney CA. Geriatric ferrets. Vet Clin Exot Anim Pract 2020;23(3):549–650.
MacPhail C. Ferret soft tissue surgery. In: Bennett A, Pye GW, eds. Surgery of Exotic Animals, 2021:277–296.
Suran JN, Latney LV, Wyre NR. Radiographic and ultrasonographic findings of the spleen and abdominal lymph nodes in healthy domestic ferrets. J Small Anim Pract 2017;58(8):444–453.
Webb JK, Graham JE, Burgess KE, Antinoff N. Presentation and survival time of domestic ferrets (*Mustela putorius furo*) with lymphoma treated with single-and multiagent protocols: 44 cases (1998–2016). J Exot Pet Med 2019;1(31):64–67.
Williams BH, Wyre NR. Neoplasia in ferrets. In: Quesenberry KE, Carpenter JW, eds. Ferrets, Rabbits and Rodents, 4th ed. Clinical Medicine and Surgery. 2021. St. Louis: Saunders, 2020:92–108.

Author Barbara Oglesbee, DVM, DABVP (Avian) and Natalie Antinoff, DVM, DABVP (Avian)

LYMPHOPLASMACYTIC ENTERITIS AND GASTROENTERITIS

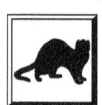

BASICS

OVERVIEW
- A form of inflammatory bowel disease characterized by lymphocyte and/or plasma cell infiltration into the lamina propria of the stomach, intestine, or both
- Lymphocytic infiltration into the lamina propria of the intestines is a common inflammatory response to many infectious agents or environmental stimuli. Lymphocytic infiltration into the lamina propria of the stomach is abnormal and usually indicates significant disease.
- Plasmacytic infiltration indicates chronicity or a more severe inflammatory reaction.
- An abnormal immune response to infectious agents or environmental stimuli may be responsible for initiating gastrointestinal inflammation. Continued exposure to antigen, coupled with self-perpetuating inflammation, may result in disease.
- The exact mechanisms, antigens, and patient factors involved in initiation and progression remain unknown.

SIGNALMENT
No sex or age predilection

SIGNS
- Anorexia
- Weight loss, muscle wasting
- Diarrhea, sometimes with blood or mucus
- Melena
- Vomiting
- Ptyalism, pawing at the mouth
- Physical examination—cachexia; thickened, ropy intestines; enlarged mesenteric lymph nodes; and splenomegaly often palpable

CAUSES AND RISK FACTORS
- Pathogenesis is most likely multifactorial.
- Gastric lesions are often associated with *Helicobacter mustelae.*
- Intestinal lesions may be associated with epizootic catarrhal enteritis (ECE), giardia, salmonella, campylobacter, cryptosporidiosis, Aleutian disease virus (ADV), or other infectious agents.
- Meat proteins, food additives, artificial coloring, preservatives, and milk proteins may play a role.

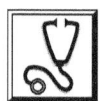

DIAGNOSIS

DIFFERENTIAL DIAGNOSIS
- Intestinal lymphosarcoma
- Infectious diseases (e.g., *H. mustelae*, ECE, ADV, giardiasis, salmonellosis, campylobacter enteritis, cryptosporidiosis, mycobacteriosis)
- Gastrointestinal foreign body
- Other infiltrative inflammatory bowel conditions (e.g., eosinophilic gastroenteritis)

CBC/BIOCHEMISTRY/URINALYSIS
- May be normal
- Nonregenerative anemia and mild leukocytosis without a left shift sometimes seen
- Hypoproteinemia from protein-losing enteropathy

OTHER LABORATORY TESTS
- Fecal direct examination, fecal flotation, zinc sulfate centrifugation many demonstrate gastrointestinal parasites
- Fecal cytology—may reveal RBC or fecal leukocytes, which can be associated with inflammatory bowel disease or invasive bacterial strains
- Fecal culture should be performed if abnormal bacteria are observed on the fecal gram's stain, or if salmonella is suspected.

IMAGING
- Survey abdominal radiographs—usually normal
- Barium contrast studies—rarely reveal mucosal abnormalities or thickened bowel loops; generally not helpful in establishing a definitive diagnosis; can be normal even in individuals with severe disease

DIAGNOSTIC PROCEDURES
- Definitive diagnosis requires biopsy and histopathology, usually obtained via exploratory laparotomy.
- Intestinal fluid can also be submitted for quantitative culture if bacterial overgrowth is suspected.
- Lymph node biopsy is indicated on enlarged mesenteric nodes.

PATHOLOGIC FINDINGS
- Grossly, stomach and intestinal appearance can range from normal to edematous, thickened, and ulcerated.
- The hallmark histopathologic finding is an infiltrate of lymphocytes and, in some cases, plasma cells in the lamina propria.
- The distribution may be patchy, so take several biopsy specimens.

TREATMENT

APPROPRIATE HEALTH CARE
- Outpatient, unless the patient is debilitated from dehydration, hypoproteinemia, or cachexia
- Patients that are dehydrated or emaciated, and those with protein-losing enteropathies or other concurrent illnesses, may require hospitalization until they are stabilized.

NURSING CARE
If the patient is dehydrated, any balanced fluid such as lactated Ringer's solution is adequate (for a patient without other concurrent disease); otherwise, select fluids on the basis of secondary diseases. If held NPO due to vomiting, provide a dextrose-containing fluid and monitor blood glucose concentration.

ACTIVITY
No need to restrict unless severely debilitated

DIET
- Highly digestible diets with novel protein sources may be useful for eliciting remission, although an allergic cause has not be documented and little information is available regarding the efficacy of these diets. If attempted, choose feline diets since ferrets have high nutritional protein and fat requirements. Foods that have been anecdotally reported to elicit remission include feline lamb and rice diets, diets consisting exclusively of one type of meat (lamb, duck, turkey), or a "natural prey diet" consisting of whole rodents or chicks. Avoid diets that contain plant-based proteins (peas, soy, and grains) since these have been associated with the development of urinary calculi. If remission is elicited, continue diet for at least 8–13 weeks; this diet may need to be fed lifelong.
- Anorexic ferrets may refuse dry foods but are often willing to eat canned cat foods or pureed meats.

CLIENT EDUCATION
Explain the difficulty in finding an underlying cause and therefore successful treatment. There is a potential for long-term therapy.

SURGICAL CONSIDERATIONS
N/A

MEDICATIONS

DRUG(S) OF CHOICE
- Treat the underlying cause (e.g., helicobacter, salmonella, giardia, etc.) if found.
- If gastric lesions are present, empirical treatment for helicobacter is indicated. The combination of amoxicillin (30 mg/kg PO q8–12h) plus metronidazole (20 mg/kg PO q8–12h) and bismuth subsalicylate (17.5 mg/kg PO q8–12h or 1 mL/kg of regular-strength preparation [262 mg/15 mL] PO q12h) is an inexpensive treatment regimen that is often effective. Treat for at least 2, and up to 3–4 weeks; q8h dosing may be needed to eliminate infection. Alternatively,

clarithromycin (12.5 mg/kg PO q8–12h) and ranitidine bismuth citrate or ranitidine HCl (24 mg/kg PO q8–12h) for 2 weeks have also been effective.
• Immunosuppressive agents: Prednisone (2 mg/kg PO q24h or divided q12h); when signs resolve, gradually taper the corticosteroid dose by 1/2 every other week to effect (usually 0.5–1 mg/kg every other day) or azathioprine (0.9 mg/kg PO q24–72h)
• Antibiotics used for immune modulating effect or to modify intestinal include metronidazole (10–15 mg/kg PO q12–24h); tylosin (25 mg/kg PO q12–24h); tetracycline 2 (0–25 mg q8–12h)
• Cobalamin for ferrets with chronic diarrhea—250 µg/kg SC weekly for 6 weeks, followed by 250 µg/kg q2w for 6 weeks, then monthly. Check cobalamin concentrations 1 month after administration to determine if continued therapy is warranted.

CONTRAINDICATIONS
N/A

PRECAUTIONS
• In ferrets with concurrent infectious diseases, use corticosteroids with caution.
• Metronidazole—can cause reversible neurotoxicity at high dosages; discontinuing the drug usually reverses the neurologic signs. Ferrets generally object to the taste.

POSSIBLE INTERACTIONS
N/A

ALTERNATIVE DRUGS
N/A

FOLLOW-UP

PATIENT MONITORING
• For resolution of clinical signs
• Severely affected patients require frequent monitoring; adjust medications during these visits.

• Check patients with less severe disease 2–3 weeks after their initial evaluation and then monthly to bimonthly until immunosuppressive therapy is discontinued.

PREVENTION/AVOIDANCE
If a food intolerance or allergy is suspected or documented, avoid that particular item and adhere strictly to dietary changes.

POSSIBLE COMPLICATIONS
• Weight loss, debilitation, and death in refractory cases
• Adverse effects of prednisone therapy

EXPECTED COURSE AND PROGNOSIS
• Variable, depending on the underlying cause
• Ferrets with mild inflammation—good-to-excellent prognosis for full recovery
• Patients with severe infiltrates, particularly if other portions of the GI tract are involved or if an underlying cause cannot be found—more guarded prognosis
• Often the initial response to therapy sets the tone for a given individual's ability to recover.

MISCELLANEOUS

ASSOCIATED CONDITIONS
Many affected ferrets also have splenomegaly (nonspecific in aged ferrets)

AGE-RELATED FACTORS
N/A

ZOONOTIC POTENTIAL
Giardia and cryptosporidiosis have zoonotic potential

PREGNANCY/FERTILITY/BREEDING
• Corticosteroids have been associated with increased incidence of congenital defects, abortion, and fetal death.
• Metronidazole is mutagenic in laboratory animals; avoid

SYNONYMS
N/A

SEE ALSO
Eosinophilic gastroenteritis
Epizootic catarrhal enteritis
Gastrointestinal and esophageal foreign bodies
Helicobacter mustelae

ABBREVIATIONS
ADV = Aleutian disease virus
ECE = epizootic catarrhal enteritis

Suggested Reading
Cazzini P, Watson MK, Gottdenker N et al. Proposed grading scheme for inflammatory bowel disease in ferrets and correlation with clinical signs. J Vet Diagn Invest 2020; 32(1):17–24.
Di Girolamo N, Selleri P. Medical and surgical emergencies in ferrets. Vet Clin Exot Anim 2016;19:431–464.
Hoefer HL. Gastrointestinal diseases of ferrets. In: Quesenberry KE, Carpenter JW, eds. Ferrets, Rabbits, and Rodents, 4th ed. Clinical Medicine and Surgery. 2021. St. Louis: Saunders, 2020:27–38.
Johnson-Delaney CA. Geriatric ferrets. Vet Clin Exot Anim Pract 2020;23(3): 549–565.
Livingstone M. Dealing with gastrointestinal disease in ferrets. In Practice 2022;44: 169–179.
Murray J, Kiupel M, Maes RK. Ferret coronavirus-associated diseases. Vet Clin North Am Exot Anim Pract 2010;13(3): 543–560.
Watson MK, Cazzini P, Mayer J et al. Histology and immunohistochemistry of severe inflammatory bowel disease versus lymphoma in the ferret (*Mustela putorius furo*). J Vet Diagn Invest 2016;28(3): 198–206.

Author Barbara Oglesbee, DVM, DABVP-Avian

MAST CELL TUMORS

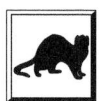

BASICS

OVERVIEW
• Neoplasia arising from mast cells
• Histamine and other vasoactive substances released from mast cell tumors—may cause erythema and edema
• Mast cell tumors in ferrets are usually benign and do not metastasize.

SIGNALMENT
• The most common skin tumor in ferrets
• Mean age reported as 4 years

SIGNS
Historical Findings
• Patient may have had skin tumor for days to months at the time of examination.
• May have appeared to fluctuate in size or appearance; may have appeared to disappear completely only to recur
• Some tumors are extremely pruritic
• Anorexia and vomiting, as seen in dogs with splenic or GI tumors, have not been reported in ferrets. However, splenic MCTs can be seen in ferrets, and GI signs should be anticipated in affected animals.

Physical Examination Findings
• Cutaneous—primarily found in the subcutaneous tissue or dermis; may be papular or nodular, solitary or multiple, and hairy or alopecic or have an ulcerated surface; slight predilection for the head and neck regions
• Tumors may appear to rupture and become covered with a dry black exudate.
• Alopecia and crusting associated with pruritic masses

CAUSES AND RISK FACTORS
Unknown

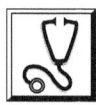

DIAGNOSIS

DIFFERENTIAL DIAGNOSIS
• Any other skin tumor, benign or malignant
• Insect bite or allergic reaction
• Splenic—benign splenomegaly due to extramedullary hematopoiesis; splenic lymphoma

CBC/BIOCHEMISTRY/URINALYSIS
Usually normal; anemia and mastocythemia seen in other mammals not reported in ferrets

OTHER LABORATORY TESTS
N/A

IMAGING
Abdominal radiography—may reveal splenomegaly in animals with rare splenic tumors

DIAGNOSTIC PROCEDURES
• Cytologic examination of fine-needle aspirate—most important preliminary diagnostic test; reveals round cells with basophilic cytoplasmic granules that do not form sheets or clumps
• Tissue biopsy—necessary for definitive diagnosis

PATHOLOGIC FINDINGS
• Histopathologic examination—consists of well-differentiated mast cells

TREATMENT

APPROPRIATE HEALTH CARE
• Surgery—to excise cutaneous tumor; aggressive surgical excision with wide margins is not necessary since these tumors rarely metastasize or recur
• Surgical excision is only effective method of treating pruritic tumors
• Splenectomy or partial splenectomy—may be necessary for splenic tumor

NURSING CARE
N/A

ACTIVITY
N/A

DIET
N/A

CLIENT EDUCATION
• Warn client that patient may develop new mast cell tumors.
• Advise client that fine-needle aspiration and cytologic examination should be performed as soon as possible on any new mass.

SURGICAL CONSIDERATIONS
• Complete surgical excision
• Submit excised mass for histologic examination to confirm diagnosis.

MEDICATIONS

DRUG(S) OF CHOICE
• Chemotherapy generally unnecessary; if rare case of metastatic MCT is encountered, consider feline protocols
• Presurgical treatment with antihistamines usually unnecessary

CONTRAINDICATIONS
N/A

PRECAUTIONS
N/A

POSSIBLE INTERACTIONS
N/A

ALTERNATIVE DRUGS
N/A

FOLLOW-UP

PATIENT MONITORING
Evaluate any new masses cytologically or histologically

PREVENTION/AVOIDANCE
N/A

POSSIBLE COMPLICATIONS
• Bleeding
• Appearance of new masses

EXPECTED COURSE AND PROGNOSIS
• Cutaneous tumors—prognosis excellent; metastasis not reported but may occur
• Splenic tumor—survival rates not reported

MISCELLANEOUS

ASSOCIATED CONDITIONS
N/A

AGE-RELATED FACTORS
N/A

ZOONOTIC POTENTIAL
N/A

PREGNANCY/FERTILITY/BREEDING
N/A

SEE ALSO
Adrenal disease (hyperadrenocorticism)
Canine distemper virus
Dermatophytosis
Ear mites
Fleas and flea infestation

ABBREVIATION
MCT = mast cell tumor

Suggested Reading
d'Ovidio D, Santoro D. Dermatologic diseases of ferrets. In: Quesenberry KE, Carpenter JW, eds. Ferrets, Rabbits and Rodents, 4th ed. Clinical Medicine and Surgery. 2021. St. Louis: Saunders, 2020:109–116.
Dulli R, Clark SD. Digital cytology in exotic practice. Vet Clin Exot Anim 2022;25:663–678.
Hoppmann E, Wilson Barron H. Ferret and rabbit dermatology. J Exot Pet Med 2007; 16:225–237.
Kanfer S, Reavill DR. Cutaneous neoplasia in ferrets, rabbits, and guinea pigs. Vet Clin North Am Exot Anim 2013;16:579–598.
MacPhail C. Ferret soft tissue surgery. In: Bennett A, Pye GW, eds. Surgery of Exotic Animals, 2021:277–296.
Williams BH, Wyre NR. Neoplasia in ferrets. In: Quesenberry KE, Carpenter JW, eds. Ferrets, Rabbits and Rodents, 4th ed. Clinical Medicine and Surgery. 2021. St. Louis: Saunders, 2020:92–108.
Author Barbara Oglesbee, DVM, DABVP (Avian)

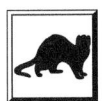

BASICS

DEFINITION
Rather than a single disease entity, megaesophagus refers to esophageal dilation and hypomotility, which may be a primary disorder or secondary to esophageal obstruction or neuromuscular dysfunction.

PATHOPHYSIOLOGY
• Esophageal motility is decreased or absent, resulting in accumulation and retention of food and liquid in the esophagus.
• Lesions anywhere along the central or peripheral neural pathways, the myoneural junction, or esophageal muscles may result in esophageal hypomotility and distention.
• Sequelae to megaesophagus may include starvation and aspiration pneumonia.

SYSTEMS AFFECTED
• Gastrointestinal—regurgitation, weight loss/cachexia
• Neuromuscular—may be manifestation of neuromuscular disease
• Respiratory—if aspiration pneumonia occurs

GENETICS
Congenital idiopathic megaesophagus has not been reported in ferrets but may exist.

INCIDENCE/PREVALENCE
True incidence unknown—sporadically seen in clinical practice as a cause of regurgitation or cachexia

GEOGRAPHIC DISTRIBUTION
Unknown

SIGNALMENT
• Only reported in adult ferrets (3–7 years old), implying an acquired form
• Congenital megaesophagus, where signs of regurgitation first appear at weaning, has not been reported in ferrets.

SIGNS

Historical Findings
• May include regurgitation of food and water, dysphagia, gagging, choking, anorexia, weight loss, and hypersalivation
• May see coughing, mucopurulent nasal discharge, and dyspnea with concurrent aspiration pneumonia
• Signs may first be noted days to months prior to presentation

Physical Examination Findings
• Related to megaesophagus—regurgitation, weight loss, halitosis, ptyalism, bruxism, bulging of the esophagus at the thoracic inlet, and pain associated with palpation of the cervical esophagus

• Related to the sequelae of megaesophagus—respiratory crackles, tachypnea, pyrexia with aspiration pneumonia; cachexia, muscle weakness and wasting from starvation; dry mucous membranes, sunken eyes from dehydration

CAUSES
• In most cases, the cause is not identified.
• Miscellaneous—esophagitis, toxicosis (lead, thallium, acetylcholinesterase inhibitors
• Esophageal obstruction—esophageal foreign body, stricture, neoplasia, and granuloma
• Neurologic and neuromuscular diseases—none well documented in ferrets; possible causes include botulism, CNS disorders, degenerative, infectious/inflammatory, neoplasia, traumatic disorders of the brainstem and spinal cord, and bilateral vagal damage (myasthenia gravis and autoimmune causes have not been identified)

RISK FACTORS
N/A

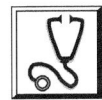

DIAGNOSIS

DIFFERENTIAL DIAGNOSIS
• Other disorders causing regurgitation
• Obstructive pharyngeal disease (foreign bodies, inflammation, neoplasia) may produce regurgitation with normal esophageal motility.
• Pharyngeal pain and dysphagia with obstructive pharyngeal disease.
• Distinguish regurgitation from dysphagia and vomiting.
• Regurgitation is a passive process with no forceful abdominal contraction, anticipatory salivation, nausea, or retching.
• Bile-stained ingesta suggests vomiting.

CBC/BIOCHEMISTRY/URINALYSIS
• Leukocytosis with secondary aspiration pneumonia, increased PCV with dehydration
• Increased AST and ALT may be seen; hypoglycemia with starvation and/or concurrent insulinoma

OTHER LABORATORY TESTS
Blood lead and cholinesterase levels to evaluate for toxicity

IMAGING

Survey Thoracic Radiographs
• Esophagus dilated with gas, fluid, or ingesta
• The trachea is often displaced ventrally by the distended esophagus.

Contrast Esophagram and Fluoroscopy
• An esophagram using either barium liquid or paste may demonstrate contrast pooling and abnormal esophageal motility.
• Fluoroscopy may demonstrate abnormal primary and secondary esophageal peristalsis.
• Contrast studies—not necessary for diagnosing most cases of megaesophagus; use with caution in animal patients with known megaesophagus because of the risk of aspiration.

DIAGNOSTIC PROCEDURES
• Endoscopy—can use to visualize a dilated esophagus, foreign bodies, neoplasia, and esophagitis; mucosal biopsy specimens and cytology samples may be obtained; esophageal foreign bodies may be removed. However, the small size of the patient and subsequent limitations on instrument size often limits the use of endoscopy.
• Muscle and nerve biopsies/histopathology—possibly useful to confirm the diagnosis of inflammatory and degenerative disorders of muscles and nerves

PATHOLOGIC FINDINGS
Dilation of both the cervical and thoracic esophagus; inflammation and ulceration of the esophageal mucosa seen with advanced disease

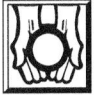

TREATMENT

APPROPRIATE HEALTH CARE
Most patients have aspiration pneumonia and/or severe debilitation requiring hospitalization.

NURSING CARE
• Correct dehydration with IV fluid therapy (maintenance = 75–100 mL/kg/day) using 0.9% saline or lactated Ringer's solution. If hypoglycemic, use 2.5% dextrose and 0.45% saline.
• Hospitalize in a warm, quiet location with a hide box to minimize stress.

ACTIVITY
Restricted due to associated weakness and lethargy

DIET
• Feed in an upright position (45–90-degree angle to the floor) and maintain the position for 10–15 minutes following feeding.
• If the patient has been anorectic, assist feed an easily digestible high-protein/high-fat diet such as Lafeber Carnivore Critical Care Diet (Lafeber Company, Cornell, IL) or Oxbow Carnivore Critical Care Diet (Oxbow Animal Health, Omaha, NE); may also add dietary supplement such as Nutri-Cal (EVSCO

Pharmaceuticals) to increase caloric content to these foods.
• A more liquid consistency may decrease regurgitation but increase aspiration pneumonia risk.
• Caloric requirements for sick ferrets have been reported to be as high as 400 kcal/kg BW per day, although this may be a high estimate.
• Patients with severe regurgitation may need parenteral feeding via a gastrotomy tube.

CLIENT EDUCATION

An underlying cause is rarely identified or corrected, and most ferrets are debilitated due to starvation, hepatic lipidosis, and aspiration pneumonia. Advise client of poor prognosis.

SURGICAL CONSIDERATIONS

• Surgery may be necessary to remove esophageal foreign bodies or neoplasia if identified
• No surgical procedures improve esophageal motility.

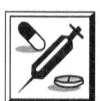

MEDICATIONS

DRUG(S) OF CHOICE

• No drugs are commonly used to treat megaesophagus alone; direct treatment at the underlying disease or associated conditions (e.g., aspiration pneumonia).
• Sucralfate (25 mg/kg PO q8h)
• Gastrointestinal antisecretory agents are helpful to treat and possibly prevent gastritis in anorectic ferrets. Ferrets continually secrete a baseline level of gastric hydrochloric acid and, as such, anorexia itself may predispose to gastric ulceration. Those successfully used in ferrets include omeprazole (4 mg/kg PO q24h), famotidine (0.25–0.5 mg/kg PO, SC, IV q24h), and cimetidine (10 mg/kg PO, SC, IM, IV q8h)
• Metoclopramide (0.2–1.0 mg/kg PO, SC, IM q6–8h) speeds gastric emptying, increases gastroesophageal sphincter tone, and is most useful when reflux esophagitis is a contributing or the primary cause; use of metoclopramide for other causes has had limited success.
• Broad-spectrum antibiotics—necessary for patients with aspiration pneumonia; parenteral antibiotics may be required for patients with severe regurgitation. Ideally,

based on culture and susceptibility testing from an airway specimen; begin with an antibiotic combination that is broad spectrum and effective against anaerobes (e.g., enrofloxacin 5–10 mg/kg IM, PO, SC q12h plus amoxicillin 20 mg/kg IM, PO q12h); alter therapy based on culture/ susceptibility results

CONTRAINDICATIONS
N/A

PRECAUTIONS
Corticosteroids may be necessary to treat conditions causing megaesophagus; use with caution in patients with aspiration pneumonia.

POSSIBLE INTERACTIONS
N/A

ALTERNATIVE DRUGS
N/A

FOLLOW-UP

PATIENT MONITORING
May use repeat thoracic radiographs, esophagrams, and fluoroscopic examinations to follow progression or resolution of megaesophagus.

PREVENTION/AVOIDANCE
Esophageal obstruction may be prevented if pets are not allowed access to rubber toys, bones, garbage, or other tempting items.

POSSIBLE COMPLICATIONS
Aspiration pneumonia, hepatic lipidosis

EXPECTED COURSE AND PROGNOSIS
• Poor to grave, with or without treatment
• Aspiration pneumonia and malnutrition are leading causes of death.

MISCELLANEOUS

ASSOCIATED CONDITIONS
• Insulinoma
• Hyperadrenocorticism
• Gastric ulcers
• *Helicobacter mustelae*

AGE-RELATED FACTORS
Regurgitation at weaning suggests congenital or obstructive megaesophagus but has not been reported in ferrets.

ZOONOTIC POTENTIAL
Determine rabies vaccination status for all patients.

PREGNANCY/FERTILITY/BREEDING
N/A

SYNONYMS
N/A

SEE ALSO
Dysphagia
Pneumonia

ABBREVIATIONS
ALT = alanine aminotransferase
AST = aspartate aminotransferase
CNS = central nervous system
PCV = packed cell volume

Suggested Reading
Blanco MC, Fox JG, Rosenthal K et al. Megaesophagus in nine ferrets. J Am Vet Med Assoc 1994;205:444–447.
Couturier J, Huynh M, Boussarie D et al. Autoimmune myasthenia gravis in a ferret. J Am Vet Med Assoc 2009;235:1462–1466.
Garner MM, Ramsell K, Schoemaker NJ et al. Myofasciitis in the domestic ferret. Vet Pathol 2007;44:25–38.
Hoefer HL. Gastrointestinal diseases of ferrets. In: Quesenberry KE, Carpenter JW, eds. Ferrets, Rabbits, and Rodents, 4th ed. Clinical Medicine and Surgery. 2021. St. Louis: Saunders, 2020:27–38.
Huynh M, Pignon C. Gastrointestinal disease in exotic small mammals. J Exot Pet Med 2013;22(2):118–131.
Johnson-Delaney CA. Geriatric ferrets. Vet Clin Exot Anim Pract 2020;23(3):549–565.
Murray J, Kiupel M, Maes RK. Ferret coronavirus-associated diseases. Vet Clin North Am Exot Anim Pract 2010;13(3):543–560.
Webb J, Graham J, Fordham M, DeCubellis J, Buckley F, Hobbs J, Berent A, Weisse C. Diagnosis and treatment of esophageal foreign body or stricture in three ferrets (*Mustela putorius furo*). J Am Vet Med Assoc 2017;251(4):451–457.
Author Barbara Oglesbee, DVM, DABVP-Avian

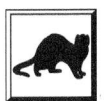

BASICS

DEFINITION
Presence of digested blood in the feces. Appears as green-black, tarry stool.

PATHOPHYSIOLOGY
Usually the result of upper gastrointestinal bleeding. However, melena can also be associated with ingested blood from the oral cavity or upper respiratory tract.

SYSTEMS AFFECTED
• Gastrointestinal—gastric ulcers, foreign body
• Hematopoietic—bleeding disorders
• Respiratory—swallowed blood

SIGNALMENT
No breed or gender predilections

SIGNS
Historical Findings
• Melena may be accompanied by anorexia, weight loss, bruxism, hypersalivation, vomiting, or regurgitation.
• Feces may be formed or diarrheic.
• Question the owner about the ferret's chewing habits and possible ingestion of foreign bodies, especially rubber toys, or foam or cloth bedding material.
• Exposure to other ferrets or new ferrets in the household

Physical Examination Findings
• Pallor of the mucous membranes
• Weight loss—indicates chronic disease
• Poor hair coat or alopecia
• Dehydration
• Fecal staining of the perineum
• Abdominal distention may be due to thickened or fluid-filled intestinal loops, masses, or organomegaly
• Mesenteric lymph nodes may be palpably enlarged.

CAUSES
• Bacterial infection—*Helicobacter mustelae* gastritis (most common cause), *Salmonella* spp., *Mycobacterium avium*-intracellulare
• Viral infection—epizootic catarrhal enteritis (common)
• Obstruction—foreign body and neoplasia (most common), intussusception
• Neoplasia—lymphoma, adenocarcinoma
• Drugs and toxins—NSAIDs, vaccine reaction
• Infiltrative—lymphoplasmacytic gastroenteritis, eosinophilic gastroenteritis

• Ingestion of blood—oropharyngeal, nasal, or sinus lesions (abscess, trauma, neoplasia, and mycotic)

Other uncommon causes
• Metabolic disorders—liver disease, renal disease
• Coagulopathy
• Stress
• Septicemia

RISK FACTORS
• Unsupervised chewing
• Exposure to other ferrets
• Vaccine reaction

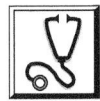

DIAGNOSIS

DIFFERENTIAL DIAGNOSIS
Differentiating Causes
• Melena and anorexia most common with *H. mustelae* or gastrointestinal foreign body
• Thickened intestinal loops and palpably enlarged mesenteric lymph nodes common with eosinophilic enterocolitis, lymphoplasmacytic enteritis, ECE, or lymphoma
• Bile-stained (green), mucous-covered diarrhea seen most commonly with ECE
• Granular, "bird seed"-like feces seen with maldigestive/malabsorptive disorders

CBC/BIOCHEMISTRY
• Regenerative anemia may be seen with chronic gastrointestinal bleeding.
• TWBC elevation with neutrophilia may be seen with bacterial enteritis.
• TWBC elevation with lymphocytosis, or normal TWBC with relative lymphocytosis, may be suggestive of lymphoma.
• Eosinophilia (as high as 35%) in some ferrets with eosinophilic gastroenteritis
• Serum albumin concentration increased with dehydration
• Hypoalbuminemia may be seen with protein loss from the intestinal tract, especially with proliferative bowel disease.
• Serum biochemistry abnormalities may suggest renal or hepatic disease; ALT elevations are usually seen with ECE.

OTHER LABORATORY TESTS
Coagulation studies—may help rule out bleeding disorders; however, very little data on normal values exist. Normal values reported (based on $n = 6$): APTT 18.4 ± 1.4 seconds; PT 10.3 ± 0.1 seconds; thrombin time 28.8 ± 8.7 seconds; whole blood clotting time 2 ± 0.5 minutes in glass

tubes. Normal values for FDP in ferrets have not been reported, so results must be interpreted from feline data.

IMAGING
Radiographic Findings
• Survey abdominal radiography may indicate intestinal obstruction, organomegaly, mass, foreign body, or ascites.
• Contrast radiography may indicate thickening of the intestinal wall, mucosal irregularities, mass, severe ileus, foreign body, or stricture.
• Abdominal ultrasonography may demonstrate intestinal wall thickening, gastrointestinal mass, foreign body, ileus, or mesenteric lymphadenopathy.

DIAGNOSTIC PROCEDURES
• Fecal cytology—may reveal RBC or fecal leukocytes, which are associated with inflammatory bowel disease or invasive bacterial strains
• Fecal culture should be performed if abnormal bacteria are observed on the fecal gram's stain, or if salmonella is suspected.

Surgical Considerations
• Exploratory laparotomy and surgical biopsy should be pursued if there is evidence of obstruction or intestinal mass, and/or for a definitive diagnosis of gastrointestinal inflammatory or infiltrative diseases or *H. mustelae* gastritis.

TREATMENT
• Treatment must be specific to the underlying cause to be successful.
• Patients with mild disease usually respond to outpatient treatment.
• Patients with moderate to severe disease usually require hospitalization and 24-hour care for parenteral medication and fluid therapy.
• Correct electrolyte and acid–base disturbances.
• If anorexic, assist feed an easily digestible high-protein/high-fat diet such as Lafeber Carnivore Critical Care Diet (Lafeber Company, Cornell, IL) or Oxbow Carnivore Critical Care Diet (Oxbow Animal Health, Omaha, NE); if these are unavailable, offer chicken baby foods; may also add dietary supplement such as Nutri-Cal (EVSCO Pharmaceuticals) to increase caloric content to these foods.
• Exploratory laparotomy to remove foreign bodies or tumors

FERRETS

FERRETS

MEDICATIONS

DRUG(S) OF CHOICE

Antibiotic Therapy

• Indicated in patients with bacterial inflammatory lesions in the gastrointestinal tract. Also indicated in patients with disruption of the intestinal mucosa evidenced by blood in the feces. Selection should be based on the results of culture and susceptibility testing when possible.

• Some choices for empirical use while waiting for culture results include trimethoprim sulfa (15–30 mg/kg PO, SC q12h), amoxicillin (20 mg/kg PO, SC q12h), or enrofloxacin (5–10 mg/kg PO, SQ, IM q12h)

• Proliferative bowel disease— chloramphenicol (50 mg/kg, IM, SQ, PO q12h)

• Giardiasis, anaerobic bacterial infections— metronidazole (20 mg/kg PO q12h)

• *H. mustelae*—the combination of amoxicillin (30 mg/kg PO q8–12h) plus metronidazole (20 mg/kg PO q8–12h) and bismuth subsalicylate (17.5 mg/kg PO q12h or 1 mL/kg of regular strength preparation [262 mg/15 mL] PO q8–12h) is a common, inexpensive treatment regimen; however, many ferrets find this unpalatable. Dosing every 8 hours may be necessary to eliminate the infection. Combine this treatment with an antisecretory agent (see below). Treat for at least 2 (often 3–4) weeks. The combination of clarithromycin (12.5 mg/kg PO q8–12h) and ranitidine bismuth citrate or ranitidine HCl (24 mg/kg PO q8–12h) for 2 weeks has also been reported to be effective in the eradication of *Helicobacter* spp. Ranitidine is no longer approved for human use in the US and can be difficult to find. The combination of clarithromycin (50 mg/kg PO q24h or divided q12h); omeprazole (4 mg/kg PO q24h); metronidazole (20 mg/kg PO q12h) for 14 days has also been used for eradication.

Gastrointestinal Antisecretory Agents

• Are helpful to treat, and possibly preventing gastritis in anorectic ferrets. Ferrets continually secrete a baseline level of gastric hydrochloric acid and, as such, anorexia itself may predispose to gastric ulceration. Those successfully used in ferrets include omeprazole (4 mg/kg PO q24h), famotidine (0.25– 0.5 mg/kg PO, SC, IV q24h), and cimetidine (10 mg/kg PO, SC, IM, IV q8h)

• Intestinal protectants—bismuth subsalicylate (17.5 mg/kg PO q12h or 1 mL/kg of regular-strength preparation [262 mg/15 mL] PO q12h), sucralfate suspension (25 mg/kg PO q8h)

Corticosteroids

• Often helpful in the treatment of inflammatory bowel diseases (treat underlying disease whenever possible)— prednisone (1.25–2.5 mg/kg PO q24h); when signs resolve, gradually taper the corticosteroid dose to (0.5–1.25 mg/kg) every other day

• Vaccine reaction—diphenhydramine (0.5–2.0 mg/kg PO, IM, IV), dexamethasone sodium phosphate (4–8 mg/kg slow IV), or prednisolone sodium succinate (22 mg/kg slow IV)

CONTRAINDICATIONS

Avoid the use of corticosteroids if an underlying infectious disease is confirmed or suspected.

PRECAUTIONS

It is important to determine the cause of diarrhea. A general shotgun antibiotic approach may be ineffective or detrimental.

POSSIBLE INTERACTIONS

N/A

ALTERNATIVE DRUGS

See specific diseases for a more detailed description of treatment.

FOLLOW-UP

PATIENT MONITORING

• PCV daily until anemia is stabilized, then weekly

• Fecal volume and character, appetite, attitude, and body weight

• If melena does not resolve, consider reevaluation of the diagnosis.

POSSIBLE COMPLICATIONS

• Septicemia due to bacterial invasion of enteric mucosal

• Dehydration due to fluid loss

MISCELLANEOUS

ASSOCIATED CONDITIONS

• Septicemia

• Lymphoma

AGE-RELATED FACTORS

• Gastrointestinal foreign bodies are more common in young ferrets (<1–2 years of age)

• Older ferrets demonstrate more severe clinical signs with ECE

• Proliferative bowel disease is seen more commonly in ferrets <1 year of age

ZOONOTIC POTENTIAL

N/A

PREGNANCY/FERTILITY/BREEDING

N/A

SEE ALSO

Epizootic catarrhal enteritis
Gastroduodenal ulcers
Helicobacter mustelae
Inflammatory bowel disease

ABBREVIATIONS

ALT = alanine aminotransferase
APTT = activated partial thromboplastin time
ECE = epizootic catarrhal enteritis
FDP = fibrin degradation product
NSAID = nonsteroidal anti-inflammatory drug
PT = prothrombin time
RBC = red blood cell count
TWBC = total white blood cell count

Suggested Reading
Di Girolamo N, Selleri P. Medical and surgical emergencies in ferrets. Vet Clin Exot Anim 2016;19:431–464.
Hoefer HL. Gastrointestinal diseases of ferrets. In: Quesenberry KE, Carpenter JW, eds. Ferrets, Rabbits, and Rodents, 4th ed. Clinical Medicine and Surgery. 2021. St. Louis: Saunders, 2020:27–38.
Huynh M, Pignon C. Gastrointestinal disease in exotic small mammals. J Exot Pet Med 2013;22(2):118–131.
Johnson-Delaney CA. Geriatric ferrets. Vet Clin Exot Anim Pract 2020;23(3):549–565.
Livingstone M. Dealing with gastrointestinal disease in ferrets. In Practice 2022; 44:169–179.
Mullen HS, Scavelli TD, Quesenberry KE. Gastrointestinal foreign body in ferrets: 25 cases (1986–1990). J Am Anim Hosp Assoc 1992;28:13–19.

Author Barbara Oglesbee, DVM, DABVP-Avian

NASAL DISCHARGE AND SNEEZING

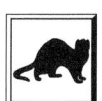

BASICS

DEFINITION
• Nasal discharges may be serous, mucoid, mucopurulent, purulent, blood-tinged, or contain frank blood (epistaxis) or food debris.
• Sneezing is the reflexive expulsion of air through the nasal cavity and is commonly associated with nasal discharge.

PATHOPHYSIOLOGY
• Secretions are produced by mucous cells of the epithelium and glands. Irritation of the nasal mucosa (by mechanical, chemical, or inflammatory stimulation) increases nasal secretion production.
• Mucosal irritation and accumulated secretions are a potent stimulus of the sneeze reflex; sneezing may be the first sign of nasal discharge. Sneezing frequency often decreases with chronic disease.

SYSTEMS AFFECTED
• Respiratory—mucosa of the upper respiratory tract, including the nasal cavities, sinuses, and nasopharynx
• Gastrointestinal—these signs may also be observed with extra nasal diseases such as swallowing disorders and esophageal or gastrointestinal diseases
• Hemic/Lymphatic/Immune—systemic diseases may cause blood-tinged nasal discharge or epistaxis due to hemostasis disorders

SIGNALMENT
• Young animals—CDV, influenza
• Older animals—nasal tumors, influenza, primary dental disease (rare)
• No age, gender predilection for other disorders

SIGNS

Historical Findings
• Nasal discharge and sneezing are commonly reported as concurrent problems. Information concerning both the initial and present character of the discharge and whether it was originally unilateral or bilateral are important historical findings.
• The response to previous antibiotic therapy may be helpful in determining secondary bacterial involvement. Bacterial infection secondary to influenza virus usually responds to treatment; however, bacterial infection secondary to dental disease or foreign body usually responds initially to antibiotic therapy but commonly will relapse or progress despite treatment. Nasal tumors, CDV infection, and fungal rhinitis typically show little response.

Physical Examination Findings
• Secretions or dried discharges on the hair around the muzzle and front limbs
• Concurrent dental disease
• Ocular discharge
• Bony involvement (tumor, fungal infection, and tooth abscess) may cause facial swelling or pain secondary to osteomyelitis
• Regional lymph node enlargement may be present
• Pyrexia (CDV, influenza, and secondary bacterial infections)

CAUSES

Unilateral discharge often is associated with nonsystemic processes:
• Foreign bodies
• Nasal tumors
• Dental-related disease—abscess (oronasal fistula, uncommon in ferrets)
• Fungal infections (cryptococcosis, blastomycosis—occur rarely)

Bilateral discharge is most common with the following:
• Infectious agents—influenza virus, CDV, mycoplasma, secondary bacterial infections
• Nasal tumors may cause unilateral discharge initially then progress to bilateral discharge as the disease extends through the nasal septum.
• Allergies have not been reported as a cause of nasal discharge in the ferret, but should be considered

Discharge may be unilateral or bilateral with the following:
• Nasal tumors
• Foreign bodies
• Hypersensitivity reaction

Sneezing without nasal discharge:
Many normal ferrets will sneeze several times a day

RISK FACTORS
• Exposure to other animals; exposure to ferrets or humans with influenza
• Dental disease
• CDV in poorly vaccinated animals
• Immunosuppression

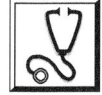

DIAGNOSIS

DIFFERENTIAL DIAGNOSIS

Differentiating Similar Causes
• Serous discharge associated with mild irritation, viral disorders, acute phase of inflammation, and possibly allergies
• Mucoid discharges associated with acute inflammation, early neoplastic conditions

• Purulent (or mucopurulent) discharges are seen with secondary bacterial or mycotic infections, nasal foreign bodies
• Serosanguinous or blood-tinged discharges are seen with destructive processes (primary nasal tumors), after violent/paroxysmal sneezing episodes (traumatic capillary rupture) associated with coagulopathies.
• The presence of other clinical signs will help to differentiate CDV from other causes. In ferrets with CDV, facial dermatitis (rash, crusts) is usually seen after the onset of nasal discharge. These signs are followed by severe respiratory signs and signs of systemic illness, progressing invariably to death.

CBC/BIOCHEMISTRY/URINALYSIS
• Elevated TWBC with inflammatory leukogram is often seen with bacterial or mycotic diseases.
• Although not specific for any cause of nasal discharge, a chemistry profile may be valuable for detecting concurrent problems and as part of a thorough evaluation before any procedure requiring anesthesia.

OTHER LABORATORY TESTS
• Fluorescent antibody test for CDV—on conjunctival or mucous membrane scrapings, or peripheral blood smears (false negatives possible)
• Bacterial culture
• PCR for mycoplasma
• Coagulation studies (not well described in ferrets)

IMAGING

Radiographic Findings
• Radiography of the nasal cavities can be helpful in cases of chronic nasal discharge, especially to rule out neoplasia, foreign body, or associated dental disease. Because of difficulties with overlying structures, the patient should be anesthetized and carefully positioned.
• The lateral view is useful in detecting any periosteal reaction over the nasal bones, for gross changes in the maxillary teeth, nasal cavity and frontal sinus, and for evaluating the air column of the nasopharynx.
• The open mouth ventro-dorsal and the intraoral view (using sheet film) are best for evaluating the nasal cavities and turbinates; disease may be localized to the affected side.
• The lateral oblique views are best for detecting maxillary teeth abnormalities.
• The rostrocaudal view is used to evaluate each frontal sinus (e.g., periosteal reaction, filling).
• CT scans are the most helpful in detecting the extent of bony changes associated with nasal tumors and fungal rhinitis.

NASAL DISCHARGE AND SNEEZING

FERRETS

DIAGNOSTIC PROCEDURES
• Rhinoscopy may be indicated in cases of chronic or recurrent nasal discharge; however, the small size of the patient makes this procedure more challenging. Bleeding disorders may be a contraindication.
• Nasal cytology—nonspecific inflammation is most commonly found.
• Cultures may be difficult to interpret due to the presence of normal nasal flora. However, the heavy growth of a single organism is usually significant. Deep cultures obtained by rhinoscopy would be most reliable.
• Biopsy of the nasal cavity is indicated in any animal with chronic nasal discharge in which neoplasia is suspected. Specimens may be obtained by direct endoscopic biopsy or rhinotomy. Multiple samples may be necessary to ensure adequate representation of the disease process.
• Periodontal probing is indicated in animals with dental calculus where tooth root abscess is suspected.

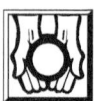

TREATMENT
• Outpatient treatment is acceptable unless the patient is exhibiting signs of systemic illness in addition to nasal discharge.
• Symptomatic treatment and nursing care are important in the treatment of ferrets with sneezing and nasal discharge. Patient hydration, nutrition, warmth, and hygiene (keeping nares clean) are important.
• If a normal diet is refused, most ferrets will accept high-calorie diets such as Eukanuba Maximum Calorie diet (Iams Co., Dayton, OH), Feline a/d (Hills Products, Topeka, KS), chicken-based baby foods, or Clinicare Feline liquid diet (Abbott Laboratories, North Chicago, IL); may also add dietary supplement such as Nutri-Cal (EVSCO Pharmaceuticals) to increase caloric content to these foods. Warming the food to body temperature or offering via syringe may increase acceptance. Administer these supplements several times a day.
• Surgery may be necessary to remove foreign bodies, obtain samples for biopsy, or to debulk tumors, abscesses, or granulomas.
• Treat-associated dental disease— extractions, gingivectomy, flap closure for

fistulas—techniques are those used in feline patients

MEDICATIONS
DRUG(S) OF CHOICE
• Nasal secretions clear more easily if the patient is well hydrated; fluid therapy should be considered if hydration is marginal.
• Decongestants or antihistamines may be used in an attempt to dry up the nasal secretions; diphenhydramine (0.5–2.0 mg/kg PO, IM, SC q8–12h) or chlorpheniramine (1–2 mg/kg PO q8–12h)
• Antibiotics for secondary bacterial infections—treat according to culture results. Choices include trimethoprim/sulfonamide (15–30 mg/kg PO, SC q12h), enrofloxacin (5–10 mg/kg PO, SC, IM q12h), amoxicillin/ clavulanate (13–25 mg/kg PO q12h), or a cephalosporin (cephalexin 15–25 mg/kg PO q8–12h).
• There are no drugs that palliatively decrease the frequency of sneezing.

CONTRAINDICATIONS
N/A

PRECAUTIONS
Topical or systemic administration of corticosteriods should be used with caution in patients with bacterial or mycotic disease.

POSSIBLE INTERACTIONS
N/A

ALTERNATIVE DRUGS
N/A

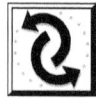

FOLLOW-UP
PATIENT MONITORING
• Observe nasal discharge; note changes in volume or character.
• Monitor CBC; should return to normal with successful treatment of infectious diseases
• Repeat cytology and cultures to monitor response to treatment.
• If the discharge is due to CDV, clinical signs will progress, eventually leading to death.

POSSIBLE COMPLICATIONS
• Loss of appetite

• Extension of primary disease into mouth, eye, or brain
• Dyspnea due to nasal obstruction

MISCELLANEOUS
ASSOCIATED CONDITIONS
• Sinusitis
• CDV
• Influenza
• Dental disease

AGE-RELATED FACTORS
N/A

ZOONOTIC POTENTIAL
Influenza virus

PREGNANCY/FERTILITY/BREEDING
N/A

SYNONYMS
N/A

SEE ALSO
Canine distemper virus
Influenza virus

ABBREVIATION
CDV = canine distemper virus

Suggested Reading
Capello V, Lennox AM. Diagnostic imaging of the respiratory system in exotic companion mammals. Vet Clin Exot Anim 2011;14:369–389.
Johnson-Delaney CA. Ferret respiratory system: clinical anatomy, physiology, and disease. Vet Clin Exot Anim 2011;14:357–367.
Kiupel M, Perpiñán D. Viral diseases of ferrets. In: Fox JG, Marini RP, eds. Biology and Diseases of the Ferret, 3rd ed. John Wiley & Sons, 2014:439–517.
Lennox A. Respiratory disorders in ferrets. Vet Clin Exot Anim 2021;24:483–493.
Perpiñán D. Respiratory diseases of ferrets. In: Quesenberry KE, Carpenter JW, eds. Ferrets, Rabbits and Rodents, 4th ed. Clinical Medicine and Surgery. 2021. St. Louis: Saunders, 2020:71–76.
Swenson SL, Koster LG, Jenkins-Moore M et al. Natural cases of 2009 pandemic H1N1 Influenza A virus in pet ferrets. J Vet Diagn Invest 2010;22(5):784–788.
Author Barbara Oglesbee DVM, DABVP (Avian)

BASICS

OVERVIEW
• The most common tumors of the digestive system are functional pancreatic islet cell tumor (insulinoma) and lymphoma. These neoplastic disorders account for a large percentage of all clinical disease seen in pet ferrets and are therefore discussed as a separate topics.
• Metastatic tumors to the liver are more common than primary tumors, especially lymphoma, islet cell tumors, and pancreatic adenocarcinomas.
• Other digestive system tumors, including tumors of the gastrointestinal tract, liver, pancreas, and salivary gland, occur sporadically in ferrets.
• The incidence of reported digestive system neoplasia in ferrets is low, such that accurate accounts of biologic behavior and response to treatment cannot be assessed.
• Reported tumor types include esophageal, gastric, or intestinal adenocarcinoma, leiomyoma, and leiomyosarcoma; hepatic hemangioma and hemangiosarcoma; hepatocellular or bile duct adenoma and adenosarcoma, bile duct cystadenoma, and cystadenocarcinoma; pancreatic adenoma and adenocarcinoma; and salivary gland adenocarcinoma.

SIGNALMENT
• Age—depend on tumor type; most likely in ferrets 4–7 years old
• Data on sex predilection not available

SIGNS
• Gastrointestinal tumors—lethargy and weakness (hind limb paresis), anorexia, vomiting, weight loss, diarrhea; gastric mass or distension may be palpable
• Hepatobiliary tumors—lethargy and weakness (hind limb paresis), anorexia, vomiting, weight loss; abdominal distension; ascites, mass, or hepatomegaly may be palpable
• Pancreatic tumors—(nonfunctional tumors) may be asymptomatic if adenomas; adenocarcinomas tend to be aggressive; see weakness, anorexia, vomiting, weight loss, and abdominal distension

CAUSES AND RISK FACTORS
• Infection with *Helicobacter mustelae* may predispose to gastric adenocarcinoma or lymphoma
• Other tumors—unknown

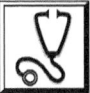

DIAGNOSIS

DIFFERENTIAL DIAGNOSIS
• Gastrointestinal lymphoma is much more common than other types of neoplasia.
• Gastrointestinal foreign body
• Infiltrative or inflammatory bowel diseases
• Infectious causes of vomiting, diarrhea (bacterial, viral, and parasitic)
• Chronic cholangiohepatitis
• Hepatic abscess

CBC/BIOCHEMISTRY/URINALYSIS
• May be normal
• May reflect dehydration or electrolyte disorders from vomiting or diarrhea
• Increased ALT, ALP, bile acids, and bilirubin, especially with hepatic or biliary neoplasia
• Anemia with chronic disease; lymphocytosis or lymphopenia reported with lymphoma
• Bilirubinuria with hepatobiliary neoplasia

OTHER LABORATORY TESTS
N/A

IMAGING
Radiography
• May demonstrate hepatomegaly, a single mass lesion, or apparent asymmetry of hepatic silhouette
• May demonstrate solitary mass or gastric distension
• Positive contrast radiography—may reveal a filling defect (stomach); may note intraluminal space occupying or annular constriction in the intestines
• Thoracic radiographs—may identify pulmonary metastases

Abdominal Ultrasonography
• May reveal a thickened wall of the stomach or bowel
• May reveal discrete mass lesion with variable echogenicity in liver

DIAGNOSTIC PROCEDURES
• Histopathologic examination—definitive diagnosis
• Suspected hepatic tumor—aspiration cytology using a 23- or 25-gauge 1–1.5-inch needle under ultrasonographic guidance
• Exploratory laparotomy—to obtain biopsy samples for definitive diagnosis and to remove tumor when possible. Always evaluate the abdominal lymph nodes, pancreas, and adrenals for evidence of disease, since adrenal

disease and insulinomas often occur concurrent with other tumor types.

PATHOLOGIC FINDINGS
Vary with tumor type

TREATMENT

SURGICAL CONSIDERATIONS
• Surgical resection—treatment of choice; may not be curative if complete removal is not possible or metastasis has occurred
• Debulking may provide palliation of obstruction
• Biopsy of local lymph nodes and normal liver for histologic evaluation is usually indicated to look for metastasis; evaluate adrenal gland and pancreas for evidence of disease
• When in doubt, follow recommendations for similar tumors in canine or feline patients.

MEDICATIONS

DRUG(S) OF CHOICE
Too few reports exist to evaluate effectiveness of chemotherapy; consult an oncologist for recommendations.

CONTRAINDICATIONS/POSSIBLE INTERACTIONS
N/A

FOLLOW-UP

EXPECTED COURSE AND PROGNOSIS
• Gastrointestinal adenocarcinomas tend to metastasize early.
• Pancreatic adenomas are generally benign but functional (insulin secreting).
• Pancreatic adenocarcinomas tend to be more aggressive and metastasize early.
• Complete surgical excision—usually curative for discrete, benign masses that can be completely resected

NEOPLASIA, DIGESTIVE SYSTEM

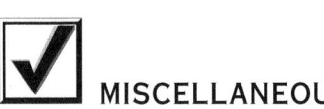
MISCELLANEOUS

SEE ALSO
Insulinoma
Lymphosarcoma

Suggested Reading
Hoefer HL. Gastrointestinal diseases of ferrets. In: Quesenberry KE, Carpenter JW, eds. Ferrets, Rabbits and Rodents, 4th ed. Clinical Medicine and Surgery. 2021. St. Louis: Saunders, 2020:27–38.
Johnson-Delaney CA. Geriatric ferrets. Vet Clin Exot Anim Pract 2020;23(3):549–650.
Livingstone M. Dealing with gastrointestinal disease in ferrets. In Practice 2022;44:169–179.
Suran JN, Latney LV, Wyre NR. Radiographic and ultrasonographic findings of the spleen and abdominal lymph nodes in healthy domestic ferrets. J Small Anim Pract 2017;58:444–453.
Williams BH, Wyre NR. Neoplasia in ferrets. In: Quesenberry KE, Carpenter JW, eds. Ferrets, Rabbits and Rodents, 4th ed. Clinical Medicine and Surgery. 2021. St. Louis: Saunders, 2020:92–108.

Author Barbara Oglesbee DVM, DABVP (Avian)

BASICS

OVERVIEW
- Integumentary neoplasms are extremely common in ferrets.
- Common tumor types reported include mast cell tumors, basal cell tumors, apocrine gland tumors of the preputial gland, squamous cell carcinomas, and adenocarcinomas
- Unlike other mammalian species, mast cell tumors in ferrets are benign.
- Fibromas and fibrosarcomas, hemangioma and hemangiosarcoma, cutaneous lymphoma, myxoma and myxosarcomas, and histiocytomas have been reported less frequently.

SIGNALMENT
- Common—fourth most common site of neoplasia in ferrets (after adrenal gland, pancreatic, and lymphoma)
- Age—depend on tumor type; most common in ferrets 4–7 years old
- Data on sex predilection not available

SIGNS
- Mast cell tumors—papular or nodular, solitary or multiple, and hairy or alopecic or have an ulcerated surface; slight predilection for the head and neck regions; tumors may appear to rupture and become covered with a dry black exudate
- Basal cell tumors—well-demarcated, firm, alopecic masses, either pedunculated or plaque-like, often pink-beige in color; may occur anywhere on the body
- Apocrine gland adenocarcinoma: most found in the perineal area (preputial gland, anal gland)—appear as raised, well-demarcated, and often ulcerated masses. These tumors are malignant and often very aggressive. Also reported in or around the ear (ceruminous gland)—often raised red, firm, or ulcerated.
- Most commonly of the preputial gland around the prepuce.
- Adenomas and adenocarcinomas—sebaceous and sweat gland adenoma/adenocarcinoma: may appear anywhere on the body, often firm, raised, multilobulated or wartlike, tan-brown in color.
- Squamous cell carcinoma—reported on the face, feet, and trunk; firm nodules or gray-white plaques described, often ulcerated
- Fibroma and fibrosarcoma—can occur anywhere on the body; well-demarcated firm mass in the dermis or subcutaneous tissues

- Hemangioma and hemangiosarcomas—hemangiomas are usually dermal and well circumscribed; hemangiosarcoma is more common on feet and legs, swollen, red, firm, and may have boney involvement
- Cutaneous lymphoma—cutaneous epitheliotropic lymphoma (mycoses fungoides) reported on feet and as generalized alopecia/erythema; may be pruritic
- Myxoma and myxosarcomas—rarely described; soft, gray/white, poorly demarcated masses
- Histiocytoma—rarely described, raised firm dermal masses, may become ulcerated

CAUSES AND RISK FACTORS
Unknown

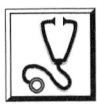

DIAGNOSIS

DIFFERENTIAL DIAGNOSIS
- Other skin tumors not listed above
- Pyoderma or mycotic dermatitis
- Abscess
- Intradermal cysts

CBC/BIOCHEMISTRY/URINALYSIS
Usually normal

OTHER LABORATORY TESTS
N/A

IMAGING
Radiographs to look for metastasis (sublumbar or mediastinal lymph nodes) or boney involvement (hemangiosarcoma, fibrosarcoma, ceruminous gland adenocarcinoma, and squamous cell carcinoma)

DIAGNOSTIC PROCEDURES
Excisional biopsy for histopathologic examination—definitive diagnosis

PATHOLOGIC FINDINGS
Vary with tumor type

TREATMENT

SURGICAL CONSIDERATIONS
- Surgical excision—generally curative for mast cell tumors, basal cell tumors, and some adenomas or hemangiomas
- Wide surgical excision or amputation recommended when possible—for hemangiosarcoma, fibrosarcoma, squamous cell carcinoma, and adenocarcinoma; biopsy local lymph nodes when possible to evaluate for metastasis

- When in doubt, follow recommendations for similar tumors in canine or feline patients.

Radiotherapy
Has been attempted in numerous tumor types, including squamous cell carcinoma, fibrosarcoma, and adenocarcinoma; consult an oncologist for recommendations

MEDICATIONS

DRUG(S) OF CHOICE
Chemotherapy has been attempted in most of the above malignant tumor types. Too few reports exist to evaluate effectiveness; consult an oncologist for recommendations.

CONTRAINDICATIONS/POSSIBLE INTERACTIONS
N/A

FOLLOW-UP
- Complete surgical excision—usually curative for mast cell tumors, basal cell tumors, and hemangiomas
- Adenocarcinomas, hemangiosarcomas, fibrosarcomas, and squamous cell carcinomas tend to recur locally, or metastasize, especially to local lymph nodes.

Suggested Reading
d'Ovidio D, Santoro D. Dermatologic diseases of ferrets. In: Quesenberry KE, Carpenter JW, eds. Ferrets, Rabbits and Rodents, 4th ed. Clinical Medicine and Surgery. 2021. St. Louis: Saunders, 2020:109–116.

Dulli R, Clark SD. Digital cytology in exotic practice. Vet Clin Exot Anim 2022;25: 663–678.

Hoppmann E, Wilson Barron H. Ferret and rabbit dermatology. J Exot Pet Med 2007;16:225–237.

Kanfer S, Reavill DR. Cutaneous neoplasia in ferrets, rabbits, and guinea pigs. Vet Clin North Am Exot Anim 2013;16:579–598.

MacPhail C. Ferret soft tissue surgery. In: Bennett A, Pye GW, eds. Surgery of Exotic Animals. Wiley-Blackwell, 2021:277–296.

Williams BH, Wyre NR. Neoplasia in ferrets. In: Quesenberry KE, Carpenter JW, eds. Ferrets, Rabbits and Rodents, 4th ed. Clinical Medicine and Surgery. 2021. St. Louis: Saunders, 2020:92–108.

Author Barbara Oglesbee, DVM, DABVP (Avian)

NEOPLASIA, MUSCULOSKELETAL, AND NERVOUS SYSTEM

BASICS

OVERVIEW
• Tumors of the musculoskeletal and nervous system are relatively uncommon in ferrets.
• The most common musculoskeletal tumors are chordoma, arising from the notochord remnant and osteoma; chondroma and chondrosarcoma, fibrosarcoma, rhabdomyosarcoma, and synovial cell sarcoma have also been reported.
• Nervous system tumors have very rarely been reported; schwannoma, neurofibrosarcoma, and ganglioneuromas are reported tumors of the peripheral nervous system; central nervous system tumors reported include granular cell tumors, meningioma, astrocytoma, and glioma.
• The reported incidence of these tumor types in ferrets is low, such that accurate accounts of biologic behavior and response to treatment cannot be assessed.

SIGNALMENT
Data on age and sex predilection not available

SIGNS
• Chordoma—most occur on tail, especially the tail tip, appearing as a smooth, round, well-demarcated mass; chordomas of the cervical vertebrae have also been reported, causing spinal cord compression and resultant weakness and ataxia caudal to the mass.
• Osteomas appear as hard, smooth, round masses on the flat bones of the head; other than the mass itself, signs are not apparent unless the mass compresses an adjacent structure.
• Chondroma, chondrosarcoma, and fibroma have all been reported on the vertebrae, intervertebral cartilage, or appendicular skeleton. Clinical signs vary with location.
• Nervous system tumors are rare; schwannomas and ganglioneuromas have been reported in the peritoneal cavity and dermis; tumors of the CNS may cause head tilt, torticollis, ataxia, seizures, and coma.

CAUSES AND RISK FACTORS
Unknown

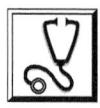

DIAGNOSIS

DIFFERENTIAL DIAGNOSIS
• For paresis, ataxia—weakness from any metabolic disease is a much more common cause of rear limb paresis
• For CNS signs—hypoglycemia (insulinoma); viral (CDV, rabies)
• For bone lesions—fungal or bacterial osteomyelitis; metastatic bone lesion from another primary site

CBC/BIOCHEMISTRY/URINALYSIS
Usually normal

OTHER LABORATORY TESTS
N/A

IMAGING
Radiography
• Osteoma—dense, bony mass on flat bones of the head
• Fibrosarcoma, chondrosarcoma—bony lysis or proliferation
• Ultrasonography may identify abdominal masses
• Thoracic radiographs—may identify pulmonary metastases
• Myelography—may establish evidence of spinal cord compression

DIAGNOSTIC PROCEDURES
• Histopathologic examination—definitive diagnosis
• Cytologic examination of bone aspirate—may yield diagnosis
• Exploratory laparotomy—to obtain biopsy samples for definitive diagnosis and to remove tumor when possible. Always evaluate the abdominal lymph nodes, pancreas, and adrenals for evidence of disease, since adrenal disease and insulinomas often occur concurrent with other tumor types.

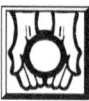

TREATMENT

SURGICAL CONSIDERATIONS
• Chordoma—usually occurs on the tip of the tail; amputation is generally curative; if in the cervical region surgical resection is indicated, may not be curative if complete removal is not possible or metastasis (rare) has occurred
• Osteoma—treatment is only necessary if causing clinical signs due to compression of adjacent structures, then surgical resection is indicated
• Fibrosarcoma, osteosarcoma—wide resection or amputation indicated when possible
• When in doubt, follow recommendations for neoplasia in canine or feline patients

MEDICATIONS

DRUG(S) OF CHOICE
Too few reports exist to evaluate effectiveness of chemotherapy; consult an oncologist for recommendations.

CONTRAINDICATIONS/POSSIBLE INTERACTIONS
N/A

FOLLOW-UP

EXPECTED COURSE AND PROGNOSIS
• Chordoma—slow growing, good prognosis if confined to tail and amputation is performed
• Osteoma—slow growing and benign; good prognosis
• Fibrosarcoma, osteosarcoma—aggressive, tend to metastasize early
• For other tumors—low numbers reported, follow guidelines for similar tumors in canine or feline patients

MISCELLANEOUS

SEE ALSO
Ataxia
Insulinoma
Paresis and paralysis

Suggested Reading
Camus M, Rech R, Choy F, Fiorello C, Howerth E. Pathology in practice. Chordoma on the tip of the tail of a ferret. J Am Vet Med Assoc 2009;235(8):949–951.
Frohlich J, Donovan T. Cervical chordoma in a domestic ferret (*Mustela putorius furo*) with pulmonary metastasis. J Vet Diagn Invest 2015;27(5):656–659.
Huynh M, Piazza S. Musculoskeletal and neurologic diseases. In: Quesenberry KE, Carpenter JW, eds. Ferrets, Rabbits and Rodents, 4th ed. Clinical Medicine and Surgery. 2021. St. Louis: Saunders, 2020:117–130.
MacPhail C. Ferret soft tissue surgery. In: Bennett A, Pye GW, eds. Surgery of Exotic Animals, 2021:277–296.
Munday J, Brown C, Richey L. Suspected metastatic coccygeal chordoma in a ferret (*Mustela putorius furo*). J Vet Diagn Invest 2004;16(5):454–458.
Williams BH, Wyre NR. Neoplasia in ferrets. In: Quesenberry KE, Carpenter JW, eds. Ferrets, Rabbits and Rodents, 4th ed. Clinical Medicine and Surgery. 2021. St. Louis: Saunders, 2020:92–108.
Author Barbara Oglesbee, DVM, DABVP (Avian)

FERRETS

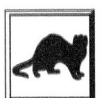

BASICS

DEFINITION
- The presence of body fat in sufficient excess to compromise normal physiologic function or predispose to metabolic, surgical, and/or mechanical problems.
- Obesity has become an extremely common, and often debilitating, problem in pet ferrets.

PATHOPHYSIOLOGY
- Increased caloric intake and/or decreased activity. Most ferrets are housed in cages that allow minimal exercise.
- Long-term corticosteroid use for common disorders such as insulinoma, IBD, and lymphoma is an extremely common cause of obesity. Large fat pads often form in the thoracic cavity, surrounding the heart and mediastinal lymph nodes. Fat can also be deposited within the lung parenchyma, resulting in dyspnea and/or exercise intolerance. Similarly, the amount of visceral fat deposition can be severe, causing lethargy and exercise intolerance.

SYSTEMS AFFECTED
- Respiratory—space-occupying effects of intrathoracic fat deposition
- Musculoskeletal—articular and locomotor problems
- Hepatobiliary—hepatic lipidosis

SIGNALMENT
More common in middle-aged and older ferrets

SIGNS
- Sites of adipose tissue to evaluate during physical examination include the intraabdominal, inguinal, and axillary regions. Excess amounts of body fat for body size; can measure as body condition score >4 on a 1–5 scale in which 1 = cachectic (>20% underweight), 2 = lean (10%–20% underweight), 3 = moderate, 4 = stout (20%–40% overweight), 5 = obese (>40% overweight)
- Dyspnea and exercise intolerance with intrathoracic and visceral fat deposition
- Lethargy and rear limb weakness are common presenting complaints. Due to their elongated body conformation, some severely obese ferrets may have difficulty lifting their body weight with their hind legs.
- Fat is commonly deposited around peripheral lymph nodes, which may be mistaken for lympadenopathy.

CAUSES AND RISK FACTOR
- Long-term corticosteroid use.
- Excessive access to highly palatable food, often combined with insufficient activity.

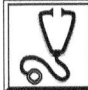

DIAGNOSIS

DIFFERENTIAL DIAGNOSIS
Differentiating Similar Signs
- Fat deposition within the lung parenchyma can mimic interstitial pneumonia radiographically
- Intraabdominal neoplasia or organomegaly
- The accumulation of fat around peripheral lymph nodes may mimic lymphadenopathy.
- Normal seasonal weight gain—many normal ferrets will gain weight and develop a thick hair coat in the fall, with subsequent loss in the spring.
- Pregnancy
- Ascites

Differentiating Causes
- Similar problems/diseases should be differentiated via history, physical examination, laboratory evaluation, and imaging.

CBC/BIOCHEMISTRY/URINALYSIS
Normal

OTHER LABORATORY TESTS
- Increased liver values with hepatic lipidosis

IMAGING
- Abdominal radiographs will differentiate visceral fat from other space-occupying masses
- Thoracic radiography—pericardial fat may mimic cardiomegaly; fat pads surrounding mediastinal lymph nodes may mimic neoplasia; and fat within the lung parenchyma may mimic interstital pneumonia
- Thoracic ultrasound and/or CT scan—very useful to differentiate fat from other masses

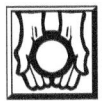

TREATMENT

DIET
- Ferrets tend to prefer sweet-tasting treats (e.g., raisins); overfeeding of these treats is the main cause of obesity in pet ferrets. Ferrets are often treated as family members, and owners have difficulty denying these treats.
- Ferrets have a short intestinal tract and decreased GI transit time (3 hours in an adult) as compared with cats and dogs. Because of this, the feeding of free-choice or multiple small meals is recommended. Generally, free-choice feeding of a high-quality ferret food will not cause obesity if the diet is not supplemented with treats. However, some ferrets will overeat and become obese if the food bowl is left full in the cage all day due to boredom and lack of exercise.
- Ferrets have a higher protein and fat requirement than dogs or adult cats—for maintenance in normal ferrets, feed a high-quality kitten, or ferret chow with animal protein listed as the first ingredient.

CLIENT EDUCATION
- Most important part of obesity therapy; must be tailored to each particular circumstance
- Discontinue feeding all sweet tasting or high-fat treats and dietary supplements.
- Most ferrets should have food available free choice if left alone in a cage for the day. Ferrets tend to become hypoglycemic relatively quickly when fasted and should not go longer than 4–6 hours without food. This is especially true in those with insulinomas.
- If possible, obese ferrets should be released from the cage for exercise and feeding at regular intervals throughout the day, thereby feeding frequent small meals with a reduced total volume of food.
- If the owner's schedule does not allow for this and food is made continuously available in the obese ferret's cage, change to a high-quality senior ferret diet and decrease the amount fed until the desired weight loss is achieved.
- When obesity is caused by owners' overfeeding of treats as a means of social interaction with the ferret, achieving weight loss can be more challenging. Many of these clients do not seek veterinary help until the ferret is morbidly obese and having difficulty ambulating. At this point, the health risks to the ferret are obvious and clients are more willing to comply.
- Recommended maintenance caloric intake has been reported to be 200–300 kcal/kg body weight per day. However, this recommendation is likely excessive for a sedentary, cage-bound pet ferret. Optimally, the owners should quantitate exactly the volume of kibble the ferret is eating per day, and caloric content of that volume should be calculated. If the ferret has become obese on a diet containing ≤200–300 kcal/kg BW/day, the total volume of food fed per day should be reduced, and the kibble should be changed to one of the many available senior ferret diets. If treats are fed, the amount of dry kibble fed should be reduced so as to not exceed 200 kcal/day. Replace sugary treats with meat-based protein treats.
- Older literature reports that ferrets need a diet containing at least 28% fat. In a sedentary ferret, this may lead to obesity. Current recommendation is a diet containing only 15%–20% fat.
- The feeding of high-fiber, carbohydrate-based cat foods is not recommended. Ferrets have a short large intestine and a limited ability to properly digest these products.

OBESITY   (CONTINUED)

FERRETS

Feeding carbohydrate-based diets may lead to the formation of cystic calculi.

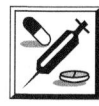

MEDICATIONS
• When possible, attempt to limit corticosteroid dosage for long-term use. If using to treat insulinoma, attempt transition or supplementation of diazoxide to reduce prednisolone dose (see insulinoma). For IBD, taper to lowest effective dose and/or add azathioprine (see IBD).

FOLLOW-UP
PATIENT MONITORING
• Lifelong follow-up and support are essential to maintain the reduced weight.
• At the initial visit, instruct clients to recognize moderate body condition score and to feed the quantity of food necessary to maintain this condition during the changing physiologic and environmental conditions of the pet's life; remind them at checkups.

MISCELLANEOUS
ASSOCIATED CONDITIONS
• Insulinoma
• IBD
• Hepatic lipidosis
• Lymphoma
• Orthopedic disorders
• Increased anesthetic risk
• Cardiovascular disorders

PREGNANCY/FERTILITY/BREEDING
Obesity may increase risk of dystocia; but because of potential risk to the fetus, do not treat pregnant animals.

SEE ALSO
Insulinoma
IBD
Lymphoma

Suggested Reading
Capello V, Lennox AM. Diagnostic imaging of the respiratory system in exotic companion mammals. Vet Clin Exot Anim 2011;14:369–389.
Johnson-Delaney CA. Geriatric ferrets. Vet Clin Exot Anim Pract 2020;23(3):549–565.
Johnson-Delaney CA. Ferret nutrition. Vet Clin Exot Anim Pract 2014;17(3):449–470.
Powers LV, Perpiñán D. Basic anatomy, physiology, and husbandry of ferrets. In: Quesenberry KE, Orcutt CJ, Mans C, Carpenter JW, eds. Ferrets, Rabbits, and Rodents, 4th ed. St. Louis, MO, USA: Elsevier, 2020:1–2.
Schoemaker NJ, van Zeeland YRA. Endocrine diseases of ferrets. In: Quesenberry KE, Carpenter JW, eds. Ferrets, Rabbits and Rodents, 4th ed.Clinical Medicine and Surgery. 2021. St. Louis: Saunders, 2020:77–91.

Author Barbara Oglesbee, DVM, DABVP (Avian)

BASICS

OVERVIEW
• Otis externa—inflammation of the external ear canal; uncommon in ferrets except in animals with ear mites
• Otitis media—inflammation of the middle ear, usually an extension of otitis externa through a ruptured tympanum (extension of otitis externa or through overaggressive cleaning); rarely occurs without a membrane being ruptured; anecdotal reports suggest that neoplasia within the middle ear is common
• Normal ferrets usually have thick, red-brown or black crusts in the outer ear—may or may not be associated with otitis

SIGNALMENT
No age or sex predilection; rare disease in ferrets

SIGNS
• Otitis externa—often a secondary symptom of an underlying disease (mites or overzealous cleaning)
• Infection—purulent and malodorous exudate
• Inflammation—exudation, pain, pruritus, and erythema

Historical Findings
• Pain
• Head shaking
• Scratching at the pinnae
• Malodorous ears

Physical Examination Findings
• Thick, red-brown, or black crusts in the outer ear—may or may not be associated with otitis; this type of material is usually a normal finding in ferret ears
• Redness and swelling of the external canal
• Exudation—may result in malodor and canal obstruction
• Vestibular signs are extremely rare (head tilt, nystagmus, anorexia, and ataxia) but indicate development of otitis media/interna.

CAUSES AND RISK FACTORS
• Otodectes cynotis mite (ear mites) infestation is common in ferrets.
• Secondary bacterial infections occasionally occur.
• Secondary mycotic infections—*Malassezia* spp.—uncommon
• Neoplasia of the ear canal (carcinoma, epithelioma) or nearby structures (salivary glands) may predispose.
• Topical drug reaction, irritation, hypersensitivity, and trauma from abrasive

cleaning techniques may occur when using topical cleaning solutions.
• Excessive moisture (e.g., from frequent cleanings with improper solutions) can lead to infection; overzealous client compliance with recommendations for ear cleanings may predispose.

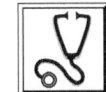

DIAGNOSIS

DIFFERENTIAL DIAGNOSIS

Differentiating Similar Signs
• Normal ferrets often have a dark, red-brown, crumbly exudate. This must be differentiated from otitis based on clinical signs, otic examination, and cytology.
• Purulent, odiferous exudate is abnormal and indicates otitis.
• The presence of even normal-appearing exudate in only one ear suggests unilateral disease.
• Alopecia and pruritus around the pinna may be caused by ferret adrenal disease, fleas, sarcoptic mange, or dermatophytes.
• Recurrent, unilateral disease—neoplasia should be strongly suspected.

CBC/BIOCHEMISTRY/URINALYSIS
May indicate a primary underlying disease

OTHER LABORATORY TESTS
N/A

IMAGING
Bullae radiographs—otitis media

DIAGNOSTIC PROCEDURES
• Microscopic examination of aural exudate—single most important diagnostic tool after complete examination of the ear canal
• Culture of exudate—to assist with antibiotic selection, most important in resistant infection
• Infections within the canal can change with prolonged or recurrent therapy; repeat examination of aural exudate is required in chronic cases.

Microscopic Examination
• Preparations—make from both canals (the contents of the canals may not be the same); spread samples thinly on a glass microscope slide; examine both unstained and modified Wright-stained samples.
• Mites—visible with oil preparations or grossly with magnification
• Type(s) of bacteria or yeast—assist in the choice of therapy
• WBCs within the exudate—active infection; systemic antibiotic therapy may be warranted

TREATMENT

APPROPRIATE HEALTH CARE
Outpatient, unless severe vestibular signs are noted

SURGICAL CONSIDERATIONS
• Indicated when neoplasia is diagnosed
• Severe, unresponsive otitis media is extremely rare in ferrets; if diagnosed, a bullae osteotomy may be indicated.

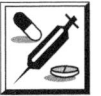

MEDICATIONS

DRUG(S) OF CHOICE

Systemic
• Antibiotics—useful in severe cases of bacterial otitis externa; mandatory when the tympanum has ruptured; trimethoprim/sulfonamide (15–30 mg/kg PO, SC q12h), enrofloxacin (10–20 mg/kg PO, SC, IM q12h), amoxicillin/clavulanate (13–25 mg/kg PO q12h), or cephalexin (15–25 mg/kg PO q8–12h)
• Corticosteroids—reduce swelling and pain; reduce wax production; anti-inflammatory dosages of prednisone (0.25–0.5 mg/kg PO q12h); use sparingly and for short durations only

Topical
• Topical therapy is necessary for resolution and control of otitis externa; however, the small size of the ear canal may hinder client compliance.
• For ear mites: Topical ivermectin: 1% ivermectin diluted 1:10 in propylene glycol, administered in ears at 400 mcg/kg q2w × 2 treatments or ivermectin (0.4 mg/kg PO, SC q14–28d) or selamectin (Revolution, Pfizer) 15 mg/kg topically q30d or Imidacloprid (10%) and moxidectin (1%) (Advantage-Multi, Bayer)—0.4 mL/animal topically q30d
• It is not necessary to clean the ears thoroughly to remove debris prior to topical administration of ivermectin since debris may aid in retention of medication in the canal. Do not use topical and parenteral ivermectin concurrently.
• If secondary bacterial or yeast infection is diagnosed, completely clean the external ear canal of debris. Thorough cleaning of the ear daily during initial therapy may be necessary with severe bacterial infections; not recommended routinely or when ear mites alone are diagnosed since cleaners are more

OTITIS EXTERNA AND MEDIA   (CONTINUED)

likely to irritate the canal and exacerbate disease; If necessary, use mild cleaners for routine cleaning or when the competence of the tympanic membrane is in question; cerumenolytics—dioctyl sodium sulfosuccinate or carbamide peroxide emulsify waxes, facilitating removal
• Generally, ingredients should be limited to those needed to treat a specific infection (i.e., antibiotics only for a bacterial infection).

CONTRAINDICATIONS
• Use extreme caution when cleaning the external ear canals of all animals with severe and chronic otitis externa because the tympanum can easily be ruptured.
• Ivermectin—do not use in pregnant jills.
• Do not use topical and parenteral or oral ivermectin concurrently.
• Ruptured tympanum—use caution with topical cleansers and medications other than sterile saline or dilute acetic acid; potential for ototoxicity is a concern; controversial

PRECAUTIONS
• Several topical medications infrequently induce contact irritation or allergic response; reevaluate all worsening cases.

ALTERNATIVE DRUGS
• Imidacloprid (10%) and moxidectin (1%) (Advantage-Multi, Bayer)—monthly spot treatment for dogs and cats; 0.4 mL applied topically every 30 days

FOLLOW-UP
PATIENT MONITORING
Repeat exudate examinations can assist in monitoring infection.

PREVENTION/AVOIDANCE
• Avoid overzealous cleaning of the ear canal.
• Control of underlying diseases

POSSIBLE COMPLICATIONS
Uncontrolled otitis externa can lead to otitis media, deafness, vestibular disease, cellulitis, facial nerve paralysis, progression to otitis interna, and rarely meningoencephalitis.

EXPECTED COURSE AND PROGNOSIS
• Otitis due to otodectes mites—prognosis is good, may recur if treated with topical preparations and owner compliance is poor
• Otitis externa—depends on underlying cause; failure to correct underlying primary cause results in recurrence.

MISCELLANEOUS
ASSOCIATED CONDITIONS
N/A

AGE-RELATED FACTORS
N/A

ZOONOTIC POTENTIAL
Potentially fungal infection

PREGNANCY/FERTILITY/BREEDING
Do not use ivermectin in pregnant jills.

SYNONYMS
N/A

SEE ALSO
Adrenal disease (hyperadrenocorticism)
Ear mites
Pruritus

Suggested Reading
d'Ovidio D, Santoro D. Dermatologic diseases of ferrets. In: Quesenberry KE, Carpenter JW, eds. Ferrets, Rabbits and Rodents, 4th ed. Clinical Medicine and Surgery. 2021. St. Louis: Saunders, 2020:109–116.
Fehr M, Koestlinger S. Ectoparasites in small exotic mammals. Vet Clin Exot Anim 2013;16:611–657.
Jekl V, Hauptman K, Knotek Z. Video otoscopy in exotic companion mammals. Vet Clin North Am Exot Anim Pract 2015;18:431–445.
Author Barbara Oglesbee, DVM, DABVP (Avian)

FERRETS

PARAURETHRAL CYSTS (UROGENITAL CYSTIC DISEASE)

BASICS

DEFINITION
Cystic structures found on the dorsal aspect of the urinary bladder or surrounding the proximal urethra in both male and female ferrets. These structures likely arise from remnants of the mesonephric or paramesonephric ducts, from the prostate, or paraprostatic tissues. Cysts are usually large, may be single or multiple, and often cause partial or complete obstruction of the urethra. Secondary bacterial infections within the cystic fluid are extremely common.

PATHOPHYSIOLOGY
• Paraurethral/urogenital cysts are associated with ferret adrenal disease and the resultant excessive production of androgens. Excessive sex steroid production causes hyperplasia of mesonephric or paramesonephric ductal tissue remnants in both sexes and prostatic or periprostatic tissues in males.
• True prostatic cysts secondary to inflammation or neoplasia are rare.
• Severe secondary bacterial infections may occur and cause chronic abscesses or prostatitis.
• Obstruction of the urethra often occurs due to extraluminal compression by the cyst or hyperplastic tissue or, with bacterial infection, may become obstructed by thick, tenacious exudate in the urine.

SYSTEMS AFFECTED
• Urinary—obstruction of the urethra, secondary bacterial cystitis
• Gastrointestinal—ferrets with large urogenital cysts may have tenesmus
• Peritoneum—focal or generalized peritonitis can develop in animals with bacterial infection of cystic fluid or abscesses

GENETICS
Unknown; however, genetics may play a role in the development of ferret adrenal disease

INCIDENCE/PREVALENCE
Urogenital cystic disease is a common cause of dysuria in ferrets.

GEOGRAPHIC DISTRIBUTION
Urogenital cystic disease and ferret adrenal disease are seen more commonly in ferrets in North America than in Europe. This may be due to genetics, early neutering practices, or differing husbandry practices.

SIGNALMENT
Predominant Sex
Seen primarily in neutered males; occasionally in female ferrets with underlying adrenal disease due to enlargement of periurethral tissues.

Mean Age and Range
More common in middle-aged animals, 3–7 years old as this is the age at which adrenal disease usually occurs.

SIGNS
Historical and Physical Examination Findings
• Presenting complaint is typically stranguria due to urethral obstruction by cysts, hyperplastic prostatic tissue, or thick exudate blocking the urethra
• Pollakiuria, tenesmus, dysuria, including intense straining or crying out when urinating
• With urethral obstruction, ferrets will have signs of uremia, including depression, lethargy, and anorexia.
• Weight loss, depression, and anorexia may be seen with secondary bacterial infections (abscesses)
• Thick, white, or yellow discharge is often visible at the urethral opening in patients with prostatic abscesses
• Bilaterally symmetric alopecia or pruritus due to adrenal disease
• Abdominal distension
• Large, turgid, painful bladder in ferrets with urethral obstruction
• Fluid-filled cysts are sometimes palpable and may be larger than the urinary bladder.

CAUSES
• Excessive androgen production due to functional adrenal hyperplasia, adenoma, or carcinomas
• Rarely, prostatic cysts are secondary to prostatic neoplasia.

RISK FACTORS
Evidence suggests that adrenal disease may be related to neutering. The gonads and adrenals arise embryonically from the urogenital ridge; some gonadal cells are likely present in the adrenals. Stimulation of these cells by pituitary gonadotropin may cause hypertrophy of these steroid-secreting cells.

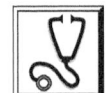

DIAGNOSIS
DIFFERENTIAL DIAGNOSIS
• For stranguria: urolithiasis, neoplasia of the bladder neck or urethra, or urethral stricture
• For mass detected in the region of the prostate: prostatic hyperplasia, prostatic neoplasia, or other abdominal mass—neoplasia, abscess, or granuloma

• Radiography and results of cytologic examination of fluid and ultrasonographic examination usually rule out these diseases. Many cysts become secondarily infected.

CBC/BIOCHEMISTRY/URINALYSIS
• Usually normal
• Hemogram may show nonregenerative anemia or leukocytosis due to secondary bacterial infection of cysts.
• Hypoglycemia may be present—usually due to concurrent insulinoma
• Urinalysis may rule out other causes of stranguria—urolithiasis (extremely common) or bacterial cystitis (uncommon). Secondary bacterial infections can lead to abscess formation in many prostatic or periprostatic cysts; exudate from these abscesses may drain into the urinary bladder or urethra. In some cases, this exudate can be thick enough to cause urethral blockage.

OTHER LABORATORY TESTS
• Elevations in plasma estradiol, androstenedione, and 17-hydroxyprogesterone combined are supportive of adrenal disease. (Available through the University of Tennessee Clinical Endocrinology Laboratory, Department of Comparative Medicine)
• Examination of cyst fluid—gross appearance can range from clear, cloudy yellow or thick, yellow to greenish, foul-smelling fluid; cytologic examination ranges from serosanguinous fluid to purulent exudate.
• Culture the fluid for bacteria.

IMAGING
Ultrasonography:
• Ultrasonography is the most useful method of imaging the prostate and demonstrating adrenal gland enlargement.
• The prostate often contains single to multiple fluid-filled cysts of varying size; fluid is hypo- or anechoic if no infection is present. With abscess formation, sediment within cysts is usually hyperechoic.
• If paraurethral cysts are present, these appear as hypo- or anechoic pockets surrounding the urethra.
• Uniform parenchymal echogenicity is seen in some ferrets
Radiography:
• Radiographs may demonstrate what appear to be two or more urinary bladders, as the cysts can be as large as or larger than the urinary bladder.
• Contrast urocystography can be used to delineate the cyst(s). Initially, both the cyst and urinary bladder will fill with contrast medium. After urinating, the cyst will retain the contrast media.

Paraurethral Cysts (Urogenital Cystic Disease)　(Continued)

DIAGNOSTIC PROCEDURES
Ultrasound-guided aspiration of cystic structures; take care to avoid rupturing an abscess

PATHOLOGIC FINDINGS
• Gross examination reveals single or multiple cysts—may be bi- or multilobulated
• Histologic examination—cyst walls usually consist of three layers: epithelium, muscle, and serosa lined with squamous epithelial cells. Areas of multifocal ulceration and necrosis are common, as is infiltration by inflammatory cells.
• Adrenal disease is always present—gross enlargement with irregular surface or discoloration of the affected gland, cysts, or differences in texture within the affected gland. Histologically, see adrenal hyperplasia, adenomas, or adenocarcinomas.

TREATMENT

APPROPRIATE HEALTH CARE
• Ferret adrenal disease may be treated with adrenalectomy or managed medically. The decision as to which form of treatment is appropriate is multifactorial including which gland is affected (left vs. right), the surgeon's experience and expertise, the severity of clinical signs, patient age, concurrent diseases, and financial issues.
• If the prostatomegaly or cyst is not causing life-threatening urethral obstruction, medical treatment may cause a sufficient reduction in size to alleviate clinical signs. Depending on the circumstances, medical treatment may be preferred; however, medical treatment is not curative, must be administered lifelong, and has no effect on adrenal tumor size or potential metastasis.
• Surgical removal of the affected adrenal gland(s), coupled with intraoperative aspiration of sterile cysts or debulking of infected cysts, is generally necessary to treat large prostatic cysts causing a life-threatening urethral obstruction. These procedures may require special surgical expertise, especially if the right adrenal gland is diseased.
• Large or multiple cysts that are abscessed, or infection with resistant bacterial pathogens may require prolonged treatment; the prognosis is poorer for complete resolution than with sterile cysts.
• Always submit samples of prostatic tissue and removed adrenal gland for histologic examination.
• If the urethra is partially or completely obstructed, hospitalization is necessary for urethral catheterization (see below).

NURSING CARE
• Fluid therapy, either subcutaneous or intravenous, depending on the state of hydration. Ferrets that are uremic require intravenous fluid therapy. Correct any acid-base disturbances as indicated by the serum biochemistry profile.
• Postoperative fluid therapy should continue for 24–48 hours.
• If the urethra is partially or completely obstructed, catheterize before surgery. Without experience, one may find urethral catheterization of male ferrets to be more difficult than for cats. The urethral opening can be difficult to visualize as it is located slightly ventral to the tip of the penis. Ferrets have a J-shaped os penis that extends to the tip of the penis, distal to the urethral opening. With practice, catheterization can be easily mastered. Catheterization should be performed under anesthesia or heavy sedation. Either a 3.5 Fr red rubber catheter or a 3 Fr ferret urethral catheter (Slippery Sam Tomcat Urethral Catheter, Smith Medical) are flexible and long enough to reach the urinary bladder. Dilation of the urethra by insertion of a 25-g IV catheter and flushing with saline before catheterization is helpful. Insert the catheter alongside the IV catheter and flush with saline as the catheter is advanced. Resistance is usually encountered at the pelvic flexure; repeated saline dilation and lubrication may be needed. Once the catheter reaches the urinary bladder, suture the catheter in place and connect a urine collection device. Ferrets with indwelling urinary catheters require an Elizabethan collar.
• Monitor urinary output - should be at least 1 to 2 mL/kg per hour; with diuresis may be as high as 140 mL per ferret per day.
• If catheterization is initially unsuccessful, decompress the bladder via cystocentesis using a 25-gauge needle. Handle the bladder carefully and perform the cystocentesis under anesthesia or rupture may occur.
• If catheterization remains unsuccessful, emergency surgery may be required to perform cystotomy with anterograde flushing, draining or debulking cysts, and adrenalectomy if possible.

ACTIVITY
Activity should be limited postoperatively.

DIET
No dietary changes are necessary.

CLIENT EDUCATION
• Removal of the affected adrenal gland(s) and drainage of the cysts at the time of surgery is often curative in ferrets with mild prostatomegaly, sterile cysts, or small abscessed cysts.

• Large or multiple cysts that are abscessed, or infection with resistant bacterial pathogens may require prolonged treatment; the prognosis is poorer for complete resolution as compared to sterile cysts.

SURGICAL CONSIDERATIONS
• Surgical removal of the affected adrenal gland(s) will cause a significant reduction in the size of hypertrophied paraurethral or prostatic tissue, usually within a few days.
• Surgical removal of the affected adrenal gland(s) is often coupled with intraoperative aspiration of sterile cysts or debulking of infected cysts. These procedures require special surgical expertise, especially if the right adrenal gland is diseased. The proximity of the right adrenal to the vena cava and the potential for vena cava invasion by malignant tumors make complete excision a high-risk procedure. Referral to a surgeon or clinician with experience is recommended when possible.
• Several techniques for adrenalectomy have been advocated, and problems may be associated with each surgical option, depending on the surgeon's expertise. Refer to the suggested reading list for a more detailed description of surgical procedures.
• Sterile cysts may be drained intraoperatively using fine-needle aspiration. Even if the fluid appears clear, submit aspirated fluid for bacterial culture and susceptibility testing. Aspiration may be insufficient to treat large, sterile cysts. Omentalization of cysts is one method used to provide sufficient drainage. Omentalization is accomplished by creating an incision into the cyst wall and suturing the omentum into the incision to absorb any fluid produced postoperatively. See the suggested reading list for details on this procedure.
• Resect or drain as many prostatic abscesses as possible; pack off the cystic tissue before draining/debriding and flush the abdomen well. Large abscesses may require marsupialization and carry a poorer prognosis.
• Some ferrets may develop peritonitis following surgery for abscesses, requiring longer-term medical management.
• If the bladder is full of purulent exudate, a cystostomy may be indicated to remove accumulated material.

MEDICATIONS

DRUG(S) OF CHOICE
GnRH analogs for medical treatment of adrenal disease:
• Treatment with a GnRH agonist is indicated even if adrenalectomy is performed

to prevent the recurrence of disease in the remaining adrenal gland.
• Leuprolide acetate is a potent gonadotropin secretion inhibitor and can begin to reduce prostate size within 12–48 hours post-administration. Smaller cysts may respond to medical treatment alone. Large prostatic cysts or abscesses will require physical debulking. This drug has become challenging to acquire and often prohibitively expensive in the US.
• Deslorelin acetate (Suprelorin-F®, Virbac Animal Health) A 4.7-mg implant is labeled for treatment of adrenal disease in ferrets in the US and a 9.4-mg implant is available in Europe. However, reduction in prostate size may take days to weeks. Large prostatic cysts or abscesses will require physical debulking.

Antibiotics:
• Indicated when a secondary bacterial infection is present. If cysts are abscessed, surgical management is also necessary. Antibiotic therapy should be based on the results of culture and susceptibility testing. Choose antibiotics that can enter the prostatic lumen such as trimethoprim/ sulfonamide (15–30 mg/kg PO, SC q12h), enrofloxacin (5–10 mg/kg PO, SC, IM q12h), or chloramphenicol (25–50 mg/kg PO, SC q12h). A minimum of 4–6 weeks of antimicrobial administration is usually necessary.

CONTRAINDICATIONS
N/A

PRECAUTIONS
N/A

ALTERNATIVE DRUGS
• Melatonin implants are available commercially (Ferretonin® 2.7-mg—ferrets < 600g) and 5.4-mg implants –most ferrets, Melatek, LLC) and have been used in ferrets with adrenal disease to alleviate alopecia and, possibly, aggressive behavior, prostatomegaly or vulvar swelling. However, effectiveness in the reduction of prostate size is questionable and the time interval required for the resolution of clinical signs limits its usefulness.
• Antiandrogen agents have been used to further reduce prostate size along with surgical and/or GnRH analog treatment. Choices include Flutamide (10 mg/kg PO q12–24h), Bicalutamide (5 mg/kg PO q12h) and Finasteride (5 mg/kg PO q24h). The use of these medications is largely anecdotal but appears to be safe and effective.

FOLLOW-UP
PATIENT MONITORING
• With surgical therapy, a reduction in cyst or prostate size is seen in 2–3 days, relieving the urethral obstruction.
• Response to therapy is evident by the remission of clinical signs, particularly hair regrowth and reduction in the size of paraurethral cysts.
• Following unilateral adrenalectomy or subtotal adrenalectomy, monitor for the return of clinical signs; tumor recurrence in the remaining adrenal gland is common. Clinical signs typically develop 1 year postoperatively.
• In ferrets with bilateral adrenalectomy, monitor for the development of Addison's disease.
• Ultrasonographic examination at 2- to 4-week intervals after adrenalectomy may be used to follow the resolution of cysts.
• With medical therapy, a reduction in prostate size may occur within days or may occur gradually occur over a period of weeks to months.

PREVENTION/AVOIDANCE
Neutering at an older age may decrease the incidence of disease.

POSSIBLE COMPLICATIONS
• Peritonitis
• Recurrence of cysts if all hyperfunctioning adrenal tissue is not removed
• Peritonitis with rupture of septic cysts

EXPECTED COURSE AND PROGNOSIS
• Sterile cysts—following adrenalectomy, cysts, or prostatic tissue should decrease in size within 1–3 days. If the urethral obstruction persists, a second adrenal tumor may be present.
• Medical therapy has shown promising results in reducing the size of prostatic tissue in ferrets with adrenal disease. Anecdotal reports suggest that in some cases, significant size reduction may occur in as little as 2–3 days; in other cases, size reduction is minimal, prolonged, or may not occur at all. Insufficient data exist to predict the outcome of long-term therapy.
• The prognosis is poorer when large prostatic abscesses are found, as complete removal is difficult and the response to antibiotic therapy is variable.

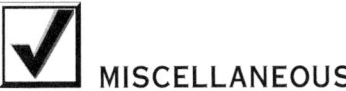

MISCELLANEOUS
ASSOCIATED CONDITIONS
• Ferret adrenal disease—always
• Insulinoma, lymphoma, and/or congestive heart failure are common in ferrets in this age range.
• Gastritis due to the overgrowth of *Helicobacter mustelae* is common in ferrets undergoing stress

AGE-RELATED FACTORS
The risk of anesthetic or surgical complications is increased in geriatric ferrets

ZOONOTIC POTENTIAL
N/A

PREGNANCY/FERTILITY/BREEDING
N/A

SYNONYMS
Paraprostatic cysts
Paraurethral cysts
Prostatic cysts

SEE ALSO
Adrenal disease (hyperadrenocorticism)
Prostatitis and prostatic abscesses

ABBREVIATIONS
FSH = follicular-stimulating hormone
GnRH = gonadotropic-releasing hormone
LH = luteinizing hormone

Suggested Reading
Bo P, Tagliavia C, Canova M, DeSilva M, Bombardi C, Grandis A. Comparative characterization of the prostate gland in intact, and surgically and chemically neutered ferrets. J Exot Pet Med 2019;31:68–74.
Di Girolamo N, Huyun M. Disorders of the urinary and reproductive systems in ferrets. In: Quesenberry KE, Carpenter JW, eds. Ferrets, Rabbits and Rodents, 4th ed. Clinical Medicine and Surgery. St. Louis: Saunders, 2020:39–54.
Di Girolamo N, Selleri P. Medical and surgical emergencies in ferrets. Vet Clin Exot Anim Pract 2016;19:431–464.
Jekl V, Hauptman K. Reproductive medicine in ferrets. Vet Clin Exot Anim Pract 2017;20:629–663.
Lennox AM, Wagner RA. Comparison of 4.7-mg deslorelin implants and surgery for the treatment of adrenocortical disease in ferrets. J Exot Pet Med 2012;21:332–335.
Powers LV, Winkler K, Garner MM et al. Omentalization of prostatic abscesses and large cysts in ferrets (*Mustela putorius furo*). J Exot Pet Med 2007;16:186–189.

FERRETS

PARAURETHRAL CYSTS (UROGENITAL CYSTIC DISEASE) (CONTINUED)

Schoemaker NJ, Van Zealand YRA. Endocrine diseases of ferrets. In: Quesenberry KE, Carpenter JW, eds. Ferrets, Rabbits and Rodents, 4th ed. Clinical Medicine and Surgery. St. Louis: Saunders, 2020:77–91.

Schoemaker NJ, van Deijk R, Muijlaert B et al. Use of a gonadotropin-releasing hormone agonist implant as an alternative for surgical castration in male ferrets (*Mustela putorius furo*). Theriogenology 2008;70:161–167.

Swiderski JK, Seim HB, MacPhail CM et al. Long-term outcome of domestic ferrets treated surgically for hyperadrenocorticism: 130 cases (1995–2004). J Am Vet Med Assoc 2008;232:1338–1343.

Wagner RA, Piché CA, Jöchle W et al. Clinical and endocrine responses to treatment with deslorelin acetate implants in ferrets with adrenocortical disease. Am J Vet Res 2005;66:910–914.

Author Barbara Oglesbee, DVM, DABVP (Avian)

FERRETS

 BASICS

DEFINITION
• Paresis—weakness of voluntary movement
• Paralysis—lack of voluntary movement
• Paraparesis—weakness of voluntary movements in pelvic limbs. Posterior paresis is an extremely common finding in ferrets with systemic disease.
• Paraplegia—absence of all voluntary pelvic limb movement

PATHOPHYSIOLOGY
• Weakness—may be caused by lesions in the upper or lower motor neuron system. In ferrets, weakness is one of the most common presenting complaints. Weakness, especially paraparesis, is usually due to the effects of systemic or metabolic disease (e.g., hypoglycemia or anemia) or severe obesity. Weakness due to structural damage to the CNS or PNS occurs less commonly.
• Evaluation of limb reflexes—determine which system (upper or lower motor neuron) is involved
• Upper motor neurons and their axons— inhibitory influence on the large motor neurons of the lower motor neuron system; maintain normal muscle tone and normal spinal reflexes; if injured, spinal reflexes are no longer inhibited or controlled and reflexes become exaggerated or hyperreflexic.
• Lower motor neurons or their processes (peripheral nerves)—if injured, spinal reflexes cannot be elicited (areflexic) or are reduced (hyporeflexic).

SYSTEMS AFFECTED
• Nervous
• Endocrine/Metabolic—hypoglycemia
• Hemic/Lymphatic—anemia

SIGNALMENT
Any age or gender

SIGNS
General Comments
Limb weakness—acute or gradual onset
• Acute onset generally seen with structural CNS or PNS damage
• Acute onset of generalized weakness or paraparesis in ferrets <1 year old is most commonly due to acute GI foreign body obstruction.
• Gradual or intermittent weakness seen with systemic or metabolic disease, severe obesity, or sometimes spinal cord damage

Historical Findings
• Ferrets with posterior paresis lose the normal arched appearance of the spine when standing or walking—spinal alignment appears flat or parallel to the ground. May progress to dragging the hind limbs, intermittently or continuously.
• Weakness may be accompanied by other signs such as lethargy, ptyalism, or stargazing, especially with metabolic diseases.
• Many focal compressive spinal cord diseases begin with ataxia and progress to weakness and finally to paralysis.

Physical Examination Findings
• Other than paresis or paralysis, usually normal with structural spinal cord damage
• Often normal in ferrets with insulinomas unless hypoglycemic at the time of physical examination
• May elicit pain on abdominal palpation with GI foreign body
• If in pain (vertebral disease, disk extrusion), the patient may resent handling and manipulation during the examination.
• With systemic or metabolic disease— weight loss, splenomegaly, depression, or dehydration may be seen
• Severe obesity may cause locomotor difficulty.

Neurologic Examination Findings
• Confirm that the problem is weakness or paralysis.
• Localize problem to either lower or upper motor neuron system.
• Paraplegia—bladder may also be paralyzed in ferrets with structural spinal cord damage

CAUSES
Metabolic Disease (most common cause of posterior paresis)
• Anemia—seen with hyperestrogenism, blood loss (esp. from GI tract), leukemia, CRF
• Hypoglycemia—from insulinomas, GI foreign bodies, severe hepatic disease, or sepsis
• Metabolic derangements associated with obstructive GI foreign bodies in ferrets <1 year old
• Cardiac disease
• Severe obesity—due to their elongated body conformation, some severely obese ferrets may have difficulty lifting their body weight with their hind legs.

Neurologic Disease—CNS or Spinal Cord Disease
CNS
• Neoplastic—any tumor of the CNS (primary or secondary)
• Infectious—canine distemper virus; rabies (rear limb ataxia may be the only clinical sign in ferrets with rabies) and any other CNS infection affecting the brain
• Inflammatory, immune-mediated— Aleutian disease virus (ADV)-induced encephalomyelitis
• Toxic—metronidazole

Spinal cord
• Traumatic—intervertebral disc herniation (rare); fracture or luxation
• Neoplastic—primary bone tumors (esp. chondroma, chondrosarcoma most common); multiple myeloma and metastatic tumors that infiltrate the vertebral body
• Vascular—hematomyelia due to the effects of hyperestrogenism, infarct (rare)
• Infectious—discospondylitis; myelitis (rare)

RISK FACTORS
N/A

 DIAGNOSIS

DIFFERENTIAL DIAGNOSIS
Weak Pelvic Limbs
• Pain or hyperesthesia elicited at site of spinal cord damage seen with trauma, IVD disease, discospondylitis, and some bone tumors (other than trauma, all are rare in ferrets).
• Lack of pain along spinal column— systemic or metabolic disease most common; vascular disease (hemorrhage, infarct), some neoplasias, CNS lesions (all rare in ferrets)
• Acute onset—most common in ferrets <1 year old with acute GI obstruction; in any age ferret with spinal cord trauma; in older ferrets with bone tumors
• Gradual onset or intermittent weakness— usually systemic or metabolic disease; possible with IVD extrusion, if extrusion is gradual; however, IVD disorders are rare in ferrets.
• Spinal reflexes—localize weakness to the cervical, thoracolumbar, or lower lumbar cord segments
• Hypoglycemia—most common cause in middle-aged to older ferrets; intermittent or episodic weakness; often see other signs: ptyalism, stargazing, tremors, retching or vomiting, diarrhea, poor hair coat, and lethargy
• Anemia—pale mucous membranes, petechia or ecchymosis, lethargy, melena, hematemesis, and swollen vulva (hyperestrogenism)
• Cardiac disease—murmurs, arrhythmias, collapse with exercise, and syncope
• Musculoskeletal disorders—typically produce lameness and a reluctance to move
• Only limbs affected—likely spinal cord dysfunction if all four limbs affected: lesion is in the cervical area or is multifocal to diffuse; only pelvic limbs affected: may be metabolic disease or spinal cord dysfunction; spinal lesion is anywhere below the second thoracic vertebra

CBC/BIOCHEMISTRY/URINALYSIS
Usually normal, unless systemic or metabolic diseases involved (e.g., hypoglycemia, electrolyte imbalance, and anemia)

FERRETS

PARESIS AND PARALYSIS   (CONTINUED)

OTHER LABORATORY TESTS
- Anemia—differentiate as nonregenerative or regenerative on the basis of the reticulocyte count or bone marrow aspirate.
- Electrolyte imbalance—correct the problem; see if weakness resolves.

IMAGING
- Spinal radiographs—lesion localized to the spinal cord; may reveal bony tumor, fracture, or luxation; disk herniation and diskospondylitis are rare findings
- Thoracic radiographs—identify neoplasia
- CT—to identify spinal lesions, organomeglay
- Abdominal ultrasonography—if gastrointestinal, hepatic, renal, adrenal, or pancreatic dysfunction suspected
- Echocardiography—if cardiac disease is suspected

DIAGNOSTIC PROCEDURES
- CSF analysis and myelography—may be helpful in establishing diagnosis. Location for CSF tap or myelography—atlanto-occipital region or L5-L6 region. Use a 22- or 20-gauge needle to inject iohexol (0.25–0.5 mL/kg). Premedication with methylprednisolone sodium succinate (10–30 mg/kg IV) may help to prevent complications from CSF tap.

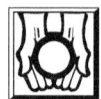

TREATMENT
Inpatient—with severe weakness or paralysis

NURSING CARE
- Bedding—move paralyzed patients away from soiled bedding, check and clean frequently to prevent urine scalding and superficial pyoderma; use padded bedding or a waterbed to help prevent decubital ulcer formation.

ACTIVITY
Restrict until spinal trauma and disk herniation can be ruled out

SURGICAL CONSIDERATIONS
Surgery for insulinoma, GI foreign bodies, fracture, IVD extrusion, and some neoplasia

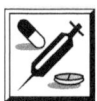

MEDICATIONS

DRUG(S) OF CHOICE
- Not recommended until the source or cause of the problem is identified.

CONTRAINDICATIONS
Corticosteroids—do not use with discospondylitis or other infectious causes of paresis/paralysis

PRECAUTIONS
Corticosteroids—associated with gastrointestinal ulceration and hemorrhage, delayed wound healing, and heightened susceptibility to infection

POSSIBLE INTERACTIONS
N/A

ALTERNATIVE DRUGS
N/A

FOLLOW-UP

PATIENT MONITORING
- Neurologic examinations—daily to monitor status
- Bladder—evacuate (via manual expression or catheterization) three to four times a day to prevent overdistension and subsequent bladder atony; once bladder function has returned, patient can be managed at home.

POSSIBLE COMPLICATIONS
- Urinary tract infection, bladder atony, urine scalding, and pyoderma; constipation, and decubital ulcer formation
- Spinal cord or neuromuscular disease—progression to weakness and possibly paralysis
- Hypoglycemia—seizures, stupor, and coma

MISCELLANEOUS

ASSOCIATED CONDITIONS
N/A

AGE-RELATED FACTORS
N/A

ZOONOTIC POTENTIAL
Rabies—rare cause of paresis/paralysis in ferrets, but when present has extreme zoonotic potential. Rabies cases must be strictly quarantined and confined to prevent exposure to humans and other animals. Local and state regulations must be adhered to carefully and completely.

PREGNANCY/FERTILITY/BREEDING
N/A

SEE ALSO
See specific diseases

Aleutian disease virus (parvovirus)
Insulinoma
Gastrointestinal and esophageal foreign bodies

ABBREVIATIONS
ADV = Aleutian disease virus
CDV = canine distemper virus
CNS = central nervous system
CRF = chronic renal failure
CSF = cerebrospinal fluid
CT = computed tomography
GI = gastrointestinal
IVD = intervertebral disc
PNS = peripheral nervous system

Suggested Reading
Di Girolamo N, Selleri P. Medical and surgical emergencies in ferrets. Vet Clin Exot Anim 2016;19:431–464.
Huynh M, Piazza S. Musculoskeletal and neurologic diseases. In: Quesenberry KE, Carpenter JW, eds. Ferrets, Rabbits and Rodents, 4th ed. Clinical Medicine and Surgery. 2021. St. Louis: Saunders, 2020:117–130.
Johnson-Delaney CA. Geriatric ferrets. Vet Clin Exot Anim 2020;23:549–565.
Kiupel M, Perpiñán D. Viral diseases of ferrets. In: Fox JG, Marini RP, eds. Biology and Diseases of the Ferret, 3rd ed. John Wiley & Sons, 2014:439–517.
Lennox AM, Gladden JN. Emergency and critical care of small mammals. In: Quesenberry KE, Carpenter JW, eds. Ferrets, Rabbits and Rodents, 4th ed. Clinical Medicine and Surgery. 2021. St. Louis: Saunders, 2020:595–608.
Mancinelli E. Neurologic examination and diagnostic testing in rabbits, ferrets and rodents. J Exot Pet Med 2015;24:52–64.
Schoemaker NJ, van Zeeland YRA. Endocrine diseases of ferrets. In: Quesenberry KE, Carpenter JW, eds. Ferrets, Rabbits and Rodents, 4th ed. Clinical Medicine and Surgery. 2021. St. Louis: Saunders, 2020:77–91.

Author Barbara Oglesbee DVM, DABVP (Avian)

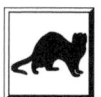

BASICS

DEFINITION
Disorders of primary hemostasis (platelet- or vessel wall mediated) that result in bleeding into the skin or mucous membranes to a degree out of proportion to the trauma

PATHOPHYSIOLOGY
• Thrombocytopenia is the most common cause of petechia or ecchymosis in ferrets. Defective platelet function causing impaired primary hemostasis (i.e., failure of platelet plug formation) has not been reported in ferrets but should be considered since little information is available on hemostasis in ferrets.
• Thrombocytopenia—caused by impaired thrombopoiesis (estrogen toxicity most common in ferrets), shortened platelet life span, or platelet sequestration
• Acquired platelet function deficits—may be associated with uremia, drugs (e.g., aspirin), dysproteinemia, or myeloproliferative disease

SYSTEMS AFFECTED
• Hemic/Lymph/Immune
• Skin/Exocrine—petechia/ecchymosis/bruising
• Respiratory—epistaxis
• Renal/Urologic—hematuria
• Gastrointestinal—melena

SIGNALMENT
• Seen most commonly in intact females with hyperestrogenism
• Other causes of thrombocytopenia and platelet function defects are not associated with age or sex predisposition.

SIGNS
• Hyperestrogenism—large vulva, serous, or purulent vaginal discharge
• Bilaterally symmetric alopecia, usually beginning at the tail base and progressing cranially with ferret adrenal disease
• Splenomegaly

CAUSES
Thrombocytopenia
• Low platelet production—hyperestrogenism (sustained estrus in intact females or ferret adrenal disease) and myelophthisis
• Sequestration of platelets in a large spleen, liver, or other sizable mass of microvasculature usually does not lead to bleeding.
• Increase in platelet use or destruction—consumptive coagulopathy
• Immune-mediated disease—anecdotally reported in ferrets

Thrombocytopathy
Acquired platelet function disorders (not well described, but possible in ferrets in a similar manner as dogs and cats)—uremia, DIC, liver disease, myeloproliferative and lymphoproliferative disease, and treatment with NSAIDs

RISK FACTORS
• Hyperestrogenism—failure to breed intact females, ovarian remnant in neutered females, ferret adrenal disease (FAD)—estrogen-secreting adrenal tumors. Evidence suggests that FAD may be related to neutering at an early age.
• Previous administration of aspirin or other NSAID

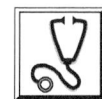

DIAGNOSIS

DIFFERENTIAL DIAGNOSIS
• Usually are not mistaken for anything else; however, injuries causing an expected amount of bleeding or bruising must be ruled out by history and physical examination.
• Evidence of any of the diseases mentioned (see Causes) should raise suspicion that it may be the underlying cause of petechiae or bruising.

CBC/BIOCHEMISTRY/URINALYSIS
• Platelets are low either by estimation on a well-made blood smear or by a direct count in patients with thrombocytopenia; normal platelet count in ferrets ($n = 5$) is 300,000 ± 46,000/μL
• RBC fragmentation suggests DIC or other vascular disease.
• Patients with myeloproliferative and lymphoproliferative diseases may be leukemic or cytopenic.
• Biochemical analysis—rule out hepatic, renal, and hormonal (e.g., FAD) causes

OTHER LABORATORY TESTS
Coagulation studies—may help rule out DIC; however, very little data on normal values exist. Normal values (based on $n = 6$): APTT 18.4 ± 1.4 seconds; PT 10.3 ± 0.1 seconds; thrombin time 28.8 ± 8.7 seconds; whole blood clotting time 2 ± 0.5 minutes in glass tubes; normal values for FDP in ferrets have not been reported, so results must be interpreted from feline data.

IMAGING
Abdominal radiography or ultrasonography may help identify splenomegaly or hepatomegaly.

DIAGNOSTIC PROCEDURES
• The buccal mucosa simplate bleeding time—long in patients with most of the thrombopathies in addition to thrombocytopenia; normal range in ferrets not reported, but presumed to be similar to dogs and cats (1.7–4.2 minutes)
• Most invasive procedures are contraindicated in patients with bleeding disorders.
• Bone marrow examination—indicated if cytopenia is detected

TREATMENT
Usually as inpatient until a definitive diagnosis is made

NURSING CARE
• Discontinue any medications that may alter platelet function (e.g., aspirin and other NSAIDs).
• Indications for whole blood transfusion are the same as those for dogs or cats. In general, most ferrets will benefit from a transfusion when the PCV falls below 15%, depending on clinical signs. Identifiable blood groups have not been demonstrated in ferrets, and transfusion reactions are unlikely, even after multiple transfusions. However, administration of dexamethasone sodium phosphate 4–6 mg/kg by slow IV injection once prior to transfusion has been recommended as a precaution. Healthy, large males with a normal PCV are the most appropriate blood donors. Up to 0.6% of donor's body weight can be safely collected (usually, 6–12 mL, depending on the size of the ferret and volume required). Collect blood from anesthetized donor ferret via the anterior vena cava or jugular vein into a syringe with 1 mL acid-citrate-dextrose anticoagulant per 7 mL of blood, or 5 units of heparin per mL of blood. (Volume of blood to be transfused is estimated in the same manner as for cats.) Administer blood within 4 hours of collection. Blood should be filtered during administration to the recipient.
• Supportive care, such as fluid therapy, warmth, and adequate nutrition

ACTIVITY
Minimize activity to reduce the risk of even minor trauma.

DIET
If normal diet is refused, most ferrets will accept high-calorie diets such as Eukanuba Maximum Calorie diet (Iams Co., Dayton, OH), Feline a/d (Hills Products, Topeka, KS), chicken-based baby foods, or Clinicare Feline liquid diet (Abbott Laboratories, North Chicago, IL); may also add dietary supplement such as Nutri-Cal (EVSCO Pharmaceuticals) to increase caloric content to these foods. Warming the food to body temperature or offering via syringe may increase acceptance.

FERRETS

PETECHIA/ECCHYMOSIS/BRUISING   (CONTINUED)

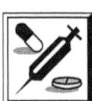

MEDICATIONS

DRUG(S) OF CHOICE
Vary with the cause of the bruising

CONTRAINDICATIONS
N/A

PRECAUTIONS
Aspirin and other NSAIDs should be avoided.

POSSIBLE INTERACTIONS
N/A

ALTERNATIVE DRUGS
N/A

FOLLOW-UP

PATIENT MONITORING
In patients with thrombocytopenia, conduct a daily platelet count until a response is noted; see specific diseases for details.

POSSIBLE COMPLICATIONS
• Death or morbidity caused by hemorrhage into the brain or other vital organs
• Shock caused by hemorrhagic hypovolemia

MISCELLANEOUS

ASSOCIATED CONDITIONS
N/A

AGE-RELATED FACTORS
None

ZOONOTIC POTENTIAL
None

PREGNANCY/FERTILITY/BREEDING
N/A

SYNONYMS
Hemorrhagic diatheses
Bleeding

SEE ALSO
Adrenal disease (hyperadrenocorticism)
Hyperestrogenism

ABBREVIATIONS
APTT = activated partial thromboplastin time
DIC = disseminated intravascular coagulation
FAD = ferret adrenal disease
FDP = fibrin degradation product
NSAID = nonsteroidal anti-inflammatory drug
PT = prothrombin time

Suggested Reading
Di Girolamo N, Huyun M. Disorders of the urinary and reproductive systems in ferrets. In: Quesenberry KE, Carpenter JW, eds. Ferrets, Rabbits and Rodents, 4th ed. Clinical Medicine and Surgery. St. Louis: Saunders, 2020:39–54.
Di Girolamo N, Selleri P. Medical and surgical emergencies in ferrets. Vet Clin Exot Anim Pract 2016;19:431–464.
Jekl V, Hauptman K. Reproductive medicine in ferrets. Vet Clin Exot Anim Pract 2017;20:629–663.
Lennox AM, Wagner RA. Comparison of 4.7-mg deslorelin implants and surgery for the treatment of adrenocortical disease in ferrets. J Exot Pet Med 2012;21:332–335.
Schoemaker NJ, Van Zealand YRA. Endocrine diseases of ferrets. In: Quesenberry KE, Carpenter JW, eds. Ferrets, Rabbits and Rodents, 4th Ed Clinical Medicine and Surgery. St. Louis: Saunders, 2020:77–91.
Wagner RA, Piché CA, Jöchle W et al. Clinical and endocrine responses to treatment with deslorelin acetate implants in ferrets with adrenocortical disease. Am J Vet Res 2005;66:910–914.
Wyre NR, Michels D, Chen S. Selected emerging diseases in ferrets. Vet Clin North Am Exot Anim Pract 2013;16(2):469–493.

Author Barbara Oglesbee, DVM, DABVP (Avian)

FERRETS

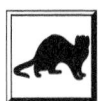

BASICS

OVERVIEW
• Abnormal accumulation of fluid within the pleural cavity
• May be due to increased production or decreased resorption of fluid
• Alterations in hydrostatic and oncotic pressures or vascular permeability and lymphatic function may contribute to fluid accumulation.

INCIDENCE/PREVALENCE
Common finding in clinical practice

SIGNALMENT
Varies with underlying cause

SIGNS
General Comments
Depend on the fluid volume, rapidity of fluid accumulation, and the underlying cause

Historical Findings
• Weakness, often manifested as rear limb paresis or paralysis
• Dyspnea
• Tachypnea
• Open mouth breathing
• Cyanosis
• Lethargy
• Inappetence
• Cough

Physical Examination Findings
• Dyspnea—respirations often shallow and rapid
• Muffled or inaudible heart and lung sounds ventrally
• Preservation of breath sounds dorsally

CAUSES AND RISK FACTORS
High Hydrostatic Pressure
• CHF—most common cause
• Intrathoracic neoplasia—(mediastinal lymphosarcoma) very common cause
• Overhydration

Vascular or Lymphatic Abnormality
• Infectious—bacterial, viral, or fungal
• Neoplasia (e.g., mediastinal lymphosarcoma, metastatic disease)
• Chylothorax (e.g., from CHF, cranial vena cava obstruction, neoplasia, fungal, diaphragmatic hernia, and trauma)
• Hemothorax (e.g., from trauma, neoplasia, and coagulopathy)
• Diaphragmatic hernia (rare)

Low Oncotic Pressure
Hypoalbuminemia—less common cause of pleural effusion in ferrets; protein-losing enteropathy, protein-losing nephropathy, and liver disease

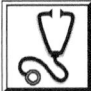

DIAGNOSIS

DIFFERENTIAL DIAGNOSIS
• Historical or physical evidence of external trauma—consider hemothorax or diaphragmatic hernia
• Fever suggests an inflammatory, infectious, or neoplastic cause.
• Murmurs, gallops, or arrhythmias combined with jugular venous distension or pulsation suggest an underlying cardiac cause.
• Decreased compressibility of the cranial thorax suggests a cranial mediastinal mass, especially lymphoma.
• Concurrent ascites suggests CHF; severe hypoalbuminemia, diaphragmatic hernia, disseminated neoplasia are unusual causes.

Fluid Analysis
Should include physical characteristics (i.e., color, clarity, odor, clots), pH, glucose, total protein, total nucleated cell count, and cytologic examination to aid in differentiating causes:
• Transudate—early CHF; rarely from hypoalbuminemia
• Modified transudate—CHF, neoplasia
• Nonseptic exudate—neoplasia, Aleutian disease virus (ADV), diaphragmatic hernia (rare cause)
• Septic exudate—pyothorax (rare)
• Hemorrhage—neoplasia, trauma, coagulopathy

CBC/BIOCHEMISTRY/URINALYSIS
• Hemogram results may be abnormal in patients with pyothorax or neoplasia.
• Severe hypoalbuminemia (generally < 1 g/dL to cause effusion) suggests protein-losing enteropathy, protein-losing nephropathy, or liver disease.
• Hyperglobulinemia (monoclonal) suggests ADV.

OTHER LABORATORY TESTS
• Cardiac disease suspected—perform heartworm ELISA (SNAP heartworm antigen test, Idexx Laboratories)—may have false negative if low worm burdens are present or in early infections
• Infection suspected—do a bacterial culture and sensitivity test and consider special stains (e.g., gram and acid-fast stains) of the fluid.
• Chyle suspected—do an ether clearance test or Sudan stain of the pleural fluid.
• Fluid analysis—cytologic examination for the presence of neoplastic or inflammatory cells

IMAGING
Radiographic Findings
• Used to confirm pleural effusion; should not be performed until after thoracocentesis

in dyspneic patients with evidence of pleural effusion on physical examination
• Evidence of pleural effusion includes separation of lung borders away from the thoracic wall and sternum by fluid density in the pleural space, fluid-filled interlobar fissure lines, loss or blurring of the cardiac and diaphragmatic borders, blunting of the lung margins at the costophrenic angles, (ventrodorsal view), and widening of the mediastinum (ventrodorsal view).
• Unilateral effusion—consider chylothorax, pyothorax; hemothorax, pulmonary neoplasia, diaphragmatic hernias, and lung lobe torsion
• Evaluate post-thoracocentesis radiographs carefully for cardiomegaly, intrapulmonary lesions, mediastinal masses, diaphragmatic hernia, lung lobe torsion, and evidence of trauma (e.g., rib fractures).

Echocardiographic Findings
• Ultrasonographic evaluation of the thorax is recommended whenever cardiac disease, a diaphragmatic hernia, or cranial mediastinal mass is suspected.
• Echocardiography is easiest to perform before thoracocentesis, provided the patient is stable.

DIAGNOSTIC PROCEDURES
Thoracocentesis—allows characterization of the fluid type and determination of potential underlying cause (following parameters extrapolated from canine and feline data):

Transudate
• Clear and colorless to pale yellow
• Protein <1.5 g/dL
• Specific gravity <1.018
• Cells <1000/mm³—mostly mesothelial cells

Modified Transudate
• Yellow or pink; may be slightly cloudy
• Protein 2.5–5.0 g/dL
• Specific gravity >1.018
• Cells 1,000–7,000/mm³ (LSA up to 100,000)—macrophage, mesothelial cell predominant cell type; few nondegenerate neutrophils erythrocytes, and lymphocytes; may contain neoplastic cells

Exudate (Nonseptic)
• Yellow or pink; cloudy; fibrin may be present
• Protein 3.0–8.0 g/dL
• Specific gravity >1.018
• Cells 5,000–20,000/mm³ (LSA up to 100,000)—nondegenerate neutrophil and macrophage predominant cell type, lymphocytes and neoplastic cells may be seen

Exudate (Septic)
• Yellow to red-brown; cloudy to opaque; may contain fibrin

PLEURAL EFFUSION

- Protein. 3.0–7.0 g/dL
- Specific gravity >1.018
- Cells 5,000–300,000/mm³—degenerate neutrophil and macrophage predominant cell type; bacteria

Hemorrhage
- Red; spun supernatant clear and sediment red
- Protein >3.0 g/dL
- Specific gravity 1.007–1.027
- Cells consistent with peripheral blood, may see macrophages with erythrophagocytosis
- Does not clot

Chyle
- Milky white; opaque
- Protein 2.5–6.0 g/dL
- Cells 1,000–20,000/mm³—lymphocytes, neutrophils, and macrophages

Exploratory Thoracotomy
- To obtain biopsy specimens of lung, lymph nodes, or pleura, if indicated

TREATMENT
- First, thoracocentesis to relieve respiratory distress. When performing thoracocentesis, be aware that the heart is located much more caudally within the thorax in the ferret compared with dogs and cats. Sedation—butorphanol (0.2–0.5 mg/kg IM) or midazolam (0.25–1.0 mg/kg IM, SC)
- If the patient is stable after thoracocentesis, outpatient treatment may be possible for some diseases. Most patients are hospitalized because they require intensive management.
- Preventing fluid reaccumulation requires treatment based on a definitive diagnosis.
- Surgery may be indicated for management of some neoplasias; other indications (diaphragmatic hernia repair, foreign body removal, and lung lobectomy for lung lobe torsion) are rare in ferrets.

MEDICATIONS
DRUG(S) OF CHOICE
- Treatment varies with specific disease
- Diuretics generally reserved for patients with diseases causing fluid retention and volume overload (e.g., CHF)

CONTRAINDICATIONS
N/A

PRECAUTIONS
- Drugs that depress respirations or decrease blood pressure
- Inappropriate use of diuretics predisposes the patient to dehydration and electrolyte disturbances without eliminating the effusion.

POSSIBLE INTERACTIONS
N/A

ALTERNATIVE DRUGS
N/A

FOLLOW-UP
PATIENT MONITORING
Radiographic evaluation is key to the assessment of treatment in most patients

PREVENTION/AVOIDANCE
N/A

POSSIBLE COMPLICATIONS
Death due to respiratory compromise

EXPECTED COURSE AND PROGNOSIS
Varies with the underlying cause, but usually guarded to poor

MISCELLANEOUS
SEE ALSO
Congestive heart failure

Heartworm disease
Lymphosarcoma

ABBREVIATIONS
ADV = Aleutian disease virus
CHF = congestive heart failure
LSA = lymphosarcoma

Suggested Reading
Capello V, Lennox AM. Diagnostic imaging of the respiratory system in exotic companion mammals. Vet Clin Exot Anim 2011;14:369–389.
Di Girolamo N, Selleri P. Medical and surgical emergencies in ferrets. Vet Clin North Am Exot Anim Pract 2016;19: 431–464.
Fitzgerald B, Dias S, Martorell J. Cardiovascular drugs in avian, small mammal, and reptile medicine. Vet Clin North Am Exot Anim Pract 2018; 21(2):399–442.
Johnson-Delaney CA. Ferret respiratory system: clinical anatomy, physiology, and disease. Vet Clin Exot Anim 2011;14: 357–367.
Kiupel M, Perpiñán D. Viral diseases of ferrets. In: Fox JG, Marini RP, eds. Biology and Diseases of the Ferret, 3rd ed. John Wiley & Sons, 2014:439–517.
Lennox A. Respiratory disorders in ferrets. Vet Clin Exot Anim 2021;24:483–493.
Morrisey JK, Malakoff RJ. Cardiovascular and other diseases of ferrets. In: Quesenberry KE, Carpenter JW, eds. Ferrets, Rabbits and Rodents, 4th ed. Clinical Medicine and Surgery. 2021. St. Louis: Saunders, 2020:5–70.
Perpiñán D. Respiratory diseases of ferrets. In: Quesenberry KE, Carpenter JW, eds. Ferrets, Rabbits and Rodents, 4th ed. Clinical Medicine and Surgery. 2021. St. Louis: Saunders, 2020:71–76.
Swenson SL, Koster LG, Jenkins-Moore M et al. Natural cases of 2009 pandemic H1N1 Influenza A virus in pet ferrets. J Vet Diagn Invest 2010;22(5):784–788.

Author Barbara Oglesbee DVM, DABVP (Avian)

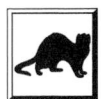

BASICS

OVERVIEW
• Most commonly bacteria and secondary to viral infection (especially influenza), aspiration of foreign material, or in debilitated ferrets.
• Fungal infections have rarely been reported
• Organisms enter the lower respiratory tract primarily by the inhalation or aspiration routes; enter less commonly by the hematogenous route; infections incite an overt inflammatory reaction

SIGNALMENT
No age or sex predilection

SIGNS
Historical Findings
• Weakness, and lethargy, often manifested as rear limb weakness
• Anorexia and weight loss
• Labored breathing
• Nasal discharge
• Fever
• Sudden death
• Cough—seen inconsistently in ferrets, even with marked pulmonary disease of any kind

Physical Examination Findings
• Fever
• Dyspnea
• Abnormal breath sounds on auscultation—increased intensity or bronchial breath sounds, crackles, and wheezes
• Weight loss
• Serous or mucopurulent nasal discharge
• Lethargy
• Dehydration

CAUSES
• Bacterial pathogens—*Streptococcus zooepidemicus, Escherichia coli, Klebsiella pneumoniae, Pseudomonas* sp., *Bordetella bronchiseptica*, and *Mycoplasma* spp. have been reported
• *Mycobacterium* sp. has been sporadically reported, these ferrets also had ocular lesion
• Anaerobic bacteria—found in pulmonary abscesses and aspiration pneumonia
• Mycotic pathogens—rare in ferrets; blastomycosis and cryptococcosis reported

RISK FACTORS
• Exposure to CDV in unvaccinated animals
• Exposure to people or ferrets with influenza virus
• Regurgitation, dysphagia, or vomiting
• Reduced level of consciousness—stupor, coma, and anesthesia
• Thoracic trauma or surgery
• Immunosuppressive therapy—chemotherapy; high-dose, long-term glucocorticoids
• Severe metabolic disorders—uremia, diabetes mellitus
• Mycotic—environmental exposure to soils rich in organic matter; exposure to bird droppings or other fecal matter possible risk factor

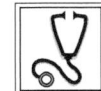

DIAGNOSIS

DIFFERENTIAL DIAGNOSIS
• Viral pneumonia—canine distemper virus and influenza virus; possibly Aleutian disease virus
• Metastatic neoplasia
• Congestive heart failure
• Mediastinal lymphoma
• Pulmonary abscess
• Intrathoracic fat accumulation
• Pleural infection—pyothorax

CBC/BIOCHEMISTRY/URINALYSIS
Inflammatory leukogram—neutrophilic leukocytosis with or without a left shift; absence does not rule out the diagnosis

OTHER LABORATORY TESTS
Florescent antibody test (IFA) for CDV—can be performed on peripheral blood or buffy coat smears, conjunctival, or mucous membrane scrapings. Vaccination will not affect the results.

IMAGING
Thoracic Radiography
• Bacterial: alveolar pattern characterized by increased pulmonary densities (margins indistinct; air bronchograms or lobar consolidation); patchy or lobar alveolar pattern with a cranial ventral lung lobe distribution
• Aspiration pneumonia—bronchoalveolar pattern most severe in the gravity-dependent lung lobes (cranial, ventral); may take up to 24 hours for the pattern to develop after acute aspiration; scrutinize for evidence of esophageal or mediastinal disease
• Mycotic—diffuse nodular interstitial and peribronchial infiltrates; nodular densities may coalesce to granulomatous masses with indistinct edges; tracheobronchial lymphadenopathy possible; large focal granulomas possible

DIAGNOSTIC PROCEDURES
• Microbiologic and cytologic examinations—aspirates, or washings; definitive diagnosis
• Samples—transtracheal washing or fine-needle lung aspiration
• Septic inflammation with degenerate neutrophils predominates
• Recent antibiotic administration—nonseptic inflammation likely
• Bacteria—may be visible microscopically; always culture specimens, even if no bacteria are seen on cytologic examination.

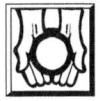

TREATMENT

APPROPRIATE HEALTH CARE
Inpatient—recommended with multisystemic signs (e.g., anorexia, high fever, weight loss, and lethargy)

NURSING CARE
• Maintain normal systemic hydration—important to aid mucociliary clearance and secretion mobilization
• Nebulization with saline—results in more rapid resolution if used in conjunction with physiotherapy and antibacterials
• Physiotherapy—chest wall coupage; always do immediately after nebulization; avoid allowing the patient to lie in one position for a prolonged time
• Oxygen therapy—for respiratory distress

MEDICATIONS

DRUG(S) OF CHOICE
• Antibiotic therapy—ideally, withhold until an airway specimen is collected. Begin with an antibiotic combination that is broad-spectrum and effective against anaerobes such as enrofloxacin (10–20 mg/kg PO, IM, IV q12h) plus: amoxicillin clavulanic acid (13–25 mg/kg PO q12h) or ampicillin clavulanic acid (20 mg/kg IV q8–12h) or doxycycline (10 mg/kg PO q12h) alter therapy based on culture/susceptibility results and continue for 10 days after resolution of clinical and radiographic signs.
• Antifungal therapy—amphotericin B—0.25 mg/IV 3×/week × 2–4 mos. Administer over 3–4 hours; best used with itraconazole (10–20 mg/kg PO q24h), ketoconazole (10–50 mg/kg PO q12–24h) or fluconazole (50mg/kg PO q12h) for severely affected patients. A dose of 0.4–0.8 mg/kg IV q7d (total dose of 7–25 mg) has been reported for the treatment of a ferret with blastomycosis.

PNEUMONIA

FERRETS

• Bronchodilators—theophylline (4.25 mg/kg PO q8–12h) or terbutaline (0.01 mg/kg SC, IM)

CONTRAINDICATIONS/POSSIBLE INTERACTIONS
• Diuretics—contraindicated
• Corticosteroids—avoid; predisposes the patient to infection
• Theophylline-derivative bronchodilators—use cautiously when combined with fluoroquinolone antibiotics and chloramphenicol; these antibiotics may prolong clearance of bronchodilators, resulting in signs of toxicity
• Anticholinergics and antihistamines—may thicken secretions and inhibit mucokinesis and exudate removal from airways

PRECAUTIONS
Antitussives—use with caution and only for short intervals to control intractable cough; potent, centrally acting agents may inhibit mucokinesis and exudate removal from airways.

FOLLOW-UP

PATIENT MONITORING
• Auscultate patient thoroughly several times daily.

• Thoracic radiographs—improve more slowly than the clinical appearance

PREVENTION/AVOIDANCE
• Vaccination against CDV
• Avoid contact with humans or other ferrets with influenza
• Identify and manage the underlying cause of aspiration pneumonia

EXPECTED COURSE AND PROGNOSIS
Prognosis—good to guarded with aggressive therapy; more guarded in young animals, patients with immunodeficiency, and patients that are debilitated or have severe underlying disease

MISCELLANEOUS

ZOONOTIC POTENTIAL
Influenza virus can be transmitted to humans.

SEE ALSO
Canine distemper virus
Influenza virus
Dyspnea and tachypnea

ABBREVIATIONS
CDV = canine distemper virus
IFA = immunoflorescent antibody test

Suggested Reading
Capello V, Lennox AM. Diagnostic imaging of the respiratory system in exotic companion mammals. Vet Clin Exot Anim 2011;14:369–389.
Di Girolamo N, Selleri P. Medical and surgical emergencies in ferrets. Vet Clin North Am Exot Anim Pract 2016;19:431–464.
Johnson-Delaney CA. Ferret respiratory system: clinical anatomy, physiology, and disease. Vet Clin Exot Anim 2011;14:357–367.
Kiupel M, Perpiñán D. Viral diseases of ferrets. In: Fox JG, Marini RP, eds. Biology and Diseases of the Ferret, 3rd ed. John Wiley & Sons, 2014:439–517.
Lennox A. Respiratory disorders in ferrets. Vet Clin Exot Anim 2021;24:483–493.
Perpiñán D. Respiratory diseases of ferrets. In: Quesenberry KE, Carpenter JW, eds. Ferrets, Rabbits and Rodents, 4th ed. Clinical Medicine and Surgery. 2021. St. Louis: Saunders, 2020:71–76.
Swenson SL, Koster LG, Jenkins-Moore M et al. Natural cases of 2009 pandemic H1N1 Influenza A virus in pet ferrets. J Vet Diagn Invest 2010;22(5):784–788.
Author Barbara Oglesbee DVM, DABVP (Avian)

PODODERMATITIS AND NAIL BED DISORDERS

BASICS

DEFINITION
Inflammation of the feet, including foot pads, nail bed, and interdigital spaces

PATHOPHYSIOLOGY
• Depends on the underlying cause
• Causes include infectious, allergic, neoplastic, and environmental diseases; autoimmune and endocrine or metabolic causes have not been described in ferrets
• Nails and nail folds—subject to trauma, infection, neoplasia, and dystrophy
• Psychogenic dermatoses not reported

SYSTEMS AFFECTED
Skin/Exocrine—primary or secondary infection (bacterial, fungal, or parasitic); neoplasia

INCIDENCE/PREVALENCE
Uncommon presenting complaint in pet ferrets

SIGNALMENT
No age or sex predilection

SIGNS
Historical Findings
• History—extremely important; determine the environment and general husbandry (e.g., unsanitary conditions, other pets affected, trauma, contact irritants, and vaccination status)
• Lesions elsewhere on the body—may aid in the diagnosis of the cause
• Licking
• Lameness
• Pain
• Swelling, erythema, exudate, or hyperkeratosis
• Deformity or sloughing of nail

CAUSES
• Viral—canine distemper virus is a common cause of pododermatitis in ferrets, usually causing hyperkeratosis.
• Parasitic—sarcoptic mange: (relatively common) two forms recognized, one involving primarily the feet another more generalized or localized to other areas of the body; demodex—very rare in ferrets
• Neoplastic—epitheliotropic lymphoma, mast cell tumor (most common) hemangioma/hemangiopericytoma, squamous cell carcinoma
• Bacterial—pyoderma, abscess
• Mycotic—dermatomycosis
• Trauma
• Immunologic—contact dermatitis has been anecdotally reported in ferrets. Cutaneous lesions resembling urticaria or histologic lesions characteristic of allergic reactions in

other species have also been anecdotally reported; however, there are no confirmed cases of atopy, food allergy, or other allergic dermatitis in ferrets.

RISK FACTORS
• Infection—trauma, unsanitary conditions
• CDV—contact of nonimmunized animals with CDV-infected animals (ferrets, dogs, or wild carnivores)

DIAGNOSIS

DIFFERENTIAL DIAGNOSIS
• CDV—pododermatitis usually follows a catarrhal phase characterized by naso-ocular discharge depression, and anorexia, followed by a characteristic, erythematous, pruritic rash on the chin and lips and spreads caudally to the inguinal area; pododermatitis is characterized by hyperkeratinization of the footpads, erythema, and swelling. CDV is uniformly fatal, and signs other than pododermatitis alone will be seen.
• Sarcoptic mange—foot lesions characterized by severe inflammation and crusting that can progress to nail and skin sloughing if untreated; generally extremely pruritic/painful
• Neoplastic—with most tumor types only one foot is affected; lymphoma may affect multiple feet; can be nodular, inflamed, swollen, or ulcerative, depending on tumor type. Mast cell tumors—raised alopecic nodules; may become ulcerated or covered with a thick black crust; may be single or multiple. Squamous cell carcinoma—usually firm and ulcerated. Hemangioma/hemangiopericytoma—swelling, red/purple discoloration
• Bacterial—swelling, diffuse, or localized depending on the underlying cause (e.g., cellulitis vs. abscess), inflammation, may be ulcerated
• Mycotic—dermatophytes rarely involve feet; partial to complete alopecia with scaling; with or without erythema; not always ringlike; may begin as small papules
• Trauma—depends on the underlying cause; usually only one digit or foot; chronic interdigital inflammation, ulceration, pyogranulomatous abscesses, draining tracts, or swelling, with or without pruritus
• Hypersensitivity/contact irritant—uncommon cause; dermatitis of the ventral interdigital surfaces is usually worse, although the whole paw may be involved; feet appear erythematous and alopecic, secondary to pruritus

CBC/BIOCHEMISTRY/URINALYSIS
• Depend on the underlying cause
• Rarely used in the initial workup

OTHER LABORATORY TESTS
• CDV—fluorescent antibody test (IFA)—can be performed on peripheral blood or buffy coat smears, conjunctival, or mucous membrane scrapings. Vaccination will not affect the results.

IMAGING
• Radiographs and ultrasound—rarely used in the initial workup; evaluate digits for bony lysis, may suggest neoplasia
• Neoplastic—depending on the underlying cause, evaluate for metastases or primary tumor site

DIAGNOSTIC PROCEDURES
• Skin scrapings, fungal culture, and cytologic examination of a stained smear of any exudate or pustule contents
• Biopsy or FNA—histopathology, rule out neoplasia
• Wood's lamp—do not use as the sole means of diagnosing or excluding dermatomycosis, owing to false negatives and misinterpretations of fluorescence
• Trial therapy—to rule out scabies; can be difficult to diagnose; skin scrapes often negative; trial course (ivermectin) may be necessary to rule out

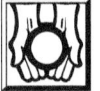

TREATMENT

APPROPRIATE HEALTH CARE
Outpatient, unless surgery is indicated

NURSING CARE
Foot soaks, hot packing, and/or bandaging may be necessary, depending on the cause.

ACTIVITY
Depends on the severity of the lesions and the underlying cause

SURGICAL CONSIDERATIONS
• Neoplasia—may require surgical excision or amputation, depending on tumor type
• Infectious—abscess—lance and drain exudate; severe infections/necrosis—may benefit from surgical debridement of devitalized tissue before medical therapy

MEDICATIONS

DRUG(S) OF CHOICE
• CDV—supportive care only, uniformly fatal
• Sarcoptic mites—ivermectin 0.2–0.4 mg/kg SC q14d for 3 to 4 doses
• Neoplasia—depends on tumor type, for example, lymphoma may respond to prednisone or other chemotherapeutic protocols

PODODERMATITIS AND NAIL BED DISORDERS (CONTINUED)

FERRETS

• Bacterial pododermatitis, abscess, cellulitis—systemic antibiotics based on culture and sensitivity; trimethoprim/sulfonamide (15–30 mg/kg PO, SC q12h), amoxicillin/clavulanate (13–25 mg/kg PO q12h) or enrofloxacin (10–20 mg/kg PO, SC, IM q12h) pending culture result
• Dermatophytosis—topical therapy—miconazole shampoo (with or without chlorhexidine) plus fluconazole (10 mg/kg PO q12h) or ketoconazole (10–15 mg/kg PO q24h) or itraconazole (10–20 mg/kg PO q24h) for 4–8 weeks
• Hypersensitivity/contact irritant—wash feet to remove substance; antihistamines—hydroxyzine (2 mg/kg PO q8h); diphenhydramine (0.5–2.0 mg/kg PO q8–12h); chlorpheniramine (1–2 mg/kg PO q8–12h); corticosteroids—prednisone (0.25–1.0 mg/kg PO q24h, divided)

CONTRAINDICATIONS
N/A

PRECAUTIONS
• Depend on the treatment protocol selected for the underlying cause; see specific drugs and their precautions
• Ivermectin—anecdotally associated with birth defects when used in pregnant jills

POSSIBLE INTERACTIONS
Depend on the underlying cause and treatment protocol selected

ALTERNATIVE DRUGS
N/A

FOLLOW-UP

PATIENT MONITORING
Depends on the underlying cause and treatment protocol selected

PREVENTION/AVOIDANCE
• Vaccination for CDV
• Environmental causes—good husbandry and preventative medical practices should avoid recurrence

POSSIBLE COMPLICATIONS
Depend on the underlying cause and treatment protocol selected

EXPECTED COURSE AND PROGNOSIS
• Success of therapy depends on finding the underlying cause
• Sarcoptes—prognosis is good to guarded depending on the severity of lesions at presentation
• Bacterial—usually good; however, treatment may be prolonged
• Dermatophytes—prognosis is good
• Neoplasia—some can be totally excised or removed; others are highly malignant and may have already spread by the time of diagnosis.

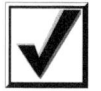

MISCELLANEOUS

ASSOCIATED CONDITIONS
N/A

AGE-RELATED FACTORS
N/A

ZOONOTIC POTENTIAL
Some causes (e.g., sarcoptic mange)

PREGNANCY
Avoid ivermectin

SYNONYMS
N/A

SEE ALSO
Alopecia, CDV; pruritus

ABBREVIATIONS
CDV = canine distemper virus
FNA = fine-needle aspiration
IFA = immunofluorescent antibody

Suggested Reading
d'Ovidio D, Santoro D. Dermatologic diseases of ferrets. In: Quesenberry KE, Carpenter JW, eds. Ferrets, Rabbits and Rodents, 4th ed. Clinical Medicine and Surgery. 2021. St. Louis: Saunders, 2020:109–116.
Hoppmann E, Wilson Barron H. Ferret and rabbit dermatology. J Exot Pet Med 2007;16:225–237.
Kiupel M, Perpiñán D. Viral diseases of ferrets. In: Fox JG, Marini RP, eds. Biology and Diseases of the Ferret, 3rd ed. John Wiley & Sons, 2014:439–517.
Morrisey JK, Malakoff RJ. Cardiovascular and other diseases of ferrets. In: Quesenberry KE, Carpenter JW, eds. Ferrets, Rabbits and Rodents, 4th ed. Clinical Medicine and Surgery. 2021. St. Louis: Saunders, 2020:5–70.
Williams BH, Wyre NR. Neoplasia in ferrets. In: Quesenberry KE, Carpenter JW, eds. Ferrets, Rabbits and Rodents, 4th ed. Clinical Medicine and Surgery. 2021. St. Louis: Saunders, 2020:92–108.

Author Barbara Oglesbee, DVM, DABVP (Avian)

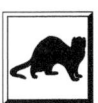 **BASICS**

DEFINITION
• Polyuria is defined as greater than normal urine production, and polydipsia as greater than normal water consumption. Assessment may be more subjective in ferrets since an extremely wide range of urine production has been reported, ranging from 26 to 140 mL/24 hr, and normal water consumption volume has been reported to be 75–100 mL/kg/24 hr.
• Polyuria and polydipsia are uncommon clinical complaints in ferrets.

PATHOPHYSIOLOGY
• Urine production and water consumption (thirst) are controlled by interactions between the kidneys, pituitary gland, and hypothalamus.
• Usually, polydipsia occurs as a compensatory response to polyuria to maintain hydration. The patient's plasma becomes relatively hypertonic and activates thirst mechanisms. Occasionally, polydipsia may be the primary process and polyuria is the compensatory response. Then, the patient's plasma becomes relatively hypotonic because of excessive water intake, and ADH secretion is reduced, resulting in polyuria.

SYSTEMS AFFECTED
• Renal/Urologic—kidneys
• Endocrine/Metabolic—pituitary gland and hypothalamus
• Cardiovascular—alterations in "effective" circulating volume

SIGNALMENT
• More likely to be seen in middle-aged to older ferrets
• No sex predilection

SIGNS
N/A

CAUSES
• Primary polyuria due to impaired renal response to ADH—renal failure, pyelonephritis, pyometra, paraurethral or prostatic abscess, hepatic failure, hypercalcemia, hypokalemia, and drugs
• Primary polyuria caused by osmotic diuresis—diabetes mellitus, post obstructive diuresis, some diuretics (e.g., mannitol and furosemide), ingestion or administration of large quantities of solute (e.g., sodium chloride, or glucose)
• Primary polyuria due to ADH deficiency—(not reported in ferrets but should be considered) traumatic, neoplastic; some drugs (e.g., alcohol)
• Primary polydipsia—such as behavioral problems, pyrexia, or pain; organic disease of

the anterior hypothalamic thirst center of neoplastic, traumatic, or inflammatory origin—not reported in ferrets but should be considered

RISK FACTORS
• Renal disease, liver disease, or adrenal disease (paraurethral or prostatic abscess; pyometra)
• Selected electrolyte disorders
• Administration of diuretics and anticonvulsants

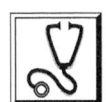 **DIAGNOSIS**

DIFFERENTIAL DIAGNOSIS
Differentiating Similar Signs
• Differentiate polyuria from an abnormal increase in the frequency of urination (pollakiuria). Pollakiuria is often associated with dysuria, stranguria, or hematuria. Patients with polyuria void large quantities of urine; patients with pollakiuria typically void small quantities of urine.
• Measuring urinary specific gravity may provide evidence of adequate urine-concentrating ability (1.030), which rules out polyuria/polydipsia.

Differentiating Causes
• If associated with progressive weight loss—consider renal failure, diabetes mellitus, hepatic failure, pyometra, and pyelonephritis
• If associated with polyphagia—consider diabetes mellitus (rare)
• If associated with bilateral alopecia and other cutaneous problems—consider concurrent adrenal disease (prostatic abscess)
• If associated with signs of nausea such as anorexia, pawing at the mouth, and bruxism (occasionally vomiting)—consider renal failure, pyelonephritis, hepatic failure, and diabetes mellitus
• If associated with swollen vulva in an intact female—consider pyometra
• If associated with abdominal distention—consider hepatic failure
• If associated with behavioral or neurologic disorder—consider hepatic failure, primary polydipsia, or concurrent insulinoma

CBC/BIOCHEMISTRY/URINALYSIS
• Serum sodium concentration may help differentiate primary polyuria from primary polydipsia. Plasma osmolarity has been reported to be 328 ± 1 mOsm/kg, rising to 366 ± 11 following 24 hours of water deprivation for normal ferrets.
• Relative hypernatremia or high serum osmolarity suggests primary polyuria.
• Hyponatremia or low serum osmolarity suggests primary polydipsia.

• Azotemia is consistent with renal causes for polyuria/polydipsia but may also indicate dehydration resulting from inadequate compensatory polydipsia. Normal creatinine is significantly lower in ferrets compared with dogs, cats, and other small mammals (normal 0.2–0.6 mg/dL); any increase in serum creatinine should be considered significant. Increased BUN is seen more commonly than increases in serum creatinine in ferrets with renal disease.
• Unexpectedly low BUN concentrations may suggest hepatic failure.
• High hepatic enzyme activities are consistent hepatic failure, pyometra, and diabetes mellitus.
• Persistent hyperglycemia is consistent with diabetes mellitus.
• Hyperkalemia, particularly if associated with hyponatremia, suggests possible iatrogenic hypoadrenocorticism or therapy with potassium-sparing diuretics.
• Hypercalcemia and hypokalemia can cause, or occur in association with, other diseases that cause polyuria/polydipsia (e.g., chronic renal failure may be associated with both).
• Hypoalbuminemia supports renal or hepatic causes of polyuria/polydipsia.
• Neutrophilia is consistent with pyelonephritis, pyometra, or hepatitis.
• Glucosuria (rare in ferrets) supports a diagnosis of diabetes mellitus or renal glucosuria; pyuria, white blood cell casts, and/or bacteriuria should prompt consideration of pyelonephritis or paraurethral cysts.

OTHER LABORATORY TESTS
• Urine culture—chronic pyelonephritis cannot be conclusively ruled out by the absence of pyuria or bacteriuria.
• Cytologic examination of lymph node aspirate may provide evidence of lymphosarcoma, which may induce polyuria by direct infiltration of renal tissues (hypercalcemic nephrotoxicity has not been reported in ferrets with lymphoma).
• Elevations in serum estradiol, androstenedione, and 17-hydroxyprogesterone combined are most diagnostic for adrenal disease. (Available through the University of Tennessee Clinical Endocrinology Laboratory, Department of Comparative Medicine)

IMAGING
Abdominal survey radiography and ultrasonography may provide additional evidence of renal (e.g., primary renal diseases and urinary obstruction), hepatic (e.g., microhepatica, hepatic infiltrate), uterine or paraurethral (e.g., pyometra, urogenital/prostatic abscess), or other disorders that can contribute to polyuria/polydipsia.

POLYURIA AND POLYDIPSIA   (CONTINUED)

FERRETS

DIAGNOSTIC PROCEDURES
N/A

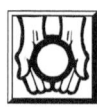

TREATMENT
- Serious medical consequence for the patient is rare if the patient has free access to water and is willing and able to drink. Until the mechanism of polyuria is understood, discourage owners from limiting access to water. Direct treatment at the underlying cause.
- Provide polyuric patients with free access to water unless they are vomiting. If polyuric patients are vomiting, give replacement maintenance (containing dextrose if insulinoma is suspected) fluids parenterally. Also, provide fluids parenterally when other conditions limit oral intake or dehydration persists despite polydipsia.
- Base fluid selection on knowledge of the underlying cause for fluid loss. In most patients, lactated Ringer's solution is an acceptable replacement fluid.
- Primary polydipsia—treat by limiting water intake to a normal daily volume. Monitor the patient closely to avoid iatrogenic dehydration.

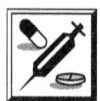

MEDICATIONS
DRUG(S) OF CHOICE
Vary with the underlying cause

CONTRAINDICATIONS
N/A

PRECAUTIONS
Until renal and hepatic failure have been excluded as potential causes for polyuria/polydipsia, use caution in administering any drug eliminated via these pathways.

POSSIBLE INTERACTIONS
N/A

ALTERNATIVE DRUGS
N/A

FOLLOW-UP
PATIENT MONITORING
- Hydration status by clinical assessment of hydration and serial evaluation of body weight
- Fluid intake and urine output—provide a useful baseline for assessing the adequacy of hydration therapy

POSSIBLE COMPLICATIONS
Dehydration

MISCELLANEOUS
ASSOCIATED CONDITIONS
- Insulinoma
- Ferret adrenal disease

AGE-RELATED FACTORS
N/A

ZOONOTIC POTENTIAL
N/A

PREGNANCY/FERTILITY/BREEDING
N/A

SYNONYMS
N/A

SEE ALSO
Diabetes mellitus
Paraurethral cysts (urogenital cystic disease)
Pyometra and stump pyometra
Renal failure
Urinary tract obstruction

ABBREVIATIONS
ADH = antidiuretic hormone
BUN = blood urea nitrogen

Suggested Reading
Di Girolamo N, Huyun M. Disorders of the urinary and reproductive systems in ferrets. In: Quesenberry KE, Carpenter JW, eds. Ferrets, Rabbits and Rodents, 4th ed. Clinical Medicine and Surgery. St. Louis: Saunders, 2020:39–54.
Di Girolamo N, Selleri P. Medical and surgical emergencies in ferrets. Vet Clin Exot Anim Pract 2016;19:431–464.
Hallman RM, Brandão J. Diagnostic imaging of the renal system in exotic companion mammals. Vet Clin Exot Anim 2020;23:195–214.
Reavill DR, Lennox AM. Disease overview of the urinary tract in exotic companion mammals and tips on clinical management. Vet Clin Exot Anim 2020;23(1):169–193.

Author Barbara Oglesbee, DVM, DABVP (Avian)

BASICS

OVERVIEW
• Proliferative bowel disease (PBD) is a characteristic infection of the distal colon caused by the spiral bacteria *Lawsonia intracellularis*. The organism is closely related to the bacterium that causes proliferative enteritis in hamsters and swine.
• May be a co-pathogen with *Campylobacter* spp., Coccidia, or other pathogens.
• Disease is characterized by large bowel diarrhea and rectal prolapse in young ferrets.

SIGNALMENT
• A relatively common disease of weaning-aged ferrets, occasionally seen in adults
• Seen primarily in ferrets 12 weeks to 6 months of age; stressed, immunosuppressed older animals also may be affected

SIGNS
Historical Findings
• Large bowel diarrhea—may be profuse and watery, but more often green in color with mucus; fresh blood usually present, small scant stools with green mucus; tenesmus and crying out when defecating
• Rectal prolapse—highly suggestive of PBD
• Severe weight loss—often losses of over 100 g within a short (2-week) period
• Ataxia, weakness, and muscle tremors
• Anorexia, abdominal discomfort, or generalized unthriftiness

Physical Examination Findings
• Partial to complete rectal prolapse is highly suggestive
• The distal colon may be palpably thickened, mesenteric lymph nodes may be enlarged
• Emaciation, muscle wasting
• Fecal and urine staining of the perineum
• Weakness, ataxia, and dehydration may be noted

CAUSES AND RISK FACTORS
• Stress, poor hygiene, concurrent disease

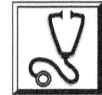

DIAGNOSIS
Presumptive diagnosis is often made on signalment, signs, and response to treatment; definitive diagnosis requires colonic biopsy or PCR on feces.

DIFFERENTIAL DIAGNOSIS
• Epizootic catarrhal enteritis (ECE) and coccidia are also common causes of diarrhea in young ferrets.

• Consider all causes of diarrhea, including systemic or metabolic disease, as well as specific intestinal disorders.
• Blood and mucus in the stool are also seen with coccidia, clostridia, campylobacter, and salmonella. All of these organisms can cause disease alone or be co-pathogens with *Lawsonia intracellularis*.
• Wasting thickened GI tract and palpable mesenteric lymph nodes—consider ECE, clostridia, campylobacter, and lymphoma.

CBC/BIOCHEMISTRY/URINALYSIS
• Leukocytosis is usually seen; differential count often demonstrates neutrophilia with a left shift
• Hypoproteinemia
• Dehydration—elevated PCV, TP, and azotemia

OTHER LABORATORY TESTS
• PCR testing for *Lawsonia intracellularis* on feces
• Fecal direct examination, fecal flotation, and zinc sulfate centrifugation may demonstrate gastrointestinal parasites.

Microbiology
• Aerobic and anaerobic fecal cultures rule out clostridia or salmonella.
• Cultures for *Lawsonia intracellularis* are not useful, since they are intracellular organisms not usually shed in the feces.
• Fecal cytology may demonstrate clostridia or other organisms, increased WBC or RBC numbers

IMAGING
Survey abdominal radiographs—usually normal

DIAGNOSTIC PROCEDURES
• Colonic biopsy would be needed for a definitive diagnosis. Organisms are intracellular (not readily shed in feces) and are demonstrated histologically using silver stains. Exploratory laparotomy may be useful rule out GI foreign bodies, neoplasia, and intestinal inflammatory diseases.
• Since this is an expensive, invasive procedure, diagnosis may be attempted based on response to empirical treatment. However, other diseases or co-pathogens (commonly present) are unlikely to respond to empirical treatment for PBD, necessitating a definitive diagnosis.
• Abdominocentesis and cytology may help determine if perforation and subsequent peritonitis have occurred.

PATHOLOGIC FINDINGS
Grossly thickened and segmented distal colon. Histopathology—mucosal cell proliferation; epithelial hyperplasia; hypertrophy of the tunica muscularis;

organisms demonstrated in epithelium using silver stains

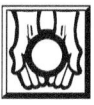

TREATMENT

APPROPRIATE HEALTH CARE
• Most patients with mild to moderate diarrhea can be treated as outpatients.
• Hospitalize when diarrhea is severe, resulting in dehydration and electrolyte imbalance; administer supportive fluids based on hydration status.

DIET
• If anorexic, assist feed an easily digestible high-protein/high-fat diet such as Lafeber Carnivore Critical Care Diet (Lafeber Company, Cornell, IL) or Oxbow Carnivore Critical Care Diet (Oxbow Animal Health, Omaha, NE); if these are unavailable, offer chicken baby foods; may also add dietary supplement such as Nutri-Cal (EVSCO Pharmaceuticals) to increase caloric content to these foods.

SURGICAL CONSIDERATIONS
• Rectal prolapse should be replaced and sutured with a purse-string closure until feces return to normal consistency.
• Owners should be advised to monitor the ferret to be sure defecation occurs while the sutures are in place.

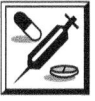

MEDICATIONS

DRUG(S) OF CHOICE
Antibiotics
• Most patients respond well to chloramphenicol palmitate (50 mg/kg PO q12h × 14d) or chloramphenicol sodium succinate (50 mg/kg PO, IM q12h × 14d)
• Metronidazole (20 mg/kg PO q12h × 10–14d) may also be effective.
• Relapses may occur when antibiotics are discontinued, requiring prolonged antibiotic therapy.

FOLLOW-UP

PATIENT MONITORING
• Monitor patients for reoccurrence of diarrhea or concurrent diseases such as GI ulceration or enteric co-pathogens.
• Response to therapy supports the diagnosis; repeat diagnostics are rarely necessary.

PREVENTION/AVOIDANCE
Avoid stress and unsanitary conditions.

PROLIFERATIVE BOWEL DISEASE

FERRETS

POSSIBLE COMPLICATIONS
Colonic ulceration, necrosis, or rupture may occur, leading to septic peritonitis.

EXPECTED COURSE AND PROGNOSIS
• Most animals with mild to moderate disease respond well to chloramphenicol therapy; chronic patients may require long-term therapy; failure to respond suggests concurrent disease; further diagnostic evaluation is indicated.
• Some ferrets have a stunted appearance following recovery

MISCELLANEOUS

ASSOCIATED CONDITIONS
• Other enteric pathogens
• Rectal prolapse

SYNONYMS
Proliferative colitis

SEE ALSO
Coccidiosis
Epizootic catarrhal enteritis
Gastrointestinal and esophageal foreign bodies
Inflammatory bowel disease

ABBREVIATIONS
ECE = epizootic catarrhal enteritis
GI = gastrointestinal
PBD = proliferative bowel disease
PCV = packed cell volume
TP = total protein

Suggested Reading
Di Girolamo N, Selleri P. Medical and surgical emergencies in ferrets. Vet Clin Exot Anim 2016;19:431–464.
Hoefer HL. Gastrointestinal diseases of ferrets. In: Quesenberry KE, Carpenter JW, eds. Ferrets, Rabbits, and Rodents, 4th ed. Clinical Medicine and Surgery. 2021. St. Louis: Saunders, 2020:27–38.
Huynh M, Pignon C. Gastrointestinal disease in exotic small mammals. J Exot Pet Med 2013;22(2):118–131.
Lennox AM, Gladden JN. Emergency and critical care of small mammals. In: Quesenberry KE, Carpenter JW, eds. Ferrets, Rabbits and Rodents, 4th ed. Clinical Medicine and Surgery. 2021. St. Louis: Saunders, 2020:595–608.
MacPhail C. Ferret soft tissue surgery. In: Bennett A, Pye GW, eds. Surgery of Exotic Animals. Wiley-Blackwell, 2021:277–296.
Miwa Y, Sladky K. Common surgical procedures of rodents, ferrets, hedgehogs, and sugar gliders. Vet Clin Exot Anim 2016;19:205–244.
Mullen HS, Scavelli TD, Quesenberry KE et al. Gastrointestinal foreign body in ferrets: 25 cases (1986–1990). J Am Anim Hosp Assoc 1992;28:13–19.
Author Barbara Oglesbee, DVM, DABVP-Avian

BASICS

DEFINITION
- Abnormally large prostate gland determined by abdominal palpation or by abdominal radiography or prostatic ultrasonography
- In ferrets, the prostate is a fusiform structure surrounding the dorsal aspect of the proximal urethra.
- Enlargement is usually due to the direct effects of excessive production of sex steroids from diseased adrenal glands. May result in diffuse prostatic enlargement or urogenital, prostatic, or periprostatic cysts; cystic structures found on the dorsal aspect of the urinary bladder or surrounding the proximal urethra. These structures likely arise from remnants of the mesonephric or paramesonephric ducts, from the prostate, or periprostatic tissues.
- Cysts can become very large, may be single or multiple, and often cause partial or complete obstruction of the urethra.
- Secondary bacterial infections within the cystic fluid are extremely common.

PATHOPHYSIOLOGY
- Prostatic hyperplasia and cyst formation are associated with ferret adrenal disease and the resultant excessive production of androgens.
- Enlargement can result from epithelial cell hyperplasia or hypertrophy, cystic change within the prostatic or periprostatic tissues, neoplasia of prostatic epithelium or stroma, or inflammatory cell infiltration (e.g., acute and chronic bacterial prostatitis and prostatic abscess).
- Obstruction of the urethra may occur due to extraluminal compression by the cyst or hyperplastic tissue, or, with bacterial infection, may become obstructed by thick, tenacious exudate in the urine.
- No information is available on the occurrence of prostatomegaly in intact ferrets without adrenal disease.

SYSTEMS AFFECTED
- Renal/Urologic—obstruction of the urethra, secondary bacterial cystitis
- Gastrointestinal—ferrets with large cysts may have tenesmus
- Peritoneum—focal or generalized peritonitis can develop in animals with bacterial infection of cystic fluid or abscesses

SIGNALMENT
Usually seen in middle-aged males, 3–7 years old

SIGNS

Historical and Physical Examination Findings
- Presenting complaint is typically stranguria due to urethral obstruction by cysts, hyperplastic prostatic tissue, or thick exudate blocking the urethra
- Pollakiuria, tenesmus, dysuria, including intense straining and crying out when urinating
- Stranguria may be confused with constipation.
- With complete obstruction, ferrets will have signs of uremia, including depression, lethargy, and anorexia.
- Weight loss, depression, and anorexia may be seen with secondary bacterial infections (abscesses)
- Thick, white or yellow discharge is often visible at the urethral opening in patients with prostatic abscesses
- Bilaterally symmetric alopecia or pruritus due to adrenal disease
- Abdominal distension
- Large, turgid, painful bladder in ferrets with urethral obstruction
- Fluid-filled cysts are sometimes palpable and may be larger than the urinary bladder.

CAUSES
- Prostatic hyperplasia, urogenital (prostatic, periprostatic) cysts—caused by excessive androgen production due to functional adrenal hyperplasia, adenoma, or carcinomas
- Neoplasia—adenocarcinoma, sarcoma, metastatic neoplasia (rare)

RISK FACTORS
Evidence suggests that adrenal disease may be related to neutering. The gonads and adrenals arise embryonically from the urogenital ridge; some gonadal cells are likely present in the adrenals. Stimulation of these cells by pituitary gonadotropin may cause hypertrophy of these steroid-secreting cells.

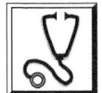

DIAGNOSIS

DIFFERENTIAL DIAGNOSIS
- For stranguria: urolithiasis, neoplasia of the bladder neck or urethra, or urethral stricture
- For mass detected in the region of the prostate: prostatic hyperplasia, prostatic neoplasia, or other abdominal mass—neoplasia, abscess, or granuloma

CBC/BIOCHEMISTRY/URINALYSIS
- CBC—usually normal in patients with sterile cysts or prostatic hyperplasia
- Leukocytosis in patients with prostatic abscess and prostatic neoplasia (occasionally)

- Urinalysis may be helpful to rule out other causes of stranguria such as urolithiasis or bacterial cystitis. However, secondary bacterial infections may cause abscess formation in prostatic or periprostatic cysts. Exudate from these abscesses may drain into the urinary bladder. This exudate can sometimes be thick enough to cause urethral blockage.

OTHER LABORATORY TESTS
- Elevations in plasma estradiol, androstenedione, and 17-hydroxyprogesterone are supportive of ferret adrenal disease (Available through the University of Tennessee Clinical Endocrinology Laboratory, Department of Comparative Medicine)
- Examination of cyst fluid—gross appearance can range from clear, cloudy yellow or thick, yellow to greenish, foul-smelling fluid; cytologic examination ranges from serosanguinous fluid to purulent exudate.
- Culture the fluid for bacteria

IMAGING
- Ultrasonography is the most useful method of imaging the prostate and demonstrating adrenal gland enlargement.
- The prostate often contains single to multiple fluid-filled cysts of varying size; fluid is hypo- or anechoic if no infection is present. With abscess formation, sediment within cysts is usually hyperechoic.
- If paraurethral cysts are present, these appear as hypo- or anechoic pockets surrounding the urethra.
- Uniform parenchymal echogenicity is seen in some ferrets

DIAGNOSTIC PROCEDURES
- Ultrasound-guided aspiration of cystic structures; take care to avoid rupturing a prostatic abscess.

TREATMENT
- Ferret adrenal disease may be treated with adrenalectomy or managed medically. The decision as to which form of treatment is appropriate is multifactorial including which gland is affected (left vs. right), the surgeon's experience and expertise, the severity of clinical signs, patient age, concurrent diseases, and financial issues.
- Removal of the affected adrenal gland(s) and drainage of the cysts at the time of surgery is often curative in ferrets with mild prostatomegaly, sterile cysts, or small abscessed cysts. These procedures require special surgical expertise, especially if the

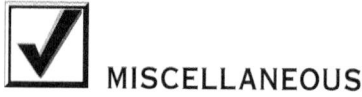
FERRETS

right adrenal gland is diseased. The proximity of the right adrenal to the vena cava and the potential for vena cava invasion by malignant tumors make complete excision a high-risk procedure. Referral to a surgeon or clinician with experience is recommended when possible.

• Fluid therapy, either subcutaneous or intravenous, depending on the state of hydration. Ferrets that are uremic require intravenous fluid therapy. Correct any acid–base disturbances as indicated by the serum biochemistry profile.

• Postoperative fluid therapy should continue for 24–48 hours.

• If the urethra is partially or completely obstructed, catheterize prior to surgery and maintain the catheter in place for 2–3 days postoperatively.

MEDICATIONS

DRUG(S) OF CHOICE

GnRH analogs for medical treatment of adrenal disease:

• Treatment with a GnRH agonist is indicated even if adrenalectomy is performed to prevent the recurrence of disease in the remaining adrenal gland.

• Leuprolide acetate is a potent gonadotropin secretion inhibitor and can begin to reduce prostate size within 12–48 hours post-administration. Smaller cysts may respond to medical treatment alone. Large prostatic cysts or abscesses will require physical debulking. This drug has become challenging to acquire and often prohibitively expensive in the US.

• Deslorelin acetate (Suprelorin-F®, Virbac Animal Health) A 4.7-mg implant is labeled for treatment of adrenal disease in ferrets in the United States and a 9.4-mg implant is available in Europe. However, reduction in prostate size may take days to weeks. Large prostatic cysts or abscesses will require physical debulking.

• If secondary bacterial infection or abscess is evident, antibiotic therapy should be based on results of culture and susceptibility testing. Choose antibiotics that can enter the prostatic lumen such as trimethoprim/sulfonamide (15–30 mg/kg PO, SC q12h), enrofloxacin (5–10 mg/kg PO, SC, IV q12h), or chloramphenicol (25–50 mg/kg PO, SC, IV q12h). A minimum of 4–6 weeks of antimicrobial administration is usually necessary.

CONTRAINDICATIONS
N/A

PRECAUTIONS
N/A

POSSIBLE INTERACTIONS
N/A

ALTERNATIVE DRUGS

• Melatonin implants are available commercially (Ferretonin® 2.7-mg-ferrets < 600g) and 5.4-mg implants—most ferrets, Melatek, LLC) and have been used in ferrets with adrenal disease to alleviate alopecia and, possibly, aggressive behavior, prostatomegaly, or vulvar swelling. However, effectiveness in the reduction of prostate size is questionable and the time interval required for the resolution of clinical signs limits its usefulness.

• Antiandrogen agents have been used to further reduce prostate size along with surgical and/or GnRH analog treatment. Choices include flutamide (10 mg/kg PO q12–24h), bicalutamide (5 mg/kg PO q12h), and finasteride (5 mg/kg PO q24h). The use of these medications is largely anecdotal but appears to be safe and effective.

FOLLOW-UP

PATIENT MONITORING

• Monitor for the development of gastritis due to the overgrowth of *Helicobacter mustelae*, common in ferrets undergoing stress.

• Following adrenalectomy, prostatic tissue should decrease in size within 1–3 days.

• With medical therapy, reduction in prostate size has been anecdotally reported to occur in as little as 2–3 days, but reports of weeks to months for a response (or no response at all) also exist.

• Abdominal ultrasonography to assess the efficacy of treatment

• Urine culture to access the efficacy of treatment in patients with abscessed cysts and bacterial cystitis

POSSIBLE COMPLICATIONS

• Urethral obstruction
• Peritonitis
• Return of prostatomegaly if all hyperfunctioning adrenal tissue is not removed or disease develops in the remaining gland

MISCELLANEOUS

ASSOCIATED CONDITIONS

• Ferret adrenal disease—always
• Insulinoma, lymphoma, and/or congestive heart failure are common in ferrets in this age range.
• Gastritis due to the overgrowth of *Helicobacter mustelae* is common in ferrets undergoing stress

AGE-RELATED FACTORS

The risk of anesthetic or surgical complications is increased in geriatric ferrets.

ZOONOTIC POTENTIAL
N/A

PREGNANCY/FERTILITY/BREEDING
N/A

SYNONYMS

Paraurethral cysts
Periprostatic cysts
Prostatic cysts

SEE ALSO

Adrenal disease (hyperadrenocorticism)
Paraurethral cysts (urogenital cystic disease)
Prostatitis and prostatic abscesses

ABBREVIATIONS

FSH = follicular-stimulating hormone
GnRH = gonadotropin-releasing hormone
LH = luteinizing hormone

Suggested Reading
Bo P, Tagliavia C, Canova M, DeSilva M, Bombardi C, Grandis A. Comparative characterization of the prostate gland in intact, and surgically and chemically neutered ferrets. J Exot Pet Med 2019;31:68–74.
Di Girolamo N, Huyun M. Disorders of the urinary and reproductive systems in ferrets. In: Quesenberry KE, Carpenter JW, eds. Ferrets, Rabbits and Rodents, 4th ed. Clinical Medicine and Surgery. St. Louis: Saunders, 2020:39–54.
Di Girolamo N, Selleri P. Medical and surgical emergencies in ferrets. Vet Clin Exot Anim Pract 2016;19:431–464.
Jekl V, Hauptman K. Reproductive medicine in ferrets. Vet Clin Exot Anim Pract 2017;20(2):629–663.
Lennox AM, Wagner RA. Comparison of 4.7-mg deslorelin implants and surgery for the treatment of adrenocortical disease in ferrets. J Exot Pet Med. 2012;21:332–335.
Powers LV, Winkler K, Garner MM et al. Omentalization of prostatic abscesses and

large cysts in ferrets (*Mustela putorius furo*). J Exot Pet Med 2007;16:186–189.

Schoemaker NJ, Van Zealand YRA. Endocrine diseases of ferrets. In: Quesenberry KE, Carpenter JW, eds. Ferrets, Rabbits and Rodents, 4th ed. Clinical Medicine and Surgery. St. Louis: Saunders, 2020:77–91.

Schoemaker NJ, van Deijk R, Muijlaert B et al. Use of a gonadotropin releasing hormone agonist implant as an alternative for surgical castration in male ferrets (*Mustela putorius furo*). Theriogenology 2008;70:161–167.

Swiderski JK, Seim HB, MacPhail CM et al. Long-term outcome of domestic ferrets treated surgically for hyperadrenocorticism: 130 cases (1995–2004). J Am Vet Med Assoc 2008;232:1338–1343.

Wagner RA, Piché CA, Jöchle W et al. Clinical and endocrine responses to treatment with deslorelin acetate implants in ferrets with adrenocortical disease. Am J Vet Res 2005;66:910–914.

Author Barbara Oglesbee, DVM, DABVP (Avian)

PRURITUS

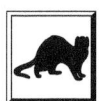

BASICS

DEFINITION
The sensation that provokes the desire to scratch, rub, chew, or lick; often an indicator of inflamed skin

PATHOPHYSIOLOGY
• Pruritus, or itching, is a primary cutaneous sensation that may be elicited from the epidermis, dermis, or mucous membranes.

SYSTEMS AFFECTED
• Skin/Exocrine
• Endocrine/Metabolic

SIGNALMENT
Variable; depends on the underlying cause

SIGNS
• The act of scratching, licking, biting, or chewing
• Evidence of self-trauma and cutaneous inflammation is often present.
• Alopecia often seen

CAUSES
• Endocrine—pruritus, often severe, occurs in approximately 30% of ferrets with adrenal disease
• Parasitic—fleas and sarcoptic mange—usually pruritic; *Otodectes cyanotis* (ear mites) occasionally pruritic; *Demodex*—very rare in ferrets, may be pruritic
• Neoplastic—cutaneous epitheliotropic lymphoma; mast cell tumor
• Bacterial/fungal—pyoderma, dermatomycosis
• Immunologic—contact dermatitis has been anecdotally reported in ferrets. Cutaneous lesions resembling urticaria or histologic lesions characteristic of allergic reactions in other species have also been anecdotally reported; however, there are no confirmed cases of atopy, food allergy, or other allergic dermatitis in ferrets.

RISK FACTORS
N/A

DIAGNOSIS

DIFFERENTIAL DIAGNOSIS
• Alopecia—diffuse/symmetrical: Over 95% of neutered ferrets with bilaterally symmetric alopecia have adrenal disease. Alopecia typically begins in the tail region and progresses cranially. In severe cases, the ferret will become completely bald. In most cases, the skin has a normal appearance, although 30% of affected ferrets are pruritic and secondary pyoderma is occasionally seen.

Other signs related to adrenal disease, such as a swollen vulva in spayed females, may be seen.
• Alopecia—focal: In most cases, a clear history of pruritus is noted; some animals may excessively lick themselves without the owner's knowledge; ear mites, scabies, dermatomycosis, bacterial pyoderma, and some cutaneous neoplasms may all cause alopecia with varying degrees of inflammation and pruritus.

Distribution of Lesions
• Ear mites—most ferrets with ear mites are not pruritic. In pruritic animals, see partial to complete alopecia caudal to the ears; waxy brown aural discharge; excoriations around the pinna
• Fleas—patchy alopecia at the tail base and in cervical and dorsal thoracic region; excoriations; secondary pyoderma sometimes seen
• Sarcoptic mange—two forms reported—generalized with diffuse alopecia and intense pruritus, and local form affecting the feet with secondary pododermatitis
• Bacterial dermatitis—usually secondary infection; primary is rare—localized or multifocal areas alopecia depending on the primary cause, lesions may appear ulcerated
• Dermatomycosis—partial to complete alopecia with scaling; with or without erythema; not always ringlike; may begin as small papules
• Mast cell tumors—often pruritic; raised alopecic nodules; may become ulcerated or covered with a thick black crust; may be single or multiple, usually found on neck and trunk

CBC/BIOCHEMISTRY/URINALYSIS
N/A

OTHER LABORATORY TESTS
• Ferret adrenal disease—elevations in plasma estradiol, androstenedione, and 17-hydroxyprogesterone combined (available through the Clinical Endocrinology Laboratory, Department of Comparative Medicine, University of Tennessee) are supportive of the diagnosis.

IMAGING
Ultrasonography—evaluate adrenal glands for evidence of ferret adrenal disease

DIAGNOSTIC PROCEDURES
• Skin scrapes, epidermal cytology, and dermatophyte cultures (with microscopic identification)—identify primary or coexisting diseases caused by parasites or other microorganisms
• Microscopic examination of ear exudate placed in mineral oil—usually a very effective means of identifying ear mites

• Wood's lamp—do not use as the sole means of diagnosing or excluding dermatomycosis, owing to false negatives and misinterpretations of fluorescence
• Skin biopsy or fine-needle aspiration—useful to diagnose cutaneous neoplasms
• Trial therapy—to rule out scabies; can be difficult to diagnose; skin scrapes often negative; trial course (ivermectin) may be necessary to rule out

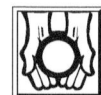

TREATMENT
More than one disease may be contributing to the itching; if treatment for an identified condition does not result in improvement, consider other causes.

SURGICAL CONSIDERATIONS
Adrenalectomy may be the preferred treatment for adrenal disease in ferrets. Consider the age of the ferret, concurrent diseases, and the owner's financial considerations when determining if medical or surgical treatment is most appropriate.

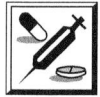

MEDICATIONS

DRUG(S) OF CHOICE
Varies with the specific cause
• Ferret Adrenal Disease–the GnRH agonist deslorelin acetate (Suprelorin-F®, Virbac Animal Health) is labeled for the treatment of adrenal disease in domestic ferrets in the United States. It is a 4.7-mg slow-release deslorelin implant reported to provide alleviation of clinical signs lasting from 8 to 20 months. Alleviation of clinical signs may be more likely in patients with adrenal hyperplasia or adenoma; adenocarcinomas may be less likely to respond. Deslorelin has no demonstrated effect on adrenal tumor growth or metastasis. In Europe, 9.4 mg deslorelin
• Ear mites—topical ivermectin: 1% ivermectin diluted 1:10 in propylene glycol, administered at 400 mcg/kg q2w × 2 treatments or ivermectin (0.4 mg/kg PO, SC q14–28d); or selamectin (Revolution, Pfizer) 15 mg/kg topically q30d
• Fleas—fipronil (Frontline, Boehringer Ingelheim) 0.2–0.4 mL/animal applied topically q30d; imidacloprid (Advantage, Bayer) 10 mg/kg topically q30d; imidacloprid and moxidectin (Advantage Multi for Cats, Bayer) 0.4 mL/animal topically q30d; selamectin (Revolution, Pfizer) 15 mg/kg topically q30d

• Sarcoptic mange—ivermectin 0.2–0.4 mg/kg SC q14d for 3 to 4 doses; selamectin (Revolution, Pfizer) 15 mg/kg topically q30d
• Bacterial folliculitis—shampoos and antibiotic therapy, preferably based on culture and susceptibility testing; good initial choices include amoxicillin/clavulanate (13–25 mg/kg PO q12h), cephalexin (15–30 mg/kg PO q12h), or trimethoprim/sulfa (15–30 mg/kg PO q12h)
• Dermatophytosis—topical therapy—miconazole shampoo (with or without chlorhexidine) plus fluconazole (10 mg/kg PO q12h) or ketoconazole (10–15 mg/kg PO q24h) or itraconazole (10–20 mg/kg PO q24h) for 4–8 weeks

Symptomatic therapy
• The efficacy of topical sprays, lotions, creams, and shampoos used in dogs and cats has not been evaluated in ferrets. Colloidal oatmeal and steroids have been anecdotally reported as the most useful topical medications.
• Corticosteroids—most effective in controlling itching; prednisone (0.25–1.0 mg/kg q24h PO divided).
• Antihistamines—use is anecdotal, generally not as effective as steroids. Hydroxyzine HCl (92 mg/kg PO q8h); diphenhydramine (0.5–2.0 mg/kg PO, SC, IM q8–12h); chlorpheniramine (1–2 mg/kg PO q8–12h)

CONTRAINDICATIONS
• Do not administer topical and oral/parenteral ivermectin simultaneously

PRECAUTIONS
Topical Antiparasitic Agents
• Sometimes the application of anything topically, including water and products containing alcohol, iodine, and benzoyl peroxide, can exacerbate itching; cool water may be soothing

• Flea shampoos, sprays, or powders—use cautiously and sparingly to minimize ingestion during grooming

Steroids
• Most well-known drug used to control itching
• Used wisely, usually safe
• Avoid long-term daily administration of oral corticosteroids.
• Short-term use seldom causes serious problems.
• In ferrets with concurrent infectious diseases, use corticosteroids with caution.

POSSIBLE INTERACTIONS
N/A

ALTERNATIVE DRUGS
N/A

FOLLOW-UP
PATIENT MONITORING
Monitor for alleviation of itching and hair regrowth

POSSIBLE COMPLICATIONS
N/A

MISCELLANEOUS
ASSOCIATED CONDITIONS
N/A

AGE-RELATED FACTORS
N/A

ZOONOTIC POTENTIAL
Some causes (e.g., sarcoptic mange)

PREGNANCY/FERTILITY/BREEDING
N/A

SEE ALSO
Adrenal disease (hyperadrenocorticism)
Dermatophytosis
Ear mites
Fleas and flea infestation

ABBREVIATIONS
FSH = follicular-stimulating hormone
GnRH = gonadotropin-releasing hormone
LH = luteinizing hormone

Suggested Reading
d'Ovidio D, Santoro D. Dermatologic diseases of ferrets. In: Quesenberry KE, Carpenter JW, eds. Ferrets, Rabbits and Rodents, 4th ed. Clinical Medicine and Surgery. 2021. St. Louis: Saunders, 2020:109–116.
Hoppmann E, Wilson Barron H. Ferret and rabbit dermatology. J Exot Pet Med 2007;16:225–237.
Schoemaker NJ, Van Zealand YRA. Endocrine diseases of ferrets. In: Quesenberry KE, Carpenter JW, eds. Ferrets, Rabbits and Rodents, 4th ed. Clinical Medicine and Surgery. St. Louis: Saunders, 2020:77–91.
Schoemaker NJ, van Deijk R, Muijlaert B et al. Use of a gonadotropin-releasing hormone agonist implant as an alternative for surgical castration in male ferrets (*Mustela putorius furo*). Theriogenology 2008;70(2):161–167.
Swiderski JK, Seim HB, MacPhail CM et al. Long-term outcome of domestic ferrets treated surgically for hyperadrenocorticism: 130 cases (1995–2004). J Am Vet Med Assoc 2008;232:1338–1343.
Wagner RA, Piché CA, Jöchle W et al. Clinical and endocrine responses to treatment with deslorelin acetate implants in ferrets with adrenocortical disease. Am J Vet Res 2005;66:910–914.

Author Barbara Oglesbee, DVM, DABVP (Avian)

PTYALISM

BASICS

DEFINITION
- Excessive production of saliva
- Pseudoptyalism is the excessive release of saliva that has accumulated in the oral cavity.

PATHOPHYSIOLOGY
- Ptyalism is an extremely common complaint in ferrets and usually associated with nausea.
- Lesions involving either the CNS or the oral cavity can cause excessive salivation.
- Diseases that affect the pharynx, esophagus, and stomach also stimulate excessive production of saliva.
- Normal saliva production may appear excessive in patients with an anatomic abnormality that allows saliva to dribble out of the mouth or a condition that affects swallowing (pseudoptyalism).

SYSTEMS AFFECTED
N/A

SIGNALMENT
- Young animals are more likely to have ptyalism caused by ingestion of a toxin, caustic agent, or foreign body.
- Older animals are more likely to have ptyalism due to nausea from GI or metabolic disease.

SIGNS

Historical Findings
- Pawing at the face or muzzle—frequently accompanies ptyalism, common sign of nausea; can also occur in patients with oral discomfort or pain
- Anorexia—seen most often in patients with oral lesions, gastrointestinal disease, and systemic disease
- Teeth grinding—seen with oral or gastrointestinal pain
- Vomiting—secondary to gastrointestinal or systemic disease
- Diarrhea or melena—seen with gastrointestinal tract disease
- Eating behavior changes—patients with oral disease may refuse to eat hard food, not chew with the affected side (patients with unilateral lesions), hold the head in an unusual position while eating, or drop prehended food.
- Other behavioral changes—irritability, aggressiveness, and reclusiveness are common, especially in patients with a painful condition or ferrets with hypoglycemia due to insulinoma.
- Dysphagia—may be seen if inability to swallow

- Neurologic signs—patients that have been exposed to causative drugs or toxins, insulinomas, and (rarely) hepatic encephalopathy

Physical Examination Findings
- May be normal in many ferrets with insulinomas or GI tract diseases
- Weight loss, muscle wasting—with GI or metabolic disease
- Abdominal palpation—may reveal GI foreign body, mesenteric lymphadenopathy, thickened intestinal tract, or splenomegaly
- Periodontal disease—inflammation may cause ptyalism
- Stomatitis, lesions of the tongue or oropharynx—ulceration and inflammation of many different causes is associated with ptyalism
- Mass in the oral cavity
- Halitosis—usually caused by oral cavity disease
- Facial pain—caused by oral cavity or pharyngeal disease
- Dysphagia—caused by oral cavity, pharyngeal, or neuromuscular disease or abnormally large retropharyngeal lymph nodes
- Salivary gland problem—inflamed, necrotic, or painful salivary glands can cause ptyalism (not yet reported in ferrets)

CAUSES

Metabolic Disorders
- Insulinoma—very common cause; hypoglycemia causes nausea characterized by ptyalism and pawing at the mouth
- Uremia
- Hepatoencephalopathy—hepatic failure

Gastrointestinal Disorders
- Gastric ulcer—very common cause
- GI foreign body—very common cause
- Infiltrative gastroenteritis—also common in ferrets; eosinophilic gastroenteritis, lymphoplasmacytic gastroenteritis, and GI lymphoma
- Infectious or parasitic gastroenteritis—ECE, salmonellosis, and giardiasis

Esophageal Disorders
- Esophageal foreign body
- Esophageal neoplasm
- Esophagitis—secondary to ingestion of a caustic agent or poisonous plant
- Megaesophagus

Oral and Pharyngeal Diseases
- Foreign body
- Neoplasm
- Gingivitis or stomatitis—secondary to periodontal disease, uremia, ingestion of a caustic agent, poisonous plant, or burns (e.g., those from biting on an electrical cord)

Salivary Gland Diseases
- Sialocele (ranula)—not yet reported in ferrets

Neurologic Disorders
- Canine distemper virus
- Rabies
- Botulism
- Disorders that cause seizures—during a seizure, ptyalism may occur because of autonomic discharge or reduced swallowing of saliva and may be exacerbated by chomping of the jaws
- Nausea associated with vestibular disease

Drugs and Toxins
- Those that are caustic (e.g., household cleaning products and some common house plants)
- Those with a disagreeable taste—many antibiotics and anthelminthics
- Those that induce hypersalivation, including organophosphate compounds, cholinergic drugs, insecticides containing boric acid, pyrethrin and pyrethroid insecticides, caffeine, and illicit drugs such as amphetamines, cocaine, and opiates

RISK FACTORS
N/A

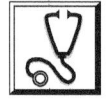

DIAGNOSIS

DIFFERENTIAL DIAGNOSIS
- Differentiating causes of ptyalism and pseudoptyalism requires a thorough history, including possible foreign body exposure, current medications, and possible toxin exposure.
- May be able to distinguish salivation associated with nausea (signs of depression, pawing at the mouth, and anorexia) from dysphagia by observing the patient
- Complete physical examination (with special attention to the oral cavity and neck) and neurologic examination are critical; wear examination gloves when rabies exposure is possible.

CBC/BIOCHEMISTRY/URINALYSIS
- CBC—often normal; leukocytosis in patients with infectious disease; lymphocytosis possible in ferrets with lymphoma; eosinophilia sometimes seen in ferrets with eosinophilic gastroenteritis
- Biochemical analysis—hypoglycemia in ferrets with insulinoma; azotemia with renal disease elevated hepatic enzyme activities with hepatic disease and ECE

FERRETS

(CONTINUED)

OTHER LABORATORY TESTS
• Fecal flotation—to screen for gastrointestinal parasitism
• Postmortem fluorescent antibody testing of the brain if rabies is suspected

IMAGING
• Survey radiography of the oral cavity, neck, and thorax when foreign body or neoplasm is suspected
• Perform abdominal radiography and abdominal ultrasonography to identify hidden conditions such as GI tract disease, hepatic disease, insulinoma, or lymphoma. Consider thoracic radiography to rule out cardiac or pulmonary disease.
• The need for further diagnostic imaging varies with the underlying condition suspected (see other topics on specific diseases).

DIAGNOSTIC PROCEDURES
• Cytologic examination of oral lesions or fine-needle aspiration of oral mass
• Biopsy and histopathology of oral lesion, salivary gland, or mass
• In order to establish a definitive diagnosis of many common GI disorders (helicobacter, ECE, and IBD) a gastric or intestinal biopsy via laparotomy is needed. Refer to sections on specific disorders for details on a definitive diagnosis.

TREATMENT
Treat the underlying cause (refer to sections pertaining to specific conditions)

MEDICATIONS
DRUG(S) OF CHOICE
• Hypoglycemia may usually be alleviated by administering honey or syrups orally, take care to avoid being bitten.

• Antiemetics—metoclopramide (0.2–1.0 mg/kg PO, SC, IM q6–8h), ondansetron (1 mg/kg PO q12–24h), or maropitant citrate (1 mg/kg SC q24h).
• Histamine H_2-receptor antagonists for animals with gastritis or gastric ulcers—omeprazole (4 mg/kg PO q24h), famotidine (0.25–0.5 mg/kg PO, SC, IV q24h), and cimetidine (10 mg/kg PO, SC, IM, IV q8h)
• Crystalloid fluids—give IV or SC to treat dehydration in anorexic animals with metabolic disease

CONTRAINDICATIONS
N/A

PRECAUTIONS
N/A

POSSIBLE INTERACTIONS
N/A

ALTERNATIVE DRUGS
N/A

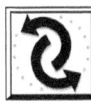

FOLLOW-UP
PATIENT MONITORING
• Depends on the underlying cause (see Causes)
• Continually monitor hydration, serum electrolytes, and nutritional status, especially in dysphagic or anorexic animals.

POSSIBLE COMPLICATIONS
• Dehydration
• Moist dermatitis

MISCELLANEOUS
ASSOCIATED CONDITIONS
N/A

AGE-RELATED FACTORS
N/A

ZOONOTIC POTENTIAL
Rabies

PREGNANCY/FERTILITY/BREEDING
N/A

SYNONYMS
Hypersalivation
Drooling
Sialorrhea

SEE ALSO
Gastroduodenal ulcers
Gastrointestinal and esophageal foreign bodies
Gingivitis and periodontal disease
Insulinoma

ABBREVIATIONS
CNS = central nervous system
ECE = epizootic catarrhal enteritis
GI = gastrointestinal
IBD = inflammatory bowel disease

Suggested Reading
Hoefer HL. Gastrointestinal diseases of ferrets. In: Quesenberry KE, Carpenter JW, eds. Ferrets, Rabbits, and Rodents, 4th ed. Clinical Medicine and Surgery. 2021. St. Louis: Saunders, 2020:27–33.
Huynh M, Pignon C. Gastrointestinal disease in exotic small mammals. J Exot Pet Med 2013;22(2):118–131.
Johnson-Delaney CA. Geriatric ferrets. Vet Clin Exot Anim Pract 2020;23(3):549–650.
Livingstone M. Dealing with gastrointestinal disease in ferrets. In Practice 2022;44:169–179.
Schoemaker NJ, van Zeeland YRA. Endocrine diseases of ferrets. In: Quesenberry KE, Carpenter JW, eds. Ferrets, Rabbits and Rodents, 4th ed. Clinical Medicine and Surgery. 2021. St. Louis: Saunders, 2020:77–91.
Author Barbara Oglesbee, DVM, DABVP (Avian)

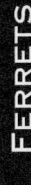

FERRETS

RABIES

FERRETS

BASICS

DEFINITION
A severe, invariably fatal, viral polioencephalitis of warm-blooded animals, including humans

PATHOPHYSIOLOGY
Virus—enters body through a wound (usually from a bite of rabid animal) or via mucous membranes; replicates in myocytes; spreads to the neuromuscular junction and neurotendinal spindles; travels to the CNS via intra-axonal fluid within peripheral nerves; spreads throughout the CNS; finally spreads centrifugally within peripheral, sensory, and motor neurons

SYSTEMS AFFECTED
• Nervous—clinical encephalitis
• Salivary glands—in ferrets infected with the raccoon rabies variant (the most common variant causing infection in ferrets), infectious virus particles are contained in the salivary glands and shed in saliva.

GENETICS
None

INCIDENCE/PREVALENCE
• Incidence of disease within infected animals, high (approaches 100%)
• Prevalence—overall low; <20 cases reported in the United States since 1954, only 2 reports exist in the United States since 1992. No reports of transmission from ferrets to humans exist.

GEOGRAPHIC DISTRIBUTION
• Worldwide
• Exceptions—British Isles, Australia, New Zealand, Hawaii, Japan, and parts of Scandinavia

SIGNALMENT
Species
• All warm-blooded animals, including dogs, cats, and humans
• United States—four strains endemic within fox, raccoon, skunk, and bat populations, all four strains can be transmitted to ferrets

Breed Predilections
None

Mean Age and Range
None

Predominant Sex
None

SIGNS
General Comments
The clinical signs of rabies in ferrets are usually mild and include anxiety, lethargy, and posterior paresis. These signs are very similar to many common diseases in ferrets. The furious form of rabies seen in other carnivores is unusual in ferrets. However, consider rabies as a differential diagnosis in any ferret displaying neurologic signs.

Historical Findings
• Change in attitude—apprehension, nervousness, anxiety; unusual shyness or aggressiveness
• Disorientation
• Muscular—rear limb paresis; incoordination; seizures; paralysis
• Erratic behavior—biting or snapping; biting at cage; wandering and roaming; excitability; irritability; viciousness (rarely reported in ferrets)

Physical Examination Findings
All or some of the historical findings

CAUSES
Rabies virus—a single-stranded RNA virus; genus *Lyssavirus*; family Rhabdoviridae

RISK FACTORS
• Lack of adequate vaccination against rabies
• Use of modified live virus rabies vaccine
• Exposure to wildlife, especially skunks, raccoons, bats, and foxes—this exposure rarely occurs in ferrets since most are indoor pets
• Bite or scratch wounds from unvaccinated dogs, cats, or wildlife
• Exposure to aerosols in bat caves

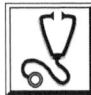

DIAGNOSIS

DIFFERENTIAL DIAGNOSIS
• Must seriously consider rabies for any ferret showing unusual mood or behavior changes or exhibiting any unaccountable neurologic signs; caution: handle with considerable care to prevent possible transmission of the virus to individuals caring for or treating the animal.
• For rear limb paresis—spinal cord damage, Aleutian disease virus, insulinoma, weakness from chronic systemic illness
• Canine distemper virus—neurologic signs may be seen without an early catarrhal phase

CBC/BIOCHEMISTRY/URINALYSIS
No characteristic hematologic or biochemical changes

OTHER LABORATORY TESTS
N/A

IMAGING
N/A

DIAGNOSTIC PROCEDURES
• DFA test of nervous tissue—rapid and sensitive test; collect brain, head, or entire body of animal that has died or has been euthanatized; chill sample immediately; submit to a state-approved laboratory for rabies diagnosis; caution: use extreme care when collecting, handling, and shipping these specimens

PATHOLOGIC FINDINGS
• Gross changes—generally absent, despite dramatic neurologic disease
• Histopathologic changes—acute to chronic polioencephalitis; large neurons within the brain may contain the classic intracytoplasmic inclusions (Negri bodies).

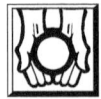

TREATMENT

APPROPRIATE HEALTH CARE
Strictly inpatient

NURSING CARE
Administer with extreme caution.

ACTIVITY
• Confine to secured quarantine area with clearly posted signs indicating suspected rabies.
• Runs or cages should be locked; only designated people should have access.
• Feed and water without opening the cage or run door.

DIET
N/A

CLIENT EDUCATION
• Thoroughly inform client of the seriousness of rabies to the animal and the zoonotic potential.
• Ask client about any human exposure (e.g., contact, bite) and strongly urge client to see a physician immediately.
• Local public health official must be notified.

SURGICAL CONSIDERATIONS
None

MEDICATIONS

DRUG(S) OF CHOICE
• No treatment
• If the diagnosis is strongly suspected, euthanasia is indicated.

CONTRAINDICATIONS
None

PRECAUTIONS
N/A

POSSIBLE INTERACTIONS
N/A

ALTERNATIVE DRUGS
N/A

FOLLOW-UP

PATIENT MONITORING
• All suspected rabies patients should be securely isolated and monitored for any development of mood change, attitude change, or clinical signs that might suggest the diagnosis.
• An apparently healthy ferret that bites or scratches a person should be monitored for a period of 10 days regardless of vaccination status; contact local public health regulatory agency for instructions on quarantining ferrets inflicting bite wounds.
• If the ferret dies during quarantine, the head should be submitted for testing as outlined above.
• An unvaccinated ferret that is bitten or exposed to a known rabid animal must be euthanized or quarantined for up to 6 months or according to local or state regulations.

PREVENTION/AVOIDANCE
• Vaccines—vaccinate according to standard recommendations and state and local requirements; all ferrets should be vaccinated at 12 weeks of age, then annually thereafter using an approved killed virus vaccine. Only use a killed vaccine approved in ferrets (in the United States the approved ferret vaccine are IMRAB 3 and IMRAB 3 TF—Merial, Athens, GA, USA); MLV vaccines have caused disease in ferrets
• Disinfection—any contaminated area, cage, food dish, or instrument must be thoroughly disinfected; use a 1:32 dilution (4 ounces per gallon) of household bleach to quickly inactivate the virus.

POSSIBLE COMPLICATIONS
• Vaccine reactions are common in ferrets and vary from pruritus and lethargy to severe reactions characterized by acute, hemorrhagic diarrhea, vomiting, collapse, and rarely death. Premedication with diphenhydramine (2 mg/kg IM) 20 minutes prior to vaccination is recommended. Monitor ferrets for 30 minutes following vaccination for adverse reaction.

EXPECTED COURSE AND PROGNOSIS
• Prognosis—grave; invariably fatal

MISCELLANEOUS

ASSOCIATED CONDITIONS
None

AGE-RELATED FACTORS
None

ZOONOTIC POTENTIAL
• Extreme
• Humans must avoid being bitten by a rabid animal or an asymptomatic animal that is incubating the disease.
• Rabies cases must be strictly quarantined and confined to prevent exposure to humans and other animals.
• Local and state regulations must be adhered to carefully and completely.

PREGNANCY/FERTILITY/BREEDING
Infection during pregnancy will be fatal to dam.

SYNONYMS
N/A

ABBREVIATIONS
DFA = direct immunofluorescent antibody
MLV = modified live virus

Suggested Reading
Greenacre CB. Incidence of adverse events in ferrets vaccinated with distemper or rabies vaccine: 143 cases (1995–2001). J Am Vet Med Assoc 2003;223:663–665.
Huynh M, Piazza S. Musculoskeletal and neurologic diseases. In: Quesenberry KE, Carpenter JW, eds. Ferrets, Rabbits and Rodents, 4th ed. Clinical Medicine and Surgery. 2021. St. Louis: Saunders, 2020:117–130.
Kiupel M, Perpiñán D. Viral diseases of ferrets. In: Fox JG, Marini RP, eds. Biology and Diseases of the Ferret, 3rd ed. John Wiley & Sons, 2014:439–517.
Mancinelli E. Neurologic examination and diagnostic testing in rabbits, ferrets and rodents. J Exot Pet Med 2015;24:52–64.
Moore GE, Glickman NW, Ward MP et al. Incidence of and risk factors for adverse events associated with distemper and rabies vaccine administration in ferrets. J Am Vet Med Assoc 2005;226(6):909–912.
Munday JS, Stedman NL, Richey LJ. Histology and immunohistochemistry of seven ferret vaccination-site fibrosarcomas. Vet Pathol 2003;40:288–293.

Author Barbara Oglesbee, DVM, DABVP (Avian)

RECTAL AND ANAL PROLAPSE

FERRETS

BASICS

OVERVIEW
• An anal prolapse (partial prolapse) is a protrusion of rectal mucosa through the external anal orifice.
• A double layer of the rectum that protrudes through the anal canal is a rectal prolapse (complete prolapse).

SIGNALMENT
• Usually young ferrets, 2–6 months of age
• Rarely occurs in adult ferrets

SIGNS
• Persistent tenesmus, may cry out when defecating
• Tubular hyperemic mass protruding from the anus
• Usually diarrhea, may see other gastrointestinal signs (vomiting, anorexia), weight loss, or dehydration

CAUSES AND RISK FACTORS
• Proliferative bowel disease (PBD)—caused by campylobacter-like organism (*Lawsonia intracellularis*) is the most common cause of rectal prolapse in young ferrets
• Coccidiosis—also a common cause of anal prolapse in young ferrets; may be co-pathogen with *Lawsonia intracellularis*
• Prostatomegaly and resultant straining to urinate or defecate may cause prolapse
• Chronic diarrhea—from epizootic catarrhal enteritis, lymphoma, infiltrative bowel diseases, giardia, or other bacterial or parasitic causes
• GI foreign body
• Rectal or anal tumors (rare)
• Tenesmus following perineal or urogenital surgery

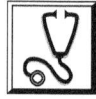

DIAGNOSIS

DIFFERENTIAL DIAGNOSIS
• Coccidia, giardia, campylobacter, and proliferative bowel disease (*Lawsonia intracellularis*) are seen in younger ferrets.
• Chronic diarrhea, prostatomegaly, and neoplasia are more likely to cause prolapse in older ferrets.

CBC/BIOCHEMISTRY/URINALYSIS
• Usually normal
• May reflect underlying cause (e.g., inflammatory leukogram with infectious disease)

OTHER LABORATORY TESTS
• PCR testing for *Lawsonia intracellularis* on feces
• Fecal direct examination, fecal flotation, and zinc sulfate centrifugation may demonstrate gastrointestinal parasites.

IMAGING
• Abdominal radiography and ultrasonography—usually normal in young ferrets with coccidia or PBD
• Abdominal radiography—may demonstrate foreign body, prostatomegaly
• Contrast radiography may indicate thickening of the intestinal wall, mucosal irregularities, mass, severe ileus, foreign body, or stricture.
• Abdominal ultrasonography may demonstrate intestinal wall thickening, gastrointestinal mass, foreign body, ileus, or mesenteric lymphadenopathy, prostatomegaly, or intussusception.

DIAGNOSTIC PROCEDURES
Exploratory laparotomy and surgical biopsy should be pursued if there is evidence of obstruction or intestinal mass and/or for definitive diagnosis of gastrointestinal inflammatory or infiltrative diseases.

PATHOLOGIC FINDINGS
Assess viability of the prolapsed tissue by surface appearance and tissue temperature—vital tissue appears swollen and hyperemic, and red blood exudes from the cut surface; devitalized tissue appears dark purple or black, and dark cyanotic blood exudes from the cut surface; ulcerations may be present.

TREATMENT

APPROPRIATE HEALTH CARE
• If prolapse is mild and does not cause straining, treating the underlying cause without replacing the mucosa may be sufficient; keep tissues moist by use of a lubricant until underlying problem resolves.
• Must identify and treat underlying cause
• Conservative medical management—gently replace prolapsed tissue through the anus with the use of lubricants; osmotic agents may help if severe swelling exists.
• Adjunctive use of a purse-string suture may aid in retention and prevent post reduction recurrence; place the suture to allow room for defecation.
• Colopexy is recommended for recurrent viable prolapses
• If the prolapse is devitalized (rare), amputation and rectal anastomosis are recommended

MEDICATIONS

DRUG(S) OF CHOICE
• Appropriate anesthetic/analgesics as needed
• Topical agents to aid in reduction—50% dextrose solution and KY Jelly
• Specific treatment for the underlying cause

CONTRAINDICATIONS/POSSIBLE INTERACTIONS
N/A

FOLLOW-UP

PATIENT MONITORING
Purse string removal in 5–7 days

POSSIBLE COMPLICATIONS
Recurrence—especially if uncontrolled underlying problem exists

MISCELLANEOUS

ASSOCIATED CONDITIONS
See Causes

SEE ALSO
Coccidiosis
Diarrhea
Dyschezia and hematochezia
Proliferative bowel disease

ABBREVIATIONS
GI = gastrointestinal
PBD = proliferative bowel disease

Suggested Reading
Di Girolamo N, Selleri P. Medical and surgical emergencies in ferrets. Vet Clin Exot Anim 2016;19:431–464.
Hoefer HL. Gastrointestinal diseases of ferrets. In: Quesenberry KE, Carpenter JW, eds. Ferrets, Rabbits, and Rodents, 4th ed. Clinical Medicine and Surgery. 2021. St. Louis: Saunders, 2020:27–38.
Huynh M, Pignon C. Gastrointestinal disease in exotic small mammals. J Exot Pet Med 2013;22(2):118–131.
Lennox AM, Gladden JN. Emergency and critical care of small mammals. In: Quesenberry KE, Carpenter JW, eds. Ferrets, Rabbits and Rodents, 4th ed. Clinical Medicine and Surgery. 2021. St. Louis: Saunders, 2020:595–608.
MacPhail C. Ferret soft tissue surgery. Surg Exot Anim 2021;24:277–296.
Miwa Y, Sladky K. Common surgical procedures of rodents, ferrets, hedgehogs, and sugar gliders. Vet Clin Exot Anim 2016;19:205–244.
Mullen HS, Scavelli TD, Quesenberry KE et al. Gastrointestinal foreign body in ferrets: 25 cases (1986–1990). J Am Anim Hosp Assoc 1992;28:13–19.

Author Barbara Oglesbee, DVM, DABVP-Avian

BASICS

DEFINITION
• Expulsion of undigested food from the esophagus through the oral cavity
• Usually implies dysphagia
• Regurgitation is a rare clinical presentation in ferrets

SYSTEMS AFFECTED
• Gastrointestinal
• Respiratory—aspiration pneumonia

SIGNALMENT
• Younger animals—esophageal foreign body
• Middle-aged to older ferrets—megaesophagus, esophagitis, neoplasia
• No sex predilection

SIGNS

Historical Findings
• Often mistaken for vomiting
• Take a thorough history to differentiate vomiting (forceful abdominal contractions) from regurgitation (passive).
• The character of the expelled ingesta and the time interval from ingestion to expulsion may also help differentiate vomiting and regurgitation.
• There may be a ravenous appetite; food may be dropped from the mouth.
• Weight loss may be profound.
• Ptyalism is common.
• Dysphagia, choking, or distress shortly after eating may be noted.
• Coughing and/or dyspnea may be the complaint when aspiration pneumonia is present.

Physical Examination Findings
• Emaciation and weakness are common.
• The cervical esophagus may bulge on expiration or with compression of the thorax.
• Fever and abnormal lung sounds on auscultation may be present in those with aspiration pneumonia.

CAUSES
• Idiopathic megaesophagus
• Megaesophagus—secondary to systemic illness or toxin
• Esophagitis
• Esophageal foreign body
• Esophageal stricture

RISK FACTORS
N/A

DIAGNOSIS

DIFFERENTIAL DIAGNOSIS

Differentiating Similar Signs
• Must distinguish from vomiting
• Signs of nausea, such as ptyalism, licking the lips, pawing at the mouth, and backing up are usually seen just prior to vomiting or retching.
• Forceful retching and involuntary abdominal contractions associated with the expulsion of digested and bile-stained ingesta or liquid support vomiting.
• Effortless expulsion of foam, liquid, or partially digested or undigested food supports regurgitation.

CBC/BIOCHEMISTRY/URINALYSIS
• Results normal in most patients
• TWBC elevation with aspiration pneumonia or esophagitis
• ALT elevation with secondary hepatic lipidosis

OTHER LABORATORY TESTS
Blood lead and cholinesterase levels to evaluate for toxicity if suspected (rare)

IMAGING

Radiographic Findings
• Survey thoracic radiographs—may reveal an esophagus dilated with gas, fluid, or ingesta (in patients with megaesophagus) or may be within normal limits; may also reveal pulmonary infiltrates consistent with aspiration pneumonia
• Contrast esophagram (with liquid barium and/or barium-coated food) may confirm obstructive disorders (foreign bodies, strictures, neoplasia, or granulomas).
• Fluoroscopy can detect pharyngeal dysfunction and esophageal motility disorders.

DIAGNOSTIC PROCEDURES
Esophagoscopy—can be useful with obstructive disorders of the esophagus and esophagitis; usually unrewarding with megaesophagus

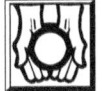

TREATMENT

APPROPRIATE HEALTH CARE
• For other causes than primary idiopathic megaesophagus, aim treatment at the primary cause.

• If no known underlying cause, treatment goals include minimizing risk of aspiration pneumonia and providing and maintaining adequate nutrition.
• Most patients with megaesophagus have aspiration pneumonia and/or severe debilitation requiring hospitalization.
• Hospitalize in a warm, quiet location with a hide box to minimize stress.

NURSING CARE
• If the patient is dehydrated, a balanced electrolyte solution may be indicated.
• Correct dehydration with IV fluid therapy (maintenance = 75–100 mL/kg/day) using 0.9% saline or LRS. If hypoglycemic, use 2.5% dextrose and 0.45% saline.

ACTIVITY
Restricted due to associated weakness and lethargy

DIET
• Feed in upright position (45- to 90-degree angle to the floor) and maintain position for 10–15 minutes following feeding.
• If the patient has been anorectic, assist feed an easily digestible high-protein/high-fat diet such as Lafeber Carnivore Critical Care Diet (Lafeber Company, Cornell, IL) or Oxbow Carnivore Critical Care Diet (Oxbow Animal Health, Omaha, NE); may also add dietary supplement such as Nutri-Cal (EVSCO Pharmaceuticals) to increase caloric content to these foods.
• A more liquid consistency may decrease regurgitation but may increase the risk of aspiration pneumonia.
• Reported caloric requirement for sick ferrets is 400 kcal/kg BW per day (this may be a high estimate)
• Patients with severe regurgitation may need parenteral feeding via gastrotomy tube.

CLIENT EDUCATION
If an underlying cause is not identifiable or corrected, most animals become debilitated due to starvation, hepatic lipidosis, and aspiration pneumonia. Advise client of poor prognosis.

SURGICAL CONSIDERATIONS
• Surgery may be necessary to remove esophageal foreign bodies or neoplasia if identified
• No surgical procedures improve esophageal motility.

FERRETS

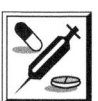

MEDICATIONS

DRUG(S) OF CHOICE
• Specific medications are recommended if regurgitation is secondary to identifiable, treatable disorders.
• Sucralfate (25 mg/kg PO q8h)
• Gastrointestinal antisecretory agents are helpful to treat and possibly prevent gastritis in anorectic ferrets. Ferrets continually secrete a baseline level of gastric hydrochloric acid and, as such, anorexia itself may predispose to gastric ulceration. Those successfully used in ferrets include omeprazole (4 mg/kg PO q24h), famotidine (0.25–0.5 mg/kg PO, SC, IV q24h), and cimetidine (10 mg/kg PO, SC, IM, IV q8h)
• Metoclopramide (0.2–1.0 mg/kg PO, SC, IM q6–8h) speeds gastric emptying, increases gastroesophageal sphincter tone, and is most useful when reflux esophagitis is a contributing or the primary cause; use of metoclopramide for other causes has had limited success.
• Broad-spectrum antibiotics—necessary for patients with aspiration pneumonia; parenteral antibiotics may be required for patients with severe regurgitation. Ideally, based on culture and susceptibility testing from an airway specimen; begin with an antibiotic combination that is broad spectrum and effective against anaerobes (e.g., enrofloxacin 5–10 mg/kg IM, PO, SC q12h, plus amoxicillin 20 mg/kg IM, PO q12h); alter therapy based on culture/susceptibility results

CONTRAINDICATIONS
N/A

PRECAUTIONS
Corticosteroids may be necessary to treat conditions causing megaesophagus; use with caution in patients with aspiration pneumonia.

POSSIBLE INTERACTIONS
N/A

ALTERNATIVE DRUGS
N/A

FOLLOW-UP

PATIENT MONITORING
Monitor for the development of aspiration pneumonia. Obtain thoracic radiographs if aspiration pneumonia is suspected—fever, cough, nasal discharge

POSSIBLE COMPLICATIONS
• Aspiration pneumonia
• Esophageal stricture following tumor or foreign body removal

EXPECTED COURSE AND PROGNOSIS
• Depends on the underlying cause
• If a cause is not identified, the prognosis is poor to grave, with or without treatment
• Aspiration pneumonia and malnutrition are likely causes of death

MISCELLANEOUS

ASSOCIATED CONDITIONS
• Insulinoma
• Gastric ulcers
• *Helicobacter mustelae*

AGE-RELATED FACTORS
N/A

ZOONOTIC POTENTIAL
Determine rabies vaccination status for all patients.

PREGNANCY/FERTILITY/BREEDING
N/A

SEE ALSO
Dysphagia
Gastrointestinal and esophageal foreign bodies
Pneumonia, aspiration

ABBREVIATIONS
ALT = alanine aminotransferase
LRS = lactated Ringer's solution
TWBC = total white blood cell count

Suggested Reading
Blanco MC, Fox JG, Rosenthal K et al. Megaesophagus in nine ferrets. J Am Vet Med Assoc 1994;205:444–447.
Couturier J, Huynh M, Boussarie D et al. Autoimmune myasthenia gravis in a ferret. J Am Vet Med Assoc 2009;235:1462–1466.
Garner MM, Ramsell K, Schoemaker NJ et al. Myofasciitis in the domestic ferret. Vet Pathol 2007;44:25–38.
Hoefer HL. Gastrointestinal diseases of ferrets. In: Quesenberry KE, Carpenter JW, eds. Ferrets, Rabbits, and Rodents (4th ed.). Clinical Medicine and Surgery. 2021. St. Louis: Saunders, 2020:27–38.
Huynh M, Pignon C. Gastrointestinal disease in exotic small mammals. J Exot Pet Med. 2013;22(2):118–131.
Johnson-Delaney CA. Geriatric ferrets. Vet Clin Exot Anim Pract 2020;23(3):549–565.
Murray J, Kiupel M, Maes RK. Ferret coronavirus-associated diseases. Vet Clin North Am Exot Anim Pract. 2010;13(3):543–603.
Webb J, Graham J, Fordham M, DeCubellis J, Buckley F, Hobbs J, Berent A, Weisse C. Diagnosis and treatment of esophageal foreign body or stricture in three ferrets (*Mustela putorius furo*). J Am Vet Med Assoc 2017;251(4):451–457.
Author Barbara Oglesbee, DVM, DABVP-Avian

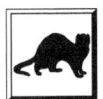

BASICS

OVERVIEW
• Slow growing, usually benign formation of cysts within renal parenchyma. One or both kidneys can be affected and can be single or several within the same kidney. Finding is usually incidental but can be clinical/pathological in some cases.
• The kidneys may become abnormally large because of the development of renal cysts or pseudocysts
• Polycystic kidney disease (PKD) is a rare, but more severe manifestation of the condition in ferrets

SIGNALMENT
• Renal cysts are a common incidental finding in middle-aged to older ferrets; reported incidence of 15% of necropsied ferrets found on ultrasound in 32%–63% of all ferrets.

SIGNS
• One or both kidneys may palpate as renomegaly or asymmetrical in size
• Renal cysts often remain undetected unless they become large and numerous enough to contribute to renal failure or abdominal enlargement; thus, patients typically are clinically normal during initial stages of cyst formation and growth and usually remain asymptomatic for life.
• May detect bosselated (lumpy) kidneys by abdominal palpation with PKD, some can be painful if capsular distension
• Most renal cysts are not painful when palpated.

CAUSES
• Renal cysts—very common; can be unilateral or bilateral, affected kidney often irregularly shaped
• Polycystic kidney disease—rare disease in ferrets characterized by bilaterally enlarged, cystic kidneys and progression to renal failure
• Hydronephrosis—can cause unilateral or bilateral renomegaly that can image/present as if large pelvic cyst; develops secondarily to ureteral obstruction (e.g., abscess, ligation, neoplasia, and urolithiasis)
• Hematoma—can occur secondarily to trauma from repeated aspiration of cysts

RISK FACTORS
• Likely congenital but not believed to be hereditary

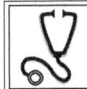

DIAGNOSIS

DIFFERENTIAL DIAGNOSIS
• Must distinguish from lymphoma, abscesses, adrenal gland neoplasia, other neoplasia/renal metastasis, ovarian cysts (if intact or improper spay), hematoma, and hydronephrosis
• Confirmation will require ultrasound/exploratory celiotomy and FNA/biopsy

CBC/BIOCHEMISTRY/URINALYSIS
• Results usually unremarkable unless patient has renal insufficiency secondary to PKD or severe bilateral renal cysts, but even with insufficiency, ferrets tend to have less dramatic azotemic responses, so assessing for isosthenuria, casts, and phosphorus and potassium abnormalities are more common.

OTHER LABORATORY TESTS
• Cytologic examination and bacterial culture of cyst fluid

IMAGING

Radiographic Findings
• Abdominal radiographs may indicate peripheral cysts or overall renomegaly
• Can use IVP to confirm presence of renomegaly, hydronephrosis, and space-occupying masses of the kidneys

Ultrasonographic Findings
Helpful to identify and differentiate renal cysts, PKD, neoplastic masses, or abscesses, and subcapsular hematoma. Renal cysts are a common incidental finding during abdominal ultrasonography.

DIAGNOSTIC PROCEDURES
• Examination of fine-needle aspirate can confirm presence of renal cyst, abscess, and neoplasia (especially lymphoma).
• If no definitive diagnosis is made by cytologic evaluation of renal aspirates, renal biopsy may be indicated.

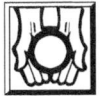

TREATMENT
• None for renal cysts. Ultrasound-guided aspiration of cystic fluid may temporarily decrease size; however, this procedure is not usually necessary and fluid is likely to reform. Spontaneous resolution of cysts is not documented in ferrets; with time, most cysts increase in size and may compress adjacent normally functioning renal parenchyma.

• Resection of renal capsule to alleviate pressure/pain or unilateral nephrectomy may be indicated.

MEDICATIONS

DRUG(S) OF CHOICE
Pain medications if indicated, be careful with NSAID options

CONTRAINDICATIONS
Avoid nephrotoxic drugs.

FOLLOW-UP

PATIENT MONITORING
• Renal cysts—perform physical examination and monitor size of cysts through ultrasound
• Monitor for signs of renal failure

POSSIBLE COMPLICATIONS
• Renal failure
• Pain

MISCELLANEOUS

ASSOCIATED CONDITIONS
• None

SEE ALSO
Hydronephrosis
Lymphosarcoma
Polyuria and polydipsia
Renal failure

ABBREVIATIONS
NSAID = nonsteroidal anti-inflammatory drug
IVP = intravenous pyelography
PKD = polycystic kidney disease

Suggested Reading
Jackson C, Rogers A, Maurer K et al. Cystic renal disease in the domestic ferret. Comp Med 2008;58(2):161–167.
Orcutt CJ. Ferret urogenital diseases. Vet Clin Exot Anim 2003;6(1):113–138.
Pollock C. Disorders of the urinary and reproductive systems. In: Quesenberry KE, Carpenter JW, eds. Ferrets, Rabbits, and Rodents: Clinical Medicine and Surgery, 3rd ed. St Louis: Elsevier, 2012:46–61.
Author Eric Klaphake, DVM, DACZM, DABVP

FERRETS

RENAL FAILURE

FERRETS

BASICS

DEFINITION
- Azotemia and urine specific gravity <1.030
- Acute renal failure (ARF) is a syndrome characterized by the sudden onset of filtration failure by the kidneys, accumulation of uremic toxins, and dysregulation of fluid, electrolyte, and acid–base balance. The most common causes of ARF in ferrets are urinary tract obstruction and NSAID toxicity.
- Chronic renal failure (CRF) results from primary renal disease that has persisted for months to years; characterized by irreversible renal dysfunction that tends to deteriorate progressively

GENERAL COMMENTS
- Chronic interstitial nephritis is common in middle-aged to older ferrets, many of which are asymptomatic. Renal failure can result from this, pyelonephritis, immune complex-mediated glomerulonephropathy, or glomerulonephritis. Nephrotic syndrome, characterized by proteinuria and hypoalbuminemia resulting in edema or ascites, is also seen in ferrets with chronic kidney disease.

SYSTEMS AFFECTED
- Renal/Urologic—impaired renal function leading to PU/PD and signs of uremia
- Nervous, gastrointestinal, musculoskeletal, and other body systems—secondarily affected by uremia
- Hemic/Lymph/Immune—anemia

GENETICS
N/A

INCIDENCE/PREVALENCE
Not well documented; however, renal failure is a common sequela to many conditions affecting ferrets (see below).

SIGNALMENT
Animals of any age can be affected, but prevalence increases with increasing age.

Predominant Sex
None

SIGNS

General Comments
Clinical signs are related to the severity of renal dysfunction and the presence or absence of complications.

Historical Findings
- ARF—sudden onset of anorexia, listlessness, vomiting (±blood), diarrhea (±blood), halitosis, ataxia, seizures, known toxin exposure, recent medical or surgical conditions, and oliguria/ anuria or polyuria

- CRF—PU/PD, anorexia, ptyalism, diarrhea, vomiting, weight loss, lethargy, poor hair coat; ataxia seizures, or coma seen in late stages. Asymptomatic animals with stable CRF may decompensate, resulting in a uremic crisis.

Physical Examination Findings
- ARF—depression, dehydration (sometimes overhydration), hypothermia, paresis, oral ulcers, fever, tachypnea, bradycardia, nonpalpable urinary bladder if oliguric
- CRF—small, irregular kidneys (or enlarged kidneys secondary to cystic kidneys or lymphoma), dehydration, cachexia, ascites, edema, mucous membrane pallor

CAUSES
- ARF: most common causes are urinary tract obstruction and NSAID toxicity. Other causes include shock, heart failure, prolonged anesthesia, or septicemia.
- ARF or CRF—glomerulonephritis, amyloidosis, pyelonephritis, cystic kidneys, nephroliths, drugs (e.g., NSAIDs, aminoglycoside, sulfonamides, chemotherapeutic agents), heavy metals, lymphoma, hypercalcemia.

RISK FACTORS
- ARF—feeding grain-free or plant-based protein diets (cystic calculi/obstruction), NSAID exposure, preexisting renal disease, dehydration, hypovolemia, hypotension, advanced age, concurrent disease, prolonged anesthesia or surgery, and administration of nephrotoxic drugs
- CRF—aging, uroliths, cystic kidneys, urinary tract infection, diabetes mellitus

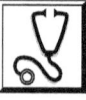

DIAGNOSIS

DIFFERENTIAL DIAGNOSIS
- For polyuria/polydipsia—iatrogenic glucocorticoid administration, pyometra, paraurethral or prostatic cysts/abscesses, hepatic failure, hypercalcemia, diabetes mellitus, post obstructive diuresis, some diuretics (e.g., mannitol and furosemide), ingestion or administration of large quantities of solute (e.g., sodium chloride or glucose), behavioral
- For renomegaly—renal neoplasia (lymphoma), cystic kidneys, hydronephrosis
- Prerenal azotemia—(decreased renal perfusion) characterized by azotemia with concentrated urine (specific gravity >1.030); correctable with fluid repletion
- Postrenal azotemia—characterized by azotemia with obstruction or rupture of the excretory system

CBC/BIOCHEMISTRY/URINALYSIS
- Nonregenerative anemia with CRF, normal or high PCV with ARF
- BUN elevation is seen more commonly than elevation in creatinine; normal creatinine concentration in ferrets is significantly lower than in dogs and cats (0.2–0.6 mg/dL); any elevation in creatinine should be considered significant
- Electrolyte and acid–base abnormalities are similar to those seen in feline patients.
- Inability to concentrate urine, mild-to-moderate proteinuria (normal protein 0–33 mg/dL), glucosuria; WBCs, RBCs; variable bacteriuria and crystalluria may be seen depending on the underlying cause

OTHER LABORATORY TESTS
- The urinary protein-to-creatinine ratio may be useful to determine the magnitude of proteinuria; however, reference values have not been established for ferrets.
- The value of using microalbuminuria assays to screen for glomerular injury has not been evaluated in ferrets.
- Serum lead or zinc concentration
- Plasma electrophoresis—elevated globulins in ferrets with ADV

IMAGING
- Abdominal radiographs may demonstrate small kidneys (or large kidneys secondary to cystic kidneys or lymphoma) in animals with CRF.
- Ultrasound reveals anechoic cavitating lesions characterized by sharply marginated smooth walls and distal enhancement in patients with cystic kidneys.
- Animals with lymphoma often have renomegaly with hypoechoic renal parenchyma.

DIAGNOSTIC PROCEDURES
- Direct or indirect blood pressure determination is indicated to monitor for hypertension (how commonly this occurs in ferrets is unknown)
- Evaluation of ultrasound-guided fine-needle aspirates of the kidney may allow differentiation of cystic kidneys from other diseases that cause renomegaly.

PATHOLOGIC FINDINGS
- Gross findings—small kidneys with a lumpy or granular surface seen in many ferrets with CRF; large, irregular kidneys with cystic kidneys or lymphoma
- Histopathologic findings—frequently nonspecific; chronic generalized nephropathy or end-stage kidneys; findings are specific for diseases causing CRF in some patients; nephrosis or nephritis seen in ferrets with ARF

(CONTINUED)

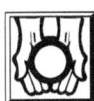

TREATMENT

APPROPRIATE HEALTH CARE
Patients with compensated CRF may be managed as outpatients; patients in ARF or uremic crisis should be managed as inpatients.

NURSING CARE
• Patients in ARF or uremic crisis—correct estimated fluid deficits with normal (0.9%) saline or balanced polyionic solution within 4–6 hours to prevent additional renal injury from ischemia; once the patient is hydrated, ongoing fluid requirements are provided by 5% dextrose or balanced electrolyte solution (approximately 75–100 mL/kg/day)
• Patients in CRF—subcutaneous fluid therapy (daily or every other day) may benefit patients with moderate to severe CRF.

ACTIVITY
Unrestricted unless hospitalized

DIET
• Dietary protein restriction is not possible in ferrets due to their high dietary protein requirements. Most renal diets contain rice or corn as a primary ingredient. Feeding diets that contain grains or plant-based proteins may lead to the development of urinary calculi in ferrets.
• If anorexic, most ferrets will accept assist feeding with an easily digestible high-protein/high-fat diet such as Lafeber Carnivore Critical Care Diet (Lafeber Company, Cornell, IL) or Oxbow Carnivore Critical Care Diet (Oxbow Animal Health, Omaha, NE); may also add dietary supplement such as Nutri-Cal (EVSCO Pharmaceuticals) to increase caloric content to these foods.
• Allow free access to fresh water at all times.

CLIENT EDUCATION
• CRF—tends to progress over months, possibly years
• ARF—inform of the poor prognosis for complete recovery, potential for morbid complications of treatment (e.g., fluid overload, sepsis, and multiple organ failure), expense of prolonged hospitalization

SURGICAL CONSIDERATIONS
Avoid hypotension during anesthesia to prevent additional renal injury.

MEDICATIONS

DRUG(S) OF CHOICE
Inadequate Urine Production (Anuric or Oliguric Renal Failure)
• Ensure patient is fluid-volume replete; provide additional isometrics fluid to achieve

mild (3%–5%) volume expansion; failure to induce diuresis by fluid replacement indicates severe parenchymal damage or underestimation of fluid deficit.
• Furosemide (1–4 mg/kg IM, IV q8–12h) and dopamine (0.01 mL/animal prn)—for ferrets with oliguric renal failure—follow feline treatment protocols
• If these treatments fail to induce diuresis within 4–6 hours, the prognosis is grave.

Uremic Crisis
• If vomiting—NPO until vomiting subsides; be certain to monitor blood glucose concentrations if NPO as many older ferrets have concurrent insulinoma; administer dextrose-containing fluids if hypoglycemia develops
• Reduce gastric acid production—H2 blockers such omeprazole (4 mg/kg PO q24h), famotidine (0.25–0.5 mg/kg PO, SC, IV q24h), and cimetidine (10 mg/kg PO, SC, IM, IV q8h)
• Mucosal protectant—sucralfate (25 mg/kg PO q6–8h)
• Antiemetics—metoclopramide (0.2–1.0 mg/kg PO, SC, IM q6–8h), ondansetron (1mg/kg PO q12–24h), or maropitant citrate (1 mg/kg SC q24h)
• Potassium chloride IV as needed to correct hypokalemia (based on cat dosages)

Compensated CRF
• Famotidine (0.25–0.5 mg/kg PO, SC IV q24h) or cimetidine (5–10 mg/kg PO, SC, IM q8h)
• Potassium gluconate (2–6 mEg/kg/day PO) to correct hypokalemia
• Intestinal phosphate binders as needed if hyperphosphatemic—use feline dosage protocols
• Epoetin alfa has been used to treat chronic anemia in ferrets (50–150 IU/kg 3 times per week until the PCV is stable, then 1–2 times a week). Monitor the PCV, and titrate the dose as needed.

CONTRAINDICATIONS
Avoid nephrotoxic agents.

PRECAUTIONS
• Modify dosages of all drugs that require renal metabolism or elimination.
• Use ACE inhibitors with caution; monitor for lethargy, weakness, or worsening of azotemia or proteinuria.

POSSIBLE INTERACTIONS
Metoclopramide may impair the effects of dopamine.

ALTERNATIVE DRUGS
Control of vomiting—chlorpromazine (0.2–0.4 mg/kg IM, SC q6–12h) can be used to treat vomiting but is associated with CNS depression, vasodilatation, and hypotension.

FOLLOW-UP

PATIENT MONITORING
• ARF—fluid, electrolyte, and acid–base balances; body weight; urine output; and clinical status; daily
• CRF—monitor at 1- to 3-month intervals, depending on therapy and severity of disease

PREVENTION/AVOIDANCE
Anticipate the potential for ARF in hemodynamically unstable patients, receiving nephrotoxic drugs, having multiple organ failure, or are undergoing prolonged anesthesia and surgery; maintenance of hydration and/or mild saline volume expansion may be preventive.

POSSIBLE COMPLICATIONS
• ARF—seizures, gastrointestinal bleeding, cardiac arrhythmias, congestive heart failure, pulmonary edema, hypovolemic shock, coma, cardiopulmonary arrest, and death
• CRF—uremic stomatitis, gastroenteritis, anemia

EXPECTED COURSE AND PROGNOSIS
• Nonoliguric ARF—milder than oliguric; recovery may occur, but the prognosis remains guarded to unfavorable.
• Oliguric ARF—extensive renal injury, is difficult to manage, and has a poor prognosis for recovery
• Anuric ARF—generally fatal
• CRF—short-term prognosis depends on severity; long-term prognosis guarded to poor because CRF tends to be progressive

MISCELLANEOUS

ASSOCIATED CONDITIONS
• Urolithiasis
• Paraurethral or prostatic cysts
• Splenomegaly
• Lymphoma

AGE-RELATED FACTORS
Increased incidence in older animals; normal renal function decreases with aging.

ZOONOTIC POTENTIAL
Leptospirosis is extremely rare in pet ferrets but may have zoonotic potential

PREGNANCY/FERTILITY/BREEDING
ARF is a rare complication of pregnancy in animals; promoted by acute metritis, pyometra, and postpartum sepsis or hemorrhage

RENAL FAILURE

SYNONYMS
Kidney failure

SEE ALSO
Polyuria and polydipsia
Renomegaly
Urinary tract obstruction

ABBREVIATIONS
ARF = acute renal failure
BUN = blood urea nitrogen
CNS = central nervous system
CRF = chronic renal failure
CRI = continuous-rate infusion
NSAID = nonsteroidal anti-inflammatory drugs
PCV = packed cell volume
PU/PD = polyuria/polydipsia
RBC = red blood cell count
WBC = white blood cell count

Suggested Reading
Di Girolamo N, Huyun M. Disorders of the urinary and reproductive systems in ferrets. In: Quesenberry KE, Carpenter JW, eds. Ferrets, Rabbits and Rodents, 4th ed. Clinical Medicine and Surgery. St. Louis: Saunders, 2020:39–54.
Di Girolamo N, Selleri P. Medical and surgical emergencies in ferrets. Vet Clin Exot Anim Pract. 2016;19:431–464.
Hallman RM, Brandão J. Diagnostic imaging of the renal system in exotic companion mammals. Vet Clin Exot Anim 2020;23:195–214.
Johnson-Delaney CA. Geriatric ferrets. Vet Clin Exot Anim Pract 2020;23(3):549–565.
Lennox AM, Gladden JN. Emergency and critical care of small mammals. In: Quesenberry KE, Carpenter JW, eds. Ferrets, Rabbits and Rodents, 4th ed. Clinical Medicine and Surgery. 2021. St. Louis: Saunders, 2020:595–608.
Reavill DR, Lennox AM. Disease overview of the urinary tract in exotic companion mammals and tips on clinical management. Vet Clin Exot Anim 2020;23(1):169–193.
Author Barbara Oglesbee, DVM, DABVP (Avian)

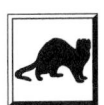

BASICS

OVERVIEW
• One or both kidneys are abnormally large as detected by abdominal palpation or radiography.
• The kidneys may become abnormally large because of the development of renal cysts or pseudocysts, abnormal cellular infiltration (e.g., inflammation, infection, and neoplasia), urinary tract obstruction, or acute tubular necrosis.

SIGNALMENT
• Renomegaly is a somewhat common physical examination finding, especially in middle-aged to older ferrets.
• Renal cysts are a common incidental finding in middle-aged to older ferrets; reported incidence of 15% of necropsied ferrets.

SIGNS
• One or both kidneys palpably large.
• If significant renal disease is present, owners may report lethargy, loss of appetite, weight loss, polyuria and polydipsia, diarrhea, vomiting, or abdominal distension.
• With significant renal disease may detect dehydration, pale mucous membranes, and cachexia.
• Renal cysts often remain undetected unless they become large and numerous enough to contribute to renal failure or abdominal enlargement; thus, patients typically are clinically normal during the initial stages of cyst formation and growth, and usually remain asymptomatic for life.
• May detect bosselated (lumpy) kidneys by abdominal palpation.
• Most renal cysts are not painful when palpated.
• Abnormally large abdomen.

CAUSES
• Renal cysts—very common; can be unilateral or bilateral, affected kidney often irregularly shaped
• Polycystic kidney disease—a rare disease in ferrets characterized by bilaterally enlarged, cystic kidneys and progression to renal failure
• Neoplasia—lymphoma most common renal tumor; may cause bilateral or unilateral renomegaly and often bosselated kidneys; other (rarely) reported tumors include renal carcinoma, transitional cell carcinoma, and cystadenocarcinoma
• Hydronephrosis—can cause unilateral or bilateral renomegaly; develops secondarily to ureteral obstruction (e.g., abscess, ligation, neoplasia, and urolithiasis)

• Infection/inflammation—Aleutian disease virus (ADV), renal abscess
• Hematoma—can occur secondarily to trauma; rare

RISK FACTORS
• The stimuli for renal cyst formation remain obscure.
• Any cause of ureteral obstruction, including uroliths, neoplasia; prostatic disease; retroperitoneal abscess, cysts, hematoma, or other mass; inadvertent ureteral ligation during ovariohysterectomy.
• Exposure to ferrets with ADV.

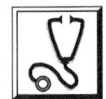

DIAGNOSIS

DIFFERENTIAL DIAGNOSIS
• Must distinguish from other abdominal masses
• Confirmation may require diagnostic imaging procedures or exploratory celiotomy

CBC/BIOCHEMISTRY/URINALYSIS
• Results are usually unremarkable unless the patient has renal insufficiency.
• Nonregenerative anemia secondary to chronic renal failure is possible
• Azotemia, hyperphosphatemia, and low urine specific gravity in patients with renal failure
• Leukocytosis is expected in patients with infectious, inflammatory, and neoplastic causes of renomegaly.
• Neoplastic cells are rarely observed in the urine of patients with renal neoplasia.

OTHER LABORATORY TESTS
• Cytologic examination and bacterial culture of cyst fluid

IMAGING

Radiographic Findings
• Abdominal radiographs to confirm renomegaly
• Can use excretory urography to confirm the presence of renomegaly, hydronephrosis, and space-occupying masses of the kidneys
• Thoracic radiography indicated to detect metastases in patients with renal neoplasia

Ultrasonographic Findings
Helpful to confirm the diagnosis and identify potential causes, such as renal cysts, neoplastic mass, abscess, and subcapsular hematoma. Renal cysts are a common incidental finding during abdominal ultrasonography.

DIAGNOSTIC PROCEDURES
• Examination of fine-needle aspirate can confirm the presence of a renal cyst, abscess, and neoplasia (especially lymphoma).

• If no definitive diagnosis is made by cytologic evaluation of renal aspirates, renal biopsy may be indicated.

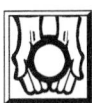

TREATMENT
• Diagnose and treat the underlying cause, if possible.
• None for renal cysts. Ultrasound-guided aspiration of cystic fluid may temporarily decrease size; however, this procedure is usually not necessary and fluid is likely to reform. Spontaneous resolution of cysts is not documented in ferrets; with time, most cysts increase in size and may compress adjacent normally functioning renal parenchyma.
• Specific treatment for hydronephrosis depends on the cause and whether there is concurrent renal failure or other disease process (e.g., neoplasia, abscess). If the obstruction is removable and sufficient renal function remains, removal of the affected kidney is not necessary.
• Treatment for renal failure may be necessary.

MEDICATIONS

DRUG(S) OF CHOICE
Vary with the cause

CONTRAINDICATIONS
Avoid nephrotoxic drugs.

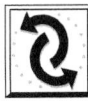

FOLLOW-UP

PATIENT MONITORING
• Renal cysts—perform a physical examination and monitor the size of cysts through ultrasound
• Monitor for signs of renal failure

POSSIBLE COMPLICATIONS
• Renal failure, depending on the underlying cause of renomegaly
• Metastasis of renal tumor

MISCELLANEOUS

ASSOCIATED CONDITIONS
• Ferret adrenal disease
• Insulinoma

SEE ALSO
Hydronephrosis
Lymphosarcoma

FERRETS

RENOMEGALY

Polyuria and polydipsia
Renal failure

ABBREVIATIONS
ADV = Aleutian disease virus

Suggested Reading
Di Girolamo N, Huynh M. Disorders of the urinary and reproductive systems in ferrets. In: Quesenberry KE, Carpenter JW, eds. Ferrets, Rabbits and Rodents, 4th ed. Clinical Medicine and Surgery. 2021. St. Louis: Saunders, 2020:39–54.
Hallman RM, Brandão J. Diagnostic imaging of the renal system in exotic companion mammals. Vet Clin Exot Anim 2020;23:195–214.
Jackson C, Rogers A, Maurer K, Lofgren J, Fox J, Marini R. Cystic renal disease in the domestic ferret. Comp Med 2008;58(2):161–167.
Orcutt CJ. Ferret urogenital diseases. Vet Clin Exot Anim 2003;6(1):113–138.
Pollock C. Disorders of the urinary and reproductive systems. In: Quesenberry KE, Carpenter JW, eds. Ferrets, Rabbits, and Rodents: Clinical Medicine and Surgery, 3rd ed. St Louis: Elsevier, 2012:46–61.
Reavill DR, Lennox AM. Disease overview of the urinary tract in exotic companion mammals and tips on clinical management. Vet Clin Exot Anim 2020;23(1):169–193.
Williams BH, Wyre NR. Neoplasia in ferrets. In: Quesenberry KE, Carpenter JW, eds. Ferrets, Rabbits and Rodents, 4th ed. Clinical Medicine and Surgery. 2021. St. Louis: Saunders, 2020:92–108.

Author Barbara Oglesbee, DVM, DABVP – Avian

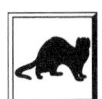

BASICS

OVERVIEW
• A bacterial disease that causes enteritis and sometimes septicemia; disease may be caused by many different serotypes of salmonella
• Salmonella—a gram-negative bacterium; colonizes the small intestine; adheres to and invades enterocytes; eventually enters and multiplies in the lamina propria and local mesentery lymph nodes; cytotoxins and enterotoxins are produced, resulting in secretory diarrhea and mucosal sloughing
• Uncomplicated gastroenteritis—organisms are stopped at the mesenteric lymph node stage; patient has only gastrointestinal tract signs
• Bacteremia and septicemia following gastroenteritis—more serious disease

SIGNALMENT
• Salmonellosis is an unusual cause of gastrointestinal tract disease in pet ferrets. Most reports are of outbreaks occurring in breeding or research colonies, or in ferrets eating rancid whole prey, undercooked meats, or poultry products.
• No age or sex predilections

SIGNS
General Comments
Disease severity varies from subclinical to mild, moderate, and severe clinical disease
• Asymptomatic carrier states—no clinical signs (rare)
• Gastroenteritis—diarrhea, often with fresh blood and/or mucus; malaise/lethargy; anorexia; vomiting; progressive dehydration; abdominal pain; tenesmus; pale mucous membranes; mesenteric lymphadenopathy; weight loss
• Gastroenteritis with bacteremia and septicemia, septic shock, or endotoxemia— pale mucous membranes; weakness; cardiovascular collapse; tachycardia; tachypnea

CAUSES AND RISK FACTORS
• Associated with feeding rancid whole prey—ferrets tend to hide whole prey food and consume later
• Associated uncooked meats and poultry products
• Salmonella serotype—virulence factors, infectious dose, and route of exposure determine course of disease; *Salmonella hadar*, *Salmonella enteritidis*, *Salmonella newport*, and *Salmonella typhimurium* reported
• Host factors that increase susceptibility— neonatal/young ferrets; immature immune system; debilitation; other concurrent disease

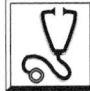

DIAGNOSIS

DIFFERENTIAL DIAGNOSIS
Salmonella is relatively rare in household ferrets. Diseases that are much more likely to cause clinical gastroenteritis include the following:
• Epizootic catarrhal enteritis—most common infectious cause
• Gastrointestinal foreign body
• *Helicobacter mustelae* gastroenteritis
• Inflammatory bowel disease— lymphoplasmacytic gastroenteritis, eosinophilic gastroenteritis
• Neoplasia, especially lymphoma; occasionally adenocarcinoma or other GI tract tumors
Also consider these less common causes of GI tract disease in pet ferrets:
• Other bacterial infections—*Campylobacter* spp., *Clostridium* spp., *Lawsonia intracellularis*, *Mycobacterium avium*-intracellulare.
• Parasitic diseases—giardia, coccidia, and *Cryptosporidium* spp.

CBC/BIOCHEMISTRY/URINALYSIS
• CBC—variable; depends on stage of illness; nonregenerative anemia or lymphopenia sometimes seen
• Hypoalbuminemia

DIAGNOSTIC PROCEDURES
• Fecal culture—special media needed; may require multiple samples
• Fecal leukocytes may be present
• Subclinical carrier states—chronic; intermittent fecal culture positive
• Note: use of antimicrobials in a patient before sampling may produce false-negative cultures.

PATHOLOGIC FINDINGS
• Gross lesions—only in severely affected patients
• Cultures of ileum, mesenteric lymph nodes

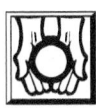

TREATMENT

APPROPRIATE HEALTH CARE
• Outpatient—uncomplicated gastroenteritis (without bacteremia) and carrier states
• Inpatient—with bacteremia/septicemia and for gastroenteritis in animals that are rapidly debilitated by diarrhea

NURSING CARE
Varies according to severity of illness—assess percentages of dehydration, body weight, ongoing fluid loss, shock, PCV/total protein, electrolytes, and acid–base status

Uncomplicated Gastroenteritis
• Supportive care—fluid and electrolyte replacement
• Parenteral, balanced, isotonic solution (lactated Ringer's)

MEDICATIONS

DRUG(S) OF CHOICE
• Antimicrobial therapy—indicated; culture and susceptibility testing/MIC necessary to assess drug-resistance problems
• Enrofloxacin—5–10 mg/kg PO, SC, IM q12h
• Chloramphenicol—20–50 mg/kg PO, SC, IM q12h
• Ciprofloxacin—10–30 mg/kg PO q12h
• Trimethoprim-sulfa—15–30 mg/kg PO, SC q12h

FOLLOW-UP

PATIENT MONITORING
• Fecal culture—repeat monthly to assess development of carrier state
• Other animals—monitor for secondary spread of infection
• Advise client to contact veterinarian if patient shows signs of recurring disease.

PREVENTION/AVOIDANCE
• Keep animals healthy—proper nutrition; clean and disinfect cages, food and water dishes frequently; store food and feeding utensils properly
• Supervise consumption of whole prey

POSSIBLE COMPLICATIONS
• Spread of infection possible within household to other animals or humans
• Development of chronic infection with diarrhea
• Recurrence of disease with stress

MISCELLANEOUS

ZOONOTIC POTENTIAL
• High potential, especially in children, elderly, immunosuppressed, and antimicrobial drug users
• Acutely ill animals may shed large numbers of salmonellae in stool.
• Isolation is needed

PREGNANCY/FERTILITY/BREEDING
• May complicate disease
• Abortion—may be a sequela to infection
• Antimicrobial therapy—take into account the effect on the fetus

SALMONELLOSIS

ABBREVIATIONS
PCV = packed cell volume

Suggested Reading
Di Girolamo N, Selleri P. Medical and surgical emergencies in ferrets. Vet Clin Exot Anim 2016;19:431–464.

Hoefer HL. Gastrointestinal diseases of ferrets. In: Quesenberry KE, Carpenter JW, eds. Ferrets, Rabbits, and Rodents, 4th ed. Clinical Medicine and Surgery. 2021. St. Louis: Saunders, 2020:27–38.

Huynh M, Pignon C. Gastrointestinal disease in exotic small mammals. J Exot Pet Med 2013;22(2):118–131.

Johnson-Delaney CA. Geriatric ferrets. Vet Clin Exot Anim Pract 2020;23(3): 549–565.

Livingstone M. Dealing with gastrointestinal disease in ferrets. In Practice 2022;44:169–179.

Author Barbara Oglesbee, DVM, DABVP-Avian

BASICS

OVERVIEW
• An uncommon, contagious parasitic skin disease of ferrets caused by infestation with the mite *Sarcoptes scabiei*, the same mite that affects dogs and cats.
• Two forms reported—local form affecting the feet with intense pruritus and secondary pododermatitis and generalized form with diffuse or focal alopecia and pruritus
• Mites are transmissible from dogs or cats to ferrets and ferret to ferret.

SIGNALMENT
• Uncommon disease of ferrets
• No age or sex predilection

SIGNS
• Foot lesions characterized by severe inflammation, swelling, and crusting that can progress to nail and skin sloughing if untreated; generally extremely pruritic/painful
• Alopecia and erythematous rash may appear in any area of the body, either focal lesions or more generalized coalescent lesions
• Nonseasonal, usually intense pruritus
• Secondary crusts, excoriations, and pyoderma may occur.
• Possible peripheral lymphadenopathy
• Multiple pet households—more than one animal (ferret or dogs) may shows signs.

CAUSES AND RISK FACTORS
• Exposure to a carrier animal before development of symptoms
• Residence in breeding colonies
• Residence at animal shelter
• Boarding

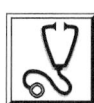
DIAGNOSIS

DIFFERENTIAL DIAGNOSIS
Differentiating Causes
• Ferret adrenal disease—bilaterally symmetric alopecia. Hair loss often begins in late winter or early spring and initially may regrow later in the year, followed by progressive alopecia the following spring. Alopecia begins in the tail region and progresses cranially. In severe cases, the ferret will become completely bald. In most cases, the skin has a normal appearance; 30% of affected ferrets are pruritic, and secondary pyoderma is occasionally seen. Other signs related to adrenal disease, such as a swollen vulva in spayed females, may be seen.
• Seasonal flank alopecia—not pruritic; seen in intact animals (or females with ovarian remnant); bilaterally symmetric alopecia begins at the tail base and progresses throughout the breeding season (March–August for females, December–July for males)
• CDV—pododermatitis usually follows a catarrhal phase characterized by naso-ocular discharge, depression, and anorexia, followed by a characteristic, erythematous, pruritic rash on the chin and lips and spreads caudally to the inguinal area; pododermatitis is characterized by hyperkeratinization of the footpads, erythema, and swelling. CDV is uniformly fatal, and signs other than pododermatitis alone will be seen.
• Neoplasia—lesions may occur on feet; however, with most tumor types only one foot is affected; lymphoma may affect multiple feet; can be nodular, inflamed, swollen, or ulcerative, depending on tumor type. Mast cell tumors—raised alopecic nodules; may become ulcerated or covered with a thick black crust; may be single or multiple, usually pruritic and found on neck and trunk
• Ear mites—most ferrets with ear mites are not pruritic. In pruritic animals, see partial to complete alopecia caudal to the ears; waxy brown aural discharge; excoriations around pinna, differentiate by otic examination and skin scrape
• Fleas—patchy alopecia at tail base and in cervical and dorsal thoracic region; excoriations; secondary pyoderma sometimes seen
• Bacterial dermatitis—usually secondary infection—localized or multifocal areas of alopecia depending on primary cause; lesions may appear ulcerated, pruritus sometimes seen; may be concurrent with scabies
• Dermatomycosis—partial to complete alopecia with scaling; with or without erythema; not always ringlike; may begin as small papules; not usually pruritic
• Demodicosis—extremely rare, has been reported in association with corticosteriod use; mites will be present on skin scrape
• Hypersensitivity/contact irritant—uncommon cause; dermatitis localized to area of contact with irritant

CBC/BIOCHEMISTRY/URINALYSIS
N/A

OTHER LABORATORY TESTS
• CDV—florescent antibody test (IFA)—can be performed on peripheral blood or buffy coat smears, conjunctival or mucous membrane scrapings. Vaccination will not affect the results
• Ferret adrenal disease—elevations serum estradiol, androstenedione, and 17-hydroxyprogesterone combined are most diagnostic (available through the University of Tennessee Clinical Endocrinology Laboratory, Department of Comparative Medicine).

IMAGING
N/A

DIAGNOSTIC PROCEDURES
• Superficial skin scrapings—mites are not always seen
• Favorable response to scabicidal treatment—common method for tentative diagnosis
• Biopsy or FNA—histopathology, rule out neoplasia
• Wood's lamp, fungal culture, and cytologic examination of stained smear of any exudate or pustule contents to rule out mycotic or bacterial infection

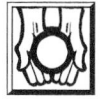
TREATMENT
• All in-contact ferrets, cats, or dogs—should be treated, even those with no clinical signs; may be asymptomatic carriers
• Thoroughly clean and treat environment; *Sarcoptes* mites can survive for up to 3 weeks.

MEDICATIONS

DRUG(S) OF CHOICE
• Ivermectin—highly effective; 0.2–0.4 mg/kg SC q14d for 3–4 doses
• Whole-body lime sulfur dip q7d may be used but less effective due to lack of owner compliance; disadvantages are bad odor and staining
• Selamectin (Revolution; Pfizer)—s15 mg/kg topically q30d
• Systemic antibiotics—may be needed to resolve any secondary pyoderma
• Symptomatic therapy to relieve pruritus—prednisone 0.25–1.0 mg/kg q24h PO divided. Antihistamines have been used anecdotally but are generally not as effective as steroids. Hydroxyzine (2 mg/kg PO q8h); diphenhydramine (0.5–2.0 mg/kg PO, IM, IV q8–12h); chlorpheniramine (1–2 mg/kg PO q8–12h)

CONTRAINDICATIONS/POSSIBLE INTERACTIONS
Ivermectin—anecdotally associated with birth defects when used in pregnant jills

FOLLOW-UP
• Topical treatments are prone to failure, owing to incomplete application of the treatment solution.
• Reinfection can occur if the contact with infected animals continues.

SARCOPTIC MANGE

FERRETS

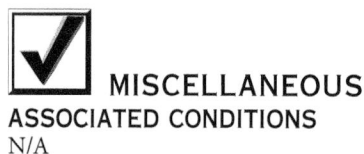

MISCELLANEOUS

ASSOCIATED CONDITIONS
N/A

ZOONOTIC POTENTIAL
People who come in close contact with an affected ferret may develop a pruritic, papular rash on their arms, chest, or abdomen; human lesions are usually transient and should resolve spontaneously after the affected animal has been treated; if the lesions persist, clients should seek advice from their dermatologist.

SEE ALSO
Adrenal disease (hyperadrenocorticism)
Canine distemper virus

Dermatophytosis
Ear mites
Fleas and flea infestation
Pododermatitis and nail bed disorders

ABBREVIATION
CDV = canine distemper virus

Suggested Reading

Fehr M, Koestlinger S. Ectoparasites in small exotic mammals. Vet Clin Exot Anim 2013;16:611–657.

Fisher M, Beck W, Hutchinson MJ. Efficacy and safety of selamectin (Stronghold/Revolution™) used off-label in exotic pets. Int J Appl Res Vet Med 2007;5:87–96.

d'Ovidio D, Santoro D. Dermatologic diseases of ferrets. In: Quesenberry KE, Carpenter JW, eds. Ferrets, Rabbits and Rodents, 4th Ed). Clinical Medicine and Surgery. 2021 ed. St. Louis: Saunders, 2020:109–116.

Hoppmann E, Wilson BH. Ferret and rabbit dermatology. J Exot Pet Med 2007;16:225–237.

Patterson MM, Kirchain SM. Comparison of three treatments for control of ear mites in ferrets. Lab Anim Sci 1999;49:655–657.

Powers LV. Bacterial and parasitic diseases of ferrets. Vet Clin Exot Anim 2009;12(3):531–561.

Author Barbara Oglesbee, DVM, DABVP (Avian)

BASICS

DEFINITION
Enlargement of the spleen; characterized as either diffuse or nodular

PATHOPHYSIOLOGY
• The spleen will often gradually increase in size with age in apparently normal ferrets; the cause of this is unknown.
• Function of the spleen includes removal of senescent and abnormal erythrocytes; filtration and phagocytosis of antigenic particles; production of lymphocytes and plasma cells; reservoir for erythrocytes and platelets; hematopoiesis, as required
• Splenomegaly is an extremely common finding in ferrets and reflects splenic functions.
• Hypersplenism is a syndrome in which red or white blood cells are removed at an abnormally high rate by the spleen, resulting in one or more cytopenias. Hypersplenism is a rare cause of splenomegaly in ferrets.

Diffuse
General pathologic mechanisms include
• Lymphoreticular hyperplasia—most common cause of splenomegaly in ferrets; hyperplasia of mononuclear phagocytes and lymphoid elements (in response to antigens); accelerated erythrocyte destruction
• Inflammatory (splenitis)—associated with infectious agents; rarely seen in ferrets

Nodular
Associated with neoplastic (most common cause) or nonneoplastic disorders (hemorrhage, infection, or inflammation)

SYSTEMS AFFECTED
N/A

SIGNALMENT
Generalized, benign splenic hyperplasia increases with age.

SIGNS

General Comments
• Reflect the underlying disease rather than splenic enlargement
• Often nonspecific

Historical Findings
Reflect underlying disease

Physical Examination Findings
• Enlarged spleen on abdominal palpation—normal finding in older ferrets; enlarged spleen may occupy up to one-third of the abdominal cavity; if extremely large, can cause abdominal distension and discomfort
• Usually diffuse, uniform enlargement palpable

• Nodular, irregular enlargement suggests neoplasia or infiltrative disease.
• Infiltrative or inflammatory disease—implied by hepatomegaly, thickened intestines, and/or enlarged mesenteric lymph nodes
• Lymphosarcoma—suggested by concurrent peripheral or mesenteric lymphadenopathy

CAUSES

Infiltration
• Extramedullary hematopoiesis—most common cause of splenomegaly; seen with chronic inflammation, infectious disease, estrogen-induced pancytopenia, chronic anemia, malignancy, insulinoma, or adrenal disease
• Lymphoid hyperplasia—chronic antigenic stimulation
• Neoplasia—lymphosarcoma most common

Hyperplasia
• Congestion—anesthetic agents; portal hypertension; right-sided heart failure
• Infection—bacterial endocarditis; other systemic infection

Nodular
• Neoplastic—malignant: hemangiosarcoma, lymphosarcoma, metastatic insulinoma; fibrosarcoma, leiomyosarcoma; benign: hemangioma, myelolipoma, leiomyoma, metastatic carcinoma
• Nonneoplastic—hematoma; abscess; rarely extramedullary hematopoiesis

Inflammation (Splenitis)
• Rare in ferrets, but may see eosinophilic splenitis with eosinophilic gastroenteritis, lymphoplasmacytic with lymphoplasmacytic enteritis, or granulomatous with mycobacteriosis

RISK FACTORS
N/A

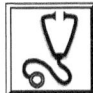

DIAGNOSIS

DIFFERENTIAL DIAGNOSIS
Other cranial organomegaly or masses

CBC/BIOCHEMISTRY/URINALYSIS
• Leukocytosis with a left shift—may indicate infectious and inflammatory conditions
• Lymphocytosis—suggests possible lymphoma
• Leukopenia—may be seen with hypersplenism (rare) or viral diseases
• Thrombocytopenia—from increased consumption secondary to hemangiosarcoma, increased destruction or sequestration (hypersplenism), or decreased production (estrogen toxicity)

• Regenerative anemia and splenomegaly—may indicate blood loss
• Eosinophilia—suggests eosinophilic gastroenteritis
• Hyperglobulinemia—from Aleutian disease virus, chronic inflammation
• Serum glucose concentration decreased with insulinoma

OTHER LABORATORY TESTS
• Elevations in serum estradiol, androstenedione, and 17-hydroxyprogesterone diagnostic of hyperadrenocorticism

IMAGING

Abdominal Radiography
• Confirm or detect splenomegaly
• May provide evidence for the underlying cause—gastrointestinal tract disease, adrenal disease, insulinoma
• Effusion—may indicate hemorrhage from splenic rupture (hemangiosarcoma, hematoma)—rare in ferrets

Thoracic Radiography
• Right and left lateral views—screen for metastasis and underlying disease (CHF)

Abdominal Ultrasonography
• Distinguishes between diffuse and nodular
• Diffuse enlargement with normal parenchyma—may be noted with congestion or cellular infiltration
• Reduced echogenicity—may be seen with lymphosarcoma
• Nodular abnormalities easily identified
• Complex, mixed echogenic pattern—hemangiosarcoma
• Can identify concurrent abdominal diseases affecting liver, kidneys, intestines, and lymph nodes

DIAGNOSTIC PROCEDURES

Fine-Needle Aspiration
• Contraindicated if hemangiosarcoma is suspected—fatal hemorrhage may occur. Rule out hemangiosarcoma (rare in ferrets) on abdominal ultrasound.
• Procedure—place patient in right lateral or dorsal recumbency; use a 23- or 25-gauge, (1- to 1.5-in) needle and 5-mL syringe; diffuse: may aspirate without ultrasonography; nodular: requires ultrasound guidance; anesthesia or tranquilization may be required
• Specimens—identify the predominant inflammatory cell type
• Neoplastic infiltrates—classified as hematopoietic, lymphatic, carcinoma, or sarcoma

Bone Marrow Aspiration
• Indicated with cytopenias before splenectomy (spleen may be the main source of circulating blood cells)

SPLENOMEGALY (CONTINUED)

• Marrow may be normal or hypercellular with hypersplenism

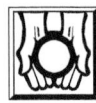

TREATMENT

Depends on the underlying cause; supportive nursing care as needed—the spleen is rarely the cause of disease.

SURGICAL CONSIDERATIONS

Splenectomy
• Indicated for hypersplenism, splenic rupture, splenic masses
• Occasionally, the spleen may become large enough to cause abdominal discomfort—partial splenectomy may alleviate discomfort. The need for total splenectomy should be carefully evaluated, especially in anemic animals, since EMH in the spleen may be a major source of hematopoiesis.
• Perform bone marrow aspirate first in ferrets with anemia or leukopenia—rule out bone marrow aplasia; spleen may be providing hematopoietic activity
• Exploratory celiotomy—permits direct evaluation of all abdominal organs for diagnosis and treatment of underlying causes of splenomegaly.

MEDICATIONS

DRUG(S) OF CHOICE
Depend on underlying disease

CONTRAINDICATIONS
N/A

PRECAUTIONS
N/A

POSSIBLE INTERACTIONS
N/A

ALTERNATIVE DRUGS
N/A

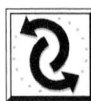

FOLLOW-UP

Antibiotics—indicated in patients that are receiving immunosuppressive therapy

POSSIBLE COMPLICATIONS
Postoperative sepsis—uncommon complication after surgery

MISCELLANEOUS

ASSOCIATED CONDITIONS
• Hyperadrenocorticism
• Insulinoma

AGE-RELATED FACTORS
The spleen may gradually enlarge with age in normal ferrets.

ZOONOTIC POTENTIAL
N/A

PREGNANCY/FERTILITY/BREEDING
N/A

SEE ALSO
Inflammatory bowel disease
Lymphosarcoma

ABBREVIATIONS
CHF = congestive heart failure
EMH = extramedullary hematopoiesis

Suggested Reading

Hoefer HL. Gastrointestinal diseases of ferrets. In: Quesenberry KE, Carpenter JW, eds. Ferrets, Rabbits and Rodents, 4th Ed). Clinical Medicine and Surgery. 2021 ed. St. Louis: Saunders, 2020:27–38.

Johnson-Delaney CA. Geriatric ferrets. Vet Clin Exot Anim Pract 2020;23(3):549–650.

Lennox AM, Gladden JN. Emergency and critical care of small mammals. In: Quesenberry KE, Carpenter JW, eds. Ferrets, Rabbits and Rodents, 4th Ed). Clinical Medicine and Surgery. 2021 ed. St. Louis: Saunders, 2020:595–608.

Miwa Y, Sladky K. Common surgical procedures of rodents, ferrets, hedgehogs, and sugar gliders. Vet Clin Exot Anim 2016;19:205–244.

Suran JN, Latney LV, Wyre NR. Radiographic and ultrasonographic findings of the spleen and abdominal lymph nodes in healthy domestic ferrets. J Small Anim Pract 2017;58:444–453.

Williams BH, Wyre NR. Neoplasia in ferrets. In: Quesenberry KE, Carpenter JW, eds. Ferrets, Rabbits and Rodents, 4th Ed Clinical Medicine and Surgery. 2021 ed. St. Louis: Saunders, 2020:92–108.

Author Barbara Oglesbee, DVM, DABVP (Avian)

FERRETS

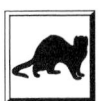

BASICS

DEFINITION
Generalized, uniform swelling of the vulvar tissue. When enlarged, the vulva can appear surprisingly large, red and inflamed, raising concern for owners.

PATHOPHYSIOLOGY
Normal secondary sex characteristic response to high levels of estrogen in the blood

SYSTEMS AFFECTED
- Reproductive
- Endocrine (adrenal)

GENETICS
Unknown

INCIDENCE/PREVALENCE
Very common in intact nonpregnant females or females with ovarian remnants; common in female ferrets with adrenal gland disease (though not all); can occasionally occur for a transient period immediately after GnRH agonist treatment (e.g., deslorelin implant) is placed in a jill

GEOGRAPHIC DISTRIBUTION
Adrenal gland disease more commonly seen in the North American ferret population

SIGNALMENT
Mean Age and Range
- If seen in ferret less than a year old, likely a normal intact female or "spayed" ferret with ovarian remnant
- If seen in ferret over 2 years of age with no previous history of such swelling, adrenal disease is more likely or attempted treatment of adrenal disease/contraception with a deslorelin implant

Predominant Sex
Female only

SIGNS
Historical Findings
- Swelling of vulva
- If chronic, lethargy may be seen
- Male ferrets attempting to mount

Physical Examination Findings
- Slight to severe swelling of the vulva
- Often yellow to green crusting on vulvar folds
- If chronic, pale mucous membranes
- Possible anemia-derived murmur/arrhthymia if chronic
- Alopecia
- Small regular scabs, sores, or ecchymotic hemorrhages of the skin

CAUSES
Functional ovary, adrenal gland neoplasia, or immediately after initial placement of deslorelin implant

RISK FACTORS
- Failure to breed intact females
- Ovarian remnant in neutered females
- Ferret adrenal disease—estrogen-secreting adrenal tumors. Evidence suggests that adrenal disease may be related to neutering at an early age.
- Transient in some deslorelin implanted jills initially after placement

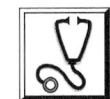

DIAGNOSIS
Visual confirmation

DIFFERENTIAL DIAGONSIS
- Rule out adrenal disease (usually seen in ferrets >2 years of age, signs not as severe and slower in onset).
- Rule out ovarian remnant in neutered animals
- Assess if deslorelin implant recently placed

CBC/BIOCHEMISTRY/URINALYSIS
If chronic, mild to severe nonregenerative anemia and thrombocytopenia
- Use caution when interpreting the PCV from ferrets in which blood was collected under isoflurane anesthesia. Artifactual lowering of the PCV, sometimes as much as 40% below the actual PCV, may occur in ferrets under isoflurane anesthesia.
- Normal PCV (46%–61%), erythrocyte count (17.0×10^6 cells/µL), and reticulocyte count (10%) are higher in ferrets than other mammals.

OTHER LABORATORY TESTS
Serum estradiol, androstenedione, and 17-hydroxyprogesterone levels (available from Clinical Endocrinology Service of the University of Tennessee College of Veterinary Medicine) to rule out adrenal disease

IMAGING
Ultrasound may detect presence of ovarian remnant or adrenal neoplasia, though lack of indication by this modality does not exclude either diagnosis

DIAGNOSTIC PROCEDURES
Histopathology of suspect ovarian remnant or abnormal adrenal gland

PATHOLOGIC FINDINGS
- Depend on underlying cause
- Adrenal disease may be caused by adrenal hyperplasia, adenoma, or adenocarcinoma. Gross examination reveals enlargement of the adrenal gland, irregular surface or discoloration of the affected gland, or cysts or differences in texture within the affected gland.

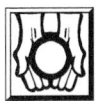

TREATMENT

APPROPRIATE HEALTH CARE
- Outpatient, unless debilitated or anemic
- If severely anemic, blood transfusion from another ferret (cross-match not critical for ferrets) may be indicated

NURSING CARE
Supportive care until source of hyperestrogenism removed

ACTIVITY
Keep very limited if anemic.

DIET
N/A

CLIENT EDUCATION
- Most ferrets in the United States are spayed prior to distribution to pet stores, and ovarian remnants are very rarely found in ferrets obtained from the primary supplier
- Seek medical attention for any ferret remaining in estrus for over 2 weeks
- Spay all intact females not used for breeding
- Discuss adrenal disease when diagnosed

SURGICAL CONSIDERATIONS
- Stabilize severely anemic ferrets (<25% PCV) with transfusions before attempting surgery.
- If intact and not planning to breed, perform routine ovariohysterectomy. Technique and approach similar to cat. DO NOT perform only an ovariectomy, as the high prevalence of adrenal disease could lead to secondary uterine pathology.
- If ovarian remnant suspected, assess regions of ovarian stumps and remove all suspicious tissue and submit for confirmatory histopathology.
- Consider dropped tissue and seeding of ovarian tissue anywhere in abdomen if no obvious tissue in normal ovarian areas
- If adrenal disease suspected, surgical removal of one or both adrenal glands may be attempted, though inadequate margins or occurrence in contralateral gland is common and medical management with a deslorelin implant (or less commonly a melatonin implant) may need to be performed concurrently.
- Removal of the right adrenal gland often involves dissection from and rebuilding of the caudal vena cava.
- A cryosurgical technique for adrenal disease has been described.

FERRETS

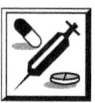

MEDICATIONS

DRUG(S) OF CHOICE

Adrenal Disease

• The GnRH agonist deslorelin acetate (Suprelorin-F®, Virbac Animal Health) is a labeled and recommended treatment in the United States for adrenal disease in domestic ferrets. It is a 4.7-mg slow-release deslorelin implant reported to provide alleviation of clinical signs lasting from 8 to 20 months. Alleviation of clinical signs may be more likely in patients with adrenal hyperplasia or adenoma; adenocarcinomas may be less likely to respond. Deslorelin has no demonstrated effect on adrenal tumor growth or metastasis. In Europe, 9.4-mg deslorelin implants are available and may be effective for up to 2–4 years.

• Melatonin implants are available commercially (Ferretonin® 2.7-mg--ferrets < 600g) and 5.4-mg implants—most ferrets, Melatek, LLC) and have been used in ferrets with adrenal disease to successfully alleviate clinical signs of alopecia, aggressive behavior, vulvar swelling, and prostatomegaly. Implants are repeated every 4 months as needed, lifelong. Alleviation of clinical signs may be more likely in patients with adrenal hyperplasia or adenoma; adenocarcinomas may be less likely to respond. Melatonin has no demonstrated effect on adrenal tumor growth or metastasis.

• Leuprolide acetate, a GnRH analog, is a potent inhibitor of gonadotropin secretion and acts to suppress LH and FSH, downregulating their receptor sites. It is available as a 1- or 4-month depot injection and may alleviate the dermal and reproductive organ signs of adrenal disease in ferrets. Reported dosages: Lupron® 30-day depot, 100–250 μg/kg IM q4w until signs resolve, then q4–8w PRN, lifelong. Larger ferrets often require the higher end of the dose range. This drug has no effect on adrenal tumor growth or metastasis. This is no longer considered the best option and has become challenging to acquire and often prohibitively expensive in the United States.

CONTRAINDICATIONS

N/A

PRECAUTIONS

N/A

ALTERNATIVE DRUGS

N/A

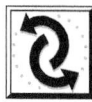

FOLLOW-UP

PATIENT MONITORING

Monitor for resolution of vulvar swelling and anemia, when present

PREVENTION/AVOIDANCE

• OHE if not planning to breed.
• Make sure entire ovary on each side is removed completely.
• There may be benefit to spaying females at an older age (often performed as early as 4–6 weeks of age in the United States), ideally before 6–8 months of age though

POSSIBLE COMPLICATIONS

• Death from hyperestrogen-induced anemia in intact, unbred jills
• The vulvar discharge may be uncomfortable to the ferret: gentle cleaning and removal may help.

EXPECTED COURSE AND PROGNOSIS

Death will occur if anemia is allowed to progress.

MISCELLANEOUS

ASSOCIATED CONDITIONS

• Adrenal disease (or early in treatment with GnRH agonist)
• Ovarian remnant or intact female

AGE-RELATED FACTORS

• Adrenal disease most likely if >2 years old, but can occur at younger ages
• Ovarian remnant or intact female likely if less than 1 year old

ZOONOTIC POTENTIAL

N/A

PREGNANCY/FERTILITY/BREEDING

Intact female—condition and management can directly impact pregnancy and breeding

SYNONYMS

None

ABBREVIATIONS

FSH = follicular-stimulating hormone
GnRH = gonadotropin-releasing hormone
LH = luteinizing hormone
OHE = ovariohysterectomy
PCV = packed cell volume
PRN = as needed

Suggested Reading

Avallone G, Forlani A, Tecilla M, Riccardi E, Belluco S, Santagostino S, Roccabianca P. Neoplastic diseases in the domestic ferret (*Mustela putorius furo*) in Italy: classification and tissue distribution of 856 cases (2000–2010). BMC Vet Res 2016;12:275–282.

Di Girolamo N, Huyun M. Disorders of the urinary and reproductive systems in ferrets. In: Quesenberry KE, Carpenter JW, eds. Ferrets, Rabbits and Rodents, 4th Ed). Clinical Medicine and Surgery ed. St. Louis: Saunders, 2020:39–54.

Di Girolamo N, Selleri P. Medical and surgical emergencies in ferrets. Vet Clin Exot Anim Pract 2016;19:431–464.

Jekl V, Hauptman K. Reproductive medicine in ferrets. Vet Clin Exot Anim Pract 20:629–663.

Schoemaker NJ, Van Zealand YRA. Endocrine diseases of ferrets. In: Quesenberry KE, Carpenter JW, eds. Ferrets, Rabbits and Rodents, 4th Ed). Clinical Medicine and Surgery ed. St. Louis: Saunders, 2020:77–91.

Author Eric Klaphake, DVM, DABVP, DACZM

BASICS

DEFINITION
Tachyarrhythmias are defined as any disturbance of the heart rhythm in which the heart rate is abnormally increased (>240 bpm in a ferret).

PATHOPHYSIOLOGY
• Most tachyarrhythmias are caused by reentry; some result from enhanced normal automaticity or abnormal mechanisms of automaticity.
• Reentry is the circular propagation of an impulse around two interconnected pathways with different conduction characteristics and refractory periods.
• With a premature beat, reentry can produce a continuous circulation of activation wavefront, producing tachyarrhythmia.
• Three conditions favor reentry: shortening of tissue refractoriness (sympathetic stimulation), lengthening of conduction pathway (hypertrophy or abnormal conduction pathways), and slowing of impulse conduction (ischemia)

SYSTEMS AFFECTED
Cardiac, respiratory, renal, ophthalmic

GENETICS
N/A

INCIDENCE/PREVALENCE
Tachyarrhythmias and sinus rhythm are the most common presenting arrhythmias when cardiac disease is present. May also manifest secondary to severe pain or end-stage systemic disease.

GEOGRAPHIC DISTRIBUTION
N/A

SIGNALMENT
Species
All ferrets are susceptible

Breed Predilections
None reported at this time

Mean Age and Range
As primary cardiac disease tends to be a more geriatric condition in ferrets, more commonly occurs in >2.5-year-old ferrets

Predominant Sex
None

SIGNS
Historical Findings
• Lethargy
• Polyuria
• Respiratory issues
• Anorexia
• Weight loss

Physical Examination Findings
• Heart rate greater than 240 bpm
• Pronounced change in heart rhythm
• Dyspnea
• Hypo/hyperthermia
• Pallor
• Ascites/pulmonary edema

CAUSES
Pain
Primary cardiac disease
Severe systemic disease
Activity/stress/fear
Medication side effect

RISK FACTORS
Primary cardiac disease, severe systemic disease, pain

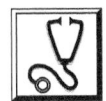

DIAGNOSIS
ECG (echocardiography)

DIFFERENTIAL DIAGNOSIS
• Pain
• Primary cardiac disease
• Other severe systemic disease
• Medication side effect

CBC/BIOCHEMISTRY/URINALYSIS
CBC may indicate severe anemia or evidence of sepsis

OTHER LABORATORY TESTS
N/A

IMAGING
Radiographs and echocardiography can provide valuable ancillary information

DIAGNOSTIC PROCEDURES
Consultation with an ACVIM specialist or cardiologist is highly recommended. (Descriptions below are from Merck Manual reference.)

ECG
• Four groups of tachyarrhythmias: visibly regular vs. irregular and having narrow vs. wide QRS complex
• Irregular, narrow QRS complex tachyarrhythmias include atrial fibrillation (AF), atrial flutter or true atrial tachycardia with variable AV conduction, and multifocal atrial tachycardia.
• Irregular, wide QRS complex tachyarrhythmias include the previous four atrial tachyarrhythmias, conducted with either bundle branch block or ventricular preexcitation, and polymorphic ventricular tachycardia (VT).
• Regular, narrow QRS complex tachyarrhythmias include sinus tachycardia, atrial flutter or true atrial tachycardia with a consistent AV conduction ratio, and paroxysmal SVTs.

• Regular, wide QRS complex tachyarrhythmias include regular, narrow QRS complex tachyarrhythmias, each with bundle branch block or ventricular preexcitation, and monomorphic VT.

PATHOLOGIC FINDINGS
• Hypertrophic or dilated cardiomyopathy
• Valvular disease
• Myocarditis
• Adult nematodes in cardiac chambers
• Endocarditis
• Ascites/pulmonary edema

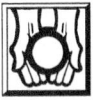

TREATMENT

APPROPRIATE HEALTH CARE
• Treat underlying cardiac disease or systemic disease as appropriate
• Treat arrhythmias as if a feline patient, no ferret-specific recommendations at this time

NURSING CARE
Treat symptomatically and for underlying etiology when appropriate.

ACTIVITY
Dependent on severity and cause, best to allow the ferret to self-regulate

DIET
Evaluating sodium levels may be appropriate.

CLIENT EDUCATION
Similar to feline guidance for clinically relevant arrhythmias

SURGICAL CONSIDERATIONS
Placement of a pacemaker may be considered, but the decision should be deferred to a boarded cardiologist

MEDICATIONS

DRUG(S) OF CHOICE
• Nonclinical tachyarrhythmias are generally not treated
• Treat the underlying cardiac or systemic disease
• Treatment regimen is usually based on feline recommendations, consult with a cardiologist before beginning treatment; digoxin (0.005–0.1 mg/kg PO q24h) has been used for supraventricular tachyarrhythmia
• Beta-blockers and calcium channel blockers can be used for supraventricular tachyarrhythmias to slow the ventricular response rate. Avoid in acute or decompensated congestive heart failure cases unless the tachyarrhythmia is itself a clinical problem and always begin with low doses of

TACHYARRHYTHMIAS

FERRETS

these drugs with the goal of only a slight rate decrease. Propranolol (0.2–1 mg/kg SC, PO q8–12h), atenolol (3.125–6.25 mg/kg PO q24), and benazepril (0.25–0.5 mg/kg PO q24h) are suggested doses for ferrets.

CONTRAINDICATIONS
N/A

PRECAUTIONS
N/A

ALTERNATIVE DRUGS
N/A

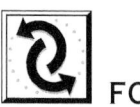

FOLLOW-UP

PATIENT MONITORING
Recheck auscultation and ECG are recommended weekly to monthly if addressing underlying causes. Repeat echocardiography if the primary cardiac disease is noted, as recommended by a cardiologist.

PREVENTION/AVOIDANCE
None known

POSSIBLE COMPLICATIONS
• Death
• Pulmonary edema
• Ascites
• Weakness
• Seizures

EXPECTED COURSE AND PROGNOSIS
Variable from incidental finding to death, depending on the underlying cause

MISCELLANEOUS

ASSOCIATED CONDITIONS
• Primary cardiac disease
• Severe generalized systemic disease
• Pain, stress, fear

AGE-RELATED FACTORS
Older ferrets are more prone to primary cardiac disease; tachyarrhythmia can occur secondarily

ZOONOTIC POTENTIAL
N/A

PREGNANCY/FERTILITY/BREEDING
None

SYNONYMS
None

ABBREVIATIONS
AF = atrial fibrillation
AV = atrioventricular
ECG = electrocardiography
SVT = supraventricular tachycardia
VT = ventricular tachycardia

INTERNET RESOURCES
http://www.merck.com/mmpe/sec07/ch075/ch075a.html Accessed 14 May, 2018.

Suggested Reading
Dudás-Györki Z, Szabó Z, Manczur F et al. Echocardiographic and electrocardiographic examination of clinically healthy, conscious ferrets. J Small Anim Pract 2011;52(1):18–25.

Fitzgerald B, Dias S, Martorell J. Cardiovascular drugs in avian, small mammal, and reptile Medicine. Vet Clin North Am Exot Anim Pract 2018;21(2):399–442.

Di Girolamo N, Selleri P. Medical and surgical emergencies in ferrets. Vet Clin North Am Exot Anim Pract 2016;19:431–464.

Malakoff RL, Laste NJ, Orcutt CJ. Echocardiographic and electrocardiographic findings in client-owned ferrets: 95 cases (1994–2009). J Am Vet Med Assoc 2012;241(11):1484–1489.

Morrisey JK, Kraus MS. Cardiovascular and other diseases of ferrets. In: KE Q, Carpenter JW, eds. Ferrets, Rabbits and Rodents, 4th Ed). Clinical Medicine and Surgery ed. St. Louis: Saunders, 2020:55–71.

van Schaik-Gerritsen KM, Schoemaker NJ, Kik MJL, Beijerink NJ. Atrial septal defect in a ferret (*Mustela putorius furo*). J Exot Pet Med 2013;22:70–75.

Van Zeeland YA, Schoemaker N. Ferret cardiology. Vet Clin Exot Anim 2022;25:541–562.

Author Eric Klaphake, DVM, DABVP, DACZM

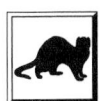

BASICS

DEFINITION
Restricted flow of urine from the urinary bladder through the external urethral orifice. Most commonly caused by urolithiasis in ferrets, but extraluminal compression by prostatic disease is also seen.

PATHOPHYSIOLOGY
• Pathophysiologic consequences depend on the degree and duration of obstruction. Complete obstruction produces a pathophysiologic state equivalent to oliguric acute renal failure.
• Perforation of the excretory pathway with extravasation of urine is functionally equivalent.

SYSTEMS AFFECTED
• Renal/Urologic
• Gastrointestinal, cardiovascular, nervous, and respiratory systems as uremia develops

SIGNALMENT
More common in males than females

SIGNS
Historical Findings
• Pollakiuria
• Intense straining and crying out when urinating
• Urine staining in the perineal area
• Urine dribbling
• Bilaterally symmetric alopecia in ferrets with adrenal disease
• Gross hematuria
• Signs of uremia develop when urinary tract obstruction is complete (or nearly complete): lethargy, dull attitude, reduced appetite, and vomiting

Physical Examination Findings
• A large, turgid, painful bladder is found on palpation with complete obstruction
• Uroliths may sometimes be palpated in the urinary bladder
• Blood, urethral plugs, or small stones may be visible at the urethral opening in ferrets with cysteine urolithiasis
• Thick, white, or yellow discharge is often visible at the urethral opening in patients with prostatic abscesses
• Purulent preputial discharge with prostatic abscesses
• Palpably enlarged prostate or periurethral cysts near the bladder; cysts may be as large or larger than the urinary bladder—can be seen in females due to the androgen effects of adrenal disease

• Bilaterally symmetric alopecia or pruritus due to adrenal disease
• Signs of severe uremia—dehydration, weakness, hypothermia, stupor, or coma occurring terminally
• Signs of perforation of the excretory pathway—leakage of urine into the peritoneal cavity causes abdominal pain and distension, fever

CAUSES
Intraluminal Causes
• Solid or semisolid structures including uroliths (most common) purulent exudate (with prostatic abscesses or urogenital cysts), urethral plugs, blood clots, and sloughed tissue fragments
• The most common type of urolith seen in the United States consist of cysteine, followed by struvite, calcium, then other, miscellaneous types.

Intramural Causes
• Periurethral cysts/prostatic cysts—seen in males and occasionally females with adrenal disease
• Prostatomegaly—hyperplasia, abscesses, or neoplasia
• Neoplasia of the bladder neck or urethra (uncommon)
• Fibrosis at a site of prior injury or inflammation can cause stricture or stenosis, which may impede urine flow or may be a site where intraluminal debris becomes lodged.
• Edema, hemorrhage, or spasm of muscular components can occur at sites of intraluminal (e.g., urethral) obstruction and contribute to persistent or recurrent obstruction to urinary flow after removal of the intraluminal material. Tissue changes might develop because of injury inflicted by the obstructing material, by the manipulations used to remove the obstructing material, or both.
• Ruptures, lacerations, and punctures—usually caused by traumatic incidents

RISK FACTORS
• Feeding ferret, cat, or dog foods that contain plant-based proteins may lead to the development of struvite urolithiasis.
• Feeding ferret, cat, or dog foods that contain soy products, grain, or legumes may lead to the development of cysteine urolithiasis.
• A genetic basis for the formation of cysteine uroliths is suspected; research is ongoing.
• Urogenital cysts, prostatic hyperplasia, or prostatic cysts are caused by excess hormone formation due to Ferret adrenal disease.

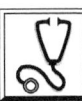

DIAGNOSIS

DIFFERENTIAL DIAGNOSIS
• Repeated unproductive straining in the litter box can be misinterpreted as constipation.
• Animals whose efforts to urinate are not observed by their owners may present for signs referable to uremia without a history of possible obstruction.
• Evaluation of any patient with azotemia should include consideration of possible postrenal causes (e.g., urinary obstruction)
• Ferrets with hyperadrenocorticism and secondary urogenital cysts or prostatomegaly generally have other clinical signs such as bilaterally symmetric alopecia.
• Once the existence of urinary obstruction is recognized, diagnostic efforts focus on detecting the presence and evaluating the severity of abnormalities secondary to obstruction and identifying the location, cause, and completeness of the impediment(s) to urine flow.

CBC/BIOCHEMISTRY/URINALYSIS
• With uroliths, the results of a hemogram are usually normal, but a stress leukogram or evidence of dehydration may be noted.
• Hemogram may show nonregenerative anemia or leukocytosis due to secondary bacterial infection of cysts in ferrets with urogenital cystic disease.
• Biochemistry analysis may reveal azotemia, hyperphosphatemia, metabolic acidosis, and hyperkalemia proportional to the duration of complete obstruction. In ferrets, BUN elevations occur before elevations in creatinine.
• Alkaline urine (pH 6.5–7.0) and crystalluria are seen in most ferrets with urolithiasis
• In ferrets with adrenal disease, paraurethral cysts may become secondarily infected, leading to abscess formation. Cysts/abscesses may drain into the urinary bladder or urethra resulting in thick purulent exudate mixed with urine in the bladder. In some cases, this exudate can be thick enough to cause urethral blockage.

OTHER LABORATORY TESTS
• Elevations in serum estradiol, androstenedione, and 17-hydroxyprogesterone are seen in ferrets with adrenal disease and associated urogenital cystic disease or prostatomegaly (available through the University of Tennessee Clinical

URETHRAL OBSTRUCTION   (CONTINUED)

Endocrinology Laboratory, Department of Comparative Medicine).
• Uroliths passed or retrieved should be sent for crystallographic analysis to determine their composition.

IMAGING

Abdominal Radiography
• Struvite uroliths are radiodense and may be detected by survey radiography.
• Cysteine uroliths are not as radiodense as compared to other types of stones; very small uroliths may be difficult to detect radiographically, especially when superimposed by the os penis.
• In ferrets with urogenital cysts, survey radiographs may reveal what appear to be two or more urinary bladders, as the cysts can be as large as or larger than the urinary bladder; contrast urocystography can be used to delineate the cyst(s).

Abdominal Ultrasonography
Ultrasonography is particularly useful for demonstrating uroliths, adrenal gland enlargement, and large prostate or urogenital cysts.

DIAGNOSTIC PROCEDURES
• Urinary catheterization has diagnostic and therapeutic value. As the catheter is inserted, the location and nature of obstructing material may be determined. Some or all of the obstructing material (e.g., small uroliths and urethral plugs) may be induced to pass out of the urethra distally for identification and analysis. Retrograde irrigation of the urethral lumen may propel intraluminal debris toward the bladder.
• Cytologic evaluation of specimens obtained from the urinary tract with the assistance of catheters may be diagnostic, particularly for carcinoma of the urethra or bladder and some prostatic cysts or abscesses.
• Ultrasound-guided aspiration of prostatic cystic structures; take care to avoid rupturing a prostatic abscess

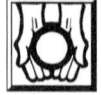

TREATMENT

APPROPRIATE HEALTH CARE
• Complete obstruction is a medical emergency that can be life threatening; treatment should usually be started immediately.
• Partial obstruction—not necessarily an emergency, but these patients may be at risk for developing complete obstruction; may cause irreversible urinary tract damage if not treated promptly
• Treat as an inpatient until the patient's ability to urinate has been restored.

• Treatment has three major components: combating the metabolic derangements associated with postrenal uremia (e.g., dehydration, hypothermia, acidosis, hyperkalemia, and azotemia); restoring and maintaining a patent pathway for urine outflow; and implementing specific treatment for the underlying cause of urine retention.

NURSING CARE
• IV administration of isotonic crystalloid based on the degree of cardiovascular compromise, dehydration, and potential for post-obstructive diuresis.
• Severe hyperkalemia (K+ >8 mmol/L, significant bradycardia/ECG changes)—administer calcium gluconate (1 mL/kg over 3–5 minutes, titrated based on ECG changes), regular insulin 0.1–0.2 U/kg IV once, and 50% dextrose bolus 1 mL/kg IV, diluted, over 5 minutes. May need continued dextrose infusion (2.5–5%) for 4–6 hours to avoid hypoglycemia. Terbutaline 0.01 mg/kg IM or IV can also be given. For more severe derangements (K+ >10 mmol/L, pH <7.1) consider sodium bicarbonate 1 mL/kg IV over 5–10 minutes.
• Monitor the electrocardiogram for evidence of hyperkalemia
• Relieve urethral obstruction by performing urinary catheterization. Without experience, one may find urethral catheterization of male ferrets to be more difficult than for cats. The urethral opening can be difficult to visualize as it is located slightly ventral to the tip of the penis. Ferrets have a J-shaped os penis that extends to the tip of the penis, distal to the urethral opening. With practice, catheterization can be easily mastered. Catheterization should be performed under anesthesia or heavy sedation. Either a 3.5 Fr red rubber catheter or a 3 Fr ferret urethral catheter (Slippery Sam Tomcat Urethral Catheter, Smith Medical) are flexible and long enough to reach the urinary bladder. Dilation of the urethra by insertion of a 25-g IV catheter and flushing with saline before catheterization is helpful. Insert the catheter alongside the IV catheter and flush with saline as the catheter is advanced. Resistance is usually encountered at the pelvic flexure; repeated saline dilation and lubrication may be needed. Once the catheter reaches the urinary bladder, suture the catheter in place and connect a urine collection device. Ferrets with indwelling urinary catheters require an Elizabethan collar.
• Monitor urinary output—should be at least 1–2 mL/kg per hour; with diuresis may be as high as 140 mL per ferret per day.
• If catheterization is initially unsuccessful, decompress the bladder via cystocentesis using a 25-gauge needle. Handle the bladder

carefully and perform the cystocentesis under anesthesia or rupture may occur.
• If catheterization remains unsuccessful, emergency surgery may be required to perform cystotomy with anterograde flushing.

SURGICAL CONSIDERATIONS
• If the urethra is blocked with calculi or debris and retrograde urohydropropulsion is unsuccessful, attempt anterograde flushing of the urethra via cystotomy.
• Remove cystic calculi via cystotomy.
• Immovable urethroliths may require urethrostomy. Ferrets have an os penis that extends from the tip of the penis to the ventral rim of the pelvis. Therefore, the urethrostomy site should be approximately 1 cm below the anus.
• Obstruction caused by urogenital cysts or prostatomegaly secondary to adrenal disease usually requires treatment with adrenalectomy and debulking of cysts. Smaller cysts or mild hyperplasia of prostatic tissue are managed medically. The decision as to which form of treatment is appropriate is multifactorial; which gland is affected (left vs. right), the surgeon's experience and expertise, the severity of clinical signs, the age of the animal, concurrent diseases, and financial issues should be considered.
• If the cysts or prostatomegaly are not causing life-threatening urethral obstruction, medical treatment for adrenal disease (see Medications, below) may cause a sufficient reduction in prostate size to alleviate clinical signs. Depending on the circumstances, medical treatment may be preferred; however, medical treatment is not curative, must be administered lifelong, and has no effect on adrenal tumor size or potential metastasis.
• Surgical removal of the affected adrenal gland(s), coupled with intraoperative aspiration of sterile cysts or debulking of infected cysts is generally necessary to treat large prostatic cysts causing a life-threatening urethral obstruction. These procedures may require special surgical expertise, especially if the right adrenal gland is diseased.
• Large prostatic abscesses require surgical resection and/or marsupialization, require special surgical expertise, and carry a poor prognosis.
• If the bladder is full of purulent exudate, a cystotomy may be indicated to remove accumulated material.

ACTIVITY
Activity should be limited postoperatively.

DIET
• If anorexic, assist feed If anorexic, assist feed an easily digestible high-protein/high-fat diet such as Lafeber Carnivore Critical Care

Diet (Lafeber Company, Cornell, IL) or Oxbow Carnivore Critical Care Diet (Oxbow Animal Health, Omaha, NE); if these are unavailable, offer chicken baby foods; may also add dietary supplement such as Nutri-Cal (EVSCO Pharmaceuticals) to increase caloric content to these foods.
• See prevention, below for long-term diet changes

CLIENT EDUCATION
Advise clients to avoid "grain-free" diets containing legumes or soy products. Feed only high-quality ferret or kitten foods containing animal-based proteins as the primary ingredients.

MEDICATIONS
DRUG(S) OF CHOICE
Sedation for Urinary Catheterization
• Procedures for relief of obstruction require sedatives or anesthetics. When substantial systemic derangements exist, start fluid administration and other supportive measures first. Careful decompression of the bladder by cystocentesis may be performed before anesthesia and catheterization. Calculate the dosage of sedative or anesthetic drug using the low end of the recommended range or give only to effect.
• Options for sedation include:
  ○ Midazolam (0.3–1.0 mg/kg IM); use 0.25–0.5 mg/kg if combined with ketamine (5–10 mg/kg IM)
  ○ Butorphanol (0.05–0.5 mg/kg IM) can be very sedating at the high end of the dosage. If combined with ketamine, midazolam, or dexmedetomidine, use the low end of the dose.
  ○ Dexmedetomidine (0.005–0.01 mg/kg IV or 0.01–0.02 mg/kg IM) can combine with ketamine and an opioid for pain management.
  ○ Alfaxalone (3–5 mg/kg IV, 5–15 mg/kg IM); use the low end of dosing if combined with other agents

Pain Management
• Do not use NSAIDs due to renal compromise. Options include butorphanol (0.05–0.5 mg/kg IM, IV), buprenorphine (0.02–0.05 mg/kg SC, IM, IV or transmucosal oral), hydromorphone (0.1–0.2 mg/kg SC, M, IV), fentanyl (loading dose of 5–10 µg/kg IV then 1.25–5 µg/kg/h IV via constant-rate infusion)

Antibiotics
• If bacterial cystitis is evident, begin oral administration of appropriate antibiotics, chosen based on bacterial culture and antimicrobial susceptibility tests.
• If bacterial prostatitis or abscess is evident, choose antibiotics that can enter the prostatic lumen such as trimethoprim/sulfonamide (15–30 mg/kg PO, SC q12h) or enrofloxacin (5–10 mg/kg PO, SC, IM q12h). A minimum of 4–6 weeks of antimicrobial administration is usually necessary.

CONTRAINDICATIONS
• Corticosteroids are contraindicated while a urinary catheter is in place. This can predispose to the development of UTI.
• Nonsteroidal anti-inflammatory medications should be initially avoided in more metabolically compromised patients.

PRECAUTIONS
Avoid drugs that reduce blood pressure or induce cardiac dysrhythmia until dehydration and hyperkalemia are resolved.

FOLLOW-UP
PATIENT MONITORING
• Assess urine production and hydration status frequently and adjust fluid administration rate accordingly.
• Verify ability to urinate adequately.

POSSIBLE COMPLICATIONS
• Death
• Injury to the urethra while trying to relieve obstruction
• Hypokalemia during post-obstruction diuresis
• Recurrence of obstruction

MISCELLANEOUS
ASSOCIATED CONDITIONS
• Ferret adrenal disease
• Insulinoma
• Bacterial cystitis

AGE-RELATED FACTORS
Both urolithiasis and prostatic disorders secondary to Ferret adrenal disease are most common in middle-aged animals.

ZOONOTIC POTENTIAL
N/A

PREGNANCY/FERTILITY/BREEDING
N/A

SYNONYMS
Urethral obstruction

SEE ALSO
Adrenal disease
Paraurethral cysts
Prostatomegaly
Urolithiasis

ABBREVIATIONS
N/A

Suggested Reading
Di Girolamo N, Huyun M. Disorders of the urinary and reproductive systems in ferrets. In: Quesenberry KE, Carpenter JW, eds. Ferrets, Rabbits and Rodents, 4th Ed). Clinical Medicine and Surgery ed. St. Louis: Saunders, 2020:39–54.
Di Girolamo N, Selleri P. Medical and surgical emergencies in ferrets. Vet Clin Exot Anim Pract 2016;19:431–464.
Garbin M, Pablo LS, Alexander AB. Management of hyperkalemia and associated complications in a ferret (*Mustela putorius furo*) with urinary obstruction requiring surgery. J Exot Pet Med 2021;39:4–7.
Hallman RM, Brandão J. Diagnostic imaging of the renal system in exotic companion mammals. Vet Clin Exot Anim 2020;23:195–214.
Hanak EB, Di Girolamo N, DeSilva U, Marschang RE, Brandao JL et al. Variation in mineral types of uroliths from ferrets (*Mustela putorius furo*) submitted for analysis in North America, Europe, or Asia over an 8-year period. J Am Vet Med Assoc 2021;259:757–763.
Lennox AM, Wagner RA. Comparison of 4.7-mg deslorelin implants and surgery for the treatment of adrenocortical disease in ferrets. J Exot Pet Med 2012;21:332–335.
Pacheco RE. Cystine urolithiasis in ferrets. Vet Clin Exot Anim 2020;23:309–319.
Reavill DR, Lennox AM. Disease overview of the urinary tract in exotic companion mammals and tips on clinical management. Vet Clin Exot Anim 2020;23(1):169–193.
Swiderski JK, Seim HB III, MacPhail CM et al. Long-term outcome of domestic ferrets treated surgically for hyperadrenocorticism: 130 cases (1995–2004). J Am Vet Med Assoc 2008;232:1338–1343.
Wagner RA, Piché CA, Jöchle W et al. Clinical and endocrine responses to treatment with deslorelin acetate implants in ferrets with adrenocortical disease. Am J Vet Res 2005;66:910–915.

Author Barbara Oglesbee, DVM, DABVP (Avian)

FERRETS

UROLITHIASIS

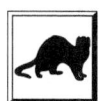

FERRETS

BASICS

DEFINITION
Formation of polycrystalline concretions (i.e., uroliths, calculi, or stones) in the urinary tract. The most common type of urolith seen in North America are composed of cysteine, followed by struvite, calcium, then other, miscellaneous types.

PATHOPHYSIOLOGY
Cysteine
• Feeding ferret, cat, or dog foods that contain legumes, soy products, or other vegetable proteins may lead to the development of cysteine urolithiasis. The dramatic increase in the percentage of ferrets with cysteine uroliths corresponds with the rise in the popularity of grain-free cat and ferret foods. A recent retrospective study of 210 North American ferrets demonstrated that developing cystine urolithiasis was 57.9 times more likely to receive a grain-free diet compared to the reference population.
• A genetic basis for the formation of cysteine uroliths is suspected and research to support this is ongoing. Supporting a genetic basis, anecdotal reports suggest that in households in which all ferrets are fed the same grain-free diets, only ½ develop cysteine urolithiasis

Sterile Struvite
• Occurs more commonly than infection-induced struvite. Ferrets fed a diet containing plant-based protein will produce alkaline urine (pH of 6.5–7), whereas ferrets fed a high-quality animal-based protein diet will produce a more acidic urine (pH near 6). The formation of MAP crystals occurs when the urine pH is above 6.4
• In addition to urinary pH, the specific type of protein fed appears to affect crystal formation. Research suggests that ferrets with urinary pH of 6–7 were less likely to form struvite uroliths when fed animal-based proteins compared with ferrets with the same urinary pH but fed diets with corn-based proteins.
• Microbial urease is not involved in the formation of sterile struvite uroliths.

SYSTEMS AFFECTED
Renal/Urologic

GENETICS
Unknown—suspected in ferrets which develop cysteine uroliths

INCIDENCE/PREVALENCE
• The percentage of ferrets with cysteine uroliths has risen dramatically in North America in the past 10 years. Until 2007, only

15% of uroliths were composed of cystine. A recent large-scale retrospective study reported 93% of the 1014 uroliths submitted from US ferrets between 2010 and 2018 were composed of cysteine, vs only 27% of uroliths submitted from European ferrets. During this same time, the popularity of grain-free diets in North America has risen.

GEOGRAPHIC DISTRIBUTION
Ubiquitous

SIGNALMENT
Species or Breed Predilections
N/A

Mean Age and Range
• Most common in middle-aged to older ferrets—3–7 years of age

Predominant Sex
Urethral obstruction is more common in males but can occur in females.

SIGNS
General Comments
Signs depend on location, size, and number of uroliths

Historical Findings
• Typical signs of urocystoliths include pollakiuria, dysuria, hematuria, urine straining in the perineal area, and urine dribbling.
• Typical signs of urethroliths include pollakiuria and dysuria, including intense straining and crying out when urinating. With complete obstruction, ferrets will have signs of uremia, including depression, lethargy, and anorexia
• Nephroliths are rare but may be associated with signs of renal insufficiency.

Physical Examination Findings
• A large, turgid, painful bladder is found on palpation with complete obstruction.
• Uroliths may sometimes be palpated in the urinary bladder.
• Blood, urethral plugs, or small stones may be visible at the urethral opening in ferrets with cysteine urolithiasis.
• Complete urine outflow obstruction—depression, dehydration, lethargy, or coma.
• Obstruction of a ureter may cause enlargement of the associated kidney.

CAUSES AND RISK FACTORS
• Feeding ferret, cat, or dog foods that contain plant-based proteins may lead to the development of struvite urolithiasis.
• Feeding ferret, cat, or dog foods that contain soy products, grain, or legumes may lead to the development of cysteine urolithiasis.
• A genetic basis for the formation of cysteine uroliths is suspected; research is ongoing.

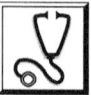

DIAGNOSIS

DIFFERENTIAL DIAGNOSIS
• Uroliths mimic other causes of pollakiuria, dysuria, hematuria, and/or outflow obstruction, the most common of which is prostatomegaly and paraurethral cysts in both male and female ferrets
• Ferrets with prostatomegaly and perurethral cysts usually have other signs of adrenal disease, especially bilaterally symmetric alopecia
• Differentiate from other causes by urinalysis, urine culture, radiography, and ultrasonography.
• For renomegaly—ureteral ligation or entrapment causing hydronephrosis, renal neoplasia; renal cysts are a common incidental finding in ferrets

CBC/BIOCHEMISTRY/URINALYSIS
• Biochemistry analysis may reveal azotemia, hyperphosphatemia, metabolic acidosis, and hyperkalemia proportional to the duration of complete obstruction. In ferrets, BUN elevations occur before elevations in creatinine.
• Alkaline urine (pH 6.5–7.0) and crystalluria are seen in most ferrets with urolithiasis
• Pyuria (normal value 0–1 WBC/hpf), hematuria (normal value 0–3 RBC/hpf), and proteinuria (normal value 0–33 mg/dL) indicate urinary tract inflammation, but these are nonspecific findings that may result from infectious and noninfectious causes of lower urinary tract disease.
• Crystalluria is usually present.

OTHER LABORATORY TESTS
• Quantitative bacterial culture of urine, preferably collected by cystocentesis
• Bacterial culture of inner portions of infection-induced struvite uroliths
• Quantitative mineral analysis of uroliths retrieved via cystotomy

IMAGING
Abdominal Radiography
• Struvite uroliths are radiodense and may be detected by survey radiography.
• Cysteine uroliths are not as radiodense as compared to other types of stones; very small uroliths may be difficult to detect radiographically, especially when superimposed by the os penis.
• In ferrets with urogenital cysts, survey radiographs may reveal what appear to be two or more urinary bladders, as the cysts can be as large as or larger than the urinary bladder; contrast urocystography can be used to delineate the cyst(s).

Abdominal Ultrasonography
Ultrasonography is particularly useful for demonstrating uroliths, adrenal gland enlargement, and large prostate or urogenital cysts.

DIAGNOSTIC PROCEDURES
N/A

PATHOLOGIC FINDINGS
N/A

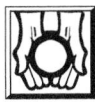

TREATMENT
APPROPRIATE HEALTH CARE
• Complete obstruction is a medical emergency that can be life-threatening; treatment should usually be started immediately.
• Partial obstruction—not necessarily an emergency, but these patients may be at risk for developing complete obstruction; may cause irreversible urinary tract damage if not treated promptly
• Treat as an inpatient until the patient's ability to urinate has been restored.
• Treatment has three major components: combating the metabolic derangements associated with postrenal uremia (e.g., dehydration, hypothermia, acidosis, hyperkalemia, and azotemia); restoring and maintaining a patent pathway for urine outflow; and implementing specific treatment for the underlying cause of urine retention.

NURSING CARE
• IV administration of isotonic crystalloid based on the degree of cardiovascular compromise, dehydration, and potential for post-obstructive diuresis.
• Severe hyperkalemia (K+ >8 mmol/L, significant bradycardia/ECG changes)—administer calcium gluconate (1 mL/kg over 3–5 minutes, titrated based on ECG changes), regular insulin 0.1–0.2 U/kg IV once, and 50% dextrose bolus 1 mL/kg IV, diluted, over 5 minutes. May need continued dextrose infusion (2.5–5%) for 4–6 hours to avoid hypoglycemia. Terbutaline 0.01 mg/kg IM or IV can also be given. For more severe derangements (K+ >10 mmol/L, pH <7.1) consider sodium bicarbonate 1 mL/kg IV over 5–10 minutes.
• Monitor the electrocardiogram for evidence of hyperkalemia
• Relieve urethral obstruction by performing urinary catheterization. Without experience, one may find urethral catheterization of male ferrets to be more difficult than for cats. The urethral opening can be difficult to visualize as it is located slightly ventral to the tip of the penis. Ferrets have a J-shaped os penis that extends to the tip of the penis, distal to the

urethral opening. With practice, catheterization can be easily mastered. Catheterization should be performed under anesthesia or heavy sedation. Either a 3.5 Fr red rubber catheter or a 3 Fr ferret urethral catheter (Slippery Sam Tomcat Urethral Catheter, Smith Medical) are flexible and long enough to reach the urinary bladder. Dilation of the urethra by insertion of a 25-g IV catheter and flushing with saline before catheterization is helpful. Insert the catheter alongside the IV catheter and flush with saline as the catheter is advanced. Resistance is usually encountered at the pelvic flexure; repeated saline dilation and lubrication may be needed. Once the catheter reaches the urinary bladder, suture the catheter in place and connect a urine collection device. Ferrets with indwelling urinary catheters require an Elizabethan collar.
• Monitor urinary output—should be at least 1–2 mL/kg per hour; with diuresis may be as high as 140 mL per ferret per day.
• If catheterization is initially unsuccessful, decompress the bladder via cystocentesis using a 25-gauge needle. Handle the bladder carefully and perform the cystocentesis under anesthesia or rupture may occur.
• If catheterization remains unsuccessful, emergency surgery may be required to perform cystotomy with anterograde flushing.
• Postoperative fluid therapy should continue for 24–48 hours.

SURGICAL CONSIDERATIONS
• If the urethra is blocked with calculi or debris and retrograde urohydropropulsion is unsuccessful, attempt anterograde flushing of the urethra via cystotomy.
• Remove cystic calculi via cystotomy.
• Immovable urethroliths may require urethrostomy. Ferrets have an os penis that extends from the tip of the penis to the ventral rim of the pelvis. Therefore, the urethrostomy site should be approximately 1 cm below the anus.

ACTIVITY
Activity should be limited postoperatively.

DIET
• If anorexic, assist feed If anorexic, assist feed an easily digestible high-protein/high-fat diet such as Lafeber Carnivore Critical Care Diet (Lafeber Company, Cornell, IL) or Oxbow Carnivore Critical Care Diet (Oxbow Animal Health, Omaha, NE); if these are unavailable, offer chicken baby foods; may also add dietary supplement such as Nutri-Cal (EVSCO Pharmaceuticals) to increase caloric content to these foods.
• See prevention, below for long-term diet changes

CLIENT EDUCATION
Advise clients to avoid "grain-free" diets containing legumes or soy products. Feed only high-quality ferret or kitten foods containing animal-based proteins as the primary ingredients.

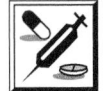

MEDICATIONS
DRUG(S) OF CHOICE
Sedation for Urinary Catheterization
• Procedures for relief of obstruction require sedatives or anesthetics. When substantial systemic derangements exist, start fluid administration and other supportive measures first. Careful decompression of the bladder by cystocentesis may be performed before anesthesia and catheterization. Calculate the dosage of sedative or anesthetic drug using the low end of the recommended range or give only to effect.
• Options for sedation include:
  ○ Midazolam (0.3–1.0 mg/kg IM); use 0.25–0.5 mg/kg if combined with ketamine (5–10 mg/kg IM)
  ○ Butorphanol (0.05–0.5 mg/kg IM) can be very sedating at the high end of the dosage. If combined with ketamine, midazolam, or dexmedetomidine, use the low end of the dose.
  ○ Dexmedetomidine (0.005–0.01 mg/kg IV or 0.01–0.02 mg/kg IM) can combine with ketamine and an opioid for pain management.
  ○ Alfaxalone (3–5 mg/kg IV, 5–15 mg/kg IM); use the low end of dosing if combined with other agents

Pain Management
• Do not use NSAIDs due to renal compromise. Options include butorphanol (0.05–0.5 mg/kg IM, IV), buprenorphine (0.02–0.05 mg/kg SC, IM, IV or transmucosal oral), hydromorphone (0.1–0.2 mg/kg SC, M, IV), fentanyl (loading dose of 5–10 μg/kg IV then 1.25–5 μg/kg/h IV via constant-rate infusion)

Antibiotics
• If bacterial cystitis is evident, begin oral administration of appropriate antibiotics, chosen based on bacterial culture and antimicrobial susceptibility tests.
• If bacterial prostatitis or abscess is evident, choose antibiotics that can enter the prostatic lumen such as trimethoprim/sulfonamide (15–30 mg/kg PO, SC q12h) or enrofloxacin (5–10 mg/kg PO, SC, IM q12h). A minimum of 4–6 weeks of antimicrobial administration is usually necessary.

UROLITHIASIS

FERRETS

CONTRAINDICATIONS
• Corticosteroids are contraindicated while a urinary catheter is in place. This can predispose to the development of UTI.

PRECAUTIONS
Avoid drugs that reduce blood pressure or induce cardiac dysrhythmia until dehydration and hyperkalemia are resolved.

ALTERNATIVE DRUGS
N/A

FOLLOW-UP

PATIENT MONITORING
Monitor for licking and chewing at incision site; Elizabethan collars are usually necessary.

PREVENTION/AVOIDANCE
• Ferrets have a much higher dietary protein requirement than dogs or cats (30–35%). Feeding a high-quality, animal protein-based ferret or kitten food that does not contain cysteine-rich legumes, grain and soy are recommended to prevent cystine urolithiasis
• Recurrent sterile struvite uroliths may be prevented by feeding a high-quality ferret or cat food.
• Increasing the water content of food and encouraging water consumption will produce dilute urine and reduce crystal concentration
• Infection-induced struvite urolithiasis may be prevented by eradicating and controlling infections by urease-producing bacteria.

POSSIBLE COMPLICATIONS
• Rupture of the bladder
• Urethral tear
• Recurrence of uroliths if diet is not improved

EXPECTED COURSE AND PROGNOSIS
• Treatment of urethroliths carries a good to guarded prognosis. If urohydropulpusion via urethral catheterization is successful in removing the obstruction, the prognosis is good.
• Urohydropulpusion via urethral catheterization can sometimes be difficult to successfully perform, and emergency procedures such as cystotomy for anterograde urohydropropulsion or perineal urethrostomy may be necessary to relieve the obstruction. Complications such as bladder or urethral rupture may occur.
• Nephroliths are usually asymptomatic if the ureters remain unobstructed, and often respond to dietary changes alone.

MISCELLANEOUS

ASSOCIATED CONDITIONS
Any disease that predisposes to bacterial urinary tract infection

AGE-RELATED FACTORS
N/A

ZOONOTIC POTENTIAL
None

PREGNANCY/FERTILITY/BREEDING
In pregnant jills close to parturition, a caesarian section should be performed at the same time as cystotomy to prevent straining and dehiscence during parturition.

SYNONYMS
Bladder stones
Urethral stones

SEE ALSO
Adrenal disease
Paraurethral cysts
Prostatomegaly

ABBREVIATIONS
BUN = blood urea nitrogen
MAP = magnesium ammonium phosphate
RBC = red blood cell count
WBC = white blood cell count

Suggested Reading
Di Girolamo N, Huyun M. Disorders of the urinary and reproductive systems in ferrets. In: Quesenberry KE, Carpenter JW, eds. Ferrets, Rabbits and Rodents, 4th Ed). Clinical Medicine and Surgery ed. St. Louis: Saunders, 2020:39–54.
Di Girolamo N, Selleri P. Medical and surgical emergencies in ferrets. Vet Clin Exot Anim Pract 2016;19:431–464.
Garbin M, Pablo LS, Alexander AB. Management of hyperkalemia and associated complications in a ferret (*Mustela putorius furo*) with urinary obstruction requiring surgery. J Exot Pet Med 2021;39:4–7.
Hallman RM, Brandão J. Diagnostic imaging of the renal system in exotic companion mammals. Vet Clin Exot Anim 2020;23:195–214.
Hanak EB, Di Girolamo N, DeSilva U, Marschang RE, Brandao JL et al. Variation in mineral types of uroliths from ferrets (*Mustela putorius furo*) submitted for analysis in North America, Europe, or Asia over an 8-year period. J Am Vet Med Assoc 2021;259:757–763.
Pacheco RE. Cystine urolithiasis in ferrets. Vet Clin Exot Anim 2020;23:309–319.
Reavill DR, Lennox AM. Disease overview of the urinary tract in exotic companion mammals and tips on clinical management. Vet Clin Exot Anim 2020;23(1):169–193.

Author Barbara Oglesbee, DVM, DABVP (Avian)

BASICS

DEFINITION
• Acute manifestation of a Type I hypersensitivity reaction (anaphylaxis) mediated through the rapid introduction of an antigen into a host having antigen-specific antibodies of the IgE subclass.
• Vaccine reactions are seen most commonly following vaccination for CDV but can also occur following rabies vaccination.
• Most adverse reactions occur within 30 minutes of vaccine administration, but can occur up to 48 hours post-vaccine

SYSTEMS AFFECTED
• Gastrointestinal—salivation, vomiting, and diarrhea
• Skin/Exocrine—pruritus, urticaria, and edema
• Cardiovascular—shock

GENETICS
N/A

INCIDENCE/PREVALENCE
• Overall incidence of 5–10%, but the risk of adverse reaction increases with prior exposure to either CDV or rabies vaccine. Risk is cumulative (i.e., increases with the number of previous vaccinations).
• Risk also increases when CDV and rabies vaccines are administered simultaneously

GEOGRAPHIC DISTRIBUTION
Worldwide

SIGNALMENT
No age or gender variation in risk

SIGNS
• Acute anaphylaxis—typically occurs within 30 minutes of administration. Collapse, hypersalivation, pale mucus membranes, diarrhea (often liquid with fresh blood), piloerection, and vomiting.
• Delayed, mild reaction—typically occurs within 24–48 hours of administration. Lethargy, pruritis, and urticariaa
• Swelling at vaccination site—swelling and formation of fibrosarcomas has been reported.

CAUSES
The first exposure of the patient to the vaccine can cause a humoral response and results in the production of IgE, which binds to the surface of mast cells; the patient is then considered to be sensitized to that antigen. The second exposure to the antigen results in cross-linking of two or more IgE molecules on the cell surface, resulting in mast cell degranulation and activation; the release of mast cell granules initiates an anaphylactic reaction.

RISK FACTORS
Previous exposure (sensitization) increases the chance of the animal developing a reaction.

DIAGNOSIS
A presumptive is based on the clinical signs and timing of vaccination.

CBC/BIOCHEMISTRY/URINALYSIS
• Because of the acute onset of signs, no tests are available that reliably predict individual susceptibility.
• May be useful to rule out other causes of clinical signs, if in doubt

IMAGING
Radiographs—usually not necessary

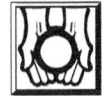

TREATMENT

APPROPRIATE HEALTH CARE
Inpatient with acute anaphylaxis
Outpatient for less severe reactions

NURSING CARE
• Emergency life support through the maintenance of an open airway, preventing circulatory collapse, and reestablishing physiologic parameters.
• Administer fluids intravenously at shock dosages to counteract hypotension
• Administer oxygen to dyspneic patients

ACTIVITY
Limited

DIET
Withhold food until reaction abates

CLIENT EDUCATION
• Inform clients of the risk of adverse reactions, especially in ferrets that have been previously vaccinated. Have clients wait in the clinic for at least 30 minutes following vaccine administration.
• If clients are reluctant to vaccinate for CDV due to previous vaccine reactions, recommend measuring antibody titers. A titer higher than 1:50 is currently considered high enough to provide immunity to CDV infection in ferrets.

SURGICAL CONSIDERATIONS
N/A

MEDICATIONS

DRUGS OF CHOICE
• Diphenhydramine (2 mg/kg IV or IM)
• Epinephrine hydrochloride (20 mcg/ kg IV, IM, SC, or intratracheally)

• Dexamethasone sodium phosphate (1–2 mg/kg IV or IM)

CONTRAINDICATIONS
N/A

PRECAUTIONS
N/A

POSSIBLE INTERACTIONS
N/A

ALTERNATIVE DRUGS
N/A

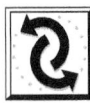

FOLLOW-UP

PATIENT MONITORING
• Keep the patient in the clinic to monitor for signs of vaccine reaction for at least 30 minutes following vaccine administration
• Monitor for development of lethargy, urticaria, or swelling for 24–48 hours
• Document the site of vaccination in the medical record for reference should fibrosarcoma develop in the future.

PREVENTION/AVOIDANCE
• Administration of diphenhydramine (2 mg/kg IM) 15–20 minutes prior to vaccination may decrease the risk of an adverse reaction.
• Do not administer CDV and rabies vaccinations simultaneously
• Use only vaccines that are approved for use in ferrets. The approved vaccines available in the US are Fervac-D (United Vaccines, Inc., Madison WI) and PureVax (Merial, Athens, GA).
• Canine or ferret tissue culture-adapted vaccines can induce disease and should never be used.

POSSIBLE COMPLICATIONS
• Death with severe vaccine reactions.

EXPECTED COURSE AND PROGNOSIS
• Most ferrets will recover with immediate treatment
• Death can occur if treatment is delayed or in severe cases.

MISCELLANEOUS

ASSOCIATED CONDITIONS
N/A

AGE-RELATED FACTORS
N/A

ZOONOTIC POTENTIAL
NA

PREGNANCY/FERTILITY/BREEDING
N/A

VACCINE REACTION

SYNONYMS
Vaccine anaphylaxis

ABBREVIATIONS
CDV = canine distemper virus

Suggested Reading
Greenacre CB. Incidence of adverse events in ferrets vaccinated with distemper or rabies vaccine: 143 cases (1995–2001). J Am Vet Med Assoc 2003;223:663–665.

Kiupel M, Perpiñán D. Viral diseases of ferrets. In: Fox JG, Marini RP, eds. Biology and Diseases of the Ferret, 3rd ed. Wiley, 2014:439–517.

Moore GE, Glickman NW, Ward MP et al. Incidence of and risk factors for adverse events associated with distemper and rabies vaccine administration in ferrets. J Am Vet Med Assoc 2005;226(6):909–912.

Munday JS, Stedman NL, Richey LJ. Histology and immunohistochemistry of seven ferret vaccination-site fibrosarcomas. Vet Pathol 2003;40:288–293.

Perpinan D, Ramis A, Tomás A. Outbreak of canine distemper in domestic ferrets (*Mustela putorius furo*). Vet Rec 2008;163:246–250.

Author Barbara Oglesbee, DVM, DABVP (Avian)

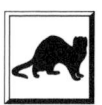

BASICS

DEFINITION
Any substance emanating from the vulvar labia

PATHOPHYSIOLOGY
May originate from several distinct sources, depending in part on the age, reproductive status of the patient, or presence of underlying diseases (e.g., ferret adrenal disease); from urinary tract, uterus, vagina, or perivulvar skin; may be normal or abnormal

SYSTEMS AFFECTED
- Reproductive
- Endocrine
- Renal/Urologic
- Skin/Exocrine

SIGNALMENT
- Estrual and postpartum females—bloody discharge not normally visible with estrus; postpartum discharge may be normal
- Postestrual, pregnant, and postpartum or spayed females—may be more serious

SIGNS
Historical Findings
- Sexually mature females (>8–12 months old)
- Swollen vulva
- Bilaterally symmetric alopecia—with adrenal disease
- Attracting males
- Parturition—with postpartum discharge
- Recent estrus—with pyometra or vaginitis

Physical Examination Findings
- Discharge may appear serosanguinous, sanguinous, clear, mucoid, or purulent
- Alopecia
- Swollen vulva
- Pruritis

CAUSES
Serosanguinous
- Urinary tract infection
- Foreign body
- Vaginal neoplasia
- Vaginal trauma
- Fetal death
- Vaginal hematoma

Purulent Exudate
- Primary vaginitis
- Secondary vaginitis—from foreign body, urinary tract infection, vaginal neoplasia, and fetal death
- Pyometra or stump pyometra
- Embryonic and fetal death
- Postpartum metritis
- Perivulvar dermatitis

Other
Acquired perivulvar dermatitis can also be mistaken for vaginal discharge

RISK FACTORS
- Ferret adrenal disease (FAD)—may predispose to vaginitis or stump pyometra
- Prolonged estrus in unbred females—hyperestrogenism predisposes patient to pyometra
- Small litter size—litters of <3 kits may be insufficient to stimulate parturition, resulting in fetal death

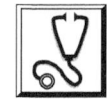

DIAGNOSIS

DIFFERENTIAL DIAGNOSES
- History and signalment—establish hormonal influences (e.g., prolonged estrus, FAD, pregnancy, and parturition)
- Source and type of the discharge—must be identified by appropriate diagnostics
- Rule out Ferret adrenal disease—FAD usually seen in ferrets >2 years of age and is associated with bilaterally symmetric alopecia. Secretion of sex steroids may cause vulvar swelling, discharge, vaginitis, pyometra, or stump pyometra
- Rule out hyperestrogenism—in unbred females remaining in estrus for >1 month—may cause vaginitis, pyometra, or bleeding disorders due to the toxic effects of estrogen on bone marrow.
- Rule out ovarian remnant in spayed females—may also cause estrogen toxicity; may predispose patient to vaginitis or stump pyometra

CBC/BIOCHEMISTRY/URINALYSIS
- Nonregenerative anemia, pancytopenia—in ferrets with hyperestrogenism
- Leukocytosis with a left shift—with pyometra or metritis
- High BUN and creatinine—with pyometra
- Urinary tract infection—may be noted

OTHER LABORATORY TESTS
- Examination of vaginal cytology may reveal numerous cornified cells or purulent exudate in ferrets with pyometra.
- Elevations in serum estradiol, androstenedione, and 17-hydroxyprogesterone to diagnose FAD as the underlying cause of discharge (available through the University of Tennessee Clinical Endocrinology Laboratory, Department of Comparative Medicine)
- High serum estrogen (estradiol) concentration to help confirm hyperestrogenism

IMAGING
- Radiography—detect a large uterus in patients with pyometra or later stages of fetal death
- Ultrasonography—determine pregnancy as early as 12 days post-breeding; may be used to detect pyometra, stump pyometra, or identify affected adrenal gland in ferrets with FAD.

DIAGNOSTIC PROCEDURES
- Vaginal bacterial culture—via guarded swab; perform before doing any other vaginal procedure
- Vaginal cytologic examination—determine if the discharge is sanguinous, serosanguinous, or purulent; the extent of cornification helps establish whether the jill is in proestrus or estrus
- Cystocentesis and bacterial culture—help rule out urinary tract infection
- Biopsy of vaginal mass—rule out neoplasia

TREATMENT
- Outpatient, unless pyometra or hyperestrogenism
- Hospitalization is required in ferrets exhibiting clinical signs related to anemia or hemorrhage due to hyperestrogenism, or for pyometra patients exhibiting anorexia, dehydration, or weakness. Supportive care, such as fluid therapy, warmth, and adequate nutrition are required for recovery in these patients.
- Blood transfusions may be required in patients with pancytopenia due to hyperestrogenism.
- Ovariohysterectomy is the treatment of choice in patients with pyometra or hyperestrogenism. This is a relatively safe procedure in ferrets with PCV >30, and no evidence of bleeding disorders. Ferrets with PCV <30 would benefit from a blood transfusion prior to surgery. Ferrets that are extremely anemic, thrombocytopenic, and with secondary infections such as pneumonia or pyometra are poor surgical risks, and should be stabilized, if possible, prior to surgery (transfusion as needed and medical treatment with hCG—see below).
- Perform celiotomy in ferrets with ovarian remnant. Ovarian tissue may be small and is located at the caudolateral pole of the kidney.
- FAD—may be treated with adrenalectomy or managed medically. The decision as to which form of treatment is appropriate is multifactorial: which gland is affected (left vs. right), surgeon's experience, severity of clinical signs, age of the animal, concurrent

VAGINAL DISCHARGE

diseases, and financial issues should be considered.
• Remove or treat any other inciting causes—foreign body; neoplasia; urinary tract infection

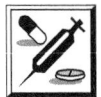

MEDICATIONS
DRUG(S) OF CHOICE
GnRH Analogs
• The GnRH agonist deslorelin acetate (Suprelorin-F®, Virbac Animal Health) is labeled for the treatment of adrenal disease in domestic ferrets in the United States. It is a 4.7-mg slow-release deslorelin implant reported to provide alleviation of clinical signs lasting from 8 to 20 months. Alleviation of clinical signs may be more likely in patients with adrenal hyperplasia or adenoma; adenocarcinomas may be less likely to respond. Deslorelin has no demonstrated effect on adrenal tumor growth or metastasis. In Europe, 9.4-mg deslorelin implants are available and may be effective for up to 2–4 years.
• Leuprolide acetate, a GnRH analog, is a potent gonadotropin secretion inhibitor and suppresses LH and FSH, downregulating their receptor sites. It is available as a 1- or 4-month depot injection and may alleviate the dermal and reproductive organ signs of adrenal disease in ferrets. Reported dosages: Lupron® 30-day depot, 100–250 μg/kg IM q4w until signs resolve, then q4–8w PRN, lifelong. Larger ferrets often require the higher end of the dose range. This drug has no effect on adrenal tumor growth or metastasis. This drug has become challenging to acquire and often prohibitively expensive in the United States.

Other Treatments for Adrenal Disease
• Melatonin implants are available commercially (Ferretonin® 2.7-mg-ferrets < 600 g) and 5.4-mg implants—most ferrets, Melatek, LLC) and have been used in ferrets with adrenal disease to alleviate alopecia and, possibly, aggressive behavior, prostatomegaly, or vulvar swelling. Implants are repeated every 4 months as needed, lifelong. Alleviation of clinical signs may be more likely in patients with adrenal hyperplasia or adenoma; adenocarcinomas may be less likely to respond. Melatonin has no demonstrated effect on adrenal tumor growth or metastasis.

For Hyperestrogenism
Administer hCG 100 IU per ferret IM to stimulate ovulation and end estrus. Signs of estrus (particularly vulvar swelling) should diminish within 3–4 days. If signs are still apparent 1 week posttreatment, repeat the injection. Treatment is only effective after day 10 of estrus.

For Metritis or Primary Vaginitis
• systemic antibiotics such as trimethoprim-sulfa (15–30 mg/kg PO q12h), enrofloxacin (5–10 mg/kg PO, IM, SC q12h), amoxicillin/clavulanate (12.5 mg/kg PO q12h), or a cephalosporin (cephalexin 15–25 mg/kg PO q8–12h).

CONTRAINDICATIONS
Many antibiotics are contraindicated during pregnancy.

PRECAUTIONS
N/A

POSSIBLE INTERACTIONS
N/A

ALTERNATIVE DRUGS
N/A

FOLLOW-UP
PATIENT MONITORING
Ultrasonography or radiography—determine uterine size and contents with pyometra or metritis

POSSIBLE COMPLICATIONS
Toxic shock—with severe pyometra or metritis

MISCELLANEOUS
ASSOCIATED CONDITIONS
• Insulinoma
• Ferret adrenal disease

AGE-RELATED FACTORS
N/A

ZOONOTIC POTENTIAL
N/A

PREGNANCY/FERTILITY/BREEDING
Many antibiotics are contraindicated during pregnancy.

SEE ALSO
Adrenal disease (hyperadrenocorticism)
Hyperestrogenism

ABBREVIATIONS
FAD = ferret adrenal disease
FSH = follicular-stimulating hormone
hCG = human chorionic gonadotropin
LH = luteinizing hormone
LHRH = luteinizing hormone-releasing hormone
PCV = packed cell volume

Suggested Reading
Di Girolamo N, Huyun M. Disorders of the urinary and reproductive systems in ferrets. In: Quesenberry KE, Carpenter JW, eds. Ferrets, Rabbits and Rodents, 4th Ed). Clinical Medicine and Surgery ed. St. Louis: Saunders, 2020:39–54.
Di Girolamo N, Selleri P. Medical and surgical emergencies in ferrets. Vet Clin Exot Anim Pract. 2016;19:431–464.
Jekl V, Hauptman K. Reproductive medicine in ferrets. Vet Clin Exot Anim Pract 2017;20:629–663.
Lennox AM, Wagner RA. Comparison of 4.7-mg deslorelin implants and surgery for the treatment of adrenocortical disease in ferrets. J Exot Pet Med 2012;21:332–335.
Schoemaker NJ, Van Zealand YRA. Endocrine diseases of ferrets. In: Quesenberry KE, Carpenter JW, eds. Ferrets, Rabbits and Rodents, 4th Ed). Clinical Medicine and Surgery ed. St. Louis: Saunders, 2020:77–91.
Schoemaker NJ, Van Deijk R, Muijlaert B et al. Use of a gonadotropin releasing hormone agonist implant as an Alternative for surgical castration in male ferrets (*Mustela putorius furo*). Theriogenol 2008;70:161–167.
Swiderski JK, Seim HB III, MacPhail CM et al. Long-term outcome of domestic ferrets treated surgically for hyperadreno-corticism: 130 cases (1995–2004). J Am Vet Med Assoc 2008;232:1338–1343.
Wagner RA, Piché CA, Jöchle W et al. Clinical and endocrine responses to treatment with deslorelin acetate implants in ferrets with adrenocortical disease. Am J Vet Res 2005;66:910–914.
Author Barbara Oglesbee, DVM, DABVP (Avian)

BASICS

DEFINITION
A complex reflex that results in the expulsion of food or fluid from the alimentary tract through the oral cavity.

PATHOPHYSIOLOGY
Vomiting can be caused by diseases of the alimentary tract or can occur secondary to toxic, neurologic, metabolic, infectious, and noninfectious causes. Vomiting is seen less frequently in ferrets than in dogs and cats with similar diseases, and when seen, usually indicates serious disease. Vomiting occurs when the vomiting center, located in the brain, is stimulated by input from various receptor sites throughout the body. Vomiting can be stimulated by peripheral receptors located in the gastrointestinal tract or in various organs. Vomiting can also be initiated directly by stimulation of the receptors in the vomiting center in animals with CNS disease. Stimulation of the chemoreceptor trigger zone by metabolic or bacterial toxins, drugs, motion sickness, or vestibulitis will also trigger vomiting.

SYSTEMS AFFECTED
• Endocrine/Metabolic—electrolyte abnormalities, prerenal azotemia, and dehydration
• Gastrointestinal
• Respiratory—aspiration pneumonia
• Nervous—altered mental attitude

SIGNALMENT
N/A

SIGNS

Historical Findings
• Signs of nausea, such as ptyalism, licking the lips, pawing at the mouth, and backing up are usually seen just prior to vomiting or retching.
• Change in diet or access to spoiled foods or garbage
• Exposure to other ferrets
• Chewing habits—missing toys, chewing on furniture (especially foam rubber)
• Changes in appetite
• Weight loss

Physical Examination Findings
• Weight loss with loss of fat stores and musculature—indicates chronic disease
• Poor hair coat—seen with chronic disease (infiltrative intestinal disease, hepatic disease, and metabolic disorders)
• Thickened bowel loops, masses, or pain on abdominal palpation
• Diarrhea or melena

• Dry, pale mucous membranes if the ferret is dehydrated

CAUSES
• Bacterial infection—*Helicobacter mustelae* (common), *Campylobacter* spp., *Salmonella* sp., *Clostridium* spp.
• Viral infection—epizootic catarrhal enteritis (ECE)—very common cause, rotavirus, parvovirus less common
• Obstruction—very common; foreign body most common cause, followed by neoplasia; intussusception rare
• Infiltrative—lymphoplasmacytic gastroenteritis, eosinophilic gastroenteritis (common diseases, occasionally causes vomiting)
• Neoplasia—lymphoma, adenocarcinoma, and insulinoma
• Parasitic causes—giardia, coccidia (both may be primary pathogens, or secondary to ECE), *Cryptosporidium* spp.
• Metabolic disorders—liver disease, renal disease, pancreatitis, metabolic acidosis, and electrolyte abnormalities (e.g., hypokalemia, hyperkalemia, hyponatremia, and hypercalcemia)
• Dietary—diet changes, eating spoiled food, dietary intolerance
• Drugs and toxins—vaccine reaction (causes acute onset of vomiting), chemotherapeutic agents, plant toxins, isoflurane anesthesia
• Nervous—(unusual cause) cerebral edema, CNS tumor, otitis media/interna

RISK FACTORS
• Exposure to other ferrets (ECE, other infectious diseases)
• Unsupervised chewing (foreign bodies)
• Stress, debility (predisposes to *Helicobacter*-induced gastritis)
• Feeding raw meat products (bacterial enteritis, cryptosporidiosis)
• Vaccine reaction
• Dietary changes

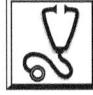

DIAGNOSIS

DIFFERENTIAL DIAGNOSIS

Differentiating Similar Signs
• Differentiate primary alimentary tract disease from disease of other organ systems.
• It is important to distinguish vomiting from regurgitation, since regurgitation is usually caused by primary esophageal disease. Vomiting is often preceded by restlessness, pawing at the mouth, hypersalivation, licking the lips, backing up, and retching. Vomitus may be digested food, mucus, or liquid with bile staining; fresh or digested blood may be present, especially with gastrointestinal

ulceration. Regurgitation is a passive act that results in the expulsion of food into the oral cavity. The contents may be tubular in shape and typically composed of undigested food. Esophageal disorders are relatively rare in ferrets but can occur concurrently with diseases of the stomach and small intestine.
• Diarrhea, abnormal stool, or significant weight loss is more suggestive of intestinal disease.
• Vomiting is an uncommon clinical sign in ferrets; when seen, a thorough diagnostic workup is indicated.

CBC/BIOCHEMISTRY/URINALYSIS
• Hemogram may be normal or reveal nonregenerative anemia secondary to chronic disease.
• Increased hematocrit and serum protein concentration seen with dehydration
• Regenerative anemia may be seen with chronic gastrointestinal bleeding.
• TWBC elevation with neutrophilia may be seen with bacterial enteritis.
• TWBC elevation with lymphocytosis, or normal TWBC with relative lymphocytosis, may be suggestive of lymphoma.
• Eosinophilia (as high as 35%) suggests eosinophilic gastroenteritis.
• Hypoalbuminemia may be seen with protein loss from the intestinal tract, especially with proliferative or infiltrative bowel disease.
• Serum biochemistry abnormalities may suggest renal or hepatic disease; ALT elevations usually seen with ECE.

OTHER LABORATORY TESTS
• Fecal direct examination, fecal flotation, zinc sulfate centrifugation many demonstrate gastrointestinal parasites.
• Fecal cytology—may reveal RBC or fecal leukocytes, which are associated with inflammatory bowel disease or invasive bacterial strains.
• Fecal culture should be performed if abnormal bacteria are observed on the fecal gram's stain, or if salmonella is suspected.

IMAGING

Radiographic Findings
• Survey abdominal radiography may indicate intestinal obstruction, organomegaly, mass, foreign body, or ascites.
• Contrast radiography may indicate thickening of the intestinal wall, mucosal irregularities, mass, severe ileus, foreign body, or stricture.
• Abdominal ultrasonography may demonstrate intestinal wall thickening, gastrointestinal mass, foreign body, ileus, mesenteric lymphadenopathy, or hepatic disease.

VOMITING   (CONTINUED)

DIAGNOSTIC PROCEDURES
• Gastroscopy to detect and remove small foreign bodies or to identify mucosal lesions. Endoscopy is superior to radiography in evaluating inflammation, erosions, and ulcers. However, the small size of the patient and subsequent limitations on instrument size often limits the use of endoscopy.
• Exploratory laparotomy and surgical biopsy should be pursued if there is evidence of obstruction or intestinal mass, and/or for definitive diagnosis of gastrointestinal inflammatory or neoplastic diseases or *H. mustelae*-induced gastritis.

TREATMENT
• Treatment must be specific to the underlying cause to be successful.
• Patients with mild disease usually respond to outpatient treatment.
• Patients with moderate to severe disease usually require hospitalization and 24-hour care for parenteral medication and fluid therapy.
• Correct electrolyte and acid–base disturbances.
• Ferrets rarely have intractable vomiting such that holding NPO for long periods is necessary. If holding NPO, monitor ferrets carefully for hypoglycemia. A fast of greater than 4 hours can be dangerous. Insulinoma is extremely common in middle-aged ferrets and may be the cause of signs of gastritis or may occur simultaneously with other causes of gastritis.
• Once vomiting has subsided, offer a bland diet such as canned chicken baby foods. If the patient has been anorectic, assist feed an easily digestible high-protein/high-fat diet such as Lafeber Carnivore Critical Care Diet (Lafeber Company, Cornell, IL) or Oxbow Carnivore Critical Care Diet (Oxbow Animal Health, Omaha, NE); may also add dietary supplement such as Nutri-Cal (EVSCO Pharmaceuticals) to increase caloric content to these foods.
• Warming the food to body temperature or offering via syringe may increase acceptance; administer these foods several times a day.

MEDICATIONS
DRUG(S) OF CHOICE
• Depend on the cause of vomiting; see specific diseases for more detailed treatment options
• Antibiotic therapy—indicated in patients with bacterial inflammatory lesions in the gastrointestinal tract. Also indicated in patients with disruption of the intestinal mucosa evidenced by blood in the feces. Selection should be based on results of culture and susceptibility testing when possible. For empirical treatment, use broad-spectrum antibiotics such as trimethoprim sulfa (15–30 mg/kg q12h), amoxicillin/clavulanate (12.5 mg/kg PO q12h), cephalexin (15–25 mg/kg PO q12h), or enrofloxacin (5–10 mg/kg PO, SQ, IM q12h).
• *H. mustelae*—the combination of amoxicillin (30 mg/kg PO q8–12h) plus metronidazole (20 mg/kg PO q8–12h) and bismuth subsalicylate (17.5 mg/kg PO q12h or 1 mL/kg of regular strength preparation [262 mg/15 mL] PO q8–12h) is a common, inexpensive treatment regimen; however, many ferrets find this unpalatable. Dosing every 8 hours may be necessary to eliminate infection. Combine this treatment with an antisecretory agent (see below). Treat for at least 2 (often 3–4) weeks. The combination of clarithromycin (12.5 mg/kg PO q8–12h) and ranitidine bismuth citrate or ranitidine HCl (24 mg/kg PO q8–12h) for 2 weeks has also been reported to be effective in the eradication of *Helicobacter* spp. Ranitidine is no longer approved for human use in the US and can be difficult to find. The combination of clarithromycin (50 mg/kg PO q24h or divided q12h); omeprazole (4 mg/kg PO q24h); metronidazole (20 mg/kg PO q12h) for 14 days has also been used for eradication
• Gastrointestinal antisecretory agents are helpful to treat and possibly prevent gastritis in anorectic ferrets. Ferrets continually secrete a baseline level of gastric hydrochloric acid and, as such, anorexia itself may predispose to gastric ulceration. Those successfully used in ferrets include omeprazole (4 mg/kg PO q24h), famotidine (0.25–0.5 mg/kg PO, SC, IV q24h), and cimetidine (10 mg/kg PO, SC, IM, IV q8h)
• Sucralfate suspension (25 mg/kg PO q8h) protects ulcerated tissue (cytoprotection) by binding to ulcer sites.
• Antiemetics should be reserved for patients with refractory vomiting that have not responded to treatment of the underlying disease. Options include metoclopramide (0.2–1.0 mg/kg PO, SC, IM q6–8h), Ondansetron (1 mg/kg PO q12–24h), or maropitant citrate (1 mg/kg SC q24h).

CONTRAINDICATIONS
• Alpha-adrenergic blockers such as chlorpromazine should not be used in dehydrated patients, since they can cause hypotension.
• Metoclopramide is contraindicated in patients with gastrointestinal obstruction and is associated with signs of restlessness and depression.

PRECAUTIONS
Antiemetics such as chlorpromazine may cause severe drowsiness and should be avoided when possible since they can mask an underlying problem.

POSSIBLE INTERACTIONS
N/A

ALTERNATE DRUGS
N/A

FOLLOW-UP
PATIENT MONITORING
Continued vomiting, fecal volume and character, appetite, attitude, and body condition

POSSIBLE COMPLICATIONS
• Reflux esophagitis
• Aspiration pneumonia
• Dehydration due to fluid loss

MISCELLANEOUS
ASSOCIATED CONDITIONS
N/A

AGE-RELATED FACTORS
• Foreign body or lymphoma may be seen in any age ferret.
• Older ferrets demonstrate more severe clinical signs with ECE.

ZOONOTIC POTENTIAL
• Cryptosporidiosis
• Giardia

PREGNANCY/FERTILITY/BREEDING
N/A

SEE ALSO
Epizootic catarrhal enteritis
Gastrointestinal and esophageal foreign bodies
Helicobacter mustelae
Inflammatory bowel disease

ABBREVIATIONS
ALT = alanine aminotransferase
CNS = central nervous system
ECE = epizootic catarrhal enteritis
TWBC = total white blood cell count

Suggested Reading
Cazzini P, Watson MK, Gottdenker N et al. Proposed grading scheme for inflammatory bowel disease in ferrets and correlation with clinical signs. J Vet Diagn Invest 2020;32(1):17–24.

Di Girolamo N, Selleri P. Medical and surgical emergencies in ferrets. Vet Clin Exot Anim 2016;19:431–464.

Doria-Torra G, Vidaña B, Ramis A, Amarilla S, Martínez J. Coronavirus infection in ferrets: antigen distribution and inflammatory response. Vet Path 2016;53(6):1180–1186.

Hoefer HL. Gastrointestinal diseases of ferrets. In: Quesenberry KE, Carpenter JW, eds. Ferrets, Rabbits, and Rodents, 4th Ed). Clinical Medicine and Surgery. 2021 ed. St. Louis: Saunders, 2020:27–38.

Huynh M, Pignon C. Gastrointestinal disease in exotic small mammals. J Exot Pet Med 2013;22(2):118–131.

Johnson-Delaney CA. Geriatric ferrets. Vet Clin Exot Anim Pract 2020;23(3):549–565.

Li T, Yoshizaki S, Kataoka M, Doan Y, Ami Y, Suzaki, Y.. . .Wakita, T. Determination of ferret enteric coronavirus genome in laboratory ferrets. Emerg Infect Dise 2017;23(9):1568–1570.

Livingstone M. Dealing with gastrointestinal disease in ferrets. In Practice 2022;44:169–179.

Murray J, Kiupel M, Maes RK. Ferret coronavirus-associated diseases. Vet Clin North Am Exot Anim Pract 2010;13(3):543–560.

Watson MK, Cazzini P, Mayer J et al. Histology and immunohistochemistry of severe inflammatory bowel disease versus lymphoma in the ferret (*Mustela putorius furo*). J Vet Diagn Invest 2016;28(3):198–206.

Author Barbara Oglesbee, DVM, DABVP-Avian

WEIGHT LOSS AND CACHEXIA

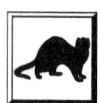

BASICS

DEFINITION
• Weight loss is considered clinically important when it exceeds 10% of the normal body weight and is not associated with fluid loss.
• Cachexia is defined as the state of extreme poor health and is associated with anorexia, weight loss, weakness, and mental depression.

PATHOPHYSIOLOGY
• Weight loss can result from many different pathophysiologic mechanisms that share a common feature—insufficient caloric intake or availability to meet metabolic needs.
• Insufficient caloric intake can be caused by (1) a high energy demand (e.g., that characteristic of a hypermetabolic state); (2) inadequate energy intake, including insufficient quantity or quality of food, or inadequate nutrient assimilation (e.g., with anorexia, dysphagia, regurgitation, or malabsorptive disorders); or (3) excessive loss of nutrients or fluid, which can occur in patients with gastrointestinal losses, glucosuria, or proteinuria.

SYSTEMS AFFECTED
Any can be affected by weight loss, especially if severe or the result of systemic disease.

SIGNALMENT
No age or sex predilections

SIGNS

Historical Findings
• Clinical signs of particular diagnostic value in patients with weight loss are whether the appetite is normal, increased, decreased, or absent.
• Historical information is very important, especially regarding type of diet, environment (chewing habits and access to potential GI foreign bodies), signs of gastrointestinal disease (including dysphagia, regurgitation, vomiting, or diarrhea), or signs of any specific disease.

Physical Examination Findings
Seek signs of systemic disease, gastrointestinal disease, neoplasia, cardiac disease, and neuromuscular disorders.

CAUSES

Malabsorptive Disorders
• Infiltrative and inflammatory bowel disease—very common
• Gastric foreign body—very common
• Gastritis—very common (especially *Helicobacter mustelae*)
• Epizootic catarrhal enteritis (ECE)—very common
• Severe intestinal parasitism (rare)

Metabolic Disorders
• Insulinoma—very common
• Cancer cachexia (lymphoma, adrenal neoplasia)—very common
• Organ failure—cardiac failure, hepatic failure, and renal failure—common
• Aleutian disease virus (parvovirus)

Excessive Nutrient Loss
• Protein-losing enteropathy (secondary to infectious or infiltrative diseases)
• Protein-losing nephropathy
• Diabetes mellitus (rare)

Anorexia
Pseudoanorexia
• Inability to smell, prehend, or chew food
• Dysphagia
• Regurgitation
• Vomiting

Dietary causes
• Insufficient quantity
• Poor quality
• Inedible food—decreased palatability

Neuromuscular Disease
• Lower motor neuron disease—rare
• CNS disease—usually associated with anorexia or pseudoanorexia—unusual

Excessive Use of Calories
• Increased physical activity
• Pregnancy or lactation
• Increased catabolism—fever, inflammation, cancer

RISK FACTORS
See Causes above

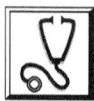

DIAGNOSIS
• Confirm weight loss by comparing the current weight to previous weights.
• If previous weights are not available, subjectively assess the patient for cachexia, emaciation, dehydration, or other clues that would confirm the owner's complaint of weight loss.
• After weight loss is confirmed, seek the underlying cause.

DIFFERENTIAL DIAGNOSIS
• Categorize the weight loss as occurring with a normal, increased, or decreased appetite.
• The list of likely differential diagnoses for a patient with weight loss despite a normal or increased appetite is usually different and much shorter than that for patients with decreased appetite or anorexia.
• Determine what the patient's appetite was at the onset of weight loss; any condition can lead to anorexia if it persists long enough for the patient to become debilitated.

• The patient's age may provide a clue as to the underlying cause (e.g., GI foreign body or helicobacter gastritis in a young ferret and neoplasia or insulinoma in a middle-aged or older ferret).
• Also seek causes of pseudoanorexia (e.g., loss of sense of smell, dysphagia, and disorders of the oral cavity, head, and neck).
• Fever suggests that the underlying cause may be infectious or inflammatory.

CBC/BIOCHEMISTRY/URINALYSIS
• Help identify infectious, inflammatory, and metabolic diseases, including organ failure.
• Especially helpful when the history and physical examination do not provide much useful information

OTHER LABORATORY TESTS
• Determined by the clinician's list of most likely differential diagnoses on the basis of the specific findings of the history and physical examination
• Fecal direct examination, fecal flotation, zinc sulfate centrifugation to rule out gastrointestinal parasites, especially in patients with diarrhea
• Fecal cytology—may reveal RBC or fecal leukocytes, which can be associated with inflammatory bowel disease or invasive bacterial strains

IMAGING
Abdominal radiography and ultrasonography should be utilized to evaluate gastrointestinal disorders, hepatic, renal, and urogenital diseases, or internal abscesses. Secondary hepatic lipidosis is best evaluated through imaging using ultrasonography.

Thoracic radiography is used initially to evaluate for cardiac and respiratory diseases. Because of the small thorax, ultrasonography can sometimes be used to localize and guide aspiration of respiratory masses. Echocardiography is used to evaluate for specific cardiac diseases.
• The need for further diagnostic imaging varies with the underlying condition suspected (see other topics on specific diseases).

DIAGNOSTIC PROCEDURES
• Vary depending on initial diagnostic findings and the suspected underlying cause of weight loss
• If gastrointestinal disease is probable but unconfirmed, examine biopsy specimens taken from the indicated portions of the gastrointestinal tract via exploratory laparotomy.
• Many indications for exploratory laparotomy exist—obtain multiple biopsy specimens from the suspected organ or organs as well as from other routinely biopsied abdominal organs such as liver, gastrointestinal tract, pancreas, and mesenteric lymph nodes.

(CONTINUED)

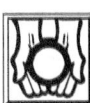

TREATMENT

• The most important treatment principle is to treat the underlying cause of the weight loss.
• Symptomatic therapy includes attention to fluid and electrolyte derangements, reduction in environmental stressors, and modification of the diet to improve palatability.
• If refusing solid food, most ferrets will accept assist feeding with an easily digestible high-protein/high-fat diet such as Lafeber Carnivore Critical Care Diet (Lafeber Company, Cornell, IL) or Oxbow Carnivore Critical Care Diet (Oxbow Animal Health, Omaha, NE); may also add dietary supplement such as Nutri-Cal (EVSCO Pharmaceuticals) to increase caloric content to these foods.
• Easily digestible, high-protein diets such as chicken baby food are often helpful in ferrets recovering from ECE or inflammatory bowel disease.
• The caloric recommendation for sick ferrets is approximately 400 kcal/kg BW per day (although this may be a high estimate).
• Techniques for providing enteral nutrition include assisted syringe-feeding or placement of nasogastric, esophagostomy, gastrostomy, or jejunostomy tubes.
• Parenteral nutrition may be provided via infusion through a polyurethane jugular catheter using a syringe pump.

MEDICATIONS

DRUG(S) OF CHOICE
Depend on the underlying cause of the weight loss; see specific topic for each condition, including anorexia.

CONTRAINDICATIONS
N/A

PRECAUTIONS
N/A

POSSIBLE INTERACTIONS
N/A

ALTERNATIVE DRUGS
• Capromorelin (Entyce) has been anecdotally used at canine doses

FOLLOW-UP

PATIENT MONITORING
The necessity for frequent patient monitoring and the methods required depend on the underlying cause of the weight loss; however, the patient should be weighed regularly and often.

POSSIBLE COMPLICATIONS
See Causes

MISCELLANEOUS

ASSOCIATED CONDITIONS
See Causes

AGE-RELATED FACTORS
N/A

ZOONOTIC POTENTIAL
N/A

PREGNANCY/FERTILITY/BREEDING
Pregnancy and lactation can be associated with weight loss due to increased calorie expenditure.

SYNONYMS
N/A

SEE ALSO
Eosinophilic gastroenteritis
Epizootic catarrhal enteritis
Gastroduodenal ulcers
Gastrointestinal and esophageal foreign bodies
Insulinoma
Lymphoplasmacytic enteritis and gastroenteritis
Lymphosarcoma

ABBREVIATIONS
CNS = central nervous system
ECE = epizootic catarrhal enteritis
GI = gastrointestinal
RBC = red blood cells

Suggested Reading
Capello V, Lennox AM. Diagnostic imaging of the respiratory system in exotic companion mammals. Vet Clin Exot Anim 2011;14:369–389.
Johnson-Delaney CA. Geriatric ferrets. Vet Clin Exot Anim Pract 2020;23(3):549–565.
Johnson-Delaney CA. Ferret nutrition. Vet Clin Exot Anim Pract 2014;17(3):449–470.
Powers LV, Perpiñán D. Basic anatomy, physiology, and husbandry of ferrets. In: Quesenberry KE, Orcutt CJ, Mans C, Carpenter JW, eds. Ferrets, Rabbits, and Rodents, 4th ed. St. Louis, MO: Elsevier, 2020:1–2.
Schoemaker NJ, van YRA Z. Endocrine diseases of ferrets. In: Quesenberry KE, Carpenter JW, eds. Ferrets, Rabbits and Rodents, 4th Ed). Clinical Medicine and Surgery. 2021 ed. St. Louis: Saunders, 2020:77–91.

Author Barbara Oglesbee, DVM, DABVP (Avian)

FERRETS

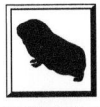

GUINEA PIGS

ABSCESSES

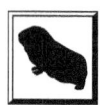

BASICS

DEFINITION
An abscess is a local collection of a liquid inflammatory product consisting of cells (leukocytes) and a thin fluid called liquor puris and liquefied tissue enclosed within a fibrous capsule.

PATHOPHYSIOLOGY
• Abscesses usually form in response to an invading pathogen or a foreign material.
• The pus within the fibrous capsule is usually thick, caseous, and does not easily drain.
• Subcutaneous abscesses often develop in guinea pigs as a result of bite wounds secondary to fighting, especially between adult boars. Bite wounds from dogs and cats may also result in abscess formation.
• Facial abscesses (e.g., mandibular) are most likely dental in origin and associated with malocclusion and odontogenic periapical infection.
• Retrobulbar abscesses are not uncommon in guinea pigs are typically odontogenic and involving the last two maxillary cheek teeth.
• Abscesses in the throat area may be caused by the penetration of a hay thistle through the oral mucosa and its subsequent migration.
• Cervical lymphadenitis is primarily caused by *Streptococcus zooepidemicus* and can develop into abscesses of the affected cervical lymph nodes. These abscesses are located in the ventral cervical region of the body.
• Abscessation secondary to bacteremia may occur anywhere on/in the body, including internal organs. Yersiniosis can lead to abscesses involving viscera.
• Bacterial pneumonia is very common in guinea pigs and may result in pulmonary abscesses.
• Plantar abscesses secondary to chronic pododermatitis are rare in guinea pigs. A diffuse plantar cellulitis is the most common presentation associated with chronic pododermatitis.

SYSTEMS AFFECTED
• Skin/Exocrine—percutaneous
• Gastrointestinal—dental abscesses
• Hepatobiliary—liver parenchyma
• Respiratory—pulmonary parenchyma

GENETICS
N/A

INCIDENCE/PREVALENCE
Most common cause of subcutaneous and submandibular swelling in guinea pigs. Odontogenic abscesses have a reported prevalence of 3.1% and skin abscesses a prevalence of 2% in a study on 1000 European guinea pigs. Another study from California reported a prevalence of 6% for skin abscesses in guinea pigs. In that report, abscesses were the most common cause behind skin nodules.

GEOGRAPHIC DISTRIBUTION
N/A

SIGNALMENT
• Adult boars are more likely to present with subcutaneous abscesses as a result of fighting.
• Odontogenic periapical abscessation is more prevalent in older individuals or animals diagnosed with a chronic vitamin C deficiency.

SIGNS

Historical Findings
• Facial and mandibular abscesses—history of dental disease, ptyalism, discharge, facial deformation, reluctance to chew, vitamin C deficiency.
• Subcutaneous abscesses—history of group housing, of biting
• Anorexia, lethargy
• A fast-growing swelling that may or may not be painful. Difficult to identify in long-haired guinea pigs

Physical Examination Findings
• Firm or fluctuant mass that may or may not be associated with an ulcerated/ necrotizing area
• Ventral cervical masses are characteristic of cervical lymphadenitis.
• Mandibular or facial swellings are likely caused by a dental abscess. The mass is usually attached to underlying bone. Other signs of dental disease may be present.
• A brief oral examination using an otoscope may identify dental malocclusion and ulceration. However, a more thorough dental examination under general anesthesia using endoscopic equipment is recommended for facial swelling and suspected dental disease.
• Pain and splinting may be elicited on abdominal palpation when visceral abscessation is present.

CAUSES
• Pyogenic bacteria:
  ∘ *Staphylococcus* spp. (in particular *S. aureus*) and *Streptococcus* spp. are often isolated from abscesses. *Pseudomonas aeruginosa, Pasteurella multocida,* and *Corynebacterium pyogenes* may also be cultured.
  ∘ *Streptococcus zooepidemicus* is the causative agent of cervical lymphadenitis; Lancefield's group C, a gram-positive coccus; *Caviibacter abscessus* (previously known as *Streptococcus moniliformis*) is uncommonly involved. *S. zooepidemicus* is considered part of the normal oral flora of guinea pigs.
  ∘ *Yersinia pseudotuberculosis* can cause abscesses of internal organs.
  ∘ Mixed infection caused by aerobic and anaerobic bacteria is the rule in dental abscessation.
• Foreign body: hay thistle, plant foreign body, and grass/clover stems
• Dental disease: reserve crown elongation, crown deformities, malocclusion, dental spurs, food impaction between teeth, vitamin C deficiencies, and periodontal pockets can lead to dental abscesses.

RISK FACTORS
• Group housing and breeding seasons
• Dental disease—higher-energy and lower-fiber diets are thought to contribute to dental malocclusion.
• Vitamin D and C deficiencies may also predispose to dental disease.
• Immunosuppression
  ∘ Vitamin C deficiency may increase susceptibility to bacterial infections.
  ∘ Corticosteroid use, neoplastic disease, underlying disease, and environmental stressors

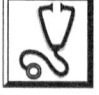

DIAGNOSIS

DIFFERENTIAL DIAGNOSIS
• Cervical lymphadenitis—results in abscesses but should be considered a particular clinical entity.
• Neoplasia—in particular, trichofolliculomas
• Cysts—intra-abdominal cysts: ovarian cysts.
• Thyroid tumors are frequently large and may be cystic. They may be confused with cervical lymphadenitis or a neck abscess.
• Hematoma/seroma

CBC/BIOCHEMISTRY/URINALYSIS
CBC—most often normal. Inflammatory leukogram frequent in case of bacteremia

OTHER LABORATORY TESTS
• Cytology and staining of abscess material to try to identify causative organism
• Culture and sensitivity of abscess material—most often, culture results are negative if swab is taken at the center of the abscess material. Better culture results may be achieved if the sample is collected at the abscess tissue interface. Aerobic culture will

also be negative when anaerobic bacteria are involved (especially for odontogenic abscesses).

IMAGING
• Radiography—useful to determine the extent of bone involvement, especially for mandibular and facial abscesses. Skull radiographs are essential to assess the severity of the dental disease and the presence of osteomyelitis.
• Ultrasonography—useful for diagnosing deeper and intra-abdominal abscesses.
• CT scan—allows more accurate assessment of dental, tympanic bulla, retrobulbar, and skull diseases

DIAGNOSTIC PROCEDURES
• Aspiration—cytologic examination reveals degenerate neutrophils with intra- and extracellular bacteria. A small number of mononuclear inflammatory cells may also be observed. Gram's stain of an aspirate smear is recommended, especially for samples obtained from dental abscesses from which bacterial cultures may not be rewarding.
• Culture—pus and abscess capsule can be submitted for culture. Submitting part of the fibrous capsule may yield better results over a sample collected in the center of the abscess. Anaerobic culture is encouraged for dental abscesses.
• Bacterial sensitivity testing is important to direct antibiotic selection.

PATHOLOGIC FINDINGS
• Exudate—degenerate neutrophils, intra- and extracellular bacteria, macrophages, and necrotic tissues
• Capsule and surrounding tissue—fibrinous inflammation, edema, congestion, fibrous connective tissue, presence of neutrophils, macrophages, lymphocytes, and plasma cells

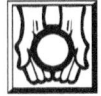

TREATMENT

APPROPRIATE HEALTH CARE
• Subcutaneous abscesses—the pus found in most guinea pig abscesses does not drain well, but lancing, draining, and flushing with hydrogen peroxide, povidone iodine, or chlorhexidine may be adequate for uncomplicated cases. The procedure may have to be repeated daily for several days.
• Cervical lymphadenitis—see corresponding chapter
• Dental abscesses—techniques described in rabbits can be used: antimicrobial wound-packing technique, marsupialization technique, AIPMMA beads. A thorough

dental examination is mandatory with teeth equilibration and resurfacing, intraoral removal of loose teeth, and cleaning of food impaction between teeth and in gingival pockets.
• Surgical removal of the abscess, including the capsule, may be necessary depending on location, cause, and treatment response.
• Systemic antibiotic therapy
• Outpatient—well-demarcated abscess without concurrent debilitating conditions

NURSING CARE
• Depends on location of the abscess, treatment elected, and concurrent conditions (e.g., dental disease, anorexia, and weight loss)
• Sepsis—aggressive fluid therapy, intravenous antibiotics
• Bandaging as needed

ACTIVITY
Restricted until resolution of the abscess

DIET
• If the patient is anorexic, assisted feeding is necessary (e.g., Critical Care for Herbivores, Oxbow Pet Products, Murdock, NE) 50–100 mL/kg/day. Alternatively, ground pellets may be used.
• Diet should primarily include hay and roughage with a limited amount of pellets. Fresh vegetables may also be offered in limited quantity. High-carbohydrate treats should be avoided.
• Guinea pigs need a dietary source of vitamin C. Higher levels should be provided to sick individuals (30–50 mg/kg daily). Vitamin C may be ground and fed directly to the pig. Vitamin C treats are also available for guinea pigs (e.g., Daily C, Oxbow Pet Products, Murdock, NE).

CLIENT EDUCATION
• Discuss diet and group housing.
• Dental abscesses can be challenging to treat and multiple follow-ups are necessary. Dental disease requires lifelong treatment.
• Cervical lymphadenitis is mildly contagious to other guinea pigs. Prognosis may be guarded. Owners should be educated on the difficulty in resolving this condition during the initial treatment period. Reoccurrence of cervical abscesses is likely in the majority of these cases.

SURGICAL CONSIDERATIONS

Subcutaneous Abscesses
• Complete removal of the entire abscess may be indicated, with care to not rupture the capsule.
• Alternatively: lancing, curettage, cleaning, and flushing. Leave abscess open. Express pus and flush once to twice daily with hydrogen

peroxide, povidone iodine, or chlorhexidine until granulation tissue forms and pus is no longer present.
• Remove any nidus of infection: foreign object, hay thistle, necrotic tissue.
• Packing the abscess with antibiotic-impregnated or iodoform gauze may help clear the infection and keep the abscess draining.
• Place on 2–3 weeks of antibiotic treatment.

Dental Abscesses
• Several techniques have been described in rabbits with good success and can be extrapolated to guinea pigs.
• Debridement and marsupialization technique:
  ○ Remove abscess in its entirety with capsule, affected bone, and teeth if possible; abscess is often associated with the bone or a tooth apex.
  ○ Curette and debride abnormal and infected tissue. Bone defects may be filled with AIPMMA beads.
  ○ Marsupialize the remaining opening to the skin.
  ○ Clean and flush every day until granulation and closure of the wound by secondary intention.
• Wound-packing technique.
• Lance, clean, and flush the abscess.
• Pack the abscess defect with strips of gauze impregnated with a selected antibiotic. Antibiotics are selected based on the oral microflora of guinea pigs, and initially may include ampicillin 30 mg/kg or clindamycin 20 mg/kg. Antimicrobial treatment should be altered depending on culture and sensitivity.
• Suture the incision.
  ○ Repeat every week until pus is no longer present and the abscess cavity is almost completely replaced by granulation tissue.
• Other techniques have been described with mixed results:
  ○ Local use of AIPMMA beads, long-lasting doxycycline gel, honey, 50% dextrose. Intraoral endoscopy-assisted drainage and local treatment if a draining tract can be localized.
• Place on long-term antibiotic treatment: 1–3 months; pain management
• Retrobulbar abscesses: an infraorbital approach used in rabbits allowing preservation of the eye is more difficult to perform in guinea pigs because the dental apices are more medial and the zygomatic process is thicker. Enucleation may be recommended in most cases.

ABSCESSES

Internal Abscesses
- Surgical removal when possible
- Long-term antibiotic treatment

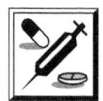

MEDICATIONS

DRUG(S) OF CHOICE

Antibiotics
- Antibiotics should be selected based on the bacterial culture and sensitivity. Pending the sensitivity results, selection is based on the common isolates reported in guinea pig abscesses and antibiotics that are safe to use in this species. Unfortunately, antibiotics with the best effect against frequent isolates, especially *Staphylococcus aureus* and *Streptococcus zooepidemicus*, can lead to antibiotic-associated dysbiosis and enterotoxemia. Treatment should be pursued for at least 2 weeks.
- Broad-spectrum antibiotics safe to use in guinea pigs include enrofloxacin (5–15 mg/kg PO q12–24h), which is ineffective against anaerobes and may be variably effective against *Streptococcus* spp., trimethoprim-sulfa (15–30 mg/kg PO q12h), and chloramphenicol (30–50 mg/kg PO q8–12h). Azithromycin (30 mg/kg PO q12–24h) is safe to use in guinea pigs and can reach a high concentration in pus through transportation by heterophils.
- For dental abscesses, antibiotic therapy including anaerobic coverage and good penetration in bones should be selected. Azithromycin, chloramphenicol, and metronidazole (10–20 mg/kg PO q12h) have good anaerobic spectrum. Penicillin G (40,000–60,000 IU/kg SC q2–7d) can also be used (see Precautions). Longer systemic antibiotic treatment is usually needed for dental abscesses: 1–3 months. Topical antibiotics in gauze packing and AIPMMA offer a wider range of selection because of reduced systemic absorption and avoidance of oral administration.

Pain Management
- Butorphanol (0.4–2.0 mg/kg SC, IM q4–12h)—short acting
- Buprenorphine (0.05–0.2 mg/kg SC, IM, transmucosal q8–12h)—longer acting opioid
- Buprenorphine SR 0.3 mg/kg q48–72h
- Meloxicam (0.5–1 mg/kg PO, SC, IM q12–24h)—also for long-term pain management for dental abscesses and dental disease
- Local anesthetics/dental blocks of bupivacaine (1 mg/kg), lidocaine (1 mg/kg), use in combination or alone—before more advanced surgery

CONTRAINDICATIONS
- Oral administration of penicillins, macrolides, lincosamides, and cephalosporins
- Use of immunosuppressive drugs such as corticosteroids
- Procaine, which is included in some penicillin preparations, can be toxic to guinea pigs.
- Extensive surgery on a debilitated animal

PRECAUTIONS
- Oral administration of antibiotics may cause antibiotic-associated enteritis, dysbiosis, and enterotoxemia.
- Procaine penicillin G has been used as an alternative therapy, but there are anecdotal reports of fatal enterotoxemia with the use of any form of penicillin, including parenteral, in guinea pigs.
- Opioids may have an effect on the gastrointestinal motility.
- Chloramphenicol—humans should wear gloves to avoid contact due to potential bone marrow toxicity.

POSSIBLE INTERACTIONS
N/A

ALTERNATIVE DRUGS
N/A

FOLLOW-UP

PATIENT MONITORING
- Monitor daily for swelling, resolution of inflammation, and improvement in clinical signs.
- Dental abscesses: recheck weekly.
- Dental disease: recheck every 4–20 weeks for dental trimming.

PREVENTION/AVOIDANCE
- Prevention of acquired dental disease by providing high-fiber and good quality food with supplemental vitamin C
- Treating and monitoring dental disease in early stage to prevent progression to more severe dental malformation and abscesses formation
- Prevention of bite wounds by limiting group housing, especially of adult boars during breeding seasons
- Isolation of sick individuals
- Providing a clean, stress-free environment

POSSIBLE COMPLICATIONS
- Sepsis
- Spreading of the infection to surrounding tissue
- Recurrence, chronic pain, extensive tissue destruction
- Dental abscesses: face deformation, tissue destruction, worsening of the preexisting dental disease, inability to eat, facial paralysis

EXPECTED COURSE AND PROGNOSIS
- Depends on organ involved, location, size, pathogenicity of organism, immune status of the animal
- Subcutaneous abscesses: good to fair prognosis
- Dental abscesses: good to guarded prognosis
- Internal abscesses: fair to grave prognosis

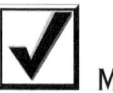

MISCELLANEOUS

ASSOCIATED CONDITIONS
- Immunosuppression
- Dental disease
- Gastrointestinal hypomotility
- Hepatic lipidosis—chronic anorexia

AGE-RELATED FACTORS
N/A

ZOONOTIC POTENTIAL
N/A

PREGNANCY/FERTILITY/BREEDING
N/A

SYNONYMS
N/A

SEE ALSO
Anorexia and pseudoanorexia
Cervical lymphadenitis
Cutaneous and subcutaneous masses
Dental malocclusion

ABBREVIATIONS
AIPMMA = antibiotic-impregnated polymethyl methacrylate
CT = computed tomography

INTERNET RESOURCES
N/A

Suggested Reading
Bohmer E. Abscesses. In: Bohmer E, ed. Dentistry in Rabbits and Rodents. Wiley Blackwell, 2015:213–241.
Capello V. Clinical technique: treatment of periapical infections in pet rabbits and rodents. J Exot Pet Med 2008;17:124–131.
Harkness JE, Murray KA, Wagner JE. In: Fox JG, Anderson LC, Loew FM, Quimby FW, eds. Laboratory Animal Medicine, 2nd ed. Ames: Academic Press, 2002:203–246.
Minarikova A, Hauptman K, Jeklova E, Knotek Z, Jekl V. Diseases in pet guinea pigs: a retrospective study in 1000 animals. Vet Record 2015;177(8):200.
Miwa Y, Sladky K. Common surgical procedures of rodents, ferrets, hedgehogs, and sugar gliders. Vet Clin Exot Anim 2016;19:205–244.

Pignon C, Mayer J. Guinea pigs. In: Quesenberry KE, Carpenter JW, eds. Ferrets, Rabbits and Rodents 4th ed. Clinical Medicine and Surgery. 2021. St. Louis: Saunders, 2020: 270–297.

Taylor WM, Beaufrere H, Mans C, Smith DA. Long-term outcome of treatment of dental abscesses with a wound-packing technique in pet rabbits: 13 cases (1998–2007). J Am Vet Assoc 2010;237(12):1444–1448.

White SD, Guzman DS, Paul-Murphy J, Hawkins MG. Skin diseases in companion guinea pigs (*Cavia porcellus*): a retrospective study of 293 cases seen at the Veterinary Medical Teaching Hospital, University of California at Davis (1990–2015). Vet Dermatol 2016;27(5):395–400.

Author Hugues Beaufrere, Dr.Med.Vet.

ALOPECIA

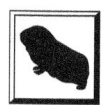

BASICS

DEFINITION
Alopecia is the partial or complete lack of hair in areas where it is normally present.

PATHOPHYSIOLOGY

Etiology
• Any disease that can affect hair follicles that results in hair loss
• Two categories of alopecia: hereditary (uncommon) and acquired
• Acquired alopecia—the guinea pig is or was capable of producing structurally normal hair; an etiology destroys the hair follicle or shaft, interferes with the growth of hair, or causes the animal discomfort leading to self-trauma and destruction of hair.
• Acquired alopecia is further divided into two categories: inflammatory and noninflammatory.

SYSTEMS AFFECTED
Skin/Exocrine

GENETICS
Congenital alopecia has been reported but is rare.

INCIDENCE/PREVALENCE
Most common dermatologic presentations

SIGNALMENT
• Hair loss may be obvious or subtle, depending on the disease process affecting the animal.
• Pattern of hair loss may be focal, multifocal, symmetric, or generalized.

SIGNS

Historical Findings
Duration and progression of lesion, presence or absence of pruritus, evidence of contagion, or nondermatologic problems

Physical Examination Findings
• The distribution of lesions (e.g., focal, multifocal, symmetric, and generalized) should be noted.
• Hair should be examined to determine if they are being shed from the hair follicle or broken off.
• Signs of secondary skin infections or ectoparasites should be noted and a careful nondermatologic physical examination should be performed. Noninflammatory
• Pattern hair loss
• No signs of inflammation
• Hyperpigmentation
• Lichenification
• Erythema

• Scaling
• Excessive shedding
• Pruritus
• Secondary skin diseases, such as a bacterial pyoderma or seborrhea

CAUSES
Noninflammatory—diseases that can directly inhibit or slow hair follicle growth:
• Neurological/behavioral
  ○ Stress—generalized hair loss
  ○ Barbering, fur chewing—anywhere but commonly on rump and perineal areas
• Nutritional deficiencies
  ○ Particularly protein deficiencies and hypovitaminosis C
• Hyperestrogenism
  ○ Cystic ovarian disease—common cause of alopecia over the back, ventrum, and flanks
  ○ Pregnancy-associated alopecia—flanks, bilaterally symmetric
• Diabetes
• Hypothyroidism (rare)
• Severe inflammatory diseases of the dermis (e.g., pruritus, deep pyoderma)
• Ectoparasites—demodicosis, *Chirodiscoides*, *Trixacarus caviae*, *Gyropus ovalis*, *Gliricola porcelli*, and *Ctenocephalides felis*
  ○ *Trixacarus caviae*—shoulders, dorsum, and flanks, may be generalized and may be associated with crusting, hyperpigmentation, and lichenification. The pruritus is intense. Parasites are readily identified in skin scrapes preparation.
  ○ *Chirodiscoides caviae*—primarily affecting the groin and axilla. Mites are present in the hair and are easily observed on collected hair.
  ○ Other ectoparasites—*Cheyletiella parasitivorax* usually produces lesions on the dorsum; *Demodex caviae* is frequently located on the head and forelegs. Lice often are associated with lesions around the ears and dorsum.
• Dermatophytosis
  ○ Can be pruritic—*Trichophyton mentagrophytes* often affects hair around the face and legs, sometimes dorsum.
• Bacterial pyoderma
  ○ Location depends on the inciting cause and may be present anywhere. Exfoliative dermatitis is reported most commonly in the ventral aspect.
• Traumatic episodes (burns)
• Allergic skin diseases (e.g., atopy, food allergy, contact, and insect hypersensitivity)
  ○ Contact hypersensitivity has been reported in guinea pigs.
• Neoplasia

RISK FACTORS
Concurrent disease, hypovitaminosis C, overcrowding, and poor husbandry

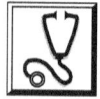

DIAGNOSIS

DIFFERENTIAL DIAGNOSIS
Pattern and degree—important in formulating differential diagnosis (see Causes, above)

CBC/BIOCHEMISTRY/URINALYSIS
Need is dependent on the underlying disease process and is useful in the diagnosis of endocrinopathies such as diabetes mellitus. CBC is often normal, except in severe pyoderma and parasite infestation.

IMAGING
Abdominal ultrasound—identifying ovarian cyst

DIAGNOSTIC PROCEDURES
• Skin scrapings for ectoparasites—deep skin scrapings are necessary to reveal *Trixacarus caviae* and *Demodex caviae*. The hair should be clipped before processing. Mineral oil can be used for slide preparation.
• Direct visualization—combing of the hair coat for fleas, mites, and lice
• Impression smears of the skin for evidence of bacterial or yeast infections
• Adhesive tape collection—for surface-living ectoparasites
• Bacterial culture and sensitivity—infected lesions are frequently contaminated with the resident microbiological flora.
• Diagnosing dermatophytosis
  ○ Wood's lamp examination (should be not relied on solely)—useful to diagnose dermatophytosis caused by *Microsporum* spp. Use is limited in guinea pigs where *Trychophyton mentagrophytes* is the most common dermatophyte and does not fluoresce when exposed to ultraviolet light.
  ○ Fungal culture on Sabouraud's agar—hair can be collected as well as samples obtained from brush techniques. Growth may be slow and take up to 1 month.
  ○ Direct microscopy/hair plucking—the edge of the lesion is the preferred collection site; fungal arthrospores and hyphae may be observed; there may be evidence of self-trauma.
• Skin biopsy—sample should contain normal and abnormal sites. Evaluate hair follicle structures, numbers, and anagen/telogen ratios. Examine for evidence of bacterial, fungal, neoplastic, or parasitic skin infections.

(CONTINUED)

TREATMENT

APPROPRIATE HEALTH CARE
• More than one disease condition may be contributing (summation of effects). Initial therapy may be indicated based on top differential diagnoses when one fails to definitively identify an inciting cause.
• Hair should be clipped around the affected area in cases of fungal and bacterial dermatitis.
• All exposed animals should be treated in case of ectoparasitic infestation. The environment may also need to be thoroughly cleaned.

Neurological/Behavioral
Preventive measures include separating affected animals, decreasing environmental stress, early weaning, correcting diet, and feeding long-stemmed hay.

Hypovitaminosis C
Correcting diet and additional supplementation until clinical signs resolve (50–100 mg/kg SC q24h). Maintain animal on daily supplementation of vitamin C (30–50 mg/kg PO q24h) after clinical signs resolve.

Alopecia Due to Ovarian Cysts
• Ovariohysterectomy
• See Ovarian Cysts

Ectoparasites—Cavy Mites and Lice Infestation
• Most common ectoparasites include mites (*Trixacarus caviae*, *Chirodiscoides caviae*), lice (*Gliricola porcelli*, *Gyropus ovalis*), and rarely (*Demodex caviae*)
• Ivermectin (0.4 mg/kg PO, SC every 7–10 days for 3–4 doses) is usually effective to treat mite infestation.
• Selamectin 15–30 mg/kg topically every 21–28 days
• Imidacloprid 10%/moxidectin 1% can also be used safely in guinea pigs at 0.1 mL/animal
• Pyrethrin-based flea powder can be used, being careful not to overdose.

Dermal Bacterial Infection
• Hair should be clipped and cleaned with disinfectants such as dilute povidone iodine or dilute chlorhexidine initially.
• Topical treatment with antimicrobial shampoos can be used in pyoderma and may be useful as adjunctive therapy in dermatophytosis. Antimicrobial shampoos include chlorhexidine and ethyl lactate shampoos.
• Therapy should be based on culture and sensitivity if possible. Broad-spectrum antibiotics safe to use in guinea pigs include trimethoprim-sulfa (15–30 mg/kg PO q12h), chloramphenicol (30–50 mg/kg PO q8–12h), azithromycin (15–30 mg/kg PO q24h), and enrofloxacin (5–20 mg/kg PO q12–24h) {Should be reserved for microbes that are resistant to tier one antibiotics}, which is ineffective against anaerobes and may be variably effective against *Streptococcus* spp.
• Treatment should be continued for 2 weeks past resolution of clinical signs.
• Avoid oral antibiotics that select against gram-positive bacteria such as penicillins, macrolides, lincoamides, and cephalosporins, as these may cause fatal enteric dysbiosis and enterotoxemina.

Dermatophytosis
• Antifungals—terbinafine (20–30 mg/kg PO q24h) is most effective for treatment of dermatophytes—all guinea pigs in the house hold should be treated
   Alternatively, use griseofulvin (15–50 mg/kg PO q24h), itraconazole (5–10 mg/kg PO q24h), treatment should be continued for 2 weeks past resolution of clinical signs.
• Affected areas should be clipped and cleaned with disinfectants such as dilute povidone iodine or dilute chlorhexidine initially.
• Antifungal shampoos—ketoconazole, miconazole, and lime sulfur shampoos
• Focal fungal lesions can also be addressed using clotrimazole cream.
• Lime sulfur dip—dip q7d for 4–6 treatments (dilute 1:40 with water)

Antipruritic Therapy
• If there are signs of severe pruritus, corticosteroids may be used. Guinea pigs tend to tolerate the use of corticosteroids well. Prednisone, prednisolone 0.25–1 mg/kg PO q12–24h. May be given on an alternate-day basis.
• Antihistamines are usually not very effective except in cases of allergic dermatitis. Hydroxyzine 2 mg/kg PO q8–12h, diphenhydramine PO, SC 2 mg/kg q8–12h.
• NSAIDs—meloxicam (0.5–1 mg/kg PO, SC, IM q24h) or carprofen (4 mg/kg SC q24h or 1–2 mg/kg PO q12h).

DIET
Guinea pigs need a dietary source of vitamin C. Higher levels should be provided to sick individuals (30–50 mg/kg daily). Vitamin C may be ground and fed directly to the pig. Vitamin C treats are also available for guinea pigs (e.g., Daily C, Oxbow Pet Products, Murdock, NE).

CLIENT EDUCATION
Most of the parasitic diseases are contagious, and other animals, including other species, may have to be treated.

MEDICATIONS

DRUG(S) OF CHOICE
See treatment section

CONTRAINDICATIONS
Oral administration of penicillins, macrolides, lincosamides, and cephalosporins

PRECAUTIONS
• Dipping and bathing guinea pigs can be stressful.
• Prevent guinea pigs from licking topical products.
• Oral administration of antibiotics may cause antibiotic-associated enteritis, dysbiosis, and enterotoxemia.

FOLLOW-UP

PATIENT MONITORING
Monitor for resolution of clinical signs and toxicity to the medications.

PREVENTION/AVOIDANCE
• Isolation and treatment of sick and in-contact individuals
• Cleaning of the environment

POSSIBLE COMPLICATIONS
• Sepsis
• Seizures with severe *Trixacarus* infestation

MISCELLANEOUS

ASSOCIATED CONDITIONS
Pruritus

ZOONOTIC POTENTIAL
• Dermatophytosis
• *Trixacarus caviae* and *Cheyletiella parasitivorax* may cause a mild dermatitis in humans.

PREGNANCY/FERTILITY/BREEDING
Griseofulvin and ivermectin are teratogenic.

SEE ALSO
Abscesses
Dermatophytosis
Fleas and flea infestation
Lice and mites
Ovarian cysts

ABBREVIATIONS
GnRH = gonadotropin-releasing hormone
hcG = human chorionic gonadotropin

INTERNET RESOURCES
www.vin.com

GUINEA PIGS

Suggested Reading
Ballweber LR, Harkness JE. Parasites of guinea pigs. In: Baker DG, ed. Flynn's Parasites of Laboratory Animals, 2nd ed. Ames: Blackwell, 2007:421–449.

Eshar D, Abram TB. Comparison of efficacy, safety, and convenience of selamectin versus ivermectin for treatment of *Trixacarus caviae* mange in pet guinea pigs (*Cavia porcellus*). J Am Vet Med Assoc 2012;241(8):1056–1058.

Palmerio BS, Roberts H. Clinical approach to dermatologic disease in exotic animals. Vet Clin North Am Exot Anim Pract 2013; 16(3):523–577.

Pignon C, Mayer J. Guinea pigs. In: Quesenberry KE, Carpenter JW, eds. Ferrets, Rabbits and Rodents, 4th ed. Clinical Medicine and Surgery. 2021. St. Louis: Saunders, 2020:270–297.

Riggs SM. Guinea pigs. In: Mitchell MA, Tully TN, eds. Manual of Exotic Pet Practice. St Louis: Saunders/Elsevier, 2009:456–473.

White SD, Sanchez-Migallon D, Paul-Murphy J. Skin diseases in companion guinea pigs (*Cavia porcellus*): a retrospective study of 293 cases seen at the Veterinary Medical Teaching Hospital, University of California at Davis (1990–2015). Vet Dermatol 2016;27:395–e100.

Authors Jessica Comolli, DVM and Rodney Schnellbacher, DVM, Dipl. ACZM

GUINEA PIGS

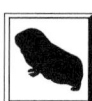

BASICS

DEFINITION

- Anorexia is the lack or loss of appetite for food. Appetite is psychologic and depends on memory and association. Hunger is physiologically aroused by the body's need for food. The existence of appetite in animals is assumed.
- The term *pseudoanorexia* is used to describe animals that have a desire for food but are unable to eat because they cannot prehend, chew, or swallow food. Pseudoanorexia due to tongue entrapment by overgrown cheek teeth is one of the most common causes of lack of food intake in guinea pigs.

PATHOPHYSIOLOGY

- Anorexia is commonly associated with malaise, pain, or systemic disease. Mechanisms by which these conditions cause anorexia in histrichomorphic rodents are not fully understood.
- Research indicates that appetite is modulated hormonally in the hypothalamus. Some hormones (e.g., leptin, cholecystokinin) induce an increased appetite; other hormones (e.g., tumor necrosis factor alpha, some interleukins) act to reduce appetite. The hypothalamus affects an increase or decrease in appetite via nervous and hormonal pathways to stimulate food intake.
- Gastric distention may cause satiety in humans, but it is doubtful that this occurs in herbivorous grazers.
- Pseudoanorexia is commonly associated with oral pain, tongue entrapment, and dyspnea.

SYSTEMS AFFECTED

- Anorexia/pseudoanorexia can be life threatening in guinea pigs. Lack of food intake can cause gastrointestinal hypomotility. Hypomotility can cause pain and nausea and can further reduce food intake, becoming a vicious cycle without veterinary intervention. Lack of food intake may lead to intestinal floral changes and overgrowth of toxin-producing bacteria. Enterotoxemia along with breakdown of intestinal mucosal barrier can result in septic or endotoxic shock and death.
- Anorexia/pseudoanorexia can cause a negative energy balance and induce hepatic lipidosis.
- Anorexia/pseudoanorexia can cause hypovitaminosis C and its effects on the immune and musculoskeletal system.

SIGNALMENT

Varies according to the underlying cause

SIGNS

Historical Findings

- Refusal to eat is a common owner complaint.
- Weight loss with chronic anorexia or subtle/undetected pseudoanorexia
- Ptyalism, halitosis, and odynophagia (painful eating)
- Decrease in the size or number of fecal pellets
- Bruxism with oral or visceral pain
- Lack of normal vocalizations
- Stiffness or hunched posture or gait can be associated with visceral or musculoskeletal pain (e.g., hypovitaminosis C)
- Dysuria and sometimes hematuria with ureteral, cystic, and urethral calculi
- Lethargy and malaise with underlying systemic disease
- Dyspnea with respiratory disease, tracheal compression, and cardiac disease
- Guinea pigs with enterotoxic shock due to anorexia/pseudoanorexia often present laterally recumbent.

Physical Examination Findings

- Observation at rest may indicate a painful posture or lameness/stiffness.
- Observation at rest and after handling may suggest overt or subtle dyspnea. Open-mouth breathing indicates a potential emergency, including heat stroke. Guinea pigs are intolerant of temperatures above 80°F.
- Observation of attitude, behavior in cage and on examination table or floor may suggest depression
- Skin turgor may be decreased with dehydration, but guinea pigs that have not eaten are often dehydrated even if not clinically detectable.
- Evidence of dermatitis, abscesses, or cutaneous neoplasia—may be sufficiently uncomfortable to cause anorexia
- Carefully examine all four feet with attention to painful conditions such as pododermatitis, ingrown nails, and cutaneous horns (arising from the pads of the feet). Examination of the legs should include palpation of joints for swelling, manipulation for signs of crepitus and/or pain, and for asymmetry in muscle mass.
- Examine the face, head, and neck by palpation and visualization for cheilitis (usually on the rostral aspect of the lips/philtrum), asymmetry to mandibles (especially the lateroventral aspect) or maxillae, pain on palpation of the jaw bones, pain on pressure of cheek against upper dental arcade (due to spurs on buccal aspect

of upper teeth), scaly eyelids (a vague sign of illness), head tilt (common with otitis media/interna), and enlarged, possibly painful submandibular or cervical lymph nodes.
- Examine the eyes for disorders that are painful or impair vision (e.g., corneal ulcers, uveitis, and exophthalmos secondary to dental abscess or neoplasia).
- Oral exam should always be part of the physical examination for the anorexic/pseudoanorexic guinea pig. Incisors should be evaluated from the front and from the side with attention to occlusion and lateral mobility of mandible. There should be adequate range of motion laterally to each side. Thorough evaluation of the cheek teeth is not easily accomplished in the awake patient. Due to small aperture of the mouth, the wiggly, uncooperative nature of the patients, and the presence of food in the mouth, examination without sedation does not rule out dental disease. Examine awake patients for evidence of tongue entrapment by the lower cheek teeth using a large otoscope cone.
- Thoracic auscultation for evidence of cardiac or pulmonary disease. Decreased breath sounds are commonly noted with pulmonary disease. Muffled heart sounds may indicate pleural effusion.
- Abdominal palpation is often extremely valuable in the diagnosis. Palpation may reveal gaseous distention of the stomach or cecum, abnormal renal size, presence of fluid, masses, palpable urinary calculi, and the presence and location of pain.
- Decreased borborygmus on abdominal auscultation with gastrointestinal hypomotility
- Quite often, examination findings are unremarkable. However, in guinea pigs with anorexia or weight loss, further evaluation is indicated to look for underlying cause(s) that are difficult to identify on physical examination.

CAUSES

Anorexia

- A true lack of appetite is caused by almost any systemic disease process.
- Gastrointestinal disease is one of the most common causes. Often manifesting itself as dynamic ileus, hypomotility can be both a cause and effect of anorexia. Rarely, a true obstruction can develop due to trichobezoar or phytobezoar. Gastric dilatation in guinea pigs is painful and debilitating.
- Pain—guinea pigs do not handle pain with stoicism. Common painful conditions include urinary calculi (especially ureteral calculi), dental disease, and orthopedic disorders

ANOREXIA AND PSEUDOANOREXIA   (CONTINUED)

• Poor nutrition—diets with inadequate coarse fiber will increase risk of hypomotility and dental disease. Inadequate vitamin C can cause joint pain and poor immune function.
• Metabolic diseases such as renal disease or hepatic disease (especially hepatic lipidosis)
• Cardiac and/or pulmonary disease (e.g., pneumonia)
• Caseous lymphadenitis and other causes of significant cervical lymphadenopathy (e.g., cavian leukemia)
• Neoplasia anywhere in the body
• Cystic ovaries

Pseudoanorexia

• Nonpainful oral disease can cause pseudoanorexia. Most often see entrapment of the tongue by lingually directed overgrowth of the lower cheek teeth.
• Neurologic and neuromuscular diseases are rare causes of anorexia.

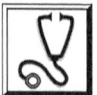

DIAGNOSIS

DIFFERENTIAL DIAGNOSIS

• Gastric hypomotility, usually caused by inappropriate diet, pain, or any systemic disorder, is a common cause of anorexia.
• Dental disease is a common cause of anorexia/pseudoanorexia.
• Anamnesis should include husbandry review, including caging, bedding, ambient temperature, and the age/responsibility of the primary caretaker. Identify how water is provided, degree of consumption, and any recent changes. Ask about the diet as fed and as eaten, and the method and frequency of vitamin C supplementation. Any recent changes in appetite or food intake should be recorded. It is ideal to have owners bring photos of the cage and brand names or samples of the dietary elements (pellets, hay, vegetables, fruits, and treats).
• Complete physical examination is an essential element in diagnosis of anorexia/pseudoanorexia. Guinea pigs often exhibit subtle signs.
• A minimum laboratory database for the anorexic/pseudoanorexic guinea pig includes a CBC, serum chemistries, and whole body radiographs. This database will help identify systemic disorders and/or nutritional issues that may be present. Further testing should be based on these results as indicated.
• In the anorexic guinea pig with gastric hypomotility, ptyalism, oral pain, and/or weight loss, obtain a sedated oral examination and skull radiographs to evaluate the oral cavity for infection, painful lesions, malocclusion, and tooth bud displacement. Skull radiographs should include multiple views including at least a lateral and right and left lateral obliques. It is also helpful to obtain DV, cranial/caudal, and a VD view. If otitis media/interna is suspected or any vestibular signs are present, tympanic bullae should be radiographically evaluated.

CBC/BIOCHEMISTRY/URINALYSIS

• Vary with different underlying causes of anorexia/pseudoanorexia.
• Increased liver enzymes may indicate hepatic lipidosis secondary to negative caloric balance.

OTHER LABORATORY TESTS

Other tests may be indicated based on a well-defined differential diagnosis list.

IMAGING

• Abdominal radiography should be part of the minimum database for the anorexic guinea pig. Radiographs are helpful in diagnosis of gastrointestinal diseases, urolithiasis, ovarian cysts, musculoskeletal diseases, and neoplasia. Abdominal ultrasonography is indicated in some cases to further investigate suspected pathology.
• Thoracic radiography is indicated to look for causes of dyspnea and to rule out occult pneumonia and heart disease. Thoracic ultrasonography, including echocardiography, is indicated to further investigate suspected pathology.
• Radiography of the skull should be performed on any guinea pig with suspected dental disease or if the cause of anorexia is uncertain. CT scans can be very helpful in further defining the extent of pathology or in rare cases where radiography is not diagnostic.
• Other imaging studies may be indicated on a case-by-case basis and should be considered as needed.

DIAGNOSTIC PROCEDURES

Vary with working or tentative diagnoses

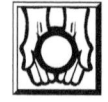

TREATMENT

• Treat underlying cause.
• All guinea pigs with a lack of effective food intake should receive supportive care with careful attention to hydration, nutrition, and pain management. Oral or parenteral vitamin C is indicated in most cases.
• Fluid support is most commonly administered via oral and subcutaneous routes. Intravenous or intraosseous fluids are reserved for the severely ill patient. Maintenance fluids are estimated at 100 mL/kg/day.
• Nutritional support is imperative. Anorexic guinea pigs are extremely prone to cascading effects of continued stasis and mortality from bacterial floral changes and enterotoxemia. Assist syringe feeding with an appropriate herbivore supplement such as Critical Care for Herbivores (Oxbow Pet Products, Murdock, NE) or Emeraid Herbivore (Lafeber Company, Cornell, IL). Care must be taken in the dyspneic or struggling patient. Tube feeding may be indicated. Both of the above products come in formulations that can be administered via esophagostomy or nasogastric tubes.
• Once the gastrointestinal tract receives fluid and high-fiber food and hypomotility begins to wane, the patient will often begin feeding on hay and its regular diet. Be sure to offer solid food in between assist-feeding sessions.
• Anorexia/pseudoanorexia is often caused by pain. Hypomotility secondary to lack of food intake can be painful. Pain management is an extremely important part of patient management.

MEDICATIONS

DRUG(S) OF CHOICE

• Varies with underlying cause
• Anorexia, regardless of the cause, contributes to or causes gastrointestinal tract hypomotility. There is no better medication for hypomotility than food; assist feed as noted above. The use of promotility agents such as metoclopromide (0.2–1.0 mg/kg PO, SC, IV q12h) or cisapride (0.5–1 mg/kg PO q8–12h) may be helpful in regaining normal motility; cisapride is available through compounding pharmacies. Constant rate infusion of metoclopramide may be necessary for prokinesis.
• For analgesia, mild opioids (e.g., buprenorphine 0.05 mg/kg SC, IM, IV or oral transmucosal q8–12h) are appropriate in the short term. Pure mu agonists tend to exacerbate hypomotility and are generally avoided. NSAIDs such as meloxicam (0.2–0.5 mg/kg PO, SC q12–24h) can be used when renal function is normal and the patient is hydrated.
• For gastric inflammation and pain, H2 receptor antagonists such as famotidine (0.5 mg/kg PO, SC, IV q24h) or ranitidine (2 mg/kg IV or 2–5 mg/kg PO q24h. Metoclopramide (0.2–1.0 mg/kg PO, SC, IVq12h) increases gastric emptying.

CONTRAINDICATIONS

• Corticosteroids should be avoided in guinea pig patients. They are never to be used to stimulate appetite.
• Antibiotics that select against gram-positive bacteria, such as oral penicillins, cephalosporins, lincosamines, or macrolides, should not be used in these animals as it can cause fatal dysbiosis and enterotoxemia.

PRECAUTIONS
Meloxicam should be used with caution in dehydrated patients and those with renal compromise.

POSSIBLE INTERACTIONS
N/A

ALTERNATIVE DRUGS
N/A

FOLLOW-UP

PATIENT MONITORING
• Body weight, amount and size of fecal pellets, clinical hydration status, urine production, attitude, reduction of pain, and voluntary food intake are parameters to observe to help determine efficacy of treatment regimen.
• Any laboratory abnormalities noted in the diagnostic workup should be evaluated for resolution.

PREVENTION/AVOIDANCE
• Depends on cause
• Maintaining a proper plan of nutrition with a high-fiber diet, thin coarse hay, and appropriate vitamin C supplementation will provide some protection against dietary-induced hypomotility and acquired dental disease.

POSSIBLE COMPLICATIONS
• Lack of food intake can be associated with dysbiosis and enterotoxemia. This is the most common cause of mortality in anorexic/pseudoanorexic guinea pigs.
• Dehydration, hypovitaminosis C, malnutrition, weight loss/cachexia, and hepatic lipidosis are common complications of anorexia/pseudoanorexia.
• Hepatic lipidosis occurs quickly in anorexic guinea pigs.

EXPECTED COURSE AND PROGNOSIS
• Depends on cause

• The longer the period of anorexia/pseudoanorexia, the more pronounced the secondary effects. The sooner the patient is treated, the better the prognosis for control of the consequences of reduced food intake.

MISCELLANEOUS

ASSOCIATED CONDITIONS
See Causes

AGE-RELATED FACTORS
Renal disease more common in older patients

ZOONOTIC POTENTIAL
N/A

PREGNANCY/FERTILITY/BREEDING
N/A

SYNONYMS
Hyporexia
Inappetence

SEE ALSO
Antibiotic-associated enterotoxemia
Dental malocclusion
Diarrhea
Dyspnea and tachypnea
Dysuria, hematuria, and pollakiuria
Exophthalmos and orbital diseases
Gastric dilation
Gastrointestinal hypomotility and gastrointestinal stasis
Hypovitaminosis C (scurvy)
Pododermatitis
Dental malocclusion
Weight loss and cachexia

ABBREVIATIONS
CT = computed tomography
DV = dorsoventral
GI = gastrointestinal
NSAID = nonsteroidal anti-inflammatory drug
VD = ventral dorsal

INTERNET RESOURCES
Veterinary Information Network (www.vin.com)
Veterinary Partner (www.veterinarypartner.com)

Suggested Reading
Bays TB. Geriatric care of rabbits, guinea pigs, and chinchillas. Vet Clin Exot Anim 2020;23:567–593.
Bohmer E. Changes in the cheek teeth. In: Bohmer E, ed. Dentistry in Rabbits and Rodents. Sussex, UK: Wiley Blackwell, 2015: 35–87, 118-212.
Bradley Bays T. Guinea pig behavior. In: Bradley Bays T, Lightfoot T, Mayer J, eds. Exotic Pet Behavior: Birds, Reptiles, and Small Mammals. St Louis: WB Saunders, 2006:207–238.
Capello V, Lennox AM, Widmer WR. Clinical Radiology of Exotic Companion Mammals. Ames: Wiley-Blackwell, 2008:168–223.
DeCubellis J. Common emergencies in rabbits, guinea pigs, and chinchillas. Vet Clin Exot Anim 2016;19:411–429.
Minarikova A, Hauptman K, Jeklova E et al. Diseases in pet guinea pigs: a retrospective study in 1000 animals. Vet Rec 2015;177(8):200.
Miwa Y, Sladky K. Common surgical procedures of rodents, ferrets, hedgehogs, and sugar gliders. Vet Clin Exot Anim 2016;19:205–244.
Pignon C, Mayer J. Guinea pigs. In: Quesenberry KE, Carpenter JW, eds. Ferrets, Rabbits and Rodents 4th ed. Clinical Medicine and Surgery. 2021. St. Louis: Saunders, 2020:270–297.
Ritzman TK. Diagnosis and clinical management of gastrointestinal conditions in exotic companion mammals (rabbits, guinea pigs, and chinchillas). Vet Clin Exot Anim 2014;17:179–194.
Author Jeffrey L. Rhody, DVM, DABVP-ECM

ANTIBIOTIC-ASSOCIATED ENTEROTOXEMIA

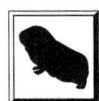

GUINEA PIGS

BASICS

DEFINITION
• Alteration of gastrointestinal bacterial flora induced by antimicrobials that allows for overgrowth of *Clostridium difficile*. This results in production of this bacterium's potent enterotoxins.

PATHOPHYSIOLOGY
• The normal bacterial flora of the large and small intestine of guinea pigs is predominately gram positive. In the normal animal, *Clostridium* spp. are found in low numbers, in a vegetative form, and not pathogenic.
• Antibiotics that alter the gram-positive flora allow overgrowth of enterotoxin-producing *Clostridium difficile* and/or *E. coli* septicemia.
• *C. difficile* enterotoxin binds to enteric mucosal cells, resulting in permeability changes or cell death, inducing secretory diarrhea, hemorrhagic typhlitis, and severe enterocolitis.

SYSTEMS AFFECTED
• Gastrointestinal system is the location of the pathology and toxin production.
• Once toxin is produced, systemic effects include hypovolemic and/or septic shock.
• Multiple organ failure can result.
• In guinea pigs, once toxin is produced, death is almost certain.

SIGNALMENT
Varies according to the underlying reason for the antibiotic therapy

SIGNS
Historical Findings
• Anorexia
• Acute, severe depression and lethargy
• Owner may report the impression their pet is painful.
• Diarrhea (liquid feces) is common.
• Bruxism and/or hunched posture or gait may be seen with visceral pain.
• Lateral recumbency indicates imminent death.
• Sudden death with fecal staining of perineum can be noted.

Physical Examination Findings
• Most affected guinea pigs are severely depressed.
• Exam findings related to the condition that resulted in antimicrobial usage may be present.
• Hypothermia can be associated with circulatory shock (septic or hypovolemic).
• Dehydration may be clinically detectable.

• Perineal area and rear legs may be stained or wet from liquid feces.
• Abdominal palpation may result in painful response. Borborygmus may be increased.
• Dyspnea or changes in character of respirations are related to shock and metabolic acidosis.
• Lateral recumbency is frequently seen and portends imminent death.
• Agonal respirations can be seen.

CAUSES
• Guinea pigs are exceptionally prone to antibiotic-induced gastrointestinal floral changes.
• Floral changes can occur with any antibiotic, but medications with a predominately gram-positive spectrum are notably more dangerous.
• Administration of beta lactam antibiotics (e.g., penicillin, ampicillin) and cephalosporins (cephalexin, cefazolin) has a profound effect on GI flora since they are excreted in the bile.
• Administration of macrolide antibiotics such as lincomycin, erythromycin, tylosin, and clindamycin has a known association with enterotoxemia. However, azithromycin can be used at 15–30 mg/kg PO q24h with relative safety.
• Chlortetracycline has also been implicated in this condition.

RISK FACTORS
Inappropriate antibiotic usage

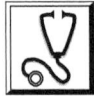

DIAGNOSIS

DIFFERENTIAL DIAGNOSIS
• Liquid diarrhea can occur with dysbiosis and infectious enteritides.
• Bacterial enteritis can be caused by *Salmonella* species, *Yersinia pseudotuberculosis*, *Clostridium perfringens*, *E. coli*, *Pseudomonas aeruginosa*, *Clostridium piliforme*, and *Listeria monocytogenes*. Most of these enteric infections cause morbidity and mortality in weanling guinea pigs.
• Protozoal diarrhea can be caused by cryptosporidium and coccidia (*Eimeria caviae*). Cryptosporidiosis is more common in weanlings, but immunosuppressed animals of any age are susceptible. Acute coccidiosis is typically seen in weanlings.
• Coronaviral enteritis may occur in weanlings.
• Idiopathic typhlitis has been reported.
• Anorexia and gastrointestinal hypomotility can induce floral changes that will result in enterotoxemia.

• Anamnesis should include review of husbandry and past medical history, especially recent administration of antibiotics.
• Complete physical examination is an essential element in diagnosis of any cause of lethargy, weight loss, pain, or anorexia.
• Guinea pigs with enterotoxemia usually demonstrate severe clinical signs and have evidence of severe illness on physical examination. Liquid diarrhea, hypothermia, severe depression, and pain are physical findings that should alert the clinician to the potential for high mortality.
• Most guinea pigs with antibiotic-associated enterotoxemia do not survive a diagnostic workup. Definitive diagnosis requires necropsy.

CBC/BIOCHEMISTRY/URINALYSIS
There are no reports of antemortem diagnostics for this condition. One can expect the results to be compatible with changes due to sepsis and shock.

OTHER LABORATORY TESTS
• *C. difficile* is difficult to isolate via culture.
• Fecal assays for *C. difficile* toxin are available but not often used clinically.

IMAGING
• Abdominal radiography is likely to demonstrate increased intestinal gas.
• Thoracic radiography may show microcardia due to hypovolemic shock.

DIAGNOSTIC PROCEDURES
Necropsy and toxin assay are often required for diagnostic confirmation.

TREATMENT

APPROPRIATE HEALTH CARE
Hospitalization is required, although successful treatment is rare. Once enterotoxemia develops, normalization of floral changes, and pathology is nearly impossible.

NURSING CARE
• Inappropriate antimicrobials (beta lactams, cephalosporins, macrolides, and chlortetracycline) should be discontinued immediately.
• Treatment of endotoxic, septic, and/or hypovolemic shock may be required. Treatment of shock follows the same principals as in dogs and cats, including fluid support (crystalloids), intravascular osmotic support (colloids), maintenance of renal blood flow (e.g., dobutamine), and antimicrobials (IV) for sepsis.
• In the stable patient, rehydration may be possible with subcutaneous fluids.

(CONTINUED) ANTIBIOTIC-ASSOCIATED ENTEROTOXEMIA

Maintenance needs are estimated at 100 mL/kg/day. Secretory diarrhea can lead to tremendous fluid losses; reevaluate hydration status frequently.
• Treatment of hypothermia with external heat source is appropriate. However, guinea pigs are obligate intranasal breathers and are prone to heat stroke. Care should be taken to avoid overheating.
• Judicious management of pain should be considered in all patients. Guinea pigs do not deal well with pain. Failure to manage pain effectively will inhibit recovery in any ill guinea pig.
• Transfaunation with feces from normal guinea pigs can be attempted orally and may be effective in mild cases.
• Transfaunation via retention enema has been reported in the rabbit with this condition; however, its efficacy in guinea pigs is unknown.

DIET
• It is prudent to avoid oral food and water supplementation in the critically ill patient. Enterotoxemia can be associated with severe pathology, including sloughing of enterocytes and pooling of splanchnic blood.
• Guinea pigs that do not eat are extremely prone to further deleterious effects of gastric hypomotility. In the stable patient, assist syringe feeding with an appropriate herbivore supplement such as Critical Care for Herbivores (Oxbow Pet Products, Murdock, NE) or Emeraid Herbivore (Lafeber Company, Cornell, IL) is appropriate for patients capable of receiving oral medications. Care must be taken in the dyspneic or struggling patient.
• Some sources recommend administration of commercial *Lactobacillus* products or live-culture yogurt to help reestablish normal microflora. However, the effectiveness of this is unknown since the microbiome of the guinea pig gastrointesinal tract has not been studied.

CLIENT EDUCATION
This condition carries with it a grave prognosis and is very painful. Treatment of critical patients should be considered heroic. Euthanasia should remain a part of the discussion with the owner until the patient is stable. Even relatively stable patients can decompensate rapidly.

SURGICAL CONSIDERATIONS
N/A

MEDICATIONS
DRUG(S) OF CHOICE
• Pain should be controlled with opioids (e.g., buprenorphine 0.05 mg/kg SC, IM, IV q8–12h). Severe pain may require mu agonists (e.g., hydromorphone 0.1mg/kg SC, IV q6–12h). NSAIDs should be avoided in face of shock, renal compromise, continuing fluid losses, and dehydration. Once stable, meloxicam (0.2–0.5 mg/kg PO, SC, IM q12–24h) can be administered.
• For gastric pain, H2 receptor antagonists such as famotidine (0.5 mg/kg PO, SC, IV q24h) or ranitidine (2 mg/kg IV or 2–5 mg/kg PO q24h. Metoclopramide (0.2–1.0 mg/kg PO, SC, IVq12h) increases gastric emptying.
• Oral or intravenous administration of chloramphenicol (30–50 mg/kg PO, SC, IV q8–12h) or metronidazole (10–20 mg/kg PO, IV q12h) may suppress further clostridial overgrowth.
• Cholestyramine (50–75 mg/kg PO) has been used to bind enterotoxins.

CONTRAINDICATIONS
• Inappropriate antimicrobials (beta lactams, cephalosporins, macrolides, and chlortetracycline)

PRECAUTIONS
Meloxicam should be avoided in patients with severe fluid losses, dehydration, shock, and renal compromise.

POSSIBLE INTERACTIONS
N/A

ALTERNATIVE DRUGS
N/A

FOLLOW-UP
PATIENT MONITORING
• Critical care monitoring for inpatients as in dogs and cats should be considered with understanding of limitations of patient size.
• An end to liquid stools in the stable patient indicates improvement.

PREVENTION/AVOIDANCE
• Do not use beta lactam, cephalosporin, or macrolide antibiotics in guinea pigs.
• Avoid use of chlortetracycline.

• While no antibiotic is free from risk on any individual patient, veterinarians should consider use of only the following antibiotics: chloramphenicol (30–50 mg/kg PO, SC, IV q8–12h), ciprofloxacin (5–25 mg/kg PO q12–24h), doxycycline (2.5–5 mg/kg PO q12h), enrofloxacin (5–20 mg/kg PO q12–24h), marbofloxacin (2–5 mg/kg PO, IM q24h), metronidazole (10–20 mg/kg PO, IV q12h), trimethoprim-sulfa (15–30 mg/kg PO q12h), or azithromycin (15–30 mg/kg PO q24h). Aminoglycoside administration is not known to be associated with enterotoxemia, but use of this class of drugs carries a relatively narrow safety margin.
• During antibiotic use, be sure food intake and stools are normal. Supplementation with high-fiber dietary assist feeding formulas such as those discussed above in Treatment section will support normal GI function.

POSSIBLE COMPLICATIONS
• If the patient survives the enterotoxemia, subsequent gastrointestinal hypomotility is likely to present further therapeutic challenges.
• Patients may require a prolonged course of assist feeding and hydration support.

EXPECTED COURSE AND PROGNOSIS
• Most guinea pigs will not survive this illness.
• Unstable patients usually die within hours of presentation.
• Stable patients can deteriorate and die within days.
• For the critically ill patient, prognosis is grave. For the stable patient, prognosis is guarded and may need to be adjusted to grave based on clinical progression.

MISCELLANEOUS
ASSOCIATED CONDITIONS
N/A

AGE-RELATED FACTORS
N/A

ZOONOTIC POTENTIAL
N/A

PREGNANCY/FERTILITY/BREEDING
N/A

GUINEA PIGS

ANTIBIOTIC-ASSOCIATED ENTEROTOXEMIA

SYNONYMS
Antibiotic-induced colitis
Dysbacteriosis
Dysbiosis
Enterotoxemia

SEE ALSO
Gastrointestinal hypomotility and gastrointestinal stasis

INTERNET RESOURCES
Veterinary Information Network (www.vin.com)

Suggested Reading
DeCubellis J. Common emergencies in rabbits, guinea pigs, and chinchillas. Vet Clin Exot Anim 2016;19:411–429.
Minarikova A, Hauptman K, Jeklova E et al. Diseases in pet guinea pigs: a retrospective study in 1000 animals. Vet Rec 2015;177(8):200.
Pignon C, Mayer J. Guinea pigs. In: Quesenberry KE, Carpenter JW, eds. Ferrets, Rabbits and Rodents (4th ed.). Clinical Medicine and Surgery. 2021. St. Louis: Saunders, 2020:270–297.
Ritzman TK. Diagnosis and clinical management of gastrointestinal conditions in exotic companion mammals (rabbits, guinea pigs, and chinchillas). Vet Clin Exot Anim 2014;17:179–194.
Young JD, Hurst WJ, White WJ, Lang CM. An evaluation of ampicillin pharmacokinetics and toxicity in guinea pigs. Lab An Sci 1987;37(5):652–656.
Author Jeffrey L. Rhody, DVM, DABVP-ECM

GUINEA PIGS

BASICS

DEFINITION
Incoordination during voluntary movement due to disruption of the sensory pathways that control proprioception

PATHOPHYSIOLOGY
There are three types of ataxia:

Cerebellar Ataxia
• The cerebellum coordinates and regulates motor activity, assists in maintaining equilibrium, and controls posture.
• Sensory impulses are transmitted via the cerebellar peduncles from the vestibular system, cerebral cortex, and spinal cord.
• The cerebellum does not initiate motor activity; therefore, paresis is not present with cerebellar dysfunction.
• Affected patients will demonstrate abnormal rate, range, or force of movement with intact strength.

Vestibular Ataxia
• The vestibular system is composed of sensory receptors in the inner ear and vestibular labyrinth that detect linear acceleration and rotational movement of the head.
• Motor activity is not initiated but is refined and coordinated via the vestibular system, by controlling muscles used to maintain head position, eye movement, and equilibrium.
• Information is transmitted to the muscles via vestibulospinal tracts, which stimulate ipsilateral extensor muscles; unilateral lesions result in a loss of ipsilateral extensor tone which forces the animal to fall or lean toward the side of the lesion as the contralateral side no longer has the opposing side to antagonize or balance extension.
• Dysfunction results in loss of balance; animals often list or fall to one side and may have head tilt.

Proprioceptive Ataxia
• Proprioceptive signals from the limbs and trunk are relayed to the brain via the spinal cord.
• Compression or injury of the spinal cord interferes with the transmission of sensory impulses, resulting in deficits in proprioception, motor dysfunction, and failure to properly place the limbs.
• The sensory tracts are superficial in the spinal cord, so proprioceptive defects may be the first sign of a lesion.
• Patients will show decreased awareness of limb position; often results in scuffing of toes, crossing of limbs, and standing on the dorsum of paws.

SYSTEMS AFFECTED
• Nervous
• Musculoskeletal—atrophy or contracture of musculature is a secondary complication

GENETICS
None

INCIDENCE/PREVALENCE
Vestibular disorders, primarily due to otitis interna/media are the most common cause of ataxia in guinea pigs and are frequently accompanied by other signs of upper respiratory infection.

GEOGRAPHIC DISTRIBUTION
None

SIGNALMENT
No age, breed, or sex predisposition

SIGNS

General Comments
• It is important to determine whether ataxia is cerebellar, vestibular, or proprioceptive and to localize the lesion based on lateralization of signs and neurologic examination.
• It is important to differentiate deficits in proprioception from generalized weakness; patients with generalized weakness will not exhibit any deficits on neurologic exam. However, this can be difficult to interpret in the debilitated guinea pig.
• Clinical signs may be acute or chronic and may be progressive or static. Onset and progression may be indicative of etiology.
• Acute or peracute onset of signs without progression or with gradual improvement is usually consistent with trauma or vascular events.
• Gradual or subacute onset with gradual improvement in response to treatment usually indicates infection.
• Slow onset and continued progression of clinical signs usually indicates a neoplastic or degenerative process.
• Static clinical signs (or signs present at birth) indicate an anomalous cause.

Historical Findings
• Owner may notice weakness, wobbliness, head tilt, wide-based stance, circling, dragging of the limbs, or inability to rise or maintain a standing position.
• Owner may notice an abnormal gait, leaning to one side, falling, or inability to stand or walk.
• There may be a known traumatic event such as being dropped or stepped on, or there may be a history of children playing with the pet.
• Inability to right itself from lying down, or an inability to get up without assistance
• Dragging of a limb
• Urine staining around perineum and/or on limbs (may be unilateral or bilateral)

• Swelling, redness, or pododermatitis of unaffected or less affected limbs may be the first sign identified and is often the result of excessive weight bearing on these limbs.
• Alopecia of the affected limbs may be present from rubbing or dragging.

Physical Examination Findings
• Mentation is usually normal.
• Pain may be present on spinal palpation in cases of trauma or injury.
• Muscle wasting may be present in patients with more gradual onset or prolonged disease.
• Patient may be tachypneic in response to pain or fear.
• Urine staining may be present around perineum and/or on limbs (may be unilateral or bilateral).
• Swelling, redness, or pododermatitis of unaffected or less affected limbs may be identified and is often the result of excessive weight bearing on these limbs.
• Alopecia of the affected limbs (particularly the dorsal aspect) may be present from rubbing or dragging.
• Gastric dilation (usually mild) may occur as a result of aerophagia; anorexia or diarrhea may be present due to inappetence from pain or an inability to access food or water.

Neurologic Examination Findings
Pain may be present on spinal palpation in cases of trauma.

Cerebellar
• Symmetric truncal ataxia
• Wide-based, hypometric gait
• Intention tremor, most evident in the head, usually exaggerated with purposeful movement
• Nystagmus may be present; usually tremorlike if it does occur, may be horizontal, rotary, or vertical
• Menace responses may be impaired, but facial nerve function and vision are normal—this is difficult to assess in guinea pigs as it is difficult to evaluate a menace response.
• Decerebellate rigidity is characterized by opisthotonus, tonic extension of the forelimbs with flexion of hind limbs, a critical state which requires emergency management.
• Paresis and muscle wasting are absent.

Vestibular
• May be central or peripheral vestibular disease
• Head tilt or turn, usually toward the side of the lesion
• Usually unilateral or asymmetric ataxia
• Falling, drifting, or circling are common features, usually toward the side of the lesion, but may be away from the lesion in central vestibular ataxia

• Nystagmus is usually present; in peripheral disease, horizontal or rotary with fast phase away from the side of the lesion; with central disease, nystagmus may be vertical, horizontal, or rotary and may change direction loss of extensor tone on the side of the lesion causes animals to fall toward the side of the lesion.
• If paresis or proprioceptive deficits are present along with a head tilt, this is a clear indicator of central vestibular disease.

Proprioceptive
• Proprioceptive deficits will be present in the affected limbs; this must be interpreted with caution as many guinea pigs will fail placing test even when completely normal.
• Deep pain is assessed by using a toe-pinch (superficial pain) or pinching of the pad/bone (deep pain); withdrawal of the limb alone is a reflex that alone does not indicate intact pain sensation; conscious response to the pinch is required to indicate spinal cord integrity.
• Neurolocalization is important.
• Cervical (C1–C6): Proprioceptive or motor deficits of all four limbs. Pain may be found on cervical palpation.
• Cervicothoracic (C6–T2): Lower-motor neuron signs to the forelimb including poor motor function and weak withdrawal with loss of reflexes
• Thoracolumbar (T3–L3): Weakness and proprioceptive abnormalities in the rear limbs with normal motor function and proprioception in the front limbs. Spinal reflexes are normal. Pain may be found on spinal palpation.
• Lumbosacral (L4–S3): Lower motor neuron signs to the rear limbs including proprioceptive abnormalities, weakness, poor withdrawal reflexes, and loss of segmental spinal reflexes. Urinary and fecal incontinence may be present.

CAUSES
Cerebellar
• Trauma/injury; an incident may have been directly observed, or there may be a history of contact with children or other pets.
• Infectious: meningitis/encephalitis— bacterial (consider spread of otitis media/ interna or upper respiratory infection); most common organisms include *Streptococcus pneumoniae, Streptococcus zooepidemicus, Staphylococcus aureus, and Bordatella bronchiseptica;* abscesses may form and act as a space-occupying mass; viral (lymphocytic choriomeningitis virus—LCM), toxoplasmosis; disseminated infection; lymphocytic choriomeningitis (LCM) virus—zoonotic disease that is naturally occurring in guinea pigs; causes meningitis and hind limb paralysis
• Neoplasia (lymphoma)

• Vascular accident
• Toxicity—lead, *Clostridium botulinum,* organophosphate are among toxins that can cause CNS or PNS signs and should be suspected if there is a possibility of ingestion or exposure
• Anomalous—although not described in guinea pigs, it is reasonable to assume that cerebellar hypoplasia or abiotrophy may occur in any species.

Vestibular (Central)
• Infectious—common organisms include *Streptococcus pneumoniae, Streptococcus zooepidemicus, Staphylococcus aureus, Bordatella bronchiseptica;* abscesses may form and act as a space-occupying mass; toxoplasmosis
• Neoplastic
• Metabolic—hyperglycemia, hypoglycemia, or electrolyte abnormalities
• Toxin—lead; metronidazole
• Inflammatory/idiopathic—not reported; may be a default when a diagnosis cannot be established

Vestibular (Peripheral)
• Infectious: Otitis interna/media is the most common cause, often associated with upper respiratory infection; common organisms include *Streptococcus pneumoniae, Streptococcus zooepidemicus, Staphylococcus aureus,* and *Bordatella bronchiseptica,* although yeast and fungal organisms are occasionally present.
• Neoplastic—rare
• Trauma
• Idiopathic—not reported; may be a default when a diagnosis cannot be established

Proprioceptive
• Trauma/injury of the spine is the most common cause of proprioceptive deficits, paresis, or paralysis in pet guinea pigs; an incident may have been directly observed, or there may be a history of contact with children or other pets.
• Neoplasia of spinal cord; none commonly reported
• CNS abscess (effects and diagnostics may mimic neoplasia)
• Vascular event
• Poliovirus—an RNA enterovirus transmitted via fecal-oral route; clinical signs include lameness and/or flaccid paralysis; rarely causes clinical signs
• LCM virus—zoonotic disease that is naturally occurring in guinea pigs; causes meningitis and hind limb paralysis
• Toxicity—lead, *Clostridium botulinum,* organophosphate are among toxins that can cause CNS or PNS signs and should be suspected if there is a possibility of ingestion or exposure

RISK FACTORS
• Otitis media/interna—upper respiratory infection, immunocompromise due to stress, overcrowding, poor ventilation
• Fractures, luxations—often the result of trauma from improper handling or housing, children, or other pets
• Spondylosis/arthritis—unknown etiology
• Hypovitaminosis C (scurvy)—nutritional

DIAGNOSIS
DIFFERENTIAL DIAGNOSIS
• Hypovitaminosis C (scurvy)
• Weakness (metabolic) may lead to similar clinical presentation
• Osteoarthritis
• Hypovitaminosis E—myopathy leading to hind limb weakness has been described in guinea pigs
• Pododermatitis
• Pregnancy

CBC/BIOCHEMISTRY/URINALYSIS
Usually normal unless infection is present; leukocytosis may be present in cases of infection; profound leukocytosis (>100,000) may occur in guinea pigs with leukemia; elevations in CK are likely in cases of trauma.

OTHER LABORATORY TESTS
• Cytology, culture, and sensitivity—if otitis media or upper respiratory infection are present, cultures may be representative of bacteria in the ear.
• Lymphocytic choriomeningitis testing— PCR, IFA, and serology are available and performed at many universities and commercial veterinary laboratories.
• Blood lead levels if ingestion is suspected
• Cholinesterase testing may be performed if organophosphate toxicity is suspected.

IMAGING
Radiography—may reveal spinal fracture or luxation, osteomyelitis, osteoarthritis, discospondylitis, and bone neoplasia. Skull radiographs may reveal bulla disease. CT—more sensitive for evaluation of brain infiltrate, spinal cord compression, or bony lesions

DIAGNOSTIC PROCEDURES
• CSF analysis can be performed via the cisterna magna; indicated if infection or neoplasia is suspected; do not attempt to aspirate but instead collect sample via capillary tube; only a few drops will be obtained
• EMG/NCV (electromyelogram/nerve conduction velocity)—not commonly performed in guinea pigs, normal values are

not established—compare to unaffected limb to establish normal

PATHOLOGIC FINDINGS
Pathology will vary with underlying etiology.

TREATMENT

APPROPRIATE HEALTH CARE
Inpatient—neurologic signs; severe infections; anorexic patients; nonambulatory patients

Outpatient—stable patients that are able to eat and drink with little or no assistance

NURSING CARE
• Fluid therapy to maintain hydration—subcutaneous generally adequate unless severe infection/sepsis
• Assisted feeding of anorexic animals
• Maintain clean, soft bedding with padding if necessary.
• Lubricate eyes if blink response is absent or diminished.
• In severe cases, turn patient every 4 hours or as needed to prevent formation of decubitus ulcers.
• Express bladder if patient unable to void without assistance
• Keep fur clean and dry.

ACTIVITY
Restrict activity, particularly in cases of trauma. Confine to a very small space initially to prevent falls or further injury.

DIET
• It is essential to maintain food intake during treatment; patients may become anorexic due to pain or neurologic signs; anorexia may lead to gastrointestinal stasis and ileus; secondary derangements of intestinal microbial populations may occur.
• Offer a wide variety of fresh leafy greens (romaine lettuce, cilantro, parsley, kale, cabbage, collard greens, mustard greens, bok choy, dandelion greens, turnip greens, spinach, and mesclun salad mixes) and high-quality grass hay. Place food and water in a position that the guinea pig is able to reach, or hand offer.
• If patient is inappetent/anorexic, it is essential to provide adequate nutritional support. Syringe feed a formulated diet such as Critical Care for Herbivores (Oxbow Pet Products, Murdock, NE) or Emeraid Herbivore (Lafeber Company, Cornell, IL) 10–15 mL/kg q6–8h. If neither product is available, a slurry can be made with blended leafy green vegetables that are high in vitamin C, or guinea pig pellets blended with water and vegetable baby food.

• Avoid high-carbohydrate foods, treats, or grains.
• Use caution when syringe feeding as aspiration pneumonia may occur in patients with central nervous system signs.

CLIENT EDUCATION
• Owners should be informed that in cases of spinal trauma or paralysis, motor function may improve gradually or may not improve at all.
• Educate clients that pets with cerebellar or vestibular ataxia may have permanent changes and may require household adaptations to prevent injury from loss of disequilibrium or loss of balance.
• Owners should keep pet in a small area with no vertical surfaces to prevent injuries or falls due to incoordination.
• Food and water must be placed in accessible locations; guinea pigs may not be able to lift head to a water bottle or feeder, so hand feeding or assistance may be necessary.

SURGICAL CONSIDERATIONS
• Endoscopic myringotomy has been used successfully. May require specialized expertise.
• Bulla osteotomy (and total ear canal ablation) may be indicated in severe cases of otitis media/interna with bulla osteitis; however, if central vestibular signs are present, prognosis may be poor.
• Surgical repair of spinal fractures or tumors should only be undertaken by an experienced orthopedic or neurologic surgeon and may be of limited value. Many cases of partial paresis or paralysis will improve without surgery; surgery in these small patients has the potential of further destabilizing the spinal cord.

MEDICATIONS
DRUG(S) OF CHOICE
• Corticosteroids are recommended in mammals with spinal trauma, but their use is controversial in guinea pigs because they are believed to be very susceptible to adverse side effects and secondary infections; however, other references cite that guinea pigs are a steroid-resistant species.
• If administered, a short-acting steroid such as methylprednisolone sodium succinate (10–30 mg/kg IV or IM is the canine dose; guinea pig dose not reported) may be preferable to minimize any long-term immunosuppression.
• Analgesics should be administered in cases of confirmed or suspected trauma; systemic meloxicam (0.5–1.0 mg/kg PO, SC, IM q24h) for its anti-inflammatory effects alone or in combination with an opioid (avoid if

corticosteroids have been administered); buprenorphine (0.05–0.2 mg/kg SC, IM, IV q8–12h), butorphanol (0.4–2.0 mg/kg SC, IM q4–12h), or tramadol (5–10 mg/kg PO q12h) for additional analgesia
• For suspected or confirmed CNS infections, use systemic antibiotics. Choose broad-spectrum antibiotics that penetrate the CNS, such as enrofloxacin (5–20 mg/kg PO q12–24h) or trimethoprim-sulfa (15–30 mg/kg PO q12h); for anaerobic infections consider chloramphenicol (30–50 mg/kg PO, SC, IM, IV q12h), florfenicol (20–25 mg/kg PO, IM, IV q12h), or metronidazole (10–20 mg/kg PO, IV q12h).

CONTRAINDICATIONS
• Avoid the use of antimicrobials that may disrupt gastrointestinal flora, which may lead to dysbiosis and fatal enterotoxemia (penicillins, macrolides, lincosamides, tetracyclines, and cephalosporins).
• Avoid the use of corticosteroids in conjunction with meloxicam or other NSAIDs.
• Corticosteroids—because of the immunosuppressive effects of corticosteroids, their use may prolong or exacerbate infection and may increase risk of systemic disease.
• Avoid the use of drugs that are potentially toxic to the central nervous system (metronidazole at high doses; aminoglycosides)

PRECAUTIONS
• Do not use steroids in conjunction with NSAIDs.
• Use caution in choosing antimicrobials.

POSSIBLE INTERACTIONS
Do not use steroids in conjunction with NSAIDs.

ALTERNATIVE DRUGS
N/A

FOLLOW-UP
PATIENT MONITORING
Serial neurologic examinations should be performed daily or more frequently initially to monitor for progression of clinical signs.

PREVENTION/AVOIDANCE
• Avoid free roaming or unsupervised activity or interactions with children or other pets.
• Treat upper respiratory infections and otitis early and aggressively to prevent dissemination to the middle and inner ear and brain.

POSSIBLE COMPLICATIONS
• Urine retention, urine scald, urinary tract infection, ascending renal infection

ATAXIA   (CONTINUED)

- Pododermatitis and osteomyelitis from excessive weight bearing of unaffected or lesser affected limbs
- Permanent paralysis, permanent head tilt
- Cerebellar changes may be permanent

EXPECTED COURSE AND PROGNOSIS
- Depends on etiology
- Head tilt, proprioceptive deficits, and cerebellar signs may persist even if underlying cause is resolved, but many patients can learn to adapt to these changes.

MISCELLANEOUS

ASSOCIATED CONDITIONS
- Nutritional deficiencies, either as a cause (hypovitaminosis C, E) or result of inability to access food
- Gastrointestinal hypomotility
- Otitis media/interna or upper respiratory infection may serve as a source for CNS infections.

AGE-RELATED FACTORS
None

ZOONOTIC POTENTIAL
LCM virus is rare but zoonotic.

PREGNANCY/FERTILITY/BREEDING
Guinea pigs with paresis or paralysis should not bred; pregnancy and parturition would put excessive strain on any injury.

SYNONYMS
None

SEE ALSO
Ataxia
Head tilt (vestibular disease)
Hypovitaminosis C (scurvy)
Otitis media and interna

ABBREVIATIONS
CK = creatine kinase
LCM = lymphocytic choriomeningitis
CNS = central nervous system
CSF = cerebrospinal fluid
CT = computed tomography
EMG = electromyelogram
IFA = immunoflorescence antibody analysis
MRI = magnetic resonance imaging
NCV = nerve conduction velocity
NSAID = nonsteroidal anti-inflammatory drug
PCR = polymerase chain reaction

Suggested Reading
Harkness JE, Turner PV, VandeWoude S, Wheeler CL. Clinical signs and differential diagnoses: nervous and musculoskeletal conditions. In: Harkness JE, Turner PV, VandeWoude S, Wheeler CL, eds. Biology and Medicine of Rabbits and Rodents, 5th ed. Ames: Wiley-Blackwell, 2010: 214–216.
Jekl V, Hauptman K, Knotek Z. Video otoscopy in exotic companion mammals. Vet Clin North Am Exot Anim Pract 2015;18:431–445.

Mancinelli E. Neurologic examination and diagnostic testing in rabbits, ferrets and rodents. J Exot Pet Med 2015;24:52–64.
Meredith AL, Richardson J. Neurologic disease of rabbits and rodents. J Exot Pet Med 2015;24:21–33.
Minarikova A, Hauptman K, Jeklova E, Knotek Z, Jekl V. Diseases in pet guinea pigs: a retrospective study in 1000 animals. Vet Rec 2015;177:200.
Miwa Y, Sladky K. Common surgical procedures of rodents, ferrets, hedgehogs, and sugar gliders. Vet Clin Exot Anim 2016;19:205–244.
Pignon C, Mayer J. Guinea pigs. In: Quesenberry KE, Carpenter JW, eds. Ferrets, Rabbits and Rodents, 4th ed.Clinical Medicine and Surgery. 2021. St. Louis: Saunders, 2020:270–297.
Rosset RA, Pignon C, Desprez I et al. Development and validation of an endoscopic myringotomy technique to treat otitis media and interna in a case series of three guinea pigs (*Cavia porcellus*). J Exot Pet Med 2020;31:31–38.

Authors Natalie Antinoff, DVM, Dipl. ABVP (Avian) and Barbara Oglesbee, DVM, Dipl. ABVP (Avian)

CARDIAC AND PERICARIDIAL DISEASE

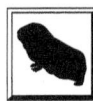

BASICS

DEFINITION

<u>Myocarditis definition:</u> Inflammatory changes in cardiomyocytes

<u>Myocardial necrosis definition:</u> Necrosis of cardiomyocytes

<u>Valvular endocardiosis definition:</u> Myxomatous change in valve structure resulting in valvular insufficiency

<u>Congenital heart disease definition:</u> Cardiac disease present at birth that may or not create clinical signs until later in life.

<u>Neoplasia:</u> Tumors of cardiac tissue or associated structures nearby that can affect cardiac function.

<u>Pericardial effusion definition:</u> Fluid present in the pericardial sac above the normal amount.

<u>Pericardial tamponade:</u> When the pressure in the pericardial sac is raised above the ability of the right atrium causing compression of this structure.

PATHOPHYSIOLOGY

• Myocarditis: Often due to bacterial infection, leads to cardiac muscle dysfunction and cardiac failure and peri- or epicarditis

• Myocardial necrosis: Often leads to fibrosis and cardiac dysfunction

• Valvular endocardiosis: Often creates audible murmur and can progress to congestive heart failure

• Congential heart disease: Often causes audible murmur and in some cases can progress to more severe disease and congestive heart failure

• <u>Neoplasia:</u> Heart base tumors are often associated with pericardial effusion. One case of ventricular septal leiomyosarcoma has been reported. It is unsure if this caused any clinical disease. Mesenchymoma of the right atrium and myocardial fibrosarcoma have also been reported.

• Pericardial disease: Right atrium compression followed by right ventricular compression; left-sided compression may also occur. Compression creates decreased cardiac output and arterial hypotension. Right-sided heart failure is usually present

SYSTEMS AFFECTED

• Cardiovascular (histopathological lesions as noted above, CHF possible, pericardial effusion possible)

• Respiratory (pleural effusion, pulmonary edema)

• Urinary (prerenal azotemia)

• All organ systems potentially at risk due to poor cardiac output and local hypoxemia in the event of CHF, systemic infection, pericardial effusion

INCIDENCE/PREVALENCE

Unknown but cases have been anecdotally reported as common; one published report of pericaridial disease

SIGNALMENT

No known sex or age predilection

SIGNS

Historical Findings

Signs related to low cardiac output

• Weakness

• Inappetence

• Depression

• Exogenous corticosteroid usage (one anecdotal report of RCM due to endomyocarditis responsive to enrofloxacin and metronidazole)

• Syncope

Signs related to congestive heart failure

• Dyspnea

• Tachypnea

• Collapse

• Abdominal distension in the presence of effusion or gastric dilation due to aerophagia

Physical Examination Findings

• Cardiac auscultation—possibly normal, murmur (intensity based on degree of valvular insufficiency), arrhythmia

• Atrial arrhythmias appear to predominate with endomyocardial fibrosis.

• Muffled heart sounds in event of pleural effusion or pericardial effusion

• Rales/crackles in lungs in event of pulmonary edema

• Pale or cyanotic mucus membranes in event of cardiogenic shock or significant peripheral hypoxia; membranes may have poor refill time

• Pulse deficits may be present in event of arrhythmia

• Hypothermia is possible due to low cardiac output

CAUSES AND RISK FACTORS

• Genetics may play a role in spontaneous cardiomyopathy (segmental necrosis of cardiac and skeletal muscles). This condition was worsened by oxygen therapy and exercise.

• Congenital heart disease has been reported in several males from a single source

• Myocardial necrosis was found to have a poor correlation to vitamin E and selenium status of guinea pigs

• Causes of pericardial disease include idiopathic pericardial effusion, hemorrhagic effusion (toxins, left atrial tear, idiopathic, iatrogenic), and fibrinous, septic effusion

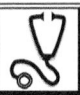

DIAGNOSIS

DIFFERENTIAL DIAGNOSIS

• Cardiac disease—dilated cardiomyopathy, hyperthyroidism (left ventricular underload), pericardial disease, neoplastic disease, congenital heart disease

• Unclassified cardiomyopathies

• Pleural effusion—dilated cardiomyopathy, neoplasia, infection (pyothorax), hemothorax (chylous effusion has not been reported)

• Muffled heart sounds—pericardial disease, pleural effusion

• Pulmonary edema—pneumonia, electrocution

• Cyanosis—severe respiratory disease

• Pale mucus membranes/poor capillary refill time—cardiogenic or noncardiogenic shock

• Cough/dyspnea—pneumonia, pulmonary abscessation/consolidation, severe upper respiratory disease, maxillary dental abscessation with obstruction of nasal passages, pleural effusion not related to heart disease (neoplasia, pyothorax, and hemothorax)

• Pulse deficits—arrhythmia, electrical alternans associated with pericardial effusion

• Jugular pulses with right-sided murmur may indicate tricuspid valve disease/right sided congestive heart failure

• Hepatomegaly—hepatic lipidosis, neoplasia

• Hypothermia—noncardiogenic shock, gastric dilatation/volvulus

CBC/BIOCHEMISTRY/URINALYSIS

• Routine blood tests and urinalysis are usually normal unless heart failure is causing hepatic congestion (increased ALT) or pre-renal azotemia

• Therapy for congestive failure can also cause abnormalities such as hypokalemia, prerenal azotemia, and exacerbation of primary renal disease.

• Disease concurrent to myocardial disease and valvular endocardiosis may affect the lab results

OTHER LABORATORY TESTS

• Endomyocardial biopsy (endomyocarditis)—not reported to have been performed in the guinea pig

• Blood culture in cases of suspected infectious disease

• Cytologyand fluid analysis of pericardial fluid, bacterial culture when indicated

DIAGNOSTIC IMAGING

Radiographic Findings

• Pericaridal disease: enlarged cardiac silhouette—heart may be globoid, tracheal

CARDIAC AND PERICARIDIAL DISEASE

elevation may be seen on lateral views, and pleural effusion may be present
• Valvular endocardiosis: enlarged cardiac silhouette—heart may be globoid (differential diagnosis is pericardial effusion, DCM, HCM, RCM
• Valvular endocardiosis: pulmonary edema and/or pleural effusion are common
• Valvular endocardiosis: possibly bicavitary effusion
• Valvular endocardiosis: possibly hepatomegaly in right-sided heart failure
• Often normal in cases of myocarditis and myocardial necrosis
• Neoplasia: enlarged cardiac silhouette in cases with pericardial effusion
• Congenital heart disease: cardiac enlargement may be noted especially if develops into cardiomyopathy pleural effusion or ascites if develops into right- sided CHF.

Echocardiographic Findings
• Echocardiogram for definitive diagnosis
• Identify pericardial fluid; mitral or tricuspid insufficiency, endomyocardial disease, neoplasia, or congenital heart disease

DIAGNOSTIC TESTS
Electrocardiography
• While normal values for EKG parameters are available for guinea pigs, this modality is not commonly used in guinea pigs unless an arrythmia is auscultated.
• Use padded alligator clips or nontraumatic flat clips with alcohol or ultrasonic gel as conductive agent
• Ventricular and supraventricular arrythmias can be noted.
• Electrical alternans may be noted with pericardial effusion.

Pleural, Pericadial, or Abdominal Fluid Analysis
• Analysis of pleural fluid is important to rule out pyothorax, neoplasia, and hemothorax.
• Analysis of peritoneal fluid will help rule out neoplastic, septic, and hemorrhagic effusions.
• Results of fluid analysis in heart disease often reveals a modified transudate.

Pathologic Findings
• Ventricular walls are thickened (endomyocarditis) or may show fibrosis in the endocardium, subendocardium, or the myocardium
• Atrial chambers may be dilated in cases of valvular insufficiency
• Valve anatomy may be abnormal. Myxomatous changes in the valves create thickened cusp edges that no longer extend to point of complete closure

• Fibrosis and mineralization can be seen in myocarditis and endomyocarditis.
• Epicarditis can be seen in experimental infection with *Borrelia*
• Myocarditis can be seen in experimental infection with *Listeria*
• Neoplasia has been reported in the interventricular septum with extension into the right ventricle, but this was microscopic lesion and not noted grossly.
• Ventricular septal defect leading to CHF was diagnosed in 5 male guinea pigs.

TREATMENT
APPROPRIATE HEALTH CARE
• Decompensated cardiac disease in guinea pigs should prompt hospitalization for stabilization.
• Mildly affected patients can be managed as outpatients.

EMERGENT CARE
• Severely dyspneic patients may need immediate oxygen therapy. Guinea pigs often struggle with oxygen masks and flow-by oxygen therapy and may decompensate rapidly. Oxygen cages are preferred.
• Hypothermia should be managed using warm water bottles or water blankets in a warmed cage environment. Absorption of parenteral medications is not reliable in patients with severe hypothermia. Intravenous access can be difficult to obtain in decompensated patients. Intraosseous catheter may be needed. Sedation and local anesthesia are recommended to place these catheters.
• Most guinea pigs benefit from mild sedation in the hospital environment (midazolam 0.2–0.4 mg/kg IM and butorphanol 0.4–2 mg/kg SC, IM)
• In cases where the risk of diagnostics is too great, consider furosemide (2–5 mg/kg SC, IM, IV, IO) and/or nitroglycerin ointment (2%) applied to the hairless area on the ear. 1/8–1/16″ of the ointment is applied. Wear gloves to avoid ointment contacting your skin.
• Avoid all stress including nearby predators and noises from other hospitalized pets. Handle the patient minimally until its condition improves to allow diagnostics (radiography first and foremost).
• Thoracocentesis can be therapeutic in cases of pleural effusion. Using techniques extrapolated from dogs and cats, draining as much fluid as possible from each hemithorax can allow patient to compensate rapidly. Use sterile technique. Many patients require

sedation beyond butorphanol/midazolam (e.g., local anesthesia, low-dose isoflurane for immobilization).
• If concerned for pericardial effusion, be careful to tap chest either with ultrasound guidance or by evaluating likely area of heart on radiographs and tap caudal to that area.

MEDICATIONS
FUROSEMIDE
• Indicated only for patients with fluid accumulation (pleural effusion, pulmonary edema, and abdominal effusion)
• Dosage: 2–5 mg/kg SC, IM, IV, IO q4–6 hours (emergent care); 1–4 mg/kg SC, IM, PO for outpatient care.
• Titrate to lowest effective dose (often 1–2 mg/kg PO q12–24 hours).
• Best if compounded to flavored suspension, but this author has used flavored injectable solution orally in some patients.
• Monitor for dehydration, azotemia, and hypokalemia
• Be aware, patients on this diuretic will usually have isosthenuric urine (~1.010).

NITROGLYCERIN OINTMENT (2%)
• A dab of this ointment on the hairless inner pinna can cause enough venous dilation to aid in reducing pulmonary edema and pleural effusion.
• Should be used in conjunction with a diuretic.
• Useful in emergent cases only.

PIMOBENDAN
• A potent positive inotropic agent with positive effects on preload and afterload
• Dose is extrapolated from the dog: (0.25 mg/kg PO q12h)
• This drug may need to be compounded into a suspension to accurately dose a guinea pig.
• Pimobendan has been used in cats with HCM to positive effect despite the lack of need for inotropic support.

ENALAPRIL
• An ACE inhibitor
• While this agent has been used in guinea pigs with CHF, RCM, and HCM its use has fallen out of favor for heart failure with many cardiologists due to lack of measurable effect in heart disease.
• Dosage: 0.3 mg/kg q12h PO
• This medication may need to be compounded into a suspension for accurate dosing for guinea pig patients.
• Enalapril and furosemide together are more likely to cause azotemia than furosemide alone.

ANTIBIOTICS

• May be beneficial if one suspects infectious cause of pleural, abdominal, or pericardial effusions or myocardial disease.

• Chloramphenicol and a combination of enrofloxacin and metronidazole have both been used anecdotally with beneficial, even curative effects.

FOLLOW-UP

VALVULAR ENDOCARDIOSIS

• Once stabilized, periodic re-evaluation using radiographs and echocardiograms can help titrate drug dosages to more precise effect.

• Frequency of re-evaluation depends on the patient's clinical signs.

• Closely observe patient at home for dyspnea, lethargy, weakness, and anorexia

• Having the owner measure the resting (sleeping) respiratory rate at home can help owner identify potential problems early. (Normal RR: 40–150 bpm; average of 80bpm)

• Periodic monitoring of renal function and serum or plasma potassium is recommended.

• Prognosis in valvular disease in guinea pigs is unknown but assumed to be like dogs and cats and is predicated upon severity of condition at diagnosis.

MYOCARDITIS AND MYOCARDIAL NECROSIS

• Most of these lesions have been reported in research studies on sacrificed animals.

• Nevertheless, it is prudent to follow-up on any clinical case with clinical signs with physical exams and tests (based on the clinical signs and/or etiology of the patient at time of diagnosis).

NEOPLASIA

• Follow-up depends on clinical signs and size, location, and suspected of tumor.

CONGENITAL HEART DISEASE

• Follow-up should include repeated echocardiograms as needed according to original diagnosis and echocardiogram. Renal function should be monitored, if appropriate, during drug therapy.

PERICARDIAL EFFUSION

• Once case of idiopathic hemorrhagic pericardial effusion with only 7cc of flood removed via pericardiocentesis was followed with echocardiograms up to 6 month post-presentation with no recurrence of signs or fluid accumulation. Guinea pig lived for 25 months post presentation.

MISCELLANEOUS

ABBREVIATIONS

ACE = angiotensin-converting enzyme
ALT = alanine aminotransferase
BPM = breaths per minute
CBC = complete blood cell count
CHF = congestive heart failure
DCM = dilated cardiomyopathy
EKG = electrocardiogram
HCM = hypertrophic cardiomyopathy

RCM = restrictive cardiomyopathy
RR = respiratory rate

Suggested Reading

Bays TB. Geriatric care of rabbits, guinea pigs, and chinchillas. Vet Clin Exot Anim 2020;23:567–593.

Caulfield JB, Shelton RW. Spontaneous cardiomyopathy in guinea pigs. Rec Adv Stud Cardiac Struct Metab 1973;2:353–360.

Dyzban LA, Garrod LE, Besso JG. Pericardial effusion and pericardiocentesis in a guinea pig (*Cavia porcellus*). J Am Anim Hosp Assoc 2001;37:21–26.

Fitzgerald BC, Dias S, Martorell J. Cardiovascular drugs in avian, small mammal, and reptile medicine. Vet Clin Exot Anim 2018;21:399–442.

Franklin JM, Guzman DSM. Dilated cardiomyopathy and congestive heart failure in a guinea pig. Exot DVM 2005;7(6):9.

Miwa Y, Sladky K. Common surgical procedures of rodents, ferrets, hedgehogs, and sugar gliders. Vet Clin Exot Anim 2016;19:205–244.

Pignon C, Mayer J. Guinea pigs. In: Quesenberry KE, Carpenter JW, eds. Ferrets, Rabbits and Rodents, 4th ed. Clinical Medicine and Surgery. 2021. St. Louis: Saunders, 2020:270–297.

Schnellbacher R, Olson EE, Mayer J. Emergency presentations associated with cardio-vascular disease in exotic herbivores. J Exot Pet Med 2012;21:316–327.

Author Jeff Rhody, DVM, DABVP (ECM)

GUINEA PIGS

CARDIOMYOPATHY, DILATED (DCM), HYPERTROPHIC (HCM), AND RESTRICTIVE (RCM)

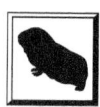 **BASICS**

DEFINITION

DCM

Heart muscle disease is characterized by weak cardiac muscles. Clinical signs are associated with ventricular pump failure and volume overload.

HCM

Hypertrophic cardiomyopathy (HCM) is a primary myocardial (heart muscle) disease defined as left ventricular (LV) concentric hypertrophy in the absence of an identifiable increase in afterload. Biatrial enlargement ensues. Systolic function is usually preserved.

RCM

Restrictive cardiomyopathy (RCM) is a myocardial disease characterized by left or biatrial enlargement and diastolic dysfunction associated with ventricular wall stiffness. The result is a restrictive pathophysiology and poor diastolic filling. Generally, ventricular compliance is impeded by endocardial, subendocardial, or myocardial fibrosis, or by an infiltrative condition. Ventricular myocardium may be slightly thickened or normal, with normal to mildly decreased ventricular volume. Systolic function is often normal or only mildly diminished.

PATHOPHYSIOLOGY

• Myocardial failure leads to decreased cardiac output and congestive heart failure.
• Arterial thromboembolism is possible and related to a clot in the dilated left atrium.

SYSTEMS AFFECTED

• Cardiovascular (left-sided CHF is common with HCM)
• Respiratory (pleural effusion, pulmonary edema)
• Urinary (prerenal azotemia)
• All organ systems are potentially at risk due to poor cardiac output and local hypoxemia

INCIDENCE/PREVALENCE

True incidence is unknown, but multiple case reports of DCM have been published and anecdotally reported; HCM and RCM are less common and only anecdotally reported in guinea pigs

SIGNALMENT

Middle-aged to older guinea pigs. No sex predilection. Congenital defects (e.g., ventricular septal defect) may lead to secondary DCM.

SIGNS

Historical Findings

Signs related to low cardiac output

• Weakness
• Inappetence
• Depression
Signs related to congestive heart failure
• Dyspnea
• Tachypnea
• Abdominal distension in the presence of effusion or gastric dilation due to aerophagia
• Collapse
Signs related to aortic thromboembolism
• Hind limb ataxia, weakness, or paralysis
• Pain

Physical Examination Findings

• Cardiac Auscultation—possibly normal, murmur (intensity based on the degree of turbulent blood flow), arrhythmia
• Muffled heart sounds in even of pleural effusion or pericardial effusion
• Rales/crackles in lungs in the event of pulmonary edema
• Diffuse ventral subcutaneous edema
• Posterior paresis/paralysis in the event of thromboembolism
• Generalized or rear-leg specific pain in the event of thromboembolism; other arterial embolic events cause clinical signs related to arterial blockage at the site of embolism.
• Pulse deficits may be present in the event of arrhythmia
• Pale or cyanotic mucus membranes in the event of cardiogenic shock or significant peripheral hypoxia; membranes may have poor refill time
• Hypothermia is possible due to low cardiac output

CAUSES AND RISK FACTORS

• Underlying risk factors are unknown. Dietary factors (decreased vitamin C, low magnesium and high phosphorus, vitamin E or selenium deficiency) may be involved.
• Exogenous corticosteroid usage (one anecdotal report of RCM due to endomyocarditis)
• Troponin mutation is linked to DCM in guinea pigs and has been implicated in HCM in cats.
• Preexisting myocarditis may be a factor in some cases of RCM.

 DIAGNOSIS

DIFFERENTIAL DIAGNOSIS

• Cardiac disease secondary to hyperthyroidism (left ventricular underload)
• Pleural effusion—dilated cardiomyopathy, neoplasia, infection (pyothorax), hemothorax (chylous effusion has never been reported)

• Muffled heart sounds—pericardial disease, pleural effusion
• Pulmonary edema—pneumonia, electrocution
• Cyanosis—severe respiratory disease
• Pale mucus membranes/poor capillary refill time—cardiogenic or non-cardiogenic shock
• Cough/dyspnea—pneumonia, pulmonary abscessation/consolidation, severe upper respiratory disease, maxillary dental abscessation with obstruction of nasal passages, pleural effusion not related to heart disease (neoplasia, pyothorax, and hemothorax)
• Pulse deficits—arrhythmia, electrical alternans associated with pericardial effusion
• Hypothermia—non-cardiogenic shock, gastric dilatation/volvulus

CBC/BIOCHEMISTRY/ URINALYSIS

• Routine blood tests and urinalysis are usually normal unless heart failure is causing hepatic congestion (increased ALT) or prerenal azotemia
• Therapy for congestive failure can also cause abnormalities such as hypokalemia, prerenal azotemia, and exacerbation of primary renal disease.
• Disease concurrent to HCM or RCM may also affect test results.

DIAGNOSTIC IMAGING

Radiographic Findings

• Enlarged cardiac silhouette—heart may be globoid (differential diagnosis is pericardial effusion)
• Pulmonary edema and/or pleural effusion are common
• Possibly bicavitary effusion
• Possibly hepatomegaly in right sided heart failure

Echocardiographic Findings

• Echocardiogram for definitive diagnosis; used to differentiate type of cardiomyopathies and pericardial effusion.
• Characteristic findings include enlarged thin ventricular walls, left atrial enlargement (with or without a clot), increased left ventricular systolic and end-diastolic dimensions, and decreased fractional shortening.
• Other findings can include mitral and/or triscuspid insufficiency and altered transaortic flow rates
• HCM—characteristic findings include enlarged thickened ventricular walls, biatrial enlargement (with or without a left atrial clot), decreased diastolic filling of the hypertrophied or rigid ventricles.

DIAGNOSTIC TESTS

Electrocardiography
- While normal values for EKG parameters are available for guinea pigs, this modality is not commonly used in guinea pigs unless an arrythmia is auscultated.
- Use padded alligator clips or nontraumatic flat clips with alcohol or ultrasonic gel as conductive agent
- Ventricular and supraventricular arrythmias can be noted.
- Electrical alternans may be noted with pericardial effusion.

Pleural or Abdominal Fluid Analysis
- Analysis of pleural fluid is important to rule out pyothorax, neoplasia, and hemothorax.
- Analysis of peritoneal fluid will help rule out neoplastic, septic, and hemorrhagic effusions.
- Results of fluid analysis in heart disease often reveal a modified transudate.

Pathologic Findings
- Heart to body ratio is increased
- DCM—Ventricular tricular walls are thin; chamber is dilate. Histopathology can show myocardial degeneration, myocardial fibrosis, and multifocal areas of myocardial necrosis.
- HCM—ventricular walls are thickened or may show fibrosis in the endocardium, subendocardium, or the myocardium (RCM); atrial chambers are dilated
- In RCM, endocardial thickening from deposition of hyaline, fibrous, and granulation tissue may be extreme. Chondroid metaplasia of the surface occurs occasionally.

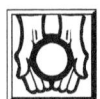

TREATMENT

APPROPRIATE HEALTH CARE
- Decompensated cardiomyopathic guinea pigs should be hospitalized for stabilization.
- Mildly affected patients can be managed as outpatients.

EMERGENT CARE
- Severely dyspneic patients may need immediate oxygen therapy. Guinea pigs often struggle with oxygen masks and flow-by-oxygen therapy and may decompensate rapidly. Oxygen cages are preferred.
- Hypothermia should be managed using warm water bottles or water blankets in a warm cage environment. Absorption of parenteral medications is not reliable in patients with severe hypothermia. Intravenous access can be difficult to obtain in decompensated patients. Intraosseous

catheter may be needed. Sedation and local anesthesia are recommended to place these catheters.
- Most guinea pigs benefit from mild sedation in the hospital environment (midazolam 0.2–0.4 mg/kg IM and butorphanol 0.4–2 mg/kg SC, IM)
- In cases where the risk of diagnostics is too great, consider furosemide (2–5 mg/kg SC, IM, IV, IO) and/or nitroglycerin ointment (2%) applied to the hairless area on the ear. 1/8–1/16″ of the ointment is applied. Wear gloves to avoid ointment contacting your skin.
- Avoid all stress including nearby predators and noises from other hospitalized pets. Handle the patient minimally until its condition improves to allow diagnostics (radiography first and foremost).
- Thoracocentesis can be therapeutic in cases of pleural effusion. Using techniques extrapolated from dogs and cats, draining as much fluid as possible from each hemithorax can allow the patient to compensate rapidly. Use a sterile technique. Many patients require sedation beyond butorphanol/midazolam (e.g., local anesthesia, low dose isoflurane for immobilization.)
- If concerned for pericardial effusion, be careful to tap chest either with ultrasound guidance or by evaluating likely area of heart on radiographs and tap caudal to that area.

MEDICATIONS

FUROSEMIDE
- Indicated only for patients with fluid accumulation (pleural effusion, pulmonary edema, and abdominal effusion)
- Dosage: 2–5 mg/kg SC, IM, IV, IO q4–6h (emergent care); 1–4 mg/kg SC, IM, PO for outpatient care.
- Titrate to lowest effective dose (often 1–2 mg/kg PO q12–24h).
- Best if compounded to flavored suspension but this author has used flavored injectable solution orally in some patients.
- Monitor for dehydration, azotemia, and hypokalemia
- Be aware, patients on this diuretic will usually have isosthenuric urine (~1.010).

NITROGLYCERIN OINTMENT (2%)
- A dab of this ointment on the hairless inner pinna can cause enough venous dilation to aid in reducing pulmonary edema and pleural effusion.
- Should be used in conjunction with a diuretic.
- Useful in emergent cases only.

PIMOBENDAN
- A potent positive inotropic agent with positive effects on preload and afterload
- Dose is extrapolated from the dog: (0.25 mg/kg PO q12h)
- This drug may need to be compounded into a suspension to accurately dose a guinea pig.
- Pimobendan has been used in cats with HCM to positive effect despite the lack of need for inotropic support.

ENALAPRIL
- An ACE inhibitor
- While this agent has been used in guinea pigs with CHF, RCM, and HCM its use has fallen out of favor for heart failure with many cardiologists due to lack of measurable effect in heart disease.
- Dosage: 0.3 mg/kg q12h PO
- This medication may need to be compounded into a suspension for accurate dosing for guinea pig patients.
- Enalapril and furosemide together are more likely to cause azotemia than furosemide alone.

ATENOLOL
- Used by many cardiologists in the presence of severe systolic anterior motion (HCM).
- Decreases papillary muscle contractility thereby reducing systolic anterior motion
- 0.2–2.0 mg/kg PO q24h

CARVEDIOL
- Carvediol is a third-generation beta blocker and alpha blocker with antioxidant effects
- Reported in 1 case to be effective along with furosemide and enalapril in a case of DCM
- Dosage: 0.2–0.4 mg/kg PO q24h

PLAVIX® (CLOPIDOGREL)
Has been used anecdotally in guinea pigs at a dosage extrapolated from cats for severe left atrial enlargement and evidence of thrombus in LA on echocardiogram.

FOLLOW-UP
- Once stabilized, periodic re-evaluation using radiographs and echocardiograms can help titrate drug dosages to a more precise effect.
- Frequency of re-evaluation depends on the patient's clinical signs.
- Closely observe the patient at home for dyspnea, lethargy, weakness, and anorexia
- Having the owner measure the resting (sleeping) respiratory rate at home can help the owner identify potential problems early. (Normal RR: 40–150 bpm; average of 80 bpm)

CARDIOMYOPATHY, DILATED (DCM), HYPERTROPHIC (HCM), AND RESTRICTIVE (RCM)   (CONTINUED)

- Periodic monitoring of renal function and serum or plasma potassium is recommended.
- Prognosis for HCM and RCM in guinea pigs is fair to guarded. However, with appropriate testing, treatment, and follow-up, some patients can be managed successfully long-term. Patients with CHF have a more guarded prognosis.

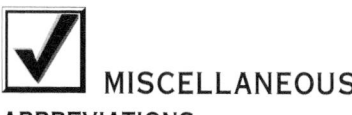

MISCELLANEOUS

ABBREVIATIONS
ACE = Angiotensin-converting enzyme
ALT = alanine aminotransferase
BPM = breaths per minute
CBC = complete blood cell count
CHF = congestive heart failure
DCM = dilated cardiomyopathy
EKG = electrocardiogram
HCM = hypertrophic cardiomyopathy
LV = left ventricle
RCM = restrictive cardiomyopathy
RR = respiratory rate

Suggested Reading
Bays TB. Geriatric care of rabbits, guinea pigs, and chinchillas. Vet Clin Exot Anim 2020;23:567–593.
Fitzgerald BC, Dias S, Martorell J. Cardiovascular drugs in avian, small mammal, and reptile medicine. Vet Clin Exot Anim 2018;21:399–442.
Franklin JM, Guzman DSM. Dilated cardiomyopathy and congestive heart failure in a guinea pig. Exot DVM 2006;7(6):9–12.
Pignon C, Mayer J. Guinea pigs. In: Quesenberry KE, Carpenter JW, eds. Ferrets, Rabbits and Rodents, 4th ed. Clinical Medicine and Surgery. 2021. St. Louis: Saunders, 2020:270–297.
Author Jeff Rhody, DVM, DABVP (ECM)

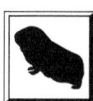

BASICS

DEFINITION
• Infection with abscessation of cervical lymph nodes; usually caused by *Streptococcus zooepidemicus*

PATHOPHYSIOLOGY
• Inflammation and enlargement of the cervical lymph nodes
• Cervical lymphadenitis is primarily caused by *Streptococcus zooepidemicus* and can develop into abscesses of the affected cervical lymph nodes. These abscesses/swollen lymph nodes are located in the ventral cervical region of the body.
• *Streptococcus zooepidemicus* is usually present in the conjunctiva and nasal cavity of guinea pigs.
• The lymphatic system may be exposed to the causative organisms from a compromised oral epithelium or the upper respiratory tract.
• The cervical lymph nodes will often become asymmetrically enlarged due to swelling and/or abscess formation.
• The pus within the fibrous capsule is usually thick, caseous, and does not easily drain.
• Multiple body systems may be affected if infection becomes systemic, including the middle ear, eyes, and lungs, resulting in conjunctivitis, labored breathing, cyanosis, hematuria, hemoglobinuria, abortions, stillbirths, arthritis, peritonitis, pericarditis, hepatitis, and/or peracute death.
• Primarily caused by *Streptococcus zooepidemicus* Lancefield's group C, but *Streptobacillus moniliformis* and *Yersinia pseudotuberculosis* have also been identified as causative agents.
• Transmission of causative organisms can occur through direct contact (e.g., skin lesions, oral mucosal compromise), aerosol, or genital contact.
• Systemic infections may develop into chronic suppurative abscesses affecting the cervical lymph nodes, lungs, liver, and reproductive tract.

SYSTEMS AFFECTED
• Cervical lymph nodes—swelling and abscessation
• Ocular—panophthalmitis, conjunctivitis
• Respiratory—pneumonia, sinusitis
• Reproductive—abortions, stillbirths
• Cardiac—pericarditis
• Liver—hepatitis
• Renal—hematuria
• Joints—arthritis
• Middle/inner ear—torticollis

GENETICS
N/A

INCIDENCE/PREVALENCE
The most common cause of asymmetrical submandibular swelling in guinea pigs

GEOGRAPHIC DISTRIBUTION
N/A

SIGNALMENT
• Affected animals are usually fed hard-stemmed hays, maintained on a wood chip substrate, and/or are diagnosed with hypovitaminosis C.
• A history of other animals within the enclosure being diagnosed with cervical lymphadenitis

SIGNS

Historical Findings
• Vitamin C deficiency
• Poor-quality hay being fed
• Wood chip substrate
• Group housing, with other animals having been diagnosed
• Previous diagnosis and treatment for cervical lymphadenitis
• Reproductive disorders in sows
• A fast-growing swelling that may or may not be painful. Difficult to identify in long-haired guinea pigs.

Physical Examination Findings
• Firm or fluctuant mass that may or may not be associated with an ulcerated/necrotizing area
• Asymmetrical ventral cervical masses
• Lameness
• Labored breathing
• Anorexia, lethargy
• Torticollis
• Pain and splinting may be elicited on abdominal palpation when visceral abscessation is present.

CAUSES
Pyogenic bacteria infection of the cervical lymph nodes:
• *Streptococcus zooepidemicus* Lancefield's group C, a gram-positive coccus, is considered the primary causative agent of cervical lymphadenitis. *Streptococcus moniliformis* is uncommonly involved.
• *Yersinia pseudotuberculosis*
• Mixed infection caused by aerobic and anaerobic bacteria is the rule in dental abscessation.

RISK FACTORS
• Abrasion of the oral mucosa
• Contact with infected animal
• Group housing
• Hard-stemmed hays/wood chip substrates
• Vitamin C deficiency
• Malocclusion/dental disease

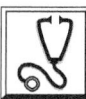

DIAGNOSIS

DIFFERENTIAL DIAGNOSIS
• Neoplasia, especially lymphoma
• Reactive lymph node
• Generalized bacterial infection other than *S. zooepidemicus*
• Hematoma/seroma

CBC/BIOCHEMISTRY/URINALYSIS
CBC—most often normal. Inflammatory leukogram is frequent in cases of bacteriemia

OTHER LABORATORY TESTS
• Cytology and staining of abscess material to identify causative organism.
• Culture and sensitivity of abscess material—most often, culture results are negative if swab is taken at the center of the abscess material. More accurate culture results may be achieved if the sample is collected at the abscess tissue interface.

IMAGING
• Rarely needed for the typical cervical lymphadenitis patient
• Radiography—useful to determine the extent of abscess formation
• Ultrasonography—useful for diagnosing deeper and intra-abdominal abscesses
• CT scan—allow better and more accurate assessment of middle/inner ear involvement of guinea pigs presenting with torticollis

DIAGNOSTIC PROCEDURES
• Aspiration—Cytology reveals degenerate neutrophils with intra- and extracellular bacteria. A small number of mononuclear inflammatory cells may also be observed. Gram's stain of an aspirate smear is recommended, especially for samples obtained from dental abscesses from which bacterial cultures may not be rewarding.
• Culture—Pus and abscess capsule can be submitted for culture. Submitting part of the fibrous capsule may yield better results than a sample collected in the center of the abscess. Anaerobic culture is encouraged for dental abscesses.
• Bacterial sensitivity is important to direct antibiotic selection.

PATHOLOGIC FINDINGS
• Exudate—degenerate neutrophils, intra and extracellular bacteria, macrophages, and necrotic tissues
• Capsule and surrounding tissue—fibrinous inflammation, edema, congestion, fibrous connective tissue, presence of neutrophils, macrophages, lymphocytes, and plasma cells

GUINEA PIGS

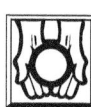

TREATMENT

APPROPRIATE HEALTH CARE
• Generously clip hair around affected area(s).
• Surgical removal of the abscess, including the capsule, is recommended for most presentations to reduce the incidence of reoccurrence. Must be aware of possible hematologic seeding of bacteria following surgical removal of abscess that may result in sepsis.
• Incising, draining, and copious flushing of the abscess site with hydrogen peroxide, povidone iodine, or chlorhexidine may be effective in a small percentage of cases without surgical intervention.
• Systemic antibiotic therapy
• Vitamin C supplementation
• Treat secondary disease conditions associated with infection.

NURSING CARE
• Flushing and treatment of treated abscess area(s) as needed.
• Sepsis—aggressive fluid therapy, intravenous antibiotics
• Bandaging as needed, although most treated areas are left open to heal by secondary intension

ACTIVITY
Restricted until recovery is complete

DIET
• If the patient is anorexic, assisted feeding is necessary (e.g., Critical Care for Herbivores, Oxbow Pet Products, Murdock, NE) or Emeraid Herbivore (Lafeber Company, Cornell, IL), 10–15 mL/kg q6–8h. If neither product is available, a slurry can be made with blended leafy green vegetables that are high in vitamin C, or guinea pig pellets blended with water and vegetable baby food.
• Diet should primarily include hay (e.g., timothy grass) and roughage with a limited amount of pellets. Fresh vegetables may also be offered in limited quantities. High-carbohydrate treats should be avoided.
• Guinea pigs need a dietary source of vitamin C. Higher levels should be provided to sick individuals (30–50 mg/kg daily). Vitamin C may be ground and fed directly to the pig. Vitamin C treats are also available for guinea pigs (e.g., Daily C, Oxbow Pet Products, Murdock, NE).

CLIENT EDUCATION
• Cervical lymphadenitis is mildly contagious to other guinea pigs. Prognosis may be guarded. Owners should be educated on the difficulty in resolving this condition during the initial treatment period. Reoccurrence of cervical abscesses is likely in the majority of these cases.
• Discuss diet, substrate, and group housing.
• Review vitamin C supplementation as key to overall health of guinea pig.

SURGICAL CONSIDERATIONS
• Surgical removal of abscessed lymph nodes with capsule is recommended as the treatment of choice in most uncomplicated cervical lymphadenitis cases.
• Surgical removal may predispose the patient to bacterial sepsis. Proper antibiotic treatment is recommended prior to surgery.
• Alternatively: lancing, curettage, cleaning, and flushing. Leave abscess open. Express pus and flush once to twice daily with hydrogen peroxide, povidone iodine, or chlorhexidine until granulation tissue forms and pus is no longer present.
• Place on 2–3 weeks of antibiotic treatment.

MEDICATIONS

DRUG(S) OF CHOICE
Antibiotics
• Antibiotics should be selected based on the bacterial culture and sensitivity. Pending the sensitivity results, selection is based on the common isolates reported in guinea pig abscesses and antibiotics that are safe to use in this species. Unfortunately, antibiotics with the best effect against frequent isolates, especially *Staphylococcus aureus* and *Streptococcus zooepidemicus*, can lead to antibiotic-associated dybiosis and enterotoxemia. Treatment should be pursued for at least 2 weeks.
• Broad-spectrum antibiotics safe to use in guinea pigs include enrofloxacin (5–20 mg/kg PO q12h), which is ineffective against anaerobes and may be variably effective against *Streptococcus* spp., Trimethoprim-sulfa (15–30 mg/kg PO q12h), and chloramphenicol (30–50 mg/kg PO, SC, IM, IV q8–12h). Azithromycin (15–30 mg/kg PO q24h) is safe to use in guinea pigs and can reach a high concentration in pus through transportation by heterophils.

Pain Management
• Butorphanol (0.4–2.0 mg/kg SC, IM q4–12h)—short acting
• Buprenorphine (0.05–0.2 mg/kg SC, IM q8–12h)—longer acting opioid
• Meloxicam (0.5–1.0 mg/kg PO, SC, IM q24h)—also for long-term pain management for dental abscesses and dental disease
• Local anesthetics/dental blocks of bupivacaine (1 mg/kg), lidocaine (1 mg/kg), use in combination or alone—before more advanced surgery

CONTRAINDICATIONS
• Oral administration of penicillins, macrolides, lincosamides, and cephalosporins
• Use of immunosuppressive drugs such as corticosteroids
• Extensive surgery on a debilitated animal

PRECAUTIONS
• Oral administration of antibiotics may cause antibiotic-associated enteritis, dysbiosis, and enterotoxemia.
• Opioids may have an effect on the gastrointestinal motility.
• Chloramphenicol—humans should wear gloves when handling this drug.

POSSIBLE INTERACTIONS
N/A

ALTERNATIVE DRUGS
N/A

FOLLOW-UP

PATIENT MONITORING
• Monitor daily for swelling, resolution of inflammation, and improvement in clinical signs.
• Recheck every 2 weeks for reoccurrence of cervical swelling for a month.
• Dental disease: recheck every 4–20 weeks for dental trimming.

PREVENTION/AVOIDANCE
• Providing high-fiber and good-quality food with supplemental vitamin C.
• Avoid wood chip substrates; commercial recycled paper substrates are recommended (e.g., Carefresh, Absorption Corp., Ferndale, WA)
• Treating and monitoring dental disease prevent oral abrasions.
• Prevent exposure to diseased animals.
• Isolation of sick individuals
• Providing a clean, stress-free environment

POSSIBLE COMPLICATIONS
• Sepsis
• Recurrence, chronic pain, extensive tissue destruction
• Systemic involvement, leading to otitis media, panopthalmitis, pneumonia, torticollis, hematuria, abortion, hepatitis, or pericarditis
• Peracute death

EXPECTED COURSE AND PROGNOSIS
• Depends on the extent and duration of the disease process and the immune status of the animal
• Noncomplicated cervical lymphadenitis—cervical swelling: fair to guarded prognosis
• Secondary disease conditions present: guarded to poor prognosis

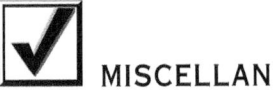

MISCELLANEOUS

ASSOCIATED CONDITIONS
- Immunosuppresion
- Dental disease
- Vitamin C deficiency
- Poor diet and husbandry
- Group housing of infected animals

AGE-RELATED FACTORS
N/A

ZOONOTIC POTENTIAL
- *Streptococcus moniliformis*
- *Yersinia pseudotuberculosis*

PREGNANCY/FERTILITY/BREEDING
Will cause abortions and stillbirths in pregnant sows

SYNONYMS
Lumps
Streptococcal lymphadnitis

SEE ALSO
Abscesses
Anorexia and pseudoanorexia
Cutaneous and subcutaneous masses
Hypovitaminosis C (scurvy)

ABBREVIATIONS
CT = computed tomography

INTERNET RESOURCES
N/A

Suggested Reading
Barrios-Arpi LM, Morales-Cauti SM. Cytomorphological characterization of lymphadenopathies in guinea pigs: study of 31 clinical cases. J Exot Pet Med 2020; 32:1–5.
Bays TB. Geriatric care of rabbits, guinea pigs, and chinchillas. Vet Clin Exot Anim 2020;23:567–593.
Johnson-Delaney C. Guinea pigs, chinchillas, degus and duprasi. In: Meredith A, Johnson-Delaney C, eds. BSAVA Manual of Exotic Pets, 5th ed. Quedgeley, Gloucester, UK: British Small Animal Veterinary Association, 2010:28–64.
Miwa Y, Sladky K. Common surgical procedures of rodents, ferrets, hedgehogs, and sugar gliders. Vet Clin Exot Anim 2016;19:205–244.
Pignon C, Mayer J. Guinea pigs. In: Quesenberry KE, Carpenter JW, eds. Ferrets, Rabbits and Rodents, 4th ed. Clinical Medicine and Surgery. 2021 ed. St. Louis: Saunders, 2020:270–297.

Author Thomas N. Tully, Jr., DVM, MS, Dipl. ABVP (Avian), Dipl. ECZM (Avian)

GUINEA PIGS

CHEILITIS

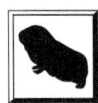

BASICS

DEFINITION
Inflammation of the mucocutaneus junction of the lips, commissures of the mouth, and nasal philtrum in guinea pigs

PATHOPHYSIOLOGY
The etiology is unknown; inflammation likely has multiple causes

SYSTEMS AFFECTED
• Respiratory
• Dermatologic

GENETICS
N/A

INCIDENCE/PREVALENCE
Most common cause of crusting around the mouth in guinea pigs

GEOGRAPHIC DISTRIBUTION
N/A

SIGNALMENT
• Affected animals are usually fed hard-stemmed hays, maintained on a wood chip substrate, and/or are diagnosed with hypovitaminosis C.
• A history of other animals within the enclosure being diagnosed

SIGNS
Historical Findings
• Nonhealing crusts, ulcers, and scabs around the lips; severity may wax and wane
• Poor husbandry
• Vitamin C deficiency
• Poor-quality hay being fed
• Group housing, with other animals having been diagnosed

Physical Examination Findings
• Crusts, ulcerations, erythema, and scab formation beginning at lip commissures and progressing around the mouth and nasal philtrum
• Lesions may progress into the mouth
• Weight loss, debility with chronic disease

CAUSES
• May begin with trauma to the lips by coarse foods or bedding
• Poor husbandry, dirty food, and water dishes may contribute.
• Nutritional deficiencies may play a role
• *Streptococcus* spp. and *Candida albicans* are common secondary infections
• May begin with trauma to the lips by coarse foods or bedding
• Poor husbandry, dirty food, and water dishes may contribute.

RISK FACTORS
• Abrasion of the oral mucosa
• Contact with infected animal
• Group housing
• Hard-stemmed hays/wood chip substrates
• Vitamin C deficiency

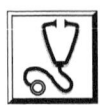

DIAGNOSIS

DIFFERENTIAL DIAGNOSIS
• Dermatophytosis
• Dental disease
• Trauma

CBC/BIOCHEMISTRY/URINALYSIS
CBC—most often normal. Inflammatory leukogram may be present

OTHER LABORATORY TESTS
N/A

IMAGING
N/A

DIAGNOSTIC PROCEDURES
• Cytology and staining of impression smears—large numbers of bacteria and inflammatory cells
• Culture and sensitivity to direct antibiotic selection.

PATHOLOGIC FINDINGS
• Biopsy and histopathology—hyperkeratosis of epidermis; infiltration with neutrophils, lymphocytes, and macrophages may be seen. Ulcers and erosions of dermis

TREATMENT

APPROPRIATE HEALTH CARE
• Outpatient

NURSING CARE
• Scrub lesions to remove crusts with dilute chlorhexidine or povidone iodine solution twice daily until lesions resolve
• Application of topical wound care solutions such as Vetericyn Plus (Innovacyn, Rialto, CA) may be helpful
• Application of ointments containing Vitamin A
• Clean and disinfect food dishes daily. Clean cages regularly

ACTIVITY
No restrictions

DIET
• If the patient is anorexic, assisted feeding is necessary (e.g., Critical Care for Herbivores, Oxbow Pet Products, Murdock, NE) or

Emeraid Herbivore (Lafeber Company, Cornell, IL), 10–15 mL/kg q6–8h. If neither product is available, a slurry can be made with blended leafy green vegetables that are high in vitamin C, or guinea pig pellets blended with water and vegetable baby food.
• Guinea pigs need a dietary source of vitamin C. Higher levels should be provided to sick individuals (30–50 mg/kg daily). Vitamin C may be ground and fed directly to the pig. Vitamin C treats are also available for guinea pigs (e.g., Daily C, Oxbow Pet Products, Murdock, NE).

CLIENT EDUCATION
• Daily cleaning and topical treatment of the wounds are necessary or will recur
• Discuss diet, substrate, and group housing.
• Review vitamin C supplementation as key to overall health of guinea pig.

SURGICAL CONSIDERATIONS
N/A

MEDICATIONS

DRUG(S) OF CHOICE
Antibiotics
• Systemic antibiotics are usually only needed in severe or chronic cases. Choose broad-spectrum antibiotics safe to use in guinea pigs: enrofloxacin (5–20 mg/kg PO q12h), trimethoprim-sulfa (15–30 mg/kg PO q12h), and chloramphenicol (30–50 mg/kg PO, SC, IM, IV q8–12h).

Pain Management
• Meloxicam (0.5–1.0 mg/kg PO, SC, IM q24h)—also for long-term pain management for dental abscesses and dental disease

CONTRAINDICATIONS
• Oral administration of penicillins, macrolides, lincosamides, and cephalosporins
• Use of immunosuppressive drugs such as corticosteroids
• Topical application of triple antibiotic ointments—may have adverse effect on GI flora if consumed

PRECAUTIONS
• Oral administration of antibiotics may cause antibiotic-associated enteritis, dysbiosis, and enterotoxemia.
• Chloramphenicol—humans should wear gloves when handling this drug.

POSSIBLE INTERACTIONS
N/A

ALTERNATIVE DRUGS
N/A

GUINEA PIGS

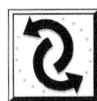 FOLLOW-UP

PATIENT MONITORING
• Monitor daily resolution of inflammation and improvement in clinical signs.
• Recheck every 2 weeks for reoccurrence

PREVENTION/AVOIDANCE
• Providing high-fiber and good-quality food with supplemental vitamin C.
• Avoid wood chip substrates; commercial recycled paper substrates are recommended (e.g., Carefresh, Absorption Corp., Ferndale, WA)
• Treating and monitoring dental disease prevent oral abrasions.
• Prevent exposure to diseased animals.
• Isolation of sick individuals
• Providing a clean, stress-free environment

POSSIBLE COMPLICATIONS
• Sepsis
• Recurrence, chronic pain, extensive tissue destruction
• Weight loss, debility

EXPECTED COURSE AND PROGNOSIS
• Depends on the extent and duration of the disease process and the immune status of the animal
• Generally requires 2–4 weeks of treatment to resolve
• Recurrence is common

 MISCELLANEOUS

ASSOCIATED CONDITIONS
• Immunosuppression
• Dental disease
• Vitamin C deficiency
• Poor diet and husbandry
• Group housing of infected animals

AGE-RELATED FACTORS
N/A

ZOONOTIC POTENTIAL
N/A

PREGNANCY/FERTILITY/BREEDING
N/A

SYNONYMS
N/A

SEE ALSO
Abscesses
Anorexia and pseudoanorexia
Dermatophytosis
Hypovitaminosis C (scurvy)

ABBREVIATIONS
N/A

INTERNET RESOURCES
N/A

Suggested Reading
Bays TB. Geriatric care of rabbits, guinea pigs, and chinchillas. Vet Clin Exot Anim 2020;23:567–593.

Johnson-Delaney C. Guinea pigs, chinchillas, degus and duprasi. In: Meredith A, Johnson-Delaney C, eds. BSAVA Manual of Exotic Pets, 5th ed. Quedgeley, Gloucester, UK: British Small Animal Veterinary Association, 2010:28–64.
Lennox AM, Capello V, Legendre LF. Small mammal denistry. In: Quesenberry KE, Carpenter JW, eds. Ferrets, Rabbits and Rodents, 4th ed. Clinical Medicine and Surgery. 2021 ed. St. Louis: Saunders, 2020:514–535.
Minarikova A, Hauptman K, Jeklova E et al. Diseases in pet guinea pigs: a retrospective study in 1000 animals. Vet Rec 2015;177(8):200–200.
Palmerio BS, Roberts H. Clinical approach to dermatologic disease in exotic animals. Vet Clin North Am Exot Anim Pract 2013;16(3):523–577.
Pignon C, Mayer J. Guinea pigs. In: Quesenberry KE, Carpenter JW, eds. Ferrets, Rabbits and Rodents, 4th ed. Clinical Medicine and Surgery. 2021 ed. St. Louis: Saunders, 2020:270–297.
Smith M. Staphylococcal cheilitis in the guinea pig. J Small Anim Pract 1977;18: 47–50.

Author Barbara Oglesbee, DVM, Dipl. ABVP (Avian)

GUINEA PIGS

CHLAMYDIOSIS

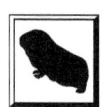

BASICS

DEFINITION
Chlamydiosis of guinea pigs (AKA Guinea pig inclusion conjunctivitis-GIPC) is caused by *Chlamydophila caviae* (formerly *Chlamydia caviae, Chlamydia psittaci*) a gram-negative intracellular bacterium. The infection is generally self-limiting and results in recovery with no residual damage.

PATHOPHYSIOLOGY
• *Chlamydophila* organisms multiply in the cytoplasm of the conjunctival epithelial cells.
• The life cycle of this organism is unique and involves two forms, the elementary body and reticulate body. The elementary bodies are metabolically inert and relatively stable in the environment. They are taken up by the host cells via endocytosis and remain in the cytoplasm in inclusion bodies. The elementary bodies then transform into reticulate bodies, which are metabolically active and divide several times within the inclusion body.
• The progeny of the reticulate body differentiate into elementary bodies and are released from the cell en mass during cell lysis or singly during the fusion of the elementary body with the cell membrane.
• Clinical signs can be observed in animals as young as 1 week of age.
• Early in the course of the infection, there is a lymphocytic infiltration but few intracytoplasmic inclusion bodies. Later in the course of the disease, there are many inclusion bodies and a heterophilic response.
• The disease is usually completely resolved 28 days after the onset of clinical signs based on cytologic examination.
• The disease may recur on a cyclical basis

SYSTEMS AFFECTED
• Ocular
• Upper respiratory tract
• Lower respiratory tract
• Genital tract—abortions

GENETICS
Unknown

INCIDENCE/PREVALENCE
Uncommonly encountered in clinical practice

GEOGRAPHIC DISRIBUTION
Widespread

SIGNALMENT
Most common in younger guinea pigs (4–8 weeks old) but may also be seen in adults

SIGNS

Historical Findings
Introduction of a new guinea pig, abortion, ocular discharge, reddened eyelids

Physical Examination Findings
Infections may be subclinical. When present, expected clinical signs include mild erythema of the eyelid margins, conjunctivitis (conjunctival hyperemia), serous to purulent exudative ocular discharge (usually bilateral), rhinitis, genital tract infection, lower respiratory tract infections, staining/secretions on the hair around the nose, eyes, or front limbs

CAUSES
Chlamydophila caviae is the primary cause. The infection can be exacerbated by *Bordetella*, streptococcal, or other secondary bacterial infections.

RISK FACTORS
• Exposure to infected animals, neonatal to subclinically infected adults
• Age (young animals 4–8 weeks of age most commonly affected)
• Poor diet: feeding diets deficient in vitamin C can lead to immunosuppression; mildly scorbutic animals may be predisposed to multiple causes of conjunctivitis
• Immunosuppression: caused by lack of vitamin C in the diet, stress, concurrent disease, and corticosteroid use

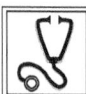

DIAGNOSIS

DIFFERENTIAL DIAGNOSIS
• Infectious cases of bacterial conjunctivitis (*Bordetella bronchiseptica, Streptococcus* spp., *Salmonella* spp., *Staphylococcus aureus*, coliforms, and *Pasteurella multocida*)
• Inflammation, allergy, or irritant (foreign body) of the eye
• Dental disease causing a fistula or infection near the eye
• Neoplasia of the eye/conjunctiva (uncommon)

CBC/BIOCHEMISTRY/URINALYSIS
An elevation in total white blood cell count is uncommon, but a shift in the proportion of heterophils to lymphocytes with an increase in heterophils and a decrease in lymphocytes is often seen. Increases in platelet numbers can also be seen with inflammation.

OTHER LABORATORY TESTS
• Antigen detection in conjunctival scrapes using immunofluorescence for specific monoclonal antibodies

• Antibody detection in serum using microimmunofluorescence
• *Chlamydophila* PCR (conjunctival swab) will test for *Chlamydophila* species but is not specific for the guinea pig strain

IMAGING
N/A

DIAGNOSTIC PROCEDURES
• Conjunctival scrape: intracytoplasmic inclusion bodies in Giemsa- or Macchiavello-stained conjunctival epithelial cells (historical)
• Cytology of exudates: swab of nasal or ocular discharge, nasal swab, recommended standard cell stain (Diff Quick), and gram stain of exudates to evaluate for both chlamydiosis and other secondary bacterial infections
• Culture of exudates: difficult to grow *Chlamydophila* organisms but may have other pathogenic bacteria present; can be difficult to obtain a good sample
• *Chalmydophilia* PCR of exudate or swab from the affected area (conjunctival or genital)

PATHOLOGIC FINDINGS
Intracytoplasmic inclusion bodies, exudate, and mixed inflammatory cell infiltration are often visible on histopathologic examination of the conjunctiva. However, bacteria of the *Chlamydiales* order are small and their inclusions are difficult to detect by standard microscopy. In many cases, macroscopic and/or histologic changes, which are pathognomic or indicative for a chlamydial infection, may not be present.

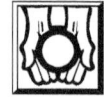

TREATMENT

APPROPRIATE HEALTH CARE
Outpatient treatment is usually acceptable.

NURSING CARE
• Clean the hair around the eyes to remove any discharge.
• No extensive care is usually necessary, as this disease is self-limiting.

ACTIVITY
No change in activity level is necessary; allow affected animals to set their own pace.

DIET
• Continue to feed an appropriate diet consisting mostly of timothy hay and supplemented with vegetables.
• Guinea pigs require an exogenous source of vitamin C supplementation which can be given at 50–100 mg/kg/day when ill.

• Encourage oral fluid intake to maintain hydration by offering water or wet vegetables.

CLIENT EDUCATION
This disease is generally self-limiting but can be exacerbated by other bacterial causes of conjunctivitis. Animals with *Chlamydophila* conjunctivitis usually recover with no residual damage.

SURGICAL CONSIDERATIONS
N/A

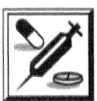

MEDICATIONS

DRUG(S) OF CHOICE
• Drug therapy is generally not required as the disease is typically self-limiting.
• If treatment is necessary, antimicrobial drugs can be implemented. Doxycycline (2.5–5 mg/kg PO q12h) for 10–14 days is the treatment of choice but has the potential to cause GI upset.
• Sulfonamide antibiotics, trimethoprim sulfa (15–30 mg/kg PO q12–24h), and ophthalmic antibiotic drops (ciprofloxacin eye drops—one drop in the affected eye twice daily) have also been effective.

CONTRAINDICATIONS
• Antibiotics that select against gram-positive bacteria such as oral penicillins, cephalosporins, lincosamines, or macrolides should not be used in these animals as it can cause fatal dysbiosis and enterotoxemia. Some topical use may be acceptable short term. Procaine, which is included in some penicillin preparations, can be toxic to guinea pigs.
• Using corticosteroids can suppress the immune system and exacerbate bacterial infections.

PRECAUTIONS
Any antibiotic can cause diarrhea, which should be monitored in these patients, and the antibiotic is discontinued if diarrhea is present. Supplementation with probiotics or guinea pig transfaunation can be considered.

POSSIBLE INTERACTIONS
None

ALTERNATIVE DRUGS
N/A

FOLLOW-UP

PATIENT MONITORING
Continue to monitor patient for a relapse via clinical signs. Guinea pigs develop short-lived immunity so may be susceptible to reinfection of the eyes or genital tract after a short time.

PREVENTION/AVOIDANCE
• Eliminate exposure to clinically affected guinea pigs.
• Improve husbandry and diet (ensure appropriate vitamin C supplementation).
• Avoid stressful situations and corticosteroid use.

POSSIBLE COMPLICATIONS
N/A

EXPECTED COURSE AND PROGNOSIS
This disease is typically self-limiting within 28 days of the appearance of clinical signs. The prognosis for recovery is good in uncomplicated cases.

MISCELLANEOUS

ASSOCIATED CONDITIONS
• Abortion
• Rhinitis and sinusitis
• Pneumonia

AGE-RELATED FACTORS
More commonly seen in younger animals

ZOONOTIC POTENTIAL
Chlamydia caviae has been documented as a cause of community-acquired pneumonia in otherwise apparently healthy and immunocompetent adults after exposure to ill guinea pigs. Although all 3 cases lived, 2 cases required ICU admission and mechanical ventilation prior to recovery. Staff handling potentially infected guinea pigs should wear appropriate personal protective equipment (PPE), such as long-sleeved lab coat and gloves to avoid exposure.

PREGNANCY/FERTILITY/BREEDING
Abortions have been reported with *Chlamydophila caviae* infection, and young born to subclinically infected adults may acquire the disease during parturition.

SYNONYMS
Guinea pig inclusion conjunctivitis (GIPC)
Chlamydia caviae
Chlamydia psittaci

SEE ALSO
Pneumonia
Rhinitis and sinusitis

ABBREVIATIONS
GI = gastrointestinal
PCR = polymerase chain reaction

INTERNET RESOURCES
"Zoonotic Chlamydiae from Mammals" fact sheet can be found at: http://www.cfsph. iastate.edu/Factsheets/pdfs/chlamydiosis.pdf
http://www.merckvetmanual.com www.vin. com

Suggested Reading
Borel N, Polkinghorne A, Pospischil A. A review on chlamydial diseases in animals: still a challenge for pathologists? Vet Pathol 2018;55(3):374–390.
Mayer J, Mans C. Rodents. In: Carpenter JW, ed. Exotic Animal Formulary, 5th ed. St Louis: Elsevier, 2018:459–479.
Pignon C, Mayer J. Guinea pigs. In: Quesenberry KE, Carpenter JW, eds. Ferrets, Rabbits and Rodents, 4th ed. Clinical Medicine and Surgery. 2021 ed. St. Louis: Saunders, 2020:270–297.
Ramakers BP, Heijne M, Lie N et al. Zoonotic *chlamydia caviae* presenting as community-acquired pneumonia. N Engl J Med 2017;377(10):992–994.
Shomer NH, Holcombe H, Harkness JE. Biology and diseases of guinea pigs. In: Anderson LC, Otto G, Pritchett-Coming KR, Whary MT, Fox JG, eds. Laboratory Animal Medicine, 3rd ed. London: Elsevier Academic Press, 2015:247–283.

Authors Christy L. Rettenmund, DVM, Dipl. ACZM and J. Jill Heatley, DVM, MS, Dipl. ABVP (Avian, Reptilian, Amphibian), Dipl. ACZM

CONJUNCTIVITIS

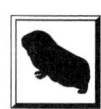

BASICS

DEFINITION
Inflammation of the conjunctiva, the vascularized mucosal membrane lining the eyelids and the rudimentary nictitating membrane (palpebral conjunctiva), and is continuous with the bulbar conjunctiva which overlies the anterior portion of the globe (bulbar conjunctiva).

PATHOPHYSIOLOGY
• Primary—infectious, environmental irritation
• Secondary to an underlying ocular or systemic disease

SYSTEMS AFFECTED
• Ophthalmic—may include cornea (keratoconjunctivitis), eyelids/periocular skin (e.g., blepharoconjunctivitis), and nasolacrimal system (dacryocystitis)
• Respiratory—upper respiratory infections and apical tooth root invasion of sinuses
• Oral cavity—related dental disease with extension to nasolacrimal system, and orbital and nasal cavities

GENETICS
N/A

INCIDENCE/PREVALENCE
Common

GEOGRAPHIC DISTRIBUTION
N/A

SIGNALMENT
Breed Predilections
Hairless guinea pigs—listeria conjunctival infection reported

Mean Age and Range
N/A

Predominant Sex
N/A

SIGNS
Historical Findings
• History of nasal discharges or sneezing
• History of previous treatment for dental disease

Physical Examination Findings
• Conjunctival hyperemia
• Chemosis
• Ocular discharge—may be serous (epiphora), mucoid or mucopurulent, "flaky" (vitamin C deficiency)
• Conjunctival follicle formation
• Blepharospasm—normal blink frequency is low (2–5 blinks/20 minutes at rest; 1–17 blinks/10 minutes of restrained time), and corneal sensation is relatively low in the normal guinea pig eye.

• Periocular alopecia or matted fur, crusting of discharges on cheeks and/or nasal rostrum
• Upper respiratory infection—sneezing, nasal discharge
• Oral cavity signs—malocclusion, elongated incisors, or cheek teeth
• Signs of pain—depression, lethargy, hiding, and hunched posture
• Symptoms of vitamin C deficiency—rough hair coat, anorexia, diarrhea, delayed wound healing, lameness, and malocclusion

CAUSES
Bacterial
• *Chlamydophila caviae*—most commonly reported; often self-limiting
• *Bordetella bronchiseptica*—in association with upper and occasionally lower respiratory disease (i.e., pneumonia)
• *Streptococcus* spp.—in association with upper respiratory disease
• *Salmonella* spp.; *Yersinia enterocolitica*; *Listeria monocytogenes*—transmission is usually from fecal contamination of feed and may also be associated with diarrhea—weanlings most susceptible
• *Pasturella* spp.

Nutritional
• Scurvy—the guinea pig cannot form its own vitamin C, due to lack of hepatic microsomal enzyme L-gulonolactone oxidase, and is susceptible to deficiency—conjunctivitis is an early sign related to defects in collagen synthesis with associated vascular fragility with petechiation of mucous membranes

Secondary to Trauma or Environmental Causes
• Conjunctival foreign body—hay, bedding—especially if unilateral
• Exposure to environmental irritants (airborne or contact)—may be related to poor hygiene of local environment (soiled bedding)
• Irritation from barbering—the dominant guinea pig chews the facial hair and whiskers of cage mates

Secondary to Adnexal Disease
• KCS—conjunctival inflammation secondary to dryness associated with reduced function of orbital lacrimal glands; discharge usually mucoid
• Entropion or aberrant hairs (trichiasis) causing mechanical irritation to cornea, conjunctiva, or both
• Nasolacrimal duct obstruction and dacryocystitis—inflammation of the canaliculi, lacrimal sac, or nasolacrimal ducts; may be associated with dental disease due to incisor or cheek tooth elongation
• Orbital disease—orbital abnormality is usually more prominent (e.g., exophthalmos)

Secondary to Other Ocular Diseases
• Irritation from corneal or conjunctival dermoid—congenital
• Ulcerative keratitis
• Anterior uveitis—lens-induced uveitis may accompany cataracts, which are common; bilateral uveitis unrelated to cataract may be indicative of systemic disease
• Glaucoma—primary (rare) or related to other intraocular disease; may be associated with osseous metaplasia of ciliary body

Ectoparasites
Frequently associated with periocular dermatitis and alopecia, dermal lichenification—conjunctivitis is due to either direct irritation or secondary to pruritus-induced periocular self-trauma
• Dermatophytosis (*Trichophyton* spp.)
• *Chirodiscoides caviae*—"fur mite"
• *Trixacarus caviae, Sarcoptes scabei*—sarcoptes mite
• Pediculosis (*Gyropus ovalis, Gliricola porcelli*)

Neoplastic/Other
• Tumors involving conjunctiva (e.g., lymphosarcoma)—rare
• Mass-like lesions—"pea eye"—displacement of orbital lacrimal gland or salivary glands into the inferior subconjunctival space

RISK FACTORS
• Recent introduction of companion guinea pig—may carry infectious agent
• Poor diet—vitamin C deficiency; lack of sufficient hay contributes to cheek teeth overgrowth
• Dental disease—malocclusion of incisors or cheek teeth resulting in overgrowth and extension of disease from oral cavity to orbit or nasolacrimal system
• Stress—especially in young guinea pigs
• Environmental stressors—crowding with associated aggression (ocular trauma from fighting, barbering from cage mates); unhygienic housing (ammonia irritation from unclean bedding)

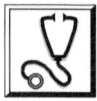

DIAGNOSIS

DIFFERENTIAL DIAGNOSIS
Must differentiate primary cause from secondary with full assessment of eye—more than one cause can occur simultaneously
• Superficial vessels (conjunctival)—originate near fornix; move with the conjunctiva; branch repeatedly; blanch quickly with topical sympathomimetic (e.g., 1:100000 epinephrine); suggests ocular surface disease (e.g., conjunctivitis, superficial keratitis, and blepharitis)

• Deep vessels (episcleral)—originate near limbus; branch infrequently; do not move with the conjunctiva; blanch slowly or incompletely with topical sympathomimetic; suggests episcleritis or intraocular disease (e.g., anterior uveitis, glaucoma)
• Discharge—mucopurulent or purulent: typical of ocular surface disorders, dacryocystitis, or blepharitis; serous or none: typical of nasolacrimal obstruction or intraocular disease
• Unilateral condition with ocular pain (blepharospasm)—typical of trauma, foreign body or aberrant hairs (e.g., dermoid), anterior uveitis, and ipsilateral dental disease
• Bilateral chronic condition—congenital problem, chronic upper respiratory tract infection, and bilateral tooth root disorders
• Low tear production—keratoconjunctivitis sicca (KCS) defined as lower than the normal STT value (<1 mm/min compared with 3.8 ± 1.3 mm/min) in conjunction with keratoconjunctivitis
• Corneal opacification, neovascularization, or fluorescein retention—keratitis
• Pupil—compare to unaffected contralateral eye—miotic pupil may accompany uveitis or corneal ulceration; dilated pupil more common in glaucoma; normal pupil size with blepharitis and conjunctivitis; dyscoria (abnormal shape of pupil) or discoloration of iris: anterior uveitis or iris neoplasia
• Aqueous flare or hyphema—anterior uveitis
• Luxated or cataractous lens—anterior uveitis or glaucoma
• IOP—high: diagnostic for glaucoma; low: suggests uveitis
• Vision loss—severe keratitis or uveitis, cataract, hyphema, or glaucoma; guinea pigs have low blink frequency and inconsistent menace response, making assessment of vision difficult
• Differentiate from conjunctival masses (e.g., "pea eye"—a subconjunctival nodule of orbital gland material that protrudes from the inferior conjunctival sac—can be unilateral or bilateral) and infiltrative disease

CBC/BIOCHEMISTRY/URINALYSIS
N/A if primary

OTHER LABORATORY TESTS
• Bacterial C&S—swab conjunctival sac with microtip culturette, taking care to avoid touching periocular fur
• Conjunctival cytology—intracytoplasmic inclusion bodies within epithelial cells with *Chlamydophila caviae*; PCR assay—for *Chlamydophila caviae*

IMAGING
• Skull radiographs—to identify dental, nasal sinus, or maxillary bone lesions
• CT—superior to radiographs to localize obstruction and characterize associated

lesions; may define extent and nature of intraocular disease
• Ocular ultrasonography—if the ocular media are opaque
• Dacryocystorhinography—radiopaque contrast material to help localize nasolacrimal duct obstruction

DIAGNOSTIC PROCEDURES
• Complete ophthalmic examination—examine intraocular structures for signs of uveitis (miosis, aqueous flare) and adnexa for foreign body, or eyelid abnormalitites (aberrant cilia, entropion); ideally use magnification
• Tear production—rule out keratoconjunctivitis sicca—phenol red thread (PRT) test may be more informative than Schirmer tear test due to low values obtained with STT in normal patients (3.8 ± 1.3 mm/ min); mean values for PRT reported: 16 and 21.26 mm/15 s
• Aerobic bacterial C&S—acquire sample ideally before any solutions are used (topical anesthetic, fluorescein stain, flush) to prevent inhibition and dilution of bacterial growth. *Staphylococcus epidermidis*, a-hemolytic *Streptococcus*, and *Corynebacterium* are common aerobic commensal isolates from normal healthy guinea pigs.
• Conjunctival cytology—may see degenerate neutrophils and intracellular bacteria with bacterial infection; may see *Chlamydia* inclusions in epithelial cells
• Fluorescein stain—rule out corneal ulceration
• Intraocular pressure—rule out glaucoma; mean of 18 mmHg reported for applanation tonometry
• Nasolacrimal flush—rule out obstruction or dacryocystitis; may dislodge foreign material; a 23-gauge lacrimal cannula or a 24-gauge Teflon intravenous catheter can be used after application of topical anesthetic; may require sedation
• Conjunctival biopsy may be appropriate in chronic, unresponsive cases; confirm dermoid histologically (rarely necessary)

PATHOLOGIC FINDINGS
• Cause of chronic conjunctivitis—inflammatory cell population may suggest cause—neutrophils (bacterial); eosinophils (allergic, parasitic); granulomatous inflammation
• Characteristic features of malignancy (anisocytosis, anisokaryosis, increase in mitotic figures)
• Normal glandular elements—lacrimal or salivary—suggests "pea eye"

 TREATMENT

APPROPRIATE HEALTH CARE
• Primary conjunctivitis—outpatient

• Remove cause of ocular irritation—extract corneal or conjunctival foreign body; keratectomy or conjunctivectomy for removal of dermoid; surgical correction of entropion; treatment of other primary ocular disease (e.g., ulcerative conjunctivitis, uveitis)
• Secondary to systemic disease—hospitalize only if critical—guinea pigs do not tolerate hospitalization well
• Appropriate dental treatment in cases of related dental disease—trimming of cheek teeth (coronal reduction) may correct or control progression of root elongation. If tooth extraction is required or tooth root abscess is diagnosed it may require referral to a veterinarian with special expertise, if feasible. In patients with extensive tooth root abscesses, aggressive debridement is indicated. Maxillary and retrobulbar abscesses can be particularly challenging.
• Therapeutic nasolacrimal flushing in dacryocystitis—may be required weekly until resolved
• General husbandry should be assessed in all ill guinea pigs—avoid crowding and provide security zones for individual pigs; ensure housing hygiene; adequate diet

NURSING CARE
• Supportive—rinse any mucoid or mucopurulent debris from eye as produced—and always before treating with topical drugs to improve absorption; minimize crusty or moist build-up on periocular fur to reduce risk of secondary dermatitis
• May require change in housing if stressful or if suspect environmental irritant
• Provide hiding box of towel for burrowing for security if hospitalized

ACTIVITY
• Primary—typically no restriction; segregate if infectious cause suspected/confirmed
• Secondary—reduce exposure to at-risk environment or contact with potential irritant

DIET
• Be certain the patient continues to eat to prevent gastrointestinal motility disorders.
• If vitamin C deficient ensure adequate supplementation
• Provide fresh or dried grasses, hay to encourage normal tooth wear

CLIENT EDUCATION
• Clean discharge from conjunctival surfaces/ cul-de-sacs before treatment
• If multiple topical medications required, use drops followed by ointments or lubricants and allow 5 minutes between different preparations
• If related to dental disease, long-term management may be required to reduce chronic recurrent disease

CONJUNCTIVITIS

GUINEA PIGS

SURGICAL CONSIDERATIONS
If mass or localized lesion, excisional biopsy recommended

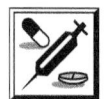

MEDICATIONS

DRUG(S) OF CHOICE
Topical antibiotics preferred over systemic if adequate to avoid GI upset or enterotoxemia

Primary Bacterial
• Ideally based on culture and sensitivity results
• Initial treatment—based on cytology and Gram's stain, or empirical with broad spectrum agent such as topical oxytetracycline or fluoroquinolone pending C&S results
• *Chlamydophila caviae*—tetracycline ointment topically q6h until signs resolve—mild infections are self-limiting and may not require treatment—avoid tetracycline systemically; enrofloxacin (5–20 mg/kg PO, SC, IM q12–24h); topical fluoroquinolone—ciprofloxacin, ofloxacin q6h
• *Bordetella bronchispetica*—chloramphenicol (30–50 mg/kg PO, SC, IM, IV q8–12h)
• *Streptococcus* spp.—enrofloxacin (5–20 mg/kg PO, SC, IM q12–24h); trimethoprim/sulfa (15–30 mg/kg PO q12h)

Vitamin C in Deficient Patients
• 20–50 mg/kg PO for maintenance
• 50–100 mg/animal PO, SQ daily in deficient patient

Anti-inflammatory Therapy
• Topical NSAID (e.g., flurbiprofen 0.03% BID-QID or ketorolac 0.5% BID-QID or 1% diclofenac BID-QID) to reduce inflammation if marked
• Systemic NSAID (e.g., meloxicam 0.5–1.0 mg/kg PO, SC, IM q12–24h)

Analgesics
• Topical nalbuphine 1.2% if corneal ulceration q8h

CONTRAINDICATIONS
• Avoid steroid containing ophthalmic preparations in cases of ulcerative keratitis; steroids may contribute to gastrointestinal stasis and exacerbate infectious disease.
• Guinea pigs have a marked, often lethal disruption of GI tract flora with antibiotic therapy (dysbiosis)—the anaerobic flora is sensitive to antibiotics with a gram-positive spectrum, particularly those with biliary excretion; disturbances of the flora caused by antibiotics may cause an over-colonization of clostridia, particulary *Clostridium difficile*—with resultant toxin elaboration
• Penicillins, ampicillin, bacitracin, erythromycin, spiramycin, lincomycin, gentamycin, clindamycin, and vancomycin at therapeutic doses carry the risk of inducing the syndrome and are contraindicated.

PRECAUTIONS
• Great care is required when considering the use of antibiotics in guinea pigs, including topical preparations.
• Low-risk antibiotics include chloramphernicol, aminoglycosides, sulphonamides, and the quinolones.
• Chloramphenicol—avoid human contact due to potential blood dyscrasia. Advise owners of potential risk.

POSSIBLE INTERACTIONS
N/A

ALTERNATIVE DRUGS
N/A

FOLLOW-UP

PATIENT MONITORING
Reevaluate short-term after initiating therapy (i.e., 5–7 days); treat until condition resolved then recheck again 5–7 days after therapy is discontinued—stain cornea with fluorescein at each recheck

PREVENTION/AVOIDANCE
• Therapy for underlying conditions
• Appropriate diet—purchase processed diets to feed before vitamin C degrades
• Correct husbandry/clean environment
• Treat new arrivals for mites and thoroughly clean environment to prevent reinfestation.

POSSIBLE COMPLICATIONS
• Keratitis—from reduced aqueous tear production, entropion, trichiasis, dermoid, or foreign body mechanical irritation
• Stenosis of nasolacrimal punctae—from chronic conjunctival inflammation
• Periocular dermatitis from persistent ocular discharges

EXPECTED COURSE AND PROGNOSIS
• Primary/Infectious—usually resolves with appropriate antibiotics or other specific treatment
• Secondary—depends on course of predisposing condition

✓ MISCELLANEOUS

ASSOCIATED CONDITIONS
Vitamin C deficiency

AGE-RELATED FACTORS
N/A

ZOONOTIC POTENTIAL
• *Bordetella*
• *Salmonella* spp.
• Dermatophytes
• *Trixacarus caviae*—sarcoptes mite

PREGNANCY/FERTILITY/BREEDING
• Use of systemic antibiotics should be used with caution in pregnant sow.
• Carriers of chronic infection (*Chlamydia*, *Bordetella*) may not be suitable for breeding.
• Do not breed patients with malocclusion.
• Avoid grisiofulvin (for dermatophytosis) in pregnant sows—teratogenic

SYNONYMS
Pink eye

SEE ALSO
Antibiotic-associated enterotoxemia
Epiphora
Exophthalmos and orbital diseases
Hypovitaminosis C (scurvy)
Pea eye

ABBREVIATIONS
C&S = culture and sensitivity results
CT = computed tomography
GI = gastrointestinal
IOP = intraocular pressure
KCS = keratoconjunctivitis sicca
NSAID = nonsteroidal anti-inflammatory drug
PCR = polymerase chain reaction
PRT = phenol red thread test
STT = Schirmer tear test

Suggested Reading
Carpenter JW. Exotic Animal Formulary, 3rd ed. St Louis: Elsevier Saunders, 2005.
Coster ME, Stiles J, Krohne SG et al. Results of diagnostic ophthalmic testing in healthy guinea pigs. JAVMA 2008;232(12):1825–1833.
Flecknell P. Guinea pigs. In: Meredith A, Redrobe S, eds. BSAVA Manual of Exotic Pets, 4th ed. Quedgeley, Gloucester: British Small Animal Veterinary Association, 2002:52–64.
Monk C. Ocular surface disease in rodents (guinea pigs, mice, rats, chinchillas). Vet Clin Exot Anim 2019;22:15–26.
Van der Woerdt A. Ophthalmologic diseases of small mammals. In: Quesenberry KE, Carpenter JW, eds. Ferrets, Rabbits and Rodents, 4th ed. Clinical Medicine and Surgery. 2021 ed. St. Louis: Saunders, 2020:583–594.
Williams D. Ocular disease in the guinea pig (*Cavia porcellus*): a survey of 1000 animals. Vet Ophthalmol 2010;13(Supplement 1):54–62.

Authors Georgina Newbold, DVM, Dipl. ACVO and A. Michelle Willis, DVM, Dipl. ACVO

CONSTIPATION (LACK OF FECAL PRODUCTION)

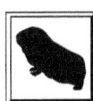

BASICS

DEFINITION
• Constipation: infrequent, incomplete, or difficult defecation
• Obstipation, where the colon is full of hard, dry feces that prevent passage of feces and gas; generally does not occur in guinea pigs
• Decreased stool production (reduced size or number of fecal pellets) or lack of stool production is a common occurrence in guinea pigs with a lack of food intake and/or gastrointestinal hypomotility.

PATHOPHYSIOLOGY
• Two distinctly different physiologic scenarios exist and are common in guinea pigs: decreased stool production and decreased ability to eliminate stool.
• Decreased ability to eliminate stool is most commonly seen as an anorectal or colorectal impaction with soft feces. Cause of this impaction, which is seen in older animals, is not known. Colorectal impactions with trichobezoars, wood shavings, or inspissated feces can lead to fatal cecal outflow obstruction or cecal bloat. Effects of cecal outflow obstruction include pain, anorexia, and potentially, fatal enterotoxemia.
• Decreased stool production is generally associated with gastrointestinal hypomotility/ stasis. Normal intestinal motility is dependent on continued ingestion of insoluble fiber. Lack of appropriate fiber intake (due to either deficient diet or lack of food intake) reduces motility. Decreased motility decreases fecal output.
• Effects of decreased fecal output can interfere with normal feces ingestion (cecotrophy) and cause vitamin B and vitamin K deficiencies.

SYSTEMS AFFECTED
• Gastrointestinal system—primary system affected; dynamic, functional ileus is the primary change
• Hepatobiliary system—chronic inappetence resulting in hepatic lipidosis
• Musculoskeletal and immune systems—can be indirectly affected by lack of adequate intake of vitamin C. However, in most cases, this requires chronic anorexia/ pseudoanorexia.
• Respiratory system—can be affected by metabolic alterations

INCIDENCE/PREVALENCE
• GI hypomotility/stasis is one of the most common clinical problems seen in the pet guinea pig.
• Colorectal impactions occur occasionally.

SIGNALMENT
• Anorectal impactions occur in older animals.
• Gastric hypomotility (stasis) and colorectal impactions can occur in guinea pigs of any age.

SIGNS

Historical Findings
Decreased ability to eliminate stools
• Lack of fecal output
• Soft, clumpy feces stuck to rear
• Odor to feces or from the perineal region
• Possibly diet low in insoluble fiber
• Owner may report the impression their pet is painful or uncomfortable.
• Normal history is possible for guinea pigs with anorectal impaction.
Decreased stool production
• Depression and lethargy (stasis or cecal obstruction)
• Owners may report a spectrum of malaise from "not acting right" to severe lethargy and lack of activity.
• Decreased appetite or complete anorexic/ pseudoanorexic.
• Reduction of size or number of fecal pellets. Occasionally, owner will report softer stools or stools of abnormal shape.
• Ptyalism, halitosis, and odynophagia (painful eating) can be associated with many causes of stasis.
• Bruxism occurs with oral or visceral pain.
• Lack of normal vocalizations
• Stiffness or hunched posture or gait can be associated with visceral or musculoskeletal pain (e.g., hypovitaminosis C).
• Dysuria is common with ureteral, cystic, and urethral calculi. Hematuria can be noted as well.
• Dyspnea can be associated with respiratory disease, tracheal compression, and cardiac disease. Pain can also alter the character of respirations.
• Guinea pigs with enterotoxic shock due to stasis usually present laterally recumbent.
• Dyspnea (stasis or cecal obstruction)
• Sudden death can occur with cecal torsions.

Physical Examination Findings
Decreased ability to eliminate stools
• Most patients show little to no abnormality other than referable to the impaction. Eversion of anal mucosa reveals a pocket of odiferous feces that may be partially desiccated. Bedding, hair, or other foreign material is present as well. The rectal mucosa may appear thickened or inflamed.
• Most guinea pigs are painful upon manipulation of the impaction.
• Mass may be observed or palpated in or near rectum.
• Some patients are obese.

• Rarely, there is abdominal enlargement. Pain may be associated with this finding.
• In the more severe cases, appetite may decrease due to pain/discomfort. Findings consistent with GI hypomotility can result.
• In many guinea pigs, anorectal impaction is an incidental finding. It can be a physical exam finding causing no clinical signs or change in stool.
Decreased stool formation
• Observation at rest may indicate a painful posture or lameness/stiffness.
• Observation at rest and after handling may suggest overt or subtle dyspnea.
• Observation of attitude, behavior in cage, and on examination table or floor may suggest depression
• Abdominal palpation is often extremely valuable in the diagnosis. Palpation may reveal gaseous distention of the stomach or cecum, abnormal renal size, ovarian cysts, tumors, palpable urinary calculi, or the presence and location of pain.
• Decreased borborygmus on abdominal auscultation with gastrointestinal hypomotility
• With severe, late-stage GI stasis or cecal bloat/torsion, animals are depressed, painful on palpation, or may present moribund, with severe gas distension of the GI tract on palpation.
• May see evidence of dermatitis, abscesses, or cutaneous neoplasia—may be sufficiently uncomfortable to cause anorexia
• Carefully examine all four feet with attention to painful conditions such as pododermatitis, ingrown nails, and cutaneous horns. Palpate joints for swelling, crepitus, and/or pain, and for asymmetry in muscle mass.
• Examine the face, head, and neck by palpation and visualization for causes of anorexia such as cheilitis, asymmetry to mandibles or maxillae, pain on palpation, scaly eyelids (a vague sign of illness), head tilt, and enlarged or painful submandibular or cervical lymph nodes.
• Examine the eyes for disorders that are painful or impair vision and may cause anorexia (e.g., corneal ulcers, uveitis, exophthalmos secondary to dental abscess or neoplasia).
• Oral exam should always be part of the physical examination for anorexic or pseudoanorexic guinea pigs. Incisors should be evaluated from the front and from the side with attention to occlusion and lateral mobility of mandible. There should be an adequate range of motion laterally to each side. Examine awake patients for evidence of tongue entrapment by the lower cheek teeth using a large otoscope cone or bivalve

CONSTIPATION (LACK OF FECAL PRODUCTION)   (CONTINUED)

speculum. Thorough evaluation of the cheek teeth is difficult in the awake patient. Due to the small aperture of the mouth, wiggly, uncooperative nature of the patients, and the presence of food in the mouth, examination without sedation does not rule out dental disease.

• Thoracic auscultation for evidence of underlying cardiac or pulmonary disease.

• Quite often, examination findings are unremarkable. However, in guinea pigs with GI stasis, further evaluation is indicated to look for underlying cause(s) that are difficult to identify on physical examination.

CAUSES AND RISK FACTORS

Anorectal or Colorectal Impaction
• The cause of anorectal impaction or cecal torsion is not known.

• The cause of colorectal impaction and cecal bloat is not known, but impactions consist of trichobezoars, bedding materials, and dried, inspissated feces.

• Mass lesions in or around the rectum may cause impaction.

Gastrointestinal Hypomotility/Stasis
GI hypomotility/stasis can begin with anorexia/pseudoanorexia, pain and physical or emotional stress (even while receiving a fiber-deficient diet). Guinea pigs can also develop GI stasis and the cause cannot be found.

Anorexia or Inappetence
• Anorexia can be due to any number of causes, including pain, systemic disease or infection, and malaise of any cause. Pseudoanorexia can be due to nonpainful oral pathology (e.g., some incisor or molar malocclusions) including dental disease, and dyspnea.

• Dyspnea can result in trouble eating, inability to breath and swallow at the same time. Aspiration of food may occur.

• Guinea pigs do not handle pain with stoicism. Any painful process can negatively influence appetite. Common causes of pain include pododermatitis, oral (e.g., dental abscessation, tongue trauma), musculoskeletal, gastrointestinal, and urinary disorders.

• Gastrointestinal disease can be painful. GI hypomotility/stasis causes pain and decreases food intake. Pain and decreased food intake exacerbate stasis and, if left untreated, can progress to GI floral changes with resultant enterotoxemia and death.

• Metabolic diseases such as renal disease, hepatic disease (especially hepatic lipidosis), and diabetes mellitus

• Cardiac and/or pulmonary disease (e.g., pneumonia)

• Caseous lymphadenitis and other causes of significant cervical lymphadenopathy (e.g., cavian leukemia)

• Neoplasia anywhere in the body

• Cystic ovaries can cause malaise and act as a space-occupying abdominal mass and decrease food intake.

• Neurologic and neuromuscular diseases are rare causes of anorexia and stasis.

Dietary and Environmental Causes
Poor nutrition may result in anorexia. Failure to ingest adequate insoluble fiber will increase the risk of hypomotility. Failure to chew coarse hay will promote dental disease. Failure to ingest adequate vitamin C can cause joint pain and poor immune function.

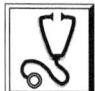

DIAGNOSIS

DIFFERENTIAL DIAGNOSIS

GI Hypomotility/Stasis
• Stasis is a syndrome involving lack of food intake, increased intestinal gas, and variable amounts of pain. In nearly all cases, it is caused by an underlying disease. Every attempt should be made to find the underlying disease.

• GI hypomotility/stasis can be confused with a GI obstruction. Bezoars have been reported in the guinea pig but are exceptionally rare compared with stasis. The accumulation of hair along with other ingesta in the stomach is not a disease but can be a symptom or consequence of GI hypomotility or stasis. Guinea pigs normally ingest hair during grooming. Healthy guinea pigs will always have some amount of hair and ingesta in the stomach. These stomach contents may be palpable and visible radiographically in the normal, healthy patient. With GI hypomotility, stomach contents are often deformable on palpation. True bezoars form concretion-like masses in the stomach that are physically too large to pass when normal GI motility returns.

• Dysbiosis due to the use of inappropriate antibiotics will cause severe illness that can be confused with advanced stasis. Guinea pigs with dysbiosis are usually presented as critically ill or moribund, with severe gas distension of the intestines and possibly true liquid diarrhea.

• Gastric hypomotility can be caused by anything that decreases food intake. Common causes include dental disease, urinary calculi (especially ureteral calculi), and orthopedic disorders.

• Gastric dilation/gastric dilatation/volvulus will cause lack of stool production, but the

patient usually presents with acute abdominal pain and bloating.

• Complete physical examination is an essential element in the diagnosis of stasis. Guinea pigs often exhibit subtle signs.

• Anamnesis should include husbandry review, including caging, bedding, ambient temperature, and the age/responsibility of the primary caretaker. Identify how water is provided and assess the degree of consumption and any recent changes. It is extremely important to ask about the diet as fed and as eaten, and the method and frequency of vitamin C supplementation. Any recent changes in appetite or food intake should be recorded. It is ideal to have owners bring photos of the cage and brand names or samples of the dietary elements (pellets, hay, vegetables, fruits, and treats).

• A minimum laboratory database for the guinea pig with stasis includes a CBC, serum chemistries, and whole-body radiographs. Further testing should be based on these results as indicated.

• In the guinea pig with stasis that demonstrates ptyalism, oral pain, and/or weight loss, it is appropriate to obtain a sedated oral examination and skull radiographs to evaluate the oral cavity. Skull radiographs should include multiple views, including at least a lateral, and right and left lateral obliques. It is also helpful to obtain DV, cranial/caudal, and VD views. If otitis media/interna is suspected or any vestibular signs are present, tympanic bullae should be radiographically evaluated.

Cecal Impactions
• Obstruction of outflow from cecum due to foreign bodies or inspissated stool
• Idiopathic typhlitis
• Antibiotic-associated enterotoxemia
• True diarrheal illnesses
• Cecal torsion

CBC/BIOCHEMISTRY/URINALYIS
• Abnormalities are not to be expected due to anorectal impaction unless there is a comorbid condition.

• With gastrointestinal stasis and cecal impaction, abnormalities vary with different underlying causes; increased liver enzymes may indicate hepatic lipidosis secondary to negative caloric balance.

OTHER LABORATORY TESTS
Vary, depending on suspected underlying cause

IMAGING
• Increased intraluminal rectal soft tissue density may be seen associated with anorectal or colorectal impaction; may be helpful in identifying comorbid conditions

• With cecal impactions, the cecum may appear gas filled, or full of fluid/ingesta; stool will not be present in colon.
• Abdominal radiography should be part of the minimum database for the guinea pig with stasis. Radiographs often show an increase in gastric gas with a notable absence of ingesta. Increased small intestinal gas (ileus) is also present; this change can be subtle. Dramatic increase in small intestinal gas should raise suspicion for severe illness (e.g., obstruction, enterotoxemia). Radiographs may also reveal underlying disorders such as urolithiasis, ovarian cysts, musculoskeletal diseases, and neoplasia. Abdominal ultrasonography is indicated in some cases to further investigate suspected pathology. Thoracic radiography is indicated to look for causes of dyspnea and to rule out occult pneumonia and heart disease. Thoracic ultrasonography including echocardiography is indicated to further investigate suspected pathology.

DIAGNOSTIC PROCEDURES
• Necropsy is required for diagnostic confirmation of cecal torsion. Hemorrhagic, edematous cecum is filled with fluid and gas.
• Histology of mass lesions

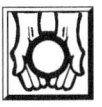

TREATMENT
NURSING CARE
Anorectal Impactions
• Successful treatment involves digital evacuation of stool and other impacted material. Sedation may be necessary for this procedure in the painful or uncooperative patient.
• Administration of subcutaneous fluids is recommended.
• Analgesics are sometimes indicated for a short-time post-evacuation.
• Vitamins B and K supplementation may be indicated in chronic cases or patients with very frequent recurrences.

GI Hypomotility/Stasis and Cecal Impactions
• Treat underlying cause if it can be identified.
• All guinea pigs with stasis should receive aggressive supportive care with careful attention to hydration, nutrition, and pain management. Oral or parenteral vitamin C is indicated in most cases.
• Fluid support is most commonly administered via oral and subcutaneous routes. Intravenous or intraosseous fluids are reserved for the severely ill patient. Maintenance needs are estimated to be 100 mL/kg/day.

• Nutritional support is imperative. When a guinea pig stops eating, GI hypomotility can progress rapidly. Anorexic guinea pigs are extremely prone to mortality from bacterial floral changes and enterotoxemia. Assisted syringe-feeding with an appropriate herbivore supplement such as Critical Care for Herbivores (Oxbow Pet Products, Murdock, NE) or Emeraid Herbivore (Lafeber Company, Cornell, IL) is appropriate in most cases. Care must be taken on the dyspneic or struggling patient. Tube feeding may be indicated. Both of the above products come in formulations that can be administered via esophagostomy or nasogastric tubes.
• Once the gastrointestinal tract receives fluid and high-fiber food and hypomotility begins to wane, the patient will often begin feeding on hay and its regular diet. Be sure to offer solid food in between assist-feeding sessions.
• Stasis can be caused by pain, but stasis is also a source of GI pain. Pain management is an extremely important part of patient management.

CLIENT EDUCATION
Anorectal impactions will recur frequently, requiring regular maintenance cleaning.

SURGICAL CONSIDERATIONS
• Surgery may be indicated for cecal foreign body obstruction, but the prognosis for surgery must be considered guarded to grave.
• Resection of mass lesions

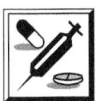

MEDICATIONS
DRUG(S) OF CHOICE
• Varies with an underlying cause
• For hypomotility—There is no better medication for hypomotility than food; assist-feed as noted above. The use of promotility agents such as metoclopromide (0.5–1.0 mg/kg PO, SC q8–12h) or cisapride (0.5–1 mg/kg PO q8–12h) may be helpful in regaining normal motility; cisapride is available through compounding pharmacies. Constant rate infusion of metoclopramide may be necessary for prokinesis.
• For analgesia, mild opioids are appropriate in the short term. Use buprenorphine (0.05 mg/kg SC, IM, IV q8–12h), as pure mu agonists tend to exacerbate hypomotility and are reserved for severe pain. NSAIDs such as meloxicam (0.2–0.5 mg/kg PO, SC q12–24h) can be used when renal function is normal and the patient is hydrated.
• For gastric inflammation and pain, H2 receptor antagonist such as Famotidine (0.5 mg/kg PO, SC, IV q24h) or ranitidine (2 mg/kg IV or 2–5 mg/kg PO q24h.

Metoclopramide (0.2–1.0 mg/kg PO, SC, IV q12h) increase gastric emptying.
• Chronic disease may result in vitamin K and B deficiencies. Vitamin K1 1–10 mg/kg PO, SC q24h; vitamin B complex supplementation (0.02–0.2 mL/kg SC, IM q24h)

CONTRAINDICATIONS
• Prokinetic agents are contraindicated in the presence of GI obstruction.
• Corticosteroids should not be used in guinea pig patients for any reason. They are never to be used to stimulate appetite.
• Oral antibiotics that select against gram-positive bacteria, such as penicillins, cephalosporins, lincosamines, or macrolides, should not be used in these animals as they can cause fatal dysbiosis and enterotoxemia.

PRECAUTIONS
Meloxicam should be used with caution in dehydrated patients and those with renal compromise.

POSSIBLE INTERACTIONS
N/A

ALTERNATIVE DRUGS
N/A

FOLLOW-UP
PATIENT MONITORING
• Patients that are presented with anorectal impactions can be monitored at home and presented at the first sign of recurrent impaction. Some owners can be instructed to successfully manage this problem at home.
• For patients with hypomotility and colorectal impactions, monitor body weight, amount and size of fecal pellets, clinical hydration status, urine production, attitude, reduction of pain, and voluntary food intake to determine the efficacy of treatment regimen.
• Any laboratory abnormalities noted in the diagnostic workup should be evaluated for resolution.

PREVENTION/AVOIDANCE
• For anorectal impactions unrelated to mass lesions, there is no way to prevent recurrences.
• For hypomotility and colorectal impactions, maintaining a proper plane of nutrition with a high-fiber diet, thin coarse hay, and appropriate vitamin C supplementation will provide some measure of protection against dietary-induced hypomotility and trichobezoar cecal obstruction. Avoid the use of wood shavings as bedding.

CONSTIPATION (LACK OF FECAL PRODUCTION)   (CONTINUED)

GUINEA PIGS

POSSIBLE COMPLICATIONS
• For anorectal impactions, complications are rarely seen. Theoretically, digital manipulation can cause damage to rectum or anus. Overzealous manipulation could cause bleeding or tear tissue.
• For hypomotility and colorectal impactions: dehydration, hypovitaminosis C, malnutrition, weight loss/cachexia, and hepatic lipidosis are common complications of anorexia associated with stasis. Hepatic lipidosis occurs quickly in anorexic guinea pigs.
• Anorexia can be associated with dysbiosis and enterotoxemia. This is the most common cause of mortality in guinea pigs with stasis.
• Post-surgical complications of rectal mass excision include incomplete closure, infection, and stricture.

EXPECTED COURSE AND PROGNOSIS
• For anorectal impactions, prognosis is good for successful treatment. Recurrences are expected.
• For hypomotility and colorectal impactions—depends on underlying cause
• The worse the clinical appearance of the patient, the greater the need for prolonged supportive care. Frequent assist-feedings may be gradually reduced to daily or BID

supplement. The sooner the patient is presented, the better the prognosis for control of stasis and its secondary effects.
• For mass lesions—variable, depending or completeness of excision and histologic findings.

MISCELLANEOUS

ASSOCIATED CONDITONS
See causes

AGE-RELATED FACTORS
Anorectal impactions are most common in older animals.

ZOONOTIC POTENTIAL
N/A

PREGNANCY/FERTILITY/BREEDING
N/A

SYNONYMS
N/A

SEE ALSO
Gastrointestinal hypomotility and gastrointestinal stasis

ABBREVIATIONS
DV = dorsoventral
GI = gastrointestinal
NSAID = nonsteroidal anti-inflammatory
VD = ventral dorsal

INTERNET RESOURCES
www.vin.com

Suggested Reading
Bohmer E. Dentistry in Rabbits and Rodents. Sussex, UK: Wiley Blackwell, 2015:35–87, 118–212.
Ness RB. Rodents. In: Carpenter JW, ed. Exotic Animal Formulary, 3rd ed. St Louis: Elsevier, 2005:377–408.
O'Rourke DP. Disease problems of guinea pigs. In: Quesenberry KE, Carpenter JW, eds. Ferrets, Rabbits, and Rodents: Clinical Medicine and Surgery, 2nd ed. Philadelphia: WB Saunders, 2004: 245–254.
Percy DH, Barthold SW. Pathology of Laboratory Rodents and Rabbits, 3rd ed. Ames: Blackwell, 2007:242.
Quesenberry KE, Donnelly TM, Hillyer EV. Biology, husbandry, and clinical techniques of guinea pigs and chinchillas. In: Quesenberry KE, Carpenter JW, eds. Ferrets, Rabbits, and Rodents: Clinical Medicine and Surgery, 2nd ed. Philadelphia: WB Saunders, 2004: 232–244.

Author Jeffrey L. Rhody, DVM, DABVP-ECM

CUTANEOUS AND SUBCUTANEOUS MASSES

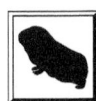

BASICS

DEFINITION
Tissue enlargement and swelling that involves the surface epithelium and/or subcuticular tissue

PATHOPHYSIOLOGY
• Trichofolliculomas are the most common cutaneous tumor diagnosed in guinea pigs.
• Plantar abscesses secondary to chronic pododermatitis are rare in guinea pigs. A diffuse plantar cellulitis with an associated swelling is the most common presentation associated with chronic pododermatitis.
• Subcutaneous abscesses often develop in guinea pigs as a result of bite wounds secondary to fighting, especially between adult boars. Bite wounds from dogs and cats may also result in abscess formation.
• Facial abscesses (e.g., mandibular), are most likely dental in origin and associated with malocclusion and tooth root infection.
• Abscesses in the throat area may be caused by the penetration of a hay thistle through the oral mucosa and its subsequent migration.
• Cervical lymphadenitis is primarily caused by *Streptococcus zooepidemicus* and can develop into abscesses of the affected cervical lymph nodes. These abscesses are located in the ventral cervical region of the body.
• Although rare, neoplasia may be associated with subcutaneous swelling in guinea pigs.
• Hypovitaminosis C can result in osteoarthritis and subsequent joint swelling.
• Swellings associated with mammary tissue—result of a bacterial infection or neoplasia
• Hematoma/seroma result from trauma or surgical procedure

SYSTEMS AFFECTED
• Skin—neoplasia
• Skeletal—dental abscesses
• Lymph—abscesses
• Subcutaneous tissue—abscesses, hematoma, seroma
• Thyroid—neoplasia
• Mammary gland—inflammation, neoplasia

GENETICS
N/A

INCIDENCE/PREVALENCE
• Cervical lymphadenitis is the most common cause of subcutaneous and submandibular swelling in guinea pigs.
• Dental disease associated with facial swelling is common.
• Group-housed animals commonly fight, resulting in subcutaneous abscesses.

• Trichofolliculimas are the most common cutaneous tumor and are found on the dorsum of the animal.
• Hypovitaminosis C can result in swellings associated with pododermatitis, osteoarthritis, and cervical lymphadenitis.
• Wet, dirty cages and trauma caused by nursing young may result in mastitis.
• Hematomas and seromas are often associated with trauma or a surgical procedure.

GEOGRAPHIC DISTRIBUTION
N/A

SIGNALMENT
• Adult boars are more likely to present with subcutaneous abscesses as a result of fighting.
• Dental abscessation is more prevalent in older individuals or animals diagnosed with a chronic vitamin C deficiency.
• Swelling associated with pododermatitis is often associated with poor substrate and/or overweight animals.

SIGNS

Historical Findings
• Facial and mandibular swelling—history of dental disease, ptyalism, discharge, face deformation, reluctance to chew, vitamin C deficiency
• Subcutaneous swelling—history of group housing, of biting resulting in abscess formation
• A fast-growing swelling that may or may not be painful located anywhere on the body
• Swollen area may be bloody and/or draining purulent material.
• Mammary gland swelling—dirty cage conditions and nursing young
• Traumatic or surgical incident

Physical Examination Findings
• Round, hairless cutaneous mass on the dorsum (e.g., trichofolliculima)
• Swollen, painful joints
• Swollen, necrotic areas on the plantar surfaces of the feet
• Firm or fluctuant mass that may or may not be associated with an ulcerated/necrotizing area
• Ventral cervical masses are characteristic of cervical lymphadenitis.
• Mandibular or facial swellings are likely caused by a dental abscess. The mass is usually attached to underlying bone. Other signs of dental disease may be present.
• Hyperemic, swollen, warm mammary glands

CAUSES
• Subcutaneous swelling associated with abscess formation is commonly caused by the following bacteria:
  ○ *Staphylococcus* spp. (in particular *S. aureus*) and *Streptococcus* spp. are often

isolated from abscesses. *Pseudomonas aeruginosa*, *Pasteurella multocida*, and *Corynebacterium pyogenes* may also be cultured.
  ○ *Streptococcus zooepidemicus* is the causative agent of cervical lymphadenitis; Lancefield's group C, a gram-positive coccus; *Streptococcus moniliformis* is uncommonly involved
  ○ *Yersinia pseudotuberculosis* can cause abscesses of internal organs.
  ○ Mixed infection caused by aerobic and anaerobic bacteria is the rule in dental abscessation.
• Subcutaneous swelling due to foreign body involvement: hay thistle, plant foreign body, grass/clover stems
• Subcutaneous facial swelling resulting from underlying dental disease: root elongation, crown deformities, malocclusion, dental spurs, food impaction between teeth, vitamin C deficiencies, and periodontal pockets can lead to dental abscesses.
• Osteoarthritis: hypovitaminosis C
• Mammary swelling: bacterial infection; wet, dirty environment
• Cutaneous swelling: trichofolliculoma
• Neoplasia: thyroid carcinoma

RISK FACTORS
• Group housing and breeding seasons
• Dental disease—higher energy and lower fiber diets are thought to contribute to dental malocclusion. Vitamin D and C deficiencies may also predispose to dental disease.
• Exposure to infected animals: cervical lymphadenitis
• Hypovitaminosis C
• Hard-stemmed diets
• Poor husbandry
• Nursing young
• Trauma
• Surgical procedure

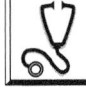

DIAGNOSIS

DIFFERENTIAL DIAGNOSIS
• Cervical lymphadenitis—results in abscesses but should be considered as a particular clinical entity
• Neoplasia—in particular, trichofolliculomas
• Thyroid tumors are frequently cystic and may be confused with cervical lymphadenitis.
• Hematoma/seroma
• Abscess
• Cyst

CBC/BIOCHEMISTRY/URINALYSIS
CBC—most often normal. Inflammatory leukogram common in cases of bacteremia

CUTANEOUS AND SUBCUTANEOUS MASSES (CONTINUED)

OTHER LABORATORY TESTS
• Cytology and staining of abscess material to identify causative organism
• Culture and sensitivity of abscess material—often, culture results are negative if swab is taken at the center of the abscess material. More accurate culture results may be achieved if the sample is collected at the abscess tissue interface.

IMAGING
• Radiography—useful to determine the extent of swellings. Skull radiographs are essential to assess the severity of the dental disease and the presence of osteomyelitis.
• Ultrasonography—useful for diagnosing thyroid cysts
• CT scan—allows more accurate assessment of dental, tympanic bulla, and skull diseases

DIAGNOSTIC PROCEDURES
• Aspiration—cytology to differentiate between hematoma/seroma, neoplasia, and abscess. Gram's staining of an aspirate smear is recommended, especially for samples obtained from dental abscesses from which bacterial cultures may not be rewarding.
• Culture—pus and abscess capsule can be submitted for culture. Submitting part of the fibrous capsule may yield better results over a sample collected in the center of the abscess. Anaerobic culture is encouraged for dental abscesses.
• Bacterial sensitivity testing is important to direct antibiotic selection.
• Biopsy of mass for diagnostic purposes (e.g., neoplasia)

PATHOLOGIC FINDINGS
• Neoplastic tissue
• Abscess: exudate—degenerate neutrophils, intra- and extracellular bacteria, macrophages, necrotic tissues
• Abscess: capsule and surrounding tissue—fibrinous inflammation, edema, congestion, fibrous connective tissue, presence of neutrophils, macrophages, lymphocytes, and plasma cells

TREATMENT

APPROPRIATE HEALTH CARE
• Seroma/hematoma: incise and flush. If active hemorrhage, provide hemostasis. Reduce subcutaneous dead space and close by primary intention.
• Neoplasia: surgical removal or debulking
• Subcutaneous abscesses: the pus found in most guinea pig abscesses does not drain well. However, lancing, draining, and flushing with hydrogen peroxide, povidone iodine, or chlorhexidine may be adequate for

uncomplicated cases. The procedure may have to be repeated daily for several days.
• Cervical lymphadenitis: surgical removal, including capsule
• Dental abscesses: techniques described in rabbits can be used: antimicrobial wound-packing technique, marsupialization technique, AIPMMA beads. A thorough dental examination is mandatory with teeth equilibration and resurfacing, intraoral removal of loose teeth, and cleaning of food impaction between teeth and in gingival pockets.
• Surgical removal of the abscess, including the capsule, may be necessary depending on location, cause, and treatment response.
• Mammary tumors: surgically remove
• Mastitis: appropriate antibiotic treatment, hot packs on affected tissue, clean environment
• Systemic antibiotic therapy

NURSING CARE
• Treatment of surgical site: keep clean, treat and bandage as necessary
• Abscess: dependent on location of the lesion, treatment elected, and concurrent conditions (e.g., dental disease, anorexia, and weight loss)
• Sepsis—aggressive fluid therapy, intravenous antibiotics
• Bandaging as needed

ACTIVITY
Restricted until resolution of the disease condition

DIET
• If the patient is anorexic, assisted feeding is necessary (e.g., Critical Care for Herbivores, Oxbow Pet Products, Murdock, NE) 50–100 mL/kg/day or Emeraid Herbivore (Lafeber Company, Cornell, IL), 10–15 mL/kg q6–8h. If neither product is available, a slurry can be made with blended leafy green vegetables that are high in vitamin C, or guinea pig pellets blended with water and vegetable baby food.
• Diet should primarily include hay and roughage with a limited amount of pellets. Fresh vegetables may also be offered in limited quantity. High-carbohydrate treats should be avoided.
• Guinea pigs need a dietary source of vitamin C. Higher levels should be provided to sick individuals (30–50 mg/kg daily). Vitamin C may be ground and fed directly to the pig. Vitamin C treats are also available for guinea pigs (e.g., Daily C, Oxbow Pet Products, Murdock, NE).

CLIENT EDUCATION
• Discuss proper diet, husbandry, and group housing.

• Inform owner of the critical need for vitamin C supplementation.
• Dental abscesses can be challenging to treat and multiple follow-ups are necessary. Dental disease requires lifelong treatment.
• Cervical lymphadenitis is mildly contagious to other guinea pigs. Prognosis may be guarded. Owners should be educated on the difficulty in resolving this condition during the initial treatment period. Reoccurrence of cervical abscesses is likely in the majority of these cases.

SURGICAL CONSIDERATIONS
Tumors
• Adequate clipping of hair around cutaneous/subcutaneous swelling
• Complete surgical removal of tumor
• Submit excised tissue for biopsy.
• Use primary intension closure.
• Treat incision site with topical antibiotic cream and bandage as needed.
• Systemic antibiotic therapy

Subcutaneous Abscesses
• Complete removal of the entire abscess may be indicated with care not to rupture the capsule.
• Alternatively: lancing, curettage, cleaning, and flushing. Leave abscess open. Express pus and flush once to twice daily with hydrogen peroxide, povidone iodine, or chlorhexidine until granulation tissue forms and pus is no longer present.
• Remove any nidus of infection: foreign object, hay thistle, necrotic tissue
• Packing the abscess with antibiotic-impregnated or iodoform gauze may help clear the infection and keep the abscess draining.
• Place on 2–3 weeks of antibiotic treatment.

Dental Abscesses
• Several techniques have been described in rabbits with good success and can be extrapolated to guinea pigs.
• Debridement and marsupialization technique:
  ◦ Remove abscess in its entirety with capsule, affected bone and teeth if possible; abscess is often attached to the bone or a tooth root.
  ◦ Curette and debride abnormal and infected tissue. Bone defects may be filled with AIPMMA beads.
  ◦ Marsupialize the remaining opening to the skin.
  ◦ Clean and flush every day until granulation and closure of the wound by secondary intention.
• Wound-packing technique:
  ◦ Lance, clean, and flush the abscess.
  ◦ Pack with strips of gauze impregnated with a selected antibiotic. Antibiotics are

(CONTINUED)   # CUTANEOUS AND SUBCUTANEOUS MASSES

selected based on the oral microflora of guinea pigs; initial treatment may include ampicillin 30 mg/kg or clindamycin 20 mg/kg. Antimicrobial treatment should be altered depending on culture and sensitivity.
  ◦ Suture the incision.
  ◦ Repeat every week until pus is no longer present and the abscess cavity is almost completely replaced by granulation tissue.
• Other techniques have been described with mixed results:
• Local use of AIPMMA beads, long-lasting doxycycline gel, honey, 50% dextrose.
• Intraoral endoscopy-assisted drainage and local treatment if a draining tract can be localized.
• Place on long-term antibiotic treatment: 1–3 months; pain management

Internal Abscesses
• Surgical removal when possible
• Long-term antibiotic treatment

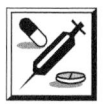

MEDICATIONS
DRUG(S) OF CHOICE
Antibiotics
• Antibiotics should be selected based on the bacterial culture and sensitivity. Pending the sensitivity results, selection is based on the common isolates reported in guinea pig abscesses and antibiotics that are safe to use in this species. Unfortunately, antibiotics with the best effect against frequent isolates, especially *Staphylococcus aureus* and *Streptococcus zooepidemicus*, can lead to antibiotic-associated dybiosis and enterotoxemia. Treatment should be pursued for at least 2 weeks.
• Broad-spectrum antibiotics safe to use in guinea pigs include enrofloxacin (5–20 mg/kg PO q12h), which is ineffective against anaerobes; trimethoprim-sulfa (15–30 mg/kg PO q12h); and chloramphenicol (30–50 mg/kg PO q8–12h). Azithromycin (15–30 mg/kg PO q24h) is safe to use in guinea pigs and can reach a high concentration in pus through transportation by heterophils.
• For dental abscesses, antibiotic therapy, including anaerobic coverage and good penetration in bones, should be selected. Azithromycin (15–30 mg/kg PO q24h), chloramphenicol (30–50 mg/kg PO, SC, IM, IV q8–12h), and metronidazole (10–20 mg/kg PO, IV q12h) have good anaerobic spectrum. Penicillin G (40,000–60,000 IU/kg SC q2–7d) can also be used (see Precautions). Longer systemic antibiotic treatment is usually needed for dental abscesses: 1–3 months. Topical antibiotics in

gauze packing and AIPMMA offer a wider range of selection because of reduced systemic absorption and avoidance of oral administration.

Pain Management
• Butorphanol (0.4–2.0 mg/kg SC, IM q4–12h)—short acting
• Buprenorphine (0.5–0.2 mg/kg SC, IM q8–12h)—longer acting opioid
• Meloxicam (0.5–1.0 mg/kg PO, SC, IM q24h—also for long-term pain management for dental abscesses and dental disease
• Local anesthetics/dental blocks of bupivacaine (1 mg/kg), lidocaine (1 mg/kg), use in combination or alone—before more advanced surgery

CONTRAINDICATIONS
• Oral administration of penicillins, macrolides, lincosamides, and cephalosporins
• Procaine, which is included in some penicillin preparations, can be toxic to guinea pigs.
• Use of immunosuppressive drugs such as corticosteroids
• Extensive surgery on a debilitated animal

PRECAUTIONS
• Oral administration of antibiotics may cause antibiotic-associated enteritis, dysbiosis, and enterotoxemia.
• Procaine penicillin G has been used as an alternative therapy, but there are multiple anecdotal reports of fatal enterotoxemia with the use of any form of penicillin, including parenteral, in guinea pigs.
• Opioids adversely affect the gastrointestinal motility.
• Chloramphenicol—humans should wear gloves when handling this drug.

POSSIBLE INTERACTIONS
N/A

ALTERNATIVE DRUGS
N/A

FOLLOW-UP
PATIENT MONITORING
• Monitor daily for swelling, resolution of inflammation, and improvement in clinical signs.
• Dental abscesses: recheck weekly
• Dental disease: recheck every 4–20 weeks for dental trimming

PREVENTION/AVOIDANCE
• Adequate supplementation of vitamin C (30–50 mg/kg PO q24h)
• Avoid trauma to the animal
• Appropriate surgical techniques to reduce incidence of seroma formation

• Prevention of acquired dental disease by providing high-fiber and good-quality food with supplemental vitamin C
• Treating and monitoring dental disease in early stage to prevent progression to more severe dental malformation and abscesses formation
• Prevention of bite wounds by limiting group housing, especially of adult boars during breeding seasons
• Isolation of sick individuals
• Providing a clean, stress-free environment

POSSIBLE COMPLICATIONS
• Sepsis
• Spreading of the infection to surrounding tissue
• Recurrence, chronic pain, extensive tissue destruction
• Dental abscesses: face deformation, tissue destruction, worsening of the preexisting dental disease, inability to eat, and facial paralysis
• Death due to septic condition associated with bacterial infection (e.g., mastitis, pododermatitis, and abscess)

EXPECTED COURSE AND PROGNOSIS
• Depends on underlying disease condition associated with the swelling, pathogenicity of organism, and immune status of the animal
• Subcutaneous abscesses: good to fair prognosis
• Neoplasia: fair to guarded prognosis
• Seroma/hemangioma: good prognosis
• Pododermatitis: good to fair prognosis
• Mastitis: fair to guarded prognosis

MISCELLANEOUS
ASSOCIATED CONDITIONS
• Immunosuppresion
• Dental disease
• Depression
• Alopecia at location of swelling
• Hepatic lipidosis—chronic anorexia

AGE-RELATED FACTORS
N/A

ZOONOTIC POTENTIAL
• *Streptococcus moniliformis*
• *Yersinia pseudotuberculosis*

PREGNANCY/FERTILITY/BREEDING
N/A

SYNONYMS
N/A

SEE ALSO
Anorexia and pseudoanorexia
Cervical lymphadenitis
Dental malocclusion
Pododermatitis

CUTANEOUS AND SUBCUTANEOUS MASSES   (CONTINUED)

ABBREVIATIONS
AIPMMA = antibiotic-impregnated polymethyl methacrylate
CBC = complete blood count
CT = computed tomography

INTERNET RESOURCES
N/A

Suggested Reading
Barrios-Arpi LM, Morales-Cauti SM. Cytomorphological characterization of lymphadenopathies in guinea pigs: study of 31 clinical cases. J Exot Pet Med 2020;32:1–5.

Bays TB. Geriatric care of rabbits, guinea pigs, and chinchillas. Vet Clin Exot Anim 2020;23:567–593.

Capello V. Clinical technique: treatment of periapical infections in pet rabbits and rodents. J Exot Pet Med 2008;17:124–131.

Johnson-Delaney C. Guinea pigs, chinchillas, degus and duprasi. In: Meredith A, Johnson-Delaney C, eds. BSAVA Manual of Exotic Pets, 5th ed. Quedgeley, Gloucester, UK: British Small Animal Veterinary Association, 2010:28–64.

Miwa Y, Sladky K. Common surgical procedures of rodents, ferrets, hedgehogs, and sugar gliders. Vet Clin Exot Anim 2016;19:205–244.

Pignon C, Mayer J. Guinea pigs. In: Quesenberry KE, Carpenter JW, eds. Ferrets, Rabbits and Rodents, 4th ed. Clinical Medicine and Surgery. 2021 ed. St. Louis: Saunders, 2020:270–297.

Riggs SM. Guinea pigs. In: Mitchell MA, Tully TN, eds. Manual of Exotic Pet Practice. St Louis: Saunders/Elsevier, 2009:456–473.

Author Thomas N. Tully, Jr., DVM, MS, Dipl. ABVP (Avian), Dipl. ECZM (Avian)

GUINEA PIGS

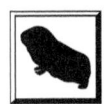

BASICS

DEFINITION

• "Malocclusion" is just a single aspect of dental disease of guinea pigs, referring to abnormalities of the clinical crowns. Since congenital or developmental abnormalities of the skull have not been documented in this species, "acquired dental disease" is a more accurate terminology.
• Acquired dental disease is a syndrome—a complex of clinical symptoms and signs, which may be associated with the syndrome alone or with related diseases (i.e., abscess).
• Thus, the more precise terminology for malocclusion in guinea pigs is acquired dental disease syndrome.

ANATOMY

• The guinea pig is a rodent species belonging to the suborder Caviomorph or Hystrycomorph ("guinea pig–like" or "porcupine-like" rodent).
• All rodent species are *Simplicidentata*. Unlike rabbits, they have one single maxillary incisor tooth for each quadrant.
• All rodent species have one pair of well-developed maxillary and mandibular incisor teeth, representing the best-known anatomical peculiarity of this order.
• Incisor teeth greatly vary in shape, color, and thickness among rodent species. Incisor teeth of rodents are covered by enamel only over the labial surface. In guinea pigs, the enamel is white; incisors have a chisel-shaped occlusal surface, and the length of the mandibular incisors is normally threefold that of the maxillary incisors.
• Incisor teeth are continually growing throughout life and are open rooted (elodont) in all rodent species.
• Dental formula of guinea pigs is 2 × 1I 0C 1P 3M = 20; as with all rodent species and rabbits, guinea pigs lack canine teeth and there is a diastema between the incisor and the premolar tooth.
• Premolar and molar teeth are anatomically indistinguishable and are usually simply called "cheek teeth" for this reason. Each quadrant includes 4 cheek teeth, for a total of 16.
• The cheek teeth of guinea pigs are open-rooted (elodont); the occlusal surface is rough and uneven due to enamel crests and dentinal grooves.
• A very important anatomical peculiarity of cheek teeth of guinea pigs is that they are curved—the mandibular with a buccal (lateral) convexity and the maxillary with a palatal (medial) convexity. This results in a 30-degree oblique occlusal plane that slants from dorsal to ventral, from lateral to medial. The clinical crowns are much shorter than reserve crowns.

PATHOPHYSIOLOGY

• Guinea pigs have elodont (continuously growing) incisors and cheek teeth (similar to rabbits), which are worn during normal chewing activity.
• The primary cause of dental disease in guinea pigs is insufficient or improper wearing of cheek teeth due to inappropriate diet, particularly a lack of crude fiber. Secondary nutritional hyperparathyroidism in satin guinea pigs may have an impact on dentition.
• Acquired malocclusion and severe deviation of incisor teeth occur most often following acquired dental disease of cheek teeth and uneven chewing. However, it may also be primary following traumatic fractures of the clinical crowns.
• Severe overgrowth of clinical crowns of cheek teeth may lead to stretching of masticatory muscles and temporomandibular joint capsule; this sometimes progresses to unilateral or bilateral subluxation of the TMJ.
• Because even a slight alteration of the sloped occlusal plane of cheek teeth is enough to hamper chewing, and a slight overgrowth of clinical crowns is enough to interfere with movements of the tongue and swallowing, guinea pigs are much more prone to reduced food intake and anorexia due to dental disease than are rabbits.

SIGNS

Historical Findings

• Guinea pigs usually present with symptoms directly related to and suggesting dental diseases, such as reduced food intake, dysphagia, or anorexia.
• In multipig households, owners may be unaware of decreased appetite in one individual, and the only presenting sign may be weight loss.
• There is usually a history of improper feeding, most particularly lack of fiber (hay).
• Malocclusion of incisor teeth is often present and may be noted by observant owners.

Physical Examination Findings

• The small size and the natural behavior make an effective oral examination, challenging, or less than optimal in the awake guinea pig.
• Complete inspection and proper diagnosis of dental disease should be performed under heavy sedation or general anesthesia.
• Oral inspection and treatment of dental disease in rodents requires specialized equipment. The tabletop mouth gag and restrainer is much easier to use than traditional mouth gags, which are difficult to keep in place due to the smaller patient size. Smaller, modified open-blade cheek dilators are available and are much more effective than those used in rabbits as they provide more effective hold on the well-developed buccal folds of guinea pigs.
• Inspection by oral endoscopy provides optimal oral visualization for all rodent species. A 14- to 18-cm-long, 2.7-mm-thick, 30-degree rigid endoscope is commonly used. Other magnification devices are helpful but not always sufficient, and many lesions can be missed without the help of stomatoscopy.
• Identify incisor abnormalities—the two most common patterns of incisor malocclusion are excessive coronal elongation of the mandibular incisors or lateral deviation. Both are usually a consequence of cheek teeth abnormalities. Primary incisor malocclusion in guinea pigs is extremely rare.
• Fractured incisors can be seen, often related to behavioral problems (e.g., chewing of cage bars).
• Identify cheek teeth abnormalities—excessive coronal elongation and malocclusion of cheek teeth is the most common pattern. Due to the peculiar orientation of their occlusal plane, mandibular crowns always elongate lingually, while maxillary crowns always orient laterally. Mandibular cheek teeth may eventually bend lingually over the tongue, hampering movement. A typical bridge-like malocclusion occurs when the first mandibular premolars occlude or even cross each other.
• Unlike rabbits, uneven occlusal planes such as "step" and "wave" mouth are not common, and spike or spur formation is seen much less frequently.
• Additional lesions frequently encountered are gingivitis and fur impaction of the gingival sulcus.
• With severe disease, stretching of the masticatory muscles and abnormal movements of temporomandibular joints occur.

CAUSES AND RISK FACTORS

Feeding diets are insufficient in crude fiber; hay provides an abrasive material to grind coronal surfaces.

DIAGNOSIS

DIFFERENTIAL DIAGNOSIS

For reduced food intake or anorexia—gastrointestinal disease, pain, and metabolic disease

CBC/BIOCHEMISTRY/URINALYSIS
Usually normal unless secondary problems or concurrent disease are present.

OTHER LABORATORY TESTS
N/A

IMAGING
• An optimal radiologic study includes five views (lateral; two obliques; ventrodorsal and rostrocaudal). Additional extraoral oblique projections, as well as additional intraoral views, may also be used.
• Modern spiral CT scanning provides excellent detail in small species such guinea pigs. Three-dimensional volume and surface renderings of the head provide tremendous information for diagnosis of dental disease or related problems such as osteomyelitis and abnormalities of the temporomandibular joint.

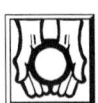

TREATMENT
The goal of treatment is restoration of dental anatomy to as close to normal as possible. Extraction of diseased teeth may be part of the dental treatment as well. In most cases, treatment provides only palliation, as effective restoration of dental anatomy to normal is not possible.

APPROPRIATE HEALTH CARE
Unless severely debilitated, treatment of dental disease is performed on an outpatient basis.

DIET
• It is absolutely imperative that the patient continues to eat during and following treatment. Most guinea pigs with dental disease present for reduced food intake or anorexia and may be unable to eat solid food for some time following coronal reduction. Anorexia will cause or exacerbate GI hypomotility, derangement of the gastrointestinal microflora, and overgrowth of intestinal bacterial pathogens.
• Syringe-feed a gruel such as Critical Care for Herbivores (Oxbow Pet Products) or Emeraid Herbivore (Lafeber Company, Cornell, IL), 10–15 mL/kg PO q8–12h. Larger volumes and more frequent feedings are often accepted; feed as much as the patient will readily accept.
• Return the patient to a solid food diet as soon as possible to encourage normal occlusion and wear. Increase the amount of tough, fibrous foods and foods containing abrasive silicates such as hay and wild grasses.

CLIENT EDUCATION
• The prognosis is directly related to the stage of dental disease and related complications.
• If significant stretching and inflammation of the masticatory muscles has occurred, or if the TMJ is affected, the patient may not be able to eat following coronal reduction.
• It is usually not possible to predict the degree of masticatory muscle or TMJ involvement prior to performing coronal reduction. The ability of the patient to eat following treatment is the best predictor of the degree of muscle or TMJ disease. Some patients will begin to eat immediately following reduction, indicating little to no muscle/TMJ involvement. For other patients, a prolonged period of assist-feeding, supportive care, and repeated coronal reduction may be required until muscle inflammation resolves. With severe TMJ disorders, the patient may never return to eating; further treatment is unrewarding and euthanasia may be indicated.
• Inform the owner that repeated coronal reduction and additional dental treatment will usually be necessary, often life-long. However, treatment is beneficial to control the progression of dental disease and related clinical signs and symptoms.

SURGICAL CONSIDERATIONS
Trimming of the Cheek Teeth (Coronal Reduction)
• Coronal reduction requires general anesthesia.
• Use a focused, directed light source and magnification loops. Adequate visualization and protection of soft tissues requires specialized equipment (see Physical Examination Findings, above)
• A rotating dental unit with a straight handpiece and small metal or silicon burs is used to reduce coronal surfaces.
• The goal of occlusal adjustment is to shorten the elongated clinical crowns and restore the proper oblique occlusal plane, which is a critical aspect of treatment in this species.
• Due to the normal curvature of cheek teeth in guinea pigs, extraction is very challenging, unless the tooth is loose secondary to periodontal infection. Unfortunately, diseased teeth fracture easily, making complete extraction difficult or unlikely.

Trimming of the Incisors (Coronal Reduction)
• Coronal reduction of incisors is usually performed in conjunction with reduction of cheek teeth, under general anesthesia. Use high-speed precision dental handpieces and burrs, or a tool for hobbyists with a diamond

cutting blade, along with metal spatulas to protect soft tissues. Do not use cutting instruments such as nail trimmers or rongeurs, as these cause iatrogenic damage to the tooth (e.g., fracture, root damage, and abscess).
• Malocclusion of incisors occurs as a result of check teeth malocclusion and is therefore usually corrected if the occlusion of the cheek teeth is corrected. Extraction is rarely needed in guinea pigs.

MEDICATIONS
DRUG(S) OF CHOICE
Antibiotics
• Antimicrobial drugs are indicated if bacterial infection is diagnosed.
• Antibiotics should be selected based on the bacterial culture and antimicrobial sensitivity but can be chosen empirically for the initial phase of treatment. A limited number of antibiotics are safe to use in guinea pigs, as many cause potentially fatal antibiotic-associated dybiosis and enterotoxemia.
• Broad-spectrum antibiotics safe to use in guinea pigs include enrofloxacin (5–20 mg/kg PO q12–24h), which is ineffective against anaerobes; trimethoprim-sulfa (15–30 mg/kg PO q12h); and chloramphenicol (30–50 mg/kg PO SC, IM, IV q8–12h). Azithromycin (50 mg/kg PO q12) is safe to use in guinea pigs and can reach a high concentration in pus through transportation by heterophils.
• For dental abscesses, antibiotic therapy including anaerobic coverage and good penetration in bones should be selected. Azithromycin, chloramphenicol, and metronidazole (10–20 mg/kg PO, IV q12h) have good anaerobic spectrum. Penicillin G (40,000–60,000 IU/kg SC q2–7d) can also be used (see Precautions).

Pain Management
• Butorphanol (0.4–2.0 mg/kg SC, IM q4–12h)—short acting
• Buprenorphine (0.05–0.2 mg/kg SC, IM, IV q8–12h)—longer acting opioid
• Meloxicam (0.5–1.0 mg/kg PO, SC, IM q12–24h)—used for long-term pain management
• Local anesthetics/dental blocks of bupivacaine (1 mg/kg), lidocaine (1 mg/kg), use in combination or alone—before more advanced surgery

CONTRAINDICATIONS
• Oral administration of penicillins, macrolides, lincosamides, and cephalosporins will cause potentially fatal enteric dysbiosis.

(CONTINUED)

• Procaine, which is included in some penicillin preparations, can be toxic to guinea pigs.
• Use of immunosuppressive drugs such as corticosteroids.
• Extensive surgery on a debilitated animal, as in the case of facial abscesses.

PRECAUTIONS
• Oral administration of antibiotics may cause antibiotic-associated enteritis, dysbiosis, and enterotoxemia.
• Procaine penicillin G has been used as an alternative therapy, but there are anecdotal reports of fatal enterotoxemia with the use of any form of penicillin, including parenteral, in guinea pigs.
• Opioids may have an effect on the gastrointestinal motility.

POSSIBLE INTERACTIONS
N/A

ALTERNATIVE DRUGS
N/A

 FOLLOW-UP

PATIENT MONITORING
• Monitor food intake following treatment. Many patients require assist-feeding with hay-based gruel. The duration of assist-feeding depends on the severity of disease and on time for improvement.
• Reevaluate and trim as needed. Evaluate the entire oral cavity with each recheck.

PREVENTION/AVOIDANCE
Provide adequate tough, fibrous hay and grasses to encourage normal wear.

POSSIBLE COMPLICATIONS
Periapical infections and abscesses, recurrence, chronic pain, or inability to chew.

EXPECTED COURSE AND PROGNOSIS
• In general, the prognosis for dental disease in guinea pigs is more guarded than in rabbits.
• Nevertheless, unless the patient is presented in very poor general condition, the prognosis is fair to good. The critical prognostic indicator following the restoration of the normal dental anatomy is a return to normal chewing. In patients with advanced involvement of the masticatory muscles and/or the temporomandibular joint, dental treatment may be unrewarding, and prognosis is poor.
• Patients that do not immediately return to eating may not wear their teeth down to the degree required to prevent repeated overgrowth. These patients often require additional coronal reduction until the soft tissues heal and the patient is able to eat enough high-fiber food to allow normal wearing.

 MISCELLANEOUS

AGE-RELATED FACTORS
N/A

ZOONOTIC POTENTIAL
N/A

PREGNANCY/FERTILITY/BREEDING
N/A

SYNONYMS
N/A

SEE ALSO
Abscesses
Anorexia and pseudoanorexia

ABBREVIATIONS
GI = gastrointestinal
TMJ = temporomandibular joint

INTERNET RESOURCES
N/A

Suggested Reading
Capello V, Gracis M. Dental Procedures. In: Lennox AM, ed. Rabbit and Rodent Dentistry Handbook. West Palm Beach: Zoological Education Network, 2005; Ames: Wiley Blackwell, 2007:213–246.
Capello V, Lennox AM. Clinical Radiology of Exotic Companion Mammals. Ames: Wiley Blackwell, 2008.
Capello V, Lennox AM. Small mammal dentistry. In: Quesenberry KE, Carpenter JW, eds. Ferrets, Rabbits and Rodents Clinical Medicine and Surgery, 3rd ed. St Louis: Elsevier Saunders, 2012:452–471.
Capello V. Diagnostic imaging of dental disease in pet rabbits and rodents. Vet Clin Exot Anim 2016;19(3):757–782.
Crossley DA. Clinical aspects of rodent dental anatomy. J Vet Dent 1995;12(4):131–135.
Legendre L. Anatomy and disorders of the oral cavity of guinea pigs. Vet Clin Exot Anim 2016;19(3):825–842.
Popesko P, Rjtova V, Horak J. A Colour Atlas of Anatomy of Small Laboratory Animals. Vol. I: Rabbit, Guinea Pig. London: Wolfe, 1992.
Authors Vittorio Capello, DVM, and Barbara Oglesbee, DVM

GUINEA PIGS

DERMATOPHYTOSIS

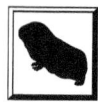

BASICS

DEFINITION
An external fungal infection, caused by *Microsporum* spp. or *Trichophyton* spp., which involves the stratum corneum layer of skin

PATHOPHYSIOLOGY
• *Trichophyton mentagrophytes* most commonly isolated (>90%); occasionally *Microsporum canis*
• May have subclinical carriers
• Young guinea pigs are most often affected due to underdeveloped immune systems and lower amounts of fungistatic fatty acids in sebum.
• Immunosuppressed animals are very susceptible.
• Direct contact and fomites are the most common methods of exposure.

SYSTEMS AFFECTED
Skin/hair

GENETICS
N/A

INCIDENCE/PREVALENCE
Common cause of hair loss in pet guinea pigs

GEOGRAPHIC DISTRIBUTION
N/A

SIGNALMENT
• Most commonly diagnosed in young and immunosuppressed animals

SIGNS
Historical Findings
• Pruritic, focal, circular areas of alopecia and dry crusty skin
• Lesion pattern usually starts on the face and ears, later spreading over the dorsum and limbs

Physical Examination Findings
• Pruritus
• Alopecia (focal circumscribed areas), often with erythematous, raised borders
• Pustules if secondary bacterial infection
• Dry, crusty skin
• Lesions most common on the face, forehead, ears, dorsum, and limbs
• May be signs of underlying disease in immunosuppressed animals
• Asymptomatic carriers common

CAUSES
• *Trichophyton mentagrophytes*; occasionally *Microsporum canis*

RISK FACTORS
• Immunosuppression
• Hypovitaminosis C
• Pregnancy and parturition
• Young animal

• Exposure to an infected animal
• High environmental temperature and humidity

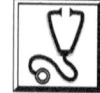

DIAGNOSIS

DIFFERENTIAL DIAGNOSIS

Noninflammatory Diseases that can Directly Inhibit or Slow Hair Follicle Growth:
• Neurological/behavioral—Stress—usually see generalized hair loss; barbering or fur chewing—alopecia can occur anywhere but commonly on rump and perineal areas
• Nutritional deficiencies—particularly protein deficiencies and hypovitaminosis C—see diffuse thinning of hair coat
• Hyperestrogenism—cystic ovarian disease—common cause of symmetric alopecia over the back, ventrum, and flanks; pregnancy-associated alopecia—flanks bilaterally
• Diabetes
• Hypothyroidism (uncommon)

Inflammatory Alopecia
Directly cause destruction or damage to the hair shaft or follicle resulting in severe inflammatory diseases of the dermis (e.g., pruritus, deep pyoderma):
• Ectoparasites
Trixacarus caviae—shoulders, dorsum, and flanks, may be generalized and associated with severe crusting, hyperpigmentation, and lichenification. The pruritus is intense.
• Parasites are readily identified in skin scrapes preparation.
Chirodiscoides caviae—primarily affecting the groin and axilla. Mites are present in the hairs and are easily observed on collected hair.
• Other ectoparasites—*Cheyletiella parasitivorax* usually produces lesions on the dorsum; *Demodex caviae* is frequently located on the head and forelegs. Lice often are associated with lesions around the ears and dorsum.
• Cheilitis—inflammation, ulcerations, scabs, and crusts at mucocutaneous junction of lips and philtrum
• Bacterial pyoderma
Location depends on the inciting cause and may be present anywhere. Exfoliative dermatitis is reported most commonly in the ventral aspect.
• Traumatic episodes (burns)
• Allergic skin diseases (e.g., atopy, food allergy, contact, and insect hypersensitivity) Contact hypersensitivity has been reported in guinea pigs.
• Neoplasia

CBC/BIOCHEMISTRY/URINALYSIS
Need is dependent on the underlying disease process. Most often normal unless a secondary disease condition is present

OTHER LABORATORY TESTS
N/A

IMAGING
N/A

DIAGNOSTIC PROCEDURES
• Wood's lamp examination (should be not relied on solely)—useful to diagnose dermatophytosis caused by *Microsporum* spp. Use is limited in guinea pigs where *Trychophyton mentagrophytes* is the most common dermatophyte and does not fluoresce when exposed to ultraviolet light.
• Fungal culture on Sabouraud's agar—hair can be collected as well as samples obtained from brush techniques. Growth may be slow and take up to 1 month.
• Direct microscopy/hair plucking—the edge of the lesion is the preferred collection site. Fungal arthrospores and hyphae may be observed. Place collected hairs and crusts on DTM.

PATHOLOGIC FINDINGS
Epidermal hyperplasia, hyperkeratosis; arthrospores may be visible

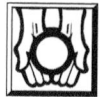

TREATMENT

APPROPRIATE HEALTH CARE
• Most animals are treated as outpatients.
• Isolate affected animals due to infectious and zoonotic potential.

NURSING CARE
• Focal areas should be clipped and cleaned with disinfectants such as dilute povidone iodine or dilute chlorexidine initially.

DIET
• Correcting dietary deficiencies and additional supplementation of vitamin C (50–100 mg/kg SC q24h) until clinical signs resolve. Maintain the animal on daily supplementation of vitamin C (30–50 mg/kg PO q24h) after clinical signs resolve. Vitamin C may be ground and fed directly to the pig. Vitamin C treats are also available for guinea pigs (e.g., Daily C, Oxbow Pet Products, Murdock, NE).

ACTIVITY
N/A

CLIENT EDUCATION
• Dermatophytosis is potentially a zoonotic disease, and other animals, including other species, may have to be treated.
• Treatment of all in-contact animal is essential
• Advise owners to clean the cage—discard bedding, thoroughly disinfect cage

(CONTINUED)

SURGICAL CONSIDERATIONS
N/A

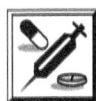

MEDICATIONS

DRUG(S) OF CHOICE
• Systemic antifungals—combined with environmental disinfection is necessary for successful treatment. All in-contact animals should be treated, even if asymptomatic.
  ◦ Terbinafine—drug of choice. More effective than other oral antifungals. Treat all in-contact guinea pigs (20 mg/kg PO q24h × 14–28 days)
  ◦ Itraconazole (5–10 mg/kg PO q24h × 14–28 days)—also effective
  ◦ Griseofulvin (15–25 mg/kg PO q24h × 4–6 weeks) Griseofulvin is teratogenic and therefore should never be administered to pregnant animals.
• Topical treatment—Useful as adjunctive treatment and may cause remission, but seldom cure
  ◦ Antimicrobial shampoos can be used in pyoderma and may be useful as adjunctive therapy in dermatophytosis. Antimicrobial shampoos include chlorhexidine and ethyl lactate shampoos.
  ◦ Antifungal shampoos—ketoconazole, miconazole, and lime sulphur shampoos
  ◦ Topical products may be effective in treating focal lesions; topical solutions/creams include clotrimazole cream (q24h × 2–4 weeks); miconazole, topical treatment (q24h × 2–4 weeks); and 1% butenafine cream (q24h × 10–20 days); take care to prevent ingestion during grooming.
  ◦ Lime sulfur dip—q7d for 4–6 treatments (dilute 1:40 with water) may be effective, but dipping is very stressful to guinea pigs.

PRECAUTIONS
• Dipping and bathing guinea pigs can be stressful.
• Prevent guinea pigs from licking topical products.

• Griseofulvin—causes bone marrow suppression in other species; not yet reported in guinea pigs, but may occur
• Itraconazole—vasculitis and hepatopathy reported in other species; not yet reported in guinea pigs, but may occur

POSSIBLE INTERACTIONS
N/A

ALTERNATIVE DRUGS
N/A

FOLLOW-UP

PATIENT MONITORING
• Monitor for resolution of clinical signs and toxicity to the medications.
• Dermatophyte culture is the only means of truly monitoring response to therapy.
• Weekly CBC is treated with griseofulvin; monitor liver enzymes if treated with ketoconazole or itraconazole

PREVENTION/AVOIDANCE
• Isolation and treatment of sick and in-contact individuals
• Cleaning of the environment

POSSIBLE COMPLICATIONS
Recurrence or lack of treatment response in the young, pregnant, or immunosuppressed patient

EXPECTED COURSE AND PROGNOSIS
Dermatophytosis—good prognosis with early-stage diagnosis
  Will recur if careful disinfection of environment and/or treatment of all in-contact animals is not performed

MISCELLANEOUS

ASSOCIATED CONDITIONS
• Pruritus
• Immunosuppression, underlying disease

AGE-RELATED FACTORS
Young guinea pigs most susceptible

ZOONOTIC POTENTIAL
Dermatophytosis is zoonotic.

PREGNANCY/FERTILITY/BREEDING
Griseofulvin is teratogenic.

SYNONYMS
Ringworm

SEE ALSO
Abscesses
Alopecia
Dermatophytosis
Flea and flea infestation
Lice and mites

ABBREVIATIONS
DTM = dermatophyte test media

INTERNET RESOURCES
N/A

Suggested Reading
Palmerio BS, Roberts H. Clinical approach to dermatologic disease in exotic animals. Vet Clin North Am Exot Anim Pract 2013;16(3):523–577.
Pignon C, Mayer J. Guinea pigs. In: Quesenberry KE, Carpenter JW, eds. Ferrets, Rabbits and Rodents, 4th ed. Clinical Medicine and Surgery. 2021. St. Louis: Saunders, 2020:270–297.
Riggs SM. Guinea pigs. In: Mitchell MA, Tully TN, eds. Manual of Exotic Pet Practice. St Louis: Saunders/Elsevier, 2009:456–473.
White SD, Sanchez-Migallon D, Paul-Murphy J. Skin diseases in companion guinea pigs (*Cavia porcellus*): a retrospective study of 293 cases seen at the Veterinary Medical Teaching Hospital, University of California at Davis (1990–2015). Vet Dermatol 2016;27:395–e100.
Author Thomas N. Tully, Jr., DVM, MS, Dipl. ABVP (Avian), Dipl. ECZM (Avian)

DIARRHEA

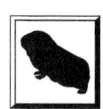

BASICS

DEFINITION
An increase in the frequency, volume, or fluidity of feces

PATHOPHYSIOLGY
• Guinea pigs feed by grazing, are hind-gut (cecal) fermenters, and are normally coprophagic or cecophagic. Proper hind-gut fermentation and gastrointestinal tract motility are dependent on the ingestion of large amounts of coarse fiber. Diets containing inadequate fiber disrupt normal cecal flora, increase the frequency of cecal stool release, and decrease transit time through the colon. The resultant feces (cecotrophs) are softer than normal. Guinea pigs are prone to this so-called cecotrophic diarrhea.
• True diarrhea, characterized by profuse, watery feces, is generally the result of severe disruption of the normal gastrointestinal flora, causing overgrowth of pathogenic bacteria.

SYSTEMS AFFECTED
• Gastrointestinal
• True diarrhea usually results in dehydration, hypovolemia, septicemia, enterotoxemia, and endotoxemia. Resulting decreased organ perfusion and consequences of shock deleteriously affect the entire body.

SIGNALMENT
• Many diarrheal diseases are more common in weanling or young animals.
• No age or gender predilection for cecotrophic diarrhea

SIGNS

Historical Findings—Diarrhea
• Signs often begin soon after arrival to a new environment
• Soft or liquid feces
• Possibly diet fed is low in insoluble fiber
• Depression and lethargy
• Owner may report the impression their pet is painful.
• Fecal staining of perineum
• Bloated abdomen
• Dyspnea
• Subcutaneous ventral swellings (edema)
• Lateral recumbency indicates imminent death
• Sudden death

Historical Findings—Cecotrophic Diarrhea
• Usually bright, alert, normal appetite
• Owners describe soft, pasty, often odiferous stools; intermittent in production and often interspersed with normal-appearing feces
• May be history of recent diet change, stress

• May be history of inappropriate diet (inadequate fiber content)

Physical Examination Findings—Diarrhea
• Degree of abnormalities depends on both type of diarrhea and severity of illness.
• Dehydration
• Perineal area and rear legs may be stained or wet from liquid feces.
• Abdominal palpation may result in painful response. Borborygmus may be increased.
• Underlying cause is often progressive, and it is not uncommon for patients with mild diarrhea and malaise to develop severe clinical signs and decompensate rapidly.
• Severely affected guinea pigs may present with agonal signs. Hypothermia is common and associated with circulatory shock (septic/hypovolemic); subcutaneous edema; may have palpable abdominal fluid wave due to ascites; dyspnea or change in character of respirations can be related to shock, metabolic acidosis, or pleural effusion; lateral recumbency portends imminent death.

Physical Exam Findings—Cecotrophic Diarrhea
• Physical examination findings are usually normal, unless reflecting underlying disease.
• Fecal pasting to fur around perineum

CAUSES AND RISK FACTORS
• Diets low in fiber are the most common cause of cecotrophic diarrhea. Nutritional causes of diarrhea usually increase volume and odor of feces but do not cause liquid feces.
• In pet guinea pigs, the most common cause of true diarrhea is enterotoxemia caused by the administration of antibiotics. Floral changes can occur with any antibiotic, but antibiotics with a predominantly gram-positive spectrum (e.g., penicillins, cephalosporins, lincomycin, erythromycin, tylosin, and clindamycin) are most likely to cause potentially fatal enteric dysbiosis.
• Most other causes of true diarrhea are infectious. Bacterial causes include *Salmonella* spp., *Yersinia pseudotuberculosis*, *Clostridium perfringens*, *E. coli*, *Pseudomonas aeruginosa*, *Clostridium piliforme*, and *Listeria monocytogenes*. Protozoal diarrhea can be caused by cryptosporidium or *Eimeria caviae*. Coronaviral enteritis may occur in weanlings.
• Guinea pigs that are anorexic for longer than 24 hours can develop gastrointestinal stasis and rapidly develop diarrhea and enterotoxemia.
• Neoplastic disease of the GI tract is a rare cause.
• Toxic causes are rare; the most commonly reported cause is aflatoxicosis.
• Idiopathic typhlitis has been reported.

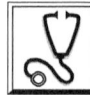

DIAGNOSIS

DIFFERENTIAL DIAGNOSIS
It is important to first differentiate true diarrhea from cecotrophic diarrhea. Cecotrophic diarrhea is characterized by soft, sometimes odiferous stools that are often intermixed with normal-appearing feces. Affected animals generally appear healthy or show signs of other underlying disorders. Guinea pigs with true diarrhea produce liquid diarrhea and quickly show signs of generalized illness.
• Liquid diarrhea can occur with dysbiosis and infectious enteritides.
• Most bacterial enteric infections cause morbidity and mortality in weanling guinea pigs.
• Protozoal diarrhea is more common in weanlings, but immunosuppressed animals of any age are susceptible. Acute coccidiosis is typically seen in weanlings.
• Coronaviral enteritis may occur in weanlings.
• Anorexia and gastrointestinal hypomotility can induce floral changes that will result in enterotoxemia.
• Anamnesis should include review of husbandry and past medical history, especially recent stressors and/or administration of antibiotics.
• Complete physical examination is an essential element in diagnosis of any cause of lethargy, weight loss, pain, or anorexia. Guinea pigs with true diarrhea are usually profoundly ill.
• Most guinea pigs with true diarrhea do not survive. Definitive diagnosis often requires necropsy.

CBC/BIOCHEMISTRY/URINALYSIS
Varies with underlying causes

OTHER LABORATORY TESTS
• Fecal direct examination (with and without Lugol's iodine), fecal floatation, and zinc sulfate centrifugation may demonstrate high protozoal burden or spore-forming bacteria.
• Fecal Gram's stain—may demonstrate large numbers of spore-forming bacteria consistent with *Clostridium* spp. or excessive numbers of gram-negative bacteria.

IMAGING
• Often unremarkable in patients with cecotrophic diarrhea
• In patients with true diarrhea, abdominal radiography is likely to demonstrate ileus with gas distension of intestinal tract; possible peritoneal effusion

• Thoracic radiography may show pleural effusion or microcardia due to hypovolemic shock.

DIAGNOSTIC PROCEDURES
Necropsy is often required for definitive diagnosis.

TREATMENT
NURSING CARE
• Successful treatment of the patient with true diarrhea is rare. Very few patients are reported to survive despite therapy and supportive care.
• Inappropriate antimicrobials (beta lactams, cephalosporins, macrolides, and chlortetracycline) should be discontinued immediately.
• Treatment of endotoxic, septic, and/or hypovolemic shock may be required. Treatment of shock follows the same principle as in dogs and cats, including fluid support (crystalloids), intravascular osmotic support (colloids), maintenance of renal blood flow (e.g., dobutamine), and antimicrobials (IV) for sepsis.
• In the stable patient, rehydration may be possible with subcutaneous fluids. Maintenance needs are estimated at 100 mL/kg/day. Secretory diarrhea can lead to tremendous fluid losses; reevaluate hydration status frequently.
• Treatment of hypothermia with an external heat source is appropriate. However, guinea pigs are obligate intranasal breathers and are prone to heat stroke. Care should be taken to avoid overheating.
• Judicious management of pain is an important component of treatment. Guinea pigs do not deal well with pain. Failure to manage pain effectively will inhibit recovery in any ill guinea pig.
• Transfaunation with feces from normal guinea pigs can be attempted orally and may be effective in mild cases.
• Transfaunation via retention enema has been reported in the rabbit with enteric dysbiosis; however, efficacy in guinea pigs is unknown.
• Cholestyramine (50–75 mg/kg) orally or rectally can be helpful to remove toxins formed by *Clostrida* spp.

DIET
• Guinea pigs that do not eat are extremely prone to further deleterious effects of gastric hypomotility. In the stable patient, assist syringe-feeding with an appropriate herbivore supplement such as Critical Care for Herbivores (Oxbow Pet Products, Murdock, NE) or Emeraid Herbivore (Lafeber

Company, Cornell, IL) is appropriate for patients capable of receiving oral medications. Care must be taken in the dyspneic or struggling patient.
• Diet change alone will often correct cecotrophic diarrhea. Feed a diet that is high in coarse fiber such as long-stemmed grass and timothy hay, high-quality timothy-based guinea pig pellets, fresh vegetables, and appropriate vitamin C supplementation.

CLIENT EDUCATION
Due to the poor prognosis and pain associated with diarrheal illnesses in guinea pigs, euthanasia should be considered for the unstable patient.

MEDICATIONS
DRUG(S) OF CHOICE
• Varies with clinical condition
• Pain should be controlled with opioids (e.g., buprenorphine 0.05 mg/kg SC, IM, IV q8–12h). Severe pain may require mu agonists (hydromorphone 0.1 mg/kg SC, IV q6–12h). NSAIDs should be avoided in face of shock, renal compromise, continuing fluid losses, and dehydration. Once stable, meloxicam (0.2–0.5 mg/kg PO, SC q12–24h) can be administered.
• Maropitant has been anecdotally used to mitigate GI pain at a dose of 1–2 mg/kg SC or slow IV q24h
• For gastric pain and reflux, H2 receptor antagonists may be helpful. Famotidine, cimetidine, or ranitidine can be used at doses appropriate for cats or dogs. Metoclopramide (0.2–1.0 mg/kg PO, SC, IM, IV q12h) may help reduce gastric reflux and increase gastric emptying.
• Oral or intravenous administration of chloramphenicol (30–50 mg/kg PO, SC, IM, IV q8–12h) or metronidazole (10–20 mg/kg PO, IV q12h) may suppress further clostridial overgrowth in patients with enterotoxemia.
• For *Eimeria caviae*—trimethoprim-sulfa (15–30 mg/kg PO q12h × 10 days). No known treatment for cryptosporidium

CONTRAINDICATIONS
• Oral medications are contraindicated in shock.
• Corticosteroids at shock doses will cause immunosuppression. They are contraindicated.
• Antibiotics that select against gram-positive bacteria such as oral penicillins, cephalosporins, lincosamines, or macrolides should not be used in these animals as it can cause fatal dysbiosis and enterotoxemia.

PRECAUTIONS
Meloxicam should be avoided in patients with severe fluid losses, dehydration, shock, and renal compromise.

FOLLOW-UP
PATIENT MONITORING
• Patients that are presented with liquid diarrhea are often critically ill or will become so soon.
• Critical care monitoring for inpatients as in dogs and cats should be considered with understanding of limitations of patient size.
• An end to liquid stools in the stable patient indicates improvement.
• Any abnormal changes noted on diagnostic testing should be periodically evaluated for resolution.

PREVENTION/AVOIDANCE
• Proper diet and environmental hygiene
• Avoid overcrowding and stressors.
• Avoid immunosuppression and administration of corticosteroids.
• While no antibiotic is free from risk on any individual patient, consider use of only the following antibiotics: chloramphenicol (30–50 mg/kg PO, SC, IM, IV q8–12h), ciprofloxacin (5–25 mg/kg PO q12h), doxycycline (2.5–5 mg/kg PO q12h), enrofloxacin (5–20 mg/kg PO q12–24h; initial dose may be administered IM), metronidazole (10–20 mg/kg PO q12h), trimethoprim-sulfa (15–30 mg/kg PO q12h), and azithromycin (15–30 mg/kg q24h)
• During antibiotic use, be sure food intake and stools are normal. Supplementation with high-fiber dietary assist-feeding formulas such as those discussed above under Treatment will support normal GI function.

POSSIBLE COMPLICATIONS
• If the patient survives the enterotoxemia, subsequent gastrointestinal hypomotility is likely to present further therapeutic challenges.
• Patients may require a prolonged course of assist-feeding and hydration support.

EXPECTED COURSE AND PROGNOSIS
• Cecotrophic diarrhea usually carries a good prognosis with appropriate diet modification.
• For the critically ill patient, prognosis is grave. For the stable patient, prognosis is guarded and may need to be adjusted to grave based on clinical progression. Most guinea pigs will not survive true diarrheal illnesses.

DIARRHEA

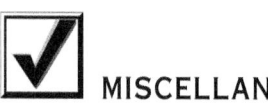

MISCELLANEOUS

AGE-RELATED FACTORS
Weanling and young animals are at greatest risk of infectious causes of true diarrhea.

SEE ALSO
Antibiotic-associated enterotoxemia
Gastrointestinal hypomotility and gastrointestinal stasis
Tyzzer's disease

INTERNET RESOURCES
Veterinary Information Network
(www.vin.com)

Suggested Reading
DeCubellis J. Common emergencies in rabbits, guinea pigs, and chinchillas. Vet Clin Exot Anim 2016;19:411–429.
Minarikova A, Hauptman K, Jeklova E et al. Diseases in pet guinea pigs: a retrospective study in 1000 animals. Vet Rec 2015;177(8):200–200.
Percy DH, Barthold SW. Pathology of Laboratory Rodents and Rabbits, 3rd ed. Ames: Blackwell, 2007:225–226, 235–236.
Pignon C, Mayer J. Guinea pigs. In: Quesenberry KE, Carpenter JW, eds. Ferrets, Rabbits and Rodents, 4th ed. Clinical Medicine and Surgery. 2021 ed. St. Louis: Saunders, 2020:270–297.
Ritzman TK. Diagnosis and clinical management of gastrointestinal conditions in exotic companion mammals (rabbits, guinea pigs, and chinchillas). Vet Clin Exot Anim 2014;17:179–194.

Author Jeffrey L. Rhody, DVM, DABVP-ECM

DYSPNEA AND TACHYPNEA

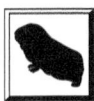

BASICS

DEFINITION
• Dyspnea: the feeling of distress associated with difficult or labored breathing leading to shortness of breath
• Tachypnea: an increased rate of respiration, not necessarily associated with labored breathing
• Open-mouth breathing is a poor prognostic indicator in guinea pigs because they are obligate nasal breathers. Open-mouth breathing can occur with severe upper or lower respiratory tract disease, resulting in complete obstruction of the nasal passages.

PATHOPHYSIOLOGY
• Primary respiratory disease can be caused by upper or lower respiratory tract problems.
• Nonrespiratory causes of dyspnea include abnormalities in pulmonary vascular tone (CNS disease, shock), pulmonary circulation (CHF), oxygenation (anemia), or ventilation (obesity, ascites, abdominal organomegaly, and musculoskeletal disease).

SYSTEMS AFFECTED
• Respiratory
• Cardiovascular
• Nervous (secondary to hypoxia)
• Gastrointestinal (secondary to inappropriate ingestion of air [bloat, secondary gastrointestinal stasis])

GENETICS
Unknown

INCIDENCE/PREVALENCE
Respiratory disease is commonly encountered in clinical practice.

GEOGRAPHIC DISRIBUTION
Widespread

SIGNALMENT
No breed, sex, or gender predilection

SIGNS

Historical Findings
Vary depending on cause: anorexia, lethargy, weight loss, nasal or ocular discharge, coughing, sneezing, exercise intolerance, wheezing/labored breathing, dyspnea, history of recent intubation or multiple attempts at intubation, poor husbandry, including inappropriate ventilation, aromatic substrate, or poor cleanliness

Physical Examination Findings
• Lethargy, weight loss, poor hair coat, pyrexia (bacterial or viral infections), and anorexia (may show signs of gastrointestinal stasis, and bloat)
• Upper respiratory tract disease: serous or mucopurulent nasal discharge, ocular

discharge, and dental disease (ptyalism, bruxism, and facial abscess)
• Upper airway obstruction: open-mouth breathing, stertor, stridor, and increased respiratory effort
• Pneumonia: abnormal breath sounds on auscultation, including crackles, wheezes, increased bronchovesicular sounds, or decreased or absent breath sounds with abscess, lung consolidation, neoplasia, or heart disease (effusion)
• Bloat if aerophagia is present.

CAUSES

Respiratory Causes
Upper respiratory tract
• Nasal passage obstruction: rhinitis or sinusitis, dental disease (maxillary tooth roots can extend into the nasal passages and lead to secondary bacterial infections or obstruction of nasal passages, tooth root abscesses can also develop), trauma (face, nose, and neck), foreign body, and neoplasia
• Common bacteria isolated from ondotogenic abscesses include *Bacteroides fragilis*, *Pasturella multocida*, and *Peptostreptococcus anaerobius*
• Laryngotracheal obstruction: foreign body, abscess, neoplasia, multiple traumatic intubation attempts leading to laryngeal edema
Lower respiratory tract
• Pneumonia: usually bacterial (*Bordetella brochiseptica* [most common], *Streptococcus pneumoniae*, *Streptobacillus moniliformis*, *Yersinia pseudotuberculosis*, *Haemophilus* spp., *Streptococcus zooepidemicus*, *Klebsiella pneumoniae*, *Pseudomonas aeruginosa*, *Pasturella multocida*, *Staphylococcus aureus*, and *Streptococcus pyogenes*) but can also be viral (adenovirus and parainfluenza virus—rare) or due to aspiration
• Neoplasia (brochogenic papillary adenoma, metastatic, and maxillary odontoma/elodontoma), pulmonary edema (cardiogenic or noncardiogenic), pulmonary contusion (trauma), allergy, intrathoracic tracheal disease (neoplasia, abscess, and foreign body)
• Extraluminal tracheal compression due to an abscess or neoplasia
• Traumatic airway rupture (uncommon)

Nonrespiratory Causes
• Anxiety, pain, fever, heat stroke, and obesity
• Abdominal distension: pregnancy, organomegaly, ascites, and gastric/cecal dilation
• Cardiac disease: CHF, cardiogenic shock, and severe arrhythmias
• Metabolic: acidosis, uremia
• Neuromuscular disease: severe CNS disease (trauma, abscess, neoplasia, and inflammation) and spinal disease (trauma)
• Hematologic: anemia

RISK FACTORS
• Poor husbandry: using substrate with aromatic oils such as pine and cedar, which can be irritating to respiratory mucosa, poor sanitation (ammonia build-up in the bedding), infrequent cage cleaning, over-crowding, improper ventilation/humidity/temperature control, inhaled irritants such as disinfectants (bleach, etc.), and smoke
• Poor diet: feeding diets deficient in vitamin C can lead to immunosuppression; diets deficient in coarse fiber (long-stemmed grass hay) can lead to dental disease
• Immunosuppression: caused by lack of vitamin C in the diet, stress, concurrent disease, corticosteroid use, age, and genetics
• Traumatic intubation, multiple intubation attempts, or inadvertent laryngeal trauma during dental procedures can cause laryngeal edema.
• Dental disease: Maxillary tooth roots can extend into the nasal passages and lead to secondary bacterial infections or obstruction of nasal passages; tooth root abscesses can also develop.

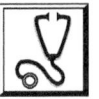

DIAGNOSIS

DIFFERENTIAL DIAGNOSIS
• Tachypnea may be present without dyspnea. It may be a physiologic response to anxiety, fear, pain, physical exertion, fever, heat stress, or acidosis.
• Dyspnea due to upper respiratory tract disease is often more pronounced with inspiration, whereas lower respiratory tract disease is often associated with increased expiratory effort.
• Tracheal mass or foreign body usually causes both inspiratory and expiratory effort.
• Pneumonia often has systemic signs of disease (anorexia, weight loss, depression, and lethargy), whereas primary cardiac disease often is associated with a murmur or arrhythmia.

CBC/BIOCHEMISTRY/URINALYSIS
• An elevation in total white blood cell count is uncommon, but a shift in proportion of heterophils to lymphocytes with an increase in heterophils and decrease in lymphocytes can occur in systemic disease, causing inflammation.
• Increases in platelet number can also be seen with inflammation.
• Chemistry panel may help to define the underlying cause with metabolic diseases.

OTHER LABORATORY TESTS
• Enzyme-linked immunosorbent assay (ELISA) and indirect immunofluorescence assays for *B. bronchiseptica* are more sensitive

than culture for detection of the organism, but they only detect antibodies and thus indicate exposure rather than active infection.
• ELISA for *S. pneumoniae*—only detects antibodies and thus indicates exposure rather than active infection
• PCR test for adenovirus is described but not readily available unless in lab animal setting

IMAGING
• Radiographs of the skull: must be done under heavy sedation or general anesthesia for optimal positioning, with a minimum of five views (lateral, two oblique laterals, anterior posterior, and ventrodorsal views) recommended, observe radiographs for bony lysis or proliferation of the turbinates and facial bones, as this can indicate chronic bacterial or neoplastic processes; tooth roots should also be assessed as they can penetrate the nasal sinuses, leading to obstruction or bacterial infection.
• CT or MRI: provide better imaging quality; may be more diagnostic than skull radiographs, especially if nasal detail is obscured by nasal discharge; can help to determine whether the cause of disease is nasal, sinus, or dental disease. CT specifically is excellent for providing bony detail, is more sensitive for area encased in bone (i.e., lungs and sinuses), and the procedure time is relatively short. However, these modalities may be cost prohibitive and not as readily available.
• Thoracic radiographs: pneumonia (alveolar pattern with increased pulmonary density which can be patchy or diffuse—air bronchograms, consolidated lung lobes), pulmonary edema, small airway disease, and cardiomegaly
• Abdominal radiographs: organomegaly, ascites, and gas-filled/distended stomach due to aerophagia or bloat
• Ultrasonography: echocardiography difficult due to small size of patient but may help determine if primary heart disease is present; abdominal ultrasound may be used for the evaluation of organomegaly, pregnancy, or masses

DIAGNOSTIC PROCEDURES
• Cytology of exudates: can use Gram stain or standard cell stain (Diff Quick)
• Culture of exudates: can be difficult to obtain a good sample, many normal commensal organisms located in the nasal passages and oral cavity, can obtain a culture with a mini tip culturette inserted into the nostril, causative agent may be located in the sinuses, which are difficult to sample
• Nasal cavity biopsy: should be performed in animals with chronic nasal discharge (especially epistaxis) if neoplasia is suspected; use endoscopy or rhinotomy to obtain sample

• Direct visualization of the pharynx or larynx: can use a 2.7-mm rigid endoscope for direct visualization, requires general anesthesia; guinea pigs have abundant soft tissue in the oral cavity, a long narrow passage between the dental arcades, and a small oral opening, making visualization difficult. However, this method may facilitate laryngeal mound sampling for cytology or culture if a lesion is visualized.
• Transtracheal wash or bronchoalveolar lavage can be difficult to perform in guinea pigs due to oral cavity anatomy, small tracheal size, and patient temperament.
• Lung aspirate can be performed with ultrasound guidance; however, diagnostic success in lung aspirates is generally regarded as low unless a specific lesion for aspiration can be identified.
• Thoracocentesis or abdominocentesis: fluid analysis and culture

PATHOLOGIC FINDINGS
N/A

TREATMENT
APPROPRIATE HEALTH CARE
Depends on the underlying cause

NURSING CARE
• Supplying an oxygen-rich environment is most important if the patient is dyspneic. Use an oxygen cage or induction chamber in a quiet environment.
• Fluid therapy to maintain normal hydration (guinea pigs fluid needs are 100 mL/kg/day)—fluid can be given IV, IO, or SC. Necessary to keep the GI tract hydrated and to aid mucocilliary clearance; may consider reductions in the maintenance fluid requirement if cardiac disease is suspected.
• Keep patients in a quiet, predator-free environment to decrease stress; always provide a hide box.
• Eliminate anxiety, pain, exertion as much as possible, as these may lead to increased respiratory effort/rate, which could worsen the patient's condition.
• Keep nares clear of nasal discharge.
• Nebulization with bland aerosols may help deliver moisture to the upper respiratory tract, and if used in conjunction with antibiotics, may lead to resolution.
• If trachea is completely obstructed, will need to attempt emergency intubation (very difficult in guinea pigs due to very small opening for intubation and redundant oral tissues) or emergency tracheostomy
• Thoracocentesis or abdominocentesis: may be diagnostic and therapeutic in patients with pleural space disease or abdominal effusion

• Surgery may be necessary to remove foreign bodies, obtain biopsy samples, or debulk tumors, abscesses, or granulomas. Maintaining adequate ventilation in these situations is difficult.

ACTIVITY
Patient's activity should be restricted as exertion can increase respiratory effort and/or rate, which can worsen obstructive airway disease.

DIET
• Anorexia can cause GI hypomotility/stasis, overgrowth of intestinal bacterial pathogens, and imbalance of GI microflora. Therefore, guinea pigs need to continue eating throughout treatment. Low-dose buprenorphine or midazolam may reduce hospital anxiety and have polyphagia effects leading to a greater likelihood that animals will eat in the hospital while having minimal cardiorespiratory effects.
• Offer a wide variety of fresh, moistened vegetables such as cilantro, parsley, romaine lettuce, dandelion greens, etc., as well as good-quality grass hay (orchard grass, western timothy).
• If the patient refuses to eat or is not maintaining condition, can syringe-feed Critical Care for Herbivores (Oxbow Pet Products, Murdock, NE) or Emeraid Herbivore (Lafeber Company, Cornell, IL) 10–15 mL/kg orally every 6–8 hours. A gruel of ground-up guinea pig pellets with vegetable baby foods, water, or fresh greens can also be used, but this is not as nutritionally complete as commercially available syringe-feeding formulas. A dyspneic guinea pig should be syringe-fed small amounts slowly and very carefully. They should be syringe-fed from the diastema rather than deep in the mouth, as gasping for air could result in inhalation of food.
• Guinea pigs require an exogenous source of vitamin C supplementation, which can be given at 50–100 mg/kg/day SC when ill.
• Encourage oral fluid intake to maintain hydration by offering water or wet vegetables.
• Aerophagia can cause hypomotility and gastrointesintal stasis.

CLIENT EDUCATION
If the underlying disease cannot be corrected (i.e., dental disease, neoplasia, and severe tissue destruction), a cure is unlikely. The treatment, depending on the cause, can be lifelong and aims to control the severe clinical signs.
    Streptococcus zooepidemicus is transmissible to other guinea pigs, and *Pasteurella* species can be transmitted to other animals.

SURGICAL CONSIDERATIONS
Anesthesia to correct dental disease or to remove foreign bodies, obtain biopsy samples, or debulk tumors, abscesses, or

granulomas may be more risky in these patients because the patient's ability to protect its airway and use the muscles that open airways is compromised by anesthesia. Sedatives may also relax the upper airway muscles, which can worsen the obstruction. Use of probiotics or prebiotics prior to surgery can be considered.

MEDICATIONS

DRUG(S) OF CHOICE
• Oxygen therapy is the most useful treatment if the patient is severely dyspneic.
• Definitive therapy is based on the primary disorder, including antibiotics, anti-inflammatories, bronchodilators, cardiac drugs, etc.

CONTRAINDICATIONS
• Oral administration of antibiotics that select against gram-positive bacteria, such as penicillins, cephalosporins, lincosamines, or macrolides, should not be used in these animals as it can cause fatal dysbiosis and enterotoxemia.
• Procaine, which is included in some penicillin preparations, can be toxic to guinea pigs.

PRECAUTIONS
• Any antibiotic can cause diarrhea, which should be monitored in these patients and the antibiotic discontinued if diarrhea is present. Supplementation with probiotics or guinea pig transfaunation can be considered.
• Corticosteroid use can suppress the immune system and exacerbate a bacterial infection. However, short-term topical or systemic corticosteroid may be considered if necessary to reduce laryngeal edema of known cause.
• Sedatives can relax the upper airway muscles, worsening the obstruction, and anesthesia decreases the patient's ability to protect its airway and use the muscles that open its airway. However, light sedation can also decrease anxiety and give muscle relaxation, which may increase the animal's ability to effectively ventilate.
• Patients with CHF or blunt force trauma to the chest are at risk for iatrogenic fluid overload leading to pulmonary edema. Respiratory rate and effort should be monitored frequently in these patients.

POSSIBLE INTERACTIONS
N/A

ALTERNATIVE DRUGS
N/A

FOLLOW-UP

PATIENT MONITORING
• Continue to monitor patient for relapse via clinical signs.
• Repeat any abnormal tests.

PREVENTION/AVOIDANCE
• Depends on the underlying disease
• Improve husbandry and diet (ensure appropriate vitamin C supplementation).
• Avoid stressful situations and corticosteroid use.
• Avoid repeated, especially blind, intubation attempts. Intubate with caution or with endoscope guidance in this species.
• Prevent dental disease by providing high-fiber foods, especially good-quality hay. Yearly veterinary exams with periodic trimming of overgrown teeth as needed

POSSIBLE COMPLICATIONS
• Depends on the underlying disease
• Relapse, progression of disease and death are common
• Bloat, GI stasis due to ingestion of air

EXPECTED COURSE AND PROGNOSIS
Prognosis is based on cause of disease, severity, and chronicity. If the underlying disease cannot be corrected (i.e., dental disease, neoplasia, cardiac disease, organomegaly, etc.), a cure is unlikely. The treatment, depending on the cause, can be lifelong and aims to control the clinical signs. Relapse, progression of disease, and death are common. A severely dyspneic or tachypneic guinea pig that does not improve over 12 hours, despite supportive care and appropriate therapy, has a guarded prognosis.

MISCELLANEOUS

ASSOCIATED CONDITIONS
• GI hypomotility/stasis
• Dental disease
• Hypovitaminosis C
• Rhinitis and sinusitis
• Pneumonia
• Stertor and stridor
• Nasal discharge and sneezing

AGE-RELATED FACTORS
N/A

ZOONOTIC POTENTIAL
Streptobacillus moniliformis is the cause of rat bite fever in humans. Guinea pigs may be a reservoir for *Streptococcus pneumoniae*, with subclinical carriage rate up to 50% in some guinea pig colonies. Close contact between pets and children could be a risk factor although relevance in human hosts is not clearly defined.

PREGNANCY/FERTILITY/BREEDING
N/A

SYNONYMS
None

SEE ALSO
Dental malocclusion
Dyspnea and tachypnea
Nasal discharge and sneezing
Pneumonia
Rhinitis and sinusitis

ABBREVIATIONS
CHF = congestive heart failure
CNS = central nervous system
CT = computed tomography
ELISA = enzyme-linked immunosorbent assay
GI = gastrointestinal
IO = intraosseous
MRI = magnetic resonance imaging
PCR = polymerase chain reaction

INTERNET RESOURCES
www.vin.com
www.merckvetmanual.com

Suggested Reading
Harkness JE, Murray KA, Wagner JE. Biology and diseases of guinea pigs. In: Fox JG, Anderson LC, Loew FM, Quimby FW, eds. Laboratory Animal Medicine, 2nd ed. San Diego: Elsevier, 2002:212–220.
Hawkins MG, Bishop CR. Disease problems of guinea pigs. In: Quesenberry KE, Carpenter JW, eds. Ferrets, Rabbits and Rodents: Clinical Medicine and Surgery, 3rd ed. St. Louis: Elsevier Saunders, 2012:298–299.
Hawkins MG, Graham JE. Emergency and critical care of rodents. Vet Clin North Am Exot Anim Pract 2007;10:501–531.
Minarikova A, Hauptman K, Jeklova E et al. Diseases in pet guinea pigs: a retrospective study in 1000 animals. Vet Rec 2015;177(8):200.
Minarikova A, Hauptman K, Knotek Z et al. Microbial flora of odontogenic abscesses in pet guinea pigs. Vet Rec 2016;179(13):331.
Riggs SM. Guinea pigs. In: Mitchell MA, Tully TN, eds. Manual of Exotic Pet Practice. St Louis: WB Saunders, 2009:456–471.
Robinson NJ, Lyons E, Grindlay D et al. Veterinarian nominated common conditions of rabbits and guinea pigs compared with published literature. Vet Sci 2017;4(4):58.

Authors Christy L. Rettenmund, DVM, Dipl. ACZM and J. Jill Heatley, DVM, MS, Dipl. ABVP (Avian, Reptilian, Amphibian), Dipl. ACZM

DYSTOCIA

GUINEA PIGS

BASICS

DEFINITION
Any difficult or abnormal parturition with or without assistance

PATHOPHYSIOLOGY
• The most common cause of dystocia in the guinea pig is the restricted size of the birth canal due to inadequate pubic symphysis relaxation at parturition secondary to mineralization of the fibrocartilaginous joint of the pubic symphysis.
  ◦ This mineralization occurs normally at 6–8 months of age in the nulliparous sow.
• The sow can begin breeding at 2–3 months of age, and breeding prior to 7 months of age prevents mineralization of the pubic symphysis.
  ◦ If the first breeding occurs after 8 months of age, there is a high probability that mineralization will occur.
• Guinea pig neonates are large relative to the dam, which can lead to complications in the delivery.
• Oversized or deformed fetuses will also cause dystocia.
  ◦ Most common pup-related cause of dystocia
• Obesity contributes to dystocia.
• Nutritional deficiencies
  ◦ Hypovitaminosis C has also been implicated as a contributing factor in dystocia, perhaps due to its effect on capillary fragility leading to excessive hemorrhage.
• Uterine inertia or uterine torsion is less common causes of dystocia.
• The average gestation period is 68 days but can range from 59 to 72 days, depending on the size of the litter.

SYSTEMS AFFECTED
Reproductive system

GENETICS
N/A

INCIDENCE/PREVALENCE
More predisposed to dystocia than other rodents due to their large pup size, narrow pelvic canals, and fusion of the pubic symphysis

GEOGRAPHIC DISTRIBUTION
N/A

SIGNALMENT
Mean Age and Range
Primiparous sows bred after 8 months of age

Historical Findings
• Mating occurred 59–78 days prior to presentation

• Mammary gland development within the last few days
• Sow has been straining for more than a 20-minute period
• Sow has been intermittently straining for over 2 hours
• Anxiety—circling, vocalizations
• Biting at the lateral body wall
• Vaginal discharge—opaque or bloody
• Anorexia
• Lethargy

Physical Examination Findings
• Sow may have body score greater than 5 out of 10
• Palpation of fetal masses in caudal abdomen. If only 1–2 fetuses present, then oversized fetuses are more likely
• Palpation of pelvic aperture; if symphysis is relaxed and separated 2–3 cm, then pups may be able to be delivered vaginally. If symphysis is firm and not separated, then cesarean section is indicated.
• Painful abdomen if uterine torsion present
• Gentle abdominal palpation to determine if uterine contractions present
• Sow is restless and irritable.
• Hunched posture, straining or lethargy and weakness if labor has been prolonged
• Vaginal discharge may be bloody or green colored.

CAUSES AND RISK FACTORS
• Most common cause is breeding of the sow after 7 months of age and pubic symphysis is unable to relax
• Oversized fetuses—often associated with small litter size
  ◦ Normal neonate is approximately 10% of sow body weight
• Malposition in birth canal
  ◦ Problems can occur when only one rear leg is presented in the birth canal, when one or both forelegs point backward, and when the head presents facing backward, sideways (ears first), or tipping downward.
  ◦ Dystocia can also develop when the back or shoulders present first at the birth canal.
• Abnormality of vaginal vault such as stricture, hyperplasia, aplasia, intraluminal, or extraluminal mass in vagina
• Uterine inertia, ineffective uterine contractions

DIAGNOSIS

DIFFERENTIAL DIAGNOSIS
• Pseudopregnancy—if fertilization fails, pseudopregnancy can occur and last 72 days. Differentiate from pregnancy by palpation, radiographs 6 weeks after mating, or abdominal ultrasound.

• Pregnancy toxemia—usually not straining or showing contractions; ketonuria present

CBC/BIOCHEMISTRY/URINALYSIS
• Hemogram—depends on length and cause of dystocia. If fetal death has occurred may see toxic heterophils; thrombocytosis with acute inflammation
• Biochemistry panel—prolonged dystocia may result in hypoglycemia, dehydration, and hypocalcemia.
  ◦ Hypocalcemia is present with uterine inertia

OTHER LABORATORY TESTS
N/A

IMAGING
• Radiography of the abdomen and pelvic area will determine number, size, and position of fetuses.
• Ultrasonography is useful for determining if fetal number and viability. Can also determine if uterine inertia is present.

DIAGNOSTIC PROCEDURES
N/A

TREATMENT

APPROPRIATE HEALTH CARE
• If pubic symphysis is relaxed, oxytocin should promote delivery within 30 minutes of administration.
• Glucose and calcium supplementation can be delivered orally if indicated by biochemistry values. Glucose can be added if intravenous fluids being administered. Do not administer calcium intravenously.

NURSING CARE
• IV access is difficult in the guinea pig; lateral saphenous vein catheters often kink; consider intraosseous catheterization if IV fluids are needed.
• Fluid therapy with balanced electrolyte solutions should be initiated in patients with evidence of dehydration. Maintenance fluid needs are 100 mL/kg/day. Subcutaneous fluids can be administered (50 mL/kg) as needed.
• Postoperative management includes assisted feeding, fluids, analgesics, and broad-spectrum antibiotics.
• Bandaging the abdomen may be warranted because incision site will be in constant contact with the cage floor.

ACTIVITY
Reduced activity in the 2-week postoperative period.

CLIENT EDUCATION
• New guinea pig owners can be educated regarding the changes that occur to the pubic symphysis as the guinea pig matures and the

importance to not breed after the sow is 7 months of age.
• Owners should be educated about proper nutrition and cautioned about the detrimental effects of overfeeding guinea pigs.

SURGICAL CONSIDERATIONS
• Cesarean section indicated if fetuses are viable and pubic symphysis is fused, if sow does not respond to oxytocin, or for oversized or malpositioned fetus.
• Ovariohysterectomy recommended to prevent further pregnancies if a fused pelvic symphysis is diagnosed and the sow is to remain with a male.
• Uterine torsion requires surgical delivery of fetuses and correction of torsion or ovariohysterectomy.

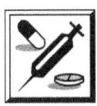

MEDICATIONS
DRUG(S) OF CHOICE
• Administer oxytocin 0.2–3.0 IU/kg IM or SC to induce uterine contractions. Can be repeated once within 15–20 minutes. If pups not delivered within 1 hour, surgical intervention is indicated.
• Pain management is essential during and following surgery. Multimodal therapy is recommended for perioperative analgesia with an anxiolytic, such as midazolam (0.4–2.0 mg/kg IM), an opioid such as butorphanol (0.4–2.0 mg/kg SC, IM q4–12h), or buprenorphine (0.05–0.2 mg/kg SC, IM q6–8h). An NSAID such as meloxicam (0.5–1 mg/kg PO, SC, IM q24h) or carprofen (4 mg/kg SC q24h or 1–2 mg/kg PO q12h–24h) can be given in the perioperative period when the animal is fully hydrated and renal perfusion is no longer compromised. Tramadol, a synthetic opioid, may also be an effective at dosages of 5–10 mg/kg PO q12h postoperatively. For severe to moderate pain pure mu opioids such as morphine (0.5–2.0 mg/kg SC, IM q2–4h) or oxymorphone (0.2–0.5 mg/kg SC, IM q40–12h) should be used; however, appetite and fecal output should be monitored as these opioids are thought to contribute to GI ileus.
• Antibiotic therapy may be indicated if vaginitis present or surgical intervention occurred and incision is difficult to maintain in a clean environment. Antimicrobial choice should be based upon the results of culture and sensitivity if surgical tissues are cultured.

CONTRAINDICATIONS
• Oxytocin is contraindicated with obstructive dystocia (fetus too large for pelvic delivery) or malposition or if longstanding fetal death.

• Oral administration of antibiotics that select against gram-positive bacteria (penicillins, cephalosporins, macrolides, and lincosamides) can cause fatal enteric dysbiosis and enterotoxaemia.
• Potentially nephrotoxic drugs (e.g., aminoglycosides, NSAIDs) in patients that are febrile or dehydrated, or have preexisting renal disease

PRECAUTIONS
• Avoid drugs that reduce blood pressure or induce cardiac dysrhythmia until dehydration is resolved.
• During surgery avoid excessive handling of gastrointestinal tissues to reduce postoperative ileus or fibrous adhesions.
• The obese sow has additional anesthetic risks.

POSSIBLE INTERACTIONS
None

ALTERNATIVE DRUGS
N/A

FOLLOW-UP
PATIENT MONITORING
• Ensure gastrointestinal motility by making sure the patient is eating, well hydrated, and passing normal feces prior to release.
• Ultrasonography to insure all fetuses have been delivered

PREVENTION/AVOIDANCE
• Breed guinea pigs prior to 8 months of age to ensure relaxation of pubic symphysis at birth.
• Avoid overfeeding the breeding sow.
• OVH to prevent future pregnancies essential

POSSIBLE COMPLICATIONS
• Loss of neonates if treatment is not provided promptly
• Postoperative gastrointestinal ileus may take days to weeks to resolve.

EXPECTED COURSE AND PROGNOSIS
• The prognosis is fair to good if neonates can be vaginally delivered.
• The prognosis is guarded if surgical cesarean section or ovariohysterectomy is required.

MISCELLANEOUS
ASSOCIATED CONDITIONS
Following delivery of pups, vaginitis, metritis, or pyometra can occur from ascending bacterial infection.

AGE-RELATED FACTORS
Dystocia due to fusion of the pelvic symphysis is due to late breeding of the nulliparous sow.

ZOONOTIC POTENTIAL
N/A

PREGNANCY/FERTILITY/BREEDING
Best to surgically sterilize guinea pig, thus preventing future pregnancies

SYNONYMS
N/A

SEE ALSO
N/A

ABBREVIATIONS
NSAIDs = nonsteroidal anti-inflammatory drugs
OVH = ovariohysterectomy

INTERNET RESOURCES
www.acbaonline.com/pdf/ACBA%20 Health%20Dystocia.pdf

Suggested Reading
Harkness JE, Turner PV, Vande Woude S et al. Specific diseases and conditions. In: Harkness JE, Turner PV, Vande Woude S et al., eds. Harkness and Wagner's Biology and Medicine of Rabbits and Rodents. Ames: Wiley-Blackwell, 2010:249–396.
Hawkins M, Bishop C. Diseases of guinea pigs. In: Carpenter J, Quesenberry K, eds. Ferrets, Rabbits, and Rodents: Clinical Medicine and Surgery, 3rd ed. St Louis: Elsevier, 2012:295–310.
Hoefer H, Latney L. Rodents: urogenital and reproductive disorders. In: Keeble E, Meredith A, eds. BSAVA Manual of Rodents and Ferrets. Gloucester: BSAVA, 2009:216–218.
Miwa Y, Sladky K. Common surgical procedures of rodents, ferrets, hedgehogs, and sugar gliders. Vet Clin Exot Anim 2016;19:205–244.
Nakamura C. Reproduction and reproductive disorders in guinea pigs. Exotic DVM 2000;2(2):11–16.
Sadar MJ, Knych HK, Drazenovich TL et al. Pharmacokinetics of buprenorphine after intravenous and oral transmucosal administration in guinea pigs (Cavia porcellus). Am J Vet Res 2018;79(3):260–266.
Authors Jessica Comolli, DVM and Rodney Schnellbacher, DVM, Dipl. ACZM

DYSURIA, HEMATURIA, AND POLLAKIURIA

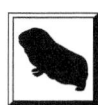

BASICS

DEFINITION
• Dysuria—difficult or painful urination
• Hematuria—the presence of blood in the urine. It is important to differentiate true hematuria from blood originating from the reproductive tract in females, and from orange, red, or red-brown colored urine caused by the excretion of dietary pigments via the urine.
• Pollakiuria—voiding small quantities of urine with increased frequency

PATHOPHYSIOLOGY
• Inflammatory and noninflammatory disorders of the lower urinary tract may decrease bladder compliance and storage capacity by damaging compliance of the bladder wall or by stimulating sensory nerve endings located in the bladder or urethra. Sensations of bladder fullness, urgency, and pain stimulate premature micturition and reduce functional bladder capacity. Dysuria and pollakiuria are generally caused by lesions of the urinary bladder and/or urethra, but these clinical signs do not exclude concurrent involvement of the upper urinary tract or disorders of other body systems.
• The most common causes of dysuria, pollakiuria, and hematuria in the guinea pig are cystitis, urolithiasis, pyometra, and dystocia.
• Urinary tract infections involving *E. coli*, *Streptococcus pyogenes*, and *Staphylococcus* spp. have been associated with pyometra, cystitis, and the presence of urinary calculi in guinea pigs. Pure cultures of *Corynebacterium renale* and *Facklamia* spp. and mixed bacterial cultures including *C. renale, Streptococcus bovis/equinus* group, and *Staphylococcus* spp. were cultured from urine of pet guinea pigs with urolithiasis, but a direct association was not confirmed. Also, *Streptococcus viridans*, *Proteus mirablis,* and mixed growth with *S. viridans, Staphylococcus* spp., *E. coli*, or *Enterococcus* spp. have been reported from cultures of some calculi.
• The etiopathogenesis of urolithiasis in guinea pigs is unclear, although the alkaline pH and high mineral content of normal guinea pig urine may favor crystal formation and precipitation. Recent reports have more commonly identified calcium carbonate calculi, but calcium oxalate and struvite have been reported.
• Guinea pigs with urolithiasis are more likely to be fed a diet high in overall percentage pellets, low in percentage hay, and less variety of vegetables and fruits. Alfalfa-based pellets and hay contain higher

concentrations of calcium, and it has been suggested this may also contribute to urinary calculi in guinea pigs.
• Inadequate water intake leading to a more concentrated urine and factors that impair complete evacuation of the bladder, such as lack of exercise, obesity, cystitis, neoplasia, or neuromuscular diseases may be associated with these signs. Without frequent urination and dilute urine, calcium crystals may precipitate from the urine within the bladder. Precipitated crystals primarily develop uroliths in guinea pigs but occasionally develop "urinary sludge" instead.
• Uroliths may also form in the kidneys or ureters, as well as the bladder.

SYSTEMS AFFECTED
• Renal/Urologic—bladder, urethra
• Reproductive—pyometra, dystocia

GENETICS
Unknown, but inherited factors have been suggested for urolithiasis

INCIDENCE/PREVALENCE
Urinary tract infections caused by hypercrystalluria and/or urolithiasis are very common problems seen in guinea pigs and may contribute to the development of these signs.

GEOGRAPHIC DISTRIBUTION
N/A

SIGNALMENT
Breed Predilections
N/A

Mean Age and Range
Can occur at any age, but middle-aged guinea pigs (2.5–5 years old) are the most common

Predominant Sex
May be seen more frequently in sows with infections, this can be due to the proximity of the urethral orifice to the anus and also due to uterine disorders.

SIGNS
Historical Findings
• Straining to urinate, small, frequent urinations and/or urinating when picked up by the owners
• Hematuria, or thick white- or tan-appearing urine
• Urine staining in the perineal area, urine scald, and moist pyoderma
• Anorexia, weight loss, lethargy, bruxism, and a hunched posture in guinea pigs with chronic or obstructive upper and lower urinary tract disease
• Gross hematuria—common in guinea pigs with urolithiasis
• Pollakiuria or stranguria; evidence of urine retention

• Hunched posture, vocalizing during urination may be associated with pain
• Abnormal posture, ataxia, or difficulty ambulating in guinea pigs with musculoskeletal or neurological disease

Physical Examination Findings
• If significant blood loss via hematuria has occurred, the patient may have pale mucous membranes or generalized paleness of the skin, face, and legs.
• Bladder palpation may demonstrate cystoliths; failure to palpate calculi does not exclude them from consideration.
• In guinea pigs with hypercrystalluria, the bladder wall may palpate thickened, and bladder contents may be sand-like.
• Large, turgid bladder (or inappropriate size remains after voiding efforts) upon palpation of the urinary bladder—can occur with pollakiuria or with uroliths
• Manual expression of the bladder may reveal hematuria or sometimes "sludgy," thick, white-tan material that has normal-appearing voided urine—this is less common in guinea pigs than in rabbits, but it does occur.
• Hematuria, stranguria, and pollakiuria may be observable if urine is voided by patient
• A large kidney may be palpable if nephritis or nephrolithiasis is present.
• Signs of uremia—dehydration, anorexia, lethargy, weakness, hypothermia, bradycardia, high rate or shallow respirations, stupor, coma, and/or seizures occur rarely, often in terminal cases, tachycardia resulting from ventricular dysrhythmias induced by hyperkalemia
• Thick, palpable uterus may be found if pyometra; pups may be palpable if dystocia is the cause.
• Organomegaly may suggest other organ system involvement or neoplasia.

CAUSES
Urinary System
• Urinary tract infection—bacterial urethritis, cystitis, pyelonephritis, nephritis; *E. coli*, *Streptococcus pyogenes*, and *Staphylococcus* spp. and occasionally anaerobes have been reported. Pure cultures of *C. renale* and *Facklamia* spp., and mixed bacterial cultures including *C. renale, Streptococcus bovis/equinus* group, and *Staphylococcus* spp. were cultured from urine of pet guinea pigs with urolithiasis, but a direct association was not confirmed. Also, *Streptococcus viridans, Proteus mirablis,* and mixed growth with *S. viridans, Staphylococcus* spp., *E. coli*, or *Enterococcus* spp. have been reported from cultures from calculi.
• Urolithiasis—anywhere within the urinary tract
• Urethral plugs—especially in boars
• Iatrogenic—for example, catheterization, overdistention of the bladder during contrast radiography or surgery

- Trauma—especially bite wounds
- Neoplasia (not common)

Reproductive System
- Endometrial hyperplasia Pyometra, vaginitis, and dystocia
- Neoplasia (uncommon)

Other Organ Systems
- Neurological/Musculoskeletal—any disease that inhibits normal posturing for urination (e.g., pododermatitis, arthritis) can lead to these signs.
- Urine scald—can cause ascending inflammation, leading to urethral spasm
- Other abdominal organomegaly may put undue pressure on the urinary system, causing straining to urinate

RISK FACTORS
- Inadequate water intake—dirty water bowls, unpalatable water, inadequate water provision, changing water sources
- Urine retention—underlying bladder pathology, neuromuscular disease, painful conditions causing a reluctance to ambulate (musculoskeletal disease, e.g., pododermatitis, arthritis), dental disease
- Inadequate cage cleaning may cause some guinea pigs to avoid urinating.
- Obesity has been suggested but not a proven cause in guinea pigs.
- Lack of exercise
- Feeding exclusively alfalfa-based diet (hay, pellets, or both)
- Calcium or vitamin/mineral supplements added to diet
- Diseases, diagnostic procedures, or treatments that (1) alter normal host urinary tract defenses and predispose to infection, (2) predispose to formation of uroliths, or (3) damage urothelium or other tissues of the lower urinary tract
- Mural or extramural diseases that compress the bladder or urethral lumen

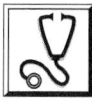

DIAGNOSIS

DIFFERENTIAL DIAGNOSIS
Differentiating from other abnormal patterns of micturition
- Rule out polyuria—increased frequency and volume of urine
- Rule out urethral obstruction—stranguria, anuria, overdistended urinary bladder, signs of postrenal uremia Differentiate causes of dysuria, pollakiuria, hematuria
- Cystitis—hematuria; bacteriuria; painful, thickened bladder
- Hypercalciuria—thick white to beige urine, sometimes streaked with fresh blood; radiopaque bladder

- Urolithiasis—hematuria, palpable uroliths in the bladder, radiopaque bladder
- Neoplasia—hematuria; palpable masses in the urethra or bladder possible; radiographs ultrasound may differentiate
- Neurogenic disorders—flaccid bladder wall; residual urine in the bladder lumen after micturition; neurologic deficits to hind legs, tail, perineum, and anal sphincter
- Iatrogenic disorders—history of catheterization, reverse flushing, contrast radiography, or surgery
- Uterine disease—female guinea pigs; guinea pigs with uterine disease often strain and expel blood when urinating, blood may mix with urine and be mistaken for hematuria

CBC/BIOCHEMISTRY/URINALYSIS
- CBC—TWBC elevations with neutrophil:lymphocyte ratio shift; toxicity of neutrophils ± bands, monocytosis suggest inflammation/infection; thrombocytosis associated with active inflammation; may be anemic if severe hematuria.
- Biochemistry panel—lower urinary tract disease complicated by urethral obstruction may be associated with azotemia. With complete (or nearly complete) obstruction, changes in electrolytes such as hyperkalemia, hypochloremia, hyponatremia may occur.
- Patients with concurrent pyelonephritis have impaired urine concentrating capacity, leukocytosis, and azotemia.
- Disorders of the urinary bladder are best evaluated with urine specimen collected by cystocentesis.
- Urinalysis including both a standard dipstick and microscopic examination of the sediment. Urinalyses data from 44 guinea pigs with urinary calculi found that the mean ± SD urine specific gravity was 1.015 ± 0.008 (range 1.004–1.046) and urine pH was 8.4 ± 0.5 (range 7.5–>9). Hematuria was the most commonly reported abnormality on urine sediment, followed by mucus and lipid droplets.
- Identification of bacteria in urine sediment suggests a urinary tract infection is causing or complicating urinary tract disease.
- Identification of neoplastic cells in urine sediment indicates urinary tract neoplasia (rare).
- Most normal guinea pigs have numerous crystals in the urine; however, hypercrystalluria should increase suspicion for causing disease.
- Calcium carbonate, calcium oxalate, and struvite crystals are all commonly seen on sediment examinations, but similar to other small animals, crystal type(s) may not predict the mineralogy of calculi present.

OTHER LABORATORY TESTS
- Prior to antibiotic use, culture the urine or bladder wall if high numbers of red or white blood cells, bacteria, or a combination of these are present on sediment examination. Collect urine via cystocentesis as free-catch samples are commonly contaminated.
- Aerobic/anaerobic bacterial urine culture and sensitivity—the most definitive means of identifying and characterizing bacterial urinary tract infection; negative urine culture results suggest a noninfectious cause, unless the patient was on concurrent antibiotics or has an anaerobic infection. There are anecdotal reports of anaerobic urinary infections in guinea pigs; therefore, choose this culture technique if anaerobic infection is suspected.
- If surgery is necessary to relieve obstruction from urolithiasis, collect and submit the calculi for analysis and culture and sensitivity, and submit a sample from the bladder wall for culture and sensitivity.
- Calculi-containing calcium carbonate requires specific methodologies to differentiate from calcium oxalate monohydrate crystals; the laboratory chosen for analysis must be able to perform these methods. Confirm the lab's ability to perform these techniques in advance, since human and some veterinary laboratories unfamiliar with exotic animal samples do not differentiate calcium oxalate from calcium carbonate.

IMAGING
- Survey abdominal radiography and abdominal ultrasound are important means of identifying and localizing causes of dysuria, pollakiuria, and hematuria.
- Urinary calculi in guinea pigs are generally radio-opaque, allowing for ease of identification using survey radiography. However, if multiple calculi or significant GI gas are present, the anatomic locations of the calculi using survey radiography alone may be obscured. The majority of obstructive urinary calculi are located in the urethra of guinea pigs but are also found in the kidneys, ureters, vagina, or sometimes in the seminal vesicles in boars. Ureteroliths are more common in guinea pigs than other rodents or rabbits.
- Contrast (negative or positive) cystography can be employed to evaluate filling defects in the bladder, or bladder masses.
- Ultrasound is useful for anatomic location of urinary calculi and for evaluating anatomic changes in the kidneys, ureters, or bladder such as hydronephrosis or hydroureter, ureteral or cystic mucosal thickening, or perforation, and for evaluating other organ systems.
- Excretory intravenous pyelograms (IVPs) are useful to further elucidate relative functional abnormalities in the kidneys or ureters.

DYSURIA, HEMATURIA, AND POLLAKIURIA (CONTINUED)

• CT/MRI are useful modalities for diagnosing urinary calculi and assessing organ architecture, more rapidly than IVP and uses significantly less contrast medium.

DIAGNOSTIC PROCEDURES
Bacterial culture/sensitivity of urine, bladder wall, or if exudates present; recommended if high numbers of RBC or WBC, bacteria, or a combination are present on urine sediment examination. If surgical urolithiasis patient, recommend bladder wall culture as generally more rewarding.

PATHOLOGIC FINDINGS
Gross lesions associated with hematuria, dysuria depend on the underlying disease. Refer to specific causes for dysuria, hematuria, and pollakiuria

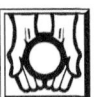

TREATMENT

APPROPRIATE HEALTH CARE
• Patients with nonobstructive urinary tract diseases are typically managed as outpatients; diagnostic evaluation may require brief hospitalization.
• Dysuria, pollakiuria, or hematuria associated with systemic signs of illness (e.g., pyrexia, depression, anorexia, and dehydration) or laboratory findings of azotemia and or leukocytosis warrant an aggressive diagnostic evaluation and initiation of supportive and symptomatic treatment.
• Guinea pigs with urinary obstruction should be hospitalized, emergency supportive, and symptomatic therapy should be provided until surgical intervention to relieve the obstruction can be performed. Medical treatment of urolithiasis has been unrewarding to date, and surgical removal of calculi is most often required. Postoperative management, including supportive and symptomatic treatment, and pain management therapies

NURSING CARE
• Subcutaneous fluids can be administered (100 mL/kg) as needed; IV access is difficult in the guinea pig; lateral saphenous vein catheters often kink; consider intraosseous (IO) catheterization if intravascular fluids are needed. Base fluid selection on evidence of dehydration, azotemia, and electrolyte imbalances. In most patients, lactated Ringer's solution or Normosol crystalloid fluids are appropriate. In obstructed patients, fluid therapy should be based on treatment modalities used in cats with obstructive urinary disease. Maintenance needs are considered to be 100 mL/kg/day.
• In females, gentle flushing of the bladder to reduce hypercrystalluria or flushing urethral calculi back into the bladder can be attempted. In females, gently flush the

bladder using a 3.5 Fr red rubber catheter under deep sedation and analgesia to attempt to remove the calculi. Catheterizing boars is much more dangerous due to the small size of the urethra; successful retropulsion of a urolith back into the bladder is unlikely.

ACTIVITY
• Long term—increase activity level by providing large exercise areas to encourage voiding and prevent recurrence.
• Activity should be reduced during the time of tissue repair if surgery is required for urinary obstruction.

DIET
• Many guinea pigs with these signs are anorectic or have decreased appetite. It is an absolute requirement that the patient continues to eat during and following treatments. Anorexia may cause or exacerbate gastrointestinal hypomotility and cause derangement of the gastrointestinal microflora and overgrowth of intestinal bacterial pathogens.
• Offer a large selection of fresh, moist greens such as cilantro, lettuces, parsley, carrots tops, dark leafy greens, and good-quality grass or Timothy hay.
• If the patient refuses these foods, syringe-feed Critical Care for Herbivores (Oxbow Pet Products, Murdock, NE) or Emeraid Herbivore (Lafeber Company, Cornell, IL) at approximately 10–15 mL/kg PO q6–8h. Larger volumes and more frequent feedings are often accepted; feed as much as the patient will readily accept. Alternatively, pellets can be ground and mixed with fresh greens, vegetable baby foods, water, or sugar-free juice to form a gruel.
• Guinea pigs have an absolute requirement for exogenous vitamin C. Provide 50–100 mg/kg/day vitamin C while hospitalized and during recovery. Vitamin C can be provided through food sources such as citrus fruits and through commercially made guinea pig pellets, or as a subcutaneous injection.

CLIENT EDUCATION
• Limiting risk factors such as obesity, sedentary life, and inappropriate diet combined with increasing water consumption is necessary to minimize or delay recurrence of lower urinary tract disease. Even with these changes, however, recurrence may occur.
• Surgical removal of urinary tract obstructions does not alter the causes responsible for their formation; limiting risk factors such as described above is necessary to minimize or delay recurrence. Even with these changes, however, recurrence is commonly reported.

SURGICAL CONSIDERATIONS
• Surgery may be required for patients with cystic hypercrystalluria or "sludge" that do not respond to medical therapy.

• Surgery is very commonly necessary to relieve obstructions if medical attempts are unsuccessful.
• Postoperative management includes assisted feeding, fluids, analgesics, and antibiotics based on culture and sensitivity results. However, recurrence of the disease is common.

MEDICATIONS

DRUG(S) OF CHOICE
• Antibiotic choice should be based upon the results of cultural and sensitivity (see Contraindications). Antibiotics commonly used include trimethoprim sulfa (15–30 mg/kg PO q12h), chloramphenicol (30–50 mg/kg PO, SC, IM, IV q8–12h), metronidazole (25 mg/kg PO q12h), and enrofloxacin (5–20 mg/kg PO q12–24h) {Should be reserved for microbes that are resistant to tier one antibiotics}.
• Reduction of inflammation and analgesia should be provided, especially if pain is causing reduced frequency of voiding; pain management is essential during and following surgery.
• Perioperative analgesic choices include butorphanol (0.4–2.0 mg/kg SC, IM, IV q4–12h) and buprenorphine (0.05–0.2 mg/kg SC, IM q6–8h). Meloxicam (0.5–1 mg/kg PO, SC q24h) and carprofen (4 mg/kg SC q24h or 1–2 mg/kg PO q12h) provide anti-inflammation as well as analgesia. Tramadol, a synthetic opioid, may also be an effective at dosages of 5–10 mg/kg PO q12h postoperatively. For severe to moderate pain pure mu opioids such as morphine (0.5–2.0 mg/kg SC, IM q2–4h) or oxymorphone (0.05–0.2 mg/kg SC, IM q6–12h) should be used; however, appetite and fecal output should be monitored as these opioids are thought to contribute to GI ileus.
• Procedures for relief of obstruction generally require administering sedatives and/or anesthetics. When substantial derangements exist, begin fluid administration and other supportive measures first. Calculate the dosage of sedative or anesthetic drug using the low end of the recommended range or give only to effect.

CONTRAINDICATIONS
• Oral administration of antibiotics that select against gram-positive bacteria (penicillins, cephalosporins, macrolides, and lincosamides) can cause fatal enteric dysbiosis and enterotoxemia.
• Potentially nephrotoxic drugs (e.g., aminoglycosides, NSAIDs) should be avoided in patients that are febrile, dehydrated, or azotemic or that are suspected of having pyelonephritis, septicemia, or preexisting renal disease.

GUINEA PIGS

(CONTINUED) # DYSURIA, HEMATURIA, AND POLLAKIURIA

- Glucocorticoids, or other immunosuppressive agents

PRECAUTIONS
- Avoid drugs that reduce blood pressure or induce cardiac dysrhythmia until any dehydration is resolved.
- If obstructed or significant renal insufficiency is evident, modify dosages of all drugs that require renal metabolism or elimination.
- If obstructed or significant renal insufficiency is evident, avoid nephrotoxic drugs (NSAIDs, aminoglycosides).

POSSIBLE INTERACTIONS
None

ALTERNATIVE DRUGS
N/A

 FOLLOW-UP

PATIENT MONITORING
- Response to treatment by clinical signs, serial physical examinations, laboratory testing, and radiographic and ultrasonic evaluations appropriate for each specific cause
- Monitor for reduction and cessation of clinical signs. Generally, a positive response occurs within a few days after instituting appropriate antibiotic and supportive therapy for lower urinary tract infections.
- Ensure gastrointestinal motility by making sure the patient is eating, well hydrated, and passing normal feces.
- Assess urine production and hydration status frequently while hospitalized, or have owners monitor daily at home, adjusting fluid administration accordingly.
- Verify the ability to urinate adequately; failure to do so may require urinary catheterization or cystocentesis to combat urine retention.
- Follow-up examination should be performed within 7–10 days of discharge from hospital, or sooner if the clinical signs are not reduced.
- Ideally, recheck of urine culture and sensitivity should be performed 3–5 days after the cessation of antibiotics when lower urinary tract infections are present.

PREVENTION/AVOIDANCE
- Prevention is based on the specific underlying cause. Limiting risk factors such as obesity, sedentary life, and inappropriate diet combined with increasing water consumption is necessary to minimize or delay recurrence of urinary tract diseases. Even with these changes, however, recurrence may occur. For animals with urolithiasis or hypercrystalluria, water is the cornerstone to any stone prevention protocol. Prevention is

targeted at increasing water intake and reducing (but not eliminating) dietary calcium. Metabolic bone disease may be induced in guinea pigs with severe dietary calcium restriction for prevention of urinary calculi. Avoid alfalfa-based diets. Diets containing a high percentage of timothy, oat, or grass hays, a lower overall percentage of pellets, and a wider variety of vegetables and fruits decrease the risk of urolith development in pet guinea pigs. It is possible that dietary inhibitors of calcium are found in greater concentration in hays than pellets.
- Hydrochlorothiazide (2 mg/kg PO q12h) is a thiazide diuretic that reduces urinary Ca^{2+}, K^+, and citrate. It is unknown if diuresis would be of benefit to guinea pigs whose urine is already considered isosthenuric. Do not use hydrochlorothiazide with severe renal disease or fluid imbalances.
- Urinary acidifiers were historically recommended based upon an assumed diagnosis of calcium oxalate calculi, but the normally alkaline urine of guinea pigs makes the use of dietary acidifiers concerning. Potassium citrate (30–75 mg/kg PO q12h) binds urinary Ca^{2+}, reduces ion activity, and alkalinizes the urine. As guinea pigs have alkaline urine even with the disease, the efficacy of this treatment is unclear. Hyperkalemia occurs, so monitor plasma K^+ closely during the treatment. Potassium citrate and hydrochlorothiazide have been used together anecdotally with some clinical success.

POSSIBLE COMPLICATIONS
- Anemia
- Urine scald; myiasis; pododermatitis
- Urinary tract obstruction with urolithiasis or hypercrystalluria

EXPECTED COURSE AND PROGNOSIS
- Depends upon the underlying disease. Generally, the prognosis for animals with uncomplicated lower urinary tract infection is good to excellent. The prognosis for patients with complicated infection is determined by the prognosis for the other urine abnormalities.
- The prognosis following surgical removal of uroliths is fair to good, but recurrence is common, and although dietary management may decrease the likelihood of recurrence, many will develop clinical disease again.

 MISCELLANEOUS

ASSOCIATED CONDITIONS
- Urolithiasis
- Pyometra, other uterine disorders

- Gastrointestinal hypomotility or dysbiosis
- Pyoderma (urine scald)

AGE-RELATED FACTORS
Frequently found in middle-aged to older guinea pigs, although it can occur in younger animals as well

ZOONOTIC POTENTIAL
N/A

PREGNANCY/FERTILITY/BREEDING
Lower urinary tract infections may ascend into the reproductive tract via the vagina. If untreated, the potential for development of vaginal or uterine infections increases.

SYNONYMS
None

SEE ALSO
Lower urinary tract infection
Urinary tract obstruction

ABBREVIATIONS
CT = computed tomography
IVP = intravenous pyelogram
RBC = red blood cells
TWBC = total white blood cell count

INTERNET RESOURCES
N/A

Suggested Reading
Hallman RM, Brandão J. Diagnostic imaging of the renal system in exotic companion mammals. Vet Clin Exot Anim 2020;23:195–214.
Hawkins MG, Ruby AL, Drazenovich TL et al. Composition and characteristics of urinary calculi from guinea pigs. J Amer Vet Med Assoc 2009;234:214–220.
Hoefer H, Latney L. Rodents: urogenital and reproductive disorders. In: Keeble E, Meredith A, eds. BSAVA Manual of Rodents and Ferrets. Gloucester: BSAVA, 2009:150–160.
Miwa Y, Sladky K. Common surgical procedures of rodents, ferrets, hedgehogs, and sugar gliders. Vet Clin Exot Anim 2016;19:205–244.
Percy D, Barthold S. Guinea pig. In: Percy D, Barthold S, eds. Pathology of Laboratory Rodents and Rabbits. Ames: Blackwell, 2001:209–247.
Pignon C, Mayer J. Guinea pigs. In: Quesenberry KE, Carpenter JW, eds. Ferrets, Rabbits and Rodents (4th ed.). Clinical Medicine and Surgery. 2021, St. Louis: Saunders; 2020. p. 270–297.
Reavill D, Lennox A. Disease overview of the urinary tract in exotic companion mammals and tips on clinical management. Vet Clin Exot Anim 2020;23:169–193.
Author Rodney Schnellbacher, DVM, Dipl. ACZM

GUINEA PIGS

EPIPHORA

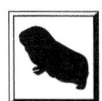

BASICS

DEFINITION
Overflow of the aqueous portion of the precorneal tear film

PATHOPHYSIOLOGY
Results from either reduction of normal flow through the nasolacrimal system or overproduction of tears (typically in response to ocular irritation), or poor eyelid function secondary to malformation or deformity

SYSTEMS AFFECTED
• Ophthalmic
• Respiratory—upper respiratory infections and apical tooth root invasion of sinuses—can cause swelling adjacent to the nasolacrimal duct
• Oral cavity—related dental disease with extension to nasolacrimal system and orbital and nasal cavities

GENETICS
A predisposition to dental malocclusion exists

INCIDENCE/PREVALENCE
Common

SIGNALMENT
Breed Predilections
Entropion—Teddy and Texel breeds
Trichiasis—Texel breed

Mean Age and Range
• Congenital deformity of adnexal tissues or nasolacrimal system—young animal
• Primary orbital or disease secondary to oral or nasal cavity disease—older patient

SIGNS
Historical Findings
• Depends on cause
• History of previous treatment for dental disease
• History of incisor overgrowth—in nearly all cases, only a symptom of cheek teeth overgrowth and generalized dental disease
• History of nasal discharge or previous upper respiratory infection

Physical Examination Findings
• Blepharospasm—ocular irritation—normal blink frequency is low (2–5 blinks/20 minutes at rest; 1–17 blinks/10 minutes of restrained time) and corneal sensation is relatively low in the normal guinea pig eye
• Periocular tear drainage "tracks"—staining on fur in medial and/or lateral canthus
• Misdirected hair onto cornea—may be associated with dermoid, entropion, trichiasis
• Conjunctivitis
• Upper respiratory infection—sneezing, nasal discharge

• Oral cavity signs—malocclusion, elongated incisors, or cheek teeth
• Signs of pain—reluctance to move, lethargy, depression, hiding, hunched posture in guinea pigs with underlying dental disease

CAUSES
Increase in Tear Production Secondary to Ocular Irritants
Congenital
• Dermoid/choristoma—normal tissue in an abnormal location; abnormal differentiation of palpebral skin; may involve the conjunctiva, cornea, sclera, or eyelid ectopically
• Entropion—neonatal Teddy or Texel breeds
• Trichiasis—Texel breeds
Acquired
• Corneal or conjunctival foreign body—from hay, grass, seed, wood shaving bedding
• Conjunctivitis
• Blepharitis
• Ulcerative keratitis
• Anterior uveitis—lens-induced may be present in patients with cataracts, which are common in guinea pigs
• Glaucoma
• Posttraumatic eyelid scarring
• Facial nerve paralysis—lagophthalmos
• Entropion
• "Pea eye"—ventral subconjunctival nodule of glandular tissue that protrudes from the inferior conjunctival cul-de-sac—may be unilateral or bilateral; can impair normal eyelid closure (lagophthalmos) and predispose to exposure keratitis

Obstruction of the Nasolacrimal Drainage System
Congenital
• Imperforate nasolacrimal punctae
• Nasolacrimal atresia—lack of distal openings into the nose
Acquired
• Foreign bodies—plant fiber; seed; sand; parasites
• Rhinitis or sinusitis—causes swelling adjacent to the nasolacrimal duct
• Incisor or cheek tooth root elongation ± abscessation involving nasolacrimal system
• Trauma, fractures—nasal or maxillary bones
• Neoplasia—of nicitians, conjunctiva, medial eyelids, nasal cavity, maxillary bone or periocular sinuses
• Dacryocystitis—inflammation of the canaliculi, lacrimal sac, or nasolacrimal duct

RISK FACTORS
• Dental disease—predisposes to nasolacrimal obstruction from apical tooth root elongation
• Poor husbandry—dirty environment can cause ocular irritation, predisposes to foreign body entrapment, self-trauma

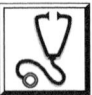

DIAGNOSIS

DIFFERENTIAL DIAGNOSIS
• Normal lacrimal secretions—bilateral, slightly milky discharge in the medial canthus—normally secreted by the healthy guinea pig eye and distributed over the coat during grooming
• Other ocular discharges (e.g., mucous or purulent)—epiphora is a serous discharge
• Eye—usually red if caused by irritation; usually quiet when caused by impaired outflow
• Acute onset, unilateral condition with blepharospasm—usually foreign body or corneal injury
• Chronic, bilateral condition—typically congenital abnormality
• Facial pain, swelling, nasal discharge, or sneezing—may indicate sinus or nasal infection or obstruction, dental disease or from neoplastic infiltration
• If purulent discharge at medial canthus—may indicate dacryocystitis

CBC/BIOCHEMISTRY/URINALYSIS
Usually normal

IMAGING
• Skull radiographs—may show nasal, sinus, or maxillary bone lesion, or evidence of dental disease
• Dacryocystorhinography—flush nasolacrimal system with radiopaque contrast material to localize obstruction
• CT—localize obstruction and characterize associated lesions

DIAGNOSTIC PROCEDURES
• Bacterial C&S testing and cytologic examination of purulent discharge from medial canthus in cases of dacryocystitis—perform prior to instilling substances on the eye
• Fluorescein stain—physiologic test for nasolacrimal patency—should reach external nares promptly; also rule out corneal ulceration

Nasolacrimal Flush
• Confirms anatomic patency of system
• May dislodge foreign material
• Apply topical anesthetic and insert 24–30 g flexible catheter into superior punctum—may require sedation to reduce mobility of patient, especially if the area is painful
• Flush diluted fluorescein stain through cannula with syringe; if fluid does not exit the inferior punctum, then obstruction is localized to the upper or lower canaliculus, the nasolacrimal sac or the inferior punctum is imperforate
• Manually obstruct lower punctum—if flushed fluid does not exit external nares,

obstruction is in the nasolacrimal duct or at its distal opening (atresia or blockage from a nasal sinus lesion)

PATHOLOGIC FINDINGS

Dermoid—most consist of stratified squamous keratinized and variably pigmented epithelium overlying an irregular dermis containing hair, sweat glands, and sebaceous glands; rarely, cartilage or bone is seen within the congenitally malpositioned tissue.

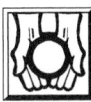

TREATMENT

APPROPRIATE HEALTH CARE

• Remove cause of irritation—removal of corneal or conjunctival foreign body; superficial keratectomy, conjunctivectomy for dermoid removal; treat primary ocular disease (e.g., conjunctivitis, ulcerative keratitis, uveitis); surgical correction of entropion (Hotz-Celsus eversion) or cicatricial eyelid abnormalities (V–Y plasty)
• Use petroleum jelly (Vaseline) or a similar lubricant to smooth aberrant hairs (trichiasis) away from the ocular surface in young animals until hairs grow to a more manageable length. Corneal lubricants (artificial tears) can protect the ocular surface from trichiasis.
• Treat primary obstructing lesion (e.g., medial canthal mass lesion, nasal or sinus mass, and apical tooth root elongation/abscessation)
• Therapeutic nasolacrimal flushing—with topical antibiotic and topical NSAID if warranted

NURSING CARE

• Supportive—rinse any mucoid or mucopurulent debris from eye as produced—and always before treating with topical drugs to improve absorption; minimize crusty or moist buildup on periocular fur to reduce risk of secondary dermatitis
• May require change in housing if stressful or if suspect environmental irritant
• Provide hiding box or towel for burrowing for security if hospitalized

ACTIVITY

• Limit following surgery for dermoid or entropion until suture removal or wound healing is complete (e.g., 10–14 days)
• Separate from cage mates during the postoperative healing phase

DIET

• Change minimally to avoid stress unless nutritionally inadequate
• If vitamin C is deficient, ensure adequate supplementation

• Provide fresh or dried grasses, hay to encourage normal tooth wear

CLIENT EDUCATION

• Nasolacrimal obstruction—recurrence is common
• Severe tooth root disease may obliterate the nasolacrimal duct; epiphora may be lifelong

SURGICAL CONSIDERATIONS

Globe manipulation—use anticholinergic treatment preoperatively to avoid vagus-induced bradyarrhythmia: atropine 0.1–0.2 mg/kg SC, IM; glycopyrrolate 0.01–0.02 mg/kg SC

MEDICATIONS

DRUG(S) OF CHOICE

• Topical broad-spectrum antibiotic ophthalmic solutions—while waiting for results of diagnostic testing (e.g., bacterial culture and susceptibility testing; diagnostic radiographs or CT); consider topical fluroquinolone (ciprofloxacin, ofloxacin), neomycin-gramicidin-polymixin B triple antibiotic, or chloramphenicol solution q4–6h
• Dacryocystitis—based on bacterial C&S test results; extended treatment (e.g., >21 days) typically required
• Topical antibiotics are preferred over systemic if adequate to avoid GI upset or enterotoxemia
• Topical NSAID (e.g., flurbiprofen 0.03% BID-QID or ketorolac 0.5% BIB-QID or 1% diclofenac BID-QID) to reduce inflammation if marked
• Systemic NSAID (e.g., meloxicam 0.5–1.0 mg/kg PO, SC, IM q24h)

CONTRAINDICATIONS

• Avoid steroid-containing ophthalmic preparations in cases of ulcerative keratitis
• Topical steroids may cause GI stasis and subsequent derangement of GI microflora and overgrowth of intestinal bacterial pathogens.
• Guinea pigs have a marked, often lethal disruption of GI tract flora with antibiotic therapy (dysbiosis)—the anaerobic flora is sensitive to antibiotics with a gram-positive spectrum, particularly those with biliary excretion; disturbances of the flora caused by antibiotics may cause an over-colonization of clostridia, particulary *Clostridium difficile*—with fatal toxin elaboration
• Penicillins, ampicillin, bacitracin, erythromycin, spiramycin, lincomycin, gentamycin, clindamycin, and vancomycin at therapeutic doses carry the risk of inducing the syndrome and are contraindicated.

PRECAUTIONS

• Great care is required when considering the use of antibiotics in guinea pigs, including topical preparations.
• If diarrhea develops, stop the administration of any antibiotic being given and reevaluate the patient and treatment protocol.

FOLLOW-UP

PATIENT MONITORING

• Reevaluate q7d until condition resolved
• Nasolacrimal obstruction—repeat nasolacrimal flushes may be required and can include antibiotics and topical NSAID.
• Problem persisting more than 7–10 days with treatment or recurs soon after cessation of treatment—indicates foreign body or nidus of infection or obstruction; requires further diagnostics (e.g., skull films, dacryocystorhinography)

PREVENTION/AVOIDANCE

• Therapy for underlying conditions
• Appropriate diet—purchase processed diets to feed before vitamin C degrades; feed grass or timothy hay to encourage proper wear of molars
• Correct husbandry/clean environment
• Do not breed guinea pigs with malocclusion, entropion

POSSIBLE COMPLICATIONS

• Recurrence—most common complication; caused by nonresolution of underlying dental disease, recurrence of ocular irritation (e.g., corneal ulceration, entropion, and environmental irritant)
• Chronic dental disease—lifelong treatment is required
• Permanent blockage of the nasolacrimal duct may occur due to scarring from chronic respiratory infection, abscess, or neoplasia

EXPECTED COURSE AND PROGNOSIS

• Depends on underlying cause—excellent: with appropriate removal of dermoid and healing of defect; good to excellent: identification and removal of foreign body or other environmental irritants; fair to poor: recurrent nasolacrimal obstruction/stenosis
• Retrobulbar tooth root abscess—depends on severity of bone involvement, underlying disease, condition of the cheek teeth, and presence of other abscesses. Fair to guarded with single isolated retrobulbar abscess, adequate surgical debridement, and medical treatment. Abscesses in the nasal passages or with multiple or severe maxillary abscesses have a guarded to poor prognosis—euthanasia may be warranted.

EPIPHORA

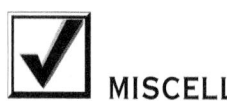

MISCELLANEOUS

ASSOCIATED CONDITIONS
Vitamin C deficiency—predisposes to bone, tooth, and conjunctival pathology

ZOONOTIC POTENTIAL
Conjunctival pathogens—*Bordetella* spp., *Salmonella* spp.

PREGNANCY/FERTILITY/BREEDING
• Do not breed patients with malocclusion.
• Use of systemic antibiotics should be used with caution in pregnant sow.

SEE ALSO
Conjunctivitis
Dental malocclusion
Pea eye
Rhinitis and sinusitis

ABBREVIATIONS
CT = computed tomography
C&S = culture and sensitivity
NSAID = nonsteroidal anti-inflammatory drug

Suggested Reading
Carpenter JW. Exotic Animal Formulary, 3rd ed. St Louis: Elsevier Saunders, 2005.
Flecknell P. Guinea pigs. In: Meredith A, Redrobe S, eds. BSAVA Manual of Exotic Pets, 4th ed. Gloucester: Quedgeley, 2002:52–64.
Kern TJ. Rabbit and rodent ophthalmology. Sem Avian Exot Pet Med 1997;6(3):138–145.
Monk C. Ocular surface disease in rodents (guinea pigs, mice, rats, chinchillas). Vet Clin Exot Anim 2019;22:15–26.
Van der Woerdt A. Ophthalmologic diseases of small mammals. In: Quesenberry KE, Carpenter JW, eds. Ferrets, Rabbits and Rodents, 4th ed). Clinical Medicine and Surgery. 2021 ed. St. Louis: Saunders, 2020:583–594.
Williams D. Ocular disease in the guinea pig (*Cavia porcellus*): a survey of 1000 animals. Vet Ophthalmol 2010;13(Supplement 1):54–62.

Authors Georgina Newbold, DVM, Dipl. ACVO and A. Michelle Willis, DVM, Dipl. ACVO

EXOPHTHALMOS AND ORBITAL DISEASES

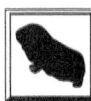

BASICS

DEFINITION
Abnormal position of the globe
- Exophthalmos—anterior displacement of a normal globe
- Enophthalmos—posterior displacement of a normal globe
- Strabismus—deviation of the globe from a correct position of gaze; not readily corrected by the patient

PATHOPHYSIOLOGY
Malposition of globe—caused by changes in volume (loss or gain) of the orbital contents or abnormal extraocular muscle function
- Exophthalmos—caused by space-occupying mass lesions posterior to the equator of the globe
- Enophthalmos—caused by reduced volume of orbital contents or by space-occupying mass lesions anterior to the equator of the globe
- Strabismus—caused by either muscular or neurological lesions affecting the tone or function of the extraocular muscles

SYSTEMS AFFECTED
- Ophthalmic
- Gastrointestinal—proximity of oral cavity to ventral orbit—malocclusion and apical root abscess extension
- Respiratory—due to proximity of orbit to nasal cavity, frontal and maxillary sinuses

GENETICS
A predisposition to dental malocclusion exists

INCIDENCE/PREVALENCE
N/A

GEOGRAPHIC DISTRIBUTION
N/A

SIGNALMENT
Breed Predilections
N/A

Mean Age and Range
- Orbital neoplasia—more common in older animals
- Exophthalmia due to dental disease—congenital malformation affects young animals; acquired apical tooth root disease can affect all ages

Predominant Sex
N/A

SIGNS
Historical Findings
- Weight loss
- Difficulty in eating or in prehension
- Drooling—"slobbers"
- Bleeding from oral cavity
- Nasal discharge or sneezing
- Anorexia
- Presence of coarse matter in stools
- Evidence of vision changes

Physical Examination Findings
Exophthalmos
- Reduced ability to retropulse globe
- Ocular discharge—serous or mucoid
- Chemosis
- Conjunctivitis
- Eyelid swelling
- Lagophthalmos—inability to close eyelids over the cornea completely when blinking
- Exposure keratitis—ulcerative or nonulcerative
- Pain on opening mouth
- Fixed protrusion of rudimentary nictitating membrane
- Fundic exam: the normal guinea pig eye has a paurangiotic retina that appears avascular on examination); may see inward deviation of posterior globe; retinal detachment; optic disc swelling
- Vision impairment caused by optic nerve compression
- Neurotropic keratitis if damage to cranial nerve V
- IOP—may see differential between affected and unaffected eyes due to external compression of globe, but rarely pathologic
- Fever and malaise—with orbital abscess or cellulitis
Enophthalmos
- Ptosis
- Elevation of nictitans
- Extraocular muscle atrophy
- Entropion—with severe disease
Strabismus
- Deviation of globe from normal position—unilateral or bilateral
- May have associated enophthalmos or exophthalmos

Oral Examination
- A complete oral exam is indicated in all guinea pigs with orbital disease—heavy sedation or general anesthesia may be required—a green food sludge is usually present in the oral cavity which hinders visualization of the dentition and presents danger of aspiration
- Specialized equipment is required—rodent dental speculum (Rodent mouth gag, Jorgensen Lab, Loveland, CO) and a set of buccal speculae (Cheek dilator, Jorgensen Labs); cotton swabs and tongue depressor to retract the tongue and examine lingual surfaces
- Incisors—overgrowth, horizontal ridges or grooves, malformation, discoloration, fractures, increased or decreased curvature, or malocclusion
- Cheek teeth—elongation, irregular crown height, spikes, curved teeth, oral ulceration or abscesses, loose or discolored teeth, halitosis or purulent discharge
- Tooth root abnormalities may be present in spite of normal-appearing crowns; skull radiographs may be necessary to identify apical root abnormalities

CAUSES
Exophthalmos
- Tooth root elongation and tooth root abscess—the guinea pig has aradicular hypsodont teeth, which grow continually due to open root apices; continuous growth must be balanced by continuous wear
- Orbital neoplasia (malignant or benign tumor)—primary or secondary to metastasis from distant site. Lymphosarcoma, periorbital lipoma, and ameloblastoma have been reported
- "Pea eye"—ventral subconjunctival nodule of glandular tissue that protrudes from the inferior conjunctival cul-de-sac—may be unilateral or bilateral; can impair normal eyelid closure (lagophthalmos) and predispose to exposure keratitis
- Orbital hemorrhage
- Salivary gland mucocele
- Harderian gland pathology—prolapse or secondary inflammation and edema of the Harderian gland or possible obstruction of the excretory ducts. Contralateral enlargement of the Harderian gland is potentially caused by inflammation passing from one orbit to the other through the optic foramen and the optic canal.
Enophthalmos
- Ocular pain
- Horner's syndrome
- Loss of orbital fat or muscle
- Severe weight loss or dehydration
- Neoplasia extending from rostral orbit
Strabismus
- Abnormal innervation to extraocular muscles
- Posttraumatic restriction of extraocular muscle motility by scar tissue
- Avulsion of extraocular muscle attachment following globe proptosis

RISK FACTORS
- Dental disease—malocclusion, inadequate coarse roughage in diet, inappropriate physical form and composition of diet
- Guinea pigs are classified as full elodonts with open-rooted systems that result in continuous growth of all teeth
- Head trauma—proptosis; strabismus

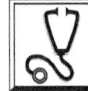

DIAGNOSIS

DIFFERENTIAL DIAGNOSIS
Exophthalmos
- Buphthalmos—enlargement of the globe due to intraocular disease; in guinea pigs

EXOPHTHALMOS AND ORBITAL DISEASES   (CONTINUED)

glaucoma can be caused by various intraocular diseases, including the seemingly benign intraocular osseous metaplasia
• Episcleritis—inflammation of the episcleral tissues can cause focal or diffuse thickening of the fibrous tunic, often mimicking a buphthalmic globe
• "Pea eye" or "fatty eye"—a ventral subconjunctival nodule protruding from the inferior cul-de-sac of one or both eyes—resulting from displacement/extension of a portion of either the orbital lacrimal or salivary glands into the subconjunctival space—may be unilateral or bilateral
• Traumatic proptosis—acute onset related to trauma to head/periocular area—eyelids typically entrapped behind globe
Enophthalmos
• Perforated/collapsed globe—acute trauma; perforation of corneal descemetocele
• Phthisis bulbi—acquired shrinkage of the globe, usually secondary to trauma and/or chronic inflammation
• Microphthalmos—congenitally smaller than normal globe which can include other anatomical abnormalities—may be blind or vision impaired—more prevalent in lethal white guinea pigs, resulting from breeding a roan X roan or a dalmation X dalmation—in these cases, there is a 1:4 chance of breeding a lethal
• Anophthalmos—congenital absence of globe—rare but reported in guinea pig
Strabismus
• Microphthalmos
• Phthisis bulbi

CBC/BIOCHEMISTRY/URINALYSIS
• Usually normal
• Leukogram—may show inflammation with orbital abscess or cellulitis

OTHER LABORATORY TESTS
N/A

IMAGING
• Skull radiographs—identify apical root abnormalities or lytic nasal, maxillary, or orbital lesions
• Orbital ultrasound—localization and characterization of space-occupying mass lesions; may guide fine-needle aspirate or biopsy, or to confirm location of normal orbital tissues (lacrimal and salivary glands—compare both orbits)
• CT scan—evaluate extent of orbital disease and determine the involvement of other cavities (nasal, oral)
• Thoracic radiographs—identify metastatic disease

DIAGNOSTIC PROCEDURES
• Resistance to globe retropulsion—confirms space-occupying mass
• Oral examination, skull radiographs, and fine-needle aspiration or biopsy of space-occupying mass lesion in orbit—perform after anesthetizing patient
• Fine-needle aspiration (use 18–20 gauge needle)—if retrobulbar mass is accessible; submit samples for aerobic, anaerobic, and fungal cultures; gram staining; and cytological evaluation
• Cytology—often diagnostic for abscess and neoplasia; guinea pig abscesses typically produce thick, paste-like purulent material
• Biopsy—indicated if fine-needle aspiration is nondiagnostic and mass lesion is accessible
• Forced duction test with strabismus—grasp conjunctiva with a fine pair of forceps following topical anesthesia; differentiates neurological disease (in which the globe moves freely) from restrictive muscle condition (in which the globe cannot be moved manually)

PATHOLOGIC FINDINGS
• Neoplasia—characteristic features of malignancy (anisocytosis, anisokaryosis, increase in mitotic figures)
• Cellulitis, abscess—inflammatory cells, intracellular bacteria
• Pea eye—normal glandular tissues

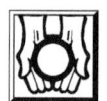

TREATMENT

APPROPRIATE HEALTH CARE
• Retrobulbar abscess—aggressive surgical debridement of orbital abscess and related affected tissues (dentition, maxilla) followed by long-term local and systemic antibiotic treatment; limited (palliative) response to antibiotic treatment alone
• Orbital neoplasm—consultation with oncologist once diagnosis is made; most are primary and malignant
• Proptosis—temporary tarsorrhaphy indicated to avoid exposure keratitis until retro-orbital swelling subsides; anti-inflammatory therapy
• Enophthalmos—depends on the cause
• Strabismus—muscle reattachment difficult

NURSING CARE
• Exophthalmos—lubrication of exposed cornea while diagnostics and treatment are carried out
• Supportive care in debilitated or anorectic patients; assisted feeding; subcutaneous or intravenous fluid therapy
• Warm compressing of periocular tissues—q6h—encourages blood flow to area—helps decrease swelling and cleans discharges

ACTIVITY
N/A

DIET
• Guinea pigs requiring radical coronal reduction, extractions, or surgical debridement of abscesses may be unable to eat solid foods for some time following surgery. Anorexia can cause or exacerbate GI hypomotility, derangement of GI microflora, and overgrowth of intestinal bacterial pathogens
• Syringe-feed a gruel such as Critical Care for Herbivores (Oxbow Pet Products, Murdock, NE) 10–15 mL/kg PO q6–8h. Alternatively, feed ground pellets mixed with fresh greens, vegetable baby foods, water, or juice to form gruel.
• Encourage oral fluid intake by offering fresh water or wetting leafy vegetables.
• Return guinea pig to solid food as soon as possible to encourage normal occlusion and wear. Increase amount of tough, fibrous foods (hay, wild grasses)

CLIENT EDUCATION
Guinea pigs with apical abscesses have generalized dental disease. Diet change and lifelong treatment, consisting of periodic teeth trimming (coronal reduction), are required.

SURGICAL CONSIDERATIONS
Retrobulbar Tooth Root Abscesses
• Abscess material is thick and paste-like, making simple drainage typically ineffective—surgical removal of the entire abscess, including the capsule is required and special expertise may be needed
• Enucleation or exenteration usually required to remove all abscess-related material. All teeth associated with the abscess should be removed and all bone involved in the abscess must be thoroughly debrided.
• The defect can be filled with AIPMMA beads—the beads release a high concentration of antibiotic into local tissues for several months. Selection of antibiotics is limited to those known to elute appropriately from bead to tissues and should be based on culture and susceptibility testing.

Orbital Neoplasms
• Early exenteration or orbitotomy
• Adjunctive chemotherapy or radiation therapy—depends on neoplasm type and extent or tissue involvement

Enucleation or Other Globe Manipulative Procedure
Use anticholinergic treatment preoperatively to avoid vagus-induced bradyarrhythmia associated with globe manipulation: atropine 0.1–0.2 mg/kg SC, IM; glycopyrrolate 0.01–0.02 mg/kg SC

MEDICATIONS

DRUG(S) OF CHOICE
• Exophthalmos (all patients)—lubricate cornea to prevent desiccation and ulceration (e.g., artificial tear ointment or gel)
• Corneal ulceration—topical antibiotic (e.g., neomycin-polymyxin-bacitracin, ciprofloxacin or ofloxacin q6–8h) and cycloplegic (e.g., atropine 1% q12–24h) to prevent infection and reduce ciliary spasm, respectively
• Antibiotics—broad spectrum pending results of culture and susceptibility testing; enrofloxacin (5–20 mg/kg PO, SC, IM q12–24h), trimethoprim/sulfa (15–30 mg/kg PO q12h), chloramphenicol (30–50 mg/kg PO, SC, IM, IV q8–12h) are safe choices
• Pain management—buprenorphine (0.05–0.2 mg/kg SQ, IM q8–12h); topical nalbuphine 1.2%—corneal ulceration
• Anti-inflammatory therapy—systemic NSAID (e.g., meloxicam 0.5–1.0 mg/kg PO, SC, IM q24h; carprofen 1–2 mg/kg PO q12h)

CONTRAINDICATIONS
• Avoid steroid-containing ophthalmic preparations—in case of corneal ulceration; steroids may cause GI stasis
• Guinea pigs have a marked, often lethal disruption of GI tract flora with antibiotic therapy (dysbiosis)—the anerobic flora is sensitive to antibiotics with a gram-positive spectrum, particularly those with biliary excretion; disturbances of the flora caused by antibiotics may cause an over-colonization of clostridia, particulary *Clostridium difficile*—with resultant toxin elaboration
• Penicillins, ampicillin, bacitricin, erythromycin, spiramycin, lincomycin, gentamycin, clindamycin, and vancomycin at therapeutic doses carry the risk of inducing the syndrome and are contraindicated.

PRECAUTIONS
• Great care is required when considering the use of antibiotics in guinea pigs, including topical preparations
• Chloramphenicol—avoid human contact due to potential blood dyscrasia. Advise owners of potential risk.

POSSIBLE INTERACTIONS
N/A

ALTERNATIVE DRUGS
N/A

FOLLOW-UP

PATIENT MONITORING
• Reevaluate q5–7d postoperatively—fluorescein stain cornea and monitor ability to cover cornea with blink response
• Dental disease—evaluate entire oral cavity and skull at each recheck and repeat skull radiographs at 3- to 6-month intervals to monitor for recurrence at the surgical site or other locations

PREVENTION/AVOIDANCE
• Appropriate diet—a diet adequate in calcium, vitamin C, and fibrous food supports strong bone and tooth development and health.
• Management of malocclusion, elongated incisors, or cheek teeth

POSSIBLE COMPLICATIONS
• Vision loss
• Loss of globe
• Permanent malposition of globe
• Death

EXPECTED COURSE AND PROGNOSIS
• Retrobulbar tooth root abscess—depends on severity of bone involvement, underlying disease, condition of the cheek teeth, and presence of other abscesses. Fair to guarded with single isolated retrobulbar abscess, adequate surgical debridement, and medical treatment. Abscesses in the nasal passages or with multiple or severe maxillary abscesses have a guarded to poor prognosis—euthanasia may be warranted
• Orbital neoplasia—fair to poor depending on tumor type, extent of involvement at presentation, and response to therapy

MISCELLANEOUS

ASSOCIATED CONDITIONS
Vitamin C deficiency—predisposes to bone and tooth pathology

AGE-RELATED FACTORS
N/A

ZOONOTIC POTENTIAL
N/A

PREGNANCY/FERTILITY/BREEDING
• Do not breed patients with malocclusion
• Use of systemic antibiotics should be used with caution in pregnant sow.

SYNONYMS
N/A

SEE ALSO
Epiphora
Dental malocclusion
Pea eye
Rhinitis and sinusitis

ABBREVIATIONS
AIPMMA = antibiotic-impregnated polymethylmethacrylate
C&S = culture and sensitivity
CT = computed tomography
IOP = intraocular pressure
NSAID = nonsteroidal anti-inflammatory drug

Suggested Reading
Carpenter JW. Exotic Animal Formulary, 3rd ed. St Louis: Elsevier Saunders, 2005.
Gasser K, Fuchs-Baumgartinger A, Tichy A et al. Investigations on the conjunctival goblet cells and on the characteristics of glands associated with the eye in the guinea pig. Vet Ophthalmol 2011;14(1):26–40.
Hittmair KM, Tichy A, Nell B. Ultrasonography of the Harderian gland in the rabbit, guinea pig, and chinchilla. Vet Ophthalmol 2014;17(3):175–183.
Kern TJ. Rabbit and rodent ophthalmology. Sem Avian Exot Pet Med 1997;6(3): 138–145.
Lennox AM, Capello V, Legendre LF. Small mammal denistry. In: Quesenberry KE, Carpenter JW, eds. Ferrets, Rabbits and Rodents, 4th ed). Clinical Medicine and Surgery. 2021 ed. St. Louis: Saunders, 2020:514–535.
Miwa Y, Sladky K. Common surgical procedures of rodents, ferrets, hedgehogs, and sugar gliders. Vet Clin Exot Anim 2016;19:205–244.
Van der Woerdt A. Ophthalmologic diseases of small mammals. In: Quesenberry KE, Carpenter JW, eds. Ferrets, Rabbits and Rodents (4th ed). Clinical Medicine and Surgery. 2021, St. Louis: Saunders; 2020. p. 583–594.
Authors Georgina Newbold, DVM, Dipl. ACVO and A. Michelle Willis, DVM, Dipl. ACVO

FLEAS AND FLEA INFESTATION

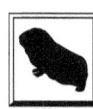

BASICS

DEFINITION
Exposure to fleas (most commonly *Ctenocephalides felis*), an ectoparasite that causes dermal inflammation at the site from which a blood meal is taken

PATHOPHYSIOLOGY
• The cat flea, *Ctenocephalides felis*, is the most common flea that feeds on guinea pigs.
• Exposure to fleas usually occurs through other animals in the house.
• Flea bites cause dermal inflammation and can result in intense pruritus.
• A large infestation can cause anemia.
• Alopecia may result from scratching associated with flea bite.

SYSTEMS AFFECTED
• Skin
• Hair

INCIDENCE/PREVALENCE
Most common in houses that have other animals, especially cats

SIGNS
Historical Findings
• Animal is itching or biting at its body.
• Pattern of hair loss is usually generalized.
• Fleas may be observed on the animal.
• Small dark droppings—"flea dirt"—may be observed under the hair coat.

Physical Examination Findings
• Hyperemic inflamed areas on skin
• Generalized alopecia
• Observation of fleas on animal
• Observation of flea droppings under fur coat or on skin
• Animal itching or biting at body

CAUSES
Ctenocephalides felis (the cat flea)

RISK FACTORS
• Cats in the house or other animals (e.g., dog)
• Lack of flea control
• Poor husbandry

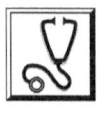

DIAGNOSIS

DIFFERENTIAL DIAGNOSIS
• Other ectoparasites—demodicosis, *Chirodiscoides*, *Trixacarus caviae*, *Gyropus ovalis*, and Gliricola porcelli
  ○ *Trixacarus caviae*—shoulders, dorsum, and flanks, may be generalized and may be associated with crusting, hyperpigmentation, and lichenification. The pruritus is intense. Parasites are readily identified in skin scrapes preparation.

  ○ *Chirodiscoides caviae*—primarily affecting the groin and axilla. Mites are present in the hair and are easily observed on collected hair.
  ○ *Other ectoparasites*—Cheyletiella parasitivorax usually produces lesions on the dorsum; Demodex caviae is frequently located on the head and forelegs. Lice often are associated with lesions around the ears and dorsum.
• Dermatophytosis—can be pruritic—Trichophyton mentagrophytes often affects hair around the face and legs, sometimes dorsum.
• Bacterial pyoderma—location depends on the inciting cause and may be present anywhere. Exfoliative dermatitis is reported most commonly in the ventral aspect.
• Traumatic episodes (burns)
• Allergic skin diseases (e.g., atopy, food allergy, contact, insect hypersensitivity)—contact hypersensitivity has been reported in guinea pigs.

CBC/BIOCHEMISTRY/URINALYSIS
With severe infestations anemia could develop, but it should resolve once the fleas are treated.

DIAGNOSTIC PROCEDURES
Combing of the hair coat for fleas

TREATMENT

APPROPRIATE HEALTH CARE
• All household animals should be on a flea control program.
• All exposed animals should be treated in case of ectoparasitic infestation. The environment may also need to be thoroughly cleaned and treated.

DIET
Normal diet with regular vitamin C supplementation

CLIENT EDUCATION
All animals in the house should be on a flea control program. Treatment of the environment may be necessary to rid the premises of flea eggs and larvae.

MEDICATIONS

DRUG(S) OF CHOICE
Flea Treatment
• Imidacloprid/moxidectin (Advantage Multi orange) 0.1 mL/kg every 30 days for three treatments.
• Selamectin (Revolution) 15–30 mg/kg topically every 21–28 days for two treatments.
• Pyrethrin-based flea powder or pet shampoo can be used, being careful not to overdose.

Antipruritic Therapy
• If there are signs of severe pruritus, corticosteroids may be used. Prednisone, prednisolone (0.25–1 mg/kg PO q12–24h). May be given on an alternate-day basis.

• Antihistamines are usually not very effective except in cases of allergic dermatitis. Hydroxyzine (2 mg/kg PO q8–12h) or diphenhydramine (2 mg/kg PO, SC q8–12h) has been used.

FOLLOW-UP

PATIENT MONITORING
Monitor for resolution of clinical signs and evidence of fleas.

PREVENTION/AVOIDANCE
• Flea control treatment of guinea pig(s) and other animals in the house
• Cleaning of the environment

POSSIBLE COMPLICATIONS
• Bacterial dermatitis due to scratching
• Alopecia associated with pruritus

MISCELLANEOUS

ASSOCIATED CONDITIONS
• Pruritus
• Alopecia

ZOONOTIC POTENTIAL
In severe infestations, fleas will bite humans.

SEE ALSO
Abscesses
Alopecia
Dermatophytosis
Lice and mites

Suggested Reading
Ballweber LR, Harkness JE. Parasites of guinea pigs. In: Baker DG, ed. Flynn's Parasites of Laboratory Animals, 2nd ed. Ames: Blackwell, 2007:421–449.
Palmerio BS, Roberts H. Clinical approach to dermatologic disease in exotic animals. Vet Clin North Am Exot Anim Pract. 2013;16(3):523–577.
Pignon C, Mayer J. Guinea pigs. In: Quesenberry KE, Carpenter JW, eds. Ferrets, Rabbits and Rodents, 4th ed). Clinical Medicine and Surgery. 2021 ed. St. Louis: Saunders, 2020:270–297.
Riggs SM. Guinea pigs. In: Mitchell MA, Tully TN, eds. Manual of Exotic Pet Practice. St Louis: Saunders/Elsevier, 2009:456–473.
White SD, Sanchez-Migallon D, Paul-Murphy J. Skin diseases in companion guinea pigs (*Cavia porcellus*): a retrospective study of 293 cases seen at the Veterinary Medical Teaching Hospital, University of California at Davis (1990–2015). Vet Dermatol 2016;27:395–e100.
Author Thomas N. Tully, Jr., DVM, MS, Dipl. ABVP (Avian), Dipl. ECZM (Avian)

GASTRIC DILATION/GASTRIC DILITATION VOLVULUS

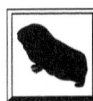

BASICS

DEFINITION
• Gastric dilation (GD)—an acute, generally fatal syndrome in which the stomach fills with gas and fluid, resulting in complex local and systemic pathologic and physiologic changes
• Gastric dilation and volvulus (GDV)—gastric dilation in the guinea pig is commonly accompanied by gastric volvulus

PATHOPHYSIOLOGY
• The cause of gastric dilation in guinea pigs is unknown.
• Guinea pigs cannot vomit due to a well-developed cardiac sphincter.
• With mechanical or physical outflow obstruction from the stomach, swallowed saliva, and gastric fluid quickly accumulate. This fluid often undergoes fermentation to produce a large volume of gas.
• Direct gastric damage and multiple systemic abnormalities can occur secondary to ischemia from rising intragastric pressures.
• Gas accumulation generally precedes volvulus; existing case reports suggest that the most common volvulus is 180 degrees.
• These changes account for the acute clinical signs, which include severe abdominal pain, hypovolemic shock, and cardiovascular failure.

SYSTEMS AFFECTED
• Gastrointestinal—gastric ischemia and necrosis; ileus
• Cardiovascular—decreased in venous return to the heart; cardiac dysrhythmias may result from myocardial ischemia, hypoxia, metabolic derangements, and release of myocardial depressant factors; hypovolemic shock; endotoxic shock; splenic congestion and reduction of lymphoid follicles have been noted
• Respiratory—pulmonary compromise may be caused by abdominal contents decreasing inspiratory diaphragmatic excursion.
• Metabolic—alterations can include simple or mixed acid–base abnormalities and hypokalemia.

GENETICS
No association has been identified.

INCIDENCE/PREVELENCE
Sporadic

SIGNALMENT
• No age, sex, or breed associations have been identified. In the few reports in the literature, it is suggested that GD/GDV may be more common in guinea pigs used as breeders. This has not been the case in the author's experience.

SIGNS

Historical Findings
• Acute onset of depression
• Reluctance to move is common
• Occasionally, owners will report a bloated belly
• Variably, there is a history of inappetence, reduced fecal pellets, and malaise for a short time prior to onset of severe clinical signs.
• Dyspnea is occasionally reported by the owner.
• Sudden death is possible.

Physical Examination Findings
• Gas-filled, tympanic cranial abdomen; auscultation with percussion may reveal gastric tympany
• Overtly depressed
• Reluctance to move and/or a painful posture
• Dyspneic guinea pigs can present with subtle breathing changes or struggling to breathe.
• Cyanotic mucus membranes are variably associated with dyspnea.
• Pain may be noted on abdominal palpation, and dyspnea may worsen with abdominal pressure. Patients often present in shock and do not react to palpation with guarding reflex.
• Heart rate may be increased due to pain or decreased due to shock. Pulse is variably palpable and may seem weak.

CAUSES AND RISK FACTORS
The cause of gastric dilation in guinea pigs is unknown.

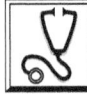

DIAGNOSIS

DIFFERENTIAL DIAGNOSIS
• Guinea pigs do not handle pain with stoicism. Any painful condition can cause severe depression and immobility. Common painful conditions include dental disease, urinary calculi, traumatic injury, hypovitaminosis C, pododermatitis, cystic ovaries, and gastrointestinal stasis.
• Patients in critical condition with advanced gastrointestinal stasis (hypomotility) or intestinal obstruction can mimic clinical picture of GD/GDV.
• Severe depression can be caused by dehydration, prolonged anorexia/pseudoanorexia, metabolic disease (including renal disease, liver disease, and diabetic ketoacidosis), gastrointestinal stasis, systemic infection, cardiovascular disease, pneumonia, and neoplasia.
• Dyspnea and changes in respiratory character can be caused by any painful condition, systemic disease resulting in metabolic acidosis, pneumonia, pleural effusion, pulmonary edema, pulmonary neoplasia (primary or metastatic), ascites, space-occupying masses in the abdomen such as large cystic ovaries, and hyperthermia (heat stroke).
• Cardiovascular shock can be caused by hypovolemia, sepsis, or endotoxic shock. Shock secondary to sepsis may occur with any bacterial infectious process. Endotoxic shock and enterotoxemia are most commonly caused by antibiotic-associated intestinal disease, gram-negative bacterial enteritis, and heat stroke.
• Anamnesis should include a review of husbandry with questions about caging, bedding, ambient temperature, and the age/responsibility of the primary caretaker. Identify how water is provided and assess degree of consumption and any recent changes in consumption. It is extremely important to ask about the diet as fed and as eaten, and the method and frequency of vitamin C supplementation. Any recent changes in appetite or food intake should be recorded.
• A minimum database for the guinea pig with suspected GD/GDV is a thorough anamnesis, complete physical examination, and an abdominal radiograph. In the acutely ill guinea pig, if radiographs demonstrate a severely dilated stomach without gas or severe ileus distal to the stomach, GD/GDV is the most likely diagnosis.
• If the radiographs are inconclusive, other laboratory testing such as CBC, serum chemistry evaluation, thoracic radiographs, and contrast gastrointestinal radiography should be considered. Stabilization and treatment for hypovolemia, shock, and pain may be necessary to allow the patient to survive the diagnostic process.

CBC/BIOCHEMISTRY/URINALYSIS
• Abnormalities vary with degree of shock, organ damage, and dysfunction.
• In one documented case of surgical derotation of a 180° clockwise volvulus, the guinea pig developed pleural effusion, hypoglycemia, hypoproteinemia, progressive interstitial edema, and died 2 days postoperatively.
• The prognosis for GD/GDV is grave. Further testing and treatment should be discussed with the understanding that if GD/GDV is present, treatment is likely to be unsuccessful.

OTHER LABORATORY TESTS
Further testing should be considered based on results of prior tests and physical condition of the patient.

GASTRIC DILATION/GASTRIC DILITATION VOLVULUS (CONTINUED)

GUINEA PIGS

IMAGING

• Abdominal radiographs in guinea pigs with GD/GDV demonstrate a large accumulation of gas in the stomach. The size of the stomach is remarkable in comparison with normal—occupying up to 50% of the volume of the abdominal cavity. The stomach may be caudally displaced, with intestines visible cranial to the stomach if volvulus is present. Generally, there is little gas accumulation in the gastrointestinal tract aboral to the stomach.

• Most guinea pigs with GI hypomotility or antibiotic-induced enterotoxemia have mild to moderate gas distension of the stomach; however, this is usually accompanied by a variable degree of gas distension of the remaining intestinal tract (intestines, cecum, and colon). Lack of significant gas distension caudal to the stomach is consistent with GD/GDV. Other conditions such as ureteral stones or orthopedic disease may be visible and useful to rule out other causes of severe pain.

• Thoracic radiographs may help rule out thoracic cavity diseases that may cause dyspnea.

• One case reportedly developed pleural effusion post-operatively.

DIAGNOSTIC PROCEDURES

Electrocardiography may help with the diagnosis of dysrhythmias.

PATHOLOGIC FINDINGS

Since mortality of guinea pigs approaches 100%, most cases of GD/GDV are confirmed with necropsy.

TREATMENT

• It should be noted that there are very few reports of successful treatment, and the author has not had success in treating this condition. Euthanasia should be considered.

• In one report, eight patients were diagnosed with GDV and 2 survived after surgery.

• Intravenous or intraosseous access is required.
  ○ Isotonic fluid replacement should be given at ~90 mL/kg/hr in order to maintain adequate central venous pressure. If blood gas analysis is performed, measures to correct the pH are appropriate.

• Gastric decompression is critical. Attempt orogastric intubation if volvulus is not evident radiographically using a well-lubricated open-ended flexible rubber tube. If a tube cannot be passed successfully into the stomach, percutaneous trocarization with a hypodermic needle can be attempted. However, percutaneous trocarization carries risk of stomach rupture and resultant abdominal contamination with GI contents.

• Upon patient stabilization and gastric decompression, surgical intervention is indicated.

CLIENT EDUCATION

The prognosis for successful treatment of GD/GDV is guarded to grave. Only one documented report of successful resolution postoperatively exists (8 cases, 2 survived). However, a few anecdotal reports suggest that with early intervention, this condition can be successfully treated with surgery.

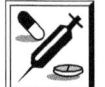

MEDICATIONS

GDV is a surgical disease complicated by severe metabolic derangements. Medical treatment alone is not indicated.

DRUG(S) OF CHOICE

• Opioids are recommended for mediation of visceral pain—hydromorphone (0.1 mg/kg SC, IV, IO) or buprenorphine (0.05 mg/kg SC, IM, IV q8–12h). While opioids may exacerbate hypomotility, adequate analgesia is imperative to stabilization.

• Endotoxic shock is generally fatal in guinea pigs. However, in GD/GDV patients, presurgical administration of antimicrobials effective against anaerobic bacteria may be helpful. Chloramphenicol (30–50 mg/kg PO, SC, IV q8–12h) or metronidazole (10–20 mg/kg PO, IV q12h) is generally safe and effective.

CONTRAINDICATIONS/ PRECAUTIONS

• Prokinetic agents are contraindicated in gastrointestinal obstruction.

• NSAIDs should be avoided in the hypovolemic patient—especially in the presence of shock.

• Corticosteroids have been advocated for use in dogs and cats with endotoxic shock. It is unlikely they would increase success in treatment of guinea pigs with GD/GDV.

• Antibiotics that select against gram-positive bacteria, such as oral penicillins, cephalosporins, lincosamines, or macrolides should not be used in these animals as they can cause fatal dysbiosis and enterotoxemia. One exception is the macrolide antibiotic azithromycin which at the proper dosage (15–30 mg/kg PO q24n) can be used with relative safety in the guinea pig.

FOLLOW-UP

• Clinical condition should be assessed as needed in the critical care/surgical phase of treatment.

• If the patient survives primary therapy, abnormal parameters noted during treatment (e.g., electrocardiogram, electrolytes) should be reevaluated prior to discharge.

PREVENTION/AVOIDANCE

• Unknown, since the cause of GD/GDV is not known

• Counsel all clients regarding proper nutrition for guinea pig pets.

POSSIBLE COMPLICATIONS

• Complications have been discussed above and can be extrapolated from knowledge of GDV in canine patients.

• Postoperative complications will likely include anorexia and gastrointestinal hypomotility.

EXPECTED COURSE AND PROGNOSIS

Many reports suggest that prognosis is very guarded. The majority of guinea pigs with GDV will die despite aggressive therapy.

MISCELLANEOUS

SYNONYMS

Bloat
Gastric tympany
Gastric volvulus

SEE ALSO

Anorexia and pseudoanorexia
Antibiotic-associated enterotoxemia
Diarrhea
Gastrointestinal hypomotility and gastrointestinal stasis

ABBREVIATIONS

GD = gastric dilation
GDV = gastric dilation and volvulus syndrome
GI = gastrointestinal
IO = intraosseous

INTERNET RESOURCES

Veterinary Information Network (www.vin.com)

Suggested Reading
DeCubellis J. Common emergencies in rabbits, guinea pigs, and chinchillas. Vet Clin Exot Anim 2016;19:411–429.
Lee KJ, Johnson WD, Lang CM. Acute gastric dilatation associated with gastric volvulusin the guinea pig. Lab An Sci 1997;27(5):685–686.
Minarikova A, Hauptman K, Jeklova E et al. Diseases in pet guinea pigs: a retrospective study in 1000 animals. Vet Rec 2015;177(8):200–200.
Miwa Y, Sladky K. Common surgical procedures of rodents, ferrets, hedgehogs, and sugar gliders. Vet Clin Exot Anim 2016;19:205–244.

Nógrádi AL, Cope I, Balogh M et al. Review of gastric torsion in eight guinea pigs (*Cavia porcellus*). Acta Vet Hung 2017;65(4):487–499.

Percy DH, Barthold SW. Pathology of Laboratory Rodents and Rabbits, 3rd ed. Ames: Blackwell, 2007:225–226, 242, 235–236.

Pignon C, Mayer J. Guinea pigs. In: Quesenberry KE, Carpenter JW, eds. Ferrets, Rabbits and Rodents, 4th ed.). Clinical Medicine and Surgery. 2021 ed. St. Louis: Saunders, 2020:270–297.

Ritzman TK. Diagnosis and clinical management of gastrointestinal conditions in exotic companion mammals (rabbits, guinea pigs, and chinchillas). Vet Clin Exot Anim 2014;17:179–194.

Author Jeffrey L. Rhody, DVM, DABVP-ECM

GASTROINTESTINAL HYPOMOTILITY AND GASTROINTESTINAL STASIS

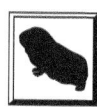

GUINEA PIGS

BASICS

DEFINITION
• Gastrointestinal hypomotility—increased gastrointestinal transit time characterized by decreased frequency of ceocolonic segmental contractions
• Gastrointestinal stasis—severe ileus with little to no caudal movement of ingesta. However, the term "GI Stasis" or "Stasis" is used commonly by most veterinary professionals and owners when referring to either GI hypomotility or GI stasis.

PATHOPHYSIOLOGY
• Guinea pigs feed by grazing and are hind-gut fermenters. Reduction of food intake for any reason, or a diet relatively low in fiber, can trigger GI hypomotility/stasis. Proper hind-gut fermentation and gastrointestinal tract motility are dependent on the ingestion of large amounts of coarse fiber. Anorexia or inadequate diets cause slowing of gastrointestinal tract motility.
• Stasis tends to be painful due to accumulation of GI gas and/or intestinal cramping. Guinea pigs do not handle pain with stoicism. Painful patients will often not eat well, exacerbating GI hypomotility/stasis.
• Affected animals suddenly or gradually refuse food; as motility slows, ingesta accumulates proximal to the colon (stomach, cecum); fecal pellets become small and scant; water is removed from fecal pellets in the colon, making the fecal pellets drier than normal.
• GI hypomotility/stasis also causes alterations in cecal fermentation, pH, and substrate production, resulting in alteration of enteric microflora populations. Bacterial floral shifts can result in overgrowth of bacterial pathogens such as *E. coli* and *Clostridium* spp. Bacterial dysbiosis can cause acute diarrhea, enterotoxemia, or ileus.
• Anorexia due to infectious or metabolic disease, pain, stress, or starvation may cause or exacerbate GI hypomotility.
• The process is often self-perpetuating; GI hypomotility and dehydration promote anorexia and exacerbation of stasis.
• Untreated stasis can be fatal.

SYSTEMS AFFECTED
• Gastrointestinal system—primary system affected; dynamic, functional ileus is the primary change
• Hepatobiliary system—chronic inappetence resulting in hepatic lipidosis
• Musculoskeletal and immune systems—can be indirectly affected by lack of adequate intake of vitamin C. However, in most cases, this requires chronic anorexia/pseudoanorexia.
• Respiratory system—can be affected by metabolic alterations

INCIDENCE/PREVALENCE
GI hypomotility/stasis is one of the most common clinical problems seen in the pet guinea pig.

SIGNALMENT
Varies according to the underlying cause

SIGNS

Historical Findings
• Guinea pigs with stasis are not eating well or are completely anorexic/pseudoanorexic.
• Owners may report a spectrum of malaise, from "not acting normal" to severe lethargy and lack of activity.
• Reduction of size or number of fecal pellets. Occasionally, owner will report softer stools.
• Bruxism occurs with oral or visceral pain.
• Lack of normal vocalizations
• Stiffness or hunched posture or gait—with visceral pain or musculoskeletal pain (e.g., hypovitaminosis C)
• Ptyalism, halitosis, and odynophagia (painful eating) can be associated with many causes of stasis.
• Dysuria is common in guinea pigs with urinary tract calculi, a common cause of GI hypomotility/stasis. Hematuria can be noted as well.
• Dyspnea can be associated with respiratory disease, tracheal compression, and cardiac disease. Pain can also alter character of respirations.
• May be history of recent illness or stressful event
• Guinea pigs with enterotoxic shock due to late-stage GI stasis usually present laterally recumbent

Physical Examination Findings
• Observation at rest may indicate a painful posture or stiffness.
• Observation at rest and after handling may suggest overt or subtle dyspnea.
• Observation of attitude, behavior in cage, and on examination table or floor may suggest depression.
• Decreased borborygmus on abdominal auscultation with gastrointestinal hypomotility
• Abdominal palpation is often extremely valuable in the diagnosis of both GI hypomotility/stasis and the underlying cause. Palpation may reveal gaseous distention of the stomach or cecum due to GI hypomotility/stasis. Underlying disorders such as abnormal renal size in patients with renoliths, the presence of fluid or round masses around the ovaries in patients with ovarian disease, palpable urinary calculi, and

the presence and location of pain may all be identified with palpation.
• With severe, late-stage GI stasis, animals are depressed, painful on palpation, or may present moribund, with severe gas distension of the GI tract on palpation.
• May see evidence of dermatitis, abscesses, or cutaneous neoplasia—may be sufficiently uncomfortable to cause anorexia
• Carefully examine all four feet with attention to painful conditions such as pododermatitis, ingrown nails, and cutaneous horns. Palpate joints for swelling, crepitus, and/or pain, and for asymmetry in muscle mass.
• Examine the face, head, and neck by palpation and visualization for causes of anorexia such as cheilitis, asymmetry to mandibles or maxillae, pain on palpation, scaly eyelids (a vague sign of illness), head tilt, enlarged or painful submandibular, or cervical lymph nodes.
• Examine the eyes for disorders that are painful or impair vision and may cause anorexia (e.g., corneal ulcers, uveitis, exophthalmos secondary to dental abscess, or neoplasia).
• Oral exam should always be part of the physical examination for anorexic or pseudoanorexic guinea pigs. Incisors should be evaluated from the front and from the side with attention to occlusion and lateral mobility of mandible. There should be adequate range of motion laterally to each side. Examine awake patients for evidence of tongue entrapment by the lower cheek teeth using a large otoscope cone or speculum. Thorough evaluation of the cheek teeth is difficult in the awake patient. Due to small aperture of the mouth, wiggly, uncooperative nature of the patients, and the presence of food in the mouth, examination without sedation does not rule out dental disease.
• Thoracic auscultation may demonstrate evidence of underlying cardiac or pulmonary disease.
• Often, examination findings are unremarkable. However, in guinea pigs with GI stasis, further evaluation is indicated to look for underlying cause(s) that are difficult to identify on physical examination.

CAUSES AND RISK FACTORS
GI hypomotility/stasis can begin with anorexia/pseudoanorexia, pain, and physical or emotional stress (especially while receiving a fiber-deficient diet). Guinea pigs can also develop GI stasis for which a cause cannot be found.

Anorexia or inappetence
• Anorexia can be due to any number of causes, including pain, systemic disease or infection, and malaise of any cause.

Pseudoanorexia can be due to nonpainful oral pathology, including dental disease and dyspnea.
• Guinea pigs do not handle pain with stoicism. Any painful process can negatively influence appetite. Common causes of pain include pododermatitis, oral (e.g., dental abscessation, tongue trauma), musculoskeletal, gastrointestinal, and urinary disorders.
• Gastrointestinal disease can be painful. GI hypomotility/stasis causes pain and decreases food intake. Pain and decreased food intake exacerbate stasis and, if left untreated, can progress to GI floral changes with resultant enterotoxaemia and death.
• Metabolic diseases such as renal disease, hepatic disease (especially hepatic lipidosis), and diabetes mellitus
• Cardiac and/or pulmonary disease (e.g., pneumonia)
• Caseous lymphadenitis and other causes of significant cervical lymphadenopathy (e.g., cavian leukemia) Neoplasia anywhere in the body
• Cystic ovaries can cause malaise and act as a space-occupying abdominal mass and decrease food intake.
• Neurologic and neuromuscular diseases are rare causes of anorexia and stasis.
Dietary and environmental causes
• Poor nutrition may result in anorexia. Failure to ingest adequate insoluble fiber will increase risk of hypomotility. Failure to chew coarse hay will promote dental disease. Failure to ingest adequate vitamin C can cause joint pain and poor immune function.

DIAGNOSIS

DIFFERENTIAL DIAGNOSIS
• GI Stasis is a syndrome involving lack of food intake, increased intestinal gas, and variable amounts of pain. In nearly all cases, it is caused by an underlying disease. Every attempt should be made to find the underlying disease.
• GI hypomotility/stasis can be confused with GI obstruction. Bezoars have been reported in the guinea pig but are exceptionally rare compared with stasis. The accumulation of hair along with other ingesta in the stomach is not a disease but can be a symptom or consequence of GI hypomotility or stasis.
• Guinea pigs normally ingest hair during grooming. Healthy guinea pigs will always have some amount of hair and ingesta in the stomach. These stomach contents may be palpable and visible radiographically in the normal, healthy patient. With GI hypomotility,

stomach contents are deformable on palpation. True bezoars form concretion-like masses in the stomach that are physically too large to pass when normal GI motility returns.
• Dysbiosis due to use of inappropriate antibiotics will cause severe illness that can be confused with advanced stasis. Guinea pigs with dysbiosis are usually presented critically ill or moribund, with severe gas distension of the intestines.
• Gastric hypomotility can be caused by anything that decreases food intake. Common causes include dental disease, urinary calculi (especially ureteral calculi), and orthopedic disorders.
• Complete physical examination is an essential element in diagnosis of GI stasis. Guinea pigs often exhibit subtle signs.
• Anamnesis should include husbandry review, including caging, bedding, ambient temperature, and the age/responsibility of the primary caretaker. Identify how water is provided and assess the degree of consumption and any recent changes. It is extremely important to ask about the diet as fed and as eaten, and the method and frequency of vitamin C supplementation. Any recent changes in appetite or food intake should be recorded. It is ideal to have owners bring photos of the cage and brand names or samples of the dietary elements (pellets, hay, vegetables, fruits, and treats).
• A minimum laboratory database for the guinea pig with GI stasis includes a CBC, serum chemistries, and whole-body radiographs. Further testing should be based on these results as indicated.
• In the guinea pig with stasis that demonstrates ptyalism, oral pain, and/or weight loss, it is appropriate to obtain a sedated oral examination and skull radiographs to evaluate the oral cavity. Skull radiographs should include multiple views, including at least a lateral, and right and left lateral obliques. It is also helpful to obtain DV, cranial/caudal, and a VD view. If otitis media/interna is suspected or any vestibular signs are present, tympanic bullae should be radiographically evaluated.

CBC/BIOCHEMISTRY/URINALYSIS
• Abnormalities vary with underlying cause.
• Increased liver enzymes may indicate hepatic lipidosis secondary to negative caloric balance.

OTHER LABORATORY TESTS
Varies, depending on suspected underlying cause

IMAGING
• Abdominal radiography should be part of the minimum database for the guinea pig with stasis. Radiographs often show an

increase in gastric gas with a notable absence of ingesta. Increased small intestinal gas (ileus) is also present; this change can be subtle. Dramatic increase in small intestinal gas should raise suspicion for severe illness (e.g., obstruction, enterotoxemia). Radiographs may also reveal underlying disorders such as urolithiasis, ovarian cysts, musculoskeletal diseases, and neoplasia. Abdominal ultrasonography is indicated in some cases to further investigate suspected pathology.
• Thoracic radiography is indicated to look for causes of dyspnea and to rule out occult pneumonia and heart disease. Thoracic ultrasonography including echocardiography is indicated to further investigate suspected pathology.
• Radiography of the skull should be performed on any guinea pig with suspected dental disease. CT scans can be very helpful in further defining the extent of pathology or in rare cases where radiography is not diagnostic.

DIAGNOSTIC PROCEDURES
Varies, depending on suspected underlying cause

TREATMENT
• Treat underlying cause if it can be identified.
• All guinea pigs with stasis should receive aggressive supportive care with careful attention to hydration, nutrition, and pain management. Oral or parenteral vitamin C is indicated in most cases.
• Fluid support is most commonly administered via oral and subcutaneous routes. Intravenous or intraosseous fluids are reserved for the severely ill patient. Maintenance needs are estimated to be 100 mL/kg/day.
• Nutritional support is imperative. When a guinea pig stops eating, GI hypomotility can progress rapidly. Anorexic guinea pigs are extremely prone to mortality from bacterial floral changes and enterotoxemia. Assisted syringe-feeding with an appropriate herbivore supplement such as Critical Care for Herbivores (Oxbow Pet Products, Murdock, NE) or Emeraid Herbivore (Lafeber Company, Cornell, IL) is appropriate in most cases. Care must be taken on the dyspneic or struggling patient. Tube feeding may be indicated. Both of the above products come in formulations that can be administered via esophagostomy or nasogastric tubes. Frequent feedings (as often as every hour) may be needed to begin to reverse hypomotility.

GASTROINTESTINAL HYPOMOTILITY AND GASTROINTESTINAL STASIS
(CONTINUED)

GUINEA PIGS

• Once the gastrointestinal tract receives fluid and high-fiber food and hypomotility begins to wane, the patient will often begin feeding on hay and its regular diet. Be sure to offer solid food in between assist-feeding sessions.
• Stasis can be caused by pain, but stasis is also a source of GI pain. Pain management is an extremely important part of patient management.

MEDICATIONS
Use parenteral medications in animals with severely compromised intestinal motility; oral medications may not be properly absorbed; begin oral medication when intestinal motility begins to return (fecal production, return of appetite, and radiographic evidence).

DRUG(S) OF CHOICE
• Varies with underlying cause
• For hypomotility—there is no better medication for hypomotility than food; assist feed as noted above. The use of promotility agents such as metoclopromide (0.5–1.0 mg/kg PO, SC, IV q12h) or cisapride (0.5–1 mg/kg PO q8–12h) may be helpful in regaining normal motility; cisapride is available through compounding pharmacies. Constant rate infusion of metoclopramide may be necessary for prokinesis.
• For analgesia, mild opioids are appropriate in the short term. Use buprenorphine (0.05 mg/kg SC, IM, IV q8–12h), as pure mu agonists tend to exacerbate hypomotility and are reserved for severe pain. NSAIDs such as meloxicam (0.2–0.5 mg/kg PO, SC q12–24h) can be used when renal function is normal and the patient is hydrated. For gastric inflammation and pain, H_2 receptor antagonists such as famotidine (0.5 mg/kg PO, SC, IV q24h) or ranitidine (2 mg/kg IV or 2–5 mg/kg PO q24h. Metoclopramide (0.2–1.0 mg/kg PO, SC, IVq12h) increases gastric emptying.

CONTRAINDICATIONS
• Prokinetic agents are contraindicated in the presence of GI obstruction.
• Corticosteroids should not be used in guinea pig patients for any reason. They are never to be used to stimulate appetite.
• Antibiotics that select against gram-positive bacteria such as oral penicillins, cephalosporins, lincosamines, or macrolides should not be used in these animals as it can cause fatal dysbiosis and enterotoxemia. One exception is the macrolide antibiotic azithromycin which can be used in guinea pigs (15–30 mg/kg PO q24) as long as the patient is not currently in stasis.

PRECAUTIONS
Meloxicam should be used with caution in dehydrated patients and those with renal compromise.

POSSIBLE INTERACTIONS
N/A

ALTERNATIVE DRUGS
N/A

FOLLOW-UP
PATIENT MONITORING
• Body weight, amount and size of fecal pellets, clinical hydration status, urine production, attitude, reduction of pain, and voluntary food intake are parameters to observe to help determine efficacy of treatment regimen.
• Any laboratory abnormalities noted in the diagnostic workup should be evaluated for resolution.

PREVENTION/AVOIDANCE
• Depends on the underlying cause
• Maintaining a proper plane of nutrition with a high-fiber diet, thin coarse hay, and appropriate vitamin C supplementation will provide some protection against dietary-induced hypomotility and acquired dental disease.

POSSIBLE COMPLICATIONS
• Dehydration, hypovitaminosis C, malnutrition, weight loss/cachexia, and hepatic lipidosis are common complications of anorexia associated with stasis.
• Anorexia can be associated with dysbiosis and enterotoxemia. This is the most common cause of mortality in guinea pigs with stasis.

EXPECTED COURSE AND PROGNOSIS
• Depends on the underlying cause
• The worse the clinical appearance of the patient, the greater the need for prolonged supportive care. Frequent assist feedings may be gradually reduced to daily or twice daily. The sooner the patient is treated, the better the prognosis for control of stasis and its secondary effects.

MISCELLANEOUS
ASSOCIATED CONDITONS
See causes

AGE-RELATED FACTORS
Renal disease more common in older patients

ZOONOTIC POTENTIAL
N/A

PREGNANCY/FERTILITY/BREEDING
N/A

SYNONYMS
Inappetence, hyporexia
Stasis

SEE ALSO
Anorexia and pseudoanorexia
Antibiotic-associated enterotoxemia
Constipation (lack of fecal production)
Dental malocclusion
Diarrhea
Dyspnea and tachypnea
Dysuria, hematuria, and pollakiuria
Gastric dilation
Hypovitaminosis C (scurvy)
Weight loss and cachexia

ABBREVIATIONS
CT = computed tomography
DV = dorsoventral
GI = gastrointestinal
NSAID = nonsteroidal anti-inflammatory drug
VD = ventral dorsal

INTERNET RESOURCES
Veterinary Information Network (www.vin.com)

Suggested Reading
Bohmer E. Dentistry in Rabbits and Rodents. Sussex, UK: Wiley Blackwell, 2015:35–87, 118–212.
DeCubellis J. Common emergencies in rabbits, guinea pigs, and chinchillas. Vet Clin Exot Anim 2016;19:411–429.
Minarikova A, Hauptman K, Jeklova E et al. Diseases in pet guinea pigs: a retrospective study in 1000 animals. Vet Rec 2015; 177(8):200–200.
Percy DH, Barthold SW. Pathology of Laboratory Rodents and Rabbits, 3rd ed. Ames: Blackwell, 2007:225–226, 235–236.
Pignon C, Mayer J. Guinea pigs. In: Quesenberry KE, Carpenter JW, eds. Ferrets, Rabbits and Rodents, 4th ed.). Clinical Medicine and Surgery. 2021 ed. St. Louis: Saunders, 2020:270–297.
Ritzman TK. Diagnosis and clinical management of gastrointestinal conditions in exotic companion mammals (rabbits, guinea pigs, and chinchillas). Vet Clin Exot Anim 2014;17:179–194.

Author Jeffrey L. Rhody, DVM, DABVP-ECM

HEAD TILT (VESTIBULAR DISEASE)

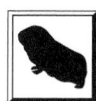

BASICS

DEFINITION
• Head tilt—the ear is held downward toward the ground and maintained in a position different than normal orientation
• Torticollis—the nose is turned toward one side and maintained in a position other than normal orientation
• Vestibular disease—disruption in the ability of the brain to recognize and respond to changes in position and to correct abnormal body position

PATHOPHYSIOLOGY
• The vestibular system is responsible for receiving and translating signals related to the orientation of the body. The receptors are the semicircular canals of the inner ear that sense rotational movements and the otoliths sense linear movements; the vestibular system receives these inputs and sends signals to the brain that direct eye movement and muscle response to maintain the body in a normal position with respect to gravity. The vestibular nuclei in the medulla and the vestibular portion of the vestibulocochlear nerve (CN VIII) provide response to the sensory input received.
• Head tilt, torticollis, and nystagmus are the most common clinical manifestations of vestibular disease.
• The most common cause of vestibular dysfunction in the guinea pig is otitis interna. Other etiologies include CNS infection or neoplasia.

SYSTEMS AFFECTED
• Nervous system—central or peripheral
• Gastrointestinal—secondary nausea, inappetence, and stasis

GENETICS
N/A

INCIDENCE/PREVALENCE
• Common

GEOGRAPHIC DISTRIBUTION
N/A

SIGNALMENT

Breed Predilections
None recognized

Mean Age and Range
None recognized; young or geriatric guinea pigs may be more susceptible to infectious otitis due to decreased immune system

Predominant Sex
N/A

SIGNS

Historical Findings
• Acute or insidious onset of rolling, torticollis, ataxia, leaning to one side, falling, or loss of balance
• Reluctance to eat or drink
• If otitis interna/media is present, findings may include drooping of pinna, scratching or pawing at ear or face (probably related to pruritus or pain), nasal or ocular discharge due to facial nerve paralysis or paresis, ocular clouding, or corneal ulcer from exposure keratitis due to diminished or absent blink from facial nerve involvement.

Physical Examination Findings
• Diarrhea may be present from inappetence, pain, and stress.
• Most nonneurologic physical examination abnormalities associated with otitis interna/media, including pain upon palpation of the bullae or temporomandibular region; facial nerve paralysis; corneal ulcer from exposure keratitis due to diminished or absent blink from facial nerve involvement; erythema of the pinna or crusts and scabs evident from scratching; exudate within the aural canal; thickened, stenotic ear canals; opaque, white, thick tympanum (difficult to visualize in the normal guinea pig)
• Nasal discharge and/or ocular discharge—due to either inability to groom, primary URI, or secondary to facial nerve paralysis

Neurologic Examination Findings
• Head tilt (ear toward the ground) or torticollis (nose pointed to one side); nystagmus (at rest or positional); leaning, falling, or rolling toward the affected side
• Peripheral nerve deficits—nystagmus (horizontal or rotary), fast phase away from the side of the lesion; facial nerve paralysis or paresis may be present; normal proprioception
• Central nervous system deficits—nystagmus (vertical, horizontal, or rotary); direction may change; proprioceptive deficits; altered mentation; possible seizures
• Facial nerve paresis or paralysis may be present in patients with otitis interna/media.

CAUSES

Peripheral Disease
• Infectious/inflammatory—otitis interna/media is the most common cause, usually bacterial; most common organisms include *Streptococcus pneumoniae, Streptococcus zooepidemicus, Staphylococcus aureus, Bordatella bronchiseptica*; may also be due to presence of yeast (*Malassezia* sp., *Candida* sp.).

• Trauma—injury to tympanum or petrous temporal bone
• Neoplastic—tumor of ear canal, bullae
• Toxin—aminoglycosides
• Metabolic—not described in guinea pigs

Central Disease
• Infectious/inflammatory—otitis interna/media with invasion into the brain is the most common cause, usually bacterial; most common organisms include *Streptococcus pneumoniae, Streptococcus zooepidemicus, Staphylococcus aureus, Bordatella bronchiseptica*; may also be due to presence of yeast (*Malassezia* sp., *Candida* sp.). Fungal agents are possible but not described in guinea pigs.
• Trauma—head trauma/injury to cerebellum, brainstem, or vestibular system
• Neoplastic—tumor of cerebellum, brainstem, and vestibular system
• Vascular—thromboembolic disease, coagulopathy, and hypertension
• Toxin—lead, metronidazole
• Degenerative—not descibed

RISK FACTORS
• Immunosuppression; glucocorticoid administration; poor nutrition; hypovitaminosis C; stress

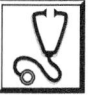

DIAGNOSIS

DIFFERENTIAL DIAGNOSIS
Otitis media/interna—characterized by peripheral disease; differentiate by careful otoscopic evaluation, bulla radiographs, CT, MRI, and sometimes response to therapy neoplasia—may demonstrate central or peripheral disease; differentiate with CT, MRI, or biopsy

CBC/BIOCHEMISTRY/URINALYSIS
• Usually normal
• Hemogram—relative heterophilia and lymphopenia are more common than leukocytosis but are not useful in differentiating infectious from inflammatory etiologies

OTHER LABORATORY TESTS
N/A

IMAGING
• Skull radiographs to evaluate for fractures, swellings suggestive of trauma, and bulla changes including thickening or sclerosis of the tympanic bullae and petrous temporal bone, fluid or soft tissue density within the bullae, or osteomyelitis. Radiographs may be normal even though disease is present.

GUINEA PIGS

• CT—more sensitive than radiographs for detection of fluid or soft tissue densities within the middle ear and to evaluate for bony changes in the bullae as well as extension of disease into the brain
• MRI—better for detection of soft tissue involvement, fluid density, vascular compromise, and invasion into the brain; less sensitive than CT for evaluation of bone involvement

DIAGNOSTIC PROCEDURES

• Otoscopic evaluation to evaluate for otitis media/interna—challenging due to the small ear canals of guinea pigs; enables visualization of the tympanum and structures behind it if damaged; also useful for collection of samples for cytology and culture and sensitivity
• Culture and sensitivity of any nasal discharge, if present, as upper respiratory infections may occur concurrently with otitis, and disease may be transmitted through the eustachian tube and extend to the peripheral or central nervous system
• Biopsy—if tumor is suspected or identified
• CSF analysis—obtain sample from cistern magna; very little fluid will be available; rather than attempt to aspirate, let fluid drip into a microtainer collection tube or collect with a capillary tube and prioritize testing; may increase risk for herniation

PATHOLOGIC FINDINGS

• Pathologic findings would be consistent with underlying etiology; may be idiopathic

TREATMENT

APPROPRIATE HEALTH CARE

Inpatient—neurologic signs; severe infections; anorexic patients; nonambulatory patients outpatient—stable patients that are able to eat and drink with little or no assistance

NURSING CARE

• Fluid therapy to maintain hydration—subcutaneous generally adequate
• Assisted feeding of anorexic animals
• Maintain clean, soft bedding
• Lubricate eyes if blink response is absent or diminished.
• In severe cases, turn the patient and bathe as needed to prevent the formation of decubitus ulcers.

ACTIVITY

Restrict activity when vestibular signs are present to prevent falls or injury; encourage ambulation and movement on flat surfaces once safe.

DIET

• It is essential to maintain food intake during treatment; patients may become anorexic due to pain or vestibular signs; anorexia may lead to gastrointestinal stasis and ileus; secondary derangements of intestinal microbial populations may occur.
• Offer a wide variety of fresh leafy greens (romaine lettuce, cilantro, parsley, kale, cabbage, collard greens, mustard greens, bok choy, dandelion greens, turnip greens, spinach, mesclun salad mixes), and high-quality grass hay. Place food and water in a position that the guinea pig is able to reach, or hand offer.
• If patient is inappetant/anorexic, it is essential to provide adequate nutritional support. Syringe-feed a formulated diet such as Critical Care for Herbivores (Oxbow Pet Products, Murdock, NE) or Emeraid Herbivore (Lafeber Company, Cornell, IL), 10–15 mL/kg q6–8h. If neither product is available, a slurry can be made with blended leafy green vegetables that are high in vitamin C, or guinea pig pellets crushed and mixed with water and vegetable baby food.
• Avoid high-carbohydrate foods, treats, or grains.
• Use caution when syringe-feeding as aspiration pneumonia may occur in patients with vestibular signs or central nervous system signs.

CLIENT EDUCATION

• Prognosis for central vestibular disorders is worse than for peripheral disorders.
• Even in cases of otitis media/interna, inform the client that it is a chronic, debilitating disease that necessitates diligent client compliance, long-term antimicrobial therapy, may be recurrent, and frequently requires surgery for complete resolution.
• Advise the client that head tilt and torticollis may persist, but in the absence or correction of underlying disease, most guinea pigs can adapt and lead a relatively normal life.

SURGICAL CONSIDERATIONS

Total ear canal ablation and bulla osteotomy may be considered for treatment of bulla disease and otitis; surgical excision of neoplastic masses or abscesses may be indicated.

MEDICATIONS

DRUG(S) OF CHOICE

• For suspected or confirmed otitis media/interna or CNS infections, use systemic antibiotics—ideally based on results of culture and sensitivity. Long-term therapy is required and should be continued for a minimum of 4–6 weeks and may require therapy for several months.
• Choose broad-spectrum antibiotics that penetrate the CNS such as enrofloxacin (5–20 mg/kg PO, SC, IM q12–24h) or trimethoprim-sulfa (15–30 mg/kg PO q12h); for anaerobic infections consider chloramphenicol (30–50 mg/kg PO, SC, IM, IV q8–12h), florfenicol (20–25 mg/kg PO, IM, IV q12h), or metronidazole (10–20 mg/kg PO, IV q12h).
• In cases of otitis, add topical antimicrobials—choose otic or ophthalmic preparations without corticosteroids such as antibiotics (gentamicin, ciprofloxacin, chloramphenicol, enrofloxacin) or antifungals (miconazole).
• For trauma, abscesses, neoplasia, and otitis—use analgesics—systemic meloxicam (0.5–1 mg/kg PO, SC, IM q24h) for its anti-inflammatory effects alone or in combination with an opioid; buprenorphine (0.05–0.2 mg/kg SC, IM q8–12h), butorphanol (0.4–2.0 mg/kg SC, IM q4–12h), or tramadol (5–10 mg/kg PO q12h) for additional analgesia. Topical DMSO can be used.
• Anxiolytics—for severe vestibular signs or seizures—midazolam (0.4–2.0 mg/kg IM) or diazepam (0.5–2.0 mg/kg IV or IM) can be used
• Meclizine (2–12 mg/kg PO q8–12h) may be useful for decreasing vestibular signs.

CONTRAINDICATIONS

• Do not use antimicrobials that may disrupt gastrointestinal flora, which may lead to dysbiosis and fatal enterotoxemia (penicillins, macrolides, lincosamides, tetracyclines, and cephalosporins).
• Avoid the use of corticosteroids in conjunction with meloxicam or other NSAIDs.
• Topical and systemic corticosteroids—guinea pigs are highly sensitive to the immunosuppressive effects of corticosteroids; their use may prolong or exacerbate infection and may increase the risk of systemic disease.
• Avoid the use of drugs that are potentially toxic to the central nervous system (metronidazole at high doses; aminoglycosides).

PRECAUTIONS

• Corticosteroids—although highly controversial, systemic prednisolone (10 mg IM or PO once) has been shown to significantly decrease the incidence of infection in experimentally induced otitis media in guinea pigs.

• Procaine penicillin G (40,000–60,000 IU SC q2–7d) has been suggested as an alternative therapy, but there are multiple reports of fatal enterotoxemia with the use of any form of penicillin, including parenteral, in guinea pigs.

POSSIBLE INTERACTIONS
• Avoid the use of NSAIDS with corticosteroids.
• Some topical medications may cause contact irritation; discontinue use if the patient is reactive to treatment.

ALTERNATIVE DRUGS
Corticosteroids are often recommended to help control CNS swelling or inflammation; use of systemic corticosteroids is controversial as guinea pigs are highly susceptible to the immunosuppressive effects, which may lead to or exacerbate bacterial infection.

FOLLOW-UP

PATIENT MONITORING
• Monitor for corneal ulceration secondary to facial nerve paralysis.
• Perform serial neurologic evaluations, initially every 24–48 hours, gradually increasing interval once progression is static or signs are improving; intervals determined by the underlying disease or rate of change

PREVENTION/AVOIDANCE
• Early and aggressive treatment of upper respiratory infections and otitis may prevent invasion by bacteria into the middle/inner ear or systemic spread.
• Proper nutrition, including appropriate vitamin C supplementation, helps minimize the risk of immunosuppression.
• Appropriate husbandry, adequate ventilation, and lack of overcrowding may decrease transmission of infectious agents and reduce stress.

POSSIBLE COMPLICATIONS
• Vestibular signs and head tilt may not resolve or may progress.
• Infections may spread through brainstem/ CNS or systemically.

• Facial nerve paralysis may be permanent and may lead to corneal ulceration and secondary URI.

EXPECTED COURSE AND PROGNOSIS
• Prognosis is variable and dependent upon underlying etiology
• Otitis media and interna may require months of systemic and topical therapy, although some cases will improve or resolve, others may be recurrent or may require surgery.
• Vestibular signs, head tilt, and facial nerve paralysis if present may persist following resolution of disease via medical or surgical means, or may improve and subsequently recur.

MISCELLANEOUS

ASSOCIATED CONDITIONS
• Upper respiratory infections
• Corneal ulcers
• Gastrointestinal stasis

AGE-RELATED FACTORS
None recognized

ZOONOTIC POTENTIAL
N/A

PREGNANCY/FERTILITY/BREEDING
N/A

SYNONYMS
Wry neck

SEE ALSO
Ataxia
Otitis media and interna

ABBREVIATIONS
CN = cranial nerve
CNS = central nervous system
CSF = cerebrospinal fluid
CT = computed tomography
DMSO = dimethyl sulfoxide
MRI = magnetic resonance imaging
NSAID = nonsteroidal anti-inflammatory drug
URI = upper respiratory infection

Suggested Reading
Bays TB. Geriatric care of rabbits, guinea pigs, and chinchillas. Vet Clin Exot Anim 2020;23:567–593.
DeCubellis J. Common emergencies in rabbits, guinea pigs, and chinchillas. Vet Clin Exot Anim 2016;19:411–429.
Harkness JE, Turner PV, VandeWoude S, Wheeler CL. *Streptococcus zooepidemicus* infections in guinea pigs. In: Harkness JE, Turner PV, VandeWoude S, Wheeler CL, eds. Biology and Medicine of Rabbits and Rodents, 5th ed. Ames: Wiley-Blackwell, 2010:382–383.
Harkness JE, Turner PV, VandeWoude S, Wheeler CL. Clinical signs and differential diagnoses: nervous and musculoskeletal conditions. In: Harkness JE, Turner PV, VandeWoude S, Wheeler CL, eds. Biology and Medicine of Rabbits and Rodents, 5th ed. Ames: Wiley-Blackwell, 2010:214–216.
Mancinelli E. Neurologic examination and diagnostic testing in rabbits, ferrets and rodents. J Exot Pet Med 2015;24:52–64.
Meredith AL, Richardson J. Neurologic disease of rabbits and rodents. J Exot Pet Med 2015;24:21–33.
Miwa Y, Sladky K. Common surgical procedures of rodents, ferrets, hedgehogs, and sugar gliders. Vet Clin Exot Anim 2016;19:205–244.
Jekl V, Hauptman K, Knotek Z. Video otoscopy in exotic companion mammals. Vet Clin North Am Exot Anim Pract 2015;18:431–445.
Pignon C, Mayer J. Guinea pigs. In: Quesenberry KE, Carpenter JW, eds. Ferrets, Rabbits and Rodents, 4th Ed). Clinical Medicine and Surgery. 2021 ed. St. Louis: Saunders, 2020:270–297.
Rosset RA, Pignon C, Desprez I et al. Development and validation of an endoscopic myringotomy technique to treat otitis media and interna in a case series of three guineapigs (*Caviaporcellus*). JEPM 2020;31:31–28.

Authors Natalie Antinoff, DVM, Dipl. ABVP (Avian) and Barbara Oglesbee, DVM, Dipl. ABVP (Avian)

GUINEA PIGS

HEAT STROKE

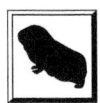

BASICS

DEFINITION
A pathologic state resulting from thermal injury to body tissues due to excessive nonphysiologic elevation in body temperature

PATHOPHYSIOLOGY
• Thermoregulation occurs in the preoptic region of the anterior hypothalamus.
• Nonpyrogenic hyperthermia is the result of the inability of the body to compensate for heat-producing mechanisms, which raises body temperature above the set point.
• Hyperthermia causes an increase in cardiac output, increased metabolic demand, decreased systemic vascular resistance, dehydration, hypovolemia, and tissue hypoxia.
• Coagulation pathways are altered and vascular endothelium throughout the body is damaged, often leading to multiple organ dysfunction, endotoxemia, and SIRS.
• Neuronal injury and cell death in the central nervous system may occur; damage to the hypothalamic thermoregulatory centers may induce permanent alteration in the ability of the body to thermoregulate.
• The effects of hyperthermia are multisystemic and often life threatening.
• Permanent enzyme alteration and cell membrane instability occur when body temperature approaches 109°F (43°C), but changes occur at temperatures around 106°F (41°C).

SYSTEMS AFFECTED
• Nervous—brain hypoxia, neuronal injury, and cellular death may occur, resulting in ischemic insult, cerebral edema, cerebellar dysfunction, focal parenchymal hemorrhage, and disruption of the thermoregulatory center.
• Gastrointestinal—ischemic insult to the gastrointestinal tract leads to gastrointestinal ulceration and sloughing of intestinal mucosa. Enterotoxemia frequently develops; these signs may be present initially or develop late in the course of disease.
• Cardiovascular—cardiovascular output increases in response to increased metabolic demand, systemic vascular resistance decreases, and dehydration and hypovolemia occur. Myocardial hemorrhage, ischemia, and necrosis may occur, leading to tachyarrhythmias and cardiogenic shock.
• Renal—the combination of thermal injury, dehydration, and hypoxia can lead to acute renal failure; rhabdomyolysis may occur and lead to dark-brownish urine production,

which can perpetuate renal tubular necrosis and renal failure.
• Hemic—disruption of the coagulation cascade by direct damage to clotting factors and indirect damage to the liver that synthesizes clotting factors may occur, predisposing the patient to coagulopathy and DIC. Thrombocytopenia may occur due to the consumption of platelets from gastrointestinal hemorrhage and may not be evident for several days. DIC may develop as a result of coagulation abnormality, platelet dysfunction or excessive consumption, sludging of blood, and disruption of vascular endothelium.
• Hepatobiliary—enterotoxemia or direct thermal damage to the liver can cause severe liver dysfunction, which may result in diminished production of clotting factors and DIC.
• Musculoskeletal—rhabdomyolysis may occur, further contributing to sludging of blood, and leading to production of dark-brownish urine that may precipitate or exacerbate renal failure.
• Metabolic—Acid–base changes such as respiratory alkalosis and metabolic acidosis occur as a result of excessive panting and shock.

GEOGRAPHIC DISTRIBUTION
• Worldwide; more common in warm climates when pets may be taken outdoors and left in sunlight and heat

SIGNS

General Comments
• A presumptive diagnosis can be made if a patient presents with a body temperature above 104°F, a history of exposure to heat or sunlight, and no overt indication of infection.
• Clinical signs may range from mild to very severe, or may be absent at the time of initial presentation (especially if the owner has taken measures to cool the guinea pig).

Historical Findings
• Often there is a history of being left outdoors in sunlight, left in a vehicle or closed warm environment, or other obvious sources of exposure to prolonged heat.
• Panting, lethargy, altered mental status, and collapse may all occur.

Physical Examination Findings
• Tachypnea, respiratory distress
• Hyperemic mucous membranes
• Hyperthermia (however, this may be absent and the patient may even be hypothermic if the owners have provided cooling measures prior to presentation)
• Weakness
• Ataxia/collapse/seizures
• Changes in mentation
• Tachycardia
• Diarrhea

• Cardiac arrhythmia
• Melena, hematochezia

CAUSES
• The cause of heatstroke is prolonged exposure to elevated temperature without adequate ventilation or other cooling mechanism.
• The most common scenario in a guinea pig is a pet taken outdoors in warm weather and left in direct sunlight (particularly in a glass enclosure).
• Lack of ventilation (such as in a glass or plastic solid-sided enclosure, even with a ventilated lid) contributes even in moderate temperatures.
• Exercise can also contribute.

RISK FACTORS
Predisposing factors include black or dark fur (absorbs rather than reflects heat), lack of acclimation to increased temperature, water deprivation, high environmental humidity, obesity, cardiovascular disease, respiratory disease, central nervous system disease, and prior episodes of heatstroke.

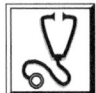

DIAGNOSIS

DIFFERENTIAL DIAGNOSIS
• Pyrexia—a lack of historical exposure to heat or inciting event, or the presence of infection can aid in differentiating
• Stress (including exam room)
• Seizure-induced hyperthermia—onset of seizures without historical exposure to excessive heat; this can also lead to heatstroke

CBC/BIOCHEMISTRY/URINALYSIS
• Important to evaluate for underlying disease and to monitor progress during recovery
• CBC—hemoconcentration initially; anemia, thrombocytopenia, leukocytosis (heterophilia), and hypoproteinemia
• Biochemistry—azotemia, elevations in ALT, AST, CPK, hypoglycemia, and electrolyte abnormalities
• Urinalysis—hematuria, casts, proteinuria, and myoglobinuria

OTHER LABORATORY TESTS
Coagulation profiles are not routinely performed on guinea pigs, but any assay of clotting parameters may be useful in monitoring for development or resolution of coagulopathy. Blood lactate levels are useful in the dog, but normal values for guinea pigs are not established.

IMAGING
Thoracic and abdominal radiographs may be helpful in evaluating for underlying disease.

DIAGNOSTIC PROCEDURES

ECG—monitoring cardiac arrhythmias and recovery

PATHOLOGIC FINDINGS

Pathologic changes are specific to organ system, and often relate to coagulation abnormalities, vascular compromise, or endotoxemia.

TREATMENT

APPROPRIATE HEALTH CARE

• Hospitalize until stabilized; often requires several days of hospitalization; however, many patients do not survive.

NURSING CARE

• External cooling should be initiated prior to or during transport whenever possible; ideally, cooling should be completed within 30–45 minutes of arrival.
• External cooling—apply cool water to skin; alcohol to footpads, ears, axilla, inguinal area; fan; avoid ice water baths
• Internal cooling—room-temperature intravenous fluids
• Discontinue cooling when body temperature reaches 103°F to prevent hypothermia.
• Fluid therapy—use crystalloids for cooling and to restore perfusion; use colloids in patients with hypotension or hypoalbuminemia or in shock (hetastarch 3–5 mL/kg bolus then 1 mL/kg/hr in conjunction with crystalloid).

ACTIVITY

Restrict activity

DIET

• It is essential to maintain food intake during treatment; patients frequently become anorexic, which may lead to gastrointestinal stasis and ileus; secondary derangements of intestinal microbial populations may occur if not already present.
• Offer a wide variety of fresh leafy greens (romaine lettuce, cilantro, parsley, kale, cabbage, collard greens, mustard greens, bok choy, dandelion greens, turnip greens, spinach, and mesclun salad mixes) and high-quality grass hay.
• If the patient is inappetant/anorexic, it is essential to provide adequate nutritional support. Syringe-feed a formulated diet such as Critical Care for Herbivores (Oxbow Pet Products, Murdock, NE) or Emeraid Herbivore (Lafeber Company, Cornell, IL) 10–15 mL/kg q6–8h. If neither product is available, a slurry can be made with blended leafy green vegetables that are high in vitamin C, or guinea pig pellets crushed and mixed with water and vegetable baby food.

• Avoid high-carbohydrate foods, treats, or grains.

CLIENT EDUCATION

• Educate the owner as to the clinical signs and conditions that cause heatstroke.
• Advise owners on how to properly cool animals.
• Most patients require hospitalization for intensive supportive care. Patients that recover initially may deteriorate over a period of days.

MEDICATIONS

DRUG(S) OF CHOICE

• GI protectants should be administered due to the risk of ischemia and bacterial translocation; H2 blockers such as famotidine (0.5 mg/kg PO, SC, IM, IV q24h) and sucralfate (25 mg/kg PO q6h)
• Antibiotics should be administered because of the risk of bacterial translocation. Choose broad-spectrum antibiotics such as enrofloxacin (5–20 mg/kg PO, SC, IM q12h) and trimethoprim-sulfa (15–30 mg/kg PO q12h); for anaerobic infections consider chloramphenicol (30–50 mg/kg PO, SC, IM, IV q8–12h) or florfenicol (20–25 mg/kg PO, IM, IV q12h) or metronidazole (10–20 mg/kg PO, IV q12h).
• Administer oxygen to critical patients and those with respiratory compromise (via oxygen cage, facemask, and nasal catheter).
• Provide dextrose to patients that are hypoglycemic (initial bolus of 0.5–1.0 mL of 50% dextrose diluted at least 1:1 with saline, followed by 2.5%–5% in fluids).
• For oliguric or anuric patients, administer furosemide once guinea pig is well hydrated (1–4 mg/kg IV).
• For ventricular arrhythmias, initiate lidocaine (2 mg/kg initial IV bolus, followed by 40–80 μg/kg/min).
• For seizures, administer diazepam (0.5–1.0 mg/kg IV; then 1.0–2.0 mg/kg/hr CRI if necessary) or phenobarbital CRI for seizure control.
• For cerebral edema, mannitol (0.5–1.5 g/kg IV over 20–30 minutes)

CONTRAINDICATIONS

• Avoid NSAIDs and antipyretic drugs such as meloxicam, carprofen, ketoprofen, and flunixin meglumine—these may increase the risk of DIC, are ineffective at cooling, and may contribute to mortality.
• Corticosteroids have been suggested, but guinea pigs are highly sensitive to the immunosuppressive effects of corticosteroids; in cases of heatstroke they may increase the risk of GI bleeding and infection, so should be avoided.

• Avoid any antimicrobials that may further disrupt GI flora (penicillin, erythromycin, lincosamides, macrolides, tetracycline, cephalosporins).

PRECAUTIONS

Do not administer furosemide until the patient is well hydrated.

FOLLOW-UP

PATIENT MONITORING

• Monitor rectal temperature continually or every 10 minutes during the first few hours until stable, then every 30–60 minutes.
• Monitor heart rate and respiratory rate every 10 minutes initially, then every 30–60 minutes.
• Monitor PCV, total protein, and blood glucose at least daily.
• Evaluate ECG daily to assess for arrhythmias; continuous ECG is ideal during the initial stages of therapy.
• Urine output—monitor urine output to enable early detection of anuric or oliguric renal failure as well as monitor response to treatment.
• Blood pressure
• Thoracic auscultation
• Biochemistry panel to evaluate for development, progression, or improvement of azotemia, hepatic changes, and electrolyte abnormalities

PREVENTION/AVOIDANCE

Avoid exposure to heat or sunlight.

POSSIBLE COMPLICATIONS

• Increased susceptibility to future episodes of heatstroke
• Diarrhea (hemorrhagic)
• Renal or other organ failure
• Enterotoxemia
• DIC
• Seizures
• Respiratory arrest
• Cardiac arrest

EXPECTED COURSE AND PROGNOSIS

The expected course of disease is variable; even patients that appear to recover initially can suffer adverse effects to the brain, gastrointestinal tract, or kidneys over time.

MISCELLANEOUS

SYNONYMS

Hyperthermia

ABBREVIATIONS

ALT = alanine aminotransferase

HEAT STROKE

AST = aspartate aminotransferase
CPK = creatine phosphokinase
CRI = constant rate infusion
DIC = disseminated intravascular coagulation
ECG = electrocardiogram
GI = gastrointestinal
NSAID = nonsteroidal anti-inflammatory drug
PCV = packed cell volume
SIRS = systemic inflammatory response syndrome

Suggested Reading
DeCubellis J. Common emergencies in rabbits, guinea pigs, and chinchillas. Vet Clin Exot Anim 2016;19:411–429.

Lennox AM, Gladden JN. Emergency and critical care of small mammals. In: Quesenberry KE, Carpenter JW, eds. Ferrets, Rabbits and Rodents, 4th ed.) Clinical Medicine and Surgery. 2021 ed. St. Louis: Saunders, 2020:595–608.
Mancinelli E. Neurologic examination and diagnostic testing in rabbits, ferrets and rodents. J Exot Pet Med 2015;24:52–64.
Minarikova A, Hauptman K, Jeklova E et al. Diseases in pet guinea pigs: a retrospective study in 1000 animals. Vet Rec 2015; 177(8):200–200.
Pignon C, Mayer J. Guinea pigs. In: Quesenberry KE, Carpenter JW, eds.

Ferrets, Rabbits and Rodents, 4th ed.). Clinical Medicine and Surgery. 2021 ed. St. Louis: Saunders, 2020:270–297.
Authors Natalie Antinoff, DVM, Dipl. ABVP (Avian) and Barbara Oglesbee, DVM, Dipl. ABVP (Avian)

HYPERCALCIURIA AND UROLITHIASIS

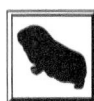

BASICS

DEFINITION
Crystal and urolith formation within the urinary tract. Crystals and uroliths may form in the urinary bladder, urethra, ureters, or renal pelvis. Most uroliths are composed of calcium salts (calcium carbonate and calcium oxalate).

PATHOPHYSIOLOGY
- Factors leading to urolithiasis in guinea pigs are unclear, although the alkaline pH and high mineral content of normal urine may favor crystal formation and precipitation.
  - One study showed that guinea pigs absorbed approximately 70% of the calcium consumed when they were fed a purified diet containing 0.9% of calcium. 62% of this calcium was excreted by the kidneys.
- Affected guinea pigs are more likely to be fed a diet high in overall percentage pellets, low in percentage hay, and less variety of vegetables and fruits
  - Alfalfa-based pellets and hay contain higher concentrations of calcium, and it has been suggested this may also contribute to urinary calculi in guinea pigs.
- Inadequate water intake leads to a more concentrated urine and factors that impair complete evacuation of the bladder, such as lack of exercise, obesity, cystitis, neoplasia, or neuromuscular diseases may be involved.
- Without frequent urination and dilute urine, calcium crystals may precipitate out from the urine within the bladder. Precipitated crystals primarily form uroliths but occasionally cause "urinary sludge" instead.
- Historical information suggested that calcium oxalate calculi were the most common uroliths identified in guinea pigs, but recent reports have more commonly identified calcium carbonate calculi.
- Bacterial urinary tract infections (involving *E. coli*, *Streptococcus pyogenes*, and *Staphylococcus* species) have been associated with the presence of urinary calculi in laboratory guinea pigs.
- Pure cultures of *Corynebacterium renale* and *Facklamia* species and mixed bacterial cultures including *C. renale*, the *Streptococcus bovis/equinus* group, and *Staphylococcus* species were found from urine of pet guinea pigs with urolithiasis, although a direct association was not confirmed.

SYSTEMS AFFECTED
- Renal/Urologic
- Gastrointestinal, neuromuscular, and cardiovascular systems may all be affected in patients with uremia.

GENETICS
Inheritance, while suspected, has not been proven.

INCIDENCE/PREVALENCE
Commonly affects middle-aged to older guinea pigs

GEOGRAPHIC DISTRIBUTION
N/A

SIGNALMENT

Breed Predilections
It has been suggested that Peruvian guinea pigs are more susceptible to urolithiasis, but this has not been proven.

Mean Age and Range
Middle-aged (2.5 years or older)

Predominant Sex
A recent study of 75 guinea pigs with urolithiasis found an equal distribution of males and females.

SIGNS

General Comments
- Some animals remain asymptomatic despite large amounts of calcium sludge accumulation in the urinary bladder
- Clinical signs are commonly associated with the size and location of the calculi.
- Bladder or urethral calculi are often associated with micturation abnormalities such as hematuria, stranguria, or dysuria and vague clinical signs such as lethargy and anorexia. If the calculus is located higher in the urinary tract, micturition abnormalities may still be present but lethargy, anorexia, weight loss, and a hunched posture may be the only clinical signs.

Historical Findings
- Pollakiuria, dysuria, and hematuria (common in guinea pigs with urolithiasis)
- Urine scalding, moist pyoderma, and staining around the perineum
- Urine appears thick, pasty, and beige to brown in color.
- Hunched posture, ataxia, difficulty ambulating, and vocalizing during urination may be associated with pain or complete or partial obstruction

Physical Examination Findings
- Hematuria, stranguria, or pollakiuria
- Abdominal palpation—
  - May detect cystoliths (most often a single large calculus)
  - A soft doughy mass within the urinary bladder may be associated with crystalluria (urine sludge).
  - Manual expression of the bladder may reveal hematuria or sometimes "sludge" (thick white-tan material), even in patients that have normal-appearing voided urine.
  - Large, turgid bladder or a painful

abdomen may be related to a partial or complete urinary obstruction.
  - A large kidney may be palpable due to obstructive nephroliths with subsequent hydronephrosis.
- Signs of uremia—dehydration, anorexia, lethargy, weakness, hypothermia, bradycardia, tachypnea, shallow respirations, stupor, or coma. Seizures occur rarely, often in terminal cases. Tachycardia results from ventricular dysrhythmias induced by hyperkalemic state.

CAUSES
- See pathophysiology

Risk Factors Contributing to Urolithiasis and Calcium "Sludge" in the Bladder
- Inadequate water intake—dirty water bowls, unpalatable water, inadequate water provision, and changing water sources
- Urine retention—underlying bladder pathology, neuromuscular disease; painful conditions causing a reluctance to ambulate, such as musculoskeletal disease (pododermatitis, arthritis) or dental disease
- Inadequate cage cleaning may cause some guinea pigs to avoid urinating.
- Obesity has been suggested as a cause but has not yet been proven.
- Lack of exercise
- Feeding exclusively alfalfa-based diet (hay, pellets, or both)
- Renal disease
- Calcium or vitamin/mineral supplements added to diet

DIAGNOSIS

DIFFERENTIAL DIAGNOSIS
- Other causes of hematuria, dysuria, and pollakiuria with or without urethral obstruction include urinary tract infection and lower tract neoplasia
- Pyometra or urinary/renal neoplasia may expel blood-tinged discharge when urinating.
  - May blend with urine and mimic hypercalciuria
- Trauma

CBC/BIOCHEMISTRY/URINALYSIS
- Hemogram—evidence of cystitis: TWBC elevations with neutrophil:lymphocyte ratio shift; toxicity of neutrophils ± bands. Monocytosis may suggest inflammation/infection. Thrombocytosis is associated with active inflammation.
- Biochemistry panel—may reflect a high calcium diet (hypercalcemia) (normal calcium range 7.8–12 mg/dL)
  - Urinary obstruction may be associated with azotemia, and also changes in electrolytes (hyperkalemia, hypochloremia, and hyponatremia).

HYPERCALCIURIA AND UROLITHIASIS (CONTINUED)

- In suspected cases of urolithiasis, urinalysis should be performed, including both a standard dipstick and microscopic examination of the sediment.
  - Urinalyses data from 44 guinea pigs with urinary calculi found that the specific gravity was 1.015 ± 0.008 (range 1.004–1.046), and urine pH was 8.4 ± 0.5 (range 7.5–>9).
  - Hematuria was the most commonly reported abnormality in urine sediment, followed by mucus and lipid droplets.
  - Calcium carbonate, calcium oxalate, and struvite crystals are all commonly seen on sediment examinations, but as with other small animals, crystal type(s) may not predict the mineralogy of calculi present.

OTHER LABORATORY TESTS
- Urinary culture—prior to antibiotic administration, culture the urine or bladder wall if high numbers of red or white blood cells, bacteria, or a combination of these are present on sediment examination.
  - Collect urine via cystocentesis as free-catch samples are commonly contaminated.
- If surgery is necessary to relieve obstruction from urolithiasis, collect and submit the calculi for analysis and culture and sensitivity, and submit the bladder wall for culture and sensitivity.
- Calculi containing calcium carbonate require specific methodologies to differentiate them from calcium oxalate monohydrate crystals. Confirm, in advance, the lab chosen for analysis's ability to perform these techniques, since human and some veterinary laboratories unfamiliar with exotic animal samples do not differentiate calcium oxalate from calcium carbonate.

IMAGING
- Obstructive calculi are usually located in the urethra of both males and females but are also found in the kidneys, ureters, vagina, or sometimes in the seminal vesicles in males.
  - Ureter obstruction is primarily identified in males.
- Urinary calculi in guinea pigs are generally radio-opaque allowing for ease of identification using survey radiography.
  - However, if multiple calculi or significant GI gas are present, the anatomic locations of the calculi using survey radiography alone may be obscured.
- Ultrasound is useful for anatomic location of the calculi and for evaluating anatomic changes in the kidneys or ureters, such as hydronephrosis, hydroureter, ureteral mucosal inflammation, or ureteral perforation.
- Excretory intravenous pyelograms (IVPs) are helpful to further elucidate relative functional abnormalities in the kidneys or ureters.

- CT/MRI imaging modalities also allow for the identification and diagnose of calculi and assessing organ architecture

DIAGNOSTIC PROCEDURES
- Urethral endoscopy can be performed to identify the location of the calculi if present in this region. Endoscopy can also be performed through a surgical incision into the bladder to attempt to identify the location of calculi within the proximal neck of the bladder.

PATHOLOGIC FINDINGS
Tissue changes may vary from intramural and/or intraluminal hemorrhage to congestion and thickening of the urethra, bladder, or ureteral mucosa in more chronic cases. Perforations of the ureter, in particular, can be indicated by chronic complete obstructions. Microscopic changes

Acutely, there may be microscopic ulceration, hemorrhage, and infiltration with heterophils. Chronic cases are characterized by infiltration of leukocytes and mononuclear cells in the lamina propria and occasionally fibroblast proliferation.

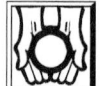

TREATMENT
APPROPRIATE HEALTH CARE
- Identify and treat any underlying cause that leads to the reluctance or inability to urinate.
- Nonobstructed animals should be provided diuresis via increased water consumption, fluid administration (intravenous or subcutaneous), and dietary modification.
- Reduce calcium in diets. Eliminate feeding foods high in calcium (alfalfa pellets) by switching to high fiber hays or pellets and feeding large volumes of fresh leafy vegetables.
- Reduce obesity and promote exercise.
- Nonobstructed animals with urolithiasis or a large amount of calcium sludge may also require voiding through urohydropropulsion.
  - Manually express the bladder to remove as much precipitate calcium as possible, monitor progress with radiographs or ultrasonography
  - Anesthesia, pain management, and smooth muscle relaxation can better improve outcomes as manual expression can be painful and traumatic.
  - Large volumes of calcium precipitate in the bladder that does not respond to medical therapy may require cystotomy for removal.
- If urolith obstruction occurs, treatment should emphasis three major components: combating the metabolic derangements associated with postrenal uremia, restoring

and maintaining a patent pathway for urine outflow, and implementing a specific treatment for the underlying cause of urine retention.
- Medical management of urethral urolith obstructions is generally unsuccessful, and surgical removal of these stones is often required.
  - Retrograde urohydropropulsion using a 3.5-Fr red rubber catheter may be attempted in sows with urethral urolithiasis under deep sedation and analgesia. However, catheterizing boars is much more dangerous because of the small size of their urethra.
- Guinea pigs with urinary obstruction should be hospitalized, and emergency supportive therapy should be provided until surgical intervention to relieve the obstruction can be performed.
- Uroliths within the bladder, ureters, or renal pelvis must be removed surgically.
  - The procedure for removing uroliths in guinea pigs is similar to small animal practice; however, care on surgical entry is paramount as guinea pigs have a large cecum.
  - After surgery, animals should be careful monitored and treated with supportive care and pain management until the patient's ability to urinate has been restored.

SURGICAL CONSIDERATIONS
- Uroliths within the bladder, ureters, renal pelvis, or urethra (that does not respond to medical therapy) require surgery.
  - Calculi removed should be submitted for analysis and culture.
  - Postoperative management includes assisted feeding, fluids, analgesics, and antibiotics based on culture and sensitivity results.
- For distal urethral uroliths in males that require a urethrotomy, the urethral incision should be left open to allow for healing via second intention to reduces the risk of strictures.

NURSING CARE
- Fluid therapy should be initiated in patients with evidence of dehydration, azotemia, or electrolyte imbalances. IV access is difficult in the guinea pigs as lateral saphenous vein catheters often kink. Consider subcutaneous fluid administration or IO catheterization. Maintenance fluid needs are estimated at 100 mL/kg/day.

ACTIVITY
- Reduced during the time of tissue repair after surgery
- Long term—increase activity level by providing large exercise areas to encourage voiding and prevent recurrence.

DIET

• Many guinea pigs with urolithiasis are anorectic or have decreased appetite. It is an absolute requirement that the patient continue to eat during and following treatments. Anorexia may cause or exacerbate gastrointestinal hypomotility and cause derangement of the gastrointestinal microflora with overgrowth of intestinal bacterial pathogens.
• Offer a large selection of fresh, moist greens such as cilantro, lettuce, parsley, carrot tops, dark leafy greens, and good-quality grass hay.
• If the patient refuses these foods, syringe-feed Critical Care for Herbivores (Oxbow Pet Products, Murdock, NE) or Emeraid Herbivore (Lafeber Company, Cornell, IL) at approximately 10–15 mL/kg PO q6–8h. Larger volumes and more frequent feedings are often accepted; feed as much as the patient will readily accept. Alternatively, pellets can be ground and mixed with fresh greens, vegetable baby foods, water, or sugar-free juice to form a gruel.
• Guinea pigs have an absolute requirement for exogenous vitamin C. Provide 50–100 mg/kg/day vitamin C while hospitalized, and during recovery. Vitamin C can be provided through food sources such as citrus fruits and through commercially made guinea pig pellets, oral supplements, or as a subcutaneous injection.
• Increased water consumption is essential to prevention and treatment of hypercalciuria. Provide multiple sources of fresh water.
• Avoid alfalfa-based diets. Animals should be fed diets containing a high percentage of timothy, oat, or grass hays, a lower overall percentage pellets, and a wider variety of vegetables and fruits. Such a diet will decrease the risk of urolith development.

CLIENT EDUCATION

• Limiting risk factors such as obesity, sedentary life, and inappropriate diet combined with increasing water consumption may delay or prevent recurrence of hypercalciuria and/or urolithiasis.

MEDICATIONS

DRUG(S) OF CHOICE

• Medical dissolution of calcium-based uroliths is ineffective in guinea pigs.
• Pain management is essential during and following surgery or if pain is causing reduced frequency of voiding. Perioperative analgesic choices include butorphanol (0.4–2.0 mg/kg SC, IM q4–12h),

buprenorphine (0.05–0.2 mg/kg SC, IM, IV q6–8h). Meloxicam (0.5–1.0 mg/kg PO, SC, IM q24h) and carprofen (4 mg/kg SC q24h or 1–2 mg/kg PO q12h). Provide anti-inflammation as well as analgesia. Tramadol, a synthetic opioid, may also be effective at dosages of 5–10 mg/kg PO q12h postoperatively. For severe to moderate pain pure mu opioids such as morphine (0.5–2.0 mg/kg SC, IM q2–4h) or oxymorphone (0.2–0.5 mg/kg SC, IM q6–12h) should be used; however, appetite and fecal output should be monitored, as these opioids are thought to contribute to GI ileus.
• Procedures for relief of obstruction generally require administering sedatives and/or anesthetics. When substantial derangements exist, begin with fluid administration and other supportive measures first. Calculate the dosage of sedative or anesthetic drug using the low end of the recommended range or give only to effect.
• Antibiotic choice should be based upon the results of culture and sensitivity (see Contraindications). Antibiotics commonly used include enrofloxacin (5–15 mg/kg PO, SC, IM q12h—this drug is basic and should therefore be diluted or injected into a subcutaneous fluid pocket to prevent tissue injury), trimethoprim sulfa (15–30 mg/kg PO q12h), chloramphenicol (30–50 mg/kg PO, SC, IM, IV q8–12h), and metronidazole (10–20 mg/kg PO, IV q12h).

CONTRAINDICATIONS

• Oral administration of antibiotics that select against gram-positive bacteria (penicillins, cephalosporins, macrolides, and lincosamides) can cause fatal enteric dysbiosis and enterotoxemia.
• Potentially nephrotoxic drugs (e.g., aminoglycosides, NSAIDs) in patients that are febrile, dehydrated, or azotemic, or that are suspected of having pyelonephritis, septicemia, or preexisting renal disease
• Glucocorticoids or other immunosuppressive agents

PRECAUTIONS

• Avoid drugs that reduce blood pressure or induce cardiac dysrhythmia until dehydration is resolved.
• Modify dosages of all drugs that require renal metabolism or elimination.
• Avoid nephrotoxic drugs (NSAIDs, aminoglycosides).

POSSIBLE INTERACTIONS

None

ALTERNATIVE DRUGS

N/A

FOLLOW-UP

PATIENT MONITORING

• Ensure gastrointestinal motility by making sure the patient is eating, well hydrated, and passing normal feces prior to release.
• Assess urine production and hydration status frequently, adjusting fluid administration rate accordingly.
• Verify the ability to urinate adequately. Failure to void may require urinary catheterization to combat urine retention or cystocentesis.

PREVENTION/AVOIDANCE

• Prevention is targeted at increasing water intake and reducing (but not eliminating) dietary calcium. Metabolic bone disease has been induced in guinea pigs with severe dietary calcium restriction for prevention of urinary calculi. For most animals, water consumption is the cornerstone of any prevention protocol.
• Avoid alfalfa-based diets. Diets containing a high percentage of timothy, oat, or grass hays, a lower overall percentage pellets, and a wider variety of vegetables and fruits decrease the risk of urolith development. It is possible that dietary inhibitors of calcium are found in greater concentration in hays than in pellets.
• Hydrochlorothiazide (2 mg/kg q12h) is a thiazide diuretic that reduces urinary calcium, potassium, and citrate. It is unknown if diuresis would be of benefit to guinea pigs whose urine is already considered isosthenuric. Do not use hydrochlorothiazide with severe renal disease or fluid imbalances.
• Urinary acidifiers were historically recommended based upon an assumed diagnosis of calcium oxalate calculi, but the normally alkaline urine of guinea pigs makes the use of dietary acidifiers concerning. Potassium citrate (30–75 mg/kg PO q12h) binds urinary calcium, reduces ion activity, and alkalinizes the urine. As guinea pigs have alkaline urine, even with disease, the efficacy of this treatment is unclear. Hyperkalemia occurs, so monitor plasma potassium closely during treatment. Potassium citrate and hydrochlorothiazide have been used together anecdotally with some clinical success.

POSSIBLE COMPLICATIONS

• Severe electrolyte imbalances
• Uremia with complete obstruction
• Urine scald
• Failure to detect or treat effectively may lead to pyelonephritis
• Pododermatitis

HYPERCALCIURIA AND UROLITHIASIS (CONTINUED)

EXPECTED COURSE AND PROGNOSIS
- The prognosis following surgical removal of uroliths is fair to good.
- Recurrence of hypercalciuria and urolithiasis is common, and although dietary management may decrease the likelihood of recurrence, many guinea pigs will develop clinical disease again.

 MISCELLANEOUS

ASSOCIATED CONDITIONS
- Urinary tract infections
- Vaginitis
- Pyometra from ascending bacterial infection of the lower urinary tract

AGE-RELATED FACTORS
This disease is frequently found in middle-aged to older guinea pigs, although it can occur in younger animals as well.

ZOONOTIC POTENTIAL
N/A

PREGNANCY/FERTILITY/BREEDING
While there is no documented evidence that urolithiasis has a hereditary component, it is generally recommended to avoid breeding these animals in the future.

SYNONYMS
Urinary stones and crystals

ABBREVIATIONS
CT = computed tomography
IVP = intravenous pyelogram
MRI = magnetic resonance imaging
NSAID = nonsteroidal anti-inflammatory drug
RBC = red blood cells
TWBC = total white blood cell count

INTERNET RESOURCES
N/A

Suggested Reading
Hallman RM, Brandão J. Diagnostic imaging of the renal system in exotic companion mammals. Vet Clin Exot Anim 2020;23:195–214.
Hawkins MG, Ruby AL, Drazenovich TL et al. Composition and characteristics of urinary calculi from guinea pigs. J Amer Vet Med Assoc 2009;234:214–220.
Hoefer H, Latney L. Rodents: urogenital and reproductive disorders. In: Keeble E, Meredith A, eds. BSAVA Manual of Rodents and Ferrets. Gloucester: BSAVA, 2009:150–160.
Miwa Y, Sladky K. Common surgical procedures of rodents, ferrets, hedgehogs, and sugar gliders. Vet Clin Exot Anim 2016;19:205–244.
Percy D, Barthold S. Guinea pig. In: Percy D, Barthold S, eds. Pathology of Laboratory Rodents and Rabbits. Ames: Blackwell, 2001:209–247.
Pignon C, Mayer J. Guinea pigs. In: Quesenberry KE, Carpenter JW, editors. Ferrets, Rabbits and Rodents (4th ed.). Clinical Medicine and Surgery. 2021, St. Louis: Saunders; 2020. p. 270–297.
Reavill D, Lennox A. Disease overview of the urinary tract in exotic companion mammals and tips on clinical management. Vet Clin Exot Anim 2020;23:169–193.
Author Rodney Schnellbacher, DVM, Dipl. ACZM

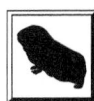

BASICS

Hyperthyroidism: A clinical disease syndrome related to hyperfunctional thyroid tissue and excessive production and release of thyroid hormone.

PATHOPHYSIOLOGY
• Hyperplastic thyroid tissue or neoplastic thyroid tissue (benign or malignant) produces and releases excessive thyroid hormone.
• Excessive thyroid hormone has adverse effects on target organs (primarily the heart and GI system).

SYSTEMS AFFECTED
• Cardiovascular: Hypertrophic cardiomyopathy results from chronically excessive thyroid hormone levels. Systemic hypertension can result (not reported in hyperthyroid guinea pigs).
• Urinary: Excessive thyroid hormone levels create high arterial pressure to the kidneys and can cause damage to kidneys while masking clinical signs and laboratory gauges of azotemia.
• Dermatologic: Thyroid disease can cause alopecia in symmetrical pattern.
• Ophthalmologic: Systemic hypertension can cause retinal detachment and loss of vision. This has not been reported in guinea pigs.
• Gastrointestinal: Hyperthyroidism can cause soft stool or diarrhea along with weight loss in the face of an adequate or increased appetite. Liver cellular leakage can occur in hyperthyroidism as evidenced by increased ALT.

INCIDENCE/PREVALENCE
• Anecdotally reported as common in pet guinea pigs
• One commercial pathology service reported a relative prevalence of 4.6% making thyroid disease the second most common pathology in cavies second to lymphoma.

SIGNALMENT
• Female guinea pigs seem to be overrepresented in some reports, but statistical significance has not been evaluated.
• Most cases of hyperthyroidism occur in guinea pigs older than 3 years of age.

SIGNS

Historical Findings
Clinical signs commonly seen in hyperthyroidism
• Hyperactivity (maybe followed by periods of inactivity and sleep)
• Resting in lateral recumbency
• Hyperesthesia
• Polydipsia
• Polyphagia
• Weight loss/possible cachexia despite normal to increased appetite
• Palpable mass in the neck
• Progressive alopecia has been reported in the German literature
• Separating themselves from others
    Clinical signs related to HCM
• Dyspnea
• Tachypnea
• Tachycardia
• Collapse
• Signs compatible with right-sided or left-sided CHF are possible.
    Clinical signs related to increased systemic blood pressure
• Blindness or partial blindness
• Dilated pupils

Physical Examination Findings
• Mass or swelling of the thyroid gland. In the guinea pig, the thyroid glands are more cranial than most companion animals. Lumps can often be found between the mandibular rami. Masses are sometimes cystic and appear as very large, fluid-filled subcutaneous swellings.
• Cardiac auscultation—possibly normal, murmur (intensity based on degree of hypertrophied ventricle(s) change in geometry).
• Muffled heart sounds (pleural effusion/pericardial effusion)
• Rales/crackles in lungs in event of pulmonary edema
• Pulse deficits may be present in event of arrhythmia
• Jugular pulses are possible due to right-sided congestive failure
• Hepatosplenomegaly possible in cases of right-sided congestive failure (passive congestion)
• Pericardial and/or abdominal effusion is possible although not reported.
• Soft stool/diarrhea
• Increased heart and respiratory rate
• Unkempt coat
• Progressive alopecia
• Anorexia in late-stage hyperthyroidism

CAUSES AND RISK FACTORS
• Females may be over-represented.
• No genetic factors noted.
• Causes include hyperplastic, benign neoplastic, and malignant thyroid tissue

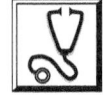

DIAGNOSIS

DIFFERENTIAL DIAGNOSIS
• Cardiac disease—any condition causing CHF
• Pleural effusion—CHF, neoplasia, infection (pyothorax), hemothorax (chylous effusion has not been reported)
• Muffled heart sounds—pleural effusion, pericardial effusion
• Pulmonary edema—CHF, pneumonia, electrocution
• Pulse deficits—arrhythmias (often tachyarrhythmias)
• Jugular pulses with right sided murmur may indicate tricuspid valve disease/right sided CHF
• Hepatomegaly—right-sided CHF, neoplasia
• Hair loss and depression—ovarian cysts, barbering (self or by others), late-stage hypothyroidism, ectoparasites, dermatophytosis, adrenal tumor
• Weight loss with good appetite—dental disease, metabolic disease, neoplasia
• Subcutaneous submandibular mass—cervical lymphadenitis, lymphoma, granuloma, mandibular salivary gland neoplasia, lymphadenopathy
• Alopecia—cystic ovaries in females, hypothyroidism
• PUPD—renal disease, diabetes mellitus
• Weight loss—dental disease, endoparasites, metabolic disease, ovarian cysts, competition for food offered
• Soft stool/diarrhea—cecal dysbiosis, recent antibiotic usage, bacterial infection

CBC/BIOCHEMISTRY/URINALYSIS
• CBC is often normal
• Serum chemistries may reveal increased ALT
• Azotemia may be due to the renal effects of hyperthyroidism or underlying, concurrent renal disease. The severity of renal compromise is often more pronounced than laboratory values would suggest. Serum creatinine concentrations often remain low in patients with preexisiting renal compromise due to the effects of systemic hypertension. Eventually, thyroid-induced hypertension will exacerbate renal dysfunction if left untreated. It should be noted that treatment for hyperthyroidism may unmask azotemia or result in clinically significant renal disease.

OTHER LABORATORY TESTS
• Cytologic evaluation of fine needle aspirates of thyroid tissue can reveal brownish or bloody fluid in cases of cystic neoplasia, and proteinaceous matrix if colloid is being produced. Exercise extreme caution when performing FNA, as significant bleeding can occur.
• Thyroid hormone levels performed on this fluid may be increased. Normal values have been reported in many sources
    ◦ TT4 1.1–5 mcg/dL
    ◦ Castrated males may have a higher median level (2.7 mcg/dL).

• Increased TT4 may also be caused by vitamin C deficiency.
• One study looked at a point-of-care analyzer for TT4 levels. Results of this study showed:
  ◦ Abaxis VetScan® analyzer with a T4/cholesterol rotor was a reliable method of looking at guinea pig TT4 levels.
  ◦ In this study, pet animals had a wider range of normal than laboratory guinea pigs
  ◦ Normal range for guinea pig TT4 was 2.26–5.82 mcg/dL
• Rare cases have normal T4 and T3 values
• Free T4 may be needed to diagnose hyperthyroidism if the total T4 is above half the low-level normal value. Normal values for free T4 have been reported to be 0.85–1.67 ng/dL (male) and 1.08–1.58 ng/dL (female).

DIAGNOSTIC IMAGING
Radiographic Findings
• Findings compatible with HCM can be seen including biatrial enlargement and evidence of ventricular enlargement.
• Skull radiographs and sedated oral exam can help rule out dental disease
• May be metastasis of adenocarcinoma to the lungs
• Evidence of thyroid gland mineralization may be noted.

Ultrasonographic Findings
• Ultrasound of thyroid masses may allow for accurate sampling for cytology or fluid to look for increased total T4 in the fluid.

Echocardiographic Findings
• Echocardiogram is the *best* way to definitively diagnose HCM.
• Effusions may be noted (analysis usually reveals modified transudate).

CT and MRI
• May have some uses in diagnosis and identifying ectopic tissue tumors in the chest and metastasis to the lungs.

Nuclear Scintigraphy
• Ideal method of identifying the location of hyperactive thyroid tissue
• This method will identify ectopic tissue in the thoracic cavity.

DIAGNOSTIC TESTS
Electrocardiography
• Use padded alligator clips or nontraumatic flat clips with alcohol or ultrasonic gel as conductive agent
• Ventricular and supraventricular arrythmias can be noted. Tachyarrhythmias are more common than bradyarrhythmias with thyroid disease.
• Electrical alternans may be noted with pericardial effusion.

Pathologic Findings
• Histopathology of the thyroid glands will reveal hyperplastic or neoplastic tissue involving the follicular cells.
• One report indicates that a majority of lesions were adenocarcinomas.
• Evaluation of the relative prevalence of hyperplasia versus adenoma or adenocarcinomas in thyroid disease has yet to be investigated.
• Most common lesions concurrent to thyroid gland pathology are pulmonary congestion and atrophy of fat
• Occasionally osseous metaplasia of the tumor

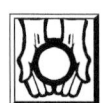

TREATMENT
APPROPRIATE HEALTH CARE
• Decompensated HCM in guinea pigs should prompt hospitalization for stabilization.
• Mildly affected patients can be managed as outpatients.

EMERGENT CARE
• Severely dyspneic patients may need immediate oxygen therapy. Guinea pigs often struggle with oxygen masks and flow-by-oxygen therapy and may decompensate rapidly. Oxygen cages are preferred. Beware of long-term 100% oxygen therapy as it may cause myocardial pathology.
• Most guinea pigs benefit from mild sedation in the hospital environment (midazolam 0.2–0.4 mg/kg SC, IM, IV and butorphanol 0.2–4 mg/kg SC, IM, IV)
• In dyspneic patients with fulminant heart failure: furosemide (2–5 mg/kg SC, IM, IV) and/or nitroglycerin ointment (2%) applied to the hairless area on the ear. For dogs and cats, ¼" of the ointment is applied. Amount should be adjusted to account for a guinea pig's small body size. Wear gloves to avoid ointment contacting your skin.
• Avoid stressors including nearby predators and noises from other hospitalized pets. Handle the patient minimally until its condition improves to allow diagnostics (radiography first and foremost).

MEDICATIONS
FOR CHF
Furosemide
• Indicated only for patients with fluid accumulation (pleural effusion, pulmonary edema, abdominal effusion, and subcutaneous ventral edema)

• Dosage: 2–5 mg/kg SC, IM, IV q4–6h (emergent care); 1–4 mg/kg PO for outpatient care.
• Titrate to lowest effective dose
• Best if compounded to flavored suspension but this author has used flavored injectable solution orally in some patients.
• Monitor for dehydration, azotemia, and hypokalemia
• Be aware, patients on this diuretic will usually have isosthenuric urine (~1.010).

Pimobendan
• A potent positive inotropic agent with positive effects on preload and afterload
• 0.25–0.4 mg/kg PO q12h
• This drug may need to be compounded into a suspension to accurately dose a guinea pig.

FOR HYPERTHYROIDISM
Surgical Treatment
Removal of all affected thyroid tissue can be curative
• Imaging recommended to detect ectopic thyroid tissue and to determine if disease appears to be uni- or bilateral.
• Some carcinomas can have a tremendous blood supply
• Removal of mass can be associated with damage to or removal of parathyroid glands.
• Recurrent laryngeal nerve passes nearby the normal thyroid gland
• Patients should always be monitored for hypocalcemia post operatively.
• Submit tissue for histopathology
• Will not be effective if functional ectopic thyroid tissue present. This ectopic tissue is often found in the thoracic cavity.
• Insufficient removal of abnormal tissue may result in only a transient response to surgery.
• Use of ketamine for anesthesia is contraindicated due to severe hypertension and tachycardia

Antithyroid Medication
• Methimazole and carbimazole are the most common drugs used. It should be compounded to administer orally or as a transdermal medication to be applied to hairless areas of the body (e.g., the pinna of the ear)
  ◦ Methimazole dose 0.5–2.0 mg/kg PO, transdermal q12–24h
  ◦ Carbimazole dose 1–2 mg/kg PO q12–24h
  ◦ Transdermal application may cause depigmentation of brown skin
  ◦ Usually begin therapy at q24h; begin q12h treatment in refractory cases
• Possible side effects include liver dysfunction, alterations in CBC (agranulocytosis), and inappetence and

depression. Side effects have not been reported in guinea pigs to date.
• In cats, hyperthyroidism can become resistant to control by these drugs over time.

Radioactive Iodine Injection (I131)
• Excellent chance of cure with minimal to no side effects.
• Identification of a nuclear medicine facility that will treat guinea pigs is not always possible.

FOLLOW-UP
• CBC/chemistry should be monitored for hematologic and hepatic changes related to antithyroid medications. Author recommends re-evaluation 1-month after onset of therapy and again every 4–6 months.
• With surgical treatment, ionized calcium level should be measured before surgery and again 2 weeks postoperatively. Calcium supplementation may be needed.
• With I-131 therapy, thyroid hormone levels should be re-evaluated 1-month post therapy. Also monitor for underlying renal disease.

• In animals with HCM, repeat radiographs and echocardiograms as indicated.
• If hypertensive, monitor blood pressure during and after therapy

MISCELLANEOUS
ABBREVIATIONS
ALT = alanine aminotransferase
CBC = complete blood cell count
CHF = congestive heart failure
DCM = dilated cardiomyopathy
EKG = electrocardiogram
GI = gastrointestinal
HCM = hypertrophic cardiomyopathy
NRC = nuclear regulatory commission
PUPD = polyuria/polydipsia
RCM = restrictive cardiomyopathy
TT4 = Total T4

Suggested Reading
Brandao J, Mayer J. Hyperthyroidism and hyperparathyroidism in guinea pigs (*Cavia porcellus*). Vet Clin Exot Anim 2013;16:407–420.

Fredholm DV, Cagle LA, Johnston MS. Evaluation of precision and establishment of reference ranges for plasma thyroxine using a point-of-care analyzer in healthy guinea pigs (*Cavia porcellus*). JEPM 2012;21:87–93.

Gibbons PM, Garner MM, Kiupel M. Morphological and immunohistochemical characterization of spontaneous thyroid gland neoplasms in guinea pigs (*Cavia porcellus*). Vet Path 2012;50(2):334–342.

Girod-Ruffer C, Muller E, Marschang RE et al. Retrospective study on hyperthyroidism in guinea pigs in veterinary practices in Germany. J Exot Pet Med 2019;29:87–97.

Kuenzel F, Hierlmeier B, Christian M et al. Hyperthyroidism in four guinea pigs: clinical manifestations, diagnosis, and treatment. JSAP 2013;54:667–671.

Mayer J, Wagner R, Taeymans O. Advanced diagnostic approaches and current management of thyroid pathologies in guinea pigs. Vet Clin Exot Anim 2010;13:509–523.

Author Jeffrey L. Rhody, DVM, DABVP-ECM

GUINEA PIGS

HYPOVITAMINOSIS C (SCURVY)

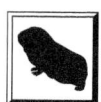

BASICS

DEFINITION
Disease caused by a deficiency of vitamin C

PATHOPHYSIOLOGY
• Guinea pigs (and primates, including humans) lack the gene required for production of L-gulonolactone oxidase, and the enzyme necessary to convert L-gulonolactone to L-ascorbic acid. They are unable to synthesize or store vitamin C, and therefore require exogenous supplementation.
• Ascorbic acid is required for hydroxylation of proline and lysine to hydroxyproline and hydroxylysine, amino acids that are important for cross-linking, and stabilizing collagen peptides.
• Collagen is required for maintaining blood vessel integrity, formation of bone, and wound healing. Deficiency results in fragile capillaries, leading to hemorrhage of the gingival mucosa, subcutis, skeletal muscle, and serosal surfaces.
• Disarray of cartilage and marrow fibrosis occurs in areas of osteogenesis, commonly at joints of long bones and ribs, leading to swelling of costochondral junctions and joints.
• The anchoring of teeth in their bony sockets may also be affected, leading to malocclusion and difficulty eating.
• Vitamin C is also involved in retention of vitamin E; secondary vitamin E deficiency may be present concurrently.

SYSTEMS AFFECTED
• Musculoskeletal—swollen, painful limb joints and an inability to extend the stifles may result in a "bunny-hop" gait; painful when touched
• Hemic/Lymphatic/Immune—swollen, hemorrhagic gums, hemorrhages on subcutis, skeletal muscle, and serosal surfaces; decreased immunity to bacterial colonization or infectious diseases
• Gastrointestinal—loosening of teeth with subsequent decrease in appetite and/or malocclusion; diarrhea; weight loss
• Skin—bruising and hemorrhage; rough hair coat

GENETICS
The lack of L-gulonolactone oxidase is present in all guinea pigs.

INCIDENCE/PREVALENCE
• Occurs in guinea pigs fed diets lacking or deficient in vitamin C

GEOGRAPHIC DISTRIBUTION
Worldwide

SIGNALMENT
• No breed or sex predilections
• Young animals are more susceptible because of a combination of rapid growth and an increased catabolism of vitamin C in guinea pigs under 4 months of age

SIGNS

Historical Findings
• Lameness; stiff "bunny-hop" gait
• Lethargy, weakness
• Anorexia
• Diet inadequate in vitamin C

Physical Examination Findings
• Joint pain and swelling in long bones and costochondral junctions
• Painful on palpation or restraint
• Bruising, bleeding, or petechia/ecchymoses of gingiva, skin
• Diarrhea
• Rough hair coat
• Weight loss

CAUSES AND RISK FACTORS
• Dietary deficiency of vitamin C
• Young animals are at greater risk because of rapidly developing bone and increased catabolism of vitamin C.
• Although guinea pig pelleted diets are fortified with ascorbic acid, the content is reduced by storage, light, heat, and moisture.
• As much as 50% of vitamin C activity may be lost within 6 weeks of storage; therefore, it is recommended to feed product within 90 days of milling.
• Vitamin C activity is diminished by water, so supplementation of drinking water may be suboptimal or ineffective; 50% of activity is lost within 24 hours.
• Some small mammal vitamin supplements do not contain adequate vitamin C levels for guinea pigs.
• Vitamin C content of vegetables varies; owners may believe they are providing adequate amounts from fruit and vegetable sources that may actually be deficient in vitamin C.
• Clinical signs can occur within 2 weeks of receiving a deficient diet.

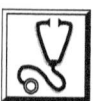

DIAGNOSIS

DIFFERENTIAL DIAGNOSIS
• Osteoarthritis
• Septic arthritis
• Rickets
• Trauma/fracture
• Anticoagulant rodenticide toxicity
• Coagulopathy
• Neoplasia

CBC/BIOCHEMISTRY/URINALYSIS
Usually normal

OTHER LABORATORY TESTS
Serum ascorbic acid levels can be performed as a confirming test, but therapy should be initiated precluding test results.

IMAGING
Radiographic findings:
• Enlarged costochondral junctions and long bone epiphyses
• Pathologic fractures may be present
• Cortical thinning
• Generalized demineralization of bones
• Periosteal separation and epiphyseal separation
• Separation of metaphysis and diaphysis

PATHOLOGIC FINDINGS
• Gross findings—hemorrhage of periosteum, periarticular tissues, subcutaneous tissues, skeletal muscle, intestine, and serosal surfaces; separation of the epiphyseal junction
• Histopathologic findings—impaired ossification of epiphyseal cartilage, microfractures, subperiosteal hemorrhage; poorly differentiated fusiform mesenchymal cells in periosteum and periarticular tissue; fragmentation of myofilaments of skeletal muscle

TREATMENT

APPROPRIATE HEALTH CARE
• It is essential to correct the underlying cause by providing adequate vitamin C and addressing dietary insufficiency.
• Inpatient—recommended for initial treatment to provide daily injections of vitamin C, fluid therapy, analgesics, and nutritional support until the patient is eating and improving
• Outpatient—appropriate during the recovery period

NURSING CARE
• Fluid therapy to maintain hydration—subcutaneous generally adequate
• Assisted feeding of anorexic animals
• Maintain clean, soft bedding
• In severe cases, turn patient and bathe as needed to prevent formation of decubitus ulcers.

ACTIVITY
Restrict activity during short-term recovery to prevent trauma and bruising, fracture, or other injuries; avoid high surfaces or potential falls; gradually encourage ambulation once clinical signs are improving (usually within 1 week of initiating treatment) to prevent muscle atrophy or contracture.

DIET
• In the acute phase, or if the patient is inappetant/anorexic, it is essential to provide adequate nutritional support. Syringe-feed a formulated diet such as Critical Care for Herbivores (Oxbow Pet Products, Murdock,

(CONTINUED)

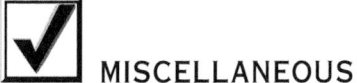

NE) or Emerald Herbivore (Lafeber Company, Cornell, IL) 10–15 mL/kg q6–8h. If neither product is available, a slurry can be made with blended leafy green vegetables that are high in vitamin C, or guinea pig pellets crushed and mixed with water and vegetable baby food.
• Provide a diet with appropriate vitamin C content. Most commercial guinea pig pellets are produced with supplemental vitamin C (minimum of 6 mg/kg/day) but must be consumed within 90 days of milling to ensure potency.
• Daily requirement for maintenance is 25–30 mg/kg; provide 50–100 mg/kg/day in deficiency.
• Oral supplementation can be provided. Several companies provide vitamin C chewable tablets for guinea pigs, which many pets will readily consume as treats.
• Children's vitamin C supplements can also be administered.
• Water supplementation can be used but must be provided in adequate amounts (200–400 mg/L) and must be changed daily.
• This method is less reliable than direct oral supplementation or dietary supplementation.

CLIENT EDUCATION
• Instruct owners to check packages of guinea pig pellets for the date of milling.
• Advise owners to avoid buying large quantities of pelleted food that cannot be consumed within the 90-day time period because 50% of vitamin C in feed is lost within 6 weeks.
• Discuss feeding fruits and vegetables with appropriate levels of vitamin C and provide the owner with information about vitamin C content of fruits and vegetables, including quantity.
• Inform owners that if water supplementation of vitamin C is to be used, they must mix fresh daily.
• Educate owners about supplements that may contain vitamin C in appropriate amounts.

SURGICAL CONSIDERATIONS
Surgery for any nonemergency reason should be postponed until resolution of clinical signs to prevent hemorrhage or delayed wound healing.

MEDICATIONS
DRUG(S) OF CHOICE
• Ascorbic acid: 50–100 mg/kg/day SC during deficiency
• Vitamin C: 50 mg/kg/day PO for deficiency, 30–50 mg/kg/day PO for maintenance/prevention, or 200–400 mg/L in drinking water daily

• For pain management, use meloxicam (0.5–1.0 mg/kg PO, SC q24h) for its anti-inflammatory effects; buprenorphine (0.05–0.2 mg/kg SC, IM, IV q8–12h), butorphanol (0.4–2.0 mg/kg SC, IM q4–12h), or tramadol (5–10 mg/kg PO q12h) can be added for additional analgesia in the acute phase of treatment.

CONTRAINDICATIONS
• Avoid the use of multivitamins to provide the appropriate dose of vitamin C, as this may lead to oversupplementation of other vitamins.

PRECAUTIONS
• High doses of vitamin C may predispose patients to oxalate or urate stone formation.
• High doses may cause false-negative urine glucose results in diabetic patients.

POSSIBLE INTERACTIONS
• High doses may cause acidification of urine, which may increase renal excretion of certain drugs such as mexiletine or quinidine, so should be used with caution in patients with cardiac disease
• Antimicrobial efficacy of certain drugs in the urine (aminoglycosides) may be reduced due to the acidification of urine
• Synergistic with deferoxamine in removing iron but may lead to increased tissue concentrations of iron

FOLLOW-UP
PATIENT MONITORING
• Radiographs can be performed at monthly intervals until no further change is evident.
• Serum ascorbic levels can be assessed for return to normal.

PREVENTION/AVOIDANCE
• Feed commercial guinea pig pellets within 90 days of milling.
• Provide a variety of vitamin C-rich vegetables daily.
• If water supplementation is provided, replace daily.

POSSIBLE COMPLICATIONS
• Osteoarthritis
• Malocclusion

EXPECTED COURSE AND PROGNOSIS
• Initial clinical response may be evident within 1 week of initiating treatment, but resolution is incomplete at this time.
• Supplementation of vitamin C should be provided for life.
• Prognosis for recovery is good, although sequelae including lameness, osteoarthritis, and dental malocclusion may occur.

✓ MISCELLANEOUS
ASSOCIATED CONDITIONS
• Dental malocclusion
• Osteoarthritis

AGE-RELATED FACTORS
Young, rapidly growing guinea pigs <4 months of age are more commonly affected.

ZOONOTIC POTENTIAL
None

PREGNANCY/FERTILITY/BREEDING
Pregnant/nursing animals may require additional vitamin C supplementation.

SYNONYMS
N/A

SEE ALSO
Anorexia and pseudoanorexia
Paresis and paralysis
Weight loss and cachexia

ABBREVIATIONS
N/A

INTERNET RESOURCES
Rothschild BM, Sebes JI. (2008) Scurvy [www document]. URL http://emedicine. medscape.com/article/413463-overview. Accessed on October 6, 2010.
  U.S. Department of Agriculture, Agricultural Research Service. 2005. USDA National Nutrient Database for Standard Reference, Release 18. Nutrient Data Laboratory Home Page, URL http://www. nal.usda.gov/fnic/foodcomp. Accessed on October 6, 2010.

Suggested Reading
Harkness JE, Turner PV, VandeWoude S, Wheeler CL. Hypovitaminosis C (scurvy) in guinea pigs. In: Harkness JE, Turner PV, VandeWoude S, Wheeler CL, eds. Biology and Medicine of Rabbits and Rodents, 5th ed. Ames: Wiley-Blackwell, 2010:316–319.
Minarikova A, Hauptman K, Jeklova E et al. Diseases in pet guinea pigs: a retrospective study in 1000 animals. Vet Rec 2015; 177(8):200–200.
Newcomer CE. Laboratory animals. In: Aiello SE, ed. The Merck Veterinary Manual, 8th ed. Whitehouse Station: Merck, 1998:1316–1339.
Pignon C, Mayer J. Guinea pigs. In: Quesenberry KE, Carpenter JW, editors. Ferrets, Rabbits and Rodents (4th Ed). Clinical Medicine and Surgery. 2021, St. Louis: Saunders; 2020. p. 270–297
Authors Natalie Antinoff, DVM, Dipl. ABVP (Avian) and Barbara Oglesbee, DVM, Dipl. ABVP (Avian)

GUINEA PIGS

LICE AND MITES

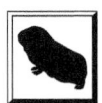

BASICS

DEFINITION
Infestation of the guinea pig by mites (*Trixacarus caviae, Chirodiscoides caviae*) and lice (*Gliricola porcelli, Gyropus ovalis*), resulting in alopecia and epidermal pathology

PATHOPHYSIOLOGY
• *Trixacarus caviae*—This sarcoptid mite is the most significant and pruritic ectoparasite of the guinea pig. The life cycle ranges from 2 to 14 days. Some cases of extreme pruritus can lead to seizures, severe self-trauma, and generalized dermatitis. Secondary bacterial infection is common. With chronicity, animals become thin and debilitated and may die.
• *Chirodiscoides caviae* is a fur mite that causes mild or no clinical signs, even with heavy infestation.
• *Gliricola porcelli* and *Gyropus ovalis* are chewing lice that adversely affect the hair coat (e.g., alopecia) but also may cause crusting of the skin.

SYSTEMS AFFECTED
• Skin
• Hair

GENETICS
N/A

INCIDENCE/PREVALENCE
• Immunosuppressed animals may be affected to a greater degree than healthy guinea pigs.
• Exposure to infested animals.

GEOGRAPHIC DISTRIBUTION
N/A

SIGNALMENT
No age or gender prediposition

SIGNS

Historical Findings
Trixacarus caviae (sarcoptic mange mite):
• History of exposure to other guinea pigs
• Lesions usually begin on the thighs and back and extend over the shoulders onto the dorsal cervical area.
• Skin may be covered with a yellow crust.
• Owners report intense itching and possibly seizure-like behavior.
• Progression to weight loss, lethargy, and general debility
Fur mites and lice (*Chirodiscoides caviae, Gliricola porcelli*, and *Gyropus ovalis*):
• May be asymptomatic
• Owners may notice rough hair coat or note the presence of lice, mites, or nits, which are visible to the naked eye.
• Alopecia
• Observation of nits, lice

• Yellow crusting of skin
• Hair loss may be obvious or subtle, depending on ectoparasite.
• Pattern of hair loss associated with specific parasite involved

Physical Examination Findings
Trixacarus caviae (sarcoptic mange mite):
• Alopecia with scales, crusting beginning on the thighs and dorsum, spreading crainially; eventually becomes generalized
• With heavy or chronic infestation, severe lichenification, erythema, scaling (skin may be friable and covered with yellow crusts)
• Intense pruritus—vigorous scratching often leads to seizurelike episodes.
• General debility—weight loss, weakness with chronic or severe infestation
• Signs of secondary skin infections should be noted and a careful nondermatological physical examination should be performed.
Fur mites and lice (*Chirodiscoides caviae, Gliricola porcelli*, and *Gyropus ovalis*):
• Mites, lice, or nits often grossly visible
• *Chirodiscoides caviae*—often found around the groin and axilla. Mites are present in the hairs and are easily observed on hair plucks.
• Excessive shedding
• Pruritus
• Secondary skin diseases, such as a bacterial pyoderma or seborrhea

CAUSES
Mites—*Trixacarus caviae* and *Chirodiscoides caviae*
Lice—*Gliricola porcelli* and *Gyropus oval*

RISK FACTORS
• Poor husbandry
• Exposure to infested animal

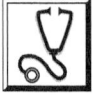

DIAGNOSIS

DIFFERENTIAL DIAGNOSIS
• Alopecia due to neurological/behavioral disorders—Stress—generalized hair loss; barbering, fur chewing—lesions can be found anywhere but commonly on rump and perineal areas
• Alopecia due to nutritional deficiencies (particularly protein deficiencies and hypovitaminosis C)—poor hair coat, generalized thinning
• Alopecia due to hyperestrogenism: Cystic ovarian disease—common cause of alopecia over the back, ventrum, and flanks; pregnancy-associated alopecia—flanks bilaterally
• Alopecia due to conditions directly causing destruction or damage to the hair shaft or follicle
• Other, uncommon ectoparasites—*Cheyletiella parasitivorax* usually produces

lesions on the dorsum; *Demodex caviae* is frequently located on the head and forelegs.
• Dermatophytosis—*Trichophyton mentagrophytes*—often affects hair around the face and legs, sometimes dorsum; can be pruritic
• Bacterial pyoderma—location depends on the inciting cause and may be present anywhere. Exfoliative dermatitis is reported most commonly in the ventral aspect.
• Traumatic episodes (burns)
• Allergic skin diseases (e.g., atopy, food allergy, contact, insect hypersensitivity)—contact hypersensitivity has been reported in guinea pigs.

CBC/BIOCHEMISTRY/URINALYSIS
Need is dependent on the underlying disease process. Most often normal except in severe pyoderma and parasite infestation. *Trixacarus caviae* will often cause a leukocytosis, monocytosis, eosinophilia, and basophilia.

OTHER LABORATORY TESTS
N/A

IMAGING
N/A

DIAGNOSTIC PROCEDURES
• Skin scrapings for ectoparasites—may be extremely painful and trigger seizures in patients severely affected by *Trixacarus caviae*. Diagnosis by characteristic signs and response to treatment. Deep skin scrapings are necessary to reveal *Trixacarus caviae* and *Demodex caviae*. The hair should be clipped before processing. Mineral oil can be used for slide preparation.
• Combing of the hair coat for mites and lice
• Impression smears of the skin for evidence of bacterial or yeast infections
• Adhesive tape collection—for surface-living ectoparasites
• Bacterial culture and sensitivity—infected lesions are frequently contaminated with the resident microbiological flora.
• Skin biopsy—sample should contain normal and abnormal sites. Evaluate hair follicle structures, numbers, and anagen/telogen ratios. Examine for evidence of bacterial, fungal, neoplastic, or parasitic skin infections.

PATHOLOGIC FINDINGS
Trixacarus caviae—orthokeratotic hyperkeratosis, eosinophilic microabscesses, and necrotic areas; cross-sections of the mites may be present.

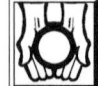

TREATMENT

APPROPRIATE HEALTH CARE
• Animals with chronic or severe infestation with *Trixacarus caviae* are often severely

debilitated and may require hospitalization for supportive care during mite treatment.
• Mildly affected animals can be treated on an outpatient basis.
• More than one disease condition may be contributing to the pruritus (summation of effects). Initial therapy may be indicated based on top differential diagnoses when one fails to definitively identify an inciting cause.
• Hair should be clipped in case of secondary bacterial dermatitis, especially around the affected area.
• All exposed animals should be treated for appropriate ectoparasite infestation. The environment may also need to be thoroughly cleaned.

NURSING CARE
Severely debilitated patients may require hospitalization for supportive care, such as fluid therapy and assisted feeding.

ACTIVITY
N/A

DIET
• Make sure the patient continues to eat to prevent gastrointestinal motility disorders.
• Guinea pigs need a dietary source of vitamin C. Higher levels should be provided to sick individuals (30–50 mg/kg PO q24h). Vitamin C may be ground and fed directly to the pig. Vitamin C treats are also available for guinea pigs (e.g., Daily C, Oxbow Pet Products, Murdock, NE).

CLIENT EDUCATION
• *Trixacarus caviae* can transiently infest humans.
• Treating all in-contact animals and cleaning and disinfecting the cage are essential to treatment success. Remove and discard all organic material from the cage (wood or paper products, bedding); disinfect cage and replace bedding with shredded paper bedding that can be discarded, and the cage thoroughly cleaned every day during the treatment period.

SURGICAL CONSIDERATIONS
N/A

MEDICATIONS
DRUG(S) OF CHOICE
• Ivermectin—0.4–0.8 SC mg/kg every 7–10 days for three doses is usually effective to treat mite infestation (less effective for chewing lice).
• Selamectin (Revolution) 15–30 mg/kg topically every 10–14 days for two treatments is usually effective for lice or mite infestation.

• Imidacloprid/moxidectin (Advantage Multi orange) 0.1 mL/kg topically once every 30 days for three treatments for lice or mite infestation.
• For chewing lice—frequent flea combing to remove nits and application of carbaryl powders (labeled for use in kittens) is often effective.
• Topical lime-sulfur dips may be helpful, but these tend to be stressful to guinea pigs.

Dermal bacterial infection—antibiotic therapy:
• Hair should be clipped cleaned with disinfectants such as dilute povidone iodine or dilute chlorexidine initially
• Topical treatment with antimicrobial shampoos can be used in pyoderma. Antimicrobial shampoos include chlorhexidine and ethyl lactate shampoos.
• Broad-spectrum antibiotics safe to use in guinea pigs include enrofloxacin (5–20 mg/kg PO, SC, IM q12h), which is ineffective against anaerobes and may be variably effective against *Streptococcus* spp., trimethoprim-sulfa (15–30 mg/kg PO q12h), chloramphenicol (30–50 mg/kg PO, SC, IM, IV q8–12h), and azithromycin (15–30 mg/kg PO q24h). Therapy should be based on culture and sensitivity if possible.
• Treatment should be continued for 2 weeks past resolution of clinical signs.

Antipruritic therapy:
• If there are signs of severe pruritus, corticosteroids may helpful. Prednisone, prednisolone (0.25–1 mg/kg PO q12–24h). May be given on an alternate-day basis.
• Antihistamines are usually not very effective except in cases of allergic dermatitis. Hydroxyzine (2 mg/kg PO q8–12h) and diphenhydramine (2 mg/kg PO, SC q8–12h) have been used.

CONTRAINDICATIONS
• Do not administer oral antibiotics that select against gram-positive bacteria such as penicillins, macrolides, lincoamides, and cephalosporins since these may cause fatal enteric dysbiosis and enterotoxemia.

PRECAUTIONS
• Dipping and bathing guinea pigs can be stressful.
• Prevent guinea pigs from licking topical products.
• Oral administration of antibiotics may cause antibiotic-associated enteritis, dysbiosis, and enterotoxemia.

POSSIBLE INTERACTIONS
N/A

ALTERNATIVE DRUGS
N/A

FOLLOW-UP
PATIENT MONITORING
Monitor for resolution of clinical signs and toxicity to medications used.

PREVENTION/AVOIDANCE
• Isolation and treatment of sick and in-contact individuals
• Cleaning of the environment is essential to treatment success.

POSSIBLE COMPLICATIONS
• Sepsis
• Seizures with severe *Trixacarus* infestation
• Reinfection may occur if contact with infected animals occurs, or if the environment is not completely cleaned.

EXPECTED COURSE AND PROGNOSIS
• Trixacarus infestation may cause severe debility. In advanced cases, the prognosis for recovery is guarded. Reinfestation is common if other in-contact animals are not treated, or the environment is not thoroughly cleaned.
• The prognosis for *Chirodiscoides caviae*, *Gliricola porcelli*, and *Gyropus oval* is good to excellent with treatment.

MISCELLANEOUS
ASSOCIATED CONDITIONS
• Pruritus
• Alopecia
• Bacterial dermatitis
• Pyoderma

AGE-RELATED FACTORS
N/A

ZOONOTIC POTENTIAL
Trixacarus caviae may cause a mild dermatitis in humans.

PREGNANCY/FERTILITY/BREEDING
Ivermectin is teratogenic.

SYNONYMS
Pediculosis—lice infestation
Scabies—mite infestation

SEE ALSO
Abscesses
Alopecia
Dermatophytosis
Fleas and flea infestation

ABBREVIATIONS
N/A

INTERNET RESOURCES
N/A

LICE AND MITES

Suggested Reading
Ballweber LR, Harkness JE. Parasites of guinea pigs. In: Baker DG, ed. Flynn's Parasites of Laboratory Animals, 2nd ed. Ames: Blackwell, 2007:421–449.
Palmerio BS, Roberts H. Clinical approach to dermatologic disease in exotic animals. Vet Clin North Am Exot Anim Pract 2013;16(3):523–577.

Pignon C, Mayer J. Guinea pigs. In: Quesenberry KE, Carpenter JW, eds. Ferrets, Rabbits and Rodents, 4th ed. Clinical Medicine and Surgery. 2021 ed. St. Louis: Saunders, 2020:270–297.
Riggs SM. Guinea pigs. In: Mitchell MA, Tully TN, eds. Manual of Exotic Pet Practice. St Louis: Saunders/Elsevier, 2009:456–473.

White SD, Sanchez-Migallon D, Paul-Murphy J. Skin diseases in companion guinea pigs (*Cavia porcellus*): a retrospective study of 293 cases seen at the Veterinary Medical Teaching Hospital, University of California at Davis (1990–2015). Vet Dermatol 2016;27: 395–e100.

Author Thomas N. Tully, Jr., DVM, MS, Dipl. ABVP (Avian), Dipl. ECZM (Avian)

GUINEA PIGS

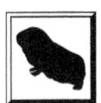

BASICS

DEFINITION
Result of microbial colonization, most commonly aerobic bacterial, of the urinary bladder and/or proximal portion of the urethra.

PATHOPHYSIOLOGY
• More frequent infection is seen in sows, which may be due to the proximity of the urethral orifice to the anus in females; increases the likelihood of infection with fecal contaminates
• Bacteria ascend the urinary tract under conditions that permit persistence, adherence to the epithelium, and subsequent colonization. Colonization requires the impairment of the mechanisms that normally defend against urinary infections. In guinea pigs, the most common etiologies that leads to urinary tract infections are hypercrystalluria and/or urolithiasis.
• Inflammation in infected tissues results in the clinical signs and laboratory test abnormalities exhibited by patient.

SYSTEMS AFFECTED
Renal/Urologic—lower urinary tract

INCIDENCE/PREVALENCE
Urinary tract hypercrystalluria and/or urolithiasis are very common problems observed in guinea pigs. Secondary bacterial cystitis is seen in many of these patients.

SIGNALMENT
Mean Age and Range
Can occur at any age, but middle-aged guinea pigs (2.5–5 years old) are most common

Predominant Sex
Disease is seen more frequently in older sows, most likely due to the proximity of the urethral orifice to the anus.

SIGNS
Historical Findings
• Straining to urinate, small, frequent urinations, and/or urinating when picked up by the owners
• Hematuria, or thick white- or tan-appearing urine.
• Gross hematuria is common in guinea pigs with urolithiasis.
• Urine staining in the perineal area, urine scald, moist pyoderma
• Anorexia, weight loss, lethargy, bruxism, a hunched posture, and vocalizing during urination may be associated with pain.

Physical Examination Findings
• In guinea pigs with hypercrystalluria, the bladder wall may be thickened on palpation, and the bladder contents may feel sand-like.
• Large, turgid bladder (or inappropriate size remains after voiding efforts) may be palpable in patients with pollakiuria or with uroliths.
• Manual expression of the bladder may reveal hematuria or sometimes "sludge" (thick white-tan material) even in patients that have normal-appearing voided urine
• Hematuria, stranguria, pollakiuria may be observable
• A large kidney may be palpable if a nephrolith or nephritis is present.
• Signs of uremia—dehydration, anorexia, lethargy, weakness, hypothermia, bradycardia, high-rate or shallow respirations; stupor, coma, and/or seizures occur rarely, often in terminal cases; tachycardia resulting from ventricular dysrhythmias induced by hyperkalemia
• Thick, palpable uterus may be found with pyometra; pups may be palpable if dystocia is the cause.
• Organomegaly may suggest other organ system involvement or neoplasia.
• If significant blood loss via hematuria has occurred, patient may have pale mucous membranes or generalized paleness of the skin, face, and legs.

CAUSES
• Any condition that causes urine stasis or incomplete emptying of the bladder predisposes to lower urinary tract infection. Common causes include urolithiasis, inadequate exercise, cage confinement, or painful conditions (reluctance to move).
• *E. coli, Streptococcus pyogenes, Staphylococcus* spp., and occasionally anaerobes have been reported to cause lower urinary tract infection. Pure cultures of *Corynebacterium renale* and *Facklamia* spp., and mixed bacterial cultures including *C. renale, Streptococcus bovis/equinus* group, and *Staphylococcus* spp. were cultured from urine of pet guinea pigs with urolithiasis, but a direct association was not confirmed. Also, *Streptococcus viridans, Proteus mirablis,* and mixed growth with *Synema viridans, Staphylococcus* spp., *E. coli,* or *Enterococcus* spp. have been reported from cultures from calculi.

RISK FACTORS
• Inadequate water intake—dirty water bowls, unpalatable water, inadequate water provision, changing water sources
• Urine retention—underlying bladder pathology, neuromuscular disease, painful

conditions causing a reluctance to ambulate (musculoskeletal disease [pododermatitis, arthritis]), dental disease
• Inadequate cage cleaning may cause some guinea pigs to avoid urinating.
• Obesity has been suggested, but not a proven cause in guinea pigs
• Lack of exercise
• Feeding exclusively alfalfa-based diet (hay, pellets or both)
• Calcium or vitamin/mineral supplements added to diet
• Diseases, diagnostic procedures, or treatments that (1) alter normal host urinary tract offenses and predispose to infection, (2) predispose to formation of uroliths, or (3) damage urothelium or other tissues of the lower urinary tract
• Mural or extramural diseases that compress the bladder or urethral lumen

DIAGNOSIS

DIFFERENTIAL DIAGNOSIS
• Female guinea pigs with pyometra or other uterine disorders many expel blood or thick, often blood-tinged vaginal discharge when urinating. This discharge may mix with urine and mimic lower urinary tract infection or urolithiasis—obtain urine sample via cystocentesis to differentiate
• Urolithiasis or hypercrystalluria without secondary bacterial cystitis
• Lower urinary tract neoplasia (uncommon in guinea pigs)
• Rule out iatrogenic disorders—history of catheterization, reverse flushing, contrast radiography, or surgery via history
• Differentiate from other causes by urinalysis, urine culture, radiography, and ultrasonography.

CBC/BIOCHEMISTRY/URINALYSIS
• CBC—TWBC elevations with neutrophil:lymphocyte ratio shift; toxicity of neutrophils ± bands, monocytosis suggest inflammation/infection; thrombocytosis associated with active inflammation; may be anemic if severe hematuria.
• Biochemistry panel—lower urinary tract disease complicated by urethral obstruction may be associated with azotemia. With complete (or nearly complete) obstruction, changes in electrolytes such as hyperkalemia, hypochloremia, and hyponatremia may occur.
• Patients with concurrent pyelonephritis have impaired urine-concentrating capacity, leukocytosis, and azotemia.

LOWER URINARY TRACT INFECTION   (CONTINUED)

- Disorders of the urinary bladder are best evaluated with a urine specimen collected by cystocentesis.
- Urinalysis including both a standard dipstick and microscopic examination of the sediment.
  - Urinalysis data from 44 guinea pigs with urinary calculi found that the mean ± SD urine specific gravity was 1.015 ± 0.008 (range 1.004–1.046) and urine pH was 8.4 ± 0.5 (range 7.5 → 9).
  - Hematuria was the most commonly reported abnormality on urine sediment, followed by mucus and lipid droplets.
  - Identification of bacteria in urine sediment suggests urinary tract infection as a cause or complication of lower urinary tract disease.
  - Identification of neoplastic cells in urine sediment indicates urinary tract neoplasia (rare).
  - Most normal guinea pigs have numerous crystals in the urine; however, hypercrystalluria should increase suspicion for causing disease.
  - Calcium carbonate, calcium oxalate, and struvite crystals are all commonly seen on sediment examinations, but similar to other small animals, crystal type(s) may not predict the mineralogy of calculi present.

OTHER LABORATORY TESTS

- Prior to antibiotic use, culture the urine or bladder wall if high numbers of red or white blood cells, bacteria, or a combination of these are present on sediment examination. Collect urine via cystocentesis since free-catch samples are commonly contaminated.
- Aerobic/anaerobic bacterial urine culture and sensitivity—the most definitive means of identifying and characterizing bacterial urinary tract infection; negative urine culture results suggest a noninfectious cause, unless the patient was on concurrent antibiotics or has an anaerobic infection. There are anecdotal reports of anaerobic urinary infections in guinea pigs; choose this culture technique if anaerobic infection suspected.
- If surgery is necessary to relieve obstruction from urolithiasis, collect and submit the calculi for analysis and culture and sensitivity, and submit sections of bladder wall for culture and sensitivity.
- Calculi containing calcium carbonate require specific methodologies to differentiate from calcium oxalate monohydrate crystals; the laboratory chosen for analysis must be able to perform these methods. Confirm the lab's ability to perform these techniques in advance, since human and some veterinary laboratories unfamiliar with exotic animal samples do not differentiate calcium oxalate from calcium carbonate.

IMAGING

- Survey abdominal radiography and abdominal ultrasound are important means of identifying and localizing causes of lower urinary tract disease.
- Urinary calculi in guinea pigs are generally radio-opaque, allowing for ease of identification using survey radiography. However, if multiple calculi or significant GI gas are present, the anatomic locations of the calculi using survey radiography alone may be obscured. The majority of obstructive urinary calculi are located in the urethra but may also be found in the kidneys, ureters, vagina, or in the seminal vesicles in boars. Ureteroliths are more common in guinea pigs than in other rodents or rabbits.
- Contrast (negative or positive) cystography can be employed to evaluate filling defects in the bladder or bladder masses.
- Ultrasound is useful for anatomic location of urinary calculi and for evaluating anatomic changes in the kidneys, ureters, or bladder such as hydronephrosis or hydroureter, ureteral or cystic mucosal thickening, or perforation, and for evaluating other organ systems.
- Excretory intravenous pyelograms (IVPs) are useful to further elucidate relative functional abnormalities in the kidneys or ureters.
- CT/MRI are useful modalities for diagnosing urinary calculi and assessing organ architecture, more rapidly than IVP and uses significantly less contrast medium.

DIAGNOSTIC PROCEDURES

Bacterial culture/sensitivity—of urine, bladder wall, or if exudates present; recommended if high numbers of RBC or WBC, bacteria, or a combination are present on urine sediment examination. If surgical urolithiasis patient, recommend bladder wall culture as this is generally more rewarding.

PATHOLOGIC FINDINGS

Gross changes may vary from thickening of the bladder mucosa with congestion in chronic cases to intramural and/or intraluminal hemorrhage in patients with acute cystitis. Microscopic changes seen in acute cases include ulceration, hemorrhage, and infiltration with heterophils. Chronic disease is characterized by infiltration of leukocytes and mononuclear cells in the lamina propria, and occasionally fibroblast proliferation. If urinary calculi are present, they can vary in size from sand-like to large concentric stones.

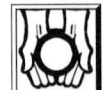 **TREATMENT**

APPROPRIATE HEALTH CARE

- Patients with nonobstructive lower urinary tract diseases are typically managed as outpatients; diagnostic evaluation may require brief hospitalization.
- Lower urinary tract disease associated with systemic signs of illness (e.g., pyrexia, depression, anorexia, and dehydration) or laboratory findings of azotemia and or leukocytosis warrant an aggressive diagnostic evaluation and initiation of supportive and symptomatic treatment.
- Guinea pigs with urinary obstruction should be hospitalized, emergency supportive and symptomatic therapy should be provided until surgical intervention to relieve the obstruction can be performed. Medical treatment of urolithiasis has been unrewarding to date, and surgical removal of calculi is most often required. Postoperative management, including supportive and symptomatic treatment, and pain management therapies

NURSING CARE

Subcutaneous fluids can be administered (100 mL/kg) as needed; IV access is difficult in the guinea pig; lateral saphenous vein catheters often kink; consider IO catheterization if intravascular fluids are needed. Base fluid selection on the underlying cause of fluid loss. In most patients, lactated Ringer's solution or Normosol crystalloid fluids are appropriate.

ACTIVITY

- Long-term—Increase activity level by providing large exercise areas to encourage voiding and prevent recurrence.
- Activity should be reduced during the time of tissue repair if surgery is required for urinary obstruction.

DIET

- Many guinea pigs with lower urinary tract disease are anorectic or have decreased appetite. It is an absolute requirement that the patient continue to eat during and following treatments. Anorexia may cause or exacerbate gastrointestinal hypomotility and cause derangement of the gastrointestinal microflora and overgrowth of intestinal bacterial pathogens.
- Offer a large selection of fresh, moist greens such as cilantro, lettuce, parsley, carrots tops, dark leafy greens, and good-quality grass hay.
- If the patient refuses these foods, syringe-feed Critical Care for Herbivores (Oxbow Pet Products, Murdock, NE) or Emeraid Herbivore (Lafeber Company, Cornell, IL) diet at approximately 10–15 mL/kg PO q6–8h. Larger volumes and more frequent feedings are often accepted; feed as much as the patient will readily accept. Alternatively, pellets can be ground and mixed with fresh greens, vegetable baby foods, water, or sugar-free juice to former gruel.

• Guinea pigs have an absolute requirement for exogenous vitamin C. Provide 50–100 mg/kg/day vitamin C while hospitalized, and during recovery. Vitamin C can be provided through food sources such as citrus fruits and through commercially made guinea pig pellets, or as a subcutaneous injection.

CLIENT EDUCATION
• Limiting risk factors such as obesity, sedentary life, and inappropriate diet combined with increasing water consumption is necessary to minimize or delay recurrence of lower urinary tract disease. Even with these changes, however, recurrence may occur.
• Surgical removal of urinary tract obstructions does not alter the causes responsible for their formation; limiting risk factors such as described above is necessary to minimize or delay recurrence. Even with these changes, however, recurrence is likely in guinea pigs.

SURGICAL CONSIDERATIONS
• Surgery may be required for patients with cystic hypercrystalluria or "sludge" that do not respond to medical therapy.
• Surgery is necessary to relieve obstructions if medical attempts are unsuccessful.
• Postoperative management includes assisted feeding, fluids, analgesics, and antibiotics based on culture and sensitivity results. However, recurrence of the disease is common.

MEDICATIONS
DRUG(S) OF CHOICE
• Antibiotic choice should be based upon the results of cultural and sensitivity (see Contraindications). Antibiotics commonly used include trimethoprim sulfa (15–30 mg/kg PO q12h), chloramphenicol (30–50 mg/kg PO, SC, IM, IV q8–12h), metronidazole (10–20 mg/kg PO, IV q12h), and enrofloxacin (5–20 mg/kg PO, SC, IM q12h—(this is a basic drug and should be diluted or injected into a subcutaneous fluid pocket to prevent tissue injury) Should be reserved for microbes that are resistant to tier one antibiotics
• Reduction of inflammation and analgesia should be provided, especially if pain is causing reduced frequency of voiding; pain management is essential during and following surgery.
• Perioperative analgesic choices include butorphanol (0.4–2.0 mg/kg SC, IM q4–12h) and buprenorphine (0.05–0.2 mg/kg SC, IM, IV q6–8h). Meloxicam (0.5–1 mg/kg PO, SC, IM q 24h) and carprofen (4 mg/kg SC q24h or 1–2 mg/kg

PO q12h) provide anti-inflammation as well as analgesia. Tramadol, a synthetic opioid, may also be an effective at dosages of 5–10 mg/kg PO q12h postoperatively. For severe to moderate pain pure mu opioids such as morphine (0.5–2.0 mg/kg SC, IM q2–4h) or oxymorphone (0.2–0.5 mg/kg SC, IM q6–12h) should be used however appetite and fecal output should be monitored as these opioids are thought to contribute to GI ileus.
• Procedures for relief of obstruction generally require administering sedatives and/or anesthetics. When substantial derangements exist, begin with fluid administration and other supportive measures first. Calculate the dosage of sedative or anesthetic drug using the low end of the recommended range or give only to effect.

CONTRAINDICATIONS
• Oral administration of antibiotics that select against gram-positive bacteria (penicillins, cephalosporins, macrolides, and lincosamides) can cause fatal enteric dysbiosis and enterotoxemia.
• Potentially nephrotoxic drugs (e.g., aminoglycosides, NSAIDs) in patients that are febrile, dehydrated, or azotemic or that are suspected of having pyelonephritis, septicemia, or preexisting renal disease
• Glucocorticoids or other immunosuppressive agents

PRECAUTIONS
• Avoid drugs that reduce blood pressure or induce cardiac dysrhythmia until any dehydration is resolved.
• If obstructed or significant renal insufficiency is evident, modify dosages of all drugs that require renal metabolism or elimination, and avoid nephrotoxic drugs (NSAIDs, aminoglycosides).

FOLLOW-UP
PATIENT MONITORING
• Monitor for reduction and cessation of clinical signs. Generally, a positive response occurs within a few days after instituting appropriate antibiotic therapy for lower urinary tract infections and supportive therapy.
• Ensure gastrointestinal motility by making sure the patient is eating, well hydrated, and passing normal feces.
• Assess urine production and hydration status frequently while hospitalized, or have owners monitor daily at home, adjusting fluid administration accordingly.
• Verify the ability to urinate adequately; failure to do so may require urinary catheterization or cystocentesis.

• Follow-up examination should be performed within 7–10 days of discharge from hospital, or sooner if the clinical signs are not reduced.
• Ideally, recheck of urine culture and sensitivity should be performed 3–5 days after the cessation of antibiotics.

PREVENTION/AVOIDANCE
• Limiting risk factors such as obesity, sedentary life, and inappropriate diet, combined with increasing water consumption, is necessary to minimize or delay recurrence of lower urinary tract disease. Even with these changes, however, recurrence may occur.
• For patients with urolithiasis or hypercrystalluria, water intake is the cornerstone to any prevention protocol. Prevention is targeted at increasing water intake and reducing (but not eliminating) dietary calcium. Metabolic bone disease may be induced in guinea pigs with severe dietary calcium restriction for prevention of urinary calculi. Avoid alfalfa-based diets. Diets containing a high percentage of timothy, oat, or grass hays, a lower overall percentage pellets, and a wider variety of vegetables and fruits decrease the risk of urolith development in pet guinea pigs. It is possible that dietary inhibitors of calcium are found in greater concentration in hays than pellets.
• Hydrochlorothiazide (2 mg/kg q12h) is a thiazide diuretic that reduces urinary Ca^{2+}, K^+, and citrate. It is unknown if diuresis would be of benefit to guinea pigs whose urine is already considered isosthenuric. Do not use hydrochlorothiazide with severe renal disease or fluid imbalances.
• Urinary acidifiers were historically recommended based upon an assumed diagnosis of calcium oxalate calculi, but the normally alkaline urine of guinea pigs makes the use of dietary acidifiers concerning. Potassium citrate (30–75 mg/kg PO q12h) binds urinary Ca^{2+}, reduces ion activity, and alkalinizes the urine. As guinea pigs have alkaline urine even with disease, the efficacy of this treatment is unclear. Hyperkalemia occurs, so monitor plasma K^+ closely during treatment. Potassium citrate and hydrochlorothiazide have been used together anecdotally with some clinical success.

POSSIBLE COMPLICATIONS
• Urine scald; myiasis; pododermatitis
• Failure to detect or treat effectively may lead to pyelonephritis.
• Development of urolithiasis

EXPECTED COURSE AND PROGNOSIS
• Generally, the prognosis for animals with uncomplicated lower urinary tract infection is good to excellent. The prognosis for

LOWER URINARY TRACT INFECTION

patients with complicated infection is determined by the prognosis for the underlying disease.

• The prognosis following surgical removal of uroliths is fair to good, but recurrence is common. Although dietary management may decrease the likelihood of recurrence, many guinea pigs will develop clinical disease again.

 MISCELLANEOUS

ASSOCIATED CONDITIONS
• Urolithiasis
• Pyometra, other uterine disorders
• Gastrointestinal hypomotility or dysbiosis

AGE-RELATED FACTORS
This disease is frequently found in middle-aged to older guinea pigs, although it can occur in younger animals as well.

PREGNANCY/FERTILITY/BREEDING
Lower urinary tract infections may ascend into the reproductive tract via the vagina. If untreated, the potential for development of vaginal or uterine infections increases.

SEE ALSO
Dysuria, hematuria, and pollakiuria
Urinary tract obstruction

ABBREVIATIONS
IO = intraosseous
IVP = intravenous pyelogram
NSAID = nonsteroidal anti-inflammatory
RBC = red blood cell
TWBC = total white blood cell count

INTERNET RESOURCES
N/A

Suggested Reading
Hallman RM, Brandão J. Diagnostic imaging of the renal system in exotic companion mammals. Vet Clin Exot Anim 2020;23:195–214.
Hawkins MG, Ruby AL, Drazenovich TL et al. Composition and characteristics of urinary calculi from guinea pigs. J Amer Vet Med Assoc 2009;234:214–220.
Hoefer H, Latney L. Rodents: urogenital and reproductive disorders. In: Keeble E, Meredith A, eds. BSAVA Manual of Rodents and Ferrets. Gloucester: BSAVA, 2009:150–160.
Percy D, Barthold S. Guinea pig. In: Percy D, Barthold S, eds. Pathology of Laboratory Rodents and Rabbits. Ames: Blackwell, 2001:209–247.
Pignon C, Mayer J. Guinea pigs. In: Quesenberry KE, Carpenter JW, eds. Ferrets, Rabbits and Rodents, 4th ed. Clinical Medicine and Surgery. 2021 ed. St. Louis: Saunders, 2020:270–297.
Reavill D, Lennox A. Disease overview of the urinary tract in exotic companion mammals and tips on clinical management. Vet Clin Exot Anim 2020;23:169–193.

Author Rodney Schnellbacher, DVM, Dipl. ACZM

BASICS

DEFINITION
Mastitis is inflammation of the mammary tissue most often caused by a bacterial infection. The affected gland becomes diffusely swollen and painful.

PATHOPHYSIOLOGY
- Sows have one mammary gland in each inguinal region.
- Mammary glands are constantly in contact with bedding and cage floor due to the short legs of the guinea pig.
- Bacteria enter the mammary gland via teat canal, cutaneous lesion, or via hematogenous spread from another site of sepsis.
- Any swelling or discharge from the gland indicates the potential for mastitis.

SYSTEMS AFFECTED
Skin/Exocrine

INCIDENCE/PREVALENCE
Common in lactating sows

SIGNALMENT
- Postpartum sow
- Lactating sow
- Can rarely occur in nonlactating females and males

SIGNS
Historical Findings
- Anorexia
- Lethargy
- Pain
- Neglect of suckling piglets
- Piglets show failure to thrive
- Death of neonates

Physical Examination Findings
- Swollen, discolored (red or purple coloration), warm and painful mammary gland(s); more chronic cases, glands become cool and cyanotic.
- Hemorrhagic or purulent fluid can be expressed from the gland
- Febrile
- Agalactia
- Discharge and caked material may or may not be obvious around the nipple
- Ulceration of teat and/or skin around mammary gland
- Abscessation of the gland(s)
- Dehydration

CAUSES AND RISK FACTORS
- Infectious—bacteria enter the mammary gland via teat canal (always in contact with bedding), cutaneous lesion (natal teeth), or via hematogenous spread from another site of sepsis.
- Pasteurella, Klebsiella, E. coli, or other coliforms, Streptococcus (alpha-hemolytic), Staphylococcus, and Pseudomonas most commonly involved.
- Trauma—inflicted by nursing piglets or exposed wire cage bottom
- Poor hygiene—wet or soiled bedding in contact with teats
- Systemic infection originating elsewhere (i.e., metritis)

DIAGNOSIS

DIFFERENTIAL DIAGNOSIS
- Galactostasis—not febrile, no leukocytosis, differentiate by cytology and culture of milk
- Sore nipples—sows with large litters may have stretched and hyperemic teats.
- Mammary neoplasia—not febrile, enlargement of the gland often asymmetrical. Common to have ulceration of the skin over the tumor.

CBC/BIOCHEMISTRY/URINALYSIS
- Leukocytosis ± left shift in acute phase
- Leukopenia in subacute phase with sepsis
- Fibrinogen elevated
- Thrombocytosis with acute inflammation
- PCV, protein, and BUN elevated if dehydrated

IMAGING
Abdominal ultrasonography is helpful to eliminate uterus as a source of sepsis.

DIAGNOSTIC PROCEDURES
- Cytology of fluid or milk expressed from the gland: heterophils, macrophages, and general inflammatory cells may be present in normal milk. Look for phagocytized bacteria and toxic heterophils.
- Culture of expressed fluid if flow does not contact the skin; otherwise, obtain samples via fine-needle aspiration to avoid contamination. Submit for aerobic and anaerobic culture.

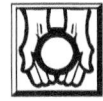

TREATMENT

APPROPRIATE HEALTH CARE
- Keep sow hospitalized until stable.
- Separate the sow from her litter.
- Sow can be an outpatient when stable

NURSING CARE
- Fluid therapy: subcutaneous isotonic fluids to address dehydration losses plus maintenance (100 mL/kg/day)
- Intravenous or intraosseous fluids if sow is septic with metritis or other infections
- Hot pack the swollen gland(s)
- Gently express fluid from the glands 2–3 times daily and apply betadine solution to nipple.

ACTIVITY
- Discontinue nursing.
  - Pups should be nursed by other lactating female or hand fed.
- Newborn guinea pigs are precocious and can eat softened pellets within a few hours of birth, as well as nibble hay within 12–24 hours.
- Milk production can be reduced by decreasing dietary pellets and greens (but continue hay ad libitum).

CLIENT EDUCATION
Discuss hygiene and cage flooring with the client.

SURGICAL CONSIDERATIONS
Abscessed or necrotic glands may require surgical debridement.

MEDICATIONS

DRUG(S) OF CHOICE
- Initiate systemic antibiotic therapy until culture results available. Treat for 7–20 days.
- Trimethoprim-sulfa if hydration normal (15–30 mg/kg PO q12h)
- Chloramphenicol (30–50 mg/kg PO, SC, IM, IV q8–12h)—potential adverse effects on nursing piglets
- Enrofloxacin (5–20 mg/kg PO, SC, IM q12h)—potential adverse effects on nursing piglets;{Should be reserved for microbes that are resistant to tier one antibiotics}.
- Anti-inflammatory medications, analgesics
  - Multimodal therapy is recommended, opioid, and NSAID: butorphanol (0.4–0.2 mg/kg SC, IM, IV q4–12h) or buprenorphine (0.05–0.2 mg/kg SC, IM q8–12h) plus meloxicam (0.5–1 mg/kg PO, SC q24h) or carprofen (4 mg/kg SC q24h or 1–2 mg/kg PO q12h). Tramadol, a synthetic opioid, may also be an effective at dosages of 5–10 mg/kg PO q12h.

CONTRAINDICATIONS
- Oral administration of antibiotics that select against gram-positive bacteria (penicillins, cephalosporins, macrolides, and lincosamides) can cause fatal enteric dysbiosis and enterotoxaemia
- Potentially nephrotoxic drugs (e.g., aminoglycosides, NSAIDs) in patients that are febrile or dehydrated or have preexisting renal disease

GUINEA PIGS

MASTITIS

FOLLOW-UP

PATIENT MONITORING
Physical exam and CBC 7–14 days after therapy, depending on severity of condition

PREVENTION/AVOIDANCE
• Improve overall hygiene of sow and pups
• Clean bedding daily.

POSSIBLE COMPLICATIONS
• Agalactia
• Piglets will need to be weaned early.
• Long-term antibiotic therapy can lead to dysbiosis.

EXPECTED COURSE AND PROGNOSIS
• Prognosis good with appropriate antibiotic treatment
• Sow may die within a few days if not treated

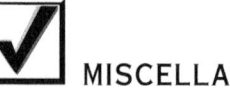

MISCELLANEOUS

ASSOCIATED CONDITIONS
Postpartum metritis

PREGNANCY/FERTILITY/BREEDING
Discontinue breeding if surgical removal of mammary gland was necessary.

SEE ALSO
Antibiotic-associated enterotoxaemia

ABBREVIATIONS
BUN = blood urea nitrogen
PCV = packed cell volume

Suggested Reading
Bertram CA, Muller K, Klopfleisch R. Genital tract pathology in female pet guinea pigs (*Cavia porcellus*): a retrospective study of 655 post-mortem and 64 biopsy cases. J Comp Path 2018;165: 13–22.

DeCubellis J. Common emergencies in rabbits, guinea pigs, and chinchillas. Vet Clin Exot Anim 2016;19:411–429.

Minarikova A, Hauptman K, Jeklova E et al. Diseases in pet guinea pigs: a retrospective study in 1000 animals. Vet Rec 2015; 177(8):200–200.

Miwa Y, Sladky K. Common surgical procedures of rodents, ferrets, hedgehogs, and sugar gliders. Vet Clin Exot Anim 2016;19:205–244.

Pignon C, Mayer J. Guinea pigs. In: Quesenberry KE, Carpenter JW, eds. Ferrets, Rabbits and Rodents, 4th Ed). Clinical Medicine and Surgery. 2021 ed. St. Louis: Saunders, 2020:270–297.

Suarez-Bonnet A, Martin de las Mulas J, M Y Millán et al. Morphological and immunohistochemical characterization of spontaneous mammary gland tumors in the guinea pig (*Cavia porcellus*). Vet Pathol 47(2) 298–305

Author Rodney Schnellbacher, DVM, Dipl. ACZM

NASAL DISCHARGE AND SNEEZING

BASICS

DEFINITION
• Nasal discharge is any liquid or evidence of dried exudate emanating from the external nares cavity and may be serous, mucoid, purulent, mucopurulent, frank blood (epistaxis), or blood tinged. The discharge may result in discoloration or crusting of the fur around the external nares.
• Sneezing: the involuntary expulsion of air through the nasal cavity, may or may not be associated with nasal discharge

PATHOPHYSIOLOGY
• Secretions are produced by the mucous cells of the epithelium, and in severe disease, damaged vessels of the epithelium. When the nasal mucosa is irritated by inflammatory, chemical, or mechanical factors, there is increased production of nasal secretions. Accumulation of secretions in and irritation of the nasal cavity can stimulate sneezing. However, sneezing frequency often decreases as the disease becomes more chronic.
• The most common cause of nasal discharge and sneezing in guinea pigs is bacterial infection. However, multiple other infectious and noninfectious etiologies can cause similar signs. The infection can spread from the nasal passages to the eye via the nasolacrimal duct, to the ear via the eustachian tube, to the lower respiratory tract via the trachea, into the bones of the face or the sinuses, or to the rest of the body via hematogenous spread.
• Dental disease or abscesses can cause destruction and/or chronic infection of the nasal turbinates or facial bones (osteomyelitis), which may result in refractory or recurrent infections.

Types of Nasal Discharge
• Serous: mild irritation, allergies, early bacterial infection, early inflammation
• Mucoid: early neoplasia, early inflammation or infection, allergies or contact irritation
• Mucopurulent/purulent: nasal foreign bodies, bacterial infections
• Serosanguineous/epistaxis: destructive processes due to neoplasia or bacterial pathogens that can cause coagulopathies, toxin, head trauma, and vitamin C deficiency

SYSTEMS AFFECTED
• Respiratory: mucosa of the upper respiratory tract (nasal cavities, sinuses, and nasopharynx)
• Ophthalmic: extension of disease via nasolacrimal duct
• Oral cavity: dental disease, tooth root abscess

• Neurologic: extension of disease via eustachian tube, causing otitis interna/media and vestibular signs
• Musculoskeletal: extension of disease into bones of the skull
• Hemic/Lymphatic/Immune: systemic disease may cause blood-tinged nasal discharge or epistaxis due to disorders of hemostasis.

GENETICS
Unknown

INCIDENCE/PREVELENCE
Respiratory disease, including nasal discharge, is commonly seen in clinical practice; dental disease is also a common cause due to elongated tooth roots.

GEOGRAPHIC DISRIBUTION
Widespread

SIGNALMENT
All ages may be affected. Younger animals are more prone to bacterial infections and/or foreign bodies, whereas in older animals, dental disease, nasal tumors, and/or bacterial infections are more common.

SIGNS

Historical Findings
Poor diet history associated with dental disease; response to previous antibiotic therapy; new substrate or overly stemmy hay introduction; lack of supervision in the house or yard; exposure to rodenticide; increased pollen or mold count; construction on the owner's house (dust, allergens); failure to clean cage regularly resulting in ammonia buildup and irritation of mucous membranes; and new introduction of other animals
  Historical clinical signs
  Nasal discharge (unilateral or bilateral), sneezing, ocular discharge, anorexia, staining of front paws, ptyalism, epistaxis, head tilt, and scratching at ears, eyelid, or ear droop

Physical Examination Findings
• Nonspecific signs such as lethargy, weight loss, and anorexia
• Serous or mucopurulent ocular or nasal discharge
• Epistaxis
• Decreased nasal airflow (unilateral or bilateral)
• Dyspnea (if complete nasal occlusion has occurred), stridor or open-mouth breathing
• Signs of dental disease such as ptyalism, facial bone deformity, and difficulty chewing
• Head tilt or facial nerve paralysis (if inner ear disease present including eyelid droop, lip droop/contracture, and ear droop)
• Alopecia or dermatitis around the nose or mouth, crusting, staining, or matting from dried secretions on the hair around the nose, eyes, or front limbs
• Bloat if aerophagia is present.

CAUSES
• Bacterial: *Bordetella brochiseptica*, *Streptococcus zooepidemicus*, *Streptococcus pneumoniae*, *Streptobacillus moniliformis*, *Yersinia pseudotuberculosis*, *Haemophilus* spp., *Klebsiella pneumoniae*, *Pseudomonas aeruginosa*, *Pasturella multocida*, *Salmonella* spp., *Staphylococcus aureus*, *Streptococcus pyogenes*, and *Citrobacter* spp.
• Viral: adenovirus and parainfluenza virus (rare)
  ○ Dental disease: maxillary tooth roots can extend into the nasal passages and lead to secondary bacterial infections or obstruction of nasal passages; tooth root abscesses can also develop. Common bacteria isolated from ondotogenic abscesses include *Bacteroides fragilis*, *Pasturella multocida*, and *Peptostreptococcus anaerobius*
• Neoplasia: nasal adenocarcinoma, fibrosarcoma, and maxillary odontoma/elodontoma
• Foreign bodies: uncommon; usually grass, hay, bedding, or seeds
• Allergens or irritants to the respiratory tract: chemicals from cleaning, smoke, dusty/dirty bedding, mold, and ammonia buildup in the cage

RISK FACTORS
• Improper husbandry: substrate with aromatic oils such as pine and cedar can be irritating to respiratory mucosa, poor sanitation, infrequent cage cleaning, overcrowding, improper ventilation/humidity/temperature control, inhaled irritants such as disinfectants (bleach, etc.), ammonia buildup on the bedding, smoke can further exacerbate this issue
• Improper diet: feeding diets deficient in vitamin C can lead to immunosuppression or feeding diets deficient in coarse fiber (long-stemmed grass hay) can lead to dental disease.
• Immunosuppression: causes include lack of vitamin C in the diet, stress, concurrent disease, corticosteroid use, age, and many other factors likely including environment and genetics.
• Dental disease: maxillary tooth roots can extend into the nasal passages and lead to secondary bacterial infections or obstruction of the nasal passages; tooth root abscesses and malocclusion can also develop.

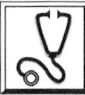

DIAGNOSIS

DIFFERENTIAL DIAGNOSIS
• Discharge may be unilateral or bilateral in cases of allergies, nasal tumors, dental disease, foreign bodies, or bacterial respiratory tract

infections. Unilateral discharge is more commonly associated with nonsystemic or local processes such as dental disease, foreign bodies, and nasal tumors.
• Rodenticide toxicity can cause epistaxis.

CBC/BIOCHEMISTRY/URINALYSIS
• An elevation in total white blood cell count is uncommon, but a shift in proportion of heterophils to lymphocytes with an increase in heterophils and decrease in lymphocytes may occur as a sequela to systemic inflammation in guinea pigs.
• Increases in platelet number can also be seen with inflammation.
• In cases with severely affected bone or soft tissue, elevations in CK or ALKP may be seen.

OTHER LABORATORY TESTS
• Enzyme-linked immunosorbent assay (ELISA) and indirect immunofluorescence assays (IFA) for *B. bronchiseptica* are more sensitive than culture for detection of the organism, but they detect antibodies and thus indicate exposure rather than active infection.
• ELISA for *S. pneumoniae*—detects antibodies and indicates exposure rather than active infection
• PCR test for adenovirus is described but not readily available unless in lab animal setting

IMAGING
• Radiographs of the skull: must be done under heavy sedation or general anesthesia for optimal positioning, with a minimum of five views (lateral, two oblique laterals, anterior posterior, and ventrodorsal views) recommended; observe radiographs for bony lysis or proliferation of the turbinates and facial bones as this can indicate chronic bacterial or neoplastic processes; tooth roots should be assessed as they can penetrate the nasal sinuses and lead to nasal passageway obstruction or bacterial infection; and the presence of foreign bodies can also be accessed. High-detail films and screens are recommended, such as those used for dental or mammography imaging.
• CT or MRI: provide better imaging quality and may be more diagnostic than skull radiographs, especially if nasal detail is obscured by nasal discharge; can help to determine whether the cause of disease is nasal, sinus, or dental disease. CT specifically is excellent for providing bony detail, is more sensitive for areas encased in bone (i.e., lungs and sinuses), and the procedure time is relatively short. However, these modalities may be cost prohibitive and are not as readily available.

DIAGNOSTIC PROCEDURES
• Cytology of nasal discharge: swab of nasal or ocular discharge; nasal swab, recommend standard cell stain (Diff Quick) and gram stain of exudates
• Culture of nasal discharge: can be difficult to obtain a good sample, many normal commensal organisms are located in the nasal passages; can obtain a culture with a mini tip culturette inserted into the nostril; causative agent may be located in the sinuses, which are difficult to sample; and many bacteria are difficult to grow. Sample may also be obtained via endoscopy or rhinotomy to reduce culture contamination, but these are more invasive procedures that are not usually indicated in uncomplicated cases.
• Nasal cavity biopsy: should be performed in animals with chronic nasal discharge (especially epistaxis) if neoplasia is suspected; use endoscopy or rhinotomy to obtain sample
• Nasal flush can be difficult to perform due to patient size
• Aspiration of lytic areas, if present, for cytology

PATHOLOGIC FINDINGS
Nasal passages, external nares, and sinuses may contain serous or mucopurulent exudate, inflammatory cells infiltrating the nasal mucosa and sinuses, neoplasia or foreign body in the nasal passages, elongation of tooth roots into nasal passages/sinuses

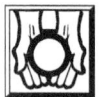

TREATMENT

APPROPRIATE HEALTH CARE
Outpatient treatment is usually acceptable unless the patient is in respiratory distress, has uncontrolled epistaxis, or has multisystemic signs of illness in addition to the nasal discharge.

NURSING CARE
• Fluid therapy to maintain normal hydration (guinea pigs fluid needs are 100 mL/kg/day)—fluid can be given IV, IO, or SC. Adequate hydration is necessary to keep the GI tract hydrated and to aid mucocilliary clearance.
• Nebulization with saline may help deliver moisture to the upper respiratory tract.
• Keep nares clear of nasal discharge.
• Keep patients in a quiet, predator-free environment to decrease stress and always provide a hide box.
• Keep environment clean, remove any environmental allergens or irritants
• Oxygen therapy if the patient is in respiratory distress or dyspneic

ACTIVITY
In most cases, no change in activity level is necessary to recommend. However, in cases of overt dyspnea, exercise-induced stridor or dyspnea, or epistaxis that is difficult to resolve, cage rest is recommended short term during the healing process.

DIET
• Anorexia can cause GI hypomotility/stasis, overgrowth of intestinal bacterial pathogens, and imbalance of GI microflora. Therefore, guinea pigs need to continue eating throughout treatment. In addition, nasal occlusion may reduce the olfactory capabilities, making the guinea pig less likely to eat. Low-dose buprenorphine or midazolam may reduce hospital anxiety and have polyphagia effects leading to a greater likelihood that animal will eat in the hospital while having minimal cardiorespiratory effects.
• Offer a wide variety of fresh, moistened vegetables such as cilantro, parsley, romaine lettuce, and dandelion greens, as well as good-quality grass hay (orchard grass, western timothy).
• If the patient refuses to eat or is not maintaining condition, can syringe-feed Critical Care for Herbivores (Oxbow Pet Products, Murdock, NE) or Emeraid Herbivore (Lafeber Company, Cornell, IL) 10–15 mL/kg orally every 6–8 hours. A gruel of ground-up guinea pig pellets with vegetable baby foods, water, or fresh greens can also be offered, but this is not as nutritionally complete as commercially available syringe-feeding formulas.
• Guinea pigs require an exogenous source of vitamin C supplementation that can be given at 50–100 mg/kg/day when ill
• Encourage oral fluid intake to maintain hydration by offering water or wet vegetables.

CLIENT EDUCATION
If the underlying disease cannot be corrected (i.e., dental disease, neoplasia, severe tissue destruction), a cure is unlikely and signs may reoccur following discontinuation of treatment (i.e., antibiotics). The treatment, depending on the cause, can be lifelong, and aims to control the severe clinical signs.

SURGICAL CONSIDERATIONS
If dental disease is the cause of the nasal discharge/sneezing, then abscess debridement, tooth trims, or tooth extractions may be necessary. If bony lesions are discovered, removal of osteomyelitic areas for culture, and histopathology is indicated if possible based on location and lesion size. Use of probiotics or prebiotics prior to surgery can be considered.

MEDICATIONS

DRUG(S) OF CHOICE
• Antimicrobial drugs are the treatment of choice if bacterial disease is suspected. Choice of antibiotic is ideally based on culture and sensitivity testing but can be chosen empirically. Long-term antibiotic therapy (4–6 weeks or even months to years) may be required with severe infection. Antibiotics commonly used include enrofloxacin (5–20 mg/kg PO, SC, IM q12–24 h—this drug has a basic pH and should be diluted or injected into a subcutaneous fluid pocket to prevent tissue injury), marbofloxacin (4 mg/kg PO q24h), pradofloxacin (5 mg/kg PO q12h), trimethoprim sulfa (15–30 mg/kg PO q12h), chloramphenicol (30–50 mg/kg PO, SC, IM, IV q8–12h), and metronidazole (10–20 mg/kg PO, q12h). Can also use enrofloxacin in combination with doxycycline (2.5–5 mg/kg PO q12h). Amikacin (5–15 mg/kg divided SC, IM, IV q8–12h) is uncommonly used as it can cause ototoxicity and neprotoxicity. The above antibiotics can also be nebulized. Combination antibiotic therapy of enrofloxacin and metronidazole is recommended for odontogenic abscesses.
• Nebulizing with saline may help moisten the upper respiratory tract.
• Topical ophthalmic solutions (ciprofloxacin or gentamicin eye drops or triple antibiotic eye ointment) can be used to treat associated conjunctivitis.
• Antihistamines can be used in guinea pigs with allergic rhinitis. Some antihistamines that have been used include chlorpheniramine maleate (0.6 mg/kg PO q24h), diphenhydramine (7.5 mg/kg PO or 1–5 mg/kg SC PRN), and ephedrine (1 mg/kg PO, IV prn). Allergic rhinitis is thought to be uncommon in guinea pigs.
• Consider pain control in cases of dental, osteomyelitic, or neoplastic related nasal discharge/sneezing—buprenorphine (0.05 mg/kg SCq 8–12 h, 0.2 mg/kg oral transmucosal q5h, 0.2 mg/kg IV q7h), butorphanol (0.4–2 mg/kg SC q4h), meloxicam (0.1–0.5 mg/kg PO, SC q24h), ketoprofen (1–3 mg/kg SC, IM q12–24 h), or carprofen (4 mg/kg SC q24h)
• Low-dose buprenorphine or midazolam may reduce hospital anxiety, combat pain and induce mild polyphagia effects leading to greater likelihood of eating in the hospital with minimal cardiorespiratory effects.
• Concurrent with antibiotic administration, provision of a probiotic or prebiotic (Florentero, Ventix Animal Heallth Corp. Burlington, ON) should be considered to reduce the risk of antibiotic-induced enteritis or clostridial overgrowth/dysbiosis

CONTRAINDICATIONS
• Antibiotics that select against gram-positive bacteria such as oral penicillins, cephalosporins, lincosamines, or macrolides should be avoided in these animals, especially orally, as it can cause fatal dysbiosis and enterotoxemia.
• Procaine, which is included in some penicillin preparations, can be toxic to guinea pigs.
• Using corticosteroids can suppress the immune system and exacerbate bacterial infections.
• Topical nasal decongestants that contain phenylephrine can worsen nasal inflammation and cause nasal ulceration and purulent rhinitis.
• Opioid use can slow down gastrointestinal transit time (butorphanol, buprenorphine).

PRECAUTIONS
• Any antibiotic can cause diarrhea or anorexia, which should be monitored in these patients and the antibiotic discontinued if diarrhea is present. Supplementation with probiotics or guinea pig transfaunation can be considered.
• The total body dose should not be exceeded topically or via nebulization due to risk of excellent systemic absorption by inflamed airways and risk for toxicity in small patients.

POSSIBLE INTERACTIONS
None

ALTERNATIVE DRUGS
Intranasal administration of ciprofloxacin or gentamicin ophthalmic drops in the nares may be given in conjunction with systemic antibiotic therapy. Guinea pigs do not like having things placed in their nose and should be restrained appropriately before intranasal treatment administration.

FOLLOW-UP

PATIENT MONITORING
Continue to monitor patient for relapse via clinical signs.

PREVENTION/AVOIDANCE
• Improve husbandry (good ventilation and appropriate substrate) and diet (ensure appropriate vitamin C supplementation).
• Avoid stressful situations and corticosteroid use.
• Prevent dental disease by providing high-fiber foods, especially good-quality hay.
• Yearly veterinary exams with periodic trimming of overgrown teeth as needed.

POSSIBLE COMPLICATIONS
• Loss of appetite
• Infection of the nasal passages and sinuses can extend to affect the eyes, ears, lungs, and musculoskeletal system.
• If nasal obstruction occurs, the patient can become dyspneic.

EXPECTED COURSE AND PROGNOSIS
Prognosis is based on cause of disease, severity, and chronicity. Mild disease may have a good prognosis with aggressive antibiotic treatment and supportive care. If the underlying disease cannot be corrected (dental disease, neoplasia, and severe tissue destruction), a cure is unlikely.

The treatment, depending on the cause, can be lifelong and aims to control the clinical signs. Neoplasia carries a grave prognosis.

MISCELLANEOUS

ASSOCIATED CONDITIONS
• GI hypomotility/stasis
• Dental disease
• Hypovitaminosis C
• Pneumonia
• Rhinitis and sinusitis

AGE-RELATED FACTORS
• Neoplasia more common in older animals
• Infectious causes more common in younger animals

ZOONOTIC POTENTIAL
Streptobacillus moniliformis is the cause of rat bite fever in humans. Guinea pigs may be a reservoir for *Streptococcus pneumoniae*, with subclinical carriage rate up to 50% in some guinea pig colonies. Close contact between pets and children could be a risk factor although relevance in human hosts is not clearly defined.

PREGNANCY/FERTILITY/BREEDING
N/A

SYNONYMS
None

SEE ALSO
Dental malocclusion
Dyspnea and tachypnea
Pneumonia
Rhinitis and sinusitis
Stertor and stridor

ABBREVIATIONS
ALKP = alkaline phosphatase
CK = creatinine kinase
CT = computed tomography
ELISA = enzyme-linked immunosorbent assay

GUINEA PIGS

GI = gastrointestinal
IFA = immunoflorescence assay
IO = intraosseous
MRI = magnetic resonance imaging

INTERNET RESOURCES
www.vin.com

Suggested Reading
Capello V, Lennox AM. Diagnostic imaging of the respiratory system in exotic companion mammals. Vet Clin Exot Anim 2011;14:369–389.
Lennox AM, Capello V, Legendre LF. Small mammal denistry. In: Quesenberry KE, Carpenter JW, eds. Ferrets, Rabbits and Rodents, 4th Ed). Clinical Medicine and Surgery. 2021 ed. St. Louis: Saunders, 2020:514–535.
Mayer J, Mans C. Rodents. In: Carpenter JW, ed. Exotic Animal Formulary, 5th ed. St Louis: Elsevier, 2018:459–479.
Minarikova A, Hauptman K, Jeklova E, Knotek Z, Jekl V. Diseases in pet guinea pigs: a retrospective study in 1000 animals. Vet Rec 2015;177(8):200.
Minarikova A, Hauptman K, Knotek Z, Jekl V. Microbial flora of odontogenic abscesses in pet guinea pigs. Vet Rec 2016;179(13):331.
Pignon C, Mayer J. Guinea pigs. In: Quesenberry KE, Carpenter JW, eds. Ferrets, Rabbits and Rodents, 4th Ed). Clinical Medicine and Surgery. 2021 ed. St. Louis: Saunders, 2020:270–297.
Riggs SM. Guinea pigs. In: Mitchell MA, Tully TN, eds. Manual of Exotic Pet Practice. St Louis: Saunders, 2009: 463–464, 466–467.
Robinson NJ, Lyons E, Grindlay D, Brennan ML. Veterinarian nominated common conditions of rabbits and guinea pigs compared with published literature. Vet Sci 2017;4(4):58.

Portions adapted from:
Oglesbee BL. Nasal discharge and sneezing. In: Oglesbee BL, ed. The 5-Minute Veterinary Consult: Ferret and Rabbit, 1st ed. Ames: Blackwell, 2006.

Authors Christy L. Rettenmund, DVM, Dipl. ACZM and J. Jill Heatley, DVM, MS, Dipl. ABVP (Avian, Reptilian, Amphibian), Dipl. ACZM

OTITIS MEDIA AND INTERNA

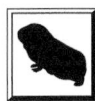

BASICS

DEFINITION
Inflammation or infection of the middle ear (otitis media) or inner ear (otitis interna)

PATHOPHYSIOLOGY
• The middle ear extends from the tympanic membrane to the inner ear and includes the eustachian tube.
• The inner ear consists of the cochlea and the vestibular system, which compose the bony labyrinth.
• Infection is frequently the result of extension of disease from the nasopharyngeal region (URI) via the eustachian tube, or extension of disease from the external ear.
• Otitis interna may also be caused by hematogenous spread from systemic infection.

SYSTEMS AFFECTED
• Nervous—peripheral nervous system may be affected, including paresis or paralysis of the facial nerve or damage to the vestibulocochlear system; central nervous system may be affected by extension of disease from the inner ear
• Ophthalmic—cornea and conjunctiva as a sequela to facial nerve damage
• Respiratory—nasal discharge and upper respiratory infection as primary disorder or secondary to facial nerve damage
• Gastrointestinal—stasis or ileus secondary to vestibular signs and anorexia

GENETICS
N/A

INCIDENCE/PREVALENCE
Necropsy studies indicate an incidence of 13%–14% of otitis interna/media, although many of these had little to no clinical signs.

GEOGRAPHIC DISTRIBUTION
N/A

SIGNALMENT
Breed Predilections
None

Mean Age and Range
All ages; juveniles may be more susceptible as immunity is developing

Predominant Sex
N/A

SIGNS
General Comments
Clinical signs will vary according to the severity and duration of disease; may range from asymptomatic to signs related to ear pain and bulla discomfort or manifestations of central nervous system involvement

Historical Findings
• Head tilt (ear held down toward ground)
• Torticollis (nose pointed to one side)
• Drooping of pinna
• Scratching or pawing at ear or face—probably related to pruritus or pain
• Leaning, circling, or rolling toward the affected side
• Inappetence or anorexia related to discomfort of the ear or pain in the temporomandibular region or due to vestibular signs
• Nasal or ocular discharge due to facial nerve paralysis or paresis
• Ocular clouding or corneal ulcer from exposure keratitis due to diminished or absent blink from facial nerve involvement

Physical Examination Findings
• Pain upon palpation of the bullae or temporomandibular region
• Corneal ulcer—from exposure keratitis due to diminished or absent blink from facial nerve involvement
• Erythema of the pinna or crusts and scabs evident from scratching
• Exudate within the aural canal—the presence of a small amount of brown waxy debris is normal
• Thickened, stenotic ear canals may be evident if otitis externa is present.
• Opaque, white, thick tympanum—difficult to visualize in the normal guinea pig without the aid of sedation
• Nasal discharge—due to either primary URI or secondary to facial nerve paralysis
• Ocular discharge—from inability to blink due to facial nerve paralysis
• External otic examination may be normal.
• Diarrhea may be present from inappetence, pain, and stress.

Neurologic Examination Findings
• Facial nerve paralysis or paresis—may be evidenced as either drooping or contracture of the muscles innervated by CN VII
• Head tilt (ear toward the ground) or torticollis (nose pointed to one side)—indicates involvement of the vestibular portion of CN VIII on the ipsilateral side
• Nystagmus (horizontal or rotary)—may be present at rest or positional; fast phase away from the affected side; can be challenging to differentiate horizontal from rotary nystagmus; vertical nystagmus indicates CNS involvement
• Leaning, falling, or rolling toward the affected side
• Normal proprioceptive responses (unless CNS involvement)

CAUSES
• Bacteria—most common organisms include *Streptococcus pneumoniae*, *Streptococcus zooepidemicus*, *Staphylococcus aureus*, *Bordatella bronchiseptica*
• Yeast—*Malassezia* spp., *Candida* spp.
• Unilateral disease—usually bacterial; consider trauma, neoplasia, foreign body

RISK FACTORS
• Hypovitaminosis C—leads to increased susceptibility to bacterial infection, probably because of immunocompromise
• Immunosuppression—(stress, concurrent disease, corticosteroid use) increases susceptibility to infection by pathogens or commensal organisms
• Upper respiratory infection—may alter mucous-producing goblet cells and contribute to damage to eustachian tube and secondary otitis

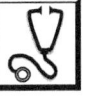

DIAGNOSIS

DIFFERENTIAL DIAGNOSIS
• Neoplasia—of either the middle/inner ear or brain; imaging of the head can aid in differentiation
• Trauma—imaging of the head and physical examination to evaluate for evidence of fracture or injury
• Cerebrovascular accident—may compromise vestibular system and lead to head tilt or torticollis

CBC/BIOCHEMISTRY/URINALYSIS
• Usually normal
• Hemogram—relative heterophilia and lymphopenia are more common than leukocytosis

OTHER LABORATORY TESTS
N/A

IMAGING
• Skull radiographs—multiple views are often required, but dorsoventral is most important to evaluate for thickening or sclerosis of the tympanic bullae and petrous temporal bone; fluid or soft tissue density within the bullae; osteomyelitis may be present; radiographs may also be normal even though disease is present
• CT—more sensitive than radiographs for detection of fluid or soft tissue densities within the middle ear and to evaluate for bony changes in the bullae as well as extension of disease into the brain
• MRI—also more sensitive than radiographs; better for detection of soft tissue involvement and invasion into the brain, but less sensitive than CT for evaluation of bone involvement

- Otoscopic evaluation—challenging due to the small ear canals of guinea pigs; enables visualization of the tympanum and structures behind it if damaged; also useful for collection of samples for cytology and culture and sensitivity; aids in performing therapeutic lavage

DIAGNOSTIC PROCEDURES

- Myringotomy—insert a 22- or 25-gauge needle using endoscopic guidance to aspirate the middle ear to obtain samples for cytology, culture, and sensitivity
- Cytologic evaluation of debris present in ear canal
- Culture and sensitivity of any nasal discharge, if present, as upper respiratory infections may occur concurrently and disease may be transmitted through the eustachian tube
- Biopsy—if tumor is suspected

PATHOLOGIC FINDINGS

- *Gross*: ruptured tympanum, purulent or caseous exudate within the middle ear cavity; fluid within the bullae, thickened sclerotic bullae
- *Histopathologic*: degenerative neutrophils with bacteria and/or yeast; osteomyelitis of bullae

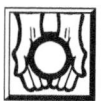

TREATMENT

APPROPRIATE HEALTH CARE

Inpatient—neurologic signs; severe infections; anorexic patients; nonambulatory patients

Outpatient—stable patients that are able to eat and drink with little or no assistance

NURSING CARE

- Fluid therapy to maintain hydration—subcutaneous generally adequate
- Culture and lavage ear canals; multiple lavages may be necessary; use 0.9% NaCl if integrity of tympanum is compromised or cannot be determined; sedation may be necessary
- Assisted feeding of anorexic animals
- Maintain clean, soft bedding
- Lubricate eyes if blink response is absent or diminished.
- In severe cases, turn patient and bathe as needed to prevent formation of decubitus ulcers.

ACTIVITY

Restrict activity when vestibular signs are present to prevent falls or injury; encourage ambulation and movement on flat surfaces once safe.

DIET

- It is essential to maintain food intake during treatment; patients may become anorexic due to pain or vestibular signs; anorexia may lead to gastrointestinal stasis and ileus; secondary derangements of intestinal microbial populations may occur.
- Offer a wide variety of fresh leafy greens (romaine lettuce, cilantro, parsley, kale, cabbage, collard greens, mustard greens, bok choy, dandelion greens, turnip greens, spinach, and mesclun salad mixes) and high-quality grass hay. Place food and water in a position that the guinea pig is able to reach, or hand offer.
- If patient is inappetent/anorexic, it is essential to provide adequate nutritional support. Syringe-feed a formulated diet such as Critical Care for Herbivores (Oxbow Pet Products, Murdock, NE) or Emeraid Herbivore (Lafeber Company, Cornell, IL), 10–15 mL/kg q6–8h. If neither product is available, a slurry can be made with blended leafy green vegetables that are high in vitamin C, nor guinea pig pellets crushed and mixed with water and vegetable baby food.
- Avoid high-carbohydrate foods, treats, or grains.
- Use caution when syringe-feeding as aspiration pneumonia may occur in patients with vestibular signs or central nervous system signs.

CLIENT EDUCATION

- Inform client that otitis media/interna is a chronic, debilitating disease that necessitates diligent client compliance, long-term antimicrobial therapy, may be recurrent, and frequently requires surgery for complete resolution.
- Advise clients that neurologic signs may persist for life, despite resolution of infection. Many guinea pigs will adapt and maintain good quality of life but may still require home care, including lubrication of eyes, and may still be predisposed to upper respiratory infections.

SURGICAL CONSIDERATIONS

- Indicated for recurrent or relapsing infections when bulla involvement is present and medical management has failed, or when neoplasia is present within the ear canal.
- Severity of clinical signs is not an indicator of the need for surgery.
- Endoscopic myringotomy has been used to successfully. May require specialized expertise.
- Bulla osteotomy and total ear canal ablation—this procedure generally carries a guarded to poor prognosis; many patients do not recover or develop intractable postoperative GI stasis. Appropriate analgesia

is essential; techniques are similar to dog and cat; drains must be avoided in guinea pigs as they may incite exudate and granuloma formation (guinea pig exudate is usually caseous and will not drain); consider the use of AIPMMA beads to improve outcome.
- Obtain samples for cytologic evaluation, culture and sensitivity, and histopathology at the time of surgery.
- AIPMMA beads provide high local concentrations of antimicrobials with little or no systemic absorption, thus sparing the guinea pig of adverse systemic effects. Limit selection of antibiotics to those for which elution data is available and base choices on results of culture and sensitivity when available. AIPMMA beads can be commercially purchased but are too large for use in the bullae of guinea pigs; they can be made by using surgical grade PMMA (Surgical Simplex; Howmedica, Rutherford, NJ or Bone Cement; Zimmer, Patient Care Division, Charlotte, NC). Add antimicrobial to powder prior to mixing with liquid; insert mixed material into a syringe and squirt out a thin line on a sterile surface, cut immediately into small spherical beads with a scalpel. Maintain aseptic technique when preparing and inserting beads; gas sterilize unused beads for future use. Antimicrobials used include gentamicin or tobramycin (1 g/20 g PMMA); amikacin (1.25 g/20 g PMMA); cefazolin, cephalothin, or ceftiofur (2 g/20 g PMMA); and clindamycin (1.5–3 g/20 g PMMA). Beads may be left in permanently or may be removed if problems or recurrent abscessation develop.

MEDICATIONS

DRUG(S) OF CHOICE

- Systemic antibiotics—ideally based on results of culture and sensitivity. Long-term therapy is required and should be continued for a minimum of 4–6 weeks and may require therapy for several months.
- Choose broad-spectrum antibiotics such as enrofloxacin (5–20 mg/kg PO q12–24h), trimethoprim-sulfa (15–30 mg/kg PO q12h); for anaerobic infections consider chloramphenicol (30–50 mg/kg PO, SC, IM, IV q8–12h), florfenicol (20–25 mg/kg PO, IM, IV q12h), or metronidazole (10–20 mg/kg PO, IV q12h).
- Topical antimicrobials—choose otic or ophthalmic preparations without corticosteroids such as antibiotics (gentamicin, ciprofloxacin, chloramphenicol, and enrofloxacin) or antifungals (miconazole)
- Analgesics—systemic meloxicam (0.5–1.0 mg/kg PO, SC, IM q24h) for its

(CONTINUED)

anti-inflammatory effects alone or in combination with an opioid; buprenorphine (0.05–0.2 mg/kg SC, IM, IV q8–12h), butorphanol (0.4–2.0 mg/kg SC, IM q4–12h), or tramadol (5–10 mg/kg PO q12h) for additional analgesia. Topical DMSO can be used.
• Anxiolytics—for severe vestibular signs or seizures—midazolam (0.25–2.0 mg/kg IM) or diazepam (0.5–2.0 mg/kg IV or IM) can be used
• Meclizine (2–12 mg/kg PO q12h) may be useful for decreasing vestibular signs.

CONTRAINDICATIONS
• Avoid the use of antimicrobials that may disrupt gastrointestinal flora, which may lead to dysbiosis and fatal enterotoxemia (penicillins, macrolides, lincosamides, and tetracyclines, and cephalosporins).
• Avoid the use of corticosteroids in conjunction with meloxicam or other NSAIDs.
• Topical and systemic corticosteroids—guinea pigs are highly sensitive to the immunosuppressive effects of corticosteroids; their use may prolong or exacerbate infection and may increase the risk of systemic disease.
• If tympanum is ruptured or integrity of tympanum cannot be assessed—avoid the use of irritating or oil-based ear preparations; use only solutions that are safe in contact with the CNS.

PRECAUTIONS
• Corticosteroids—although highly controversial, systemic prednisolone (10 mg IM or PO once) has been shown to significantly decrease the incidence of infection in experimentally induced otitis media in guinea pigs.
• Procaine penicillin G (40,000–60,000 IU SC q7d) has been suggested as an alternative therapy, but there are anecdotal reports of fatal enterotoxemia with the use of any form of penicillin, including parenteral, in guinea pigs.

POSSIBLE INTERACTIONS
• Avoid the use of NSAIDs with corticosteroids.
• Some topical medications may cause contact irritation; discontinue use if patient is reactive to treatment.

ALTERNATIVE DRUGS
N/A

 FOLLOW-UP

PATIENT MONITORING
• Monitor ear canals and tympanum for clinical improvement at 10–14 day intervals; more frequently if clinical condition is declining

• Evaluate bullae radiographs at 4–6 week intervals to assess changes, or if performing follow-up CT/MRI studies, at 8–12 week intervals to evaluate for improvement
• Monitor for corneal ulceration secondary to facial nerve paralysis.

PREVENTION/AVOIDANCE
• Early and aggressive treatment of upper respiratory infections and otitis may prevent invasion into the middle/inner ear or systemic spread.
• Proper nutrition, including appropriate vitamin C supplementation, helps minimize the risk of immunosuppression.
• Appropriate husbandry, adequate ventilation, and lack of overcrowding may decrease transmission of infectious agents and reduce stress.

POSSIBLE COMPLICATIONS
• Facial nerve paralysis may be permanent and may lead to corneal ulceration and secondary URI.
• Vestibular signs may not resolve.
• Bulla osteitis and osteomyelitis may develop.
• Infections may spread to the brainstem/CNS.

EXPECTED COURSE AND PROGNOSIS
• Otitis media and interna may require months of systemic and topical therapy; although some cases will improve or resolve, others may be recurrent or may require surgery.
• Surgical intervention may be required; surgery should be considered for severe cases with bulla involvement that have proven refractory to medical treatment.
• Vestibular signs and facial nerve paralysis may persist following resolution of disease via medical or surgical means, or may improve and subsequently recur.

 MISCELLANEOUS

ASSOCIATED CONDITIONS
• Upper respiratory infections
• Corneal ulcers
• "Dry eye"
• Gastrointestinal stasis
• Dental disease

AGE-RELATED FACTORS
None

ZOONOTIC POTENTIAL
None

PREGNANCY/FERTILITY/BREEDING
Avoid the use of drugs that cross the placenta in pregnant animals.

SYNONYMS
Wry neck
Middle and inner ear infection

SEE ALSO
Ataxia
Head tilt (vestibular disease)

ABBREVIATIONS
AIPMMA = antibiotic-impregnated polymethyl methacrylate
CN = cranial nerve
CNS = central nervous system
DMSO = dimethyl sulfoxide
URI = upper respiratory infection

INTERNET RESOURCES
N/A

Suggested Reading
Bennett RA. Antibiotic-impregnated PMMA beads: use and misuse. Proc Western Vet Conf 2008.
Hammond G, Sullivan M, Posthumus J, King A. Assessment of three radiographic projections for detection of fluid in the rabbit tympanic bulla. Vet Radiol Ultrasound 2010;51(1):48–51.
Jekl V, Hauptman K, Knotek Z. Video otoscopy in exotic companion mammals. Vet Clin North Am Exot Anim Pract 2015;18:431–445.
Minarikova A, Hauptman K, Jeklova E, Knotek Z, Jekl V. Diseases in pet guinea pigs: a retrospective study in 1000 animals. Vet Rec 2015;177:200.
Miwa Y, Sladky K. Common surgical procedures of rodents, ferrets, hedgehogs, and sugar gliders. Vet Clin Exot Anim 2016;19:205–244.
Pignon C, Mayer J. Guinea pigs. In: Quesenberry KE, Carpenter JW, eds. Ferrets, Rabbits and Rodents, 4th Ed). Clinical Medicine and Surgery. 2021 ed. St. Louis: Saunders, 2020:270–297.
Rosset RA, Pignon C, Desprez I et al. Development and validation of an endoscopic myringotomy technique to treat otitis media and interna in a case series of three guineapigs (*Caviaporcellus*). JEPM 2020;31:31–28.

Author Natalie Antinoff, DVM, Dipl. ABVP (Avian)

OVARIAN CYSTS

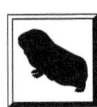

BASICS

DEFINITION
Ovarian cysts are classified according to tissue of origin within the ovary, and there are three forms documented in the guinea pig:
• Cystic rete ovarii—most common type—develop from the mesonephric tubules in the hilar region of the ovary and are devoid of germ cells.
• Follicular cysts are derived from secondary follicles that fail to ovulate or undergo atresia.
• Parovarian cysts are vestigial remnants of the mesonephric and paramesonephric ducts.

PATHOPHYSIOLOGY
• Cystic rete ovarii are the most common ovarian cysts. These are nonfunctional serous cysts that develop spontaneously throughout the estrous cycle, even during the early reproductive period.
• Follicular cysts occur less frequently and always coincide with cystic rete ovarii. These frequently secrete estrogen in normal or excessive amounts, leading to irregular estrous cycles, persistent estrus, and infertility.
• Parovarian cysts are rare in guinea pigs. These give rise to vesicular structures located in the mesosalpinx or mesovarium.
• Cysts range in diameter from <0.04 to 7 cm, with a linear relationship between prevalence and size as the animal ages.
• Cysts may be single or multilocular and are usually filled with clear fluid.
• Single or multiple pregnancies do not appear to influence cyst prevalence or size.
• Fertility is reduced in affected females over 15 months of age.
• Potentially serious uterine disorders (cystic endometrial hyperplasia, mucometra, endometritis, leiomyomas, and other uterine neoplasia) usually occur in conjunction with cysts.

SYSTEMS AFFECTED
Reproductive

GENETICS
Strain-specific differences in incidence are noted, but inherited factors associated with this disease have not been investigated.

INCIDENCE/PREVALENCE
N/A

GEOGRAPHIC DISTRIBUTION
N/A

SIGNALMENT

Breed Predilections
• Published reports in laboratory animals include Hartley and Abyssinian strains, and crosses of these two strains. Case reports of pet guinea pig populations do not specify any strains and include genetically mixed animals.

Mean Age and Range
• Literature reports that between 66% and 75% of sows, between 3 months and 5 years, have been diagnosed with ovarian cysts.
• Sows 2–4 years of age are more commonly affected and serous cysts can spontaneously develop throughout their estrus cycle.
• As sow age increase, so does the size of the ovarian cyst.
• Both ovaries are usually affected, although for unilateral cases the right ovary typically is more commonly afflicted

Predominant Sex
Females only

Historical Findings
• Can be asymptomatic
• Nonpruritic progressive hair loss over the flanks and abdomen
• Decreased fertility in older sows
• Mounting and other sexual behaviors
• Vaginal bleeding
• Anorexia

Physical Examination Findings
• "Pear" appearance to the body conformation because of abdominal enlargement caudal to the thorax.
• Bilateral symmetrical truncal alopecia
• Palpable large discrete rounded masses in cranial to middle abdomen
• Weight loss or poor body condition occurs when large cysts cause discomfort from the space-occupying mass leading to decreased appetite.
• Vaginal bleeding may be noted.

CAUSES
• The precise cause of development of cystic rete ovarii or follicular cysts is unknown.
• The pathogenesis may be related to the secretory activity of the cells lining the rete tubules. The tubules have no outlet when fluid accumulates and expand into cysts, which cause pressure atrophy of the adjacent ovarian parenchyma. Activation of these cells and excessive secretions may be under hormonal influence.
• Remnants of these embryonic structures persist, and later in life, as fluid accumulates in these blind ducts, they enlarge and appear as large fluid-filled cysts.
• Cystic dilatation of the rete ovarii in guinea pigs appears to be a function of aging.
• Defects in the inhibin-FSH system have been shown to increase the incidence of cystic rete ovarii in guinea pigs.
• The pathogenesis of follicular cysts is uncertain, but it is thought that luteinizing hormone levels are insufficient to luteinize the follicle, thus creating a mature follicle that becomes cystic.

• There was speculation that estrogenic substances in the diet, particularly moldy hay, cause cystic ovaries; however, no proof for this theory is available.

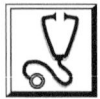

DIAGNOSIS

DIFFERENTIAL DIAGNOSIS
• Neoplasia—ovarian tumors. Granulosa cell tumors often present with signs of persistent estrus.
• Dermatological disorders known to cause alopecia such as ectoparasites, dermatophytes, or hypersensitivities
• Uterine neoplasia, metritis, or abortion can also cause vaginal bleeding.

CBC/BIOCHEMISTRY/URINALYSIS
Hemogram—increased numbers of Kurloff cells if cystic follicles present. Kurloff cells are influenced by elevated estrogen levels.

OTHER LABORATORY TESTS
Cytological examination of the cystic fluid obtained by FNA produces a clear acellular fluid.

IMAGING
• The most useful diagnostic tool is ultrasonography of the cranial abdomen to identify cysts. Ultrasonographic features of the <0.04- to 7-cm-diameter fluid-filled cysts included compartmentalization and connection to the ovary, presence of a well-defined margin, absence of internal echo, distal acoustic enhancement, and peripheral refractive zones.
• A thorough examination of the uterus is warranted to identify endometrial hyperplasia, mucometra, endometritis, or neoplastic changes associated with fibroleiomyomas.
• Plain radiography is nondiagnostic because of the similar opacity of ovarian cysts, abdominal neoplasms, and trichobezoars.

DIAGNOSTIC PROCEDURES
• FNA of the cysts can be done with ultrasound guidance or by immobilizing the cyst against the lateral abdominal wall.
• Aseptic fine-needle aspiration of the cysts produces a clear fluid.
• Aspiration of cystic fluid is not necessary for diagnosis, but if surgery is not an option then it will also reduce the size of the cysts and provide relief of abdominal distention.

PATHOLOGIC FINDINGS
• Cysts of the rete ovarii in guinea pigs are concentrated in the hilar region of the ovary and are in continuity with one another.
• 80%–90% of the ovarian parenchyma is replaced by epithelial lined cysts (cystic rete ovarii).

• Follicular cysts are large with a thin wall made up of several layers of granulosa cells and containing a large amount of fluid; they do not contain an oocyte.
• Microscopic appearance of the large ovarian cysts suggests reproductive performance in these guinea pigs should be compromised.

TREATMENT

APPROPRIATE HEALTH CARE
• Stabilize the patient if dehydrated or painful.
• Discuss options with client for OVH to remove cystic ovaries and uterus. Surgical removal of uterus is recommended because secondary changes often cause pathology in the uterus. If guinea pig has additional medical conditions or if surgery is not an option, then percutaneous aspiration of the large cysts can be performed as a temporary and palliative therapy.
• Hormonal medical therapy has been used to cause luteinization of ovarian follicular cysts; however, for nonfunctional serous cysts or parovarian cysts results are only temporary or typically nonresponsive.

SURGICAL TREATMENT
The treatment of choice is OVH because it provides resolution of the current problem and prevents recurrence.

NURSING CARE
• Fluid therapy should be initiated with evidence of dehydration. Subcutaneous fluids can be administered (100 mL/kg) as needed.
• Postoperative management includes assisted feeding, fluids, analgesics, and broad-spectrum antibiotics.
• Bandaging the abdomen may be warranted because incision site will be in constant contact with the cage floor.

ACTIVITY
• Restricted activity in the 2-week postoperative period to allow incision to heal
• If nonsurgical treatment elected, keep female separated from the boars

DIET
N/A

CLIENT EDUCATION
• If the client selects palliative care with aspiration of cystic fluid or hormonal therapy, it is important to educate the client to be aware of early signs of discomfort as the cysts enlarge, and the high probability of concurrent uterine disorders, including neoplsias.
• Clients need to be advised to keep older intact sows separate from the boars.

SURGICAL CONSIDERATIONS
• OVH surgery is recommended treatment and prevention.
• Older obese sows have increased anesthetic risk.
• Postoperative management includes assisted feeding, fluids, and analgesics.

MEDICATIONS

DRUG(S) OF CHOICE
• Hormone therapy can provide temporary resolution. Several treatments have been successful; (usually in follicular cysts):
  ◦ Leuprolide acetate (100 μg/kg SC) once every 3 weeks will provide temporary suppression of gonadotropin stimulation.
  ◦ Gonadotropin-releasing hormone (GnRH; 25 μg/treatment IM) every 2 weeks for two injections
  ◦ Human chorionic gonadotropin (hCG; 1000 USP IM) repeated in 7–10 days for three treatments, although hCG has been associated with hypersensitivity reactions
  ◦ Deslorelin implant (4.7 mg implant SC between the shoulder blades)—one guinea pig study showed that treatment did not significantly reduce ovarian cysts size during a 16 week period.
• Pain management is essential during and following surgery. Multimodal therapy is recommended for perioperative analgesia with an anxiolytic, such as midazolam (0.4–2.0 mg/kg IM), an opioid such as butorphanol (0.4–2.0 mg/kg SC, IM q4–12h), or buprenorphine (0.05–0.2 mg/kg SC, IM q6–8h). An NSAID such as meloxicam (0.5–1 mg/kg PO, SC, IM q24h) or carprofen (4 mg/kg SC q24h or 1–2 mg/kg PO q12h–24h) can be given in the perioperative period when the animal is fully hydrated and renal perfusion is no longer compromised. Tramadol, a synthetic opioid, may also be an effective at dosages of 5–10 mg/kg PO q12h postoperatively. For severe to moderate pain pure mu opioids such as morphine (0.5–2.0 mg/kg SC, IM q2–4h) or oxymorphone (0.2–0.5 mg/kg SC, IM q40–12h) should be used however appetite and fecal output should be monitored as these opioids are thought to contribute to GI ileus.
• Procedures for ultrasonography or percutaneous aspiration generally require administering sedatives. When substantial derangements exist, begin with fluid administration and other supportive measures first. Calculate the dosage of sedative using the low end of the recommended range or give only to effect.

CONTRAINDICATIONS
• Oral administration of antibiotics that select against gram-positive bacteria (penicillins, cephalosporins, macrolides, and lincosamides) can cause fatal enteric dysbiosis and enterotoxaemia.
• Glucocorticoids, or other immunosuppressive agents

PRECAUTIONS
• Aseptic technique is essential for FNA or aspiration of cystic fluid through percutaneous approach.
• If aspiration procedure done without ultrasound guidance, then manually trap the large cyst against the lateral body wall to avoid other viscera.
• During surgery, avoid excessive handling of gastrointestinal tissues to reduce postoperative ileus or fibrous adhesions.

POSSIBLE INTERACTIONS
None

ALTERNATIVE DRUGS
N/A

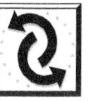

FOLLOW-UP

PATIENT MONITORING
• Ensure gastrointestinal motility by making sure the patient is eating, well hydrated, and passing normal feces.
• Assess urine production and hydration status frequently, adjusting fluid administration rate accordingly.

PREVENTION /AVOIDANCE
N/A

POSSIBLE COMPLICATIONS
Postoperative gastrointestinal ileus may take days to weeks to resolve.

EXPECTED COURSE AND PROGNOSIS
The prognosis following surgical removal of ovaries and uterus is fair to good.

MISCELLANEOUS

ASSOCIATED CONDITIONS
It is common to have uterine disorders associated with cystic ovaries such as endometrial hyperplasia, mucometra, endometritis, or fibroleiomyomas.

AGE-RELATED FACTORS
• This disease is commonly found in middle-aged to older guinea pigs, although it can occur in younger animals as well.
• Direct correlation between increasing age and increasing size of the ovarian cysts

OVARIAN CYSTS   (CONTINUED)

GUINEA PIGS

ZOONOTIC POTENTIAL
N/A

PREGNANCY/FERTILITY/BREEDING
• Single or multiple pregnancies did not appear to influence cyst prevalence or size.
• Fertility is reduced in affected females over 15 months of age.

SYNONYMS
Cystic ovaries
Cystic rete ovarii
Follicular cysts

ABBREVIATIONS
FNA = fine-needle aspiration
FSH = follicular-stimulating hormone
GnRH = gonadotropin-releasing hormone
hCG = human chorionic gonadotropin
NSAID = nonsteroidal anti-inflammatory drug
OVH = ovariohysterectomy

INTERNET RESOURCES
N/A

Suggested Reading
Bertram CA, Muller K, Klopfleisch R. Genital tract pathology in female pet guinea pigs (*Cavia porcellus*): a retrospective study of 655 post-mortem and 64 biopsy cases. J Comp Path 2018;164:12–22.
Laik-Schandelmaier C, Klopfleisch R, Schöniger S et al. Spontaneously arising tumours and tumour-like lesions of the cervix and uterus in 83 pet guinea pigs (*Cavia porcellus*). J Comp Path 2017;156:339–351.
Minarikova A, Hauptman K, Jeklova E et al. Diseases in pet guinea pigs: a retrospective study in 1000 animals. Vet Rec. 2015;177(8):200.
Pignon C, Mayer J. Guinea pigs. In: Quesenberry KE, Carpenter JW, eds. Ferrets, Rabbits and Rodents, 4th Ed). Clinical Medicine and Surgery. 2021 ed. St. Louis: Saunders, 2020:270–297.
Pilny A. Ovarian cystic disease in guinea pigs. Vet Clin North Am Exot Anim Pract. 2014;17:69–75.
Schuetzenhofer G, Goericke-Pesch S, Wehrend A. Effects of deslorelin implants on ovarian cysts in guinea pigs. Schweiz Arch Tierheilkd 2011;153:416–417.
Veiga-Parga T, LaPerle KM, Newman SJ. Spontaneous reproductive pathology in female guinea pigs. J Vet Diag Invest 2016;28(6):656–661.

Author Rodney Schnellbacher, DVM, Dipl. ACZM

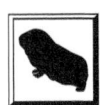

BASICS

DEFINITION
- Paresis—partial paralysis; loss of power of voluntary movement
- Paralysis (plegia)—loss of voluntary motor function
- Mono (paresis or plegia)—one limb affected
- Hemi—both limbs on the same side of the body
- Para—both pelvic limbs affected
- Quadri- or tetra—all four limbs affected

PATHOPHYSIOLOGY
- May be caused by lesions of the central or peripheral nervous system
- Central nervous system (CNS) consists of the brain and spinal cord. Cell bodies and nuclei located within the brain are responsible for initiating movement, and axons transmit impulses to various locations throughout the spinal cord.
- Peripheral nervous system consists of the sensory and motor neurons that innervate the various muscle groups; impulses to the limbs are received from the spinal cord via transmission through the ventral nerve roots into spinal nerves and to peripheral nerves.
- Collections of lower motor neurons and divergence to the peripheral nerves of the limbs occur in the cervical intumescence and the lumbar intumescence.
- Upper motor neurons maintain muscle tone and normal spinal reflexes by controlling or inhibiting lower motor neurons; when injured, spinal reflexes are no longer inhibited, which results in loss or decrease of voluntary movement and hyperreflexia.
- Lower motor neurons and peripheral nerves maintain muscle tone and control spinal reflexes; damage to the lower motor neuron results in loss or decreased movement and diminished or absent reflexes.
- Spinal reflexes do not involve conscious awareness of the stimulation. Rather, they are an evaluation of peripheral nerve function and local spinal cord segments.
- Muscle wasting will occur from disuse in as little as 5–7 days.

SYSTEMS AFFECTED
- Nervous
- Musculoskeletal—atrophy or contracture of musculature is a secondary complication.

GENETICS
None

INCIDENCE/PREVALENCE
N/A

GEOGRAPHIC DISTRIBUTION
None

SIGNALMENT
Breed Predilections
None

Mean Age and Range
None

Predominant Sex
None

SIGNS
General Comments
- It is important to differentiate paresis or paralysis from generalized weakness; patients with generalized weakness will not exhibit any deficits on neurologic exam. However, this can be difficult to interpret in the debilitated guinea pig.
- Clinical signs may be acute or chronic and may be progressive or static. Onset and progression may be indicative of etiology.
- Acute or peracute onset of signs without progression or with gradual improvement is usually consistent with trauma or vascular events.
- Gradual or subacute onset with gradual improvement in response to treatment usually indicates infection.
- Slow onset and continued progression of clinical signs usually indicates a neoplastic or degenerative process.
- Static clinical signs (or signs present at birth) indicates an anomalous cause.

Historical Findings
- Owner may notice an abnormal gait, leaning to one side, falling, or inability to stand or walk.
- There may be a known traumatic event such as being dropped or stepped on, or there may be a history of children playing with the pet.
- Inability to right itself from lying down, or an inability to get up without assistance
- Dragging of a limb
- Urine staining around perineum and/or on limbs (may be unilateral or bilateral)
- Swelling, redness, or pododermatitis of unaffected or less affected limbs may be the first sign identified and is often the result of excessive weight bearing on these -limbs.
- Alopecia of the affected limbs may be present from rubbing or dragging.

Physical Examination Findings
- Mentation is usually normal.
- Pain on spinal palpation may be present in cases of trauma or injury.
- Muscle wasting may be present in patients with more gradual onset or prolonged disease.
- Patient may be tachypneic in response to pain.

- Urine staining may be present around perineum and/or on limbs (may be unilateral or bilateral).
- Swelling, redness, or pododermatitis of unaffected or less affected limbs may be identified and is often the result of excessive weight bearing on these limbs.
- Alopecia of the affected limbs may be present from rubbing or dragging.
- Gastric dilation (usually mild) may occur as a result of aerophagia; anorexia or diarrhea may be present due to inappetence from pain or an inability to access food or water.

NEUROLOGIC EXAMINATION FINDINGS
- Pain may be present on spinal palpation in cases of trauma.
- Upper motor neuron lesions: decrease or absence of voluntary motor movement with normal or increased reflexes
- Lower motor neuron lesions: decrease or absence of voluntary motor movement with diminished or absent reflexes
- Prioprioceptive deficits will be present in the affected limbs; this must be interpreted with caution as many guinea pigs will fail to right limbs even when completely normal.
- Deep pain is assessed by using a toe-pinch (superficial pain) or pinching of the pad/bone (deep pain); withdrawal of the limb is a reflex that alone does not indicate intact pain sensation; conscious response to the pinch is required to indicate spinal cord integrity.
- Neurolocalization is important.
- Cervical (C1–C6)—proprioceptive or motor deficits of all four limbs. Pain may be found on cervical palpation.
- Cervicothoracic (C6–T2)—lower-motor neuron signs to the forelimb, including poor motor function and weak withdrawal with loss of reflexes
- Thoracolumbar (T3–L3)—weakness and proprioceptive abnormalities in the rear limbs with normal motor function and proprioception in the front limbs. Spinal reflexes are normal. Pain may be found on spinal palpation.
- Lumbosacral (L4–S3)—lower motor neuron signs to the rear limbs, including proprioceptive abnormalities, weakness, poor withdrawal reflexes, and loss of segmental spinal reflexes. Urinary and fecal incontinence may be present.

CAUSES
- Trauma/injury is the most common cause of paresis or paralysis in pet guinea pigs; an incident may have been directly observed, or there may be a history of contact with children or other pets.
- Meningitis/encephalitis—bacterial (consider spread of otitis media/interna or upper respiratory infection); viral

PARESIS AND PARALYSIS

(lymphocytic choriomeningitis virus [LCMV]), disseminated infection
• Neoplasia (brain or spinal cord)
• CNS abscess (effects and diagnostics may mimic neoplasia)
• Cerebrovascular accident
• Toxoplasmosis
• Poliovirus—an RNA enterovirus transmitted via fecal-oral route; clinical signs include lameness and/or flaccid paralysis; rarely causes clinical signs
• LCMV—zoonotic disease that is naturally occurring in guinea pigs; causes meningitis and hind limb paralysis
• Toxicity—lead, *Clostridium botulinum*, organophosphate are among toxins that can cause CNS or PNS signs and should be suspected if there is a possibility of ingestion or exposure

RISK FACTORS
• Hypovitaminosis C (scurvy)
• Fractures, luxations often the result of trauma from improper handling or housing, children, or other pets
• Spondylosis/arthritis

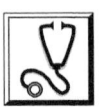

DIAGNOSIS

DIFFERENTIAL DIAGNOSIS
• Hypovitaminosis C (scurvy)
• Weakness (metabolic) may lead to similar clinical presentation.
• Osteoarthritis
• Hypovitaminosis E—myopathy leading to hind limb weakness has been described in guinea pigs
• Pododermatitis
• Pregnancy

CBC/BIOCHEMISTRY/URINALYSIS
Usually normal unless infection is present; leukocytosis may be present in cases of infection; profound leukocytosis (>100,000) may occur in guinea pigs with leukemia; elevations in CK are likely in cases of trauma

OTHER LABORATORY TESTS
• LCMV testing—PCR, IFA, and serology are available and performed at many universities and commercial veterinary laboratories.
• Blood lead levels if ingestion is suspected
• Cholinesterase testing may be performed if organophosphate toxicity is suspected.

IMAGING
• Radiography—may reveal spinal fracture or luxation, osteomyelitis, osteoarthritis, discospondylitis, and bone neoplasia. Skull radiographs may reveal bulla disease.

• CT or MRI—more sensitive for evaluation of brain infiltrate, spinal cord compression, or bony lesions

DIAGNOSTIC PROCEDURES
• CSF analysis can be performed via the cisterna magna; indicated if infection or neoplasia is suspected; do not attempt to aspirate but instead collect sample via capillary tube; only a few drops will be obtained
• EMG/NCV (electromyelogram/nerve conduction velocity)—not commonly performed in guinea pigs, compare to unaffected limb to establish normal

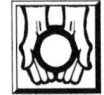

TREATMENT

APPROPRIATE HEALTH CARE
• Inpatient—neurologic signs; severe infections; anorexic patients; nonambulatory patients
• Outpatient—stable patients that are able to eat and drink with little or no assistance

NURSING CARE
• Fluid therapy to maintain hydration—subcutaneous generally adequate unless severe infection/sepsis
• Assisted feeding of anorexic animals
• Maintain clean, soft bedding with padding if necessary.
• Lubricate eyes if blink response is absent or diminished.
• In severe cases, turn patient every 4 hours or as needed to prevent formation of decubitus ulcers.
• Express bladder if patient is unable to void without assistance.
• Keep fur clean and dry.

ACTIVITY
Restrict activity, particularly in cases of trauma. Confine to a very small space initially to prevent falls or further injury.

DIET
• It is essential to maintain food intake during treatment; patients may become anorexic due to pain or neurologic signs; anorexia may lead to gastrointestinal stasis and ileus; secondary derangements of intestinal microbial populations may occur.
• Offer a wide variety of fresh leafy greens (romaine lettuce, cilantro, parsley, kale, cabbage, collard greens, mustard greens, bok choy, dandelion greens, turnip greens, spinach, and mesclun salad mixes) and high-quality grass hay. Place food and water in a position that the guinea pig is able to reach, or hand offer.
• If patient is inappetant/anorexic, it is essential to provide adequate nutritional

support. Syringe-feed a formulated diet such as Critical Care for Herbivores (Oxbow Pet Products, Murdock, NE) or Emerald Herbivore (Lafeber Company, Cornell, IL), 10–15 mL/kg q6–8h. If neither product is available, a slurry can be made with blended leafy green vegetables that are high in vitamin C, nor guinea pig pellets crushed and mixed with water and vegetable baby food.
• Avoid high-carbohydrate foods, treats, or grains.
• Use caution when syringe feeding, as aspiration pneumonia may occur in patients with central nervous system signs.

CLIENT EDUCATION
Owners should be informed that in cases of spinal trauma or paralysis, motor function may improve gradually or may not improve at all.

SURGICAL CONSIDERATIONS
Surgical repair of spinal fractures or trauma should only be undertaken by an experienced orthopedic or neurologic surgeon and may be of limited value. Many cases of partial paresis or paralysis will improve without surgery; surgery in these small patients has the potential of further destabilizing the spinal cord.

MEDICATIONS
DRUG(S) OF CHOICE
• Corticosteroids are recommended in mammals with spinal trauma, but their use is controversial in guinea pigs because they are believed to be very susceptible to adverse side effects and secondary infections; however, other references cite that guinea pigs are a steroid-resistant species.
• If administered, a short-acting steroid such as methylprednisolone sodium succinate (10–30 mg/kg IV or IM is the canine dose—guinea pig dose not reported) may be preferable to minimize any long-term immunosuppression.
• Analgesics should be administered in cases of confirmed or suspected trauma; systemic meloxicam (0.5–1.0 mg/kg PO, SC, IM q24h) for its anti-inflammatory effects alone or in combination with an opioid (avoid if corticosteroids have been administered); buprenorphine (0.05–0.2 mg/kg SC, IM, IV q8–12h), butorphanol (0.4–2.0 mg/kg SC, IM q4–12h), or tramadol (5–10 mg/kg PO q12h) for additional analgesia
• For suspected or confirmed CNS infections, use systemic antibiotics. Choose broad-spectrum antibiotics that penetrate the CNS, such as enrofloxacin (5–20 mg/kg PO, SC, IM q12–24h) or trimethoprim-sulfa (15–30 mg/kg

PO q12h); for anaerobic infections consider chloramphenicol (30–50 mg/kg PO, SC, IM, IV q12h), florfenicol (20–25 mg/kg PO, IM, IV q12h), or metronidazole (10–20 mg/kg PO, IV q12h).

CONTRAINDICATIONS
• Avoid the use of antimicrobials that may disrupt gastrointestinal flora, which may lead to dysbiosis and fatal enterotoxemia (penicillins, macrolides, lincosamides, and tetracyclines, and cephalosporins).
• Avoid the use of corticosteroids in conjunction with meloxicam or other NSAIDs.
• Topical and systemic corticosteroids—guinea pigs are highly sensitive to the immunosuppressive effects of corticosteroids; their use may prolong or exacerbate infection and may increase risk of systemic disease.
• Avoid the use of drugs that are potentially toxic to the central nervous system (metronidazole at high doses; aminoglycosides).

PRECAUTIONS
Do not use steroids in conjunction with NSAIDs.
Use caution in choosing antimicrobials.

POSSIBLE INTERACTIONS
Do not use steroids in conjunction with NSAIDs.

FOLLOW-UP

PATIENT MONITORING
Serial neurologic examinations should be performed daily or more frequently initially to monitor for progression of clinical signs.

PREVENTION/AVOIDANCE
Avoid free roaming or unsupervised activity or interactions with children or other pets.

POSSIBLE COMPLICATIONS
• Urine retention, urine scald, urinary tract infection, and ascending renal infection

• Pododermatitis and osteomyelitis from excessive weight bearing of unaffected or lesser affected limbs
• Permanent paralysis

EXPECTED COURSE AND PROGNOSIS
• Depends on etiology
• For patients with hypovitaminosis C, full recovery can be expected in most cases, although if fractures are present, there may be improper healing without primary repair.
• The loss of deep pain perception carries a poor prognosis for recovery.

MISCELLANEOUS

ASSOCIATED CONDITIONS
• Nutritional deficiencies, either as a cause (hypovitaminosis C, E) or result of inability to access food
• Gastrointestinal hypomotility
• Otitis media/interna or upper respiratory infection may serve as a source for CNS infections.

AGE-RELATED FACTORS
None

ZOONOTIC POTENTIAL
LCMV is rare but zoonotic.

PREGNANCY/FERTILITY/BREEDING
Guinea pigs with paresis or paralysis should not breed; pregnancy and parturition would put excessive strain on any injury.

SYNONYMS
None

SEE ALSO
Ataxia
Head tilt (vestibular disease)
Hypovitaminosis C (scurvy)
Otitis media and interna

ABBREVIATIONS
CK = creatine kinase
CNS = central nervous system
CSF = cerebral spinal fluid
CT = computed tomography
EMG = electromyelogram
IFA = indirect immunofluorescene assay
LCMV = lymphocytic choriomeningitis virus
MRI = magnetic resonance imaging
NCV = nerve conduction velocity
NSAID = nonsteroidal anti-inflammatory drug
PCR = polymerase chain reaction

Suggested Reading
Bays TB. Geriatric care of rabbits, guinea pigs, and chinchillas. Vet Clin Exot Anim 2020;23:567–593.
DeCubellis J. Common emergencies in rabbits, guinea pigs, and chinchillas. Vet Clin Exot Anim 2016;19:411–429.
Harkness JE, Turner PV, VandeWoude S, Wheeler CL. Clinical signs and differential diagnoses: nervous and musculoskeletal conditions. In: Harkness JE, Turner PV, VandeWoude S, Wheeler CL, eds. Biology and Medicine of Rabbits and Rodents, 5th ed. Ames: Wiley-Blackwell, 2010:214–216.
Lennox AM, Gladden JN. Emergency and critical care of small mammals. In: Quesenberry KE, Carpenter JW, eds. Ferrets, Rabbits and Rodents, 4th Ed). Clinical Medicine and Surgery. 2021 ed. St. Louis: Saunders, 2020:595–608.
Mancinelli E. Neurologic examination and diagnostic testing in rabbits, ferrets and rodents. J Exot Pet Med 2015;24:52–64.
Meredith AL, Richardson J. Neurologic disease of rabbits and rodents. J Exot Pet Med 2015;24:21–33.
Minarikova A, Hauptman K, Jeklova E, Knotek Z, Jekl V. Diseases in pet guinea pigs: a retrospective study in 1000 animals. Vet Rec 2015;177:200.
Miwa Y, Sladky K. Common surgical procedures of rodents, ferrets, hedgehogs, and sugar gliders. Vet Clin Exot Anim 2016;19:205–244.
Pignon C, Mayer J. Guinea pigs. In: Quesenberry KE, Carpenter JW, eds. Ferrets, Rabbits and Rodents, 4th Ed). Clinical Medicine and Surgery. 2021 ed. St. Louis: Saunders, 2020:270–297.

Author Natalie Antinoff, DVM, Dipl. ABVP (Avian)

GUINEA PIGS

PEA EYE

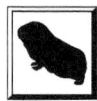

GUINEA PIGS

BASICS

DEFINITION
A nodule or nodular cluster protruding from the inferior conjunctival cul-de-sac

PATHOPHYSIOLOGY
The nodule is an anterior protrusion of orbital glandular tissue (Harderian, lacrimal, or salivary gland) into the subconjunctival space; location is typically ventral or ventromedial to globe—may suggest weakness or of ventral aspect of periorbital facial border; characteristics of glandular hypertrophy not identified, thus protruding tissue apparently normal

SYSTEMS AFFECTED
Ophthalmic

GENETICS
Genetic predisposition suspected

INCIDENCE/PREVALENCE
Unknown

SIGNALMENT
Breed Predilections
American shorthair

SIGNS
Historical Findings
• Acute onset—may have no associated abnormalities
• History of facial/ periocular trauma or inflammation

Physical Examination Findings
• Unilateral or bilateral protrusion of tissue ventral to globe
• Lagophthalmos—incomplete coverage of globe during blink—protruding subconjunctival tissue can prevent lower lid movement over, and thus appropriate coverage of, ventral globe and cornea
• Keratitis—ulcerative or nonulcerative, typically in ventral cornea
• Corneal opacification—from exposure-related scarring and degeneration
• Epiphora—irritation from corneal and conjunctival exposure and irritation

CAUSES
• Unknown—heritable etiology suspected, for example, congenital weakness of ventral periorbital fascia with anterior displacement of large glands through "rent"
• Prior trauma to periorbita—gland protrusion through rent

RISK FACTORS
• Heredity
• Previous orbital inflammatory disease

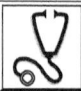

DIAGNOSIS

DIFFERENTIAL DIAGNOSIS
• Orbital neoplasia—slower progression; pea eye can be acute onset
• Orbital fat prolapse—often more yellow in color versus pink-white appearance of pea eye
• Lacrimal, Harderian, or salivary gland mucocele—signs of inflammation
• Orbital abscess—signs of inflammation, pain
• Facial nerve paralysis—with lid laxity; absence of normal palpebral response
• "Fatty eye"—lipid deposition in the conjunctiva of the lower eyelid in over-conditioned animals

CBC/BIOCHEMISTRY/URINALYSIS
• Normal in pea eye, neoplasia
• Leukogram—may demonstrate inflammation with orbital abscess

IMAGING
Orbital ultrasound—evaluate orbital structures, gland position, presence of abscess

DIAGNOSTIC PROCEDURES
• Palpebral response—stimulate periocular skin at lateral canthus to stimulate blink to determine if lid excursion can move inferior lid over ventral cornea—rule out facial nerve paralysis
• Fluorescein stain—rule out corneal ulceration
• Fine-needle aspiration (use 18–20 gauge needle) of subconjunctival tissue—submit samples for aerobic, anaerobic, and fungal cultures; gram staining; and cytological evaluation
• Cytology—may reveal acinar cells from normal glandular tissue, mucinous or lipid secretions from glands; often diagnostic for abscess and neoplasia—guinea pig abscesses typically produce thick, paste-like purulent material
• Biopsy—indicated if needle aspiration is nondiagnostic

PATHOLOGIC FINDINGS
• Pea eye—normal glandular characteristics observed
• Neoplasia—characteristics of malignancy
• Abscess—inflammatory cells, bacteria

TREATMENT

APPROPRIATE HEALTH CARE
• Prevent corneal exposure/desiccation—apply topical lubricant/gel q4–6h

• Surgery—limited information on surgical options; in cases where keratitis or discomfort is noted, or if frequent lubrication is not possible, consider lateral canthoplasty/permanent lateral tarsorrhaphy—reduces palpebral fissure size and pulls inferior lid dorsally to reduce ventral corneal exposure
• Consider attempt at definitive surgical treatment (i.e., partial gland excision)—refer to specialist with appropriate instrumentation—no reports on success rates/side effects

NURSING CARE
Prevent corneal exposure/desiccation—apply topical lubricant/gel q4–6h

ACTIVITY
Limit postoperatively until wound healing is complete if surgical options elected

CLIENT EDUCATION
• Avoid breeding of affected animals
• Monitor corneal health

MEDICATIONS

DRUG(S) OF CHOICE
• Lubricate cornea—prevent desiccation and ulceration (e.g., artificial tear ointment or gel q4–6h)
• Corneal ulceration or postoperative prophylaxis—topical antibiotic (e.g., neomycin-polymyxin-bacitracin, ciprofloxacin, or ofloxacin q6–8h) and cycloplegic (e.g., atropine 1% q12–24h) to prevent infection and reduce ciliary spasm, respectively, topical nalbuphine 1.2% q8h

FOLLOW-UP

PATIENT MONITORING
• No treatment—monitor for evidence of irritation and corneal changes (ulceration, keratitis, and degeneration).
• Surgery—reassess postoperatively at periodic intervals to ensure treatment goals are met (corneal health stable) and that gland does not reprolapse.

PREVENTION/AVOIDANCE
Avoid breeding affected animals.

POSSIBLE COMPLICATIONS
Exposure keratoconjunctivitis

EXPECTED COURSE AND PROGNOSIS
Depends on extent of lagophthalmos and corneal effects

(CONTINUED)

 MISCELLANEOUS

PREGNANCY/FERTILITY/BREEDING
Avoid breeding affected animals.

SYNONYMS
Cherry eye
Fatty eye

SEE ALSO
Exophthalmos and orbital diseases

Suggested Reading
Flecknell P. Guinea pigs. In: Meredith A, Redrobe S, eds. BSAVA Manual of Exotic Pets, 4th ed. Quedgeley, Gloucester: BSAVA, 2002:52–64.
Kern TJ. Rabbit and rodent ophthalmology. Sem Avian Exot Pet Med 1997;6(3):138–145.
Williams D. Ocular disease in the guinea pig (*Cavia porcellus*): a survey of 1000 animals. Vet Ophthalmol 2010;13(Supplement 1): 54–62.
Van der Woerdt A. Ophthalmologic diseases of small mammals. In: Quesenberry KE, Carpenter JW, eds. Ferrets, Rabbits and Rodents, 4th Ed). Clinical Medicine and Surgery. 2021 ed. St. Louis: Saunders, 2020:583–594.

Authors Georgina Newbold, DVM, Dipl. ACVO and A. Michelle Willis, DVM, Dipl., ACVO

PERINEAL SAC IMPACTION

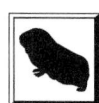

BASICS

DEFINITION
• The perineal sac is a pouch of skin containing two perineal glands that are located caudal to the urethral orifice and cranial to the anus. The perineal sacs of male guinea pigs are very large. Soiled bedding combined with inguinal sebaceous secretions can become attached to the scrotum and anus, enter the sac, and result in inguinal gland infections and fecal impaction.

PATHOPHYSIOLOGY
• Perineal scent glands are testosterone dependent. Sebum production increases at 4–5 weeks of age as puberty ensues with dominant males producing more sebum.
• During scent marking, secretions are deposited around the perineal region surface.
• Guinea pigs are coprophagic or cecophagic.
  ∘ During defecation, cecotrophs can be trapped in the perineal sac; impactions consist of soft cecal feces while harder fecal pellets can still be expressed.
• Boars can become debilitated because the blockage interferes with normal digestive processes.
• Although the underlying etiology is unknown, it is thought to be due to poor nutrition, inability to ingest cecotrophs, and atrophy of rectal muscles.
• Atrophy may be hormonally mediated, as disease is most common in older, intact boars.

SYSTEMS AFFECTED
• Skin/Exocrine
• Gastrointestinal

GENETICS
N/A

INCIDENCE/PREVALENCE
• Impaction is most often encountered in older boars between 3 and 5 years in age; however, occasionally young boars may develop an impaction.
• Rarely seen in sows
• Neutered males rarely if ever experience impaction.

GEOGRAPHIC DISTRIBUTION
N/A

SIGNS

Historical Findings
• Anorexia
• Irritability
• Weight loss
• Scooting
• Straining to defecate
• Constipation

• Lethargy, inappetence
• Pain, bruxism, relentlessness, and vocalization
• Passing large amounts of foul-smelling soft stool

Physical Examination Findings
• Perineal pruritus
• Perineal discharge

CAUSES
• As a boar ages, the muscle of the anus stretches and atrophies, thereby affecting the boar's ability to properly expel fecal pellets from the anus.
• Poor nutrition and inability to produce or ingest proper cecotrophs
• Marking habits and poor personal hygiene
• Debris such as shavings, hay, and hair can lead to or exacerbate impactions.

RISK FACTORS
Concurrent dental or GI disease, hypovitaminosis C, overcrowding, poor husbandry

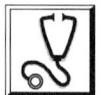

DIAGNOSIS

DIFFERENTIAL DIAGNOSIS
• Perineal sacculitis
• Perineal gland abscessation
• Neoplasia

CBC/BIOCHEMISTRY/URINALYSIS
• CBC—normal or relative neutrophilia
• Serum chemistry profile—may point to underlying cause or system affected
• Assess overall health

OTHER LABORATORY TESTS
N/A

IMAGING
Radiographs—useful in identifying dental disease or gastrointestinal disease that may cause abnormal motility and cecotroph formation

DIAGNOSTIC PROCEDURES

History and Palpation
Visualization of fecal mass or debris in the perineal sac

Secretions
• Normal perineal gland excretes clear oily secretion
• Perineal sacculitis—secretions become creamy to yellow

Cytologic Examination
• Look for signs of inflammation, infection, neoplasia
• Normal cytology—small amount of neutrophil and bacteria; however, if severe neutrophilia or a large number of bacteria are

seen, inflammation and infection should be suspected

Culture and Sensitivity
Aerobic and anaerobic bacterial culture—sterile, deep sample from affected tissue or exudate; susceptibility testing to direct antibiotic therapy

PATHOLOGIC FINDINGS
N/A

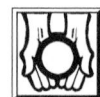

TREATMENT

NURSING CARE
• Gentle expression of contents from impaction or sacculitis
• Application of an antibiotic and corticosteroid ointment for inflammation and infection
• The perineal sac is a collecting place for all sorts of debris (hair, cage shavings, and hay) and should be cleaned out on a regular basis in older boars. Use mineral oil, warm water soaks and/or flushes, mild antiseptic shampoo, and cotton tip applicators. The folds of the anus should be retracted enough to visualize the anal sacs.

ACTIVITY
N/A

DIET
• Guinea pigs need a dietary source of vitamin C. Higher levels should be provided to sick individuals (30–50 mg/kg PO q24h). Vitamin C may be ground and fed directly to the patient. Vitamin C treats are also available for guinea pigs (e.g., Daily C, Oxbow Pet Products, Murdock, NE).
• Timothy and alfalfa hay promote normal GI flora, transit time, and fecal consistency.

CLIENT EDUCATION
• The perineal sac is a collecting place for all sorts of debris (hair, cage shavings, and hay) and should be cleaned on a regular basis in older boars. Use mineral oil, warm water soaks and/or flushes, mild antiseptic shampoo, and cotton tip applicators. When cleaning, the folds of the anus should be retracted enough to visualize the perineal sac.
• Feed a diet that promotes normal GI flora, transit time, and feces (e.g., timothy hay)

SURGICAL CONSIDERATIONS
• If necessary, establish drainage in abscesses, clean and flush anal sacs, and apply topical antibiotic.
• If abscesses recur, consider anal sac excision.
• Neutering—decreases secretion, reduces pressure on the muscles causing perineal gland atrophy

MEDICATIONS

DRUG(S) OF CHOICE

Antimicrobial Therapy
• Topical antibiotics—triple antibiotic (neomycin, polymyxin B sulfates, and bacitracin zinc) without hydrocortisone
• Topical antiseptics—Silvasorb gel (Medline Industries, Mundeline, IL); dilute betadine solution
• Broad-spectrum antibiotics can be used if there is a severe infection.
• Therapy should be based on culture and sensitivity, if possible.
  ◦ Antibiotics that are safe to use in guinea pigs includes trimethoprim-sulfa (15–30 mg/kg PO q12h), and chloramphenicol (30–50 mg/kg PO, SC, IM, IV q8–12h), enrofloxacin (5–20 mg/kg PO, SC, IM q12–24h), which is ineffective against anaerobes and may be variably effective against *Streptococcus* spp. {Should be reserved for microbes that are resistant to tier one antibiotics}.

Analgesic Therapy
• Pain management—multimodal therapy is recommended; opioid such as butorphanol (0.4–2.0 mg/kg SC, IM q4–12h) or buprenorphine (0.05–0.2 mg/kg SC, IM q6–8h); NSAID such as meloxicam (0.5–1 mg/kg PO, SC, IM q24h) or carprofen (4 mg/kg SC q24h or 1–2 mg/kg PO q12h–24h). Tramadol, a synthetic opioid, may also be an effective at dosages of 5–10 mg/kg PO q12h.

CONTRAINDICATIONS
Oral administration of penicillins, macrolides, lincosamides, and cephalosporins, as these may cause fatal enterotoxaemia

PRECAUTIONS
Ingestion of topical or oral administration of antibiotics may cause antibiotic-associated enteritis, dysbiosis, and enterotoxaemia.

POSSIBLE INTERACTIONS
N/A

ALTERNATIVE DRUGS
N/A

FOLLOW-UP

PATIENT MONITORING
Monitor for resolution of clinical signs and toxicity to the medications.

PREVENTION/AVOIDANCE
• Routine examination of the anal area
• The perineal sac should be cleaned out on a regular basis in older boars or in patients that have had prior history of impaction.
• Proper nutrition (vitamin C and B supplementation, timothy, and alfalfa hay) to promote normal GI flora, transit time, and feces
• Periodic dental examination and trimmings
• Neutering

POSSIBLE COMPLICATIONS
Scent gland impactions can result in discomfort, which can lead to anorexia and a debilitated condition.

EXPECTED COURSE AND PROGNOSIS
Most impactions will require lifelong maintenance cleaning.

MISCELLANEOUS

ASSOCIATED CONDITIONS
N/A

AGE-RELATED FACTORS
More prevalent in older male intact guinea pigs

ZOONOTIC POTENTIAL
N/A

PREGNANCY/FERTILITY/BREEDING
N/A

SYNONYMS
Cecal impaction
Scent gland impaction

SEE ALSO
Anorexia and pseudoanorexia
Constipation (lack of fecal production)
Diarrhea

ABBREVIATIONS
N/A

INTERNET RESOURCES
N/A

Suggested Reading
Bays TB. Geriatric care of rabbits, guinea pigs, and chinchillas. Vet Clin Exot Anim 2020;23:567–593.
Donnelly TM. Perineal sac impaction or rectal impaction. In: Mayer J, Donnelly TM, eds. Clinical Veterinary Advisor Birds and Exotic Pets. St. Louis: Elsevier, 2013:271–272.
Meredith A. Skin diseases and treatment of guinea pigs. In: Paterson S, ed. Skin Diseases of Exotic Pets. Ames: Blackwell, 2006:232–250.
Minarikova A, Hauptman K, Jeklova E et al. Diseases in pet guinea pigs: a retrospective study in 1000 animals. Vet Rec 2015;177(8):200–200.
Pignon C, Mayer J. Guinea pigs. In: Quesenberry KE, Carpenter JW, eds. Ferrets, Rabbits and Rodents, 4th Ed). Clinical Medicine and Surgery. 2021 ed. St. Louis: Saunders, 2020:270–297.
Ritzman TK. Diagnosis and clinical management of gastrointestinal conditions in exotic companion mammals (rabbits, guinea pigs, and chinchillas). Vet Clin Exot Anim 2014;17:179–194.
Author Rodney Schnellbacher, DVM, Dipl. ACZM

GUINEA PIGS

POLYURIA AND POLYDIPSIA

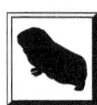

BASICS

DEFINITION
Polyuria is greater than normal urine production, and polydipsia is greater than normal water consumption. The average water intake of the guinea pig is approximately 10–15 mL/100 g BW/day.

　　Guinea pigs fed large amounts of high-moisture leafy vegetables will drink less water than those on a diet primarily of hay and/or pellets. Urine production reported for rodents is approximately 3.3–4.2 mL/100 g BW/day; values are not available specifically for guinea pigs.

PATHOPHYSIOLOGY
• Urine production and water consumption are controlled by interactions between the hypothalamus, pituitary gland, and kidneys.
• Polydipsia generally occurs as a response to polyuria to maintain circulating fluid volume. The patient's plasma becomes hypertonic, activating thirst mechanisms.
• Occasionally, polyuria may occur as a response to polydipsia. The patient's plasma becomes relatively hypotonic because of excessive water intake and ADH secretion, resulting in polyuria.

SYSTEMS AFFECTED
• Renal/Urologic
• Reproductive
• Endocrine/Metabolic
• Hepatic
• Cardiovascular—alterations in circulating fluid volume

GENETICS
N/A

INCIDENCE/PREVALENCE
N/A

GEOGRAPHIC DISTRIBUTION
N/A

SIGNALMENT

Breed Predilections
N/A

Mean Age and Range
Spontaneous diabetes mellitus generally affects young individuals (3–6 mos), but this disease is infrequently seen in pet guinea pigs.

Predominant Sex
N/A

SIGNS
N/A

CAUSES

Primary Polyuria
• Upper urinary tract disease—renal failure, pyelonephritis

• Lower urinary tract disease—infection, urolithiasis, neoplasia, anatomic, or neurologic problem
• Pyometra
• Hepatic failure
• Hypokalemia
• Osmotic diuresis—diabetes mellitus (most commonly reported in laboratory guinea pigs), post obstructive diuresis, ingestion, or administration of large quantities of solute (sodium chloride, glucose)
• Ingestion of nephrotoxic plants (e.g., lilies)
• Iatrogenic—administration of nephrotoxic drugs (aminoglycosides, NSAIDs), diuretics (furosemide and mannitol), corticosteroids, anticonvulsants (phenytoin), alcohol
• Hyperthyroidism
• Diabetes insipidus—central, renal
• ADH deficiency (not reported in guinea pigs)
• Traumatic, neoplastic

Primary Polydipsia
• Psychogenic drinking; behavioral problems (especially boredom), pyrexia, pain
• Diseases of the anterior hypothalamic thirst center of neoplastic, traumatic, or inflammatory origin (not reported in guinea pigs, but should be considered)

RISK FACTORS
• Renal or hepatic disease
• Selected electrolyte disorders
• Administration of diuretics, anticonvulsants, steroids, and nephrotoxic drugs
• Exposure to nephrotoxic plants (lilies)

DIAGNOSIS

DIFFERENTIAL DIAGNOSIS

Differentiating Similar Signs
• Differentiate polyuria from an abnormal increase in frequency of urination (pollakiuria). Pollakiuria is often associated with dysuria, stranguria, or hematuria.
• Patients with polyuria void large quantities of urine; patients with pollakiuria generally void small quantities of urine.
• Measuring urine specific gravity may provide evidence of adequate urine concentrating capacity (>1.025).

Differentiating Causes
• If associated with progressive weight loss—consider renal failure, hepatic failure, pyometra, neoplasia, pyelonephritis, diabetes mellitus, and hyperthyroidism
• If associated with hypercrystalluria—consider nephrolithiasis or renal failure
• If associated with polyphagia—consider diabetes mellitus, hyperthyroidism
• Young animals may develop diabetes mellitus secondary to infections.

• If associated with recent estrus in an intact female guinea pig—consider pyometra
• If associated with fever in an intact female guinea pig—consider pyometra
• If associated with abdominal distension—consider hepatic failure and neoplasia
• If associated with bilateral, symmetrical alopecia, weight loss, polydipsia—consider hyperadrenocorticism (Cushings syndrome—rare in guinea pigs but reported)
• If post obstructive, diuresis can cause polyuria
• Diabetes insipidus—central vs. renal
• Hypokalemia
• Iatrogenic—corticosteroids, anticonvulsants, and nephrotoxic drugs

CBC/BIOCHEMISTRY/URINALYSIS
• CBC—elevated TWBC ± heterophilia may suggest inflammation, infection; elevated platelet counts suggest inflammation
• Relative hypernatremia suggests primary polyuria; hyponatremia suggests primary polydipsia
• Elevations in BUN (>9–31 mg/dL) and creatinine (>0.6–2.2 mg/dL) are consistent with renal causes but may also indicate prerenal causes such as dehydration resulting from inadequate compensatory polydipsia.
• Hypoalbuminemia supports renal or hepatic disease.
• Patients with concurrent pyelonephritis have impaired urine-concentrating capacity, leukocytosis, and azotemia.
• Elevated hepatic enzymes suggest hepatic insufficiency.
• Hyperglycemia suggests diabetes mellitus, stress.
• Urinalysis including both a standard dipstick and microscopic examination of the sediment should be performed, preferably from a cystocentesis sample. If voided, assume sample contamination.
　　○ Glucosuria and ketonuria may be identified with diabetes mellitus. Ketonuria can also be associated with starvation or prolonged anorexia, especially during pregnancy.
　　○ Bacteriuria, pyuria (>0–1 WBC/hpf)
　　○ Hematuria (>0–3 RBC/hpf), and proteinuria indicate urinary inflammation if the sample is collected via cystocentesis but can include reproductive tract inflammation if collected via a free-catch sample; but these findings are not specific to differentiate infectious and noninfectious causes of lower urinary tract disease.
　　○ Most normal guinea pigs have numerous crystals in the urine; however, hypercrystalluria should increase suspicion for causing clinical signs.
　　　○ Calcium carbonate, calcium oxalate, and struvite crystals are all commonly

seen on sediment examinations, but similar to other small animals, crystal type(s) may not predict the mineralogy of calculi present.

○ Urine osmolality—high urine osmolality suggests primary polyuria; low osmolality suggests polydipsia.

○ Identification of neoplastic cells in urine sediment indicates urinary tract neoplasia (rare).

OTHER LABORATORY TESTS

• Prior to antibiotic use, culture the urine or bladder wall if pyuria, hematuria, bacteriuria, or a combination of these are present on sediment examination.

• Aerobic/anaerobic bacterial urine culture and sensitivity—the most definitive means of identifying and characterizing bacterial urinary tract infection; negative urine culture results suggest a noninfectious cause, unless the patient was on concurrent antibiotics or has an anaerobic infection. There are anecdotal reports of anaerobic urinary infections in guinea pigs, and so choose this culture technique if anaerobic infection is suspected. Chronic pyelonephritis cannot be completely ruled out by negative pyuria or bacteriuria.

• If surgery is necessary to relieve obstruction from urolithiasis, collect and submit the calculi for analysis and culture and sensitivity and submit a tissue sample from the bladder wall for culture and sensitivity.

• T4 testing may be useful for diagnosing and monitoring hyperthyroidism, however blood concentrations can be unreliable and difficult to interpret.

○ Reference intervals for normal thyroxine concentrations in the healthy guinea pig have been described in one study

  ○ Ranged from 14.2 to 66.9 nmol/L (1.1–5.2 mg/dL); with a median value of 27.0 nmol/L (2.1 mg/dL)

○ TSH stimulation test or nuclear scintigraphy may be useful.

• Basal serum cortisol concentrations and ACTH stimulation testing have been validated in guinea pigs and can be used to evaluate for hyperadrenocorticism.

IMAGING

Abdominal radiography and ultrasonography may provide additional evidence for renal disease (e.g., primary renal disease, urolithiasis), hepatic disease, pancreatic disease, reproductive disease (e.g., pyometra), or endocrine diseases (hyperadrenocorticism).

DIAGNOSTIC PROCEDURES

Testing for psychogenic polydipsia is similar to other companion animals; however, temporary hospitalization and PCV/TS testing is warranted while withholding water

to ensure that clinical dehydration does not occur during testing.

PATHOLOGIC FINDINGS

Will depend upon the underlying cause.

Moderate to marked fatty infiltration of the pancreas occurs frequently with increasing age but is not necessarily linked to increased susceptibility to diabetes mellitus.

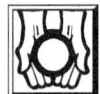

TREATMENT

APPROPRIATE HEALTH CARE

• Patients with uncomplicated PU/PD that appear otherwise normal are typically managed as outpatients; diagnostic evaluation may require brief hospitalization.

• Diseases associated with systemic signs of illness (e.g., pyrexia, depression, anorexia, and dehydration) or laboratory findings of azotemia and or leukocytosis warrant an aggressive diagnostic evaluation and initiation of supportive and symptomatic treatment.

• Guinea pigs with urinary obstruction should be hospitalized, and emergency supportive and symptomatic therapy should be provided until surgical intervention to relieve the obstruction can be performed.

• Medical treatment of urolithiasis has been unrewarding to date, and surgical removal of calculi is most often required. Postoperative management, including supportive and symptomatic treatment and pain management therapies—see chapter on hypercalciuria and urolithiasis

NURSING CARE

• Ensure patient has adequate water available at all times until the causes for the PU/PD are understood.

• Subcutaneous fluids can be administered (100 mL/kg) as needed; IV access is difficult in the guinea pig; lateral saphenous v catheters often kink; consider IO catheterization if intravascular fluids are needed. Base fluid selection on the underlying cause of fluid loss. In most patients, lactated Ringer's solution or Normosol crystalloid fluids are appropriate. Maintenance fluid rate is considered to be approximately 100 mL/kg/day.

ACTIVITY

Activity should be reduced during the time of tissue repair if surgery is required for any disease.

DIET

• Many guinea pigs with PU/PD develop inappetence. Be certain that the guinea pig is eating or provide assisted syringe feeding of an herbivore critical care diet if anorectic to

prevent the development or exacerbation of GI dysmotility/GI stasis.

• Increasing water content in foods or via oral or parenteral fluids may increase fluid intake.

• Provide multiple sources of fresh water, including supplementing fresh water with small amounts of pure fruit juice (no added sugars), high water content vegetables, or soaking or misting fresh vegetables before offering.

• Following treatment, dietary changes to lower calcium intake (especially if eating high alfalfa diets) may help prevent or delay recurrence of urolithiasis. Offer a high-fiber, low-calcium hay source such as timothy, oat, or grass hays and timothy-based guinea pigs pellets, as well as a large volume and variety of fresh vegetables—see chapter on hypercalciuria and urolithiais

CLIENT EDUCATION

• Limit risk factors and increase water consumption until the cause of the PU/PD is identified.

• Surgical removal of urinary tract calculi does not alter the causes responsible for their formation; limiting risk factors such as described above is necessary to minimize or delay recurrence. Even with these changes, however, recurrence is likely.

SURGICAL CONSIDERATIONS

If urolithiasis is present, surgery is the treatment of choice, since medical dissolution is ineffective in guinea pigs.

MEDICATIONS

DRUG(S) OF CHOICE

Based upon cause of underlying disease

CONTRAINDICATIONS

• Oral administration of antibiotics that select against gram-positive bacteria (penicillins, cephalosporins, macrolides, and lincosamides) can cause fatal enteric dysbiosis and enterotoxaemia.

• Potentially nephrotoxic drugs (e.g., aminoglycosides, NSAIDs) should be avoided in patients that are febrile, dehydrated, or azotemic or that are suspected of having pyelonephritis, septicemia, or preexisting renal disease.

• Glucocorticoids or other immunosuppressive agents

PRECAUTIONS

Until underlying renal or hepatic disease has been excluded, use caution in administering any drug eliminated by these pathways.

POSSIBLE INTERACTIONS

N/A

GUINEA PIGS

ALTERNATIVE DRUGS
N/A

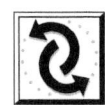

FOLLOW-UP

PATIENT MONITORING
• Hydration status by clinical assessment of dehydration and serial evaluation of body weight
• Fluid intake and urine output—provide a useful baseline for assessing adequacy of hydration therapy

PREVENTION/AVOIDANCE
Will depend upon disease

POSSIBLE COMPLICATIONS
• Dehydration
• GI hypomotility/GI stasis
• Urine scald
• Pododermatitis, myiasis if sedentary

EXPECTED COURSE AND PROGNOSIS
Will depend upon the underlying cause of these signs

MISCELLANEOUS

ASSOCIATED CONDITIONS
• Bacterial urinary tract infections
• Hypercrystalluria, urolithiasis

AGE-RELATED FACTORS
• Diabetes mellitus in laboratory guinea pigs is generally identified between 3 and 6 months of age.

ZOONOTIC POTENTIAL
N/A

PREGNANCY/FERTILITY/BREEDING
Pyometra can affect fertility or decisions regarding suitability of this patient for future breeding.

SYNONYMS
N/A

SEE ALSO
Dysuria, hematuria, and pollakiuria
Gastrointestinal hypomotility and gastrointestinal stasis
Pyometra and nonneoplastic endometrial disorders
Urinary tract obstruction

ABBREVIATIONS
ADH = antidiuretic hormone
BUN = blood urea nitrogen
GI = gastrointestinal
PCV = packed cell volume
PU/PD = polyuria/polydipsia
RBC = red blood cell
TS = total solids
TWBC = total white blood cells
WBC = white blood cells

INTERNET RESOURCES
N/A

Suggested Reading
Bays TB. Geriatric care of rabbits, guinea pigs, and chinchillas. Vet Clin Exot Anim 2020;23:567–593.
DeCubellis J. Common emergencies in rabbits, guinea pigs, and chinchillas. Vet Clin Exot Anim 2016;19:411–429.
Hallman RM, Brandão J. Diagnostic imaging of the renal system in exotic companion mammals. Vet Clin Exot Anim 2020;23:195–214.
Mayer J, Wagner R, Taeymans O. Advanced diagnostic approaches and current management of thyroid pathologies in guinea pigs. Vet Clin Exot Anim 2010;13:509–523.
Minarikova A, Hauptman K, Jeklova E et al. Diseases in pet guinea pigs: a retrospective study in 1000 animals. Vet Rec 2015;177(8):200–200.
Percy D, Barthold S. Guinea pig. In: Percy D, Barthold S, eds. Pathology of Laboratory Rodents and Rabbits. Ames: Blackwell, 2001:209–247.
Pignon C, Mayer J. Guinea pigs. In: Quesenberry KE, Carpenter JW, eds. Ferrets, Rabbits and Rodents, 4th Ed). Clinical Medicine and Surgery. 2021 ed. St. Louis: Saunders, 2020:270–297.
Reavill D, Lennox A. Disease overview of the urinary tract in exotic companion mammals and tips on clinical management. Vet Clin Exot Anim 2020;23:169–193.
Author Rodney Schnellbacher, DVM, Dipl. ACZM

BASICS

DEFINITION
Inflammation or infection of the alveoli of the lungs caused by virulent bacteria, viruses, mycoses, or foreign bodies resulting in disease of varying degrees of severity, ultimately leading to pulmonary dysfunction

PATHOPHYSIOLOGY
• The most common cause is bacteria that enter the respiratory tract via inhalation, aspiration, or hematogenous routes.
• The development of pneumonia depends on several factors, including number of organisms and their virulence, host defense/resistance mechanisms, and inoculation site.
• Bacteria incite an inflammatory reaction causing leukocytes to infiltrate the airways and alveoli. This can lead to lung lobe consolidation, atelectasis, tissue necrosis, ischemia, or abscess formation.

SYSTEMS AFFECTED
Respiratory system—primary or secondary infections

GENETICS
Unknown

INCIDENCE/PREVELENCE
Very common disease encountered in clinical practice. Based on a recent veterinary survey, literature review, and single retrospective hospital case review, prevalence of guinea respiratory disease may be overrepresented in the literature compared to actual prevalence. Guinea pigs affected by respiratory disease account for approximately 6% of observed cases in UK veterinary respondents, and 4% of guinea pigs presented to hospital in the Czech Republic, but maybe over represented in the literature with a citation case rate of 15%.

GEOGRAPHIC DISRIBUTION
Widespread

SIGNALMENT
No breed, sex, or gender predilection

SIGNS
Historical Findings
• Anorexia
• Lethargy
• Weight loss
• Nasal or ocular discharge
• Coughing
• Sneezing
• Exercise intolerance
• Wheezing/labored breathing
• Dyspnea

Physical Examination Findings
• Lethargy

• Weight loss
• Dehydration
• Fever
• Tachypnea
• Serous or mucopurulent ocular or nasal discharge
• Coughing
• Sneezing
• Abnormal breath sounds on auscultation, including crackles, wheezes, increased brochovesicular sounds, or decreased or absent breath sounds with abscess or neoplasia
• Dyspnea
• Bloat if aerophagia is present
• Torticollis
• If patient is dehydrated and/or anorexic, can see GI hypomotility with scant dry feces, gas-filled intestinal loops or firm stomach/cecum, hunched posture, rough hair coat
• Abortion and stillbirths
• Physical examination and clinical signs may appear relatively normal as guinea pigs are adept at hiding signs of illness.

CAUSES
• Bacterial—*Bordetella brochiseptica* (most common), *Streptococcus pneumoniae*, *Streptobacillus moniliformis*, *Yersinia pseudotuberculosis*, *Haemophilus species*, *Streptococcus zooepidemicus*, *Klebsiella pneumoniae*, *Pseudomonas aeruginosa*, *Pasturella multocida*, *Staphylococcus aureus*, and *Streptococcus pyogenes*
• Viral—adenovirus and parainfluenza virus (rare)
• Aspiration pneumonia—generally considered uncommon as guinea pigs do not vomit, but may be seen following force feeding or administration of oral medication.

RISK FACTORS
• Husbandry—poor nutrition, vitamin C deficiency, using substrate with aromatic oils such as pine and cedar, which can be irritating to respiratory mucosa, poor sanitation, infrequent cage cleaning, overcrowding, improper ventilation/humidity/temperature control, inhaled irritants such as disinfectants (bleach, smoke, etc.), ammonia buildup on the bedding
• Environment—close contact with other sick guinea pigs or subclinical carriers may spread infection, contact with other species that are subclinical carriers (such as dogs and rabbits)
• Age—neonatal and/or young guinea pigs have immature immune systems
• Health status—debilitated, geriatric animals, those with concurrent disease, stress, corticosteroid use, or a recent history of corticosteroid use

• Dental disease—malocclusion can predispose to points on the crowns of the teeth that can penetrate oral mucosa and provide an entry point for bacteria, periapical or tooth root abscess
• Disease agent factors—serotype of bacteria, infectious dose, virulence factors

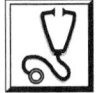

DIAGNOSIS

DIFFERENTIAL DIAGNOSIS
• Rhinitis
• Sinusitis
• Pulmonary adenocarcinoma or other neoplasia
• Pulmonary abscess
• Foreign body (bronchial or nasal)
• Congestive heart failure
• Dyspnea due to abdominal distension or thoracic effusion
• Heat stress

CBC/BIOCHEMISTRY/URINALYSIS
An elevation in total white blood cell count is uncommon, but a shift in proportion of heterophils to lymphocytes with an increase in heterophils and decrease in lymphocytes is expected. Increases in platelet number can also be seen with inflammation.

OTHER LABORATORY TESTS
• Enzyme-linked immunosorbent assay (ELISA) and indirect immunofluorescene assays (IFA) for *B. bronchiseptica* are more sensitive than culture for detection of the organism, but only detect antibodies and thus indicate exposure rather than active infection.
• ELISA for *S. pneumoniae*—only detects antibodies and thus indicates exposure rather than active infection
• PCR test for adenovirus is described but not readily available unless in lab animal setting

IMAGING
Thoracic radiographs—alveolar pattern with increased pulmonary density, which can be patchy or diffuse (air bronchograms and consolidated lung lobes may also be present)

DIAGNOSTIC PROCEDURES
• Culture of exudates and cytology—can provide definitive diagnosis, difficult to culture adenovirus or *Bordetella*
• Transtracheal wash or bronchoalveolar lavage can be difficult to perform in guinea pigs due to oral cavity anatomy, small tracheal size, and patient temperament.
• Lung aspirate can be performed with ultrasound guidance.
• Thoracocentesis: fluid analysis, cytology, and culture.

PNEUMONIA (CONTINUED)

GUINEA PIGS

PATHOLOGIC FINDINGS
• Gross: lung congestion with firm lung tissue, consolidation of lung tissue, multifocal white nodules with caseous exudate
• Histologic: suppurative/pyogranulomatous bronchopneumonia, pulmonary consolidation with emphysema and petechia, necrotizing bronchitis and bronchiolitis, leukocytic infiltration, fibrinous or fibrinopurulent bronchopneumonia, and basophilic intranuclear inclusion bodies in the case of adenovirus

TREATMENT
APPROPRIATE HEALTH CARE
Patient should be hospitalized if having respiratory difficulty or has multisystemic signs of illness

NURSING CARE
• Oxygen therapy—if the patient is in respiratory distress. Intubation or an emergency tracheotomy may be required if patient becomes apneic.
• Nebulization with saline or antibiotics may help deliver moisture to the upper respiratory tract.
• Fluid therapy to maintain normal hydration (guinea pigs fluid needs are 100 mL/kg/day)—fluid can be given IV, IO, or SC. Necessary to keep the GI tract hydrated and to aid mucocilliary clearance.
• Keep patients in a quiet environment with no predator species in the vicinity to decrease stress, provide a hide box.

ACTIVITY
Patient's activity should be restricted.

DIET
• Anorexia can cause GI hypomotility/stasis, overgrowth of intestinal bacterial pathogens, and imbalance of GI microflora. Guinea pigs must continue to eat during hospitalization and treatment. Low-dose buprenorphine or midazolam may reduce hospital anxiety and have polyphagia effects leading to a greater likelihood that animal will eat in the hospital while having minimal cardiorespiratory effects.
• Offer a wide variety of fresh, moistened vegetables such as cilantro, parsley, romaine lettuce, and dandelion greens as well as good-quality grass hay (orchard grass, western timothy).
• If the patient refuses to eat, can syringe-feed Critical Care for Herbivores (Oxbow Pet Products, Murdock, NE) or Emeraid Herbivore (Lafeber Company, Cornell, IL) 10–15 mL/kg orally every 6–8 hours. Can also make a gruel of ground-up guinea pig pellets with vegetable baby foods, water, or fresh

greens, but this is not as nutritionally complete as commercially made syringe-feeding formulas.
• Guinea pigs require an exogenous source of vitamin C supplementation, which can be given at 50–100 mg/kg/day when ill.
• Encourage oral fluid intake to maintain hydration by offering water or wet vegetables.
• Aerophagia can cause hypomotility gastrointestinal stasis.

CLIENT EDUCATION
• Significant morbidity and mortality can be associated with pneumonia, especially in the face of severe hypoxia.
• High morbidity is seen if the patient becomes septic or develops pulmonary abscesses.
• *Streptococcus zooepidemicus* is transmissible to other guinea pigs and guinea pigs can transmit *Pasturella* to other animals.

SURGICAL CONSIDERATIONS
None

MEDICATIONS
DRUG(S) OF CHOICE
• Antimicrobial drugs are the treatment of choice. Choice of antibiotic ideally based on culture and sensitivity testing but can be chosen empirically. Long-term antibiotic therapy (4–6 weeks or even months to years) may be required with severe infection. Antibiotics used most commonly include enrofloxacin (5–20 mg/kg PO, SC, IM q12–24h; this drug has a basic pH and should be diluted or injected into a subcutaneous fluid pocket to prevent tissue injury), marbofloxacin (4 mg/kg PO q24h), pradofloxacin (5 mg/kg PO q12h), trimethoprim sulfa (15–30 mg/kg PO q12–24h), chloramphenicol (30–50 mg/kg PO, SC, IM, IV q8–12h), and metronidazole (10–20 mg/kg PO, q12h). Can also use enrofloxacin in combination with doxycycline (2.5–5 mg/kg PO q12h).
• Nebulization with aminophylline (50 mg/kg), antibiotics (amikacin or enrofloxacin 1 mL in 9 mL of sterile water), terbutaline (4–10 mg/kg); acetylecysteine (2% solution nebulization over 30–60 minutes prn)—can irritate the airways so should be proceeded by a bronchodilator, used sparingly in cases of severe congestion, and used with caution
• Bronchodilators: aminophylline (50 mg/kg PO, SC), theophylline (4–10 mg/kg PO q8–12h), terbutaline (5 mg/kg PO q12h; can be nebulized). Terbutaline and theophylline used in combination can cause cardiac arrythmias.
• For sedation—diazepam (0.5–5 mg/kg IM) or midazolam (0.4–2 mg/kg IM) combined

with buprenorphine (0.05 mg/kg SC, 0.2 mg/kg oral transmucosal q5h, 0.2 mg/kg IV q7h) can be used; many other sedation protocols exist. Low dose buprenorphine or midazolam may reduce hospital anxiety, combat pain, and induce mild polyphagia leading to greater likelihood of eating in the hospital with minimal cardiorespiratory effects.
• Concurrent with antibiotic administration, provision of a probiotic or prebiotic (Florentero, Ventix Animal Heallth Corp. Burlington, ON) should be considered to reduce the risk of antibiotic-induced enteritis or clostridial overgrowth/dysbiosis.
• Parenteral antibiotics are preferred initially due to increased drug delivery to tissues (lung) while reducing the likelihood of antibiotic-induced dysbiosis.

CONTRAINDICATIONS
• Oral administration of antibiotics that select against gram-positive bacteria, such as penicillins, cephalosporins, lincosamines, or macrolides, should not be used in these animals as it can cause fatal dysbiosis and enterotoxemia.
• Procaine, which is included in some penicillin preparations, can be toxic to guinea pigs.
• Using corticosteroids can suppress the immune system and exacerbate the infection.

PRECAUTIONS
• Any antibiotic can cause diarrhea, which should be monitored in these patients and the antibiotic discontinued if diarrhea is present. Supplementation with probiotics or guinea pig transfauntation can be considered.
• Terbutaline and theophylline used in combination can cause cardiac arrythmias.

POSSIBLE INTERACTIONS
None

ALTERNATIVE DRUGS
N/A

FOLLOW-UP
PATIENT MONITORING
• Continue to monitor patient for relapse via clinical signs.
• Thoracic radiographs—radiographic changes lag behind clinical improvement
• Follow-up cultures if indicated

PREVENTION/AVOIDANCE
• Improve husbandry and diet (ensure appropriate vitamin C supplementation)
• Avoid stressful situations, exposure to infected animals (rabbits, dogs), corticosteroid use
• Prevent dental disease by providing high-fiber foods, especially good-quality hay.

Yearly veterinary exams with periodic trimming of overgrown teeth as needed.
• Commercially available vaccines for *B. bronchoseptica* (porcine *B. bronchiseptica* and human *B. pertussis*) offer some protection in experimentally infected guinea pigs.

POSSIBLE COMPLICATIONS
Possible complications include sepsis, thoracic effusion, pulmonary fibrosis, gastrointestinal stasis, bloat, antibiotic induced dysbiosis/enteritis, and death.

EXPECTED COURSE AND PROGNOSIS
• Prognosis is based on severity and chronicity of disease. Mild disease has a good prognosis with aggressive antibiotic treatment and supportive care but may be more guarded in younger animals, immunocompromised animals, debilitated/geriatric patients, or those with severe underlying disease. Chronic or widespread infection or pulmonary abcesses have a guarded to grave prognosis.
• Pneumonia can be difficult to resolve and often there is reoccurrence of clinical signs.

MISCELLANEOUS

ASSOCIATED CONDITIONS
GI hypomotility/stasis
Dental disease
Hypovitaminosis C
Rhinitis and sinusitis
Sepsis

AGE-RELATED FACTORS
Young animals may be more susceptible due to an immature immune system and thus would have a poorer prognosis.

ZOONOTIC POTENTIAL
Streptobacillus moniliformis is the cause of rat bite fever in humans; *Yersinia pseudotuberculosis* is a zoonotic disease but is rare in guinea pigs. Guinea pigs may be a reservoir for *Streptococcus pneumoniae,* with subclinical carriage rate up to 50% in some guinea pig colonies. Close contact between pets and children could be a risk factor although relevance in human hosts is not clearly defined.

PREGNANCY/FERTILITY/BREEDING
• Dams can pass *Yersinia pseudotuberculosis* to their young.
• *Bordetella bronchiseptica* may be associated with stillbirths, infertility, and abortion.

SYNONYMS
None

SEE ALSO
Dental malocclusion
Dyspnea and tachypnea
Nasal discharge and sneezing
Rhinitis and sinusitis

ABBREVIATIONS
ELISA = enzyme-linked immunosorbent assay
GI = gastrointestinal
IFA = indirect immunofluorescene assay
PCR = polymerase chain reaction

INTERNET RESOURCES
www.vin.com

Suggested Reading
Capello V, Lennox AM. Diagnostic imaging of the respiratory system in exotic companion mammals. Vet Clin Exot Anim 2011;14:369–389.

DeCubellis J. Common emergencies in rabbits, guinea pigs, and chinchillas. Vet Clin Exot Anim 2016;19:411–429.
Harkness JE, Murray KA, Wagner JE. Biology and diseases of guinea pigs. In: Fox JG, Anderson LC, Loew FM, Quimby FW, eds. Laboratory Animal Medicine, 2nd ed. San Diego: Elsevier, 2002:212–220,222.
Mayer J, Mans C. Rodents. In: Carpenter JW, ed. Exotic Animal Formulary, 5th ed. St Louis: Elsevier, 2018:459–479.
Minarikova A, Hauptman K, Jeklova E, Knotek Z, Jekl V. Diseases in pet guinea pigs: a retrospective study in 1000 animals. Vet Rec 2015;177(8):200.
Pignon C, Mayer J. Guinea pigs. In: Quesenberry KE, Carpenter JW, eds. Ferrets, Rabbits and Rodents, 4th Ed). Clinical Medicine and Surgery. 2021 ed. St. Louis: Saunders, 2020:270–297.
Robinson NJ, Lyons E, Grindlay D, Brennan ML. Veterinarian nominated common conditions of rabbits and guinea pigs compared with published literature. Vet Sci 2017;4(4):58.
Riggs SM. Guinea pigs. In: Mitchell MA, Tully TN, eds. Manual of Exotic Pet Practice. St Louis: Saunders, 2009: 466–467.

Authors Christy L. Rettenmund, DVM, Dipl. ACZM and J. Jill Heatley, DVM, MS, Dipl. ABVP (Avian, Reptilian, Amphibian), Dipl. ACZM

PODODERMATITIS (BUMBLEFOOT)

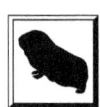

BASICS

DEFINITION
Avascular necrosis followed by abscessation, cellulitis, osteomyelitis, and synovitis involving the plantar or palmar aspect of the feet

PATHOPHYSIOLOGY
• Avascular necrosis occurs due to constant pressure applied to the skin and soft tissue pressed between the bones of the foot and a hard surface.
• Any condition that disrupts normal locomotion or alters the padding of the plantar and palmar surface of the foot may lead to the formation of pressure sores.
• Increased pressure often occurs due to obesity or decreased weight bearing on the contralateral foot.
• Prolonged contact with wire, abrasive, hard, wet, or urine- and feces-soaked surface can lead to superficial dermatitis followed by deep pyoderma and necrosis.
• Necrosis of these tissues is followed by sloughing, ulceration, abscess formation, and secondary bacterial infection.
• Untreated can lead to severe osteomyelitis and synovitis
• Locomotion may be abnormal, especially if osteomyelitis or synovitis is present.
• As the condition progresses it often become irreversible.
• Chronic cases may progress to lymphadenopathy, arthritis, tendinitis, and amyloid accumulation in kidney, liver, adrenal glands, spleen, and pancreatic islets.

SYSTEMS AFFECTED
• Skin/Exocrine
• Muscular/Skeletal

INCIDENCE/PREVALENCE
• Relatively common in guinea pigs
• Front feet are the most vulnerable to this condition
• Animals with poor husbandry and sanitation higher prevalence
• Higher incidence seen in obese animals
• No age or sex predilections

SIGNALMENT
Variable depends on the underlying cause

SIGNS

Historical Findings
Husbandry—underlying cause is usually related to poor husbandry
• Poor sanitation
• Small wire cages or hard, noncompliant surfaces
• Grass and straw bedding can also cause microabrasion and foot punctures.

◦ Medical problems—any medical problem that leads to an abnormal stance or gate
• Obesity
• Musculoskeletal disorders causing sedentary life or uneven weight bearing on the contralateral limbs
• Joint pain and reluctance to move due to hypovitaminosis C
• Urinary tract or gastrointestinal disease that causes polyuria or diarrhea leading to urine scald or pasting of feces on feet and perineal region
• Any palmar or plantar cutaneous wound can lead to secondary bacterial infection.

Physical Examination Findings
• Anorexia, depression, lameness, reluctance to move, lack of tolerance, vocalization, weight loss, and hiding
• Evidence of erythema, inflammation, and ulceration
• Staging
• Early, asymptomatic disease (Grade I)—palmar and plantar dermatitis with erythema
• Mild disease (Grade II)—erythema with soft tissue swelling
• Moderate disease (Grade III)—ulceration
• Severe disease (Grade IV)—abscess, inflammation of tendons or deeper tissues
• Severe, irreversible disease (Grade V)—osteomyelitis, synovitis, and tendonitis

CAUSES
• Pressure sores, avascular necrosis caused by entrapment of soft tissues of the limb between bone and hard surfaces
• Excoriation, friction, or constant moisture on the skin and soft tissues caused by feces, urine, or water coating the feet
• Pyogenic bacteria—secondary infection with *Staphylococcus aureus* (the most common causative agent), *Pseudomonas* spp., *Escherichia coli*, *Streptococcus* spp., *Proteus* spp., *Bacteroides* spp., and *Pasteurella multocida*
• Overgrowth of claws causing abnormal foot position

RISK FACTORS
Concurrent disease, hypovitaminosis C, overcrowding, poor husbandry

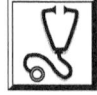

DIAGNOSIS

DIFFERENTIAL DIAGNOSIS
• Scurvy (hypovitaminosis C)
• Neoplasia
• Granuloma
• Other musculoskeletal diseases
• Bacteremia

CBC/BIOCHEMISTRY/URINALYSIS
• CBC—normal to leukocytosis with neutrophil:lymphocyte ratio shift; may observe toxicity changes ± bands, monocytosis suggest inflammation/infection; thrombocytosis associated with active inflammation
• Serum chemistry profile—may point to underlying cause or system affected

DIAGNOSTIC PROCEDURES

Fine-Needle Aspiration
• May reveal abscess with caseous exudate in patients with a secondary bacterial infection
• High nucleated cell count with primary degenerative neutrophils with lesser numbers of macrophages and lymphocytes
• Rule out neoplasia or granulomas

Biopsy
• Rule out neoplasia and granuloma
• Should be of abnormal and normal tissue
• High nucleated cell count with primary degenerative neutrophils with lesser numbers of macrophages and lymphocytes

Culture and Sensitivity
• Aerobic and anaerobic bacterial culture
• Sterile, deep sample from affected tissue or exudate
• Susceptibility testing verifying correct antibiotic therapy to isolate

PATHOLOGIC FINDINGS
Focal plantar or palmar erythema, alopecia, scabs, and epidermal cracks; parakeratotic hyperkeratosis, inflammatory cells

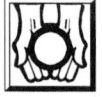

TREATMENT

APPROPRIATE HEALTH CARE
• Outpatient—early disease (erythema, alopecia)
• Inpatient—surgical procedures; daily debridement and bandaging
• It is essential to remove/correct the underlying cause for long-term success.
• Dry, soft, clean hay, pine shavings, or shredded paper bedding
• Overgrown nails should be trimmed.
• Bedding alone may be effective in early disease, Grades I and II

NURSING CARE
Severe disease, Grades III–IV—wounds should be cleaned and hair clipped around the lesions; resolution generally requires extensive, long-term care including bandaging, flushing, debriding, long-term topical and systemic antibiotics, topical antiseptics, appropriate pain control, and vitamin C supplementation.

GUINEA PIGS

Hydrotherapy and/or low-level laser therapy has been helpful adjunct treatments.

Bandaging
• Bandaging—depends on the severity of the disease; necessary for open wounds or after debridement
• If ulceration or wound appears infected, disinfectants such as povidone iodine or dilute chlorhexidine are appropriate; however, multiple and continuous use of these disinfectants can delay wound healing.
• Once infection is controlled, hydrocolloidal wound dressing can be applied over ulceration.
• Depending on the severity of the disease, frequent bandage changes may be required.

Low-Level Laser Therapy
• Helps to modulate cellular processes by accelerating angiogenesis, stimulating vasodilation, and increasing lymphatic drainage (see manufactures settings for treatment)

ACTIVITY
• Restrict until adequate healing of tissues has taken place.
• Long term—encourage activity; prolonged inactivity may cause or exacerbate pododermatitis

DIET
• Make sure that the patient continues to eat throughout treatment to avoid gastrointestinal motility disorders.
• Guinea pigs need a dietary source of vitamin C. Higher levels should be provided to sick individuals (30–50 mg/kg PO q24h). Vitamin C may be ground and fed directly to the pig. Vitamin C treats are also available for guinea pigs (e.g., Daily C, Oxbow Pet Products, Murdock, NE).

CLIENT EDUCATION
• Discuss need to correct or prevent risk factors
• Correcting underlying disease and husbandry is central for a successful outcome.
  ○ Discuss appropriate bedding material; do not house on wire flooring.
• Severe disease, involving bone and tendon, carries a guarded to poor prognosis for complete resolution; most will require multiple surgical debridements and multiple follow-up visits.
• Recurrences are common, especially if the underlying causes cannot be corrected.
• Healed lesions are predisposed to ulceration and recurrent pododermatitis.

SURGICAL CONSIDERATIONS
• Debride all visibly necrotic tissue.
• Treat as open wound—flush and debride wound daily initially, followed by twice weekly to weekly debridement as healing

occurs. Irrigate wound with dilute antiseptic solution (chlorhexidine or iodine) daily until healthy granulation bed forms, followed by hydrocolloidal wound dressings or silver sulfadiazine cream until re-epithelialization occurs. Follow debridement with application of soft, padded bandages. Bandages must be changed immediately if they become wet.
• Remove any foreign objects(s) or nidus of infection.
• Place on long-term antibiotic therapy; appropriate pain management

MEDICATIONS
DRUG(S) OF CHOICE
Analgesic and Anti-Inflammatory Drug Therapy
• Partial mu agonist or kappa agonist are generally safe to use in guinea pigs, buprenorphine (0.05–0.2 mg/kg PO, SC, IM, IV q8–12h or 0.2 mg/kg oral transmucosal q5h) and butorphanol (0.4–2.0 mg/kg SC, IM q4–12h). Tramadol, a synthetic opioid, may also be an effective at dosages of 5–10 mg/kg PO q12h postoperatively. For severe to moderate pain pure mu opioids such as morphine (0.5–2.0 mg/kg SC, IM q2–4h) or oxymorphone (0.2–0.5 mg/kg SC, IM q4–12h) should be used; however, appetite and fecal output should be monitored as these opioids are thought to contribute to GI ileus.
• Nonsteroidal anti-inflammatory drugs such as meloxicam (0.5–1 mg/kg PO, SC q 24h) or carprofen (4 mg/kg SC q24h or 1–2 mg/kg PO q12h) may be used to reduce inflammation and for analgesia.

Antibiotic Therapy
• Antimicrobial drugs ideally based on results of the culture and susceptibility. Long term use broad-spectrum antibiotic (4–8 weeks).
• Trimethoprim sulfa (15–30 mg/kg PO q12h)
• Chloramphenicol (30–50 mg/kg PO, SC, IM, IV q8–12h)
• Azithromycin (15–30 mg/kg PO q12–24h)
• Metronidazole (10–20 mg/kg PO q12h)
• Enrofloxacin (5–20 mg/kg PO, SC, IM q12–24h) {Should be reserved for microbes that are resistant to tier one antibiotics}—ineffective against anaerobes and may be variably effective against *Streptococcus* spp.

CONTRAINDICATIONS
• Oral administration of penicillins, macrolides, lincosamides, and cephalosporins due to potentially fatal enteric dysbiosis
• The use of corticosteroids (systemic or topical preparations) can severely exacerbate infection.

• Topical application of antibiotic ointment or creams—the guinea pig may ingest these; may cause enteric dysbiosis

PRECAUTIONS
• NSAIDs—meloxicam should be avoided in patients with compromised renal function.
• Chloramphenicol—avoid human contact with chloramphenicol due to potential blood dyscrasia. Advise owners of potential risks.
• Hydrotherapy can be stressful to guinea pig patients.
• Oral administration of any antibiotic may cause antibiotic-associated enteritis, dysbiosis, and enterotoxaemia; discontinue use if diarrhea or anorexia occurs.

FOLLOW-UP
PATIENT MONITORING
Monitor for resolution of clinical signs and toxicity to the medications.

PREVENTION/AVOIDANCE
• Provide adequate vitamin C supplementation (30–50 mg/kg PO q24h).
• Provide clean, appropriate surface substrates; clean soiled substrates daily to prevent prolonged sitting on soiled litter; avoid wet bedding (rain, spilled water bowls or bottles).
• Prevent obesity.
• Encourage exercise; provide large spaces to encourage movement.

POSSIBLE COMPLICATIONS
• Irreversible osteomyelitis, synovitis, and tendonitis
• Amputation of effected limb
• Development of pododermatitis on other feet due to increase in weight bearing
• Chronic cases may progress to lymphadenopathy, arthritis, tendinitis, and amyloid accumulation in kidney, liver, adrenal glands, spleen, and pancreatic islets.

EXPECTED COURSE AND PROGNOSIS
Variable, depends on severity

MISCELLANEOUS
ASSOCIATED CONDITIONS
• Scurvy (hypovitaminosis C)
• Bacteremia
• Osteomyelitis, synovitis, tendonitis
• Pyoderma

SYNONYMS
Bumblefoot
Ulcerative pododermatitis

PODODERMATITIS (BUMBLEFOOT)   (CONTINUED)

SEE ALSO
Abscesses

ABBREVIATIONS
GI = gastrointestinal
NSAID = nonsteroidal anti-inflammatory

Suggested Reading
Meredith A. Skin diseases and treatment of guinea pigs. In: Paterson S, ed. Skin Diseases of Exotic Pets. Ames: Blackwell, 2006:232–250.
Miwa Y, Sladky K. Common surgical procedures of rodents, ferrets, hedgehogs, and sugar gliders. Vet Clin Exot Anim 2016;19:205–244.

Palmerio BS, Roberts H. Clinical approach to dermatologic disease in exotic animals. Vet Clin North Am Exot Anim Pract. 2013 Sep;16(3):523–577.
Paterson S. Skin disease and treatment of guinea pigs. In: Paterson S, ed. Skin Diseases of Exotic Pets. Ames: Blackwell, 2006:222–250.
Pignon C, Mayer J. Guinea pigs. In: Quesenberry KE, Carpenter JW, eds. Ferrets, Rabbits and Rodents, 4th Ed). Clinical Medicine and Surgery. 2021 ed. St. Louis: Saunders, 2020:270–297.
Riggs SM. Guinea pigs. In: Mitchell MA, Tully TN, eds. Manual of Exotic Pet

Practice. St Louis: Saunders/Elsevier, 2009:456–473.
White SD, Sanchez-Migallon D, Paul-Murphy J. Skin diseases in companion guinea pigs (*Cavia porcellus*): a retrospective study of 293 cases seen at the Veterinary Medical Teaching Hospital, University of California at Davis (1990–2015). Vet Dermatol 2016;27:395–e100.

Author Rodney Schnellbacher, DVM, Dipl. ACZM

PREGNANCY TOXEMIA

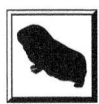

BASICS

DEFINITION
In guinea pigs there are two patterns of pregnancy toxemia that occur in advanced pregnancy and can be clinically indistinguishable:
• Pregnancy ketosis is the metabolic form due to a negative energy balance and the catabolism of fat.
• Preeclampsia is a circulatory disorder in which the gravid uterus causes compression of the aorta caudal to the renal vessels and results in uteroplacental ischemia, hypertension, and possible terminal DIC.

PATHOPHYSIOLOGY
• Pregnancy ketosis occurs 2 weeks prior to parturition or the week following parturition when energy requirements for sustaining fetal development and lactation can exceed the energy intake.
• The sow catabolizes fat to provide energy, resulting in metabolic acidosis and ketosis.
• The metabolic changes include the following:
   ◦ Accumulation of ketone bodies in the blood: acetoacetate, 3-hydroxybutyrate, and acetone.
   ◦ Increase in nonesterified fatty acids and hepatic triglycerides
   ◦ Decreased hepatic glycogen and plasma glucose concentrations
• Preeclampsia occurs in the last 2 weeks of gestation when the gravid uterus is heavy and compresses blood vessels and nerves leading to hypertension as well as vascular and neurological dysfunction.

SYSTEMS AFFECTED
Reproductive

GENETICS
While suspected, inherited factors associated with this disease have not been proven.

INCIDENCE/PREVALENCE
The disease is common in late-term obese guinea pigs with large fetal loads.

GEOGRAPHIC DISTRIBUTION
N/A

SIGNALMENT
• Late-term primiparous obese sow
• Late-term sow carrying more than four fetuses
• Obese sow in first week of lactation following parturition, often with several pups

Breed Predilections
N/A

Mean Age and Range
N/A

Predominant Sex
Sows only

SIGNS

Historical Findings
• Onset of signs is acute.
• Death may occur without premonitory signs
• Overweight sow becomes anorexic in last 2 weeks of gestation or first week postpartum
• Lethargy
• Dyspnea
• Anorexia
• Adipsia
• Salivation
• Incoordination
• Hypersensitivity
• Muscle spasms
• Paralysis
• Convulsions
• Coma

Physical Examination Findings
• Sow may be in shock and/or recumbent
• Profuse salivation
• Ketone odor to breath
• Ataxia and weakness
• Hypertension with preeclampsia
• Hypotension with pregnancy ketosis

CAUSES

Pregnancy Ketosis
• Late-term pregnancy creates an increased metabolic energy demand, and when there is failure to keep up with the demand, pregnancy ketosis occurs.
• Inadequate diet that is too low in energy relative to demands of pregnancy and lactation. When carbohydrates are unavailable or insufficient, fat becomes the predominant body fuel and excessive amounts of ketones are formed as a metabolic by-product.

Preeclampsia
Insufficient blood flow to the uterus when the gravid uterus compresses the aorta and renal blood vessels and nerves leading to hypertension, systemic dysfunctions (vascular, neurological, hepatic, or renal), uterine ischemia, and DIC

RISK FACTORS
• Obesity
• Change in diet
• Lack of exercise
• Environmental changes or stressors
• Large fetal load
• Heat stress
• Primiparity
• Mastitis
• Metritis

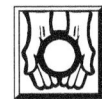

DIAGNOSIS

DIFFERENTIAL DIAGNOSIS
• Late-term abortion
• Heat stress
• Hypovolemic shock from other causes

CBC/BIOCHEMISTRY/URINALYSIS
• CBC—anemia, thrombocytopenia, and hyperlipidemia
• Biochemistry panel—hypoglycemia, elevated AST, ALT, and GGT
• Electrolytes and blood gases—metabolic acidosis, hyperkalemia, hyponatremia, and hypochloremia
• Urinalysis—aciduria (pH 5–6), proteinuria, and ketonuria

OTHER LABORATORY TESTS
N/A

IMAGING
• Ultrasonographic imaging of the liver often shows signs of hepatic lipidosis

DIAGNOSTIC PROCEDURES
• Diagnosis can be made by signalment and clinical signs but difficult to differentiate which form of toxemia is present
• Indirect blood pressure can help to differentiate preeclampsia (hypertension) from pregnancy ketosis (hypotension).
• Place cuff around the crus of the pelvic limb. Cuff size should follow recommendations: cuff width = limb circumference × 0.4

PATHOLOGIC FINDINGS
• Gross lesions include reduced gastric content, enlarged tan liver, adrenomegaly, excessive body fat, dead fetuses
• Histological confirmation of hepatic lipidosis
• Uterine infarction, hemorrhage and placental necrosis occur with preeclampsia.
• Disseminated intravascular coagulation with ischemia of the uterus

TREATMENT

APPROPRIATE HEALTH CARE
• Fluid therapy is used to correct abnormalities in volume, electrolytes, and acid–base status.
• A bolus infusion of isotonic crystalloids can be administered IV or IO at 10–15 mL/kg, followed by colloids such as 6% hetastarch at 5 mL/kg over 10 minutes until systolic blood pressure is over 40 mmHg. Then continue IV crystalloids and colloids at slow IV administration until systolic blood pressure

returns to normal range of approximately 90 mmHg.
• If suspect ketosis or hypotension, immediate IV administration of fluids as above supplemented with glucose and corticosteroids. Add calcium gluconate when IV fluid administration rate is slow (see Medications below for dosages).
• For ketosis, nutrition is a critical part of the treatment protocol. Herbivore critical care via syringe or gavage feeding (gastric, nasogastric, and esophagostomy tube) should be used for dietary maintenance.
• If sow is hypertensive, then immediate cesarean section is indicated. Poor prognosis for sow but may be able to recover the pups.
• Treatment is rarely successful

NURSING CARE
• Immediate therapy includes subcutaneous fluids (50–100 mL/kg) and oral glucose while preparing to place IV or IO catheter.
• IV access is difficult in the guinea pig, especially if hypotensive; lateral saphenous vein catheters often kink; consider IO catheterization for intravascular fluids. Base fluid selection on evidence of dehydration, acid–base, and electrolyte imbalances. Add glucose to the fluids. Administer colloids with crystalloids if sow is hypotensive.

ACTIVITY
• Minimize stress
• Exercise throughout pregnancy and in postpartum period

DIET
• It is an absolute requirement that pregnant and lactating sows continue to eat and to avoid sudden dietary changes.
• In addition to pellets, offer a large selection of fresh, moist greens such as cilantro, parsley, carrot tops, dark leafy greens, and good-quality grass hay.
• If the sow stops eating, syringe-feed Critical Care for herbivores (Oxbow Animal Health, Murdock, ME) at approximately 26 g of dry product per kg body weight per day. Dry product is mixed with approximately twice the volume of water and is fed in small portions every 6–8 hours. Larger volumes and more frequent feedings are often accepted; feed as much as the sow will readily accept.
  Alternatively, pellets can be ground and mixed with fresh greens, vegetable baby foods, water, or sugar-free juice to form a gruel.

CLIENT EDUCATION
• Antibiotic therapy may be indicated to prevent metritis or pyometra or if incision is difficult to maintain in a clean environment.
• Decrease risk factors such as obesity, sedentary life, sudden diet changes, change in feeding routine, or other stressors.

• Do not breed sows that are overweight.
• Anorexia during pregnancy is a serious clinical sign and should be treated as an emergency.

SURGICAL CONSIDERATIONS
• Immediate cesarean section may be recommended if sow is hypertensive or shows other signs of uterine ischemia. Prognosis is poor to grave.
• Client may consider OVH at time of cesarean section to avoid future breeding of the sow. Procedure may be faster especially if fetuses are dead or necrotic.
• Postoperative management includes assisted feeding, fluids, analgesics, and antibiotics to prevent metritis.

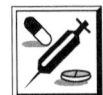

MEDICATIONS
DRUG(S) OF CHOICE
• IV administration of fluids (crystalloids and colloids) with glucose (1 mL/kg 50% glucose diluted 50% with saline), calcium gluconate (50 mg/kg), and dexamethasone SP (1–4 mg/kg)
• Pain management is essential during and following surgery. Multimodal therapy is recommended for perioperative analgesia with an anxiolytic, opioid, and NSAID: midazolam (0.4–2.0 mg/kg IM), butorphanol (0.4–2.0 mg/kg SC, IM, IV q4–12h), or buprenorphine (0.05–0.2 mg/kg SC, IM q8–12h) plus meloxicam (0.5–1 mg/kg PO, SC q24h) or carprofen (4 mg/kg SC q24h or 1–2 mg/kg PO q12h). Tramadol, a synthetic opioid, may also be an effective at dosages of 5–10 mg/kg PO q12h postoperatively. For severe to moderate pain pure mu opioids such as morphine (0.5–2.0 mg/kg SC, IM q2–4h) or oxymorphone (0.2–0.5 mg/kg SC, IM q6–12h) should be used; however, appetite and fecal output should be monitored as these opioids are thought to contribute to GI ileus.
• Antibiotic therapy may be indicated to prevent metritis or pyometra or if incision is difficult to maintain in a clean environment.

CONTRAINDICATIONS
• Oral administration of antibiotics that select against gram-positive bacteria (penicillins, cephalosporins, macrolides, and lincosamides) can cause fatal enteric dysbiosis and enterotoxaemia.
• NSAIDs are contraindicated within 24 hours of glucocorticoid administration or in sows that are febrile, dehydrated, or azotemia or that are suspected of having pyelonephritis, septicemia, or preexisting renal disease.

PRECAUTIONS
• The sow in preeclampsia or pregnancy ketosis has additional anesthetic risks.
• During surgery avoid excessive handling of gastrointestinal tissues to reduce postoperative ileus or fibrous adhesions.

POSSIBLE INTERACTIONS
None

ALTERNATIVE DRUGS
N/A

FOLLOW-UP
PATIENT MONITORING
• If pups survive, they may need to be raised without maternal care to avoid lactation demands on the sow.
• Ensure gastrointestinal motility by making sure the patient is eating, well hydrated, and passing normal feces prior to release from hospitalization.
• Follow-up examination should be performed within 5–7 days of discharge from hospital, or sooner if the sow does not return to eating.

PREVENTION/AVOIDANCE
• Prevention is based upon proper nutritional support and access to fresh water at all times for the pregnant sow.
• Avoid dietary changes during pregnancy.
• Minimize stress during pregnancy, such as transportation, changes in husbandry, and rough handling.
• Avoid overfeeding adult animals, especially breeding sows.
• For the obese guinea pig, it is critical to plan a gradual reduction in calories and institute an exercise plan.

POSSIBLE COMPLICATIONS
• Sows being treated for ketosis often die from acute enteritis due to dysbiosis and poor body condition.
• Preeclampsia can lead to uterine ischemia and DIC.

EXPECTED COURSE AND PROGNOSIS
• Pregnancy toxemia is an emergency, and if untreated, the sow can die within hours to days of detection.
• The prognosis for pregnancy toxemia is guarded to grave.

MISCELLANEOUS
ASSOCIATED CONDITIONS
• Gastrointestinal hypomotility or dysbiosis
• Metritis, pyometra, and metritis can be the predisposing stressors to the sow.

AGE-RELATED FACTORS
N/A

ZOONOTIC POTENTIAL
N/A

PREGNANCY/FERTILITY/BREEDING
If sow survives, it is recommended to avoid future breeding.

SYNONYMS
- Pregnancy ketosis
- Preeclampsia

ABBREVIATIONS
ALT = alanine aminotransferase
AST = aspartate aminotransferase
DIC = disseminated intravascular coagulation
GGT = gamma glutamyl transferase
IO = intraosseous
NSAID = nonsteroidal anti-inflammatory drug
OVH = ovariohysterectomy

INTERNET RESOURCES
N/A

Suggested Reading
Bertram CA, Muller K, Klopfleisch R. Genital tract pathology in female pet guinea pigs (*Cavia porcellus*): a retrospective study of 655 post-mortem and 64 biopsy cases. J Comp Path 2018;164:12–22.
DeCubellis J. Common emergencies in rabbits, guinea pigs, and chinchillas. Vet Clin Exot Anim 2016;19:411–429.
Golden JG, Hughes HC, Lang CM. Experimental toxemia in the pregnant guinea pig (*Cavia porcellus*). Lab Anim Sci 1980;30:174–179.
Laik-Schandelmaier C, Klopfleisch R, Schöniger S et al. Spontaneously arising tumours and tumour-like lesions of the cervix and uterus in 83 pet guinea pigs (*Cavia porcellus*). J Comp Path 2017;156:339–351.
Minarikova A, Hauptman K, Jeklova E et al. Diseases in pet guinea pigs: a retrospective study in 1000 animals. Vet Rec 2015;177(8):200.
Miwa Y, Sladky K. Common surgical procedures of rodents, ferrets, hedgehogs, and sugar gliders. Vet Clin Exot Anim 2016;19:205–244.
Pignon C, Mayer J. Guinea pigs. In: Quesenberry KE, Carpenter JW, eds. Ferrets, Rabbits and Rodents, 4th Ed). Clinical Medicine and Surgery. 2021 ed. St. Louis: Saunders, 2020:270–297.
Veiga-Parga T, LaPerle KM, Newman SJ. Spontaneous reproductive pathology in female guinea pigs. J Vet Diag Invest 2016;28(6):656–661.

Authors Jessica Comolli, DVM and Rodney Schnellbacher, DVM, Dipl. ACZM

PRURITUS

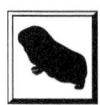

BASICS

DEFINITION
The sensation that provokes the desire to scratch, rub, chew, or lick; often an indicator of inflamed skin

PATHOPHYSIOLOGY
• The skin is abundant in sensory nerves and receptors responsible for transmitting sensory input to the central nervous system such as touch, temperature, pain, and pruritus.
• Pruritus stimulates various kinds of self-trauma, including scratching, which in turn relieves some of the sensation of itching. Self-trauma may perpetuate pruritus by contributing to skin inflammation.
• Some endogenous and chemical mediators induce the sensation of itch. Histamine induces pruritus in guinea pigs as in other mammals. Other modulators of pruritus, some of which have been demonstrated in guinea pigs, include histamine-releasing mediators (e.g., leukotrienes, prostaglandins, and serotonin), proteases (released by infectious agents, mast cells, inflammation, and tissue damage), peptides, and chemical mediators present in arthropod saliva and from plants.
• Other factors, such as boredom, anxiety, and stress, may exacerbate pruritus.
• Summation of effects occurs when the pruritic stimuli add up to reach the pruritus threshold.

SYSTEMS AFFECTED
• Skin/Exocrine
• Endocrine/Metabolic
• Nervous—intense pruritus can lead to seizures in guinea pigs

INCIDENCE/PREVALENCE
One of the most common dermatologic presentations. A study in California reported a prevalence of 50% for skin diseases. The most common dermatologic diseases were pododermatitis (47% of guinea pigs with skin diseases) and mites/lice infestation (14% of guinea pigs with skin diseases).

SIGNALMENT
Variable, depends on the underlying cause

SIGNS

Historical Findings
• The action of scratching, licking, rubbing, biting, or self-mutilating is often observed.
• Other guinea pigs, pets, or owners may have cutaneous signs associated with contagious dermatologic diseases.
• Behavioral changes may occur: anorexia, lethargy, lack of tolerance, vocalization, weight loss, and hiding.

Physical Examination Findings
Evidence of self-trauma, erythema, excoriation, broken hair, alopecia, hyperpigmentation, and lichenification

CAUSES
• Ectoparasites
  ○ *Trixacarus caviae*—this sarcoptid mite is the most significant and pruritic ectoparasite of the guinea pig. The life cycle ranges from 2 to 14 days. Some cases of extreme pruritus can lead to seizures, severe self-trauma, and generalized dermatitis. Secondary bacterial infection is common.
  ○ Other mites reported to infest guinea pigs that can cause pruritus include *Chirodiscoides caviae*, *Demodex caviae*, *Myocoptes musculinus*, *Sarcoptes scabiei*, *Notoedres muris*, and *Cheyletiella parasitivorax*. *Chirodiscoides caviae*, the second most common mite after *Trixacarus caviae*, is usually subclinical, but heavy infestation can lead to pruritus and alopecia, especially in the posterior part of the body. *Cheyletiella parasitivorax* is most commonly identified on guinea pigs that have been in contact with rabbits.
  ○ Lice—*Gliricola porcelli* and *Gyropus ovalis* are common biting lice of guinea pigs. The infestation is usually subclinical unless a heavy infestation is present, especially around the ears and on the back.
  ○ Fleas—*Ctenocephalides felis* is most commonly seen in guinea pigs housed with dogs and cats.
• Bacteria—bacterial skin infections are common in guinea pigs and cause a mild to severe pruritus. *Staphylococcus aureus*, responsible for an exfoliative dermatitis, and *Staphylococcus epidermidis* are common isolates. Other bacteria reported to cause pyoderma in guinea pigs include *Treponema* spp., *Streptococcus* spp., *Fusobacterium* spp., and *Corynebacterium* spp.
• Fungus—dermatophytosis caused by *Trichophyton mentagrophytes* and *Microsporum canis* may cause pruritus in guinea pigs.
• Hypersensitivity—contact hypersensitivity has been reported in guinea pigs.

RISK FACTORS
Concurrent disease, hypovitaminosis C, overcrowding, and poor husbandry. Some mites, such as *Chirodiscoides caviae*, have been shown to be more common in guinea pigs in pet shops than in privately owned animals.

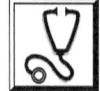

DIAGNOSIS

DIFFERENTIAL DIAGNOSIS

Nonpruritic Alopecia/Distribution of Lesions
• Dermatophytosis is most often nonpruritic—around the face and legs, sometimes dorsum

• Cystic ovarian disease—common cause of alopecia over the back, ventrum, and flanks
• Pregnancy-associated alopecia—flanks bilaterally
• Protein deficiency and other nutritional deficiencies—uncommon, generalized
• Stress—generalized hair loss
• Barbering, fur chewing—anywhere but commonly on rump and perineal areas
• Hereditary alopecia—generalized
• Cushing's disease (rare)/generalized or flanks/dorsum
• Hyperthyroidism/generalized or flanks/dorsum

Pruritic Alopecia/Distribution of Lesions
• *Trixacarus caviae*—shoulders, dorsum, and flanks, may be generalized and associated with crusting, hyperpigmentation, and lichenification. The pruritus is intense. Parasites are readily identified in skin scrapes preparation.
• *Chirodiscoides caviae*—often found around the groin and axilla. Mites are present in the hairs and are easily observed on hair plucks.
• Other ectoparasites—*Cheyletiella parasitivorax* usually produces lesions on the dorsum; *Demodex caviae* is frequently located on the head and forelegs. Lice often produce lesions around the ears and dorsum.
• Dermatophytosis can be pruritic—*Trichophyton mentagrophytes* often affects hair around the face, legs, and sometimes dorsum.
• Bacterial pyoderma—location depends on the inciting cause and may be present anywhere. Exfoliative dermatitis is reported most commonly in the ventral aspect.
• Contact dermatitis—ventral aspect, paws

CBC/BIOCHEMISTRY/URINALYSIS
The need to perform these diagnostic tests depends on the underlying disease process.
   Most often normal except in severe pyoderma and parasite infestation.

IMAGING
• Radiographs—identifying concomitant pathology or dental disease that may cause moist dermatitis secondary to ptyalism
• Abdominal ultrasound—identifying ovarian cyst

DIAGNOSTIC PROCEDURES

Ectoparasites Diagnosis
• Skin scraping—invaluable. Deep skin scrapings are necessary to reveal *Trixacarus caviae* and *Demodex caviae*. The hair should be clipped before processing. Mineral oil can be used for slide preparation.
• Hair plucking—used to identify fur mites such as *Chirodiscoides caviae*, *Cheyletiella parasitivorax*, and lice
• Adhesive tape collection—for surface-living ectoparasites

(CONTINUED)

• Coat brushing—for fleas and *Cheyletiella parasitivorax*

Bacterial Infections
Bacterial culture—infected lesions are frequently contaminated with the resident microbiological flora. Intact pustules should be sampled sterilely instead. Pus or sample of an abscess wall can also be submitted for culture.

Fungal Infections
• Wood's lamp—useful to diagnose dermatophytosis caused by *Microsporum* spp. Use is limited in guinea pigs where *Trychophyton mentagrophytes* is the most common dermatophyte and does not fluoresce when exposed to ultraviolet light.
• Direct microscopy/Hair plucking—the edge of the lesion is the preferred collection site. Fungal arthrospores and hyphae may be observed.
• Fungal culture—hair can be collected as well as samples obtained from brush techniques. Growth may be slow and take up to 1 month.

Others
• Impression cytology—may be useful to identify cellular infiltrate and bacterial organisms
• Skin biopsy—very useful in autoimmune and neoplastic processes; may be useful in mite infestations, endocrine, and fungal diseases

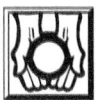

TREATMENT
APPROPRIATE HEALTH CARE
• More than one cause may be contributing to the pruritus (summation of effects). Trial therapy may be indicated when one fails to identify an inciting cause.
• Hair should be clipped in case of fungal and bacterial dermatitis.
• All in-contact animals should be treated in case of ectoparasites infestation. The environment will also need to be thoroughly cleaned.

DIET
Guinea pigs need a dietary source of vitamin C. Higher levels should be provided to sick individuals (30–50 mg/kg PO q24h). Vitamin C may be ground and fed directly to the pig. Vitamin C treats are also available for guinea pigs (e.g., Daily C, Oxbow Pet Products, Murdock, NE).

CLIENT EDUCATION
Most of the parasitic diseases are contagious, and other animals, including other species, may have to be treated.

MEDICATIONS
DRUG(S) OF CHOICE
Antipruritic Therapy
• Corticosteroids may be used in case of severe pruritus. Prednisone, prednisolone (0.25–1 mg/kg PO q12–24h). May be given on an alternate-day basis.
• Antihistamines—usually not very effective except in allergic dermatitis. Hydroxyzine (2 mg/kg PO q8–12h) and diphenhydramine (2 mg/kg PO, SC q8–12h) have been used.

Antiparasitic Therapy
• Ivermectin 0.2–0.8 SC mg/kg every 7–10 days for three doses is usually effective to treat mite infestation.
• Selamectin 15–30 mg/kg spot-on every 10 days for one to two treatments to treat mites or lice
• Imidacloprid and moxidectin (Advantage Multi) 0.1 mL/animal topically once every 30 days for three treatments for lice or mite infestation.
• Carbaryl or pyrethrin-based flea powder (labeled for use in kittens) can be used, being careful not to overdose.

Antimicrobial Therapy
• Topical treatment with antimicrobial shampoos can be used in pyoderma and may be useful as adjunctive therapy in dermatophytosis. Antimicrobial shampoos include chlorhexidine and ethyl lactate shampoos. Antifungal shampoos that may be used are ketoconazole, miconazole, and lime sulfur shampoos. Some topical products (griseofulvin 1.5%, enilconazole 0.2%) may also be used. Focal fungal lesions can also be addressed using clotrimazole cream.
• Broad-spectrum antibiotics safe to use in guinea pigs include enrofloxacin (5–15 mg/kg PO, SC, IM q12–24h), which is ineffective against anaerobes and may be variably effective against *Streptococcus* spp.; trimethoprim-sulfa (15–30 mg/kg PO q12h); chloramphenicol (30–50 mg/kg PO, SC, IM, IV q8–12h); and azithromycin (30 mg/kg PO q12–24h). Therapy should be based on culture and sensitivity if possible.
• Antifungals—terbinafine (20–30 mg/kg PO q24h) is most effective for treatment of dermatophytes—all guinea pigs in the household should be treated
   Alternatively, use griseofulvin (15–50 mg/kg PO q24h), itraconazole (5–10 mg/kg PO q24h), Treatment should be continued for 2 weeks past resolution of clinical signs.

CONTRAINDICATIONS
• Oral administration of penicillins, macrolides, lincosamides, and cephalosporins due to potentially fatal enteric dysbiosis
• Corticosteroids are contraindicated in the treatment of demodicosis and pyoderma.
• Fipronil is usually not recommended in guinea pigs but has been used safely in this species.
• Griseofulvin is teratogenic and therefore should never be administered to pregnant animals.

PRECAUTIONS
• Dipping and bathing guinea pigs can be stressful.
• Prevent guinea pigs from licking topical products.
• Oral administration of antibiotics may cause antibiotic-associated enteritis, dysbiosis, and enterotoxemia.

FOLLOW-UP
PATIENT MONITORING
Monitor for resolution of clinical signs and toxicity to the medications.

PREVENTION/AVOIDANCE
• Isolation and treatment of sick and in-contact individuals
• Cleaning of the environment

POSSIBLE COMPLICATIONS
• Sepsis
• Seizures with severe *Trixacarus* infestation

MISCELLANEOUS
ASSOCIATED CONDITIONS
Alopecia

ZOONOTIC POTENTIAL
• Dermatophytosis
• *Trixacarus caviae* and *Cheyletiella parasitivorax* may cause a mild dermatitis in humans.

PREGNANCY/FERTILITY/BREEDING
Griseofulvin and ivermectin are teratogenic.

SEE ALSO
Abscesses
Alopecia
Dermatophytosis
Fleas and flea infestation
Lice and mites
Seizures

GUINEA PIGS

Suggested Reading

Ballweber LR, Harkness JE. Parasites of guinea pigs. In: Baker DG, ed. Flynn's Parasites of Laboratory Animals, 2nd ed. Ames: Blackwell, 2007:421–449.

Meredith A. Skin diseases and treatment of guinea pigs. In: Paterson S, ed. Skin Diseases of Exotic Pets. Ames: Blackwell, 2006:232–250.

Minarikova A, Hauptman K, Jeklova E, Knotek Z, Jekl V. Diseases in pet guinea pigs: a retrospective study in 1000 animals. Vet Rec 2015;177(8):200.

Pignon C, Mayer J. Guinea pigs. In: Quesenberry KE, Carpenter JW, eds. Ferrets, Rabbits and Rodents, 4th Ed). Clinical Medicine and Surgery. 2021 ed. St. Louis: Saunders, 2020:270–297.

Palmerio BS, Roberts H. Clinical approach to dermatologic disease in exotic animals. Vet Clin North Am Exot Anim Pract. 2013;16(3):523–577.

Riggs SM. Guinea pigs. In: Mitchell MA, Tully TN, eds. Manual of Exotic Pet Practice. St Louis: Saunders/Elsevier, 2009:456–473.

White SD, Sanchez-Migallon D, Paul-Murphy J. Skin diseases in companion guinea pigs (*Cavia porcellus*): a retrospective study of 293 cases seen at the Veterinary Medical Teaching Hospital, University of California at Davis (1990–2015). Vet Dermatol 2016;27:395–e100.

Author Hugues Beaufrère, Dr. Med. Vet.

PYOMETRA AND NONNEOPLASTIC UTERINE DISORDERS

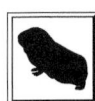

BASICS

DEFINITION
• Pyometra develops when bacteria invade abnormal endometrial tissue, leading to intraluminal accumulation of purulent exudate.
• Endometrial disorders—common nonneoplastic endometrial disorders of guinea pigs include cystic endometrial hyperplasia, endocervical hyperplasia, uterine inflammation, endometritis, metritis, endometrial hemorrhage, and mucometra.

PATHOPHYSIOLOGY
• Endometrial disorders can result in mild vaginal discharge to significant uterine hemorrhage.
• Endometrial secretions provide excellent media for bacterial growth; bacteria ascend from the vagina through the cervix or may be transmitted from the male during copulation.
• Vaginitis can ascend into uterine infections, endometritis, and pyometra.
• Hematogenous spread of bacteria to the uterus can occur but has not been reported in guinea pigs.
• Cystic rete ovarii can affect the uterus resulting in concurrent cystic, hyperplastic and neoplastic disorders.

SYSTEMS AFFECTED
Reproductive

INCIDENCE/PREVALENCE
• Uterine disorders, including hyperplasia and neoplasia, have an incidence of over 77% in sows >6 years old.
• Ovarian cysts are seen in >75% of sows >6 years of age
• Uterine inflammation is most common in younger sows, age 7–24 months.

SIGNALMENT
• Intact females both breeding and nonbreeding
• Spayed females with vaginitis

Predominant Sex
Sows only

SIGNS
Historical Findings
• Early phases of disease sows may be asymptomatic.
• Sows may fail to become pregnant.
• Hematuria is the most common presenting complaint, but blood originates from the uterus and gets mixed with the urine upon micturition. Frank blood often noted at the end of micturition and can be intermittent or cyclic.
• Vaginal discharge can be intermittent or continuous.

• May have signs of pseudopregnancy—lactation for 1–2 weeks.
• Signs of systemic illness, progressing to septicemia and shock can be observed in sows with closed cervical pyometra.
• Breeding sows with history of small litter size, increased number of stillborn or resorbed fetuses, infertility, dystocia, and abandonment of pups
• Polydipsia and polyuria may be seen with chronic pyometra.

Physical Examination Findings
• Abdominal swelling
• Palpable, large uterus
• Serosanguineous to purulent, blood-tinged vaginal discharge
• Blood-tinged perineal staining
• Lethargy
• Anorexia
• Mammary gland enlargement may be firm, or fluid filled.
• Mammary tumors may be concurrent
• Mastitis may be associated
• Febrile
• Pale mucous membranes, tachycardia if significant blood loss
• Sow may be in shock and/or recumbent

CAUSES
• Common bacteria in pyometra and endometritis—*Bordetella bronchiseptica*, *Streptococcus* spp. (especially hemolytic *Streptococcus*), *Corynebacterium pyogenes*, *Staphylococcus aureus*, *E. coli*, *Chlamydophila*, *Arcanobacterium pyogenes*, and *Salmonella*
• Cystic ovaries are common in guinea pigs and often concurrent with cystic, hyperplasitic and neoplastic disorders.

RISK FACTORS
• Intact uterus and ovaries
• Risk increases with age greater than 18 months
• Risk increases with sterile mating or sows mounting each other.

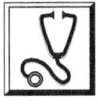

DIAGNOSIS

DIFFERENTIAL DIAGNOSIS
• Late-term abortion
• Pregnancy
• Uterine neoplasia
• Vaginitis

CBC/BIOCHEMISTRY/URINALYSIS
CBC—TWBC may be normal, or if septic there may be heterophilia or toxic heterophils noted.

CBC—regenerative or nonregenerative anemia if chronic uterine hemorrhage has occurred with endometritis

Thrombocytosis with acute inflammation

Biochemistry panel—azotemia with dehydration; increased BUN, ALT, GGT with sepsis

Electrolytes and blood gases: metabolic acidosis, hyperkalemia, hyponatremia, and hypochloremia

Urinalysis collected by ultrasound-guided cystocentesis—lack of hematuria confirms source of hemorrhage is more likely uterine or vaginal

Urinalysis—aciduria (pH 5–6), proteinuria, ketonuria with sepsis from pyometra

OTHER LABORATORY TESTS
• Cytology of vaginal discharge—lack of neoplastic cells and presence of polymorphonuclear cells and bacteria
• Culture and sensitivity of uterine endometrial or purulent contents obtained during OVH to direct antibiotic therapy
• Histopathologic examination of uterus following OVH for definitive diagnosis. Neoplasia may be an underlying cause of the mucometra or pyometra.

IMAGING
Radiography
Large soft tissue structure can be observed in the caudal abdomen

Ultrasonography
• Assess the size of the uterus and nature of the uterine contents.
• Rule out pregnancy.

DIAGNOSTIC PROCEDURES
• Diagnosis can be made by signalment and clinical signs, but difficult to differentiate which form of uterine disorder is present
• Neoplasia is often not ruled out until histopathology of uterus is completed

PATHOLOGIC FINDINGS
• Gross lesions include enlarged uterus
• Uterine endometrium friable and hemorrhagic or fluid-filled uterus with purulent material or mucus
• Reduced gastric content, enlarged tan liver if hepatic lipidosis has occurred with chronic anorexia, adrenomegaly, and excessive body fat
• Cystic rete ovarii often concomitant with endometritis and endometrial hyperplasia

TREATMENT

APPROPRIATE HEALTH CARE
• Fluid therapy is used to correct abnormalities in volume, electrolytes, and acid–base status. Caution not to exacerbate a concurrent anemia.
• In cases of pyometra and sepsis, antimicrobial therapy should be initiated immediately (culture and sensitivity should be obtained).

PYOMETRA AND NONNEOPLASTIC UTERINE DISORDERS (CONTINUED)

○ Intravenous administration is recommended if a catheter is in place.
• OVH is the treatment of choice for any uterine abnormalities.
• Endometrial disorders may be associated with endocrine changes associated with cystic ovaries, which can be treated with GnRH, leuprolide, or surgical removal.

NURSING CARE
• For pyometra, immediate therapy includes subcutaneous fluids (100 mL/kg) while preparing to place IV or IO catheter.
• IV access is difficult in the guinea pig, especially if hypotensive; lateral saphenous vein catheters often kink; consider IO catheterization of the femur for intravascular fluids. Base fluid selection on evidence of dehydration, acid–base, and electrolyte imbalances. Administer colloids with crystalloids if sow is hypotensive.
• Anorexia is a nonspecific sign that can be life threatening in the guinea pig and must be addressed with forced feeding, especially in the perioperative period. If the guinea pig was anorexic prior to treatment and OVH, then forced feeding is often required for days to weeks in the postoperative period.
• Analgesia is indicated in any disorder causing inflammation or pain.

ACTIVITY
Minimize stress

DIET
• It is an absolute requirement that sows continue to eat and to avoid sudden dietary changes.
• In addition to pellets, offer a large selection of good-quality grass hay plus fresh, moist greens such as cilantro, parsley, carrot tops, and dark leafy greens.
• If the sow stops eating, syringe-feed Critical Care for Herbivores (Oxbow Animal Health, Murdock, NE) diet at approximately 26 grams of dry product per kg body weight per day. Dry product is mixed with approximately twice the volume of water and is fed in small portions every 6–8 hours. Larger volumes and more frequent feedings are often accepted; feed as much as the sow will readily accept. Alternatively, pellets can be ground and mixed with fresh greens, vegetable baby foods, water, or sugar-free juice to form a gruel.
• Fresh water needs to be available at all times.

CLIENT EDUCATION
• OVH is the treatment of choice for most uterine disorders; medical treatment is usually insufficient to resolve the infection.
• Antibiotic therapy is indicated in the perioperative period, and the guinea pig needs to be monitored for signs of dysbiosis.

Watch for soft stools, diarrhea, and sudden change in appetite.
• Analgesia is indicated in any disorder causing inflammation or pain.

SURGICAL CONSIDERATIONS
• OVH is recommended.
• Enlarged uterus may be friable, adhesions may accompany pyometra.
• Remove the entire cervix to maximize removal of infected and inflamed tissue.
• Minimize tissue handling and keep tissues moist during surgery to minimize adhesions.
• Consider use of hemoclips to reduce tissue handling and adhesion formation.
• Use subcuticular sutures to minimize irritation of the incision because abdomen often is in contact with the cage floor.
• Lavage the abdominal cavity if any leakage of the infected uterus occurs.
• Postoperative management includes assisted feeding, fluids, analgesics, and antibiotics.

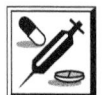

MEDICATIONS
DRUG(S) OF CHOICE
• Antibiotics will be administered empirically pending results of culture and sensitivity. Use broad-spectrum antibiotics such as trimethoprim-sulfa (15–30 mg/kg PO q12h), chloramphenicol (30–50 mg/kg PO, SC, IM, IV q8–12h) or enrofloxacin (5–20 mg/kg PO q12–24h) {Should be reserved for microbes that are resistant to tier one antibiotics}.
• Pain management is essential during and following surgery. Multimodal therapy is recommended for perioperative analgesia with an anxiolytic, such as midazolam (0.4–2.0 mg/kg IM), an opioid such as butorphanol (0.4–2.0 mg/kg SC, IM q4–12h), or buprenorphine (0.05–0.2 mg/kg SC, IM q6–8h). An NSAID such as meloxicam (0.5–1 mg/kg PO, SC, IM q24h) or carprofen (4 mg/kg SC q24h or 1–2 mg/kg PO q12h–24h) can be given in the perioperative period when the animal is fully hydrated and renal perfusion is no longer compromised. Tramadol, a synthetic opioid, may also be an effective at dosages of 5–10 mg/kg PO q12h postoperatively. For severe to moderate pain pure mu opioids such as morphine (0.5–2.0 mg/kg SC, IM q2–4h) or oxymorphone (0.2 -0.5 mg/kg SC, IM q40–12h) should be used however appetite and fecal output should be monitored as these opioids are thought to contribute to GI ileus.

CONTRAINDICATIONS
• Oral administration of antibiotics that select against gram-positive bacteria (penicillins, cephalosporins, macrolides, and

lincosamides) can cause fatal enteric dysbiosis and enterotoxaemia.
• NSAIDs are contraindicated in sows that are febrile, dehydrated, or azotemic or that are suspected of having pyelonephritis, septicemia, or preexisting renal disease.

PRECAUTIONS
• During surgery, avoid excessive handling of gastrointestinal tissues to reduce postoperative ileus or fibrous adhesions.
• Chloramphenicol—avoid human contact with chloramphenicol due to potential blood dyscrasia. Advise owners of potential risks.

FOLLOW-UP
PATIENT MONITORING
• Ensure gastrointestinal motility by making sure the patient is eating, well hydrated, and passing normal feces prior to release from hospitalization.
• Follow-up examination should be performed within 5–7 days of discharge from hospital, or sooner if the sow does not return to eating.
• Monitor for signs of pain (hunched posture, teeth grinding, and reluctance to move).
• Clean bedding is critical because region of abdominal incision is usually in contact with cage floor.

PREVENTION/AVOIDANCE
• Discontinue breeding of the sow when older than 3–4 years.
• OVH for nonbreeding sows

POSSIBLE COMPLICATIONS
• Peritonitis and sepsis in sows with endometritis or pyometra
• Postoperative adhesions may lead to chronic gastrointestinal motility disorders or pain.

EXPECTED COURSE AND PROGNOSIS
• Good prognosis if uterine infection is detected early and addressed with timely OVH
• Guarded prognosis if sow is septic or has been experiencing prolonged anorexia prior to examination

MISCELLANEOUS
ASSOCIATED CONDITIONS
• Uterine neoplasia
• Cystic ovaries
• Mastitis

AGE-RELATED FACTORS
Risk increases with age greater than 18 months.

PREGNANCY/FERTILITY/BREEDING
Pyometra or endometrial disorders greatly reduce fertility; therefore, treatment of choice is OVH.

SEE ALSO
Mastitis
Ovarian cysts

ABBREVIATIONS
ALT = alanine aminotransferase
BUN = blood urea nitrogen
GGT = gamma glutamyl transferase
GnRH = gonadotropic-releasing hormone
OVH = ovariohysterectomy
NSAID = nonsteroidal anti-inflammatory drug
TWBC = total white blood cell count

Suggested Reading
Bertram CA, Muller K, Klopfleisch R. Genital tract pathology in female pet guinea pigs (*Cavia porcellus*): a retrospective study of 655 post-mortem and 64 biopsy cases. J Comp Path 2018;164:12–22.

Bishop CR. Reproductive medicine of rabbits and rodents. Vet Clin North Am Exot Anim Pract 2002;5(507–535):vi.

Hawkins M, Bishop C. Diseases of guinea pigs. In: Carpenter J, Quesenberry K, eds. Ferrets, Rabbits, and Rodents: Clinical Medicine and Surgery, 3rd ed. St Louis: Elsevier, 2012:295–310.

Hoefer H, Latney L. Rodents: urogenital and reproductive disorders. In: Keeble E, Meredith A, eds. BSAVA Manual of Rodents and Ferrets. Gloucester: BSAVA, 2009:150–160.

Keller LS, Griffith JW, Lang CM. Reproductive failure associated with cystic rete ovarii in guinea pigs. Vet Pathol 1987;24(4):335–339.

Laik-Schandelmaier C, Klopfleisch R, Schöniger S et al. Spontaneously arising tumours and tumour-like lesions of the cervix and uterus in 83 pet guinea pigs (*Cavia porcellus*). J Comp Path 2017;156:339–351.

Minarikova A, Hauptman K, Jeklova E et al. Diseases in pet guinea pigs: a retrospective study in 1000 animals. Vet Rec 2015;177(8):200.

Miwa Y, Sladky K. Common surgical procedures of rodents, ferrets, hedgehogs, and sugar gliders. Vet Clin Exot Anim 2016;19:205–244.

Nakamura C. Reproduction and reproductive disorders in guinea pigs. Exotic DVM 2000;2:11.

Veiga-Parga T, LaPerle KM, Newman SJ. Spontaneous reproductive pathology in female guinea pigs. J Vet Diag Invest 2016;28(6):656–661.

Author Rodney Schnellbacher, DVM, Dipl. ACZM

RHINITIS AND SINUSITIS

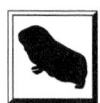

BASICS

DEFINITION
• Rhinitis—inflammation of the mucous membranes of the nose
• Sinusitis—inflammation of the paranasal sinuses

PATHOPHYSIOLOGY
• Various causes that can be infectious or noninfectious, acute or chronic
• Most common cause of rhinitis/sinusitis in guinea pigs is bacterial infection. The infection can spread from the nasal passages to the eye via the nasolacrimal duct, to the ear via the eustachian tube, to the lower respiratory tract via the trachea, into the bones of the face or the sinuses, or to the rest of the body via hematogenous spread.
• Dental disease or abscesses can cause destruction of the nasal turbinates or facial bones.

SYSTEMS AFFECTED
• Respiratory—upper respiratory tract disease
• Ophthalmic—extension of disease via nasolacrimal duct
• Oral cavity—dental disease, tooth root abscess
• Neurologic—extension of disease via eustachian tube causing otitis interna/media and vestibular signs
• Musculoskeletal—extension of disease into bones of the skull

GENETICS
Unknown

INCIDENCE/PREVELENCE
Respiratory disease is commonly seen in clinical practice; dental disease is also a common cause due to elongated tooth roots. Based on a recent veterinary survey, literature review, and single retrospective hospital case review, prevalence of guinea respiratory disease may be overrepresented in the literature compared to actual prevalence. Guinea pigs affected by respiratory disease account for approximately 6% of observed cases in UK veterinary respondents, and 4% of guinea pigs presented to hospital in the Czech Republic, but maybe over represented in the literature with a citation case rate of 15%.

GEOGRAPHIC DISRIBUTION
Widespread

SIGNALMENT
No breed, sex, or gender predilection

SIGNS

Historical Findings
• Vary depending on cause
• Anorexia and weight loss
• Lethargy
• Nasal or ocular discharge, sneezing, and staining of front paws
• Ptyalism
• Epistaxis
• Head tilt, scratching at ears

Physical Examination Findings
• Lethargy
• Weight loss
• Anorexia
• Serous or mucopurulent ocular or nasal discharge
• Epistaxis
• Decreased nasal airflow (unilateral or bilateral)
• Sneezing
• Signs of dental disease including ptyalism, facial bone deformity
• Head tilt or facial nerve paralysis if inner ear disease present
• Bloat is aerophagia is present

CAUSES
• Bacterial—*Bordetella brochiseptica*, *Streptococcus zooepidemicus*, *Streptococcus pneumoniae*, *Streptobacillus moniliformis*, *Yersinia pseudotuberculosis*, *Haemophilus* spp., *Klebsiella pneumoniae*, *Pseudomonas aeruginosa*, *Pasturella multocida*, *Salmonella* spp., *Staphylococcus aureus*, *Streptococcus pyogenes*, and *Citrobacter* spp.
• Viral—adenovirus and parainfluenza virus (rare)
• Dental disease—maxillary tooth roots can extend into the nasal passages and lead to secondary bacterial infections or obstruction of nasal passages; tooth root abscesses can also develop. Common bacteria isolated from ondotogenic abscesses include *Bacteroides fragilis*, *Pasturella multocida*, and *Peptostreptococcus anaerobius*
• Neoplasia—nasal adenocarcinoma, fibrosarcoma, and maxillary odontoma/elodontoma
• Foreign bodies—uncommon, usually grass or seeds
• Allergens or irritants to the respiratory tract—chemicals from cleaning, smoke, dusty/dirty bedding, mold, and ammonia buildup in the cage. Allergic rhinitis specifically to equine dander has been reported.

RISK FACTORS
• Poor husbandry—using substrate with aromatic oils such as pine and cedar, which can be irritating to respiratory mucosa; poor sanitation and infrequent cage cleaning; overcrowding; improper ventilation/humidity/temperature control; inhaled irritants such as disinfectants (bleach, etc.); ammonia buildup on the bedding; smoke
• Poor diet—feeding diets deficient in vitamin C can lead to immunosuppression; diets deficient in coarse fiber (long-stemmed grass hay) can lead to dental disease
• Immunosuppression—caused by lack of vitamin C in the diet, stress, concurrent disease, corticosteroid use, or age
• Dental disease—maxillary tooth roots can extend into the nasal passages and lead to secondary bacterial infections or obstruction of the nasal passages; tooth root abscesses and malocclusion can also develop
• Disease agent factors—serotype of bacteria, infectious dose, and virulence factors

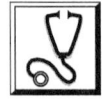

DIAGNOSIS

DIFFERENTIAL DIAGNOSIS
• Facial swelling or asymmetry—neoplasia, dental disease, and abscess
• Head tilt, facial nerve paralysis—otitis media/interna
• Ocular discharge—conjunctivitis, irritation, abscess, and incisor root elongation
• Nasal discharge, sneezing—pneumonia, upper respiratory tract infection

CBC/BIOCHEMISTRY/URINALYSIS
An elevation in total white blood cell count is uncommon, but a shift in proportion of heterophils to lymphocytes with an increase in heterophils and decrease in lymphocytes is expected. Increases in platelet number can also be seen with inflammation.

OTHER LABORATORY TESTS
• Enzyme-linked immunosorbent assay (ELISA) and indirect immunofluorescene assays (IFA) for *B. bronchiseptica* are more sensitive than culture for detection of the organism, but only detect antibodies and thus indicate exposure rather than active infection.
• ELISA for *S. pneumoniae*—only detects antibodies and thus indicates exposure rather than active infection
• PCR test for adenovirus is described but not readily available unless in lab animal setting

IMAGING
• Radiographs of the skull—must be done under heavy sedation or general anesthesia for optimal positioning. Recommend a minimum of five views (lateral, two oblique

GUINEA PIGS

laterals, anterior posterior, and ventrodorsal). Observe radiographs for bony lysis or proliferation of the turbinates and facial bones, as this can indicate chronic bacterial or neoplastic processes. Tooth roots should also be assessed, as they can penetrate the nasal sinuses, leading to obstruction or bacterial infection.

• CT or MRI—provides better imagining quality and may be more diagnostic than skull radiographs, especially if nasal detail is obscured by nasal discharge. Advanced imaging can help to determine whether the cause of disease is nasal, sinus, or dental disease. CT specifically is excellent for providing bony detail, is more sensitive for areas encased in bone (i.e., lungs and sinuses), and the procedure time is relatively short. These modalities may be cost prohibitive and not as readily available.

• Thoracic radiographs—indicated with bacterial rhinitis/sinusitis since subclinical pneumonia is common. Would expect to see an alveolar pattern with increased pulmonary density that can be patchy or diffuse (air bronchograms, consolidated lung lobes).

DIAGNOSTIC PROCEDURES

• Cytology of exudates—swab of nasal or ocular discharge, nasal swab, recommend standard cell stain (Diff Quick), and gram stain of exudates

• Culture of exudates—a sample can be obtained using a mini tip culturette inserted into the nostril. However, it can be difficult to obtain a good sample since the causative agent may be located in the sinuses, which are difficult to sample; many bacteria are difficult to grow on culture, and many normal commensal organisms are located in the nasal passages

• Nasal cavity biopsy—should be performed in animals with chronic nasal discharge (especially epistaxis) if neoplasia is suspected; use endoscopy or rhinotomy to obtain sample

• Oral endoscopy—thorough examination of the oral cavity and teeth

PATHOLOGIC FINDINGS

Nasal passages, external nares, and sinuses may contain serous or mucopurulent exudate, inflammatory cells infiltrating the nasal mucosa and sinuses, neoplasia, or foreign body in the nasal passages. Elongation of tooth roots into nasal passages/sinuses may contribute.

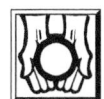

TREATMENT

APPROPRIATE HEALTH CARE
Depends on the underlying cause

NURSING CARE

• Oxygen therapy if the patient is in respiratory distress or dyspneic. Intubation or an emergency tracheotomy may be required if patient becomes apneic.

• Nebulization with saline may help deliver moisture to the upper respiratory tract.

• Keep nares clear of nasal discharge

• Fluid therapy to maintain normal hydration (guinea pigs fluid needs are 100 mL/kg/day)—fluid can be given IV, IO, or SC. Necessary to keep the GI tract hydrated and to aid mucocilliary clearance

• Keep patients in a quiet environment with no predator species in the vicinity to decrease stress, provide a hide box

• Keep environment clean, remove any environmental allergens or irritants

ACTIVITY

No change in activity level, allow the animal to set their own pace

DIET

• Anorexia can cause GI hypomotility/stasis, overgrowth of intestinal bacterial pathogens, and imbalance of GI microflora, so guinea pigs need to continue eating throughout treatment. Low-dose buprenorphine or midazolam may reduce hospital anxiety and have polyphagia effects leading to a greater likelihood that animal will eat in the hospital while having minimal cardiorespiratory effects.

• Offer a wide variety of fresh, moistened vegetables such as cilantro, parsley, romaine lettuce, and dandelion greens as well as good-quality grass hay (orchard grass, western timothy).

• If the patient refuses to eat, can syringe-feed Critical Care for Herbivores (Oxbow Pet Products, Murdock, NE) or Emeraid Herbivore (Lafeber Company, Cornell, IL) 10–15 mL/kg orally every 6–8 hours. Can also make a gruel of ground-up guinea pig pellets with vegetable baby foods, water, or fresh greens, but this is not as nutritionally complete as commercially made syringe-feeding formulas.

• Guinea pigs require an exogenous source of vitamin C supplementation, which can be given at 50–100 mg/kg/day when ill.

• Encourage oral fluid intake to maintain hydration by offering water or wet vegetables.

• Aerophagia can cause hypomotility gastrointestinal stasis.

CLIENT EDUCATION

If the underlying disease cannot be corrected (i.e., dental disease, neoplasia, and severe tissue destruction), a cure is unlikely. The treatment, depending on the cause, can be lifelong and aims to control the severe clinical signs.

SURGICAL CONSIDERATIONS

If dental disease is the cause of the rhinitis/sinusitis, then abscess debridement, tooth trims, or tooth extractions may be necessary. Use of probiotics or prebiotics prior to surgery can be considered.

MEDICATIONS

DRUG(S) OF CHOICE

• Antimicrobial drugs are the treatment of choice. Choice of antibiotic is ideally based on culture and sensitivity testing but can be chosen empirically. Long-term antibiotic therapy (4–6 weeks or even months to years) may be required with severe infection. Antibiotics used most commonly include enrofloxacin (5–20 mg/kg PO, SC, IM q12–24h; this drug has a basic pH and should be diluted or injected into a subcutaneous fluid pocket to prevent tissue injury), marbofloxacin (4 mg/kg PO q24h), pradofloxacin (5 mg/kg PO q12h), trimethoprim sulfa (15–30 mg/kg PO q12–24h), chloramphenicol (30–50 mg/kg PO, SC, IM, IV q8–12h), and metronidazole (10–20 mg/kg PO q12h). Can also use enrofloxacin in combination with doxycycline (2.5–5 mg/kg PO q12h). Combination antibiotic therapy of enrofloxacin and metronidazole is recommended for odontogenic abscesses.

• Consider pain control in cases of dental related rhinitis. Can use buprenorphine (0.05 mg/kg SC q8–12h, 0.2 mg/kg oral transmucosal q5h, 0.2 mg/kg IV q7h), meloxicam (0.5–1 mg/kg PO, SC q24h), ketoprofen (1–3 mg/kg SC, IM q12–24h), or carprofen (4 mg/kg SC q24h).

• Low-dose buprenorphine or midazolam may reduce hospital anxiety, combat pain, and induce mild polyphagia effects leading to greater likelihood of eating in the hospital with minimal cardiorespiratory effects.

• Concurrent with antibiotic administration, provision of a probiotic or prebiotic (Florentero, Ventix Animal Heallth Corp. Burlington, ON) should be considered to reduce the risk of antibiotic-induced enteritis or clostridial overgrowth/dysbiosis

• Parenteral antibiotics may be preferred for intractable rhinitis or sinusitis, particularly initially, for increased delivery of the drug to affected tissues (bone) while also reducing the likelihood of antibiotic induced dysbiosis.

CONTRAINDICATIONS

• Antibiotics that select against gram-positive bacteria such as oral penicillins, cephalosporins, lincosamines, or macrolides should not be used in these animals as it can cause fatal dysbiosis and enterotoxemia.

RHINITIS AND SINUSITIS

GUINEA PIGS

• Procaine, which is included in some penicillin preparations, can be toxic to guinea pigs.
• Using corticosteroids can suppress the immune system and exacerbate the infection.

PRECAUTIONS
Any antibiotic can cause diarrhea, which should be monitored in these patients and the antibiotic discontinued if diarrhea is present. Supplementation with probiotics or guinea pig transfaunation can be considered.

POSSIBLE INTERACTIONS
None

ALTERNATIVE DRUGS
• Nebulization with saline may help humidify the airways.
• Antihistamines such as diphenhydramine (1–5 mg/kg SC) have also been used in guinea pigs. Allergic rhinitis is thought to be uncommon in guinea pigs.

FOLLOW-UP

PATIENT MONITORING
Continue to monitor patient for relapse via clinical signs.

PREVENTION/AVOIDANCE
• Improve husbandry and diet (ensure appropriate vitamin C supplementation).
• Avoid stressful situations and corticosteroid use.
• Prevent dental disease by providing high-fiber foods, especially good-quality hay. Yearly veterinary exams with periodic trimming of overgrown teeth as needed.
• Commercially available vaccines for *B. bronchoseptica* (porcine *B. bronchiseptica* and human *B. pertussis*) offer some protection in experimentally infected guinea pigs.

POSSIBLE COMPLICATIONS
• Infection of the nasal passages and sinuses can extend to affect the eyes, ears, lungs, and musculoskeletal system.
• If nasal obstruction occurs, the patient can become severely dyspneic, since guinea pigs are obligate nasal breathers.

EXPECTED COURSE AND PROGNOSIS
Prognosis is based on cause of disease, severity, and chronicity. Mild disease may have a good prognosis with aggressive antibiotic treatment and supportive care. If the underlying disease cannot be corrected (dental disease, neoplasia, and severe tissue destruction), a cure is unlikely. The treatment, depending on the cause, can be lifelong and aims to control the clinical signs. Neoplasia carries a grave prognosis.

MISCELLANEOUS

ASSOCIATED CONDITIONS
GI hypomotility/stasis
Dental disease
Hypovitaminosis C
Pneumonia

AGE-RELATED FACTORS
• Neoplasia more common in older animals
• Infectious causes more common in younger animals

ZOONOTIC POTENTIAL
Streptobacillus moniliformis is the cause of rat bite fever in humans. Guinea pigs may be a reservoir for *Streptococcus pneumoniae*, with subclinical carriage rate up to 50% in some guinea pig colonies. Close contact between pets and children could be a risk factor although relevance in human hosts is not clearly defined.

PREGNANCY/FERTILITY/BREEDING
• Dams can pass *Yersinia pseudotuberculosis* to their young.
• *Bordetella bronchiseptica* may be associated with stillbirths, infertility, and abortion.

SYNONYMS
None

SEE ALSO
Dental malocclusion
Dyspnea and tachypnea
Nasal discharge and sneezing
Pneumonia

ABBREVIATIONS
CT = computed tomography
ELISA = enzyme-linked immunosorbent assay
GI = gastrointestinal
IFA = indirect immunofluorescene assay
MRI = magnetic resonance imaging

INTERNET RESOURCES
www.vin.com

Suggested Reading
Harkness JE, Murray KA, Wagner JE. Biology and diseases of guinea pigs. In: Fox JG, Anderson LC, Loew FM, Quimby FW, eds. Laboratory Animal Medicine, 2nd ed. San Diego: Elsevier, 2002:212–220, 222, 237–238.
Hawkins MG, Bishop CR. Disease problems of guinea pigs. In: Quesenberry KE, Carpenter JW, eds. Ferrets, Rabbits and Rodents: Clinical Medicine and Surgery, 3rd ed. St. Louis: Elsevier Saunders, 2012:298–299.
Hawkins MG, Graham JE. Emergency and critical care of rodents. Vet Clin North Am Exot Anim Pract 2007;2007(10):501–531.
Mayer J, Mans C. Rodents. In: Carpenter JW, ed. Exotic Animal Formulary, 5th ed. St Louis: Elsevier, 2018:459–479.
Minarikova A, Hauptman K, Jeklova E, Knotek Z, Jekl V. Diseases in pet guinea pigs: a retrospective study in 1000 animals. Vet Rec 2015;177(8):200.
Minarikova A, Hauptman K, Knotek Z, Jekl V. Microbial flora of odontogenic abscesses in pet guinea pigs. Vet Rec 2016;179(13):331.
Riggs SM. Guinea pigs. In: Mitchell MA, Tully TN, eds. Manual of Exotic Pet Practice. St Louis: Saunders, 2009: 463–464, 466–467.
Robinson NJ, Lyons E, Grindlay D, Brennan ML. Veterinarian nominated common conditions of rabbits and guinea pigs compared with published literature. Vet Sci 2017;4(4):58.

Authors Christy L. Rettenmund, DVM, Dipl. ACZM and J. Jill Heatley, DVM, MS, Dipl. ABVP (Avian, Reptilian, Amphibian), Dipl. ACZM

BASICS

DEFINITION
• A sudden, uncontrolled, transient increase in electrical discharge in the brain, resulting in loss or alteration of consciousness, altered muscled tone, muscle twitching, jaw chomping, and sometimes urination/defecation/salivation
• Generalized (grand-mal) seizures are tonic-clonic, where muscle tone is extremely increased (tonus) alternating with relaxation (clonus), or paddling of the limbs is present; this is the more common type of seizure in guinea pigs.
• Partial motor seizures demonstrate asymmetrical signs, focal twitching, or isolated tonic-clonic movements of the facial muscles or limbs.
• There are three phases to a seizure, although all three may not be identified or recognized. The pre-ictal phase (aura) precedes the seizure by minutes or hours and may be manifested as apprehension, anxiety, pacing, or agitation.
   The actual seizure (ictus) is characterized by the classic twitching or tonic-clonic movement, and generally lasts only a few minutes. There is a post-ictal phase during which the animal may appear disoriented, ataxic, or blind and which may last for a few minutes or many hours.

PATHOPHYSIOLOGY
• Seizures are always a sign of brain dysfunction (cerebrum).
• Seizures are classified by their cause as either extracranial or intracranial in origin.
• Excessive discharges in aggregates of neurons occur from the seizure focus, the area of the brain where the seizure originates. The spread of the abnormal electrical impulses to other parts of the brain results in the activity associated with the seizure.
• Seizures may arise from a single focus or from multiple foci in the brain simultaneously.
• A seizure event may lower the threshold for depolarization, making it easier for additional seizures to occur in close proximity to the original seizure.

SYSTEMS AFFECTED
Nervous

GENETICS
N/A

INCIDENCE/PREVALENCE
N/A

GEOGRAPHIC DISTRIBUTION
None

SIGNALMENT
No breed, age, or sex predilections have been identified.

SIGNS
General Comments
• Onset, duration, and frequency of seizures are often helpful in identifying etiology or narrowing the list of differential diagnoses.
• Acute onset with frequent severe seizures is generally more consistent with toxin, vascular event, or infectious agent.
• Gradual onset with progressive increase in frequency or duration may be suggestive of a metabolic or neoplastic process.
• Intermittent episodes with no deficits or abnormalities between episodes is most likely idiopathic.

Historical Findings
• Owners may notice a pre-ictal (aura) period during which the patient is restless, anxious, or hyperexcitable; this may last for several minutes or hours or may not be detected at all.
• The actual ictal phase of the seizure usually lasts 1–2 minutes. Owners will recognize loss of consciousness, paddling, twitching, irregular jaw movements, or sometimes urination or defecation.
• Following the seizure, the guinea pig may not recognize the owner or its surroundings and may appear dull and disoriented for a period of minutes to hours.
• It is important to ascertain any history of potential toxin exposure (including changes in food or new foods offered) or trauma.

Physical Examination Findings
• Physical examination findings will vary depending on the underlying cause.
• Some patients may have recovered from the seizure and may be completely normal upon presentation.
• Animals in the post-ictal phase may be disoriented, stuporous, have visual deficits, may circle, or may demonstrate other changes in mentation.
• Exudate may be present in ears or at tympanum in cases of otitis media/interna.
• Severe dental disease and cheek tooth overgrowth may be present in guinea pigs suffering from seizures related to nutrition, hypoglycemia, or hepatic disease.
• Ectoparasites may be present on the fur; lice and mite infestations have been associated with pruritis severe enough to induce seizure activity; the etiology is unknown.

CAUSES
Extracranial Causes
• Metabolic derangements—hypoglycemia, pregnancy toxemia, hepatic disease, hypocalcemia, severe uremia, electrolyte disturbances; heatstroke
• Toxins—organophosphates, lead, strychnine, other pesticides—question owners carefully about potential exposure; medications (metronidazole)
• Nutritional—vitamin E deficiency, thiamine deficiency (although unreported in guinea pigs); starvation (secondary to malocclusion)
• Infectious (parasitic)—severe louse or mite infestations have been reported to cause seizures in guinea pigs; the mechanism is unknown but believed to be related to the extreme intense pruritus

Intracranial Causes
• Degenerative—not described in guinea pigs
• Anomalous—not reported in guinea pigs
• Neoplastic—CNS lymphosarcoma, any CNS primary or metastatic neoplasm
• Infectious/Inflammatory—encephalitis secondary to infection: viral (lymphocytic choriomeningitis virus, and rabies virus), bacterial (focal abscess or generalized CNS infection; common organisms include *Streptococcus pneumonia*, *Pasteurella multocida*, and *Staphylococcus aureus*); may be extension of infection from respiratory tract or ear, protozoal (toxoplasmosis)
• Idiopathic—epilepsy, often a diagnosis made by elimination of other etiologies
• Trauma—head injury
• Vascular—infarct; secondary to arrhythmias or cardiac disease

RISK FACTORS
• Malocclusion—may predispose to nutritional deficiencies that may lead to metabolic disturbances
• Otitis media/interna, upper respiratory infection—may be a precursor for extension of disease into the brain
• Pregnancy—may lead to development of hypoglycemia, hyperglycemia, hypocalcemia, and pregnancy toxemia
• Free roaming in home or yard, unsupervised activity, and pesticide use
• Cardiac disease may predispose to vascular events

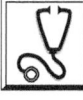
DIAGNOSIS

DIFFERENTIAL DIAGNOSIS
• Otitis media/interna may cause circling and head tilt that may be misidentified as seizure activity.
• Cerebellar or vestibular ataxia may be incorrectly described as a seizure, but also may be a post-ictal finding

SEIZURES

GUINEA PIGS

• Severe metabolic derangements and changes in mentation could be mistaken for a post-ictal state.

CBC/BIOCHEMISTRY/URINALYSIS
• May be reflective of underlying metabolic disease
• Otherwise may be normal
• CK may be elevated as a result of seizure activity.

OTHER LABORATORY TESTS
• Cytology, culture, and sensitivity—if otitis media or upper respiratory infection are present, cultures may be representative of bacteria in the ear.
• Lymphocytic choriomeningitis testing—PCR, IFA, and serology are available and performed at many universities and commercial veterinary diagnostic laboratories.
• Blood lead levels if ingestion is suspected
• Cholinesterase testing may be performed if organophosphate toxicity is suspected.

IMAGING
Radiography—may reveal fracture or other evidence of trauma. Skull radiographs may reveal bulla disease.
   CT or MRI—more sensitive for evaluation of brain infiltrate

DIAGNOSTIC PROCEDURES
• CSF analysis can be performed via the cisterna magna; indicated if infection or neoplasia is suspected; do not attempt to aspirate but instead collect sample via capillary tube; only a few drops will be obtained
• Electroencephalogram—not commonly performed in guinea pigs, normal values not established—compare to unaffected guinea pig to establish normal

PATHOLOGIC FINDINGS
Pathology will vary with underlying etiology.

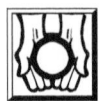

TREATMENT

APPROPRIATE HEALTH CARE
• If etiology can be identified, treat accordingly.
• Inpatient—any patient with repeated seizure episodes or ongoing seizure activity should be hospitalized for seizure management. Other patients that should be treated on an inpatient basis are those with neurologic signs; severe infections; anorexic patients; nonambulatory patients
• Outpatient—stable patients that are able to eat and drink with little or no assistance

NURSING CARE
• Fluid therapy to maintain hydration—subcutaneous generally adequate unless severe infection/sepsis; however, if continued seizure

activity is present or likely, an intravenous catheter is indicated
• Assisted feeding of anorexic animals
• Maintain clean, soft bedding with padding if necessary.
• Lubricate eyes if blink response is absent or diminished.
• In severe cases, turn patient every 4 hours or as needed to prevent formation of decubitus ulcers.
• Express bladder if patient unable to void without assistance.
• Keep fur clean and dry.

ACTIVITY
Restrict activity if any neurologic signs persist until certain that the patient is ambulatory and able to appropriately navigate. Confine to a very small space initially to prevent falls or injury; pad cage floor or walls if necessary.

DIET
• It is essential to maintain food intake during treatment; patients may become anorexic due to pain, fear, or neurologic signs; anorexia may lead to gastrointestinal stasis and ileus; secondary derangements of intestinal microbial populations may occur
• Offer a wide variety of fresh leafy greens (romaine lettuce, cilantro, parsley, kale, cabbage, collard greens, mustard greens, bok choy, dandelion greens, turnip greens, spinach, and mesclun salad mixes) and high-quality grass hay. Place food and water in a position that the guinea pig is able to reach, or hand offer.
• If patient is inappetent/anorexic, it is essential to provide adequate nutritional support. Syringe feed a formulated diet such as Critical Care for Herbivores (Oxbow Pet Products, Murdock, NE) or Emeraid Herbivore (Lafeber Company, Cornell, IL) 10–15 mL/kg q6–8h. If neither product is available, a slurry can be made with blended leafy green vegetables that are high in vitamin C, nor guinea pig pellets blended with water and vegetable baby food.
• Avoid high-carbohydrate foods, treats, or grains, which may cause gas production and stasis in the gastrointestinal tract.
• Use caution when syringe feeding, as aspiration pneumonia may occur in patients with central nervous system signs.

CLIENT EDUCATION
• Educate clients that pets with seizures may have recurrence of seizures even if the etiology is appropriately treated.
• Anticonvulsant therapy aids in controlling signs, but dosages may need to be adjusted over time.
• Owners should keep a seizure diary for tracking progression of seizures or response to medication.

SURGICAL CONSIDERATIONS
Bulla osteotomy (and total ear canal ablation) is indicated in severe cases of otitis media/interna with bulla osteitis; however, if infection has already disseminated to the brain and is contributing to seizures, prognosis is poor.

MEDICATIONS

DRUG(S) OF CHOICE
• If hypoglycemic, administer 50% dextrose IV, IO, orally, or rectally, 1–2 mL/kg diluted 1:1 with saline or lactated Ringer's solution to achieve normoglycemia
• Diazepam—administer 0.5–1.0 mg/kg IV or IO for actively seizuring patients; repeat every 5 minutes if seizures respond but reoccur; repeat up to three times; can be administered rectally at double the dose if vascular access is not established
• Midazolam can also be used in place of diazepam if vascular access is not established; administer 0.5–2.0 mg/kg IM
• If seizures are refractory to benzodiazepines, administer phenobarbital 2–10 mg/kg IV, IO, or IM
• If seizures are still not controlled, or if they respond to the above treatment but continue to reoccur, begin CRI of diazepam (1–2 mg/kg/hr) or phenobarbital (2–8 mg/kg/hr) or a combination of the two.
• For long-term seizure management, phenobarbital (2–5 mg/kg q8–12h) or potassium bromide (KBr; 30 mg/kg q24h; loading dose 100 mg/kg q24h for 3–5 days) can be continued orally.
• If cerebral edema is suspected as a result of prolonged seizure activity, administer mannitol 1 g/kg IV over 15–20 minutes.
• Steroid use can be considered if cerebral edema is suspected, but is controversial in guinea pigs and should be avoided in cases where infection is suspected (methylprednisolone sodium succinate 30 mg/kg IV or IM; dexamethasone sodium phosphate 1 mg/kg IV or IM).
• For suspected or confirmed CNS infections, use systemic antibiotics. Choose broad-spectrum antibiotics that penetrate the CNS, such as enrofloxacin (5–20 mg/kg PO, SC, IM q12h), trimethoprim-sulfa (15–30 mg/kg PO q12h); for anaerobic infections, consider chloramphenicol (30–50 mg/kg PO, SC, IM, IV q8–12h), florfenicol (20–25 mg/kg PO, IM, IV q12h), or metronidazole (10–20 mg/kg PO, IV q12h).

CONTRAINDICATIONS
• Avoid the use of antimicrobials that may disrupt gastrointestinal flora, which may lead to dysbiosis and fatal enterotoxemia

(penicillins, macrolides, lincosamides, tetracyclines, and cephalosporins).
• Avoid the use of corticosteroids in conjunction with meloxicam or other NSAIDs.
• Corticosteroids—because of the immunosuppressive effects of corticosteroids, their use may prolong or exacerbate infection and may increase risk of systemic disease.
• Avoid the use of drugs that are potentially toxic to the central nervous system (metronidazole at high doses; aminoglycosides).

PRECAUTIONS
• Respiratory depression and gastrointestinal hypomotility may occur as a result of phenobarbital use.
• Gastrointestinal stasis may occur with the use of KBr.

POSSIBLE INTERACTIONS
• Phenobarbital may increase the effects of other CNS depressants and may decrease the effects of chloramphenicol, metronidazole, and corticosteroids.
• Diazepam should not be given with cimetidine, ketoconazole, metoprolol, or propranolol as the combination may increase metabolism of diazepam and may cause excessive sedation. Antacids may slow the rate, but not the extent of oral absorption; administer 2 hours apart to avoid this potential interaction.
• Do not use steroids in conjunction with NSAIDs.

FOLLOW-UP
PATIENT MONITORING
• Evaluate CBC/biochemistry/urinalysis prior to initiating anticonvulsant therapy to establish baseline, subsequently monitor every 6 months or as dictated by underlying disease.
• Measure phenobarbital levels 2–3 weeks after initiation of therapy, then every 6 months.
• Measure KBr levels 2–3 months after initiation of therapy, then at 3 months, and every 6 months thereafter.
• Therapeutic levels for phenobarbital and KBr have not been established in guinea pigs; however, it is important to monitor for excessively high levels. Standard values for dogs are a starting point; however, if the

seizures are under control but the level is below the therapeutic range, there is no indication for increasing the dose.
• Owners should keep a journal of seizure activity to enable tracking progression of seizures or response to medication.

PREVENTION/AVOIDANCE
• Avoid free roaming or unsupervised activity or interactions with children or other pets.
• Treat upper respiratory infections and otitis early and aggressively to prevent dissemination to the middle and inner ear and brain.

POSSIBLE COMPLICATIONS
• Progression of seizure activity and status epilepticus may lead to death.
• Hyperthermia and/or hypoglycemia may develop with prolonged seizures.
• Gastrointestinal stasis and/or ulcers may develop if patient is unable to eat due to altered mentation.
• Permanent changes in mentation can occur as a result of prolonged seizure activity.
• A "seizure focus" may become established in the brain, resulting in future seizures even if the underlying etiology is resolved.

EXPECTED COURSE AND PROGNOSIS
• Depends on etiology
• Seizures may reoccur even if underlying cause is resolved, as the underlying disease may have established a "seizure focus" in the brain.
• Untreated status epilepticus or repeated uncontrollable seizures carries a poor prognosis.

MISCELLANEOUS
ASSOCIATED CONDITIONS
• Pregnancy—pregnancy toxemia
• Dental disease
• Otitis media/interna
• Upper respiratory infection

AGE-RELATED FACTORS
None

ZOONOTIC POTENTIAL
Lymphocytic choriomeningitis virus is rare but zoonotic.

PREGNANCY/FERTILITY/BREEDING
Pregnant sows are susceptible to hypoglycemia, ketosis, and pregnancy toxemia.

SYNONYMS
N/A

SEE ALSO
Ataxia
Otitis media and interna
Paresis and paralysis
Pregnancy toxemia

ABBREVIATIONS
CK = creatine phosphokinase
CNS = central nervous system
CRI = constant rate infusion
CSF = cerebrospinal fluid
CT = computed tomography
IFA = indirect immunofluorescence assay
KBr = potassium bromide
MRI = magnetic resonance imaging
PCR = polymerase chain reaction

Suggested Reading
Bays TB. Geriatric care of rabbits, guinea pigs, and chinchillas. Vet Clin Exot Anim 2020;23:567–593.
DeCubellis J. Common emergencies in rabbits, guinea pigs, and chinchillas. Vet Clin Exot Anim 2016;19:411–429.
Harkness JE, Turner PV, VandeWoude S, Wheeler CL. Clinical signs and differential diagnoses: nervous and musculoskeletal conditions. In: Harkness JE, Turner PV, VandeWoude S, Wheeler CL, eds. Biology and Medicine of Rabbits and Rodents, 5th ed. Ames: Wiley-Blackwell, 2010:214–216.
Lennox AM, Gladden JN. Emergency and critical care of small mammals. In: Quesenberry KE, Carpenter JW, eds. Ferrets, Rabbits and Rodents, 4th Ed). Clinical Medicine and Surgery. 2021 ed. St. Louis: Saunders, 2020:595–608.
Mancinelli E. Neurologic examination and diagnostic testing in rabbits, ferrets and rodents. J Exot Pet Med 2015;24:52–64.
Meredith AL, Richardson J. Neurologic disease of rabbits and rodents. J Exot Pet Med 2015;24:21–33.
Minarikova A, Hauptman K, Jeklova E, Knotek Z, Jekl V. Diseases in pet guinea pigs: a retrospective study in 1000 animals. Vet Rec 2015;177:200.
Pignon C, Mayer J. Guinea pigs. In: Quesenberry KE, Carpenter JW, eds. Ferrets, Rabbits and Rodents, 4th Ed). Clinical Medicine and Surgery. 2021 ed. St. Louis: Saunders, 2020:270–297.
Author Natalie Antinoff, DVM, Dipl. ABVP (Avian)

GUINEA PIGS

STERTOR AND STRIDOR

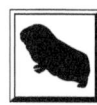

BASICS

DEFINITION
• Stertor—a low-pitched inspiratory snoring sound, sometimes due to obstruction of the larynx or upper airways (nasal passages, trachea, and pharynx)
• Stridor—a higher pitched inspiratory or expiratory sound often due to obstruction of the nasal, laryngeal, pharyngeal passages, or the trachea; occurs when erratic air currents attempt to force their way through narrowed breathing passages
• Both are abnormally loud breath sounds resulting from air passing through a narrowed upper airway and meeting resistance due to partial obstruction.

PATHOPHYSIOLOGY
Guinea pigs are obligate nasal breathers, so obstruction of the nasal passages, larynx, or pharynx may cause stertor or stridor. Airway obstruction can cause turbulence through a narrowed airway, leading to increased respiratory sounds. If the obstruction is severe, there is an increase in the effort of the respiratory muscles, which increases the turbulence of inspired air. This will increase inflammation and edema of the tissues around the obstruction leading to further obstruction of the airways.

SYSTEMS AFFECTED
Respiratory

GENETICS
Unknown

INCIDENCE/PREVALENCE
Respiratory disorders, including upper and lower infectious respiratory disease, and disorders secondary to dental disease are very common in pet guinea pigs.

GEOGRAPHIC DISTRIBUTION
Widespread

SIGNALMENT
• Tumor—usually seen in older animals
• No breed or sex predilection for other causes

SIGNS

Historical Findings
• Vary depending on cause
• Anorexia
• Lethargy
• Weight loss
• Nasal or ocular discharge
• Staining of the front paws
• Sneezing
• Epistaxis
• Ptyalism
• Bruxism
• Wheezing/labored breathing

• Dyspnea
• History of recent intubation or multiple attempts at intubation

Physical Examination Findings
• Lethargy
• Weight loss
• Tachypnea
• Serous or mucopurulent ocular discharge
• Unilateral or bilateral serous, hemorrhagic, or mucopurulent nasal discharge
• Crusting of discharge around the nose or on the front limbs
• Signs of dental disease (bruxism, anorexia, and ptyalism)
• Audible breath sounds from a distance
• Sneezing, increased upper airway sounds
• Increased respiratory effort
• Dyspnea
• Bloat if aerophagia is present

CAUSES
• Bacterial causes—*Bordetella bronchiseptica* (most common), *Streptococcus pneumoniae*, *Streptobacillus moniliformis*, *Yersinia pseudotuberculosis*, *Streptobacillus moniliformis*, *Haemophilus* spp., *Klebsiella pneumonia*, *Streptococcus zooepidemicus*, *Pseudomonas aeruginosa*, *Pasturella multocida*, *Staphylococcus aureus*, and *Streptococcus pyogenes*
• Dental disease—maxillary tooth roots can extend into the nasal passages and lead to secondary bacterial infections or obstruction of nasal passages; tooth root abscesses can also develop. Common bacteria isolated from ondotogenic abscesses include *Bacteroides fragilis*, *Pasturella multocida*, and *Peptostreptococcus anaerobius*
• Trauma to the face, nose, neck (i.e., bite wounds, crushing injuries, or falls)
• Airway tumors—brochogenic papillary adenoma, nasal adenocarcinoma (few reports)
• Foreign bodies—uncommon
• Allergens or irritants to the respiratory tract—chemicals from cleaning, smoke, dusty/dirty bedding, mold, and ammonia buildup on bedding
• Multiple intubation attempts or recent intubation leading to laryngeal edema/ inflammation
• Other causes—lower respiratory tract disease, rhinitis, sinusitis, anxiety, or nonrespiratory causes of dyspnea

RISK FACTORS
• Poor husbandry—using substrate with aromatic oils such as pine and cedar, which can be irritating to respiratory mucosa, poor sanitation, infrequent cage cleaning, overcrowding, improper ventilation/ humidity/temperature control, inhaled irritants such as disinfectants (bleach, etc.), ammonia buildup on the bedding, smoke

• Poor diet—feeding diets deficient in vitamin C can lead to immunosuppression; deficient in coarse fiber (long-stemmed grass hay) can lead to dental disease
• Immunosuppression—caused by lack of vitamin C in the diet, stress, concurrent disease, corticosteroid use, and age
• Traumatic intubation or multiple intubation attempts can cause laryngeal edema.
• Dental disease—maxillary tooth roots can extend into the nasal passages and lead to secondary bacterial infections or obstruction of nasal passages; tooth root abscesses can also develop
• Anxiety, pain, or any respiratory or cardiovascular disease that increases ventilation

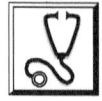

DIAGNOSIS

DIFFERENTIAL DIAGNOSIS
Use careful auscultation of the nose, pharynx, larynx, and trachea to differentiate sounds arising from the upper airway from those in the lower airway. Identify the point of maximal intensity of the abnormal sound to differentiate between inspiratory and expiratory effort as well as location. Once this has been accomplished, attempt to determine the cause.

CBC/BIOCHEMISTRY/URINALYSIS
An elevation in total white blood cell count is uncommon, but a shift in proportion of heterophils to lymphocytes with an increase in heterophils and decrease in lymphocytes is expected. Increases in platelet number can also be seen with inflammation.

OTHER LABORATORY TESTS
• Enzyme-linked immunosorbent assay (ELISA) and indirect immunofluorescence assays (IFA) for *B. bronchiseptica* are more sensitive than culture for detection of the organism, but these only detect antibodies and thus indicate exposure rather than active infection.
• ELISA for *S. pneumoniae*—only detects antibodies and thus indicates exposure rather than active infection

IMAGING
• Radiographs of the skull—must be done under heavy sedation or general anesthesia for optimal positioning. Recommend a minimum of five views (lateral, two oblique laterals, anterior posterior, and ventrodorsal). Observe radiographs for bony lysis or proliferation of the turbinates and facial bones, as this can indicate chronic bacterial or neoplastic processes. Tooth roots should also be accessed, as they can penetrate the nasal sinuses leading to obstruction or bacterial infection.

(CONTINUED)

• CT or MRI—provides better imaging quality; may be more diagnostic than skull radiographs, especially if nasal detail is obscured by nasal discharge. Advanced imaging can help to determine whether the cause of disease is nasal, sinus, or dental disease. CT specifically is excellent for providing bony detail, is more sensitive for areas encased in bone (i.e., lungs and sinuses), and the procedure time is relatively short. These modalities may be cost prohibitive and not as readily available.
• Thoracic radiographs—indicated with bacterial rhinitis/sinusitis since subclinical pneumonia is common. Would expect to see an alveolar pattern with increased pulmonary density, which can be patchy or diffuse (air bronchograms, consolidated lung lobes)

DIAGNOSTIC PROCEDURES
• Cytology of exudates—can use gram stain or standard cell stain (Diff Quick)
• Culture of exudates—a sample can be obtained using a mini tip culturette inserted into the nostril. However, it can be difficult to obtain a good sample since the causative agent may be located in the sinuses, which are difficult to sample; many bacteria are difficult to grow on culture; and many normal commensal organisms are located in the nasal passages.
• Nasal cavity biopsy—should be performed in animals with chronic nasal discharge (especially epistaxis) if neoplasia is suspected; use endoscopy or rhinotomy to obtain sample
• Direct visualization of the pharynx or larynx—can use a 2.7-mm rigid endoscope for direct visualization, requires general anesthesia; guinea pigs have abundant soft tissue in the oral cavity, a long narrow passage between the dental arcades, and a small oral opening, making visualization difficult

PATHOLOGIC FINDINGS
N/A

TREATMENT

APPROPRIATE HEALTH CARE
Patient should be hospitalized if in respiratory distress or has multisystemic signs of illness.

NURSING CARE
• Oxygen therapy if the patient is in respiratory distress. Not always needed in patients with partial airway obstruction.
• Fluid therapy to maintain normal hydration (guinea pig fluid needs are 100 mL/kg/day)—fluid can be given IV, IO, or SC. Necessary to keep the GI tract hydrated and to aid mucocilliary clearance.
• Keep patients in a quiet environment with no predator species in the vicinity to decrease stress, provide a hide box

• Eliminate anxiety, pain, exertion as much as possible as these may lead to increased ventilation, which could worsen the patient's condition.
• Keep nares clear of nasal discharge.
• If airway is completely obstructed will need to attempt emergency intubation (very difficult in guinea pigs due to very small opening for intubation and redundant oral tissues) or emergency tracheostomy

ACTIVITY
Patient's activity should be restricted as exertion can increase ventilation, which can worsen obstructive airway disease.

DIET
• Anorexia can cause GI hypomotility/stasis, overgrowth of intestinal bacterial pathogens, and imbalance of GI microflora, so guinea pigs need to continue eating throughout treatment. Low-dose buprenorphine or midazolam may reduce hospital anxiety and have polyphagia effects leading to a greater likelihood that animal will eat in the hospital while having minimal cardiorespiratory effects.
• Offer a wide variety of fresh, moistened vegetables such as cilantro, parsley, romaine lettuce, and dandelion greens, as well as good-quality grass hay (orchard grass, western timothy).
• If the patient refuses to eat, can syringe-feed Oxbow Critical Care for Herbivores or Lafeber's Critical Care for Herbivores 10–15 mL/kg orally every 6–8 hours. Can also make a gruel of ground-up guinea pig pellets with vegetable baby foods, water, or fresh greens, but this is not as nutritionally complete as commercially made syringe-feeding formulas.
• Guinea pigs require an exogenous source of vitamin C supplementation, which can be given at 50–100 mg/kg SC q24h when ill, or 30–50 mg/kg PO q24h maintenance
• Encourage oral fluid intake to maintain hydration by offering water or wet vegetables
• Aerophagia can cause hypomotility and gastrointesintal stasis.

CLIENT EDUCATION
If the underlying disease cannot be corrected (i.e., dental disease, neoplasia, and severe tissue destruction), a cure is unlikely. The treatment, depending on the cause, can be lifelong and aims to control the severe clinical signs. *Streptococcus zooepidemicus* is transmissible to other guinea pigs and *Pasturella* can be transmitted to other species.

SURGICAL CONSIDERATIONS
Anesthesia to correct dental disease may be more risky in these patients because the ability of the patient to protect its airway and use the muscles that open its airway is compromised by anesthesia. Sedatives may

also relax the upper airway muscles, which can worsen the obstruction.

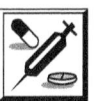

MEDICATIONS

DRUG(S) OF CHOICE
• Antimicrobial drugs may cause improvement if patient has bacterial rhinitis or sinusitis. Choice of antibiotic ideally based on culture and sensitivity testing but can be chosen empirically. Long-term antibiotic therapy (4–6 weeks or even months to years) may be required with severe infection. Use of broad-spectrum antibiotics most useful. Antibiotics used most commonly include enrofloxacin (5–20 mg/kg PO, SC, IM q12–24h; this drug has a basic pH and should be diluted or injected into a subcutaneous fluid pocket to prevent tissue injury) or trimethoprim sulfa (15–30 mg/kg PO q12–24h). If suspect an anaerobic infection, which are associated with tooth root abscesses, can use chloramphenicol (30–50 mg/kg PO, SC, IM, IV q8–12h) or metronidazole (10–20 mg/kg PO q12h). Combination antibiotic therapy of enrofloxacin and metronidazole is recommended for odontogenic abscesses.
• Steroids may be indicated if severe laryngeal edema or inflammation is present postintubation (prednisone 0.5–2.2 mg/kg PO, SC, IM, or prednisolone 1–2 mg/kg PO, SC q12–24h)
• Bronchodilators may help posttraumatic intubation. Can use theophylline (4–10 mg/kg PO q8–12h) or terbutaline (5 mg/kg PO q12h).
• Meloxicam (0.5–1.0 mg/kg PO, SC q24h) can also be used for laryngeal edema.
• Low dose buprenorphine or midazolam may reduce hospital anxiety, combat pain, and induce mild polyphagia effects leading to greater likelihood of eating in the hospital with minmal cardiorespiratory effects.
• Concurrent with antibiotic administration, provision of a probiotic or prebiotic (Florentero, Ventix Animal Heallth Corp. Burlington, ON) should be considered to reduce the risk of antibiotic induced enteritis or clostridial overgrowth/dysbiosis
• Parenteral antibiotics may be preferred

CONTRAINDICATIONS
• Oral administration of antibiotics that select against gram-positive bacteria such as penicillins, cephalosporins, lincosamines, or macrolides should not be used in these animals as it can cause fatal dysbiosis and enterotoxemia.
• Procaine, which is included in some penicillin preparations, can be toxic to guinea pigs.

PRECAUTIONS
• Any antibiotic can cause diarrhea, which should be monitored in these patients and the antibiotic discontinued if diarrhea is present. Supplementation with probiotics or guinea pig transfaunation can be considered.
• Corticosteroid use can suppress the immune system and exacerbate a bacterial infection. Can be used if absolutely necessary to reduce laryngeal edema of known cause.
• Sedatives can relax the upper airway muscles, worsening the obstruction; anesthesia decreases the patient's ability to protect its airway and use the muscles that open its airway.

POSSIBLE INTERACTIONS
N/A

ALTERNATIVE DRUGS
Buprenorphine (0.05 mg/kg SC q8–12h, 0.2 mg/kg oral transmucosal q5h, 0.2 mg/kg IV q7h) can be used for pain control, sedation, and to increase appetite. Midazolam (0.5–2 mg/kg IM) can also be used as a sedative.

FOLLOW-UP

PATIENT MONITORING
Continue to monitor patient for relapse via clinical signs.

PREVENTION/AVOIDANCE
• Improve husbandry and diet (ensure appropriate vitamin C supplementation).
• Avoid stressful situations and corticosteroid use.
• Prevent dental disease by providing high-fiber foods, especially good-quality hay. Yearly veterinary exams with periodic trimming of overgrown teeth as needed.

POSSIBLE COMPLICATIONS
Serious complications can ensue while attempting to manage the obstruction, which may require an emergency tracheostomy and mechanical ventilation. Patients should have close observational monitoring because a complete obstruction could occur at any time, even if the patient seems relatively stable.

Anesthetic agents and sedatives could worsen the obstruction.

EXPECTED COURSE AND PROGNOSIS
Prognosis is based on cause of disease, severity, and chronicity. Mild disease due to rhinitis or sinusitis may have a good prognosis with aggressive antibiotic treatment and supportive care. If the underlying disease cannot be corrected (i.e., dental disease, neoplasia, and severe tissue destruction), a cure is unlikely. The treatment, depending on the cause, can be lifelong and aims to control the clinical signs.

MISCELLANEOUS

ASSOCIATED CONDITIONS
GI hypomotility/stasis
Dental disease
Hypovitaminosis C
Rhinitis and sinusitis
Pneumonia

AGE-RELATED FACTORS
N/A

ZOONOTIC POTENTIAL
Streptobacillus moniliformis is the cause of rat bite fever in humans. Guinea pigs may be a reservoir for *Streptococcus pneumoniae,* with subclinical carriage rate up to 50% in some guinea pig colonies. Close contact between pets and children could be a risk factor although relevance in human hosts is not clearly defined.

PREGNANCY/FERTILITY/BREEDING
• Dams can pass *Yersinia pseudotuberculosis* to their young.
• *Bordetella bronchiseptica* may be associated with stillbirths, infertility, and abortion.

SYNONYMS
None

SEE ALSO
Dental malocclusion
Dyspnea and tachypnea

Nasal discharge and sneezing
Pneumonia
Rhinitis and sinusitis

ABBREVIATIONS
CT = computed tomography
ELISA = enzyme-linked immunosorbent assay
GI = gastrointestinal
IFA = indirect immunofluorescence assay
MRI = magnetic resonance imaging

INTERNET RESOURCES
www.vin.com

Suggested Reading
Harkness JE, Murray KA, Wagner JE. Biology and diseases of guinea pigs. In: Fox JG, Anderson LC, Loew FM, Quimby FW, eds. Laboratory Animal Medicine, 2nd ed. San Diego: Elsevier, 2002:212–220.
Hawkins MG, Bishop CR. Disease problems of guinea pigs. In: Quesenberry KE, Carpenter JW, eds. Ferrets, Rabbits, and Rodents: Clinical Medicine and Surgery, 3rd ed. St. Louis: Elsevier Saunders, 20012:298–299.
Hawkins MG, Graham JE. Emergency and critical care of rodents. Vet Clin North Am Exot Anim Pract 2007;2007(10):501–531.
Mayer J, Mans C. Rodents. In: Carpenter JW, ed. Exotic Animal Formulary, 5th ed. St Louis: Elsevier, 2018:459–479.
Minarikova A, Hauptman K, Jeklova E, Knotek Z, Jekl V. Diseases in pet guinea pigs: a retrospective study in 1000 animals. Vet Rec 2015.177(8):200.
Minarikova A, Hauptman K, Knotek Z, Jekl V. Microbial flora of odontogenic abscesses in pet guinea pigs. Vet Rec 2016;179(13):331.
Riggs SM. Guinea pigs. In: Mitchell MA, Tully TN, eds. Manual of Exotic Pet Practice. St Louis: Saunders, 2009:456–471.
Robinson NJ, Lyons E, Grindlay D, Brennan ML. Veterinarian nominated common conditions of rabbits and guinea pigs compared with published literature. Vet Sci 2017; 4(4):58.

Authors Christy L. Rettenmund, DVM, Dipl. ACZM and J. Jill Heatley, DVM, MS, Dipl. ABVP (Avian, Reptilian, Amphibian), Dipl. ACZM

BASICS

DEFINITION
• Infectious disease caused by *Clostridium piliforme*, a sporulating obligate intracellular bacterium
• Target organs are small intestines, cecum, liver, and cardiac muscle

PATHOPHYSIOLOGY
• Infected animals shed spores in the feces.
• Spores are quite hardy and can survive for over 1 year.
• Pathological changes can be noted as soon as 2 days post experimental inoculation.
• Guinea pig ingests the spores and organism invades the small intestine and cecum.
• Clinical disease is associated with poor hygiene, poor immunity, and/or stress.
• Inapparent carriers are possible based on seroconversion survey.
• Vertical transmission has been reported.

SYSTEMS AFFECTED
• Gastrointestinal system—lesions in ileum and cecum
• Hepatic
• Cardiac—myocytes can become necrotic late in the course of the disease.

SIGNALMENT
Tyzzer's disease is most commonly a disease of weanling guinea pigs.

SIGNS

Historical Findings
• All are nonspecific
• Signs often begin soon after arrival to a laboratory or pet store.
• Anorexia
• Depression and lethargy
• Owner may report the impression their pet is painful
• Diarrhea (liquid feces) is common
• Fecal staining of perineum
• Bloated abdomen
• Dyspnea
• Ventral subcutaneous edema
• Lateral recumbency indicates imminent death.
• Sudden death

Physical Examination Findings
• May present agonal or with sudden death
• Hypothermia is common and associated with circulatory shock (septic or hypovolemic)
• Dehydration may be clinically detectable.
• Subcutaneous edema has been reported.
• Perineal area and rear legs may be stained or wet from liquid feces.
• Abdominal palpation may result in painful response.

• May have palpable abdominal fluid wave due to ascites
• Dyspnea or change in character of respirations can be related to shock, metabolic acidosis, or pleural effusion.
• Agonal respirations can be seen.
• Lateral recumbency portends imminent death.

CAUSES AND RISK FACTORS
• Infection due to ingestion of spores of *Clostridium piliforme* or in utero transmission of bacteria
• Clinical illness is predisposed to by stress, poor diet (notably diets low in insoluble fiber), poor environmental hygiene, overcrowding, immunosuppression, and concurrent disease.
• Variable susceptibility to infection between individuals has been noted after oral inoculation of healthy guinea pigs.

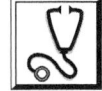

DIAGNOSIS

DIFFERENTIAL DIAGNOSIS
• Liquid diarrhea can also occur with dysbiosis and infectious enteritides.
• Bacterial enteritis can be caused by *Salmonella* species, *Yersinia pseudotuberculosis*, *Clostridium perfringens*, *E. coli*, *Pseudomonas aeruginosa*, and *Listeria monocytogenes*. Most of these enteric infections also cause morbidity and mortality in weanling guinea pigs. Some cases of Tyzzer's disease have been associated with *E. coli* or intestinal spirochetosis. The pathologic significance of this finding is unknown.
• Protozoal diarrhea can be caused by cryptosporidium and coccidia (*Eimeria caviae*). Cryptosporidiosis is more common in weanlings, but immunosuppressed animals of any age are susceptible. Acute coccidiosis is typically seen in weanlings.
• Coronaviral enteritis may occur in weanlings.
• Idiopathic typhlitis has been reported.
• Anorexia and gastrointestinal hypomotility can induce floral changes that will result in enterotoxemia.
• Anamnesis should include review of husbandry and past medical history, especially recent stressors and/or administration of antibiotics.
• Complete physical examination is an essential element in diagnosis of any cause of lethargy, weight loss, pain, or anorexia. Guinea pigs with Tyzzer's disease are usually profoundly ill due to effects of diarrhea, increased fluid accumulation in body cavities, liver damage, and perhaps septicemia.

• Most guinea pigs with Tyzzer's disease do not survive. Definitive diagnosis requires necropsy.

CBC/BIOCHEMISTRY/URINALYSIS
• There are no reports of antemortem diagnostics for this condition. Expect results to be compatible with changes due to liver damage, sepsis, and shock. Hypoalbuminemia has not been reported; however, this may be the cause of serous fluid accumulation in subcutaneous tissues and body cavities.

OTHER LABORATORY TESTS
• *C. piliforme* is difficult to isolate via culture since it is an intracellular pathogen.
• Serologic assays for *C. piliforme* have shown seroconversion in both clinically affected and clinically normal animals.

IMAGING
• Abdominal radiography is likely to demonstrate ileus and may show peritoneal effusion.
• Thoracic radiography may show microcardia due to hypovolemic shock or pleural effusion.

DIAGNOSTIC PROCEDURES
Necropsy is required for diagnostic confirmation. Intracellular bacteria are identified using Warthin-Starry or Giemsa stains.

PATHOLOGIC FINDINGS
• Gastrointestinal—gross lesions are often not present but can include edema and hemorrhage in the wall of the cecum, lower ileum, and proximal colon. Microscopically, lesions are necrotic and villi can be blunted and fused. Nests of organisms compatible with *C. piliforme* are diagnostic.
• Liver can appear mottled. Small foci of necrosis and inflammation are noted microscopically.

TREATMENT
• Successful treatment is rare. Very few patients are reported to survive despite aggressive therapy and supportive care.
• Treatment of endotoxic, septic, and/or hypovolemic shock may be required. Treatment of shock follows the same principals as in dogs and cats, including fluid support (crystalloids), intravascular osmotic support (colloids), maintenance of renal blood flow (e.g., dobutamine), and antimicrobials (IV) for sepsis.
• In the stable patient, hydration should be maintained with SC fluid administration. Maintenance in guinea pigs is estimated to be

TYZZER'S DISEASE (CONTINUED)

100 mL/kg/day. Diarrhea from clostridial infections can lead to tremendous fluid losses.
• Treatment of hypothermia with external heat source is appropriate. However, guinea pigs are obligate intranasal breathers and are prone to heat stroke. Care should be taken to avoid overheating.
• It is prudent to avoid oral food and water supplementation in the critically ill patient.
• Guinea pigs that do not eat are extremely prone to further deleterious effects of gastric hypomotility. In the stable patient, assist-syringe-feeding with an appropriate herbivore supplement such as Critical Care for Herbivores (Oxbow Pet Products, Murdock, NE) or Emeraid Herbivore (Lafeber Company, Cornell, IL) is appropriate for patients capable of receiving oral medications. Care must be taken in the dyspneic or struggling patient.
• Judicious management of pain should be considered in all patients. Guinea pigs do not deal well with pain. Failure to manage pain effectively will inhibit recovery in any ill guinea pig.

CLIENT EDUCATION
This condition carries with it a grave prognosis and is very painful. Treatment of critical patients should be considered heroic.

Euthanasia should remain a part of the discussion with the owner until the patient is stable.

SURGICAL CONSIDERATIONS
N/A

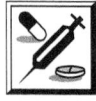

MEDICATIONS
DRUG(S) OF CHOICE
• Varies with clinical condition
• Pain should be controlled with opioids (e.g., buprenorphine 0.05 mg/kg SC, IM, IV q8–12h). Severe pain may require mu agonists (hydromorphone 0.1 mg/kg SC, IV q6–12h). NSAIDs should be avoided in face of shock, renal compromise, continuing fluid losses, and dehydration. Once stable, meloxicam (0.2–0.5 mg/kg PO, SC q12–24h) can be administered.
• Maropitant has been anecdotally used to mitigate GI pain at a dose of 1–2 mg/kg SC or slow IV q24h.
• Most antibiotics used to treat *Clostridium* spp. in other species are contraindicated in guinea pigs, due to potentially fatal enteric dysbiosis. Metronidazole (10–20 mg/kg PO, IV q12h) or doxycycline (2.5–5 mg/kg PO q12–24h) may be appropriate in guinea pigs. Long-acting injectable form of doxycyline, if available, can be attempted for animals that

cannot take oral medications. Chlortetracyline should not be used as it is a known cause of antibiotic-associated enterotoxemia.

CONTRAINDICATIONS
• Oral medications are contraindicated in shock.
• Corticosteroids at shock doses will cause immunosuppression and are contraindicated.
• Antibiotics that alter the normal gram-positive intestinal flora (beta lactams, cephalosporins, macrolides, and chlortetracycline) can cause fatal enterotoxemia.

PRECAUTIONS
Meloxicam should be avoided in patients with severe fluid losses, dehydration, shock, and renal compromise.

POSSIBLE INTERACTIONS
N/A

ALTERNATIVE DRUGS
N/A

FOLLOW-UP
PATIENT MONITORING
• Patients that are presented with liquid diarrhea are often severely ill or will become so soon.
• Critical care monitoring for inpatients as in dogs and cats should be considered with understanding of limitations of patient size.
• An end to liquid stools in the stable patient indicates improvement.
• Any pathologic changes noted on tests should be periodically evaluated for resolution (e.g., radiographs for effusions, liver enzymes, and albumin levels).

PREVENTION/AVOIDANCE
• Proper diet and environmental hygiene
• Avoid overcrowding and stressors.
• Avoid immunosuppression and administration of corticosteroids.
• Perform necropsy to identify infection as a potential cause of death of individuals in any large population of guinea pigs.

POSSIBLE COMPLICATONS
• If the patient survives the infection, gastrointestinal hypomotility is a likely sequela.
• Patients may require a prolonged course of assist feeding and hydration support.

EXPECTED COURSE AND PROGNOSIS
• Most guinea pigs will not survive this illness.

• Unstable patients usually die within hours of presentation.
• Stable patients can deteriorate and die within days.

MISCELLANEOUS
ASSOCIATED CONDITIONS
N/A

AGE-RELATED FACTORS
Weanling and young animals are at greatest risk of clinical disease.

ZOONOTIC POTENTIAL
N/A

PREGNANCY/FERTILITY/BREEDING
N/A

SYNONYMS
Bacillus piliformis infection
Clostridium piliforme infection

SEE ALSO
Diarrhea
Gastrointestinal hypomotility and gastrointestinal stasis

INTERNET RESOURCES
Veterinary Information Network (www.vin.com)

Suggested Reading
Boot R, Walvoort HC. Vertical transmission of *Bacillus piliformis* infection (Tyzzer's disease) in a guinea pig: case report. Lab Anim 1984;18:195–199.
Minarikova A, Hauptman K, Jeklova E et al. Diseases in pet guinea pigs: a retrospective study in 1000 animals. Vet Rec 2015;177(8):200–200.
Pignon C, Mayer J. Guinea pigs. In: Quesenberry KE, Carpenter JW, eds. Ferrets, Rabbits and Rodents, 4th Ed). Clinical Medicine and Surgery. 2021 ed. St. Louis: Saunders, 2020:270–297.
Ritzman TK. Diagnosis and clinical management of gastrointestinal conditions in exotic companion mammals (rabbits, guinea pigs, and chinchillas). Vet Clin Exot Anim 2014;17:179–194.
Waggie KS, Thornburg LP, Grove KJ et al. Lesions of experimentally induced Tyzzer's disease in Syrian hamsters, guinea pigs, mice and rats. Lab Anim 1987;21:155–160.
Waggie KS, Wagner JE, Kelley ST. Naturally occurring *Bacillus piliformis* infection (Tyzzer's disease) in guinea pigs. Lab Anim Sci 1986;36(5):504–506.
Author Jeffrey L. Rhody, DVM, DABVP-ECM

URINARY TRACT OBSTRUCTION

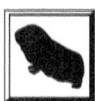

BASICS

DEFINITION
Restricted flow of urine from the kidneys through the urinary tract to the external urethral orifice

PATHOPHYSIOLOGY
• Excess resistance to urine flow through the urinary tract develops because of lesions affecting the excretory pathway, which cause increased pressure on the urinary system proximal to the obstruction and may cause abnormal distension of this space with urine.
  ○ Ensuing pathophysiologic consequences depend on the site, degree, and duration of obstruction.
  ○ Complete obstruction produces a pathophysiologic state equivalent to oliguric renal failure.
• Currently, most common cause of urinary tract obstruction in the guinea pig is calcium carbonate urolithiasis.
  ○ Calcium oxalate (historically the most common) and struvite urinary calculi have also been reported frequently.
• Factors leading to urolithiasis in guinea pigs are unclear, although the alkaline pH and high mineral content of normal guinea pig urine may favor crystal formation and precipitation.
• Bacterial urinary tract infections (involving *E. coli*, *Streptococcus pyogenes*, and *Staphylococcus* species) have been associated with the presence of urinary calculi in laboratory guinea pigs.
• Affected guinea pigs are more likely to be fed a diet high in overall percentage pellets, low in percentage hay, and less variety of vegetables and fruits. Alfalfa-based pellets and hay contain higher concentrations of calcium, and it has been suggested this may also contribute to urinary calculi in guinea pigs.
• Inadequate water intake leading to a more concentrated urine and factors that impair complete evacuation of the bladder, such as lack of exercise, obesity, cystitis, neoplasia, or neuromuscular diseases may be involved. Without frequent urination and dilute urine, calcium crystals may precipitate out from the urine within the bladder. Precipitated crystals primarily form uroliths but occasionally cause "urinary sludge" instead.
• Uroliths may also form in the kidneys or ureters as well as the bladder.

SYSTEMS AFFECTED
• Renal/Urologic
• Gastrointestinal, neuromuscular, and cardiovascular systems may all be affected in patients with uremia.

GENETICS
While suspected, inherited factors associated with this disease have not been proven.

INCIDENCE/PREVALENCE
Commonly affects middle-aged to older guinea pigs

GEOGRAPHIC DISTRIBUTION
N/A

SIGNALMENT

Breed Predilections
It has been suggested that Peruvian guinea pigs are more susceptible to urolithiasis, however, has not been proven.

Mean Age and Range
Middle-aged (2.5 years or older)

Predominant Sex
A recent study of 75 guinea pigs with urolithiasis found an equal distribution of males and females.

SIGNS

Historical Findings
• Pollakiuria (common) or stranguria; evidence of urine retention
• Gross hematuria—common in guinea pigs with urolithiasis
• Hunched posture, vocalizing during urination may be associated with pain
• Abnormal posture, ataxia, or difficulty ambulating in guinea pigs with musculoskeletal or neurological disease
• Urine scald, moist pyoderma
• Signs of uremia that develop when urinary tract obstruction is complete (or nearly complete)—anorexia, weight loss, lethargy, bruxism, tenesmus, and hunched posture

Physical Examination Findings
• Large, turgid bladder (or inappropriate size remains after voiding efforts) upon palpation of the urinary bladder
  ○ Maybe painful on abdominal palpation
• Manual expression of the bladder may reveal hematuria or sometimes "sludge" (thick white-tan material), even in patients that have normal-appearing voided urine.
• May detect cystoliths on palpation, but not always palpable
• A large kidney may be palpable if a nephrolith is present.
• Hematuria, stranguria, or pollakiuria may be observable
• Signs of uremia—dehydration, anorexia, lethargy, weakness, hypothermia, bradycardia, high rate or shallow respirations, stupor, or coma; seizures occur rarely, often in terminal cases, tachycardia resulting from ventricular dysrhythmias induced by hyperkalemia
• Thick, palpable uterus may be found if pyometra; pups may be palpable if dystocia is the cause

CAUSES

Intraluminal Causes
• Solid or semi-solid structures, especially calcium carbonate uroliths or precipitated calcium; abscess material, blood clots, sloughed soft tissue fragments

Intramural Causes
• Neoplasia of urethra, bladder neck—rare
• Fibrosis at site of injury can cause stenosis or stricture, which can impede urine flow or may be a site where intraluminal materials become lodged.
• Ruptures, lacerations, and punctures most commonly caused by traumatic incidents
• Renal/Urologic: bacterial cystitis, pyelonephritis, nephritis; urolithiasis

Extramural Causes
Reproductive: pyometra, vaginitis, urine scald, dystocia
  Neoplasia—lymphoma in abdomen causing pressure on the urinary tract

Risk Factors Contributing to Urolithiasis and Calcium "Sludge" in the Bladder
• Inadequate water intake—dirty water bowls, unpalatable water, inadequate water provision, and changing water sources
• Urine retention—underlying bladder pathology, neuromuscular disease; painful conditions causing a reluctance to ambulate, such as musculoskeletal disease (pododermatitis, arthritis) or dental disease
• Inadequate cage cleaning may cause some guinea pigs to avoid urinating.
• Obesity has been suggested as a cause but has not yet been proven.
• Lack of exercise
• Feeding exclusively alfalfa-based diet (hay, pellets or both)
• Renal disease
• Calcium or vitamin/mineral supplements added to diet

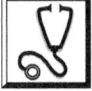

DIAGNOSIS

DIFFERENTIAL DIAGNOSIS
• Neoplasia—renal/urologic or abdominal tumors causing pressure on the urinary tract; lymphosarcoma most commonly reported; differentiate with imaging and biopsy as warranted
• Dystocia, pyometra—history and physical examination findings
• Trauma—history and physical examination findings of trauma

CBC/BIOCHEMISTRY/URINALYSIS
• Hemogram—TWBC elevations with neutrophil:lymphocyte ratio shift; toxicity of neutrophils ± bands, monocytosis may suggest

URINARY TRACT OBSTRUCTION

inflammation/infection; thrombocytosis associated with active inflammation
• Biochemistry panel—lower urinary tract disease complicated by urethral obstruction may be associated with azotemia. With complete (or nearly complete) obstruction, changes in electrolytes such as hyperkalemia, hypochloremia, and hyponatremia may occur.
• Urinalysis including both a standard dipstick and microscopic examination of the sediment. Urinalyses data from 44 guinea pigs with urinary calculi found that the mean ± SD urine specific gravity was 1.015 ± 0.008 (range 1.004–1.046) and urine pH was 8.4 ± 0.5 (range 7.5–>9.0).
  ◦ Hematuria was the most commonly reported abnormality on urine sediment, followed by mucus and lipid droplets.
• Calcium carbonate, calcium oxalate, and struvite crystals are all commonly seen on sediment examinations, but similar to other small animals, crystal type(s) may not predict the mineralogy of calculi present.

OTHER LABORATORY TESTS
• Prior to antibiotic use, culture the urine or bladder wall if high numbers of red or white blood cells, bacteria, or a combination of these are present on sediment examination. Collect urine via cystocentesis as free-catch samples are commonly contaminated.
• If surgery is necessary to relieve obstruction from urolithiasis, collect and submit the calculi for analysis and culture and sensitivity, and submit the bladder wall for culture and sensitivity.
  ◦ Calculi-containing calcium carbonate require specific methodologies to differentiate from calcium oxalate monohydrate crystals; the laboratory chosen for analysis must be able to perform these methods. Confirm the lab's ability to perform these techniques in advance, since human and some veterinary laboratories unfamiliar with exotic animal samples do not differentiate calcium oxalate from calcium carbonate.

IMAGING
• Be certain to include the perineal region in both radiographic views. Obstructive calculi are most commonly located in the distal urethra of both males and females but are also reported in the kidneys, ureters, vagina, or sometimes in the seminal vesicles.
• Urinary calculi in guinea pigs are generally radio-opaque allowing for ease of identification using survey radiography.
  ◦ However, if multiple calculi or significant GI gas are present, the anatomic locations of the calculi using survey radiography alone may be obscured.
• Ultrasound is useful for anatomic location of the calculi and for evaluating anatomic

changes in the kidneys or ureters, such as hydronephrosis or hydroureter, ureteral mucosal inflammation, or perforation.
• Excretory intravenous pyelograms (IVPs) are useful to further elucidate relative functional abnormalities in the kidneys or ureters.
• CT and MRI imaging are useful modalities for diagnosing calculi and assessing organ architecture, more rapidly than IVP and uses significantly less contrast medium.

DIAGNOSTIC PROCEDURES
• Urethral endoscopy can be performed to identify the location of the calculi if present in this region. Cystoscopy can also be performed through a surgical incision into the bladder to attempt to identify the location of calculi within the proximal neck of the bladder.

PATHOLOGIC FINDINGS
On gross examination, urinary calculi can vary in size from sand like to large concentric stones. Tissue changes may vary from thickening of the urethra, bladder, or ureteral mucosa with congestion in more chronic cases to intramural and/or intraluminal hemorrhage. Perforations of the ureter in particular can be identified with chronic, complete obstructions. Microscopic changes seen in acute cases there may be ulceration, hemorrhage, and infiltration with heterophils.
  Chronic cases are characterized by infiltration of leukocytes and mononuclear cells in the lamina propria, and occasionally fibroblast proliferation.

TREATMENT
APPROPRIATE HEALTH CARE
• Treatment has three major components: combating the metabolic derangements associated with postrenal uremia; restoring and maintaining a patent pathway for urine outflow; and implementing a specific treatment for the underlying cause of urine retention.
• Medical treatment of urolithiasis in guinea pigs has been unrewarding to date, and surgical removal of the calculi is most often required.
• Complete obstruction is a medical emergency that can be life threatening. Guinea pigs with urinary obstruction should be hospitalized, and emergency supportive therapy should be provided until surgical intervention to relieve the obstruction can be performed.
• Partial obstruction may or may not be an emergency, but these patients may be at

greater risk for complete obstruction; may cause irreversible urinary tract damage if not treated promptly.
• Treat as inpatient until the patient's ability to urinate has been restored.

NURSING CARE
• Fluid therapy should be initiated in patients with evidence of dehydration, azotemia, and electrolyte imbalances. Subcutaneous fluids can be administered (50 mL/kg) as needed. IV access is difficult in the guinea pig; lateral saphenous vein catheters often kink; consider IO catheterization if intravascular fluids are needed. Maintenance fluid needs are estimated at 100 mL/kg/day. Fluid therapy should be based on treatment modalities used in cats with obstructive urinary disease.
• In females, gentle flushing of the urethral calculi back into the bladder can be attempted. Gently flush the bladder using a 3.5 Fr red rubber catheter under deep sedation and analgesia to attempt to remove the calculi.
• Catheterizing boars is much more dangerous due to the small size of the urethra; successful retropulsion of a urolith back into the bladder is unlikely.
• In females, calculi are commonly found in the distal urethra, near the urethral orifice. Some may be removed manually via the distal urethral opening. After sedation, the urethral opening can be dilated by use of a Lone Star Retractor System® (CooperSurgical, Inc. Trumbull, CT) and the stone removed with hemostats.

ACTIVITY
• Reduced during the time of tissue repair after surgery
• Long term—increase activity level by providing large exercise areas to encourage voiding and prevent recurrence.

DIET
• Many guinea pigs with urinary tract obstruction are anorectic or have decreased appetite. It is an absolute requirement that the patient continue to eat during and following treatments. Anorexia may cause or exacerbate gastrointestinal hypomotility and cause derangement of the gastrointestinal microflora with overgrowth of intestinal bacterial pathogens.
• Offer a large selection of fresh, moist greens such as cilantro, lettuce, parsley, carrot tops, dark leafy greens, and good-quality grass hay.
• If the patient refuses these foods, syringe feed Critical Care for Herbivores (Oxbow Pet Products, Murdock, NE) or Emeraid Herbivore (Lafeber Company, Cornell, IL) at approximately 10–15 mL/kg PO q6–8h. Larger volumes and more frequent feedings are often accepted; feed as much as the

patient will readily accept. Alternatively, pellets can be ground and mixed with fresh greens, vegetable baby foods, water, or sugar-free juice to form a gruel.
• Guinea pigs have an absolute requirement for exogenous vitamin C. Provide 50–100 mg/kg/day vitamin C while hospitalized, and during recovery. Vitamin C can be provided through food sources such as citrus fruits and through commercially made guinea pig pellets, oral supplements, or as a subcutaneous injection.

CLIENT EDUCATION
• Surgical removal of urinary tract obstructions does not alter the causes responsible for their formation; limiting risk factors such as obesity, sedentary life, and inappropriate diet combined with increasing water consumption is necessary to minimize or delay recurrence. Even with these changes, however, recurrence is likely.

SURGICAL CONSIDERATIONS
• Surgery is necessary to relieve obstructions if medical attempts are unsuccessful. Submit the calculi for analysis and culture and submit the bladder wall for culture and sensitivity.
• Calculi located within the penile urethra or near the urethral opening in females can be removed via urethostomy by making a longitudinal incision over the calculus. The incision is left open to heal by second intention.
• Postoperative management includes assisted feeding, fluids, analgesics, and antibiotics based on culture and sensitivity results. However, recurrence of the disease is common.

MEDICATIONS
DRUG(S) OF CHOICE
• Medical dissolution of calcium-based uroliths is ineffective in guinea pigs.
• Pain management is essential during and following surgery or if pain is causing reduced frequency of voiding. Perioperative analgesic choices include butorphanol (0.4–2.0 mg/kg SC, IM q4–12h) and buprenorphine (0.05–0.2 mg/kg SC, IM, IV q6–8h). Meloxicam (0.5–1.0 mg/kg PO, SC, IM q24h) and carprofen (4 mg/kg SC q24h or 1–2 mg/kg PO q12h) provide anti-inflammation as well as analgesia. Tramadol, a synthetic opioid, may also be an effective at dosages of 5–10 mg/kg PO q12h postoperatively. For severe to moderate pain, pure mu opioids such as morphine (0.5–2.0 mg/kg SC, IM q2–4h) or oxymorphone (0.2–0.5 mg/kg SC, IM

q6–12h) should be used; however, appetite and fecal output should be monitored as these opioids are thought to contribute to GI ileus.
• Procedures for relief of obstruction generally require administering sedatives and/or anesthetics. When substantial derangements exist, begin with fluid administration and other supportive measures first. Calculate the dosage of sedative or anesthetic drug using the low end of the recommended range or give only to effect.
• Antibiotic choice should be based upon the results of culture and sensitivity (see Contraindications). Antibiotics commonly used included trimethoprim sulfa (15–30 mg/kg PO q12h), chloramphenicol (30–50 mg/kg PO, SC, IM, IV q8–12h), metronidazole (10–20 mg/kg PO, IV q12h), and enrofloxacin (5–15 mg/kg PO, SC, IM q12h—this is a basic drug and should be diluted or injected into a subcutaneous fluid pocket to prevent tissue injury) {Should be reserved for microbes that are resistant to tier one antibiotics}.

CONTRAINDICATIONS
• Oral administration of antibiotics that select against gram-positive bacteria (penicillins, cephalosporins, macrolides, and lincosamides) can cause fatal enteric dysbiosis and enterotoxemia.
• Potentially nephrotoxic drugs (e.g., aminoglycosides, NSAIDs) in patients that are febrile, dehydrated, or azotemic or that are suspected of having pyelonephritis, septicemia, or preexisting renal disease
• Glucocorticoids or other immunosuppressive agents

PRECAUTIONS
• Avoid drugs that reduce blood pressure or induce cardiac dysrhythmia until dehydration is resolved.
• Modify dosages of all drugs that require renal metabolism or elimination.
• Avoid nephrotoxic drugs (NSAIDs, aminoglycosides).

POSSIBLE INTERACTIONS
None

ALTERNATIVE DRUGS
N/A

FOLLOW-UP
PATIENT MONITORING
• Ensure gastrointestinal motility by making sure the patient is eating, well hydrated, and passing normal feces prior to release.
• Assess urine production and hydration status frequently, adjusting fluid administration rate accordingly.

• Verify the ability to urinate adequately; failure to do so may require urinary catheterization to combat urine retention, or cystocentesis.

PREVENTION/AVOIDANCE
• Prevention is targeted at increasing water intake and reducing (but not eliminating) dietary calcium. Metabolic bone disease has been induced in guinea pigs with severe dietary calcium restriction for prevention of urinary calculi. For most animals, water consumption is the cornerstone to any prevention protocol.
• Avoid alfalfa-based diets. Diets containing a high percentage of timothy, oat, or grass hays, a lower overall percentage pellets, and a wider variety of vegetables and fruits decrease the risk of urolith development. It is possible that dietary inhibitors of calcium are found in greater concentration in hays than in pellets.
• There are no reports of dissolution of calcium carbonate urolithiasis with special diets.
• Hydrochlorothiazide (2 mg/kg q12h) is a thiazide diuretic that reduces urinary Ca^{2+}, K^+, and citrate. It is unknown if diuresis would be of benefit to guinea pigs whose urine is already considered isosthenuric. Do not use hydrochlorothiazide with severe renal disease or fluid imbalances.
• Urinary acidifiers were historically recommended based upon an assumed diagnosis of calcium oxalate calculi, but the normally alkaline urine of guinea pigs makes the use of dietary acidifiers concerning. Potassium citrate (10–30 mg/kg PO q12h) binds urinary Ca^{2+}, reduces ion activity, and alkalinizes the urine. As guinea pigs have alkaline urine even with disease, the efficacy of this treatment is unclear. Hyperkalemia occurs, so monitor plasma K^+ closely during treatment. Potassium citrate and hydrochlorothiazide have been used together anecdotally with some clinical success.

POSSIBLE COMPLICATIONS
• Severe electrolyte imbalances, uremia with complete obstruction
• Urine scald
• Failure to detect or treat effectively may lead to pyelonephritis
• Pododermatitis

EXPECTED COURSE AND PROGNOSIS
• The prognosis following surgical removal of uroliths is fair to good, but recurrence is common, and although dietary management may decrease the likelihood of recurrence, many guinea pigs will develop clinical disease again.

URINARY TRACT OBSTRUCTION (CONTINUED)

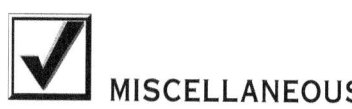

MISCELLANEOUS

ASSOCIATED CONDITIONS
- Urinary tract infections
- Vaginitis, pyometra from ascending bacterial infection of the lower urinary tract

AGE-RELATED FACTORS
This disease is frequently found in middle-aged to older guinea pigs, although it can occur in younger animals as well.

ZOONOTIC POTENTIAL
N/A

PREGNANCY/FERTILITY/BREEDING
While there is no documented evidence that urolithiasis has a hereditary component, it is generally recommended to avoid breeding these animals in the future.

SYNONYMS
Urolithiasis

SEE ALSO
Dysuria, hematuria, and pollakiuria
Lower urinary tract infection

ABBREVIATIONS
CT = computed tomography
MRI = magnetic resonance imaging
IVP = intravenous pyelogram
NSAID = nonsteroidal anti-inflammatory drug
RBC = red blood cells
TWBC = total white blood cell count

INTERNET RESOURCES
N/A

Suggested Reading
Hallman RM, Brandão J. Diagnostic imaging of the renal system in exotic companion mammals. Vet Clin Exot Anim 2020;23:195–214.
Hawkins MG, Ruby AL, Drazenovich TL et al. Composition and characteristics of urinary calculi from guinea pigs. J Amer Vet Med Assoc 2009;234:214–220.
Hoefer H, Latney L. Rodents: urogenital and reproductive disorders. In: Keeble E, Meredith A, eds. BSAVA Manual of Rodents and Ferrets. Gloucester: BSAVA, 2009:150–160.
Miwa Y, Sladky K. Common surgical procedures of rodents, ferrets, hedgehogs, and sugar gliders. Vet Clin Exot Anim 2016;19:205–244.
Percy D, Barthold S. Guinea pig. In: Percy D, Barthold S, eds. Pathology of Laboratory Rodents and Rabbits. Ames: Blackwell, 2001:209–247.
Pignon C, Mayer J. Guinea pigs. In: Quesenberry KE, Carpenter JW, eds. Ferrets, Rabbits and Rodents, 4th Ed). Clinical Medicine and Surgery. 2021 ed. St. Louis: Saunders, 2020:270–297.
Reavill D, Lennox A. Disease overview of the urinary tract in exotic companion mammals and tips on clinical management. Vet Clin Exot Anim 2020;23:169–193.
Author Rodney Schnellbacher, DVM, Dipl. ACZM

VAGINAL DISCHARGE

BASICS

DEFINITION
• Any substance emanating from the vulvar labia
  ◦ Abnormal discharge can be purulent, hemorrhagic, or serosanguineous.
  ◦ Normal discharge occurs at the time of copulation and post copulation
    ◦ During copulation the vagina is filled with a clear foamy mucus.
    ◦ Following copulation, a waxy vaginal plug forms.

PATHOPHYSIOLOGY
• Discharge may originate from multiple sources because several systems eliminate through the vagina—uterus, urinary tract, vagina, vestibule, or perivulvar skin.
  ◦ Endometrial disorders can result in mild vaginal discharge to uterine hemorrhage.
  ◦ Endometrial secretions provide excellent media for bacterial growth; bacteria ascend from the vagina through the cervix and can lead to purulent discharge—see chapter on pyometra
  ◦ Mid- and late-term abortion results in significant uterine hemorrhage.
  ◦ Dystocia will result in serosanguineous discharge—see chapter on dystocia
  ◦ Cystitis can cause hematuria—see chapter on dysuria, hematuria, and pollakiuria
  ◦ Impaction of bedding material in the vaginal vestibule may cause vaginitis;
• The normal vaginal or copulatory plug forms immediately after breeding and is expelled from the vagina several hours after mating. The plug is formed from seminal fluids and becomes enclosed within a cover of epithelial cells sloughed from the vaginal wall.

SYSTEMS AFFECTED
• Urogenital
• Skin

GENETICS
N/A

INCIDENCE/PREVALENCE
• Uterine disorders, including hyperplasia and neoplasia, have an incidence of over 77% in sows >6 years old.
• Ovarian cysts are seen in >75% of sows >6 years of age
• Uterine inflammation is most common in younger sows, age 7–24 months.

GEOGRAPHIC DISTRIBUTION
N/A

SIGNALMENT
• Intact females both breeding and nonbreeding
• Spayed females with vaginitis

Breed Predilections
N/A

Mean Age and Range
Uterine inflammation is seen in younger sows, under 2 years, whereas hyperplasia and neoplasia are seen in older sows, with a >75% incidence in those over 6 years of age.

Predominant Sex
Sows only

SIGNS

Historical Findings
• Early phases of disease may have no clinical signs.
• Hematuria is the most common presenting complaint because blood originating from the uterus gets mixed with the urine upon micturition. Frank blood is often noted at the end of micturition and can be intermittent or cyclic.
  ◦ True hematuria due to cystitis is easy to distinguish because entire stream of urine is bloody
• Vaginal discharge or perineal staining
• Polydypsia and polyuria may be seen with chronic pyometra.
• Pyometra—may have signs of systemic illness, progressing to septcemia and shock
• Breeding sows with a history of small litter size, increased number of stillborn or resorbed fetuses, mid- or late-term abortion, infertility, dystocia, or abandonment of pups may have endometritis and intermittent vaginal discharge.
• Cystic ovaries can affect the uterus with concurrent cystic endometrial hyperplasia, mucometra, endometritis in appropriate placental tissue, or neoplasia
• Failure to become pregnant
• Normal discharge occurrence post breeding

Physical Examination Findings
• Serosanguineous to purulent vaginal discharge
• Perineal staining
• Lethargy
• Anorexia
• Abdominal swelling
• Palpable large uterus
• Fever
• Mammary gland enlargement may be firm or fluid filled.
• Mastitis may be present.
• Mammary tumors may or may not be present.
• Pale mucous membranes, tachycardia if significant blood loss
• Pyometra, sow may be in shock and/or recumbent

CAUSES
• Impacted bedding in perineal folds or perivulvar dermatitis can occur due to poor husbandry.
• Common bacteria reported in pyometra—*Bordetella bronchiseptica*, *Streptococcus* spp. (especially hemolytic *Streptococcus*), *Corynebacterium pyogenes*, *Staphylococcus aureus*, *E. coli*, *Chlamydophila*, *Arcanobacterium pyogenes*, and *Salmonella*
• Cystic ovaries are common in guinea pigs and often concurrent with cystic endometrial hyperplasia, mucometra, endometritis in appropriate placental tissue, or leiomyomas
• Cystitis—see chapter dysuria, hematuria, and pollakiuria
• Breeding

RISK FACTORS
• Intact sexual status
• Risk increases with age greater than 18 months
• Risk increases with sterile mating or sows mounting each other

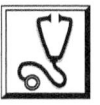

DIAGNOSIS

DIFFERENTIAL DIAGNOSIS
• Normal breeding vaginal discharge or plug
• Pregnancy
• Dystocia or abortion
• Uterine neoplasia
• Perivulvar dermatitis—bedding or feces impacted in the perineal folds
• Hematuria—use ultrasound-guided cystocentesis to collect urine; differentiates true hematuria from blood expelled from the uterus
• Serosanguineous or purulent discharge frequent with pyometra, endometritis, or vaginitis

CBC/BIOCHEMISTRY/URINALYSIS
• CBC—TWBC may be normal, or if sow is septic there may be heterophilia and toxic changes in the heterophils.
• If uterine hemorrhage has occurred there may be regenerative or nonregenerative anemia.
• Increase percentage of Kurloff cells with cystic ovaries
• Thrombocytosis occurs with acute inflammation.
• Biochemistry panel—azotemia with severe dehydration; elevated BUN, ALT, GGT with sepsis
• Electrolytes and blood gases: metabolic acidosis, hyperkalemia, hyponatremia, and hypochloremia
• Urinalysis collected by ultrasound-guided cystocentesis—lack of hematuria or leukocytes confirms source of hemorrhage

and/or inflammation is more likely uterine or vaginal
• Urinalysis—aciduria (pH 5–6), proteinuria, and ketonuria with sepsis from pyometra

OTHER LABORATORY TESTS
• Cytology of vaginal discharge—lack of neoplastic cells and presence of polymorphonuclear cells and bacteria
• Culture and sensitivity of uterine endometrial or purulent discharge or from contents obtained during OVH to direct antibiotic therapy
• Histopathologic examination of uterus following OVH for definitive diagnosis. Neoplasia may be an underlying cause of pyometra.

IMAGING
Radiography
• Large soft tissue opacity consisting of the uterus in the caudal abdomen can be associated with dystocia, abortion, endometritis, and pyometra.
• If discharge is associated with abortion, in last trimester (approximately 6 weeks of gestation) detect presence of fetal calcification.
• Most common uterine neoplastic disorders are leiomyoma, ademomas, and leiomyosarcomas. Tumors rarely metastasize (less than 10% incidence of metastasis, primarily to the lungs, has been reported); however, thoracic radiographs should be considered.

Ultrasonography
• Assess the size of the uterus and nature of the uterine contents
• Neoplasia usually confined to uterine horn. Fine-needle aspiration for cytology and assess for cystic ovarian changes
• Rule out pregnancy
• Guided cystocentesis to rule out true hematuria

DIAGNOSTIC PROCEDURES
• Diagnosis can be made by signalment and clinical signs, but it may be difficult to differentiate which form of uterine disorder is present.
• Neoplasia often not ruled out until histopathology of uterus is completed
• Vaginal cytology

PATHOLOGIC FINDINGS
• Gross lesions may include reduced gastric content, enlarged tan liver if hepatic lipidosis has occurred, adrenomegaly, excessive body fat, or dead fetuses.
• When ovariohysterectomy is treatment of choice, histological exam will differentiate endometritis or pyometra versus cystic endometical hyperplasia and neoplasia.

• Cystic rete ovarii often concomitant with endometritis, cytstic endometrial hyperplasia and leiomyoma.

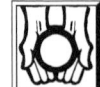

TREATMENT
APPROPRIATE HEALTH CARE
• Fluid therapy is used to correct abnormalities in volume, electrolytes, and acid–base status.
  ◦ Caution must be made not to exacerbate a concurrent anemia.
• In cases of pyometra and sepsis, antimicrobial therapy should be initiated immediately (culture and sensitivity should be obtained).
  ◦ Intravenous administration is recommended if a catheter is in place.
• OVH is the treatment of choice for any uterine abnormalities.
• Endometrial disorders may be associated with endocrine changes associated with cystic ovaries, which can be treated with hormone therapy or surgical removal
• Vaginitis requires 10–14 days of antibiotics based on culture and sensitivity as well as 5–7 days of NSAIDs to reduce inflammation.
• Analgesia is indicated with surgery or disorders causing inflammation or pain.

NURSING CARE
• Immediate therapy includes subcutaneous fluids (100 mL/kg) while preparing to place IV or IO catheter
• IV access is difficult in the guinea pig, especially if hypotensive; lateral saphenous vein catheters often kink; consider IO catheterization of the femur for intravascular fluids. Base fluid selection on evidence of dehydration, acid–base, and electrolyte imbalances. Administer colloids with crystalloids if sow is hypotensive.
• Anorexia is a nonspecific sign that can be life threatening in the guinea pig and must be addressed with forced feeding, especially in the perioperative period. If the guinea pig was anorexic prior to treatment and OVH, then forced feeding is often required for days to weeks in the postoperative period.

ACTIVITY
Minimize stress

DIET
• It is an absolute requirement that sows continue to eat and to avoid sudden dietary changes.
• In addition to pellets, offer a large selection of good-quality grass hay plus fresh, moist greens such as cilantro, parsley, carrot tops, and dark leafy greens.
• If the sow stops eating, syringe-feed Critical Care for Herbivores (Oxbow Animal Health, Murdock, ME) at approximately 26 grams of dry product per kg body weight per day. Dry product is mixed with approximately twice the volume of water and is fed in small portions every 6–8 hours. Larger volumes and more frequent feedings are often accepted; feed as much as the sow will readily accept. Alternatively, pellets can be ground and mixed with fresh greens, vegetable baby foods, water, or sugar-free juice to form a gruel.
• Fresh water needs to be available at all times.

CLIENT EDUCATION
• OVH is the treatment of choice for most uterine disorders; medical treatment is usually insufficient to resolve the infection.
• Antibiotic therapy is indicated in the perioperative period, and the guinea pig needs to be monitored for signs of dysbiosis (soft stools, diarrhea, and sudden change in appetite).
• Analgesia is indicated in any disorder causing inflammation or pain.

SURGICAL CONSIDERATIONS
• OVH is recommended if source of vaginal discharge is determined to be uterine.
• Enlarged uterus may be friable, adhesions may accompany pyometra
• Remove the entire cervix to maximize removal of infected and inflamed tissue
• Minimize tissue handling and keep tissues moist during surgery to minimize adhesions.
• Consider use of hemoclips to reduce tissue handling and adhesion formation.
• Use subcuticular sutures to minimize irritation of the incision because abdomen often is in contact with the cage floor.
• Lavage the abdominal cavity if any leakage of the infected uterus occurs.
• Postoperative management includes assisted feeding, fluids, analgesics, and antibiotics.

MEDICATIONS
DRUG(S) OF CHOICE
• Antibiotics will be administered empirically pending results of culture and sensitivity. Pending sensitivity results, use broad-spectrum antibiotics such as trimethoprim-sulfa, chloramphenicol, and enrofloxacin (should be reserved for microbes that are resistant to tier one antibiotics).
• Pain management is essential during and following surgery. Multimodal therapy is recommended for perioperative analgesia with an anxiolytic, such as midazolam (0.4–2.0 mg/kg IM), an opioid such as butorphanol (0.4–2.0 mg/kg SC, IM q4–12h), or buprenorphine (0.05–0.2 mg/kg

SC, IM, IV q6–8h). An NSAID such as meloxicam (0.5–1 mg/kg PO, SC, IM q24h) or carprofen (4 mg/kg SC q24h or 1–2 mg/kg PO q12h) can be given in the perioperative period when the animal is fully hydrated and renal perfusion is no longer compromised. Tramadol, a synthetic opioid, may also be an effective at dosages of 5–10 mg/kg PO q12h postoperatively.

CONTRAINDICATIONS

• Oral administration of antibiotics that select against gram-positive bacteria (penicillins, cephalosporins, macrolides, and lincosamides) can cause fatal enteric dysbiosis and enterotoxemia.
• NSAIDs are contraindicated in sows that are febrile, dehydrated, or azotemic or that are suspected of having pyelonephritis, septicemia, or preexisting renal disease.

PRECAUTIONS

• During surgery, avoid excessive handling of gastrointestinal tissues to reduce postoperative ileus or fibrous adhesions.
• Chloramphenicol—avoid human contact with chloramphenicol due to potential blood dyscrasia. Advise owners of potential risks.

POSSIBLE INTERACTIONS

None

ALTERNATIVE DRUGS

N/A

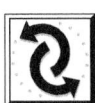

FOLLOW-UP

PATIENT MONITORING

• Ensure gastrointestinal motility by making sure the patient is eating, well hydrated, and passing normal feces prior to release from hospitalization.
• Follow-up examination should be performed within 5–7 days of discharge from hospital, or sooner if the sow does not return to eating.
• Monitor for signs of pain (hunched posture, teeth grinding, and reluctance to move). Remote observation is most reliable.

• Clean bedding is critical because region of abdominal incision is usually in contact with cage floor.
• Vaginitis can recur or progress to endometritis or pyometra if not properly treated. Follow-up examination within 2 weeks after course of treatment.

PREVENTION/AVOIDANCE

Discontinue breeding of the sow when older than 3–4 years.

POSSIBLE COMPLICATIONS

• Peritonitis and sepsis in sows with endometritis or pyometra
• Postoperative adhesions may lead to chronic gastrointestinal motility disorders or pain.

EXPECTED COURSE AND PROGNOSIS

• Good prognosis if uterine infections or abortion are detected early and addressed with timely OVH
• Guarded prognosis if sow is septic or has been experiencing prolonged anorexia prior to examination
• Good prognosis for perineal dermatitis

MISCELLANEOUS

ASSOCIATED CONDITIONS

• Uterine neoplasia
• Cystic ovaries
• Mastitis

AGE-RELATED FACTORS

Risk increases with age

ZOONOTIC POTENTIAL

N/A

PREGNANCY/FERTILITY/BREEDING

N/A

SYNONYMS

None

SEE ALSO

ABBREVIATIONS

ALT = alanine aminotransferase

BUN = blood urea nitrogen
GGT = gamma glutamyl transferase
NSAIDS = nonsteroidal anti-inflammatory drugs
OVH = ovariohysterectomy
TWBC = total white blood cell count

INTERNET RESOURCES

N/A

Suggested Reading
Bertram CA, Muller K, Klopfleisch R. Genital tract pathology in female pet guinea pigs (*Cavia porcellus*): a retrospective study of 655 post-mortem and 64 biopsy cases. J Comp Path 2018;164:12–22.
Bishop CR. Reproductive medicine of rabbits and rodents. Vet Clin North Am Exot Anim Pract 2002;5:507–535.
Hoefer H, Latney L. Rodents: urogenital and reproductive disorders. In: Keeble E, Meredith A, eds. BSAVA Manual of Rodents and Ferrets. Gloucester: BSAVA, 2009:150–160.
Laik-Schandelmaier C, Klopfleisch R, Schöniger S et al. Spontaneously arising tumours and tumour-like lesions of the cervix and uterus in 83 pet guinea pigs (*Cavia porcellus*). J Comp Path 2017;156:339–351.
Minarikova A, Hauptman K, Jeklova E et al. Diseases in pet guinea pigs: a retrospective study in 1000 animals. Vet Rec. 2015;177(8):200.
Miwa Y, Sladky K. Common surgical procedures of rodents, ferrets, hedgehogs, and sugar gliders. Vet Clin Exot Anim 2016;19:205–244.
Pignon C, Mayer J. Guinea pigs. In: Quesenberry KE, Carpenter JW, eds. Ferrets, Rabbits and Rodents, 4th Ed). Clinical Medicine and Surgery. 2021 ed. St. Louis: Saunders, 2020:270–297.
Veiga-Parga T, LaPerle KM, Newman SJ. Spontaneous reproductive pathology in female guinea pigs. J Vet Diag Invest 2016;28(6):656–661.

Author Rodney Schnellbacher, DVM, Dipl. ACZM

WEIGHT LOSS AND CACHEXIA

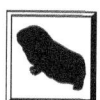

BASICS

DEFINITION
• Weight loss is considered significant when it reaches 10% of the normal body weight.
• Cachexia is a complex metabolic syndrome defined as generalized wasting and loss of body mass that is usually associated with a chronic disease process and is often not reversible by increasing caloric intake alone.
• Cachexia is not the same as starvation; in a state of starvation the body is able to slow down metabolism to compensate for the loss of nutrients; with cachexia the rate of calorie consumption by the body is normal or increased.
• Malnutrition is the earliest stage of cachexia.

PATHOPHYSIOLOGY
• In a normal physiologic state, the CNS aids in maintaining body weight by balancing hunger and satiety.
• Weight loss can occur via one of three primary mechanisms: insufficient caloric intake, increased metabolic demand, or excessive loss or malabsorption of nutrients.
• During serious illness, there is an increase in catabolism and nitrogen loss created by the underlying pathology. Normal caloric intake is insufficient to compensate for these changes.

SYSTEMS AFFECTED
• Ultimately, all body systems are affected.
• The initial body systems affected may be indicative of the underlying disease process.

SIGNALMENT
There are no breed, age, or sex predilections.

SIGNS
Historical Findings
• Initial clinical signs may be associated with the underlying disease.
• There is a difference between appetite and food intake. Owners may report that the guinea pig shows interest in food, or spends a long time at the food bowl, but is actually consuming less food than normal.
• Drooling may be present.
• Small, firm feces or diarrhea may be identified by the owner.
• It is imperative to clarify whether appetite and food intake are normal, increased, or decreased and whether fecal output is normal, increased, or decreased. Many owners may not recognize decrease in food intake if multiple guinea pigs are housed in one enclosure.

• There may be a history of changes in brand or type of food offered; it is important to discern this piece of information if not volunteered by the owner.

Physical Examination Findings
• There will be loss of epaxial musculature as well as overall loss of body mass.
• Other physical examination findings are generally related to the underlying disease process.
• With hyperthyroidism: mass or swelling of the thyroid gland. In the guinea pig, the thyroid glands are more cranial than most companion animals. Lumps can often be found between the mandibular rami. Masses are sometimes cystic and appear as very large, fluid filled subcutaneous swellings. Tachycardia, heart murmur, is common.
• Oral evaluation may reveal overgrown incisor teeth, overgrown or maloccluded cheek teeth, tongue entrapment by cheek teeth, oral ulcers, or abscesses.
• Examination of the face and head may reveal cervical abscesses, facial swellings, ocular or nasal discharge, exudate in the ear canals, pain on palpation of the bullae or jaw, or facial nerve paralysis (all dependent on and reflective of the underlying etiology).
• Gastric distention/bloat or decreased gastrointestinal sounds may be present, as hypomotility may be a primary or secondary problem.
• Urine staining of the legs or difficulty urinating may be present.
• Pododermatitis may be found on one or multiple feet due to lack of movement.
• Perform a comprehensive physical examination to evaluate for the presence of any underlying disease.

CAUSES
Insufficient Calorie Intake
Dietary causes
• Competition for food from other guinea pigs in the same enclosure—may not be recognized by the owners
• Poor nutritional quality of food or inappropriate diet
• Food deprivation
• Insufficient hay and fiber and excessive simple carbohydrate can lead to production of gas within the GI tract and subsequent ileus and anorexia.
Non-dietary causes
• Dental disease is probably the most common clinical cause of weight loss, and untreated or unrecognized dental disease can rapidly lead to cachexia due to an inability to prehend or chew food.
• Bulla osteitis/otitis/facial nerve paralysis may lead to discomfort upon movement of

the temporomandibular joint, vestibular signs, or inappetence from pain.
• Caseous lymphadenitis is an outwardly recognizable etiology that may cause discomfort with eating or swallowing.
• Gastrointestinal stasis/bloat/ileus—whether secondary to another disease or the primary problem, patients with stasis are reluctant to eat.
• Pregnancy and pregnancy toxemia—lack of appropriate food during gestation and lactation can lead to pregnancy toxemia, subsequently leading to anorexia.
• Cystic calculi—painful; may lead to inappetence from discomfort or urinary obstruction
• Metabolic disease may cause generalized malaise and lack of appetite.

Increased Metabolic Demand
• Hyperthyroidism and thyroid tumors
• Any infectious etiology leads to increased caloric needs; common infectious etiologies include bulla osteitis/otitis/facial nerve paralysis, caseous lymphadenitis
• Metabolic diseases such as renal, hepatic, or
• CNS diseases can induce a catabolic state due to their increased nutritional demand on the patient.
• Pregnancy and pregnancy toxemia—lack of appropriate food during gestation and lactation can lead to pregnancy toxemia, which causes increased metabolic demand in conjunction with a decreased appetite.

Loss or Malabsorption of Nutrients
• Gastrointestinal stasis/bloat/ileus is common as a primary or secondary abnormality; in cases of ileus, the gastrointestinal tract fails to absorb nutrients, and the cecum may not produce adequate fermentation or vitamins
• Metabolic diseases such as renal and hepatic diseases can cause loss via protein-losing nephropathy or enteropathy.
• Dysbiosis can easily be induced with antimicrobial use but also with stress or diet changes.

RISK FACTORS
Pregnant sows are at increased risk.

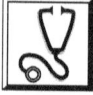

DIAGNOSIS
• Compare present weights with previous weights, if available.
• Palpate for muscle wasting.

DIFFERENTIAL DIAGNOSIS
Muscle wasting from neuropathy or traumatic injury—this should be recognizable based on other clinical signs or history

CBC/BIOCHEMISTRY/URINALYSIS
- CBC may reveal profound lymphocytosis if cavian leukemia is present; leukocytosis if other infections are present, or may be normal. Anemia is almost always present with cachexia.
- Biochemistry profile may show azotemia or hepatic enzyme elevations indicative of renal or hepatic disease; CK is likely to be elevated from muscle catabolism

OTHER LABORATORY TESTS
- Thyroid hormone levels performed on this fluid may be increased. Normal values have been reported in many sources
  - TT4 1.1-5. mcg/dl
  - Castrated males may have a higher median level (2.7 mcg/dL).
- Additional laboratory testing can be performed if an underlying etiology cannot be identified and should be based on suspicion of disease.

IMAGING
- Abdominal and thoracic radiography should be performed in the absence of a clear etiology, to evaluate for an underlying disease. If disease is still not identified, abdominal ultrasound may be useful.
- Radiographs of the skull and bullae should be performed to evaluate the occlusion of the teeth as well as the bullae.

DIAGNOSTIC PROCEDURES
- Cytologic evaluation of fine-needle aspirates of thyroid tissue can reveal brownish or bloody fluid in cases of cystic neoplasia, and proteinaceous matrix if colloid is being produced. Exercise extreme caution when performing FNA, as significant bleeding can occur.
- Endoscopic evaluation of the oral cavity may help to identify overgrown cheek teeth, oral abscesses, and oral ulcers that might otherwise not be detected.

PATHOLOGIC FINDINGS
This will vary depending upon the underlying etiology.

TREATMENT
- Early intervention in the patient with weight loss can prevent the subsequent development of cachexia.
- For primary nutritional or dietary-based weight loss and malnutrition (in the absence of cachexia), proper dietary supplementation is appropriate treatment.
- If malnutrition is secondary to a disease process, then nutritional support must be combined with treatment of the underlying disease.

- Initiate feeding immediately if weight loss approaches 10% of starting body weight. The maintenance energy requirement of the guinea pig is 136 Kcal/BWkg

APPROPRIATE HEALTH CARE
- Fluid therapy to maintain hydration—subcutaneous generally adequate unless severe infection/sepsis
- Assisted feeding of anorexic animals
- Maintain clean, soft bedding with padding if necessary

ACTIVITY
Restrict activity to prevent excessive caloric demand, but do encourage normal walking movements to help maintain muscle strength and memory.

DIET
- It is essential to maintain food intake during treatment; anorexia may lead to gastrointestinal stasis and ileus; secondary derangements of intestinal microbial populations may occur.
- Offer a wide variety of fresh leafy greens (romaine lettuce, cilantro, parsley, kale, cabbage, collard greens, mustard greens, bok choy, dandelion greens, turnip greens, spinach, and mesclun salad mixes) and high-quality grass hay. Place food and water in a position that the guinea pig is able to reach, or hand offer.
- Provide adequate nutritional support. Syringe feed a formulated diet such as Critical Care for Herbivores (Oxbow Pet Products, Murdock, NE) or Emerald Herbivore (Lafeber Company, Cornell, IL), 10–15 mL/kg q6–8h. If neither product is available, a slurry can be made with blended leafy green vegetables that are high in vitamin C, or guinea pig pellets blended with water and vegetable baby food.
- Avoid high-carbohydrate foods, treats, or grains.
- Use caution when syringe-feeding as aspiration pneumonia may occur.

CLIENT EDUCATION
- Client must be informed that if dental disease is present, it is a lifelong problem that will require periodic tooth trimming.
- Educate client to evaluate for actual food consumption rather than an interest in food alone.
- Maintain a good healthy normal weight.

SURGICAL CONSIDERATIONS
Surgery should be avoided in cachexic patients, although placement of a feeding tube should be considered, if necessary. In guinea pigs, a pharyngostomy tube is preferable to nasogastric.

MEDICATIONS
DRUG(S) OF CHOICE
- It is essential to address and treat the underlying cause; medications should be dictated by the etiology.
- Dextrose 3%–5% inhibits protein catabolism, decreases urinary nitrogen loss by 50%, and blocks hepatic glycogenesis, so should be administered in intravenous fluids
- Lipid administration has been shown to dramatically improve recovery in cachexic patients but must be administered along with glucose and proteins. Cachexia and tumor growth can be decreased by the addition of fish oil derivatives as a replacement for carbohydrates (use fish oil at 50% of the recommended carbohydrate requirements).

PRECAUTIONS
Glucocorticoids are used in humans to stimulate appetite, but caution must be used in guinea pigs—because of the immunosuppressive effects of corticosteroids, their use may prolong or exacerbate infection and may increase risk of systemic disease.

FOLLOW-UP
PATIENT MONITORING
Monitor weight daily initially until a clear trend in weight gain can be established, then continue monitoring at least weekly.

Follow-up CBC and biochemistry results as indicated to monitor for resolution of disease

PREVENTION/AVOIDANCE
- Always provide appropriate food choices.
- Avoid breeding unless already on a high nutritional plane.

POSSIBLE COMPLICATIONS
Refeeding syndrome is a possibility.

EXPECTED COURSE AND PROGNOSIS
If treated early, prior to the onset of cachexia, prognosis is good. However, prolonged cachexia dramatically decreases the potential for survival.

MISCELLANEOUS
ASSOCIATED CONDITIONS
See Causes and Risk Factors

GUINEA PIGS

WEIGHT LOSS AND CACHEXIA   (CONTINUED)

PREGNANCY/FERTILITY/BREEDING

The increased metabolic demand during pregnancy will predispose a patient to weight loss, pregnancy toxemia, and over time, cachexia.

SEE ALSO

Anorexia and pseudoanorexia
Cervical lymphadenitis
Dental malocclusion
Gastrointestinal hypomotility and gastrointestinal stasis
Hyperthyroidism
Pregnancy toxemia

ABBREVIATIONS

CK = creatine phosphokinase
CNS = central nervous system
GI = gastrointestinal

Suggested Reading

Bays TB. Geriatric care of rabbits, guinea pigs, and chinchillas. Vet Clin Exot Anim 2020;23:567–593.

DeCubellis J. Common emergencies in rabbits, guinea pigs, and chinchillas. Vet Clin Exot Anim 2016;19:411–429.

Lennox AM, Capello V, Legendre LF. Small mammal denistry. In: Quesenberry KE, Carpenter JW, eds. Ferrets, Rabbits and Rodents, 4th Ed). Clinical Medicine and Surgery. 2021 ed. St. Louis: Saunders, 2020:514–535.

Mayer J, Wagner R, Taeymans O. Current management of thryroid pathologies in guinea pigs. Vet Clin Exotic Anim 2010;13:509–523.

Minarikova A, Hauptman K, Jeklova E et al. Diseases in pet guinea pigs: a retrospective study in 1000 animals. Vet Rec 2015;177(8):200–200.

Miwa Y, Sladky K. Common surgical procedures of rodents, ferrets, hedgehogs, and sugar gliders. Vet Clin Exot Anim 2016;19:205–244.

Pignon C, Mayer J. Guinea pigs. In: Quesenberry KE, Carpenter JW, eds. Ferrets, Rabbits and Rodents, 4th Ed). Clinical Medicine and Surgery. 2021 ed. St. Louis: Saunders, 2020:270–297.

Ritzman TK. Diagnosis and clinical management of gastrointestinal conditions in exotic companion mammals (rabbits, guinea pigs, and chinchillas). Vet Clin Exot Anim 2014;17:179–194.

Author Natalie Antinoff, DVM, Dipl. ABVP (Avian)

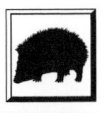

HEDGEHOGS

ALOPECIA AND QUILL LOSS

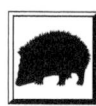

BASICS

DEFINITION
• The loss or absence of hair or quills. Can range from focal or patchy to widespread.
• Quills (spines) are modified hairs on the dorsal aspect of the body consisting of modified keratin. Hedgehogs have 5,000–7,000 spines, which serve as their main defense against predators.
• "Quilling" is a term used for the normal shedding and replacement of quills, similar to shedding. At age 6–8 weeks, then again at age 4–6 months, hedgehogs undergo a major quilling process, replacing smaller, softer baby quills with adult quills. This process can last several weeks and the animals tend to be less social, irritable, and often have a decreased appetite. Normal shed quills have a ball at the base and new quills should emerge within a few days. Smaller, shorter quilling episodes are normal and occur lifelong.

PATHOPYSIOLOGY
• Dependent on the cause
• All causes manifest as a disruption in growth of hair from the follicle due to infection, trauma, obstruction, immunogenic causes, and/or changes to the growth cycle

SYSTEMS AFFECTED
Skin/Exocrine

GENETICS
There is no known genetic predisposition for many of the underlying causes of alopecia.

INCIDENCE/PREVALENCE
Quill loss and skin disease are one of the most common health problems in African Pigmy Hedgehogs, with mite infestation is the most common cause.

GEOGRAPHIC DISTRIBUTION
N/A

SIGNALMENT
Gender and age predisposition are dependent on the specific condition causing the alopecia. Mite infestation is more common in older, stressed animals.

SIGNS
History
• May have a history of pruritis
• Recent stress or systemic disease will predispose to mite infestation
• Recent exposure to other hedgehogs, history of flea infestation in other household pets

Physical Examination Findings
• Quill loss is more common than loss of hair on the abdomen; can appear as focal, patchy, or diffuse thinning

• Dry flaky skin, crusting, seborrhea, erythema, and lichenification seen with mite infestation and/or dermatophyte infection
• Hyperkeratosis at the base of quills and on the face and ears with mite infestation
• Quills may fall off during physical examination
• Mites may be visible without magnification and appear as a white, flaky powder
• Weight loss, general debility
• Excoriations, erythema
• Obesity—can cause separation in the distance between quills, mimicking alopecia

CAUSES
• Ectoparasites are the most common cause. *Caparinia* spp, a nonburrowing psoroptid mite, is most common, but *Chorioptes* spp and sarcoptid species are also seen.
  ○ Ear mites *Notoedres* or *Otodectes* sp can cause alopecia around the face and ears
  ○ Fleas can sometimes cause quill and hair loss
• Dermatophytes—*Trichophyton erinacei*, *Trichophyton mentagrophytes*, and *Microsporum* spp most common. Other species include *Arthroderma benhamiae* and *Paecilomyces Variotii*. Dermatophytes can occur alone or in association with mite infestation. Fungal growth is facilitated by changes caused by mite infestation. Fungal spores are found in mite droppings.
• Metabolic/Nutritional—debility, underlying disease predispose to mite infestation and dermatophytosis; diets low in protein can cause barbering
• Bacterial—usually secondary to scratching; *Staphylococcus* sp. Is the most common.
• Husbandry/Environmental/Stress—contact dermatitis, urine scald
• Neoplasia—cutaneous lymphoma, mast cell tumors, cutaneous hemangiosarcoma, and histiocytic sarcoma are most commonly reported
• Trauma—environmental/cage rubbing/bite wounds, self-mutilation
• Endocrinopathy and immune-mediated causes not yet reported

RISK FACTORS
Inadequate husbandry and nutrition, underlying metabolic disease predispose to mite infestations and dermatophytes.

DIAGNOSIS

DIFFERENTIAL DIAGNOSIS
• Differentiate from normal "quilling" or shedding. Shed quills have a small ball at the base; skin appears normal and new quills will begin to form within a few days.
• Obesity—can cause separation in the distance between quills, mimicking alopecia

• Ectoparasites—hyperkeratosis at quill base, flaky skin, quills fall off during physical examination.
• Bacterial—usually secondary to pruritis, see excoriations, erythema
• Neoplasia—cutaneous lymphoma, oral squamous cell carcinoma, mast cell tumors, cutaneous hemangiosarcoma, and histiocytic sarcoma are most commonly reported.

CBC/BIOCHEMISTRY/URINALYSIS
Important to identify underlying causes, especially in hedgehogs with mites and/or dermatophytosis as most affected hedgehogs have an underlying disability.

OTHER LABORATORY TESTS
• Skin scraping—superficial for most mites—highest population around ears and face
• Dermatophyte testing, either PCR or fungal culture. Fungal culture results are often delayed due to the long growth time required. Begin treatment while awaiting results. False negatives are common, especially with PCR testing, as most laboratories do not test for all species commonly infecting hedgehogs
• Bacterial culture and sensitivity testing, if a secondary bacterial infection is suspected

IMAGING
In systemically ill patients, radiographs may help confirm the presence of organomegaly, dystrophic mineralization, or the presence of masses.

DIAGNOSTIC PROCEDURES
• Skin scrapings and dermatophyte cultures should be included as part of the minimum database.
• Skin biopsies for histopathologic evaluation may be indicated.
• Response to therapy as a trial

PATHOLOGIC FINDINGS
Results of diagnostic tests and histopathology will vary depending on the cause of the alopecia.

TREATMENT

APPROPRIATE HEALTH CARE
• Treatment will vary depending on the causative factor in each individual case.

NURSING CARE
• Unless systemically ill, almost all cases of alopecia are treated on an outpatient basis.

ACTIVITY
In most cases, activity restriction is not necessary.

DIET

Supplementation is appropriate if anorexic or if dietary deficiencies are identified as the cause of alopecia.

CLIENT EDUCATION

• Review of appropriate husbandry for the species in question
• For infectious causes, environmental disinfection—infested bedding and toys/furnishings can serve as fomites.
• Awareness of zoonotic potential with dermatophytes

SURGICAL CONSIDERATIONS

• Skin biopsies where indicated
• Repair of traumatic wounds
• Removal of masses if appropriate

MEDICATIONS

DRUG(S) OF CHOICE

• For ectoparasites: 10% imidacloprid/1.0% moxidectin spot on (0.1 mL/kg as a single treatment); selamectin (6–18 mg/kg topically q30d); fluralaner (Bravecto, Merck 15 mg/kg PO once); and ivermectin (0.2–0.4 mg/kg PO, SC, q7–14d × 3–5 treatments
• For dermatophytes—topical treatment with ketoconazole shampoo (bathe 1–2 times daily for 2–4 weeks), miconazole (apply a small amount to the affected skin 1–2 times daily for 2–4 weeks), clotrimazole cream (apply a small amount to the affected skin 1–2 times daily for 2–4 weeks), butenafine cream (apply a small amount to the affected skin 1–2 times daily for 2–4 weeks); oral, systemic treatment: terbinafine (100 mg/kg PO q12h × 4–6wks), ketoconazole (10 mg/kg PO q24h × 6–8wks), itraconazole (5–10 mg/kg PO q12–24h × 4–6wks)
• For bacterial dermatitis, select appropriate antibiotics based on safety and bacterial culture and sensitivity. Antibiotics commonly used include cephalexin (25 mg/kg PO q12h), amoxicillin/clavulanic acid (12.5–25 mg/kg PO q12h), enrofloxacin (5–10 mg/kg PO q12h), trimethoprim-sulfa (30 mg/kg PO q12h)
• Antihistamines—diphenhydramine (1–2 mg/kg PO, IM q8–12) or hydroxyzine (1–2 mg/kg PO q8–12) may be used for allergic dermatitis.
• Pain management—meloxicam (0.2 mg/kg PO, SC q24h), tramadol (2–5 mg/kg PO q8–12h), or buprenorphine (0.02–0.05 mg/kg IM, SQ, PO q6–12h) may be used for painful conditions/inflammation.
• For sedation—ketamine (20–30 mg/kg IM) + midazolam (1 mg/kg IM) or alfaxalone (1–3 mg/kg IM + midazolam (0.5–1 mg/kg IM) ± butorphanol (0.2 mg/kg IM) add alfaxalone (1 mg/kg IM) boluses PRN

CONTRAINDICATIONS

• Steroids may be used as an anti-inflammatory agent although nonsteroidal anti-inflammatories are preferred. The use of steroids is contraindicated in patients with dermatophyte infections.

PRECAUTIONS

• The use of griseofulvin should be avoided in pregnant animals and in patients with immune system suppression.

POSSIBLE INTERACTIONS

N/A

ALTERNATIVE DRUGS

Fluralaner (15 mg/kg PO once) reported to be effective with one dose; safety and toxicity not studied

FOLLOW-UP

PATIENT MONITORING

• Varies with each cause of alopecia
• Patients with ectoparasites should be evaluated 2 weeks and 4 weeks after starting therapy.
• All patients should be monitored for potential adverse effects of medications.

PREVENTION/AVOIDANCE

Appropriate husbandry, caging, substrate, sanitation, and population density

POSSIBLE COMPLICATIONS

Possible adverse effects of long-term medication, depending on the cause and treatment of the alopecia

EXPECTED COURSE AND PROGNOSIS

• Most cases of alopecia will resolve with appropriate therapy.
• Some ectoparasite infestations may be difficult to resolve and can require long-term therapy. Evaluation for underlying systemic disease is indicated.
• Environmental decontamination in the case of dermatophyte and some ectoparasite infections is important to prevent spread or reinfection.

MISCELLANEOUS

ASSOCIATED CONDITIONS

Mite infestation and dermatophytosis are most severe in animals with underlying disorders

AGE-RELATED FACTORS

Middle-aged to older animals more likely to be obese

ZOONOTIC POTENTIAL

• Hedgehogs can be asymptomatic carriers of *Salmonella*. Use gloves and careful handwashing after handling.
• Dermatophytosis

PREGNANCY/FERTILITY/BREEDING

N/A

SYNONYMS

Hair loss

SEE ALSO

Dermatophytosis
Ectoparasites

ABBREVIATIONS

N/A

INTERNET RESOURCES

Exotic DVM forum for eDVM readers: www.pets.groups.yahoo.com/group/ExoticDVM
Veterinary Information Network: www.vin.com

Suggested Reading
Chin J, Mans C. Small mammals: hedgehogs. In: Mayer J, Donnelly T, eds. Clinical Veterinary Advisor: Birds and Exotic Pets. St. Louis, MO: Saunders, 2013:338–343.
Ivey E, Carpenter J. African hedgehogs. In: Quesenberry KE, Carpenter JW, eds. Ferrets, Rabbits, and Rodents: Clinical Medicine and Surgery, 3rd ed. St Louis, MO: Saunders:339–353.
Johnson DH. African pygmy hedgehogs. In: Johnson-Delaney C, Meredith A, eds. BSAVA Manual of Exotic Pets, A Foundation Manual. Quedgeley, Gloucester: British Small Animal Veterinary Association, 2010:139–147.
Johnson DH. Geriatric hedgehogs. Vet Clin Exot Anim Pract 2020;23(3):615–637.
Keeble E, Koterwas B. Selected emerging diseases of pet hedgehogs. Vet Clin Exot Anim Pract 2020;23(2):443–458.
Lennox AM. Emergency and critical care procedures in sugar gliders (*Petaurus breviceps*), African hedgehogs (*Atelerix albiventris*), and prairie dogs (*Cynomys* spp). Vet Clin North Am Exot Anim Pract 2007;10:533–555.

Author Amanda Steinagel, DVM

HEDGEHOGS

ANOREXIA AND PSEUDOANOREXIA

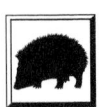

BASICS

DEFINITION
• Decreased/loss of appetite and/or refusal to eat food. The link between the body's need for food, hunger, and memories are important. Animals are assumed to have an appetite.
• May involve the mechanical inability and/or an issue that prevents the normal ability to prehend, chew, and/or swallow food. This is termed pseudoanorexia.

PATHOPHYSIOLOGY
• Anorexia is most often associated with systemic disease but can be caused by many different mechanisms.
• Appetite is controlled the central nervous system (CNS). More specifically, receptors of the hypothalamus receive neurotransmitters that cause a reaction that leads to hunger.
• Inflammatory, infectious, neoplastic, and metabolic causes can affect appetite/hunger.
• Pseudoanorexia typically involves oral pain and the inability to chew due to dental disease or oral neoplasia (oral squamous cell carcinoma).
• Inflammatory, infectious, metabolic, or neoplastic diseases can cause inappetence, probably as a result of the release of a variety of chemical mediators.

SYSTEMS AFFECTED
Gastrointestinal, any other system could be affected based upon the illness that is causing the lack of appetite.

GENETICS
N/A

INCIDENCE/PREVALENCE
N/A

GEOGRAPHIC DISTRIBUTION
N/A

SIGNALMENT
Animal of any age or gender; depends on the underlying cause

SIGNS

Historical Findings
• Decreased appetite/no appetite
• Inability to prehend food
• Decreased fecal output
• Varying degrees of lethargy, for example, not using exercise wheel
• Other signs vary depending on the underlying cause.

Physical examination findings
• Lethargy
• Dehydration
• Weight loss or gain (ascites, abdominal mass, and others)
• Thin/emaciated

Physical Examination Findings
• Weight loss or gain (as in abdominal masses)
• Decreased activity level
• In pseudoanorexia, there may be excessive drooling, halitosis, and dysphagia.
• Physical examination findings are dependent on the cause

CAUSES
Almost any disease process can lead to anorexia.
• Gastrointestinal—gastroenteritis—*Salmonella* spp., gastrointestinal obstruction (neoplasia, foreign body), parasitic disease
• Urogenital—urinary tract disease, renal failure, pyometra, pregnancy
• Respiratory: pneumonia, upper respiratory infection
• Metabolic—nutritional/dietary, hepatic disease, renal disease
• Neurological—wobbly hedgehog syndrome, vestibular disease
• Dental disease
• Cardiovascular disease—congestive heart failure
• Trauma
• Pain
• Neoplasia—oral squamous cell carcinoma

Pseudoanorexia
• *Oral abscess or neoplasia*
• *Periodontal disease, caries, tarter accumulation*

RISK FACTORS
• Poor husbandry
• Inappropriate diet

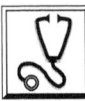

DIAGNOSIS

DIFFERENTIAL DIAGNOSIS
• First differentiate between anorexia and pseudoanorexia.
• Many differentials exist, diagnostics are needed to determine causes.

CBC/BIOCHEMISTRY/URINALYSIS
• Hypoproteinemia and hypoalbuminemia can result from protein loss caused by anorexia/starvation; also may be due to hemorrhage or parasitism.
• Due to the extensive list of causes of anorexia, any abnormalities in standard diagnostic tests are important in determining the cause of anorexia.

OTHER LABORATORY TESTS
• Fecal exam (direct and floatation)
• Bacterial culture and susceptibility testing (e.g., may need to swab oral cavity or obtain a rectal swab if diarrhea present)
• Cytology of thoracic or abdominal fluid or mass, if present

IMAGING
• Radiographs may show gastroenteritis, gastrointestinal obstruction, organomegaly, neoplasia, pulmonary disease, cardiovascular disease, urogenital disease, and others. Dental or skull imaging is helpful to determine if there is underlying dental disease. Abdominal/thoracic ultrasound may be needed to further investigate radiographic abnormalities.

DIAGNOSTIC PROCEDURES
A good oral exam under general anesthesia using cheek dilators and specula made for rodents may be necessary (Jorgenson laboratories, Inc., Loveland, CO). A small rigid endoscope can be helpful in performing a complete oral exam. The oral exam will help to identify oral abscess, gingivitis/stomatitis, ulcers, dental disorders, or masses.

PATHOLOGIC FINDINGS
Variable, depending on the cause of the anorexia

TREATMENT

APPROPRIATE HEALTH CARE
• If anorexia is complete and lasting greater than 24 hours, inpatient medical care is appropriate. Many anorexic hedgehogs present in critical condition and will need to be stabilized before diagnostics can be performed.
• If the anorexia is acute and the cause is determined early, outpatient medical care is acceptable.

NURSING CARE
• Ensure that the patient is kept warm—between 80 and 85°F (27 and 29°C). Topor occurs when the environmental temperature falls below 65°F (18°C).
• Fluid therapy is used to correct hydration following standard protocols (5%–10% of body weight administered in SQ boluses). Fluids should be kept warm to prevent hypothermia and can be warmed by placing the prepared syringe in a warm water bath prior to administration. Administration via a 22–25-gauge butterfly needle can reduce stress on the patient by minimizing restraint.
• For critical patients, administer fluid therapy via IV or intraosseous (IO) catheter. In addition to crystalloids, the patient may need colloids such as hetastarch at 10 mL/kg IO per day in several small boluses. Maintenance requirement is 100 mL/kg/day

ACTIVITY

Based on the cause of anorexia, activity may or may not need to be restricted. Most small mammals that do not feel well will be less active of their own accord.

DIET

• It is imperative that the animal receive nutritional support if it is not eating. Supplementation with a liquid diet may be required, such as Oxbow Carnivore Care (Oxbow Enterprises, Inc., Murdock, NE) or Emeraid Omnivore (Lafeber's, Cornell, IL) supplements such as Ensure (Abott Nutrition, Columbus, OH).

• A diet change should never be made abruptly in the anorexic patient. If the diet is inappropriate, wait until the patient is stable and eating again, then convert to an appropriate diet.

CLIENT EDUCATION

Educate owners about proper husbandry (caging, diet) and the need for regular examinations. The author recommends a wellness examination every 6 months.

SURGICAL CONSIDERATIONS

If surgery is required, or if oral exam, dental procedures, blood, or other sample collection requires general anesthesia, always observe these precautions:

• A 4 hour fast prior to surgery is recommended. A longer fasting period may be indicated for gastrointestinal surgery.

• It is essential to maintain core body temperature; use of a Bair Hugger (Arizant Health Care, Eden Prairie, MN), water circulating heating pad, or other warming device is crucial.

• Minimize alcohol used during preparation of any sample site (e.g., for blood collection, needle aspirates), as alcohol can increase loss of body heat.

MEDICATIONS

DRUG(S) OF CHOICE

The cause of anorexia should be identified before dispensing any medication.

If the Animal is Painful

• Buprenorphine (0.02–0.05 mg/kg SQ, IM, PO q6–8h)

• Meloxicam (0.2 mg/kg PO q24h)

For Bacterial Infection

Treat with antibiotics based on culture and sensitivity results. Broad spectrum antibiotics that are well tolerated include: cephalexin (25 mg/kg PO q12h), amoxicillin/clavulanic acid (12.5–25 mg/kg PO q12h), enrofloxacin (5–10 mg/kg PO q12h), trimethoprim-sulfa (30 mg/kg PO q12h)

For Gastric Pain or Ileus

• Promotility agents such as metoclopramide (0.5 mg/kg PO, SQ, IV q12h) or cisapride (0.5 mg/kg PO q8–12h) may be used for severe ileus.

• Maropitant (1–2 mg/kg PO, SQ q24h) may be used to decrease vomiting and help with gastroenteritis

• Anti-acid medications such as famotidine (1 mg/kg SQ, PO q24h) and omeprazole (0.5–1 mg/kg SQ, PO q24h)

As an Appetite Stimulant

• Capromorelin (1–3 mg/kg PO q24h), anecdotally effective, no published data regarding dose or efficacy.

For Sedation

• Ketamine (20–30 mg/kg IM) + midazolam (1 mg/kg IM) or alfaxalone (1–3 mg/kg IM + midazolam (0.5–1 mg/kg IM) ± butorphanol (0.2 mg/kg IM) add alfaxalone (1 mg/kg IM) boluses PRN

CONTRAINDICATIONS

• The cause of anorexia should be identified before dispensing any medication.

• Promotility agents, such as metoclopramide and cisapride, are not recommended for use with suspected gastrointestinal obstruction

PRECAUTIONS

• Use caution in dispensing drugs that have been compounded in-house; may achieve better results using a compounding pharmacy or a liquid form of the drug

POSSIBLE INTERACTIONS

N/A

ALTERNATIVE DRUGS

N/A

FOLLOW-UP

PATIENT MONITORING

• Weigh daily (owner should buy a gram scale if needed).

PREVENTION/AVOIDANCE

Depends on the cause of the anorexia

POSSIBLE COMPLICATIONS

• Severe dehydration

• May progress to cachexia, death

EXPECTED COURSE AND PROGNOSIS

The long-term prognosis will be based largely on the identification and correction of the underlying cause. In older patients, the prognosis worsens due to age-related complications and the possibility of multiple causes of anorexia.

MISCELLANEOUS

ASSOCIATED CONDITIONS

Many possibilities based on underlying cause

AGE-RELATED FACTORS

N/A

ZOONOTIC POTENTIAL

• Hedgehogs can be asymptomatic carriers of *Salmonella*. Use gloves and careful handwashing after handling.

PREGNANCY/FERTILITY/BREEDING

• Pregnancy may be a cause of anorexia. The pregnant hedgehog needs specified care and treatment to ensure the proper nutrition is acquired during pregnancy.

SYNONYMS

Inappetence

SEE ALSO

Dental disease
Diarrhea

ABBREVIATIONS

N/A

INTERNET RESOURCES

www.vin.com

Suggested Reading

Ivey E, Carpenter J. African hedgehogs. In: Quesenberry KE, Carpenter JW, eds. Ferrets, Rabbits, and Rodents: Clinical Medicine and Surgery, 3rd ed. St Louis, MO: Saunders, 2012:411–427.

Johnson DH. Geriatric hedgehogs. Vet Clin Exot Anim Pract 2020;23(3):615–637.

Keeble E, Koterwas B. Selected emerging diseases of pet hedgehogs. Vet Clin Exot Anim Pract 2020;23(2):443–458.

Lennox AM. Emergency and critical care procedures in sugar gliders (*Petaurus breviceps*), African hedgehogs (*Atelerix albiventris*), and prairie dogs (*Cynomys* spp). Vet Clin North Am Exot Anim Pract 2007;10:533–555.

Author Amanda Steinagel, DVM

ATAXIA

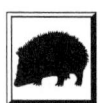

BASICS

DEFINITION
- A sign of sensory dysfunction that produces incoordination of the limbs, head, and/or trunk
- Three clinical types—sensory (proprioceptive), vestibular, and cerebellar. In hedgehogs, sensory is most common. All produce changes in limb coordination, but vestibular and cerebellar ataxia also produce changes in head and neck movement.

PATHOPHYSIOLOGY
- Sensorimotor: caused by spinal cord lesions, manifested by weakness of movement, scuffing of toes, incomplete limb extension, knuckling wobbly gait, easy falling, difficulty rising. The most common cause of this is Wobbly Hedgehog syndrome (WHS), characterized by progressive nerve demyelination leading to paralysis, weight loss, and eventually death. Similar signs can be due to intervertebral disc disease (IVDD), trauma, and neoplasia
- Cerebellar: characterized by defects in rate, range, force, and direction of movement of limbs; inability to maintain head in proper position so that it oscillates, hypermetria or hypometria, direction cannot be maintained and the animal falls easily, often in an exaggerated way.
- Vestibular: loss of balance with preservation of strength. If unilateral, the abnormality is asymmetrical, if bilateral, it is symmetrical.

SYSTEMS AFFECTED
- Nervous; spinal cord (and brain stem), cerebellum, vestibular system
- Neuromuscular
- Respiratory—with otitis interna/media

GENETICS
Due to regional disease prevalence of Wobbly Hedgehog syndrome, a genetic predisposition is suspected

INCIDENCE/PREVALENCE
Ataxia is one of the most common presenting complaints in pet hedgehogs.

GEOGRAPHIC DISTRIBUTION
Wobbly Hedgehog syndrome (WHS) is seen more commonly in North America.

SIGNALMENT
IVDD and neoplasia is more common in older animals; WHS is most common in hedgehogs 18–24 months of age.

SIGNS
Historical Findings
- Owner may report that the animal is limping, not walking normally, has a head tilt, or is showing nonspecific signs.
- Investigate the possibility of a cage accident (stuck in bars) or other trauma, such as being dropped.
- Progressive lameness beginning the rear limbs and extending forward with WHS

Physical Examination Findings
- WHS—initially, unable to ball up. Progresses to rear limb ataxia, weakness, and paralysis. In late stages, tetraparesis, weight loss, and general debility.
- Loss of CP, paresis, paralysis in rear limbs with IVDD, spinal trauma, or neoplasia
- Abnormal gait; if only one limb affected consider lameness, if rear limbs only are affected may be due to weakness
- Falling over; all or both ipsilateral limbs affected—cerebellar
- Head tilt—vestibular. Look for discharge or blood from ears.
- Evidence of trauma
- Other signs seen as a consequence of ataxia include anorexia, dehydration, and decreased activity (not using wheel, spending a lot of time in hide box)

CAUSES
- Tupor—a hibernation-like state which occurs when the environmental temperature falls below 65°F (18°C).
- Wobbly Hedgehog syndrome (WHS)—usually in younger animals; gradual progression, often beginning with inability to ball up, progressing from rear to front
- IVDD—more acute onset, rear legs only involved
- Spondylosis—acute or gradual onset; usually does not progress to front legs or severe debility
- Trauma to the brain, ear, or spinal cord—may have been noted in history, more acute onset
- Infectious: otitis, encephalitis, viral infections; may be a sequela to rhinitis and URI; see circling, head tilt, nystagmus
- Neoplastic—reported neoplasms involving the nervous system include histiocytic sarcoma, ganglioglioma, gemistocytic astrocytoma, oligodendroglioma, anaplastic astrocytoma, microglioma, oligoastrocytoma, meningioma, and lymphoma; usually older animals, more rapid progression as compared to WHS
- Poisoning, including lead (rare)

RISK FACTORS
- For trauma—inappropriate caging or handling
- Unknown for WHS and IVDD

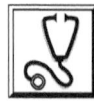

DIAGNOSIS

DIFFERENTIAL DIAGNOSIS
It is important to differentiate ataxia from weakness. Many systemic diseases may cause weakness that resembles ataxia.

CBC/BIOCHEMISTRY/URINALYSIS
Can be normal unless there is an infectious cause or metabolic disorder

OTHER LABORATORY TESTS
Bacterial culture and sensitivity testing from ear swab in patients with signs of otitis and vestibular disorder

IMAGING
- Skull radiographs to identify or rule out ear pathology
- Full-body radiographs; identify IVDD, spondylosis, spinal injury, injury that would explain lameness (versus ataxia); identify neoplasia, cardiopulmonary disease, or abdominal masses that may explain difficulty ambulating
- CT—provides superior imaging

DIAGNOSTIC PROCEDURES
- Culture and sensitivity of ear swab if vestibular syndrome suspected, especially if discharge present
- Necropsy—the diagnosis of WHS can only be made by histological examination of the nervous system.

PATHOLOGIC FINDINGS
For WHS: vacuolization of the white matter tract of the cerebrum, cerebellum, brain stem, and throughout the spinal cord.

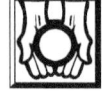

TREATMENT

APPROPRIATE HEALTH CARE
As long as the patient is eating and drinking, outpatient care is appropriate; often depends on severity and acuteness of clinical signs

NURSING CARE
- Ensure that the patient is kept warm—between 80 and 85°F (27 and 29°C). Topor occurs when the environmental temperature falls below 65°F (18°C).
- Fluid therapy is used to correct hydration following standard protocols (5%–10% of body weight administered in SQ boluses). Fluids should be kept warm to prevent hypothermia and can be warmed by placing the prepared syringe in a warm water bath prior to administration. Administration via a 22–25-gauge butterfly needle can reduce stress on the patient by minimizing restraint.
- For critical patients, administer fluid therapy via IV or intraosseous (IO) catheter. In addition to crystalloids, the patient may need colloids such as hetastarch at 10 mL/kg IO per day in several small boluses. Maintenance requirement is 100 mL/kg/day

(CONTINUED)

ACTIVITY

Exercise should be restricted. Remove ramps, exercise wheels; limit to one level of the cage.

DIET

• It is imperative that the animal receive nutritional support if it is not eating. Supplementation with a liquid diet may be required, such as Oxbow Carnivore Care (Oxbow Enterprises, Inc., Murdock, NE) or Emeraid Exotic Carnivore (Lafeber's, Cornell, IL), is essential.

CLIENT EDUCATION

• WHS is uniformly fatal. The progression of the disease varies from weeks to months and will become immobile within 9–15 months following the onset of ataxia
• Supportive care, including assisted feeding, frequent bedding changes, padding, and cleanliness are important components of home nursing care.

SURGICAL CONSIDERATIONS

N/A

MEDICATIONS

DRUG(S) OF CHOICE

• If convulsions or torticollis present: midazolam (0.5–2 mg/kg IM, IV, IO) or diazepam (0.5–2 mg/kg IM, IV, IO)
• For pain: meloxicam (0.2 mg/kg PO q24h), tramadol (2–5 mg/kg PO q8–12h), or buprenorphine (0.02–0.05 mg/kg IM, SQ, PO q6–12h)
• If an infectious cause is suspected (e.g., otitis interna/externa, encephalitis), cephalexin (25 mg/kg PO q12h), enrofloxacin (5–10 mg/kg PO q12h), or (amoxicillin/clavulanic acid 12.5–25 mg/kg PO q8–12h)
• For sedation—ketamine (20–30 mg/kg IM) + midazolam (1 mg/kg IM) or alfaxalone (1–3 mg/kg IM + midazolam (0.5–1 mg/kg IM) ± butorphanol (0.2 mg/kg IM) add alfaxalone (1 mg/kg IM) boluses PRN

CONTRAINDICATIONS

• N/A

PRECAUTIONS

• Do not use trimethoprim-sulfa if liver or kidney failure is suspected.

POSSIBLE INTERACTIONS

N/A

ALTERNATIVE DRUGS

N/A

FOLLOW-UP

PATIENT MONITORING

• Monitor for signs of pain or worsening of neurological abnormalities

PREVENTION/AVOIDANCE

• Ensure a safe cage environment. If the pet is being allowed to run free in the household, monitor closely to avoid exposure to toxins and to avoid injury.

POSSIBLE COMPLICATIONS

Depends on the underlying cause

EXPECTED COURSE AND PROGNOSIS

• Depends on the underlying cause. WHD and neoplasia are progressive and fatal

MISCELLANEOUS

ASSOCIATED CONDITIONS

Dysphagia
Weight loss

AGE-RELATED FACTORS

• Older animals—Neoplasia, IVDD
• Younger animals—WHS

ZOONOTIC POTENTIAL

• Hedgehogs can be asymptomatic carriers of Salmonella. Use gloves and careful handwashing after handling.

PREGNANCY/FERTILITY/BREEDING

N/A

SYNONYMS

• Degenerative myelopathy
• Spongiform leukoencephalopathy

SEE ALSO

• Anorexia

ABBREVIATIONS

CT = computed tomography
IVDD = intravertebral disc disease
URI = upper respiratory infection
WHS = Wobbly Hedgehog Syndrome

INTERNET RESOURCES

www.vin.com

Suggested Reading
Berg CC, Doss GA, Guevar J. Neurologic examination of healthy adult African pygmy hedgehogs (*Atelerix albiventris*). J Am Vet Med Assoc 2021;258(9): 971–976.
Díaz-Delgado J, Whitley DB, Storts RW, Heatley JJ, Hoppes S, Porter BF. The pathology of wobbly hedgehog syndrome. Vet Pathol 2018;55(5):711–718.
Ivey E, Carpenter J. African hedgehogs. In: Quesenberry KE, Carpenter JW, eds. Ferrets, Rabbits, and Rodents: Clinical Medicine and Surgery, 3rd ed. St Louis, MO: Saunders, 2012:411–427.
Johnson DH. Geriatric hedgehogs. Vet Clin Exot Anim Pract 2020;23(3):615–637.
Keeble E, Koterwas B. Selected emerging diseases of pet hedgehogs. Vet Clin Exot Anim Pract 2020;23(2):443–458.
Lennox, A.M. (2007). Emergency and critical care procedures in sugar gliders (*Petaurus breviceps*), African hedgehogs (*Atelerix albiventris*), and prairie dogs (*Cynomys* spp) Vet Clin North Am Exot Anim Pract 10: 533–555.

Authors Amanda Steinagel, DVM and Barbara Oglesbee, DVM, DABVP (Avian)

HEDGEHOGS

CARDIOMYOPATHY

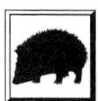

BASICS

DEFINITION
• Dilated cardiomyopathy (DCM)—the most commonly reported heart disease in African Pigmy Hedgehogs. Heart muscle disease characterized by weak cardiac muscles. Clinical signs are associated with left ventricular pump failure and volume overload.
• Hypertrophic cardiomyopathy—primary myocardial (heart muscle) disease defined as left ventricular (LV) concentric hypertrophy in the absence of an identifiable increase in afterload. Biatrial enlargement ensues. Systolic function is usually preserved. Not reported in Hedgehogs

PATHOPHYSIOLOGY
• The specific cause is unknown.
• Myocardial failure leads to decreased cardiac output and congestive heart failure.
• Arterial thromboembolism has been reported in a hedgehog secondary to DCM, with clots in both left and right atrium

SYSTEMS AFFECTED
• Cardiovascular
• Respiratory (pleural effusion, pulmonary edema)
• Urinary (prerenal azotemia)
• All organ systems are potentially at risk due to poor cardiac output and local hypoxemia.

INCIDENCE/PREVALENCE
• On post-mortem examination, DCM has been reported in up to 40% of African Pigmy Hedgehogs

SIGNALMENT
• More common in older animals (avg. 3 years of age), but has been reported in patients as young as 1 year.
• Males may be more commonly affected

SIGNS

Historical Findings
• Sudden death, with no obvious premonitory signs
• Increased respiratory rate/effort, dyspnea, and tachypnea,
• Abdominal distension with ascites
• Some hedgehogs may be asymptomatic.
• Weakness, lethargy, exercise intolerance
• Syncope

Physical Examination Findings
• Cardiac auscultation—possibly normal, murmur (intensity based on degree of turbulent blood flow), arrhythmia
• Muffled heart sounds in even of pleural effusion or pericardial effusion
• Rales/crackles in lungs in event of pulmonary edema

• Pulse deficits may be present in event of arrhythmia
• Pale or cyanotic mucus membranes in event of cardiogenic shock or significant peripheral hypoxia; membranes may have poor refill time
• Hypothermia is possible due to low cardiac output
• Tachycardia (>280 bpm)
• Dyspnea/tachypnea (>60 bpm)
• Abdominal distension, ascites, splenomegaly, and hepatomegaly
• Generalized weakness
• Poor body condition

CAUSES
• Cause of dilated cardiomyopathy is unknown and is considered idiopathic
• A genetic basis has been proposed. Import restrictions in the United States have resulted in a limited genetic pool in captive bred hedgehogs

RISK FACTORS
• Incidence increases with age

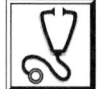

DIAGNOSIS

DIFFERENTIAL DIAGNOSIS
• Innocent heart murmur
• Cardiac disease secondary to valvular disease
• Pleural effusion—neoplasia, trauma, pulmonary hemorrhage, and pneumothorax
• Dyspnea—primary pulmonary disease (abscess, pneumonia) most common; neoplasia (heart based tumors, metastatic neoplasia), and pleural effusion
• Ascites, abdominal distension—consider hypoproteinemia, severe liver disease, ruptured bladder, peritonitis, abdominal neoplasia, and abdominal hemorrhage
• Muffled heart sounds—pericardial disease, pleural effusion
• Pale mucus membranes/poor capillary refill time—cardiogenic or noncardiogenic shock
• Hypothermia—non-cardiogenic shock, torpor
• Weakness—Wobbly hedgehog syndrome, other systemic disease

CBC/BIOCHEMISTRY/URINALYSIS
• Routine blood tests and urinalysis are usually normal unless heart failure is causing hepatic congestion (increased ALT) or prerenal azotemia
• May help to rule out other underlying disease conditions
• Treatment for congestive failure can cause abnormalities such as hypokalemia, prerenal azotemia, and exacerbation of primary renal disease.

OTHER LABORATORY TESTS
N/A

IMAGING
• Radiography—enlarged cardiac silhouette, pulmonary edema, and/or pleural effusion, possibly bi-cavitary effusion, hepatomegaly in RSHF
• Echocardiogram for definitive diagnosis—typical findings include thin ventricular walls, enlarged left ventricular end-systolic and end-diastolic dimensions, left atrial enlargement, and reduced fractional shortening
• Abdominal ultrasound—ascites, organomegaly with RSHF, rule out other causes of abdominal distension

DIAGNOSTIC PROCEDURES
• Electrocardiography—limited information on usefulness is available
• Thoraco- or abdominocentesis—analysis of pleural fluid is important to rule out pyothorax, neoplasia, and hemothorax. Analysis of peritoneal fluid will help rule out neoplastic, septic, and hemorrhagic effusions. Results of fluid analysis in heart disease often reveal a modified transudate.

PATHOLOGIC FINDINGS
• Gross post-mortem findings include cardiomegaly, hepatomegaly, pulmonary edema or congestion, pleural effusion, and/or ascites
• Histologic abnormalities are usually found in the left ventricular myocardium and included myodegeneration, myonecrosis, atrophy, hypertrophy, and myofiber disarray

TREATMENT

APPROPRIATE HEALTH CARE
• Decompensated patients should be hospitalized for stabilization.
• Mildly affected patients can be managed as outpatients.

NURSING CARE
• Oxygen therapy for patients in respiratory distress. Place in an oxygen cage or, if not available, most rolled-up hedgehogs will fit into an upturned facemask used for large dogs.
• Hypothermia should be managed using warm water bottles or water blankets in a warm cage environment—keep between 80 and 85°F (27 and 29°C). Torpor occurs when the environmental temperature falls below 65°F (18°C). Absorption of parenteral medications is not reliable in patients with severe hypothermia.

• If pleural effusion is present, thoracocentesis has both diagnostic and therapeutic benefits.
• Supportive care, including correction of dehydration; administer 5%–10% of body weight administered in SQ boluses). Fluids should be kept warm to prevent hypothermia and can be warmed by placing the prepared syringe in a warm water bath prior to administration.
• For critical patients, administer fluid therapy via IV or intraosseous (IO) catheter. Maintenance requirement is 100 mL/kg/day

ACTIVITY
Restrict activity—remove exercise wheels, ramps from cage

DIET
• Provide adequate nutrition; dyspneic animals may be reluctant to eat and may need assisted feeding with a diet such as Oxbow Critical Care Herbivore (Oxbow Enterprises, Inc., Murdock, NE) or Emeraid Exotic Herbivore (Lafeber's, Cornell, IL).

CLIENT EDUCATION
• CHF is not curable and will progress. Inform client that cardiac disease is difficult to manage, and prognosis for longer term survival is poor; aim of treatment is palliative as long as quality of life can be maintained.

SURGICAL CONSIDERATIONS
N/A

MEDICATIONS
DRUG(S) OF CHOICE
• Furosemide is recommended at the lowest effective dose to eliminate pulmonary edema and pleural effusion. If fulminate cardiac failure is evident, administer furosemide at 2.5–5 mg/kg q6–12h IV, IO, IM. Initially, furosemide should be administered parenterally. Long-term therapy should be continued orally at 1–2 mg/kg PO q12–24h.
• Titrate to the lowest effective dose, predisposes the patient to dehydration, prerenal azotemia, and electrolyte disturbances.
• Nitroglycerin (1/16–1/18-inch strip topically) in conjunction with diuretics in the management of acute, decompensated heart failure
• Enalapril (0.5–1 mg/kg PO q12–24h)
• Pimobenden (0.3 mg/kg PO q12–24h).
• Digoxin (0.005–0.01 mg/kg PO q12–24)
• Beta blockers—propanolol, atenolol, carvediol, or metoprolol have been used anecdotally (0.2–1 mg/kg PO q8–12)

CONTRAINDICATIONS
• Digoxin should be avoided in uncontrolled paroxysmal ventricular tachycardia.

PRECAUTIONS
• Treatment regimens have been extrapolated from canine or feline doses and should be used with caution and careful patient monitoring.
• ACE inhibitors and digoxin must be used cautiously in patients with renal disease.
• Overzealous diuretic therapy may cause dehydration and hypokalemia.
• Beta-blockers and calcium channel blockers are negative inotropes and may adversely affect myocardial function. Use these medications with caution.

POSSIBLE INTERACTIONS
• The use of a calcium channel blocker in combination with a beta blocker should be avoided as clinically significant bradyarrhythmias can develop in other small animals and are likely to also occur in hedgehogs.

ALTERNATIVE DRUGS
The use of vasodilators, diuretics, and antiarrhythmic drugs in dogs and cats has been extrapolated for use in Hedgehogs, but no data exists on their risks vs. benefits.

FOLLOW-UP
PATIENT MONITORING
• Cardiac disease is likely to be progressive; therefore, frequent recheck evaluation is recommended.
• Monitor response to therapy and adjust drug dosages as indicated.
• Radiographs should be repeated 1 week after treatment is started.
• Periodic monitoring of renal function and serum or plasma potassium is recommended
• Monitor patient weight.
• Monitor intake of food and water.

PREVENTION/AVOIDANCE
Unknown

POSSIBLE COMPLICATIONS
• Disease is likely to be progressive.
• Sudden death due to arrhythmias
• Subsequent acute renal failure from renal tubular necrosis and/or interstitial nephritis. Can be worsened by long-term diuretic and ACE-inhibitor use.
• Hepatic lipidosis
• Thrombotic disease/vascular thromboembolism
• Dehydration
• Anorexia

EXPECTED COURSE AND PROGNOSIS
Congestive heart failure is progressive, and the owner should be advised that treatments are palliative to increase patient comfort and control clinical signs.

MISCELLANEOUS
ASSOCIATED CONDITIONS
• Lower respiratory disease
• Renal disease

ZOONOTIC POTENTIAL
• Hedgehogs can be asymptomatic carriers of *Salmonella*. Use gloves and careful handwashing after handling.

PREGNANCY/FERTILITY/BREEDING
N/A

SYNONYMS
Heart disease
Heart failure

SEE ALSO
Pneumonia

ABBREVIATIONS
ACE = angiotensin-converting enzyme
CHF = congestive heart failure
DCM = dilated cardiomyopathy
EKG = electrocardiogram
HCM = hypertrophic cardiomyopathy
LV = left ventricle
L-CHF = left-sided congestive heart failure
R-CHF = right-sided congestive heart failure

Suggested Reading
Black PA, Marshall C, Seyfried AW, Bartin AM. Cardiac assessment of African hedgehogs (*Atelerix albiventris*). JZWM 2011;42(1):49–53.
Fitzgerald BC, Dias S, Martorell J. Cardiovascular drugs in avian, small mammal, and reptile medicine. Vet Clin Exot Anim 2018;21:399–442.
Johnson DH. Geriatric hedgehogs. Vet Clin Exot Anim Pract 2020;23(3):615–637.
Lennox AM. Emergency and critical care procedures in sugar gliders (*Petaurus breviceps*), African hedgehogs (*Atelerix albiventris*), and prairie dogs (*Cynomys* spp). Vet Clin North Am Exot Anim Pract. 2007;10:533–555.
McLaughlin A, Strunk A. Common emergencies in small rodents, hedgehogs, and sugar gliders. Vet Clin Exot Anim Pract 2016;19(2):465–499.
Raymond JT, Garner MM. Cardiomyopathy in captive African hedgehogs (*Atelerix albiventris*). J Vet Diagn Invest 2000;12(5):468–472.

Authors Amanda Steinagel, DVM and Barbara Oglesbee, DVM, Dipl. ABVP (Avian)

HEDGEHOGS

CONJUNCTIVITIS

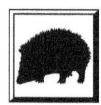

BASICS

DEFINITION
• Inflammation of the conjunctiva. The conjunctiva is the mucous membrane that surrounds the exposed portion of the ocular globe.
• The conjunctiva is made of the bulbar portion (anterior portion of the globe) and the palpebrae and third eyelid (palpebral portion)

PATHOPHYSIOLOGY
• Primary conjunctivitis may be caused by infection, exposure, trauma, and/or allergic causes.
• Secondary conjunctivitis may be caused by dental disease, upper respiratory tract infections, glaucoma, neoplasia, and/or uveitis.

SYSTEMS AFFECTED
• Ophthalmic—may include cornea (keratoconjunctivitis), eyelids/periocular skin (e.g., blepharoconjunctivitis), and nasolacrimal system (dacryocystitis)
• Respiratory—upper respiratory infections
• Oral—apical tooth root abscesses

GENETICS
N/A

INCIDENCE/PREVALENCE
Common

GEOGRAPHIC DISTRIBUTION
N/A

SIGNALMENT
• No specific age or breed predilection.

SIGNS
Historical Findings
• Previous dental disease. Exophthalmos, facial asymmetry, masses with dental abscesses.
• Owner may note trauma. May also describe a previous upper respiratory tract infection. Nasal or ocular discharge and/or sneezing.
• Periocular alopecia or crusting.
• Red, irritated eyes
• Pain

Physical Examination Findings
• Conjunctival hyperemia
• Chemosis
• Ocular discharge (purulent, mucopurulent, and serous)
• Corneal ulceration
• Chemosis
• Periocular alopecia and crusting
• Dental disease/abscesses
• Upper respiratory infection—sneezing, nasal discharge
• Signs of pain—depression, lethargy, and hiding,

CAUSES
• Bacterial infections—*Staphylococcus* spp., *Pasturella multocida*, *Pseudomonas* spp., and *Moraxella* spp. are the most common.
• Trauma—foreign body, chemical irritation, exposure
• Dental disease—tooth root disease, abscesses
• Allergic disease
• Anterior uveitis
• Glaucoma
• Neoplasia

RISK FACTORS
• Systemic bacterial infection or inflammatory disease
• Immunocompromise—corticosteroid use, stress
• Neoplasia
• Trauma
• Dental disease

DIAGNOSIS

DIFFERENTIAL DIAGNOSIS
• Important to differentiate from intra-ocular or retrobulbar disease.
• Any condition that causes conjunctivitis could be considered a differential—infectious, neoplasia, trauma, primary ocular disease, and/or dental disease.

CBC/BIOCHEMISTRY/URINALYSIS
• Typically, no significant abnormalities are noted unless other underlying systemic disease is present.

OTHER LABORATORY TESTS
• Bacterial C&S—swab conjunctival sac with microtip culturette
• Conjunctival cytology

IMAGING
• Skull radiographs—may be useful to evaluate for neoplasia, dental disease, and foreign bodies. The patient should be sedated/anesthetized for these procedures to allow for optimal positioning. Lateral views are best for detection of bony lysis of the nasal sinuses, periosteal reaction, and tooth root involvement. Ventrodorsal views are ideal for evaluation of the nasal cavity and turbinates. Lateral oblique views are best for root disease. The rostrocaudal view is ideal for evaluation of the frontal sinus (periosteal reaction).
• CT may be used for better quality imaging. Provides more detail of the nasal passages, sinuses, and dental disease.
• Orbital ultrasound may be useful in identifying reasons for exophthalmos to identify dental, nasal sinus, or maxillary bone lesions

DIAGNOSTIC PROCEDURES
• Complete ophthalmic examination—examine intraocular structures for signs of uveitis (miosis, aqueous flare) and adnexa for foreign body, or eyelid abnormalitites (aberrant cilia, entropion); ideally use magnification
• Schirmer tear test—any value lower than 5 mm/min is considered abnormal.
• Fluorescein staining—determination if a corneal ulcer is present and possibly how severe based on staining pattern.
• Tonometry—determination of ocular pressure, normal intraocular pressure is approximately 10–20 mmHg.

PATHOLOGIC FINDINGS
• Cause of chronic conjunctivitis—inflammatory cell population may suggest cause—neutrophils (bacterial); eosinophils (allergic, parasitic); granulomatous inflammation
• Characteristic features of malignancy (anisocytosis, anisokaryosis, increase in mitotic figures)

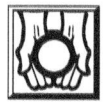

TREATMENT

APPROPRIATE HEALTH CARE
• Primary conjunctivitis—outpatient
• Remove cause of ocular irritation—extract corneal or conjunctival foreign body;

NURSING CARE
• Supportive—rinse any mucoid or mucopurulent debris from eye as produced—and always before treating with topical drugs to improve absorption; minimize crusty or moist build-up on periocular fur to reduce risk of secondary dermatitis
• May require change in housing if stressful or if suspect environmental irritant
• Provide hiding box for security if hospitalized

ACTIVITY
• Primary—typically no restriction; segregate if infectious cause suspected/confirmed
• Secondary—reduce exposure to at-risk environment or contact with potential irritant

DIET
Be certain the patient continues to eat to prevent gastrointestinal motility disorders.

CLIENT EDUCATION
• Clean discharge from conjunctival surfaces/cul-de-sacs before treatment
• If multiple topical medications required, use drops followed by ointments or lubricants and allow 5 minutes between different preparations

• Explain the possibility of chronicity of disease or reoccurrence, especially if dental disease or neoplasia is the cause.

SURGICAL CONSIDERATIONS
If mass or localized lesion, excisional biopsy recommended

MEDICATIONS
DRUG(S) OF CHOICE
• Antibiotics—(based on culture and sensitivity results)—cephalexin (25 mg/kg PO q12h), amoxicillin/clavulanic acid (12.5–25 mg/kg PO q12h), enrofloxacin (5–10 mg/kg PO q12h), trimethoprim-sulfa (30 mg/kg PO q12h), chloramphenicol (30–50 mg/kg PO q12), azithromycin (20 mg/kg PO q24h)
• Antihistamines may be used for rhinitis/inflammation. diphenhydramine (1–2 mg/kg PO, IM q8–12) or hydroxyzine (1–2 mg/kg PO q8–12) may be used for allergic disease.
• Topical antibiotic ophthalmic solutions/ointments—ciprofloxacin, ofloxacin, gentamycin, neomycin/polymyxin B sulfates/bacitracin zinc, others topically q4–6h
• Topical pain management—atropine 1% solution q12–24h
• Topical non-steroidal anti-inflammatory solutions/ointments—flurbiprofen 0.03% or diclofenac 1% q12–24h
• Pain management—meloxicam (0.2 mg/kg PO q24h), tramadol (2–5 mg/kg PO q8–12), or buprenorphine (0.03–0.05 mg/kg IM, SQ, PO q6–12h) may be used for painful conditions/inflammation.
• For sedation—ketamine (20–30 mg/kg IM) + midazolam (1 mg/kg IM) or alfaxalone (1–3 mg/kg IM + midazolam (0.5–1 mg/kg IM) ± butorphanol (0.2 mg/kg IM) add alfaxalone (1 mg/kg IM) boluses PRN

CONTRAINDICATIONS
• Avoid steroid containing ophthalmic preparations in cases of ulcerative keratitis; may exacerbate infectious disease.

PRECAUTIONS
• Chloramphenicol—avoid human contact due to potential blood dyscrasia. Advise owners of potential risk.

POSSIBLE INTERACTIONS
N/A

ALTERNATIVE DRUGS
N/A

FOLLOW-UP
PATIENT MONITORING
Reevaluate short-term after initiating therapy (i.e., 5–7 days); treat until condition resolved then recheck again 5–7 days after therapy is discontinued—stain cornea with fluorescein at each recheck

PREVENTION/AVOIDANCE
• Therapy for underlying conditions
• Correct husbandry/clean environment

POSSIBLE COMPLICATIONS
• Reoccurrence is common especially if the cause is dental disease or neoplasia.

EXPECTED COURSE AND PROGNOSIS
• Primary/Infectious—usually resolves with appropriate antibiotics or other specific treatment
• Secondary—depends on course of predisposing condition

MISCELLANEOUS
ASSOCIATED CONDITIONS
Dental disease
Neoplasia

AGE-RELATED FACTORS
N/A

ZOONOTIC POTENTIAL
• Hedgehogs can be asymptomatic carriers of *Salmonella*. Use gloves and careful handwashing after handling.

PREGNANCY/FERTILITY/BREEDING
• N/A

SYNONYMS
Pink eye

SEE ALSO
Exophthalmos and orbital diseases
Dental Disease

ABBREVIATIONS
C&S = culture and sensitivity results
CT = computed tomography
GI = gastrointestinal
IOP = intraocular pressure
KCS = keratoconjunctivitis sicca
NSAID = nonsteroidal anti-inflammatory drug
STT = Schirmer tear test

Suggested Reading
Chin J, Mans C. Small mammals: hedgehogs. In: Mayer J, Donnelly T, eds. Clinical Veterinary Advisor: Birds and Exotic Pets. St. Louis, MO: Saunders, 2013:338–343.
Ivey E, Carpenter J. African hedgehogs. In: Quesenberry KE, Carpenter JW, eds. Ferrets, Rabbits, and Rodents: Clinical Medicine and Surgery, 3rd ed. St. Louis, MO: Saunders, 2012:339–353.
Johnson DH. Geriatric hedgehogs. Vet Clin Exot Anim Pract 2020;23(3):615–637.
Lennox AM. Emergency and critical care procedures in sugar gliders (*Petaurus breviceps*), African hedgehogs (*Atelerix albiventris*), and prairie dogs (*Cynomys* spp). Vet Clin North Am Exot Anim Pract 2007;10:533–555.

Author Amanda Steinagel, DVM

HEDGEHOGS

CUTANEOUS AND SUBCUTANEOUS MASSES

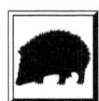

BASICS

DEFINITION
• Abnormal tissue growth or swelling that involves the epithelium and/or subcutaneous tissues

PATHOPHYSIOLOGY
• Any process that elicits an inflammatory response resulting in accumulation of inflammatory products and fluid in or under the skin
• Infection and the resultant accumulation of inflammatory or purulent material
• Neoplastic processes and growth of tumors

SYSTEMS AFFECTED
• Skin/Exocrine
• Other systems may be affected, depending on the type of mass present.

GENETICS
N/A

INCIDENCE/PREVALENCE
Subcutaneous and cutaneous masses are common presentations. The incidence of neoplasia in general is high in hedgehogs.

GEOGRAPHIC DISTRIBUTION
N/A

SIGNALMENT
Masses in general are more common in older animals regardless

SIGNS
Physical Examination Findings
• Abscesses—swelling that may be fluctuant, possible ulceration, purulent material on aspiration
• Tumors or growths
• Thin, emaciated
• Abdominal distension, organomegaly
• Oral abnormalities—missing teeth, ptyalism, oral masses, and abscesses

CAUSES
• Dental disease/Abscessation—apical or tooth root abscess, severe dental tartar, and gingivitis. Typically, bacteria involved in dental abscess includes *Streptococcus* spp., *Fusobacterium* spp., *Actinomyces* spp., and *Arcanobacterium* spp.
• Neoplasia—sarcoma, carcinoma (oral squamous cell carcinoma), adenocarcinoma (mammary gland carcinoma), mast cell tumors, lipoma, and liposarcoma
• Trauma

RISK FACTORS
Exposure to infectious agents, inadequate husbandry

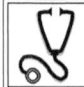

DIAGNOSIS

DIFFERENTIAL DIAGNOSIS
• Abscess
• Neoplasia
• Ingrown quills
• Trauma

CBC/BIOCHEMISTRY/URINALYSIS
• Anemia and/or leukemia may be present if the mass is neoplastic.
• Chemistry abnormalities based on the body system affected but hypercalcemia and hyperbilirubinemia are common findings with neoplastic processes. May be normal if benign masses are present.

OTHER LABORATORY TESTS
N/A

IMAGING
• Three-view survey radiographs and/or ultrasonographic imaging should be used to screen for potential metastasis if malignant neoplasia is suspected. Radiographs may also be used to evaluate bony structures for osteomyelitis in cases of neoplasia or abscess.
• CT—better quality imaging.
• Abdominal ultrasound—to assess hepatic, urogenital, gastrointestinal, lymphatic, and/ or splenic system abnormalities/enlargement. May aid in fine needle aspiration of intraabdominal masses or lymph nodes.

DIAGNOSTIC PROCEDURES
The most useful tools in diagnosing the cause of subcutaneous and cutaneous swellings include fine-needle aspirates and cytology, biopsy and histopathology, and bacterial cultures if indicated for abscesses or secondary infections. Biopsy and histopathology generally provide a more accurate means of diagnosis than fine-needle aspirates, as many swellings and masses do not exfoliate well and only an acellular sample is obtained by aspiration.

PATHOLOGIC FINDINGS
Variable depending on the etiology

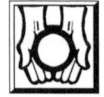

TREATMENT

APPROPRIATE HEALTH CARE
Many cases can be treated on an outpatient basis unless debilitated or requiring postoperative monitoring.

NURSING CARE
Supportive care including thermal regulation, fluid administration, and assisted feeding for stabilization of debilitated patients.

Postoperative supportive care for patients treated surgically.

ACTIVITY
Activity restriction is usually not necessary except as indicated postoperatively for patients treated surgically.

DIET
Supportive care and dietary concerns may need to be addressed based on severity of disease

CLIENT EDUCATION
• Discussion of treatment, prognosis, and management based on tumor type/ malignancy
• Mammary adenocarcinoma and oral squamous cell carcinoma tend to be locally invasive and carry a poor prognosis.
• Annual wellness examinations are important to assess for obvious masses or abnormalities

SURGICAL CONSIDERATIONS
• Surgical removal of masses or removal/ debridement of abscesses are the treatments of choice. Where neoplasia is suspected, every attempt should be made to excise masses completely with wide margins.

MEDICATIONS

DRUG(S) OF CHOICE
• Antibiotics—(based on culture and sensitivity results)—cephalexin (25 mg/kg PO q12h), amoxicillin/clavulanic acid (12.5–25 mg/kg PO q12h), enrofloxacin (5–10 mg/kg PO q12h), trimethoprim-sulfa (30 mg/kg PO q12h), chloramphenicol (30–50 mg/kg PO q12)
• Pain management—meloxicam (0.2 mg/kg PO q24h), tramadol (2–5 mg/kg PO q8–12), or buprenorphine (0.03–0.05 mg/kg IM, SQ, PO q6–12h) may be used for painful conditions/inflammation.
• For sedation—ketamine (20–30 mg/kg IM) + midazolam (1 mg/kg IM) or alfaxalone (1–3 mg/kg IM + midazolam (0.5–1 mg/kg IM) ± butorphanol (0.2 mg/kg IM) add alfaxalone (1 mg/kg IM) boluses PRN

CONTRAINDICATIONS
• Corticosteroid use is not recommended to treat infectious disease.

PRECAUTIONS
N/A

POSSIBLE INTERACTIONS
N/A

ALTERNATIVE DRUGS
• Chemotherapy—currently no data is available on the efficacy of the in hedgehogs.

FOLLOW-UP

Reevaluate patients within 1–2 weeks for resolution of clinical signs and for surgical follow-up as indicated.

PATIENT MONITORING

Reevaluate at least once every 3–4 months for recurrence of neoplastic conditions.

PREVENTION/AVOIDANCE

Optimize husbandry to avoid injury and exposure to infectious agents.

POSSIBLE COMPLICATIONS

• Metastasis or local recurrence of neoplastic lesions following surgical removal is possible.
• Some infections and abscesses may be resistant to treatment and require long-term therapy.

EXPECTED COURSE AND PROGNOSIS

• Variable, depending on cause. In general, good with abscess or ingrown quills, guarded to poor with most neoplastic disorders.

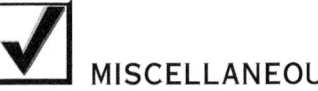

MISCELLANEOUS

ASSOCIATED CONDITIONS

• Immunosuppression
• Dental disease

AGE-RELATED FACTORS

Neoplasias are more common in older animals.

ZOONOTIC POTENTIAL

• Hedgehogs can be asymptomatic carriers of *Salmonella*. Use gloves and careful handwashing after handling.

PREGNANCY/FERTILITY/ BREEDING

N/A

SYNONYMS

• Cancer
• Neoplasia

SEE ALSO

• Neoplasia

ABBREVIATIONS

• CBC = complete blood count
• CT = computed tomography

INTERNET RESOURCES

Veterinary Information Network: www.vin.com
Exotic DVM forum for eDVM readers: www.pets.groups.yahoo.com/group/ExoticDVM

Suggested Reading

Chin J, Mans C. Small mammals: hedgehogs. In: Mayer J, Donnelly T, eds. Clinical Veterinary Advisor: Birds and Exotic Pets. St. Louis, MO: Saunders, 2013:338–343.

Ivey E, Carpenter J. African hedgehogs. In: Quesenberry KE, Carpenter JW, eds. Ferrets, Rabbits, and Rodents: Clinical Medicine and Surgery, 3rd ed. St Louis, MO: Saunders, 2012:411–427.

Johnson DH. Geriatric hedgehogs. Vet Clin Exot Anim Pract 2020;23(3):615–637.

Keeble E, Koterwas B. Selected emerging diseases of pet hedgehogs. Vet Clin Exot Anim Pract 2020;23(2):443–458.

Lennox AM. Emergency and critical care procedures in sugar gliders (*Petaurus breviceps*), African hedgehogs (*Atelerix albiventris*), and prairie dogs (*Cynomys* spp). Vet Clin North Am Exot Anim Pract 2007;10:533–555.

Author Amanda Steinagel, DVM

DENTAL DISEASE

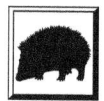

BASICS

OVERVIEW

Definition
• Syndrome affecting the oral cavity including teeth and associated structures.
• May result in periapical abscesses, which is the accumulation of inflammatory cells at the apex of a tooth.

PATHOPHYSIOLOGY
• Dental disease in hedgehogs is primarily associated with inappropriate diets that are too soft and carbohydrate rich. These diets often lead to the development of periodontal disease, caries, and tartar accumulation
• Severe periodontal disease may lead to boney involvement and abscessation.
• Trauma to the teeth may result in pulp exposure and infection.

SYSTEMS AFFECTED
• Oral cavity
• Ocular—secondary to peri-apical abscesses

INCIDENCE/PREVALENCE
• Incidence increases with age
• No sex predilection

SIGNS

Historical Findings
• Historical signs often include hyporexia or anorexia, weight loss, discharge or moisture around the mouth, and changes in the dietary items preferred (trending toward softer items).
• Altered feeding and chewing behavior may be observed by owners that should be evaluated further for evidence of dental disease and pain.
• Swellings or mass lesions around the cheeks and eyes may be noted initially by caregivers.

Physical Examination Findings
• Inspection of the oral cavity while awake is challenging in hedgehogs; therefore, proper diagnosis of dental disease must be performed under deep sedation or general anesthesia.
• Common findings include gingivitis, dental discoloration, tartar and calculus, periodontitis, and mass lesions.
• Pytalism
• Exophthalmos, ocular discharge, and nasal discharge
• Muscle wasting, weight loss

CAUSES AND RISK FACTORS
• Diets that lack hard or abrasive elements (chitinous exoskeletons), contain only soft items and are rich in carbohydrates.
• Periapical or tooth root abscess—*Streptococcus* spp., *Fusobacterium* spp., *Actinomyces* spp., and *Arcanobacterium* spp.

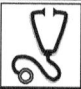

DIAGNOSIS

DIFFERENTIAL DIAGNOSIS
• Normal incisor gap—the upper incisors are normally wide set in African Pigmy Hedgehogs
• For oral ulceration and swelling—squamous cell carcinoma is the most common neoplasia in Hedgehogs and commonly occur in the oral cavity
• For anorexia—gastrointestinal disease, pain, and metabolic disease

CBC/BIOCHEMISTRY/URINALYSIS
• Usually normal unless secondary infection or other underlying metabolic disease is present

OTHER LABORATORY TESTS
• Culture/cytology of dental abscesses

IMAGING
• Culture/cytology of dental abscesses
• Radiographs may be useful to evaluate for neoplasia, dental disease, and foreign bodies. The patient should be sedated/anesthetized for these procedures to allow for optimal positioning. Lateral views are best for detection of bony lysis of the nasal sinuses, periosteal reaction, and tooth root involvement. Ventrodorsal views are ideal for evaluation of the nasal cavity and turbinates. Lateral oblique views are best for root disease. The rostrocaudal view is ideal for evaluation of the frontal sinus (periosteal reaction).
• Modern CT scans provide excellent detail in small species like hedgehogs

TREATMENT
The goal of treatment is the resolution of bacterial infection, and removal of diseased, damaged, or painful teeth.

APPROPRIATE HEALTH CARE
• Thorough dental evaluation and dental surgery should be performed under general anesthesia with appropriate analgesia.
• Provide supportive care, such as fluid therapy and assist-feeding, in patients that are not eating.
• Use of antimicrobials should, ideally, be based on the result of culture and sensitivity testing.

SURGICAL CONSIDERATIONS

Dental Extractions
• Teeth are extracted with careful dissection of the periodontal ligament using small (25-gauge) contoured needles or appropriately sized dental elevators.

• The most frequent complications are fractures of the teeth or root and fractures of the maxilla or mandible especially when osteomyelitis and/or nutritional osteodystrophy are present.
• Dental disease requiring extraction of teeth typically carries a guarded prognosis due to the difficulty and complications associated with extraction.

MEDICATIONS

DRUG(S) OF CHOICE
• Antibiotics—(based on culture and sensitivity results)—cephalexin (25 mg/kg PO q12h), amoxicillin/clavulanic acid (12.5–25 mg/kg PO q12h), enrofloxacin (5–10 mg/kg PO q12h), trimethoprim-sulfa (30 mg/kg PO q12h), and chloramphenicol (30–50 mg/kg PO q12)
• Pain management—meloxicam (0.2 mg/kg PO q24h), tramadol (2–5 mg/kg PO q8–12), or buprenorphine (0.03–0.05 mg/kg IM, SQ, PO q6–12h) may be used for painful conditions/inflammation.
• For sedation—ketamine (20–30 mg/kg IM) + midazolam (1mg/kg IM) or alfaxalone (1–3 mg/kg IM + midazolam (0.5–1 mg/kg IM) ± butorphanol (0.2 mg/kg IM) add alfaxalone (1 mg/kg IM) boluses PRN

CONTRAINDICATIONS
Extensive surgery on a debilitated animal

PRECAUTIONS
• Chloramphenicol may cause aplastic anemia in susceptible people. Clients and staff should use appropriate precautions when handling this drug.

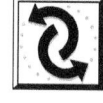

FOLLOW-UP

PATIENT MONITORING
• Monitor appetite and the ability to eat following treatment. Some patients may require assist feeding. The duration of assist-feeding depends on the severity of disease.
• Important to monitor for weight loss. Daily weights are recommended.

PREVENTION/AVOIDANCE
Provision of an appropriate diet with a variety of textures and items of differing hardness.

POSSIBLE COMPLICATIONS
Iatrogenic maxilla/mandibular fracture, recurrence, chronic pain, or inability to chew.

EXPECTED COURSE AND PROGNOSIS
• Oral abscesses typically carry a fair prognosis if they respond to medical therapy.

HEDGEHOGS

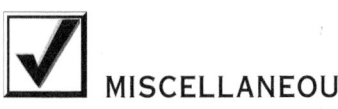

MISCELLANEOUS

ASSOCIATED CONDITIONS
- Exopthalmous
- Abscessation
- Hepatic lipidosis

AGE-RELATED FACTORS
Older patients have a higher incidence of dental disease.

ZOONOTIC POTENTIAL
- Hedgehogs can be asymptomatic carriers of *Salmonella*. Use gloves and careful handwashing after handling.

PREGNANCY/FERTILITY/BREEDING
N/A

SYNONYMS
N/A

SEE ALSO
- Anorexia
- Exopthalmous and orbital disease
- Neoplasia

Suggested Reading
Chaprazov T, Dimitrov R, Yovcheva KS, Uzenova K. Oral and dental disorders in pet hedgehogs. Turk J Vet Anim Sci 2014;38(1):1–6.
Evans EE, Souza MJ. Advanced diagnostic approaches and current management of internal disorders of select species (rodents, sugar gliders, hedgehogs). Vet Clin Exot Anim Pract 2010;13(3):453–469.
Johnson DH. Geriatric hedgehogs. Vet Clin Exot Anim Pract 2020;23(3):615–637.
Lennox AM, Miwa Y. Anatomy and disorders of the oral cavity of miscellaneous exotic companion mammals. Vet Clin Exot Anim Pract 2016;19(3):929–945.

Author Amanda Steinagel, DVM

DERMATOPHYTOSIS

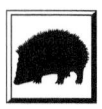

BASICS

DEFINITION
A cutaneous fungal infection affecting the cornified regions of the nails, hair, and superficial layers of the skin

PATHOPHYSIOLOGY
• Exposure to or contact with a dermatophyte may result in active infection with skin inflammation, scaling, and hair loss or may result in a latent infection or prolonged asymptomatic carrier state. Stress, immune compromise, or the use of medications such as corticosteroids may prolong infection. The incubation period for dermatophyte infection is typically 1–4 weeks. Dermatophytes grow in the keratinized layers of the skin, hair, and nails but do not thrive in living tissue.
• Dermatophyte infection often occurs in association with mite infestation. Fungal growth is facilitated by changes caused by mite infestation. Fungal spores are found in mite droppings.
• Many Hedgehogs are asymptomatic carriers

SYSTEMS AFFECTED
Skin/Exocrine

GENETICS
N/A

INCIDENCE/PREVALENCE
Quill loss and skin disease are one of the most common health problems in African Pigmy Hedgehogs, with mite infestation the most common cause.

GEOGRAPHIC DISTRIBUTION
Ubiquitous

SIGNALMENT
• More common in older animals debilitated by concurrent disease or immunosuppression

SIGNS
History
• May have a history recent stress or systemic disease

Physical Examination Findings
• Quill loss is more common than loss of hair on the abdomen; can appear as focal, patchy, or diffuse thinning
• Dry flaky skin, crusting, seborrhea, erythema, and lichenification
• Quills may fall off during physical examination
• Weight loss, general debility
• Excoriations, erythema

CAUSES
• *Trichophyton erinacei, Trichophyton mentagrophytes,* and *Microsporum* spp most common. Other species include *Arthroderma*

benhamiae and *Paecilomyces Variotii.* Dermatophytes can occur alone or in association with mite infestation. Fungal growth is facilitated by changes caused by mite infestation. Fungal spores are found in mite droppings.

RISK FACTORS
Poor husbandry, overcrowding, poor sanitation, and inappropriate nutrition increase the risk of infection with dermatophytes. Immune-suppressing disease or medications predispose animals to dermatophytosis and increase the potential for more severe and protracted infections.

DIAGNOSIS

DIFFERENTIAL DIAGNOSIS
• Ectoparasites—*Caparinia* spp, a nonburrowing psoroptid mite is most common, but *Chorioptes* spp and sarcoptid species are also seen.
  ○ Ear mites *Notoedres* or *Otodectes* sp can cause alopecia around the face and ears
  ○ Fleas can sometimes cause quill and hair loss
• Metabolic/Nutritional—debility, underlying disease predispose to mite infestation and dermatophytosis; diets low in protein can cause barbering
• Bacterial—usually secondary to scratching; *Staphylococcus* sp. most common.
• Husbandry/Environmental/Stress—contact dermatitis, urine scald
• Neoplasia—cutaneous lymphoma, mast cell tumors, cutaneous hemangiosarcoma, and histiocytic sarcoma are most commonly reported
• Trauma—environmental/cage rubbing/bite wounds, self-mutilation
• Endocrinopathy and immune-mediated causes not yet reported

CBC/BIOCHEMISTRY/URINALYSIS
In systemically ill pets or those with refractory dermatophytosis, serum biochemistries, complete blood count, and urinalysis may help identify underlying problems that are contributing factors in the development of dermatophytosis.

OTHER LABORATORY TESTS
• Dermatophyte testing—either PCR or fungal culture. Fungal culture results are often delayed due to the long growth time required. Begin treatment while awaiting results. False negatives are common, especially with PCR testing, as most laboratories do not test for all species commonly infecting hedgehogs

IMAGING
In systemically ill patients, radiographs may help confirm the presence of organomegaly, dystrophic mineralization, or the presence of masses.

DIAGNOSTIC PROCEDURES
• Skin scrapings and dermatophyte cultures should be included as part of the minimum database.
• Wood's lamp illumination is useful only for identification of *Microsporum.* Both false-positive and false-negative results are possible, so this technique should only be used in conjunction with other screening tools.
• Response to treatment with antifungal medication
• Skin biopsy may be indicated in refractory cases.

PATHOLOGIC FINDINGS
Folliculitis, perifolliculitis, and/or furunculosis are common. Hyperkeratosis, pyogranulomatous inflammation, and epidermal pustules may also be observed. While some fungal hyphae may be observed with routine H&E staining, special stains are typically needed for better visualization of the fungal organisms.

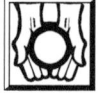

TREATMENT

APPROPRIATE HEALTH CARE
Treatment with appropriate topical or systemic antifungal medications on an outpatient basis is usually appropriate.

NURSING CARE
Quarantine may be considered in some cases due to the zoonotic potential of dermatophyte infections.

ACTIVITY
Activity restriction is not indicated.

DIET
As long as adequate nutrition is provided, diet changes are not indicated. If griseofulvin is used to treat the infection, consumption of a fatty meal improves absorption of the medication.

CLIENT EDUCATION
• Advise clients of the zoonotic potential of dermatophytes.
• In multipet households, treatment of the environment and all individuals in the collection may be necessary.
• 1:10 dilute bleach has demonstrated efficacy in environmental decontamination.
• Asymptomatic carriers exist, some individuals may have spontaneous resolution of lesions, and some cases of dermatophytosis may be recurrent in nature.

SURGICAL CONSIDERATIONS
N/A

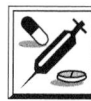

MEDICATIONS

DRUG(S) OF CHOICE
- Topical medications
  - Topical antifungals/shampoos—ketoconazole (bathe 1–2 times daily for 2–4 weeks), miconazole (apply a small amount to the affected skin 1–2 times daily for 2–4 weeks), clotrimazole cream (apply a small amount to the affected skin 1–2 times daily for 2–4 weeks), butenafine cream (apply a small amount to the affected skin 1–2 times daily for 2–4 weeks)
  - Lyme sulfur dips—diluted 1:40 with warm water, bathe once weekly for 4–6 weeks. May need to consider soaking cotton balls and using to sponge onto the hedgehog, since bathing may be stressful.
- Oral medications
  - Terbinafine (100 mg/kg PO q12h × 4–6 wk)
  - Ketoconazole (10 mg/kg PO q24h × 6–8 wks)
  - Itraconazole (5–10 mg/kg PO q12–24h × 4–6 wks)
- Environmental decontamination to prevent spread or reinfection.

CONTRAINDICATIONS
- Griseofulvin is not recommended for use with pregnant animals due to teratogenic properties. May also cause bone marrow suppression in other species but has not been reported in hedgehogs.

PRECAUTIONS
- Ketoconazole and itraconazole use may cause vasculitis and hepatopathy, but this has not been reported in hedgehogs.
- Corticosteroid use is not recommended to treat infectious disease

POSSIBLE INTERACTIONS
N/A

ALTERNATIVE DRUGS
N/A

FOLLOW-UP

PATIENT MONITORING
Repeat fungal cultures are recommended toward the end of treatment as some animals may clinically improve but remain culture positive. Treatment should be continued until a negative culture result is obtained.

PREVENTION/AVOIDANCE
Spread to other animals and reinfection can be reduced by quarantine of infected pets until dermatophyte cultures are negative. Any new animals introduced to the collection should also undergo a quarantine period to prevent introduction of organisms.

POSSIBLE COMPLICATIONS
- Recurrence, especially if concurrent mite infestation is not treated.

EXPECTED COURSE AND PROGNOSIS
Most animals will respond to treatment and clear dermatophyte infections. Persistent or refractory infections can be a problem in debilitated patients or multipet situations.

MISCELLANEOUS

ASSOCIATED CONDITIONS
Mites

AGE-RELATED FACTORS
More common in young animals or older, debilitated animals

ZOONOTIC POTENTIAL
- Hedgehogs can be asymptomatic carriers of *Salmonella*. Use gloves and careful handwashing after handling.
- Dermatophyte infections can be transmitted to humans.

PREGNANCY/FERTILITY/BREEDING
N/A

SYNONYMS
Ringworm

SEE ALSO
Alopecia
Ectoparasites

ABBREVIATIONS
N/A

INTERNET RESOURCES
Exotic DVM forum for eDVM readers: www.pets.groups.yahoo.com/group/ExoticDVM
Veterinary Information Network: www.vin.com

Suggested Reading
Chin J, Mans C. Small mammals: hedgehogs. In: Mayer J, Donnelly T, eds. Clinical Veterinary Advisor: Birds and Exotic Pets. St. Louis, MO: Saunders, 2013:338–343.
Ivey E, Carpenter J. African hedgehogs. In: Quesenberry KE, Carpenter JW, eds. Ferrets, Rabbits, and Rodents: Clinical Medicine and Surgery, 3rd ed. St Louis, MO: Saunders:339–353.
Johnson DH. African pygmy hedgehogs. In: Johnson-Delaney C, Meredith A, eds. BSAVA Manual of Exotic Pets, A Foundation Manual. Quedgeley, Gloucester: British Small Animal Veterinary Association, 2010:139–147.
Johnson DH. Geriatric hedgehogs. Vet Clin Exot Anim Pract 2020;23(3):615–637.
Keeble E, Koterwas B. Selected emerging diseases of pet hedgehogs. Vet Clin Exot Anim Pract 2020;23(2):443–458.
Lennox AM. Emergency and critical care procedures in sugar gliders (*Petaurus breviceps*), African hedgehogs (*Atelerix albiventris*), and prairie dogs (*Cynomys* spp). Vet Clin North Am Exot Anim Pract 2007;10:533–555.

Author Amanda Steinagel, DVM

HEDGEHOGS

DYSPNEA AND TACHYPNEA

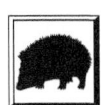

BASICS

DEFINITION
• Dyspnea is the stressful response/feeling associated with difficult or labored breathing.
• Tachypnea is an increased respiratory rate but may not be associated with labored breathing.
• Open-mouth breathing is a medical emergency.

PATHOPHYSIOLOGY
• Primary respiratory disease can be caused by upper or lower respiratory tract problems.
• Nonrespiratory causes of dyspnea include abnormalities in pulmonary vascular tone (CNS disease, shock), pulmonary circulation (CHF), oxygenation (anemia), or ventilation (obesity, ascites, abdominal organomegaly, musculoskeletal disease).

SYSTEMS AFFECTED
• Respiratory
• Cardiovascular
• Nervous (secondary to hypoxia)
Common—incidence of respiratory disease ranged from 14% to 25% in retrospective necropsy reports

SIGNALMENT
• Young animals—typically bacterial infections
• Middle aged-older animals—dental disease, neoplasia, and bacterial infections

SIGNS
Historical Findings
• Vary depending on the cause
• Anorexia, lethargy, and weight loss
• Nasal or ocular discharge, coughing, and sneezing
• History of dental disease
• Poor husbandry, including inappropriate ventilation, poor cleanliness, or inappropriate diet
• Obesity

Physical Examination Findings
• Lethargy, weight loss
• Upper respiratory tract disease: serous or mucopurulent nasal discharge, ocular discharge, dental disease (ptyalism, bruxism, and facial abscess)
• Obesity or abdominal distension
• Pneumonia: abnormal breath sounds on auscultation, including crackles, wheezes, increased bronchovesicular sounds, or decreased or absent breath sounds with abscess, lung consolidation, neoplasia, or heart disease (effusion)

CAUSES
Respiratory Causes
Upper respiratory tract
• Nasal passage obstruction: rhinitis or sinusitis. Common bacterial pathogens include *Pasturella multocida*, *Bordetella bronchiseptica*, and *Corynebacterium* sp.
• Trauma to the face, nose, and neck
• Neoplasia—especially squamous cell carcinoma (most common neoplasia in pet hedgehogs)
• Dental disease—periapical or tooth root abscess, severe dental tartar, and gingivitis. Typically, bacteria involved in dental abscesses include *Streptococcus spp.*, *Fusobacteriu* spp., *Actinomyces* spp., and *Arcanobacterium* spp.
• Laryngotracheal obstruction: foreign body, abscess, neoplasia
Lower respiratory tract
• Pneumonia: usually bacterial (*Bordetella brochiseptica Pasteurella multocida,* and *Corynebacterium* sp.) but can also be viral (Skunk adenovirus, African Pygmy Hedgehog adenovirus—rare) or due to aspiration
• Neoplasia—bronchoalveolar carcinoma; metastatic lung tumors
• Obesity—lipid pneumonia has been reported in severely obese hedgehogs
• Pulmonary edema (cardiogenic or noncardiogenic), pulmonary contusion (trauma), allergy, and intrathoracic tracheal disease (neoplasia, abscess, and foreign body)
• Extraluminal tracheal compression due to an abscess or neoplasia
• Traumatic airway rupture (uncommon)

Nonrespiratory Causes
• Cardiac disease: CHF (common)
• Abdominal distension: obesity, organomegaly, and ascites
• Neuromuscular disease: severe CNS disease (trauma, abscess, neoplasia, inflammation), spinal disease (trauma)
• Hematologic: anemia

RISK FACTORS
• Dental disease
• Immunosuppression—stress, geriatric age, concurrent disease, and corticosteroid use
• Poor husbandry
• Poor diet
• Obesity

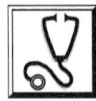

DIAGNOSIS

DIFFERENTIAL DIAGNOSIS
• Normal noises—hedgehogs have poor eyesight and hearing and rely heavily on their sense of smell. They often create a loud snuffling noise when investigating a new environment.
  ◦ Normal defensive "hiss"
  ◦ Anting or self-anointing behavior—when encountering a new smell, hedgehogs will produce copious amounts of thick, foamy saliva and spread it on their quills. Direct contact with the object creating the odor is not necessary. It is believed that this is a defensive mechanism.
• Dyspnea due to upper respiratory tract disease is often more pronounced with inspiration, whereas lower respiratory tract disease is often associated with increased expiratory effort.
• Tracheal mass or foreign body usually causes both inspiratory and expiratory effort.
• Pneumonia often has systemic signs of disease (anorexia, weight loss, depression, and lethargy), whereas primary cardiac disease often is associated with a murmur or arrhythmia.

CBC/BIOCHEMISTRY/URINALYSIS
• Complete blood count may support but cannot confirm or rule out respiratory disease.
• Biochemistry panel is useful to identify predisposing underlying disease.

OTHER LABORATORY TESTS
Culture and susceptibility testing for bacterial pathogens may be helpful in directing antibiotic therapy. May be difficult to interpret due to the high probability of culturing a commensal or opportunistic organism. Typically, the heavy growth of one organism is significant.

IMAGING
• Radiographs of the skull: must be done under heavy sedation or general anesthesia for optimal positioning, with a minimum of five views (lateral, two oblique laterals, anterior posterior, and ventrodorsal views) recommended, observe radiographs for bony lysis or proliferation of the turbinates and facial bones, as this can indicate chronic bacterial or neoplastic processes
• CT or MRI: provide better imaging quality; may be more diagnostic than skull radiographs, especially if nasal detail is obscured by nasal discharge; can help to determine whether the cause of disease is nasal, sinus, or dental disease. CT specifically is excellent for providing bony detail, is more sensitive for area encased in bone (i.e., lungs and sinuses), and the procedure time is relatively short. However, these modalities may be cost prohibitive and not as readily available.

DYSPNEA AND TACHYPNEA

- Thoracic radiographs: pneumonia (alveolar pattern with increased pulmonary density which can be patchy or diffuse—air bronchograms, consolidated lung lobes), pulmonary edema, small airway disease, cardiomegaly
- Abdominal radiographs: organomegaly, ascites, gas-filled/distended stomach due to aerophagia or bloat
- Ultrasonography: echocardiography difficult due to small size of patient but may help determine if primary heart disease is present; abdominal ultrasound may be used for the evaluation of organomegaly, pregnancy, or masses

DIAGNOSTIC PROCEDURES

- Cytology of exudates: can use Gram stain or standard cell stain (Diff Quick)
- Nasal cavity biopsy: should be performed in animals with chronic nasal discharge (especially epistaxis) if neoplasia is suspected; use endoscopy or rhinotomy to obtain the sample
- Direct visualization of the pharynx or larynx: can use a 2.7-mm rigid endoscope for direct visualization, requires general anesthesia;
- Transtracheal wash or bronchoalveolar lavage can be difficult to perform due to small tracheal size.
- For thoracic masses—aspirate can be performed with ultrasound guidance
- Thoracocentesis or abdominocentesis: fluid analysis and culture

PATHOLOGIC FINDINGS

Variable, depending on the cause

TREATMENT

APPROPRIATE HEALTH CARE

Depends on the underlying cause

NURSING CARE

- Supplying an oxygen-rich environment is most important if the patient is dyspneic. Use an oxygen cage or induction chamber in a quiet environment.
- Ensure that the patient is kept warm— between 80 and 85°F (27 and 29°C). Topor occurs when the environmental temperature falls below 65°F (18°C).
- Fluid therapy is used to correct hydration following standard protocols (5%–10% of body weight administered in SQ boluses). Fluids should be kept warm to prevent hypothermia and can be warmed by placing the prepared syringe in a warm water bath prior to administration. Administration via a 22–25-gauge butterfly needle can reduce stress on the patient by minimizing restraint.
- Fluid therapy to maintain normal hydration (fluid needs estimated to be

100 mL/kg/day)—fluid can be given IV, IO, or SC. Necessary to aid mucocilliary clearance; may consider reductions in the maintenance fluid requirement if cardiac disease is suspected.
- Keep nares clear of nasal discharge.
- Nebulization with bland aerosols may help deliver moisture to the upper respiratory tract, and if used in conjunction with antibiotics, may lead to resolution.
- If trachea is completely obstructed, will need to attempt emergency intubation or emergency tracheostomy
- Thoracocentesis or abdominocentesis: may be diagnostic and therapeutic in patients with pleural space disease or abdominal effusion
- Surgery may be necessary to remove foreign bodies, obtain biopsy samples, or debulk tumors, abscesses, or granulomas. Maintaining adequate ventilation in these situations is difficult.

ACTIVITY

Patient's activity should be restricted as exertion can increase respiratory effort and/or rate, which can worsen obstructive airway disease.

DIET

- It is imperative that the animal receive nutritional support if it is not eating. Supplementation with a liquid diet may be required, such as Oxbow Carnivore Care (Oxbow Enterprises, Inc., Murdock, NE) or Emeraid Exotic Carnivore (Lafeber's, Cornell, IL) is essential.
- Gradual caloric restriction in obese patients

CLIENT EDUCATION

- If the underlying disease cannot be corrected (i.e., dental disease, neoplasia, and severe tissue destruction), a cure is unlikely. The treatment, depending on the cause, can be lifelong and aims to control the severity of clinical signs.
- Most neoplasms are malignant, and treatment is generally palliative

SURGICAL CONSIDERATIONS

Anesthesia to correct dental disease or to remove foreign bodies, obtain biopsy samples, or debulk tumors, abscesses, or granulomas may be high risk in these patients. Sedatives may also relax the upper airway muscles, which can worsen the obstruction.

MEDICATIONS

DRUG(S) OF CHOICE

- Oxygen therapy is the most useful treatment if the patient is severely dyspneic.
- Definitive therapy is based on the primary disorder, including antibiotics, anti-inflammatories, bronchodilators, cardiac drugs, etc.

CONTRAINDICATIONS

- Depend on underlying cause

PRECAUTIONS

- Corticosteroid use can suppress the immune system and exacerbate a bacterial infection.
- Patients with CHF or blunt force trauma to the chest are at risk for iatrogenic fluid overload leading to pulmonary edema. Respiratory rate and effort should be monitored frequently in these patients.

POSSIBLE INTERACTIONS
N/A

ALTERNATIVE DRUGS
N/A

FOLLOW-UP

PATIENT MONITORING

- Continue to monitor patient for relapse via clinical signs.
- Repeat any abnormal tests.

PREVENTION/AVOIDANCE

- Depends on the underlying disease
- Improve husbandry and diet
- Avoid stressful situations and corticosteroid use.
- Keep in a well-ventilated, clean environment. Clean bedding frequently to prevent the buildup of ammonia fumes.
- Provide a high-quality diet.
- Manage dental disease by performing regular dental exams and treating disease early

POSSIBLE COMPLICATIONS

- Anorexia
- Extension of disease into the mouth, ears, eyes, lower respiratory tract, and/or brain

EXPECTED COURSE AND PROGNOSIS

Prognosis is based on cause of disease, severity, and chronicity. If the underlying disease cannot be corrected (i.e., dental disease, neoplasia, cardiac disease, organomegaly, etc.), a cure is unlikely. The treatment, depending on the cause, can be lifelong and aims to control the clinical signs. Relapse, progression of disease, and death are common. A severely dyspneic or tachypneic patient that does not improve over 12 hours, despite supportive care and appropriate therapy, has a guarded prognosis.

MISCELLANEOUS

ASSOCIATED CONDITIONS

- Neoplasia
- Dental disease
- Obesity

DYSPNEA AND TACHYPNEA   (CONTINUED)

AGE-RELATED FACTORS
N/A

ZOONOTIC POTENTIAL
• Hedgehogs can be asymptomatic carriers of *Salmonella*. Use gloves and careful handwashing after handling.
• In general, infectious agents producing sinusitis and rhinitis in hedgehogs are nonzoonotic; however, any animal disease is of concern to immunocompromised humans.

PREGNANCY/FERTILITY/BREEDING
N/A

SYNONYMS
None

SEE ALSO
Dental disease
Neoplasia
Obesity
Congestive heart failure

ABBREVIATIONS
CHF = congestive heart failure
CNS = central nervous system
CT = computed tomography

INTERNET RESOURCES
www.vin.com
www.merckvetmanual.com

Suggested Reading
Del Aguila G, Torres CG, Carvallo FR, Gonzalez CM, Cifuentes FF. Oral masses in African pygmy hedgehogs. J Vet Diagn Invest 2019;31(6):864–867.
Heatley JJ, Mauldin GE, Cho DY. A review of neoplasia in the captive African hedgehog (*Atelerix albiventris*). Semin Avian Exot Pet Med;14(3):182–192.
Johnson DH. Hedgehogs and sugar gliders: respiratory anatomy, physiology, and disease. Vet Clin Exot Anim Pract 2011;14(2):267–285.
Johnson DH. Geriatric hedgehogs. Vet Clin Exot Anim Pract 2020;23(3):615–637.
Lennox AM. Emergency and critical care procedures in sugar gliders (*Petaurus breviceps*), African hedgehogs (*Atelerix albiventris*), and prairie dogs (*Cynomys* spp). Vet Clin North Am Exot Anim Pract 2007;10:533–555.
Lightfoot TL. Therapeutics of African pygmy hedgehogs and prairie dogs. Vet Clin Exot Anim Pract 2000;3(1):155–172.
McLaughlin A, Strunk A. Common emergencies in small rodents, hedgehogs, and sugar gliders. Vet Clin Exot Anim Pract 2016;19(2):465–499.
Raymond JT, Garner MM. Cardiomyopathy in captive African hedgehogs (*Atelerix albiventris*). J Vet Diagn Invest 2000;12(5):468–472.

Authors Amanda Steinagel, DVM and Barbara Oglesbee, DVM, DABVP (Avian)

HEDGEHOGS

DYSURIA AND HEMATURIA

BASICS

DEFINITION
• Dysuria—difficult or painful urination
• Pollakiuria—voiding small quantity of urine with increased frequency
• Hematuria—the presence of blood in urine. It is important to differentiate true hematuria from blood originating from the reproductive tract in females.

PATHOPHYSIOLOGY
• Dysuria and pollakiuria are caused by lesions of the urinary bladder and/or urethra as well as outflow obstruction and provide evidence of lower urinary tract disease.
• Hematuria occurs secondary to inflammation and loss of endothelial integrity in the lower urinary tract. Must distinguish from blood originating from the reproductive tract in females.

SYSTEMS AFFECTED
Renal/Urologic—bladder, urethra

GENETICS
N/A

INCIDENCE/PREVALENCE
Common

GEOGRAPHIC DISTRIBUTION
Worldwide

SIGNALMENT
• Infection and neoplasia seen more commonly in middle-aged to older adults
• Cystitis and hematuria (due to mixing with blood from the reproductive tract) more common in females

SIGNS
Historical Findings
• Hematuria
• Straining to urinate—owners may mistake for constipation
• Urine staining in the perineum
• Anorexia, weight loss, lethargy, tooth grinding, tenesmus, in animal with chronic or obstructive lower urinary tract disease

Physical Examination Findings
• May be normal
• Abdominal palpation may induce pain, especially when the bladder is palpated.
• A large urinary bladder may be palpable in patients with partial or complete urethral obstruction.
• Masses causing obstruction of the urethra may be palpable.

CAUSES
• Urinary tract infection—bacterial
• Urolithiasis—calcium carbonate, calcium oxalate reported in hedgehogs
• Neoplasia—of urinary or reproductive tract
• Accessory gland enlargement reported causing urethral obstruction in one male hedgehog
• Trauma

RISK FACTORS
• Mural or extramural diseases that compress the bladder or urethral lumen. The most common cause is neoplasia.
• Inadequate water intake—dirty bowls, inappropriate water availability, changing water sources, and unpalatable water
• Urine stasis—inadequate exercise/strict cage confinement, painful musculoskeletal/orthopedic conditions
• Urine retention—neurological abnormalities (upper motor neuron bladder), bladder pathology (congenital, neoplasia)
• Obesity
• Diet—high calcium, magnesium, and/or phosphorus-containing diets can predispose to urolithiasis
• Inappropriate husbandry—dirty environment may cause the hedgehog to avoid urinating and defecating in the environment
• Penile injury—trauma, neoplasia

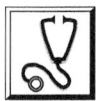

DIAGNOSIS

DIFFERENTIAL DIAGNOSIS
Differentiate from other abnormal patterns of micturition:
• Rule out polyuria—frequency and volume of urine
• Rule out urethral obstruction—stranguria, anuria, overdistended urinary bladder, and signs of postrenal uremia
Differentiate cause of dysuria and hematuria:
• Rule out urinary tract infection—hematuria, bacteriuria; painful, thickened bladder
• Rule out urolithiasis—hematuria, radiopaque bladder, nonproductive straining
• Rule out neoplasia—hematuria; ultrasound may differentiate
• Rule out neurogenic disorders—flaccid bladder wall; residual urine in bladder lumen after micturition; other neurologic deficits to hind legs, tail perineum, and anal sphincter
• Rule out uterine disease—females with uterine disease often strain and expel blood or purulent exudate when urinating; may mix with urine and be mistaken for hematuria/pyuria.

CBC/BIOCHEMISTRY/URINALYSIS
• Results may be normal.
• Leukocytosis may be seen with a lower urinary tract infection, but this finding is rare. Azotemia may be present with lower urinary tract obstruction or primary renal disease.
• Disorders of the urinary bladder are best evaluated with a urine specimen collected by cystocentesis.
• Pyuria, hematuria, and proteinuria indicate urinary tract inflammation, but these are nonspecific findings that may result from infectious and noninfectious causes of lower urinary tract disease.
• Identification of bacteria in urine sediment suggests that urinary tract infection is causing or complicating lower urinary tract disease. Identification of neoplastic cells in urine sediment indicates urinary tract neoplasia.

OTHER LABORATORY TESTS
Quantitative urine culture—the most definitive means of identifying and characterizing bacterial urinary tract infection; negative urine culture results suggest a noninfectious cause. Administration of antibiotics prior to urine culture may confound the meaning of a negative urine culture.

IMAGING
Ultrasonography of the urinary tract and uterus, abdominal radiography, and contrast cystography are important means of identifying and localizing causes of dysuria and pollakiuria. With increasing access to computed tomography and magnetic resonance imaging, these modalities may play an increasing role in the diagnosis of lower urinary tract disease.

PATHOLOGIC FINDINGS
Depends on the underlying cause

TREATMENT
APPROPRIATE HEALTH CARE
• Patients with nonobstructive lower urinary tract diseases are typically managed as outpatients; diagnostic evaluation may require brief hospitalization.
• Dysuria and pollakiuria associated with systemic signs of illness (e.g., pyrexia, depression, anorexia, and dehydration) or laboratory findings of azotemia or leukocytosis warrant aggressive diagnostic evaluation and initiation of supportive and symptomatic treatment.
• Treatment depends on the underlying cause and specific sites involved.

DYSURIA AND HEMATURIA

NURSING CARE

• Ensure that the patient is kept warm—between 80 and 85°F (27 and 29°C). Topor occurs when the environmental temperature falls below 65°F (18°C).

• Fluid therapy is used to correct hydration following standard protocols (5%–10% of body weight administered in SQ boluses). Fluids should be kept warm to prevent hypothermia and can be warmed by placing the prepared syringe in a warm water bath prior to administration. Administration via a 22–25-gauge butterfly needle can reduce stress on the patient by minimizing restraint.

• For critical patients, administer fluid therapy via IV or intraosseous (IO) catheter. In addition to crystalloids, the patient may need colloids such as hetastarch at 10 mL/kg IO per day in several small boluses. Maintenance requirement is 100 mL/kg/day

DIET

• It is imperative that the animal receive nutritional support if it is not eating. Supplementation with a liquid diet may be required, such as Oxbow Carnivore Care (Oxbow Enterprises, Inc., Murdock, NE) or Emeraid Omnivore (Lafeber's, Cornell, IL) supplements such as Ensure (Abott Nutrition, Columbus, OH).

• A diet change should never be made abruptly in the anorexic patient. If the diet is inappropriate, wait until the patient is stable and eating again, then convert to an appropriate diet.

CLIENT EDUCATION

Educate owners about proper husbandry (caging, diet) and the need for regular examinations. The author recommends a wellness examination every 6 months.

SURGICAL CONSIDERATIONS

• Surgery may be required for patients with cystic calculi or neoplasia. One report exists of perineal urethrostomy in a male hedgehog with urethral obstruction.

• Postoperative management includes assisted feeding, fluids, analgesics, and antibiotics based on culture and sensitivity results.

MEDICATIONS

DRUG(S) OF CHOICE

• Depends on the underlying cause

• If bacterial cystitis is demonstrated, begin treatment with broad-spectrum antibiotic such as amoxicillin/clavulanic acid (12.5–25 mg/kg PO q12h), enrofloxacin (5–10 mg/kg PO q12h), trimethoprim-sulfa (30 mg/kg PO q12h), chloramphenicol (30–50 mg/kg PO q12), azithromycin (20 mg/kg PO q24), modify antibacterial treatment based on the result of urine culture and sensibility testing.

• Pain management—meloxicam (0.2 mg/kg PO q24h), tramadol (2–5 mg/kg PO q8–12), or buprenorphine (0.03–0.05 mg/kg IM, SQ, PO q6–12h) may be used for painful conditions/inflammation.

• Urethral dilation: Prazosin (0.5 mg/kg PO q8–12 for 3–5 days)

• For sedation—ketamine (20–30 mg/kg IM) + midazolam (1 mg/kg IM) or alfaxalone (1–3 mg/kg IM + midazolam (0.5–1 mg/kg IM) ± butorphanol (0.2 mg/kg IM) add alfaxalone (1 mg/kg IM) boluses PRN

CONTRAINDICATIONS

• Potentially nephrotoxic drugs (e.g., aminoglycosides, NSAIDs) in patients that are febrile, dehydrated, or azotemic or that are suspected of having pyelonephritis, septicemia, or preexisting renal disease

PRECAUTIONS

• Cautious fluid therapy until patency of the urethra is established

POSSIBLE INTERACTIONS

N/A

ALTERNATIVE DRUGS

N/A

FOLLOW-UP

PATIENT MONITORING

Response to treatment by clinical signs, serial physical examination, laboratory testing, and radiographic and ultrasonic evaluation appropriate for each specific cause

PREVENTION/AVOIDANCE

• Depends on the underlying cause

• Increase water consumption for the remainder of the animal's life

• Place patient on an appropriate diet

• Increase exercise

• Provide good hygiene

POSSIBLE COMPLICATIONS

• Urine scald dermatitis/pododermatitis from abnormal urination in the environment is possible.

• Failure to identify and treat lower urinary tract infections may lead to pyelonephritis

EXPECTED COURSE AND PROGNOSIS

• Good to guarded depending on the underlying cause

• Most neoplasms (up to 85%) are malignant and carry a poor prognosis

MISCELLANEOUS

ASSOCIATED CONDITIONS

• Obesity

• Neoplasia

AGE-RELATED FACTORS

Uroliths and neoplasia are more common in middle-aged to older animals.

ZOONOTIC POTENTIAL

• Hedgehogs can be asymptomatic carriers of *Salmonella*. Use gloves and careful handwashing after handling.

PREGNANCY/FERTILITY/BREEDING

N/A

SYNONYMS

N/A

SEE ALSO

Obesity

Reproductive disorders

ABBREVIATIONS

NSAID = nonsteroidal anti-inflammatory drug

Suggested Reading

Ivey E, Carpenter J. African hedgehogs. In: Quesenberry KE, Carpenter JW, eds. Ferrets, Rabbits, and Rodents: Clinical Medicine and Surgery, 3rd ed. St. Louis, MO: Saunders, 2012:339–353.

Johnson DH. Geriatric hedgehogs. Vet Clin Exot Anim Pract 2020;23(3):615–637.

Koizumi I, Kondo H. A case of preputial cystostomy performed on an African pygmy hedgehog (*Atelerix albiventris*) with urethral obstruction. J Exot Pet Med 2019;1(30):1–6.

Lennox AM. Emergency and critical care procedures in sugar gliders (*Petaurus breviceps*), African hedgehogs (*Atelerix albiventris*), and prairie dogs (*Cynomys* spp). Vet Clin North Am Exot Anim Pract 2007;10:533–555.

McLaughlin A, Strunk A. Common emergencies in small rodents, hedgehogs, and sugar gliders. Vet Clin Exot Anim Pract 2016;19(2):465–499.

Reavill D, Lennox A. Disease overview of the urinary tract in exotic companion mammals and tips on clinical management. Vet Clin North Am Exot Anim Pract 2020;23(1):169–193.

Authors Amanda Steinagel, DVM and Barbara Oglesbee, DVM, DABVP (Avian)

BASICS

DEFINITION
The presence of parasites such as mites, lice, or fleas on the skin, fur, or in the hair follicles

PATHOPHYSIOLOGY
• The presence of large numbers of ectoparasites in the hair follicles exceeds the capacity of the immune system to tolerate the infestation, leading to furunculosis and often to secondary bacterial infection.
• Dermatophyte infection often occurs in association with mite infestation. Fungal growth is facilitated by changes caused by mite infestation. Fungal spores are found in mite droppings.

SYSTEMS AFFECTED
Skin, in severe cases psychological/ neurologic

GENETICS
N/A

INCIDENCE/PREVALENCE
Mites are one of the most common presenting complaints in pet hedgehogs.

GEOGRAPHIC DISTRIBUTION
N/A

SIGNALMENT
No age or sex predilection

IGNS
History
• Recent stress or systemic disease will predispose to mite infestation
• Dermatophyte infection may either predispose or occur concurrently

Physical Examination Findings
• Quill loss is more common than loss of hair on the abdomen; can appear as focal, patchy, or diffuse thinning
• Dry flaky skin, crusting, seborrhea, erythema, and lichenification seen with mite infestation and/or dermatophyte infection
• Hyperkeratosis at the base of quills and on the face and ears with mite infestation
• Quills may fall off during physical examination
• Mites may be visible without magnification and appear as a white, flaky powder
• Weight loss, general debility
• Excoriations, erythema common

CAUSES
• Ectoparasites are the most common cause. *Caparinia* spp., a nonburrowing psoroptid mite is the most common ectoparasite in pet hedgehogs, but *Chorioptes* spp. and Sarcoptid species are also seen.
• Ear mites—*Notoedres* or *Otodectes* sp.
• Fleas and ticks

RISK FACTORS
Inadequate husbandry and nutrition and underlying metabolic disease predispose to mite infestations.

DIAGNOSIS

DIFFERENTIAL DIAGNOSIS
• Dermatophytes—*Trichophyton erinacei, Trichophyton mentagrophytes,* and *Microsporum* spp. most common. Other species include *Arthroderma benhamiae* and *Paecilomyces Variotii.* Dermatophytes can occur alone or in association with mite infestation. Fungal growth is facilitated by changes caused by mite infestation. Fungal spores are found in mite droppings.
• Metabolic/Nutritional—debility, underlying disease predispose to mite infestation and dermatophytosis; diets low in protein can cause barbering
• Bacterial—usually secondary to scratching; *Staphylococcus* sp. most common.
• Husbandry/Environmental/Stress—contact dermatitis, urine scald
• Neoplasia—cutaneous lymphoma, mast cell tumors, cutaneous hemangiosarcoma, and histiocytic sarcoma are most commonly reported
• Trauma—environmental/cage rubbing/bite wounds, self-mutilation
• Endocrinopathy and immune-mediated causes not yet reported

CBC/BIOCHEMISTRY/URINALYSIS
In debilitated or systemically ill patients, CBC, serum biochemistry, and urinalysis should be included in the minimum database where possible to evaluate for concurrent medical conditions.

OTHER LABORATORY TESTS
• Skin scraping—superficial for most mites—highest population around ears and face
• Dermatophyte testing—most hedgehogs with mite infestation have concurrent dermatophytosis. Use either PCR or fungal culture. Fungal culture results are often delayed due to the long growth time required. Begin treatment while awaiting results. False negatives are common, especially with PCR testing, as most laboratories do not test for all species commonly infecting hedgehogs
• Bacterial culture and sensitivity testing, if a secondary bacterial infection is suspected

IMAGING
In systemically ill patients, radiographs may help confirm the presence of organomegaly, dystrophic mineralization, or the presence of masses.

DIAGNOSTIC PROCEDURES
• Skin scrapings and dermatophyte cultures should be included as part of the minimum database.
• Skin biopsies for histopathologic evaluation may be indicated.
• Response to therapy as a trial.

PATHOLOGIC FINDINGS
• Varies depending on the type of ectoparasite present

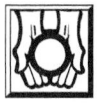

TREATMENT

APPROPRIATE HEALTH CARE
• Most cases of ectoparasite infestation will be treated on an outpatient basis.

NURSING CARE
Systemically ill or debilitated animals should be hospitalized for appropriate supportive care, including hand feeding, and fluids until stabilized.

ACTIVITY
Activity restriction is typically not necessary.

DIET
If nutrition is adequate, no changes are indicated.

CLIENT EDUCATION
Prophylactic treatment of in-contact animals in multipet households is advised.

Environmental decontamination is often necessary, including frequent cage cleaning and bedding changes. Emphasize appropriate nutrition and husbandry.

SURGICAL CONSIDERATIONS
N/A

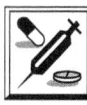

MEDICATIONS

DRUG(S) OF CHOICE
• 10% Imidacloprid/1.0% moxidectin spot on (0.1 mL/kg as a single treatment)
• Selamectin (6–18 mg/kg topically q30d)
• Ivermectin (0.3–0.4 mg/kg SQ, IM q14d for 3–5 treatments)
• Fluralaner (15 mg/kg PO once) reported to be effective with one dose
• For secondary bacterial dermatitis, select appropriate antibiotics based on safety and bacterial culture and sensitivity. Antibiotics commonly used include amoxicillin/clavulanic acid (12.5–25 mg/kg PO q12h), enrofloxacin (5–10 mg/kg PO q12h), trimethoprim-sulfa (30 mg/kg PO q12h), and chloramphenicol (30–50 mg/kg PO q12h)
• Pain management—meloxicam (0.2 mg/kg PO q24h), tramadol (2–5 mg/kg PO q8–12),

ECTOPARASITES

or buprenorphine (0.03–0.05 mg/kg IM, SQ, PO q6–12h) may be used for painful conditions/inflammation.

PRECAUTIONS

• Steroids may be used as an anti-inflammatory agent although nonsteroidal anti-inflammatories are preferred. The use of steroids is contraindicated in patients with dermatophyte infections.

POSSIBLE INTERACTIONS

N/A

ALTERNATIVE DRUGS

N/A

FOLLOW-UP

PATIENT MONITORING

Examination of multiple skin scrapings or follow-up skin cytology, as well as clinical resolution of the presenting complaints, is used to monitor progress.

PREVENTION/AVOIDANCE

• Appropriate husbandry and sanitation
• Avoid exposure to carrier animals.

POSSIBLE COMPLICATIONS

Debility, weight loss, death if untreated

EXPECTED COURSE AND PROGNOSIS

Most ectoparasite infections will improve or resolve within 2–4 weeks. If there is no improvement, make sure that there is compliance with drug administration, cage

disinfection, and other husbandry recommendations and use appropriate diagnostic tests to screen for possible underlying medical conditions.

MISCELLANEOUS

ASSOCIATED CONDITIONS

• Dermatophytes
• Mite infestation and dermatophytosis are most severe in animals with underlying disorders

AGE-RELATED FACTORS

N/A

ZOONOTIC POTENTIAL

• Hedgehogs can be asymptomatic carriers of *Salmonella*. Use gloves and careful handwashing after handling.
• Dermatophytosis

PREGNANCY/FERTILITY/BREEDING

N/A

SYNONYMS

N/A

SEE ALSO

Alopecia
Dermatophytes

ABBREVIATIONS

N/A

INTERNET RESOURCES

Exotic DVM forum for eDVM readers: www.pets.groups.yahoo.com/group/ExoticDVM
Veterinary Information Network: www.vin.com

Suggested Reading
Chin J, Mans C. Small mammals: hedgehogs. In: Mayer J, Donnelly T, eds. Clinical Veterinary Advisor: Birds and Exotic Pets. St. Louis, MO: Saunders, 2013:338–343.
Ivey E, Carpenter J. African hedgehogs. In: Quesenberry KE, Carpenter JW, eds. Ferrets, Rabbits, and Rodents: Clinical Medicine and Surgery, 3rd ed. St Louis, MO: Saunders:339–353.
Johnson DH. African pygmy hedgehogs. In: Johnson-Delaney C, Meredith A, eds. BSAVA Manual of Exotic Pets, A Foundation Manual. Quedgeley, Gloucester: British Small Animal Veterinary Association, 2010:139–147.
Johnson DH. Geriatric hedgehogs. Vet Clin Exot Anim Pract 2020;23(3):615–637.
Keeble E, Koterwas B. Selected emerging diseases of pet hedgehogs. Vet Clin Exot Anim Pract 2020;23(2):443–458.
Lennox AM. Emergency and critical care procedures in sugar gliders (*Petaurus breviceps*), African hedgehogs (*Atelerix albiventris*), and prairie dogs (*Cynomys* spp). Vet Clin North Am Exot Anim Pract 2007;10:533–555.
Author Amanda Steinagel, DVM and Barbara Oglesbee DVM, DABVP (Avian)

EXOPHTHALMOS AND ORBITAL DISEASES

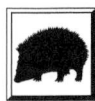

BASICS

DEFINITION
- Abnormal position of the globe
- Exophthalmos—anterior displacement of a normal globe
- Enophthalmos—posterior displacement of a normal globe

PATHOPHYSIOLOGY
- Malposition of the globe—caused by changes in volume (loss or gain) of the orbital contents or abnormal extraocular muscle function
- Exophthalmos—caused by space-occupying mass lesions posterior to the equator of the globe
- Enophthalmos—caused by the reduced volume of orbital contents or by space-occupying mass lesions anterior to the equator of the globe
- Hedgehogs are predisposed to protrusion and exophthalmos due to the shallow anatomy of the orbit and large palpebral fissures.

SYSTEMS AFFECTED
- Ophthalmic
- Respiratory—due to proximity of orbit to nasal cavity, frontal and maxillary sinuses
- Oral Cavity—proximity of oral cavity to ventral orbit—malocclusion and apical root abscess extension

INCIDENCE/PREVALENCE
- Trauma occurs frequently due to shallow orbit.
- Exophthalmos or peri-orbital swelling are common secondary to dental disease

GEOGRAPHIC DISTRIBUTION
N/A

SIGNALMENT
- No gender predilection.
- Older animals more prone to dental related abscesses

SIGNS

Historical Findings
- Sudden onset exophthalmos—trauma (e.g., orbital hemorrhage, proptosis)
- Chronic, progressive exophthalmos—neoplasia or tooth root abscess
- Weight loss, difficulty in eating or in prehension, anorexia—dental disease

Physical Examination Findings
Exophthalmos
- Proptosis—peri-ocular hemorrhage
- Dental disease—hypersalivation; bleeding from oral cavity; periocular swelling
- Facial abscess-periocular swelling may be present in the retrobulbar space, associated with auditory structures, or oral/dental disease.
Enophthalmos
- Ptosis
- Elevation of nictitans
- Extraocular muscle atrophy
- Entropion—with severe disease
Oral examination
- Specialized equipment is required—rodent dental speculum (Rodent mouth gag, Jorgensen Lab, Loveland, CO) and a set of buccal speculae (Cheek dilator, Jorgensen Labs); cotton swabs and tongue depressor to retract the tongue and examine lingual surfaces
- Heavy sedation or general anesthesia may be required.
- Tooth root abnormalities may be present in spite of normal-appearing crowns; skull radiographs may be necessary to identify apical root abnormalities if index of suspicion is high for dental involvement

CAUSES
Exophthalmos
- Orbital hemorrhage/proptosis—trauma to orbital structures
- Neoplasia of orbital structures
- Dental disease—orbital extension of dental disease
- Trauma-bite-induced retrobulbar abscess
Enophthalmos
- Ocular pain—retraction of globe
- Horner's syndrome
- Neoplasia extending from rostral orbit displacing globe posteriorly

RISK FACTORS
- Head trauma—proptosis
- Dental disease—caries of molars can predispose to tooth root abscesses; can be due to inappropriate physical form and composition of diet

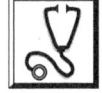

DIAGNOSIS

DIFFERENTIAL DIAGNOSIS
Exophthalmos
- Conformational—prominence of the globe is a normal feature—evaluate bilateral symmetry; observe grossly from a position above the head of the patient
- Buphthalmos—enlargement of the globe due to intraocular disease (i.e., glaucoma)—uncommon in hedgehogs
- Traumatic proptosis—acute onset related to trauma to head/periocular area
Enophthalmos
- Perforated/collapsed globe—acute trauma, perforation of corneal descemetocele
- Phthisis bulbi—acquired shrinkage of the globe, usually secondary to trauma and/or chronic inflammation
- Microphthalmos—congenitally smaller than normal globe, which can include other anatomical abnormalities—may be blind or vision impaired
- Anophthalmos—congenital absence of globe—rare, reported in other small mammals

CBC/BIOCHEMISTRY/URINALYSIS
Usually normal; WBC count may be elevated with orbital abscesses

OTHER LABORATRY TESTS
N/A

IMAGING
- Orbital ultrasound—localize and characterize space-occupying mass lesions; guide aspirate or biopsy diagnostic procedures
- Skull radiographs—orbital and dental assessment
- CT—evaluate extent of orbital disease and determine involvement of other cavities (nasal, oral)

DIAGNOSTIC PROCEDURES
- Resistance to globe retropulsion—confirms space-occupying mass
- Tonometry—rule out glaucoma; rebound tonometer best suited to small eyes of rodent and provides accurate assessment of IOP (reported mean 10–20 mmHg)
- Oral examination, skull radiographs, and fine-needle aspiration or biopsy of space-occupying mass lesion in orbit—perform after anesthetizing patient
- Fine-needle aspiration (use 20–22 gauge needle)—if retrobulbar mass is accessible; submit samples for aerobic, anaerobic, and fungal cultures; Gram's staining; and cytological evaluation
- Cytology—often diagnostic for abscess and neoplasia
- Biopsy—indicated if needle aspiration is nondiagnostic and mass lesion is accessible

PATHOLOGIC FINDINGS
- Neoplasia—characteristic features of malignancy (anisocytosis, anisokaryosis, increase in mitotic figures)
- Cellulitis, abscess—inflammatory cells, intracellular bacteria

TREATMENT

APPROPRIATE HEALTH CARE
- Proptosis—enucleation is indicated.
- Retrobulbar abscess—aggressive surgical debridement of orbital abscess and related

EXOPHTHALMOS AND ORBITAL DISEASES   (CONTINUED)

affected tissues (dentition, maxilla) followed by long-term local and systemic antibiotic treatment; limited (palliative) response to antibiotic treatment alone

NURSING CARE
• Exophthalmos—lubrication of exposed cornea while diagnostics and treatment are carried out
• Supportive care in debilitated or anorectic patients; assisted feeding; subcutaneous or intravenous fluid therapy

ACTIVITY
N/A

DIET
Minimize changes in diet during treatment and recovery; may require syringe-feeding if anorectic or during the perioperative period

CLIENT EDUCATION
• Enucleation is necessary with proptosis
• Educate clients on the appropriate diet to avoid recurrent dental disease.

SURGICAL CONSIDERATIONS
• Enucleation/exenteration—careful dissection and evaluation during surgery is paramount to avoid excessive hemorrhage.

MEDICATIONS

DRUG(S) OF CHOICE
• Exophthalmos—lubricate exposed cornea to prevent desiccation and ulceration (e.g., artificial tear ointment or gel)
• Corneal ulceration—topical antibiotic (e.g., neomycin-polymyxin-bacitracin, ciprofloxacin, or ofloxacin q6–8h) and cycloplegic (e.g., atropine 1% q12–24h) to prevent infection and reduce ciliary spasm, respectively
• Antibiotics—(based on culture and sensitivity results)—cephalexin (25 mg/kg PO q12h), amoxicillin/clavulanic acid (12.5–25 mg/kg PO q12h), enrofloxacin (5–10 mg/kg PO q12h), trimethoprim-sulfa (30 mg/kg PO q12h), chloramphenicol (30–50 mg/kg PO q12)
• Pain management—meloxicam (0.2 mg/kg PO q24h), tramadol (2–5 mg/kg PO q8–12),

or buprenorphine (0.03–0.05 mg/kg IM, SQ, PO q6–12h) may be used for painful conditions/inflammation.
• Topical pain management—atropine 1% solution q12–24h
• Topical nonsteroidal anti-inflammatory solutions/ointments—flurbiprofen 0.03% or diclofenac 1% q12–24h
• For sedation—ketamine (20–30 mg/kg IM) + midazolam (1 mg/kg IM) or alfaxalone (1–3 mg/kg IM + midazolam (0.5–1 mg/kg IM) ± butorphanol (0.2 mg/kg IM) add alfaxalone (1 mg/kg IM) boluses PRN

CONTRAINDICATIONS
• Avoid steroid-containing ophthalmic preparations—in case of corneal ulceration

PRECAUTIONS
N/A

POSSIBLE INTERACTIONS
N/A

ALTERNATIVE DRUGS
N/A

FOLLOW-UP

PATIENT MONITORING
• Dental abscess—evaluate the entire oral cavity and skull at each recheck and repeat skull radiographs at 3–6-month intervals to monitor for recurrence at the surgical site or other locations

PREVENTION/AVOIDANCE
Educate owners on proper diet.

POSSIBLE COMPLICATIONS
• Vision loss
• Loss of globe
• Permanent malposition of globe
• Death

EXPECTED COURSE AND PROGNOSIS
• Retrobulbar tooth root abscess—depends on severity of bone involvement, underlying disease, condition of the teeth, and presence of other abscesses. Fair to guarded with single isolated retrobulbar abscess, adequate surgical

debridement, and medical treatment. Abscesses in the nasal passages or with multiple or severe maxillary abscesses have a guarded to poor prognosis—euthanasia may be warranted

MISCELLANEOUS

ASSOCIATED CONDITIONS
N/A

AGE-RELATED FACTORS
N/A

ZOONOTIC POTENTIAL
• Hedgehogs can be asymptomatic carriers of *Salmonella*. Use gloves and careful handwashing after handling.

PREGNANCY/FERTILITY/BREEDING
N/A

SYNONYMS
N/A

SEE ALSO
Conjunctivitis
Neoplasia

ABBREVIATIONS
CT = computed tomography
IOP = intraocular pressure
WBC = white blood cell

Suggested Reading
Chaprazov T, Dimitrov R, Yovcheva KS, Uzenova K. Oral and dental disorders in pet hedgehogs. Turk J Vet Anim Sci 2014;38(1):1–6.
Evans EE, Souza MJ. Advanced diagnostic approaches and current management of internal disorders of select species (rodents, sugar gliders, hedgehogs). Vet Clin Exot Anim Pract 2010;13(3):453–469.
Johnson DH. Geriatric hedgehogs. Vet Clin Exot Anim Pract 2020;23(3):615–637.
Lennox AM, Miwa Y. Anatomy and disorders of the oral cavity of miscellaneous exotic companion mammals. Vet Clin Exot Anim Pract 2016;19(3):929–945.
Author Amanda Steinagel, DVM

FEMALE REPRODUCTIVE TRACT DISORDERS

BASICS

OVERVIEW
• Neoplastic disorders are most common and include ovarian granulosa cell tumor, uterine adenomas, uterine adenocarcinoma, uterine endometrial stromal sarcoma, uterine leiomyoma/leiomyosarcoma, uterine spindle cell sarcoma, vaginal spindle cell sarcoma, vaginal tunic neurofibrosarcoma, mammary adenocarcinoma, mammary papillary adenoma
• Pyometra—develops when bacterial invasion of abnormal endometrium leads to intraluminal accumulation of purulent exudate.
• Common endometrial disorders include endometiral hyperplasia (most common), endometrial venous aneurysms, endometriosis, endometritis, hydrometra, and mucometra.
• Most endometrial disorders can result in significant uterine hemorrhage.

PATHOPHYSIOLOGY
• Sexual mature/reproductively active females are between 6 and 8 months old.
• Gestation typically lasts between 34 and 38 days.
• Pseudopregnancy may occur. It typically lasts between 10 and 15 days. It is commonly followed by hydrometra, pyometra, mucometra, or endometrial hyperplasia.
• Bacterial infection of the uterus is common as the normal endometrial secretions are an ideal media for growth and may act as a nidus for infection. Bacterial will move from the vagina into the partially open or open cervix during either transition from proestrus to estrus, during intercourse, or via hematogenous means

SIGNALMENT
• Intact females
• Highest incidence middle-aged to older females

SIGNS
Historical Findings
• Hematuria—most common presenting complaint. Not true hematuria since blood originates from the uterus but is released during micturition. Hematuria is often reported as intermittent or cyclic; usually occurs at the end of micturition
• With mild or early endometrial disease may have no clinical signs
• Serosanguinous to purulent, blood-tinged vaginal discharge

Physical Examination Findings
• Uterus—may be palpably large; careful palpation may allow determination of size

• Serosanguinous to purulent, blood-tinged vaginal discharge
• Blood-stained perineum
• Enlarged mammary glands—one or multiple, may be firm and multilobulated (mammary tumors)
• Pale mucous membranes, tachycardia in patients that have had significant uterine hemorrhage
• Depression, lethargy, anorexia in patients with pyometra or uterine hemorrhage

CAUSES AND RISK FACTORS
• Intact sexual status
• Risk increases with age
• Common bacteria involved in pyometra include *Pasteurella* spp. and *Staphylococcus* spp.

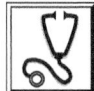

DIAGNOSIS

DIFFERENTIAL DIAGNOSIS
• Pregnancy
• Lower urinary tract disorders

CBC/BIOCHEMISTRY/URINALYSIS
• Often unremarkable. An elevated white blood cell count may be noted with pyometra. Anemia may be noted with severe uterine hemorrhage. Azotemia may be noted with dehydration, primary kidney disease, and/or septicemia.
• Urinalysis—sample collected by ultrasound-guided cystocentesis to differentiate hematuria from uterine bleeding

OTHER LABORATORY TESTS
• Cytologic examination of vaginal discharge—polymorphonuclear cells and bacteria
• Bacterial culture and sensitivity—vaginal discharge, uterine wall, and contents after surgical removal
• Histopathologic examination of uterus following ovariohysterectomy—necessary for definitive diagnosis

IMAGING
Radiography
• Detect a large uterus
• Rule out pregnancy

Ultrasonography
• Assess size of uterus and nature of uterine contents
• Rule out pregnancy

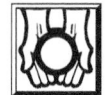

TREATMENT

APPROPRIATE HEALTH CARE
Inpatient in patients with pyometra, or uterine hemorrhage; can be life threatening

NURSING CARE
• Ensure that the patient is kept warm—between 80 and 85°F (27 and 29°C). Topor occurs when the environmental temperature falls below 65°F (18°C).
• Fluid therapy is used to correct hydration following standard protocols (5%–10% of body weight administered in SQ boluses). Fluids should be kept warm to prevent hypothermia and can be warmed by placing the prepared syringe in a warm water bath prior to administration. Administration via a 22–25-gauge butterfly needle can reduce stress on the patient by minimizing restraint.
• For critical patients, administer fluid therapy via IV or intraosseous (IO) catheter. In addition to crystalloids, the patient may need colloids such as hetastarch at 10 mL/kg IO per day in several small boluses. Maintenance requirement is 100 mL/kg/day

ACTIVITY
Depending on the cause, activity may or may not need to be restricted. Most small mammals that do not feel well will be less active of their own accord.

DIET
• It is imperative that the animal receive nutritional support if it is not eating. Supplementation with a liquid diet may be required, such as Oxbow Carnivore Care (Oxbow Enterprises, Inc., Murdock, NE) or Emeraid Omnivore (Lafeber's, Cornell, IL) supplements such as Ensure (Abott Nutrition, Columbus, OH). A diet change should never be made abruptly in the anorexic patient. If the diet is inappropriate, wait until the patient is stable and eating again, then convert to an appropriate diet.

CLIENT EDUCATION
• Inform client that ovariohysterectomy is indicated with any uterine disorder.

SURGICAL CONSIDERATIONS
• Ovariohysterectomy preferred treatment for all uterine disorders

MEDICATIONS

DRUG(S) OF CHOICE
• Antibiotics—indicated for all patients with pyometra or endometritis. Empirical, pending results of bacterial culture and sensitivity testing—enrofloxacin (5–10 mg/kg PO q12), trimethoprim-sulfa (30 mg/kg PO q12h), amoxicillin clavulanic acid (12.5–25 mg/kg PO q12h)
• Pain management—buprenorphine (0.02–0.05 mg/kg SQ, IM, IV q6–8h), hydromorphone (0.1 mg/kg SQ, IM, IV

FEMALE REPRODUCTIVE TRACT DISORDERS   (CONTINUED)

q4–6h), meloxicam (0.2 mg/kg PO, SQ q24h), and tramadol (2–4 mg/kg PO q12h)
• For sedation—ketamine (20–30 mg/kg IM) + midazolam (1 mg/kg IM) or Alfaxalone (1–3 mg/kg IM + midazolam (0.5–1 mg/kg IM) ± butorphanol (0.2 mg/kg IM) add alfaxalone (1 mg/kg IM) boluses PRN

CONTRAINDICATIONS
• Corticosteroids—associated with gastrointestinal ulceration and hemorrhage, delayed wound healing, and heightened susceptibility to infection

PRECAUTIONS
• Chloramphenicol—avoid human contact with chloramphenicol due to potential blood dyscrasia. Advise owners of potential risks.
• Meloxicam and other NSAIDs—use with caution in patients with compromised renal function

ALTERNATIVE DRUGS
N/A

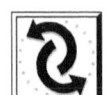

FOLLOW-UP

PATIENT MONITORING
• Monitor for signs of pain, especially after ovariohysterectomy. Assist feeding may be needed if the hedgehog is not eating well on her own following surgery

POSSIBLE COMPLICATIONS
• Peritonitis, sepsis in patients with endometritis or pyometra
• Hemorrhage, possible death in females with bleeding uterine disorders

EXPECTED COURSE AND PROGNOSIS
• Good prognosis with timely ovariohysterectomy for most uterine disorders, including adenocarcinoma that has not metastasized
• Guarded prognosis with vigorous vaginal hemorrhage; emergency stabilization and hysterectomy is indicated to control hemorrhage.
• Poor with all neoplastic disorders

MISCELLANEOUS

ASSOCIATED CONDITIONS
• Obesity

AGE-RELATED FACTORS
Risk increases with age

ZOONOTIC POTENTIAL
• Hedgehogs can be asymptomatic carriers of *Salmonella*. Use gloves and careful handwashing after handling.

SEE ALSO
Neoplasia
Dysuria and hematuria

Suggested Reading
Ivey E, Carpenter J. African hedgehogs. In: Quesenberry KE, Carpenter JW, eds. Ferrets, Rabbits, and Rodents: Clinical Medicine and Surgery, 3rd ed. St. Louis, MO: Saunders, 2012:339–353.
Johnson DH. Geriatric hedgehogs. Vet Clin Exot Anim Pract 2020;23(3):615–637.
Juan-Sallés C, Garner MM. Cytologic diagnosis of diseases of hedgehogs. Vet Clin Exot Anim Pract 2007;10(1):51–59.
Lennox AM. Emergency and critical care procedures in sugar gliders (*Petaurus breviceps*), African hedgehogs (*Atelerix albiventris*), and prairie dogs (*Cynomys* spp). Vet Clin North Am Exot Anim Pract 2007;10:533–555.
Reavill DR, Lennox AM. Disease overview of the urinary tract in exotic companion mammals and tips on clinical management. Vet Clin Exot Anim 2020;23(1):169–193.
Authors Amanda Steinagel, DVM and Barbara Oglesbee, DVM, DABVP (Avian)

HEDGEHOGS

HEAD TILT (VESTIBULAR DISEASE)

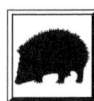

BASICS

DEFINITION
• Head tilt—change in the angle of the head that deviates from the normal position.
• Vestibular disease—disruption in the ability of the brain to recognize and respond to changes in body position and to correct this abnormality; this could be either peripheral or central.

PATHOPHYSIOLOGY
• The vestibular system is responsible for receiving and translating signals related to the orientation of the body. The receptors are the semicircular canals of the inner ear that sense rotational movements and the otoliths sense linear movements; the vestibular system receives these inputs and sends signals to the brain that direct eye movement and muscle response to maintain the body in a normal position with respect to gravity. The vestibular nuclei in the medulla and the vestibular portion of the vestibulocochlear nerve (CN VIII) provide response to the sensory input received.
• Head tilt, torticollis, and nystagmus are the most common clinical manifestations of vestibular disease.

SYSTEMS AFFECTED
• Nervous system—central or peripheral
• Gastrointestinal—secondary nausea, inappetence

INCIDENCE/PREVALENCE
• Uncommon

GEOGRAPHIC DISTRIBUTION
N/A

SIGNALMENT
No gender predilection; young or geriatric hedgehogs may be more susceptible to infectious otitis due to decreased immune system

SIGNS
Historical Findings
• Acute or insidious onset of rolling, torticollis, ataxia, leaning to one side, falling, or loss of balance
• Reluctance to eat or drink
• If otitis interna/media is present, findings may include scratching or pawing at ear or face; may be historical or concurrent nasal or ocular discharge.

Physical Examination Findings
• With otitis interna/media—erythema of the pinna or crusts and scabs evident from scratching; exudate within the aural canal; thickened, stenotic ear canals
• Nasal discharge and/or ocular discharge—if concurrent URI

• Head tilt, nystagmus (at rest or positional); leaning, falling, or rolling toward the affected side
• Central nervous system deficits—nystagmus (vertical, horizontal, or rotary); direction may change; proprioceptive deficits; altered mentation; possible seizures

CAUSES
Peripheral Disease
• Infectious/inflammatory—otitis interna/media is the most common cause, usually bacterial; most common organisms include *Streptococcus* spp. and *Staphylococcus* spp.
• Trauma—injury to tympanum or petrous temporal bone; head trauma/injury to cerebellum, brainstem, or vestibular system
• Neoplastic—tumor of ear canal, cerebellum, brainstem, and vestibular system
• Vascular—thromboembolic disease, coagulopathy, and hypertension
• Toxin—lead, metronidazole
• Degenerative—not described

RISK FACTORS
• Immunosuppression; glucocorticoid administration; stress
• Trauma

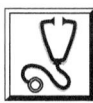

DIAGNOSIS

DIFFERENTIAL DIAGNOSIS
• Otitis media/interna—characterized by peripheral disease; differentiate by careful otoscopic evaluation, bulla radiographs, CT, MRI, and sometimes response to therapy
• Neoplasia—may demonstrate central or peripheral disease; differentiate with CT, or biopsy if accessible

CBC/BIOCHEMISTRY/URINALYSIS
• Usually normal

OTHER LABORATORY TESTS
N/A

IMAGING
• Radiographs may be useful to evaluate for neoplasia, trauma, cardiovascular disease, and inner ear disease/bullae changes. The patient should be sedated/anesthetized for these procedures to allow for optimal positioning. CT may be used for better quality imaging.

DIAGNOSTIC PROCEDURES
• Otoscopic evaluation to evaluate for otitis media/interna—challenging due to the small ear canals
• Culture and sensitivity of any nasal discharge, if present, as upper respiratory infections may occur concurrently with otitis, and disease may be transmitted through the eustachian tube and extend to the peripheral or central nervous system

• Biopsy or FNA and cytology—if accessible tumor is suspected or identified

PATHOLOGIC FINDINGS
• Pathologic findings would be consistent with underlying etiology; may be idiopathic

TREATMENT

APPROPRIATE HEALTH CARE
• Inpatient—neurologic signs; severe infections; anorexic patients; nonambulatory patients
• Outpatient—stable patients that are able to eat and drink with little or no assistance

NURSING CARE
• Supportive care such as fluid therapy, eye lubrication, rotating the patient, cleaning the environment, and assist feeding may be required based on the severity of disease and the underlying cause.

ACTIVITY
Restrict activity when vestibular signs are present to prevent falls or injury; encourage ambulation and movement on flat surfaces once safe.

DIET
• It is essential to maintain food intake during treatment; patients may become anorexic due to pain or vestibular signs. Assist feeding may be required. Carnivore care (Oxbow Pet Products, Murdock, NE) or Emeraid Omnivore (Lafeber Company, Cornell, IL) are common diets used.

CLIENT EDUCATION
• Prognosis for central vestibular disorders is worse than for peripheral disorders.
• Neurological signs may not resolve even after treatment of the underlying cause.
• May need to restrict activity or provide additional supportive care at home based on the severity of neurological signs.

SURGICAL CONSIDERATIONS
Total ear canal ablation and bulla osteotomy may be considered for treatment of bulla disease and otitis; surgical excision of neoplastic masses or abscesses may be indicated.

MEDICATIONS

DRUG(S) OF CHOICE
• For suspected or confirmed otitis media/interna or CNS infections, use systemic antibiotics—ideally based on results of culture and sensitivity.
• Choose antibiotics that penetrate the CNS such as enrofloxacin (5–10 mg/kg PO q12h),

HEDGEHOGS

HEAD TILT (VESTIBULAR DISEASE)

trimethoprim-sulfa (30 mg/kg PO q12hq), chloramphenicol (30–50 mg/kg PO q12h), for anaerobic infections consider chloramphenicol (50 mg/kg PO, SC, IM, IV q12h), azithromycin (20 mg/kg PO q 24), and/or amoxicillin clavulanic acid (12.5–25 mg/kg PO q8–12h)
• In cases of otitis, add topical antimicrobials—choose otic or ophthalmic preparations without corticosteroids such as antibiotics (gentamicin, ciprofloxacin, chloramphenicol, and enrofloxacin)
• Pain management—meloxicam (0.2 mg/kg PO q24h), tramadol (2–5 mg/kg PO q8–12h), and/or buprenorphine (0.03–0.05 mg/kg IM, SQ, PO q6–12h)
• For nausea—maropitant (1–2 mg/kg SC, PO q24h) or metoclopramide (0.5–1 mg/kg PI, SC, IV q8–12h)

CONTRAINDICATIONS
• Avoid the use of drugs that are potentially toxic to the central nervous system (metronidazole at high doses; aminoglycosides).

PRECAUTIONS
• Corticosteroids—avoid in animals with infectious disease

POSSIBLE INTERACTIONS
• N/A

ALTERNATIVE DRUGS
Corticosteroids are often recommended to help control CNS swelling or inflammation.

FOLLOW-UP

PATIENT MONITORING
• Perform serial neurologic evaluations, initially every 24–48 hours, gradually increasing the interval once progression is static or signs are improving; intervals determined by the underlying disease or rate of change

PREVENTION/AVOIDANCE
• Early and aggressive treatment of upper respiratory infections and otitis may prevent invasion by bacteria into the middle/inner ear or systemic spread.
• Proper nutrition helps minimize the risk of immunosuppression.

POSSIBLE COMPLICATIONS
• Vestibular signs and head tilt may not resolve or may progress.
• Infections may spread through brainstem/CNS or systemically.

EXPECTED COURSE AND PROGNOSIS
• Prognosis is variable and dependent upon underlying etiology
• Otitis media and interna may require months of systemic and topical therapy; although some cases will improve or resolve, others may be recurrent or may require surgery.
• Vestibular signs, head tilt, and facial nerve paralysis if present may persist following the resolution of disease, or may improve and subsequently recur.

MISCELLANEOUS

ASSOCIATED CONDITIONS
• Upper respiratory infections

AGE-RELATED FACTORS
None recognized

ZOONOTIC POTENTIAL
• Hedgehogs can be asymptomatic carriers of *Salmonella*. Use gloves and careful handwashing after handling.

PREGNANCY/FERTILITY/BREEDING
N/A

SYNONYMS
Wry neck

SEE ALSO
Ataxia

ABBREVIATIONS
CN = cranial nerve
CNS = central nervous system
CT = computed tomography
NSAID = nonsteroidal anti-inflammatory drug
URI = upper respiratory infection

Suggested Reading
Berg CC, Doss GA, Guevar J. Neurologic examination of healthy adult African pygmy hedgehogs (*Atelerix albiventris*). J Am Vet Med Assoc 2021;258(9):971–976.
Evans EE, Souza MJ. Advanced diagnostic approaches and current management of internal disorders of select species (rodents, sugar gliders, hedgehogs). Vet Clin Exot Anim Pract 2010;13(3):453–469.
Johnson DH. African pygmy hedgehogs. In: Johnson-Delaney C, Meredith A, eds. BSAVA Manual of Exotic Pets, A Foundation Manual. Quedgeley, Gloucester: British Small Animal Veterinary Association, 2010:139–147.
Johnson DH. Geriatric hedgehogs. Vet Clin Exot Anim Pract 2020;23(3):615–637.
Wissink-Argilaga N. Veterinary care of African pygmy hedgehogs. In Pract 2020;42(3):151–158.
Author Amanda Steinagel, DVM

NASAL DISCHARGE AND SNEEZING

BASICS

DEFINITION
• Nasal discharge results from inflammation of the nasal cavity and sinuses—may be serous, purulent, mucoid, mucopurulent, serosanguinous, or hemorrhagic.
• Sneezing is the involuntary expulsion of air through the nostrils and may be associated with nasal discharge

PATHOPHYSIOLOGY
• Normal serous secretions are produced by the epithelial cells lining the nasal mucosa. These cells can increase secretion production with irritation of the mucosa either by mechanical, chemical, or inflammatory stimulation.
• Typically, serous discharge is associated with allergic disease, acute inflammation, and early bacterial infection. Mucoid discharge may be caused by severe allergic disease or contact irritation, neoplasia, and early bacterial infections. Purulent or mucopurulent discharge typically involves bacterial or fungal infection, nasal foreign bodies, and possibly neoplasia. Serosanguinous discharge may be associated with neoplasia, severe bacterial or fungal infections, and clotting disorders.

SYSTEMS AFFECTED
• Respiratory—nasal mucosa, sinuses, and oropharynx commonly, extension to the trachea and lungs are possible with pneumonia
• Ophthalmic—extension to the eyes via the nasolacrimal duct
• Otic—extension of infection via the Eustachian tube to the middle/inner ear
• Neurological—extension of infection via the eustachian tube may cause vestibular signs due to otitis interna
• Musculoskeletal—osteomyelitis involving bones of the skull

INCIDENCE/PREVALENCE
Common—incidence of respiratory disease ranged from 14% to 25% in retrospective necropsy reports

SIGNALMENT
• Young animals—typically bacterial infections
• Middle aged-older animals—dental disease, neoplasia, and bacterial infections

SIGNS

Historical Findings
• Nasal discharge and sneezing. Nasal discharge may be unilateral or bilateral. This may be important in determining the underlying cause.
• Previous response to antibiotic therapy. Typically, bacterial infections, dental disease, and foreign bodies will respond to antibiotics but may relapse after finishing treatment. Neoplasia will not resolve with antibiotic therapy.
• Ocular discharge
• Vestibular signs
• Increased respiratory rate/effort, lethargy, anorexia

Physical Examination Findings
• Dried nasal discharge noted around nares and/or medial aspect of the paws
• Nasal discharge—serous, purulent, mucoid, mucopurulent, serosanguinous, or hemorrhagic.
• Concurrent dental disease—tooth root impaction, abscesses, dental tartar, gingivitis, and gingival hyperplasia. May also see ptyalism, anorexia, ocular discharge, and exophthalmos with dental disease.
• Bony lysis/osteomyelitis—tooth root abscesses, neoplasia, others. Typically causes pain and obvious facial swelling
• Ocular discharge—serous, purulent, and mucopurulent. Other clinical signs include conjunctivitis, blepharospasm, and exophthalmos.
• Lethargy, anorexia
• Vestibular signs—rolling, ataxia, head tilt, and/or nystagmus with severe inner ear disease.
• Dyspnea—respiratory distress may be noted with severe upper respiratory tract infections and/or involvement of the lower respiratory tract, such as tracheitis or pneumonia.
• Auscultation findings variable and include increased to decreased or absent airway noise

CAUSES
• Pyogenic bacteria—*Pasturella multocida*, *Bordetella bronchiseptica*, and *Corynebacterium* sp. most common pathogens. *Staphylococcus aureus*, *Moraxella catarrhalis*, *Pseudomonas aeruginosa*, *Mycobacterium* spp., *Fusobacterium* spp., *Actinomyces* spp., and *Arcanobacterium* spp. have also been reported.
• Viral—Skunk adenovirus, African Pygmy Hedgehog adenovirus recently reported
• Mycotic—rare; disseminated histoplasmosis reported in one hedgehog
• Dental disease—periapical or tooth root abscess, severe dental tartar, and gingivitis. Typically, bacteria involved in dental abscesses include *Streptococcus* spp., *Fusobacterium* spp., Actinomyces spp., and *Arcanobacterium* spp.
• Foreign objects—food, bedding material, chew toys
• Obesity—lipid pneumonia has been reported in severely obese hedgehogs
• Allergic disease—dust, ammonia (urine build up in the environment), use of cat litters/clumping litters, plant material
• Neoplasia—oral squamous cell carcinoma, odontogenic fibroma or fibrosarcoma; primary lung tumor—bronchoalveolar carcinoma; metastatic lung tumors

• Typically, unilateral nasal discharge is associated with noninfectious causes such as foreign bodies, dental disease, and neoplasia.

RISK FACTORS
• Dental disease
• Immunosuppression—stress, geriatric age, concurrent disease, corticosteroid use
• Poor husbandry
• Poor diet
• Obesity

DIAGNOSIS

DIFFERENTIAL DIAGNOSIS
• Normal "snuffling" noises—hedgehogs have poor eyesight and hearing and rely heavily on their sense of smell. They often create a loud snuffling noise when investigating a new environment. This is often accompanied by a small amount normal, serous nasal discharge.
• Normal defensive "hiss"
• Anting or self-anointing behavior—when encountering a new smell, hedgehogs will produce copious amounts of thick, foamy saliva and spread it on their quills. Direct contact with the object creating the odor is not necessary. It is believed that this is a defensive mechanism.
• Trauma—may be history or evidence of an injury
• Careful attention to breathing pattern and auscultation may help differentiate between upper and lower respiratory disease.

CBC/BIOCHEMISTRY/URINALYSIS
• Complete blood count may support but cannot confirm or rule out respiratory disease.
• Biochemistry panel is useful to identify predisposing underlying disease.

OTHER LABORATORY TESTS
• Culture and susceptibility testing for bacterial pathogens may be helpful in directing antibiotic therapy. May be difficult to interpret due to the high probability of culturing a commensal or opportunistic organism. Typically, heavy growth of one organism is significant

IMAGING
• Radiography may be useful to evaluate for neoplasia, dental disease, and foreign bodies. The patient should be sedated/anesthetized for these procedures to allow for optimal positioning. Lateral views are best for detection of bony lysis of the nasal sinuses, periosteal reaction, and tooth root involvement. Ventrodorsal views are ideal for evaluation of the nasal cavity and turbinates. Lateral oblique views are best for root disease. The rostrocaudal view is ideal for evaluation of the frontal sinus (periosteal reaction).

HEDGEHOGS

NASAL DISCHARGE AND SNEEZING

• CT or MRI: provide better imaging quality; may be more diagnostic than skull radiographs, especially if nasal detail is obscured by nasal discharge; can help to determine whether the cause of disease is nasal, sinus, or dental disease. CT specifically is excellent for providing bony detail, is more sensitive for areas encased in bone (i.e., lungs and sinuses), and the procedure time is relatively short. However, these modalities may be cost-prohibitive and not as readily available.

DIAGNOSTIC PROCEDURES
• Response to antibiotic therapy as a trial
• FNA for cytology or biopsy for histopathology—useful for suspected neoplasia
• Rhinoscopy—may be useful for visualization of the nasal passages, for removal of foreign bodies and/or sample nasal tumors, and patient size makes this challenging.

TREATMENT
APPROPRIATE HEALTH CARE
• Inpatient—severe debilitating disease or respiratory distress. Respiratory distress is a medical emergency requiring oxygen supplementation
• Discharge stable patients

NURSING CARE
• Patients in respiratory distress require oxygen therapy.
• Ensure that the patient is kept warm—between 80 and 85°F (27 and 29°C). Topor occurs when the environmental temperature falls below 65°F (18°C).
• Supportive care, including correction of dehydration and hypovolemia, and assisted feeding
• Keep the nares clean

DIET
• It is imperative that the animal receive nutritional support if it is not eating. Supplementation with a liquid diet may be required, such as Oxbow Carnivore Care (Oxbow Enterprises, Inc., Murdock, NE) or Emeraid Exotic Carnivore (Lafeber's, Cornell, IL) is essential.
• Gradual caloric restriction in obese patients

CLIENT EDUCATION
• Explain the possibility of chronicity of disease or reoccurrence, especially if dental disease is the cause.
• Most neoplasms are malignant, and treatment is generally palliative

SURGICAL CONSIDERATIONS
• Foreign body removal
• Biopsy/Histopathology
• Mass removal, debulking procedures, and/or abscess removal

MEDICATIONS
DRUG(S) OF CHOICE
• Antibiotics—ideally based on culture and sensitivity results—cephalexin (25 mg/kg PO q12h), amoxicillin/clavulanic acid (12.5–25 mg/kg PO q12h), enrofloxacin (5–10 mg/kg PO q12h), trimethoprim-sulfa (30 mg/kg PO q12h), chloramphenicol (30–50 mg/kg PO q12h), and azithromycin (20 mg/kg PO q24)
• Nebulization may be helpful—sterile water or saline alone may be beneficial to moisten airways. Other commonly nebulized agents include enrofloxacin (2–10 mg/mL of sterile saline); acetylcysteine, as a mucolytic (50 mg as a 2% solution diluted with saline), or aminophylline (3 mg/mL of sterile saline)
• Antihistamines may be used for rhinitis/inflammation. diphenhydramine (1–2 mg/kg PO, IM q8–12) or hydroxyzine (1–2 mg/kg PO q8–12) may be used for allergic disease/inflammatory rhinitis.
• Ophthalmic topical treatment—ciprofloxacin, ofloxacin, triple antibiotic ointments, and solutions may be used to treat secondary conjunctivitis.
• Pain management—meloxicam (0.2 mg/kg PO q24h), tramadol (2–5 mg/kg PO q8–12h), or buprenorphine (0.03–0.05 mg/kg IM, SQ, PO q6–12h) may be used for painful conditions/inflammation

CONTRAINDICATIONS
• Corticosteroid use in patients with infectious disease.

PRECAUTIONS
All therapeutic agents should be used with caution in debilitated, dehydrated patients. Ideally, vascular abnormalities (dehydration, hypotension) are addressed prior to initiating therapy.

POSSIBLE INTERACTIONS
N/A

ALTERNATIVE DRUGS
N/A

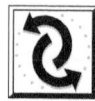

FOLLOW-UP
PATIENT MONITORING
Dyspneic patients are often reluctant to eat or drink. Patients should be monitored carefully to ensure adequate intake.

PREVENTION/AVOIDANCE
• Keep in a well-ventilated, clean environment. Clean bedding frequently to prevent the buildup of ammonia fumes.
• Provide a high-quality diet.

• Manage dental disease by performing regular dental exams and treating disease early

POSSIBLE COMPLICATIONS
• Anorexia
• Extension of disease into the mouth, ears, eyes, lower respiratory tract, and/or brain
• Dyspnea/Respiratory distress

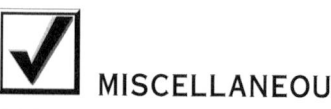

MISCELLANEOUS
ASSOCIATED CONDITIONS
Neoplasia
Dental disease
Obesity

ZOONOTIC POTENTIAL
• Hedgehogs can be asymptomatic carriers of *Salmonella*. Use gloves and careful handwashing after handling.
• In general, infectious agents producing sinusitis and rhinitis in hedgehogs are nonzoonotic; however, any animal disease is of concern to immunocompromised humans.

PREGNANCY/FERTILITY/BREEDING
N/A

SYNONYMS
N/A

SEE ALSO
Dental disease
Neoplasia
Obesity

Suggested Reading
Del Aguila G, Torres CG, Carvallo FR, Gonzalez CM, Cifuentes FF. Oral masses in African pygmy hedgehogs. J Vet Diagn Invest 2019;31(6):864–867.
Heatley JJ, Mauldin GE, Cho DY. A review of neoplasia in the captive African hedgehog (*Atelerix albiventris*). Semin Avian Exot Pet Med;14(3):182–192.
Johnson DH. Geriatric hedgehogs. Vet Clin Exot Anim Pract 2020;23(3):615–637.
Johnson DH. Hedgehogs and sugar gliders: respiratory anatomy, physiology, and disease. Vet Clin Exot Anim Pract 2011;14(2):267–285.
Lightfoot TL. Therapeutics of African pygmy hedgehogs and prairie dogs. Vet Clin North Am Exot Anim Pract 2000;3(1):155–172.
Madarame H, Uchiyama J, Tamukai K, Katayama Y, Osawa N, Suzuki K, Mizutani T, Ochiai H. Complete genome sequence of an adenovirus-1 isolate from an African pygmy hedgehog (*Atelerix albiventris*) exhibiting respiratory symptoms in Japan. Microbiol Resour Announc 2019;8(40):e00695-19.

Authors Amanda Steinagel, DVM and Barbara Oglesbee, DVM, DABVP (Avian)

BASICS

OVERVIEW
• Neoplasia is the most common disorder reported in African Pigmy Hedgehogs. Virtually any organ system can be affected, and more than one type may occur simultaneously.
• The most commonly affected systems are the integumentary, hemolymphatic, digestive, endocrine, and reproductive systems
• Most neoplasms in Hedgehogs are malignant.

SYSTEMS AFFECTED
• Hemolymphatic
• Integumentary
• Reproductive
• Digestive
• Endocrine
• Neurological
• Renal
• Respiratory

GENETICS
• Due to importation bans leading to a limited genetic pool for captive African Pigmy Hedgehogs, a genetic predisposition is suspected.

INCIDENCE/PREVALENCE
• Most common disorder of pet hedgehogs. Retrospective studies report a prevalence of neoplasia ranging from 29% to 52%

SIGNALMENT
• Average age of onset is 3.5 years, but reports exist in patients under one year of age.
• No sex predilection reported

SIGNS

Historical Findings
• Nonspecific signs, such as lethargy, weight loss, and anorexia common
• Tumors or growths

Physical Examination Findings
• Depend on the organ system affected
• Thin, emaciated
• Abdominal distension, organomegaly
• Palpable masses
• Dyspnea
• Oral abnormalities—missing teeth, ptyalism, oral masses, or ulceration
• Musculoskeletal/neurological abnormalities—ataxia, hindlimb paresis, decreased muscle mass, and conscious proprioceptive deficits

CAUSES
• Hemolymphatic—lymphosarcoma (common), eosinophilic leukemia, myelogenous leukemia, multicentric epitheliotropic lymphoma, splenic lymphoma, disseminated histiocytic sarcoma

• Integumentary—fibrosarcoma, hemangiosarcoma, histiocytic sarcoma, lipoma, liposarcoma, malignant fibrous histiocytoma, mast cell tumor, plasmacytoma, sebaceous gland carcinoma, T-cell lymphoma
• Digestive—oral/oronasal squamous cell carcinoma, colonic mucinous adenocarcinoma, gastric adenocarcinoma, hepatocellular carcinoma, intestinal adenocarcinoma, intestinal lymphoma, large intestine plasmacytoma, odontogenic fibroma, oral fibrosarcoma
• Endocrine—adrenal cortical carcinoma, malignant neuroendocrine tumor, pancreatic islet cell carcinoma, parathyroid adenoma, pheochromocytoma, pituitary adenoma, thyroid adenoma/carcinoma
• Reproductive—ovarian granulosa cell tumor, uterine adenomas, uterine adenocarcinoma, uterine endometrial stromal sarcoma, uterine leiomyoma/leiomyosarcoma, uterine spindle cell sarcoma, vaginal spindle cell sarcoma, vaginal tunic neurofibrosarcoma, penile myxoma mammary adenocarcinoma, mammary papillary adenoma
• Musculoskeletal—osteoma/lumbar parosteal sarcoma, rib/skull osteoma, osteosarcoma, maxilla osteochondroma
• Nervous system—histiocytic sarcoma, ganglioglioma, gemistocytic astrocytoma, oligodendroglioma, anaplastic astrocytoma, microglioma, oligoastrocytoma, meningioma, and lymphoma
• Respiratory—bronchoalveolar carcinoma

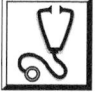

DIAGNOSIS

DIFFERENTIAL DIAGNOSIS
• For paresis, ataxia—Wobbly hedgehog syndrome, IVDD, spondylosis, trauma, encephalitis, vestibular disease, and generalized weakness from systemic disease
• For weight loss—cardiomyopathy, gastroenteritis, infectious disease, and dental disorders
• For abdominal distension—hepatic lipidosis, congestive heart failure, and pyometra
• For dyspnea—congestive heart failure, pneumonia

CBC/BIOCHEMISTRY/URINALYSIS
• Anemia and/or leukemia may be present.
• Chemistry abnormalities based on body system affected but hypercalcemia and hyperbilirubinemia are common findings.
• Useful to rule out or diagnose concurrent metabolic disorders

IMAGING
• Radiographs—assessment for metastatic disease, intraabdominal masses, and thoracic masses

• Ultrasonography assessment for metastatic disease, intraabdominal masses, and thoracic masses
• CT scanning—superior detail

DIAGNOSTIC PROCEDURES
• Histopathologic examination—definitive diagnosis
• Cytologic examination—may yield diagnosis
• Bone marrow aspiration—for diagnosis of hematopoietic neoplasia and staging

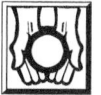

TREATMENT

NURSING CARE
• Ensure that the patient is kept warm—between 80 and 85°F (27 and 29°C). Topor occurs when the environmental temperature falls below 65°F (18°C).
• Supportive care such as fluid therapy, assist feeding, and cleaning of bedding

ACTIVITY
Restriction is usually not necessary; most patients will self-regulate.

DIET
• It is imperative that the animal receive nutritional support if it is not eating. Supplementation with a liquid diet may be required, such as Oxbow Carnivore Care (Oxbow Enterprises, Inc., Murdock, NE) or Emeraid Exotic Carnivore (Lafeber's, Cornell, IL) is essential.

CLIENT EDUCATION
• Most neoplasms are malignant, and treatment is generally palliative

SURGICAL CONSIDERATIONS
• Surgical excision is recommended when possible. Margins based on tumor type and malignancy.
• When in doubt, follow recommendations for neoplasia in canine or feline patients

MEDICATIONS

DRUG(S) OF CHOICE
• Too few reports exist to evaluate the effectiveness of chemotherapy; consult an oncologist for recommendations.
• Pain control may be helpful with palliative care—meloxicam (0.2 mg/kg PO q24h), tramadol (2–5 mg/kg PO q8–12h), or buprenorphine (0.03–0.05 mg/kg IM, SQ, PO q6–12h)
• Corticosteroids—prednisolone (0.5–2 mg/kg PO q12–24h)
• For sedation—ketamine (20–30 mg/kg IM) + midazolam (1 mg/kg IM) or Alfaxalone

(1–3 mg/kg IM) + midazolam (0.5–1 mg/kg IM) ± butorphanol (0.2 mg/kg IM) add alfaxalone (1 mg/kg IM) boluses PRN

CONTRAINDICATIONS/POSSIBLE INTERACTIONS
Do not use NSAIDs and corticosteroids concurrently

FOLLOW-UP

EXPECTED COURSE AND PROGNOSIS
• Most neoplasms (up to 85%) are malignant and carry a poor prognosis

ASSOCIATED CONDITIONS
• Hepatic lipidosis
• Weight loss

AGE-RELATED FACTORS
The risk of neoplasia increases with age

ZOONOTIC POTENTIAL
• Hedgehogs can be asymptomatic carriers of *Salmonella*. Use gloves and careful handwashing after handling.

PREGNANCY/FERTILITY/BREEDING
N/A

SYNONYMS
Cancer
Tumors

SEE ALSO
• Wobbly Hedgehog syndrome
• Cutaneous and subcutaneous masses

ABBREVIATIONS
CT = computed tomography
IVDD = Intervertebral disc disease

Suggested Reading
Del Aguila G, Torres CG, Carvallo FR, Gonzalez CM, Cifuentes FF. Oral masses in African pygmy hedgehogs. J Vet Diagn Invest 2019;31(6):864–867.
Heatley JJ, Mauldin GE, Cho DY. A review of neoplasia in the captive African hedgehog (*Atelerix albiventris*). Semin Avian Exot Pet Med 2005;14(3):182–192.
Johnson DH. Geriatric hedgehogs. Vet Clin Exot Anim Pract 2020;23(3):615–637.
Juan-Sallés C, Garner MM. Cytologic diagnosis of diseases of hedgehogs. Vet Clin Exot Anim Pract 2007;10(1):51–59.
Authors Amanda Steinagel, DVM and Barbara Oglesbee, DVM, DABVP (Avian)

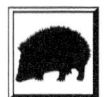

BASICS

DEFINITION
• The presence of body fat in sufficient excess to compromise normal physiologic function or predispose to metabolic, surgical, and/or mechanical problems. Obesity has become an extremely common, and often debilitating, problem in pet hedgehogs.

PATHOPHYSIOLOGY
• Most obese hedgehogs are fed an inappropriate high-fat, caloric-dense diet. Hedgehogs are voracious eaters and prone to obesity in captivity. In the wild, African Pygmy hedgehogs are insectivores and omnivores, feeding primarily on insects, amphibians, small reptiles, bird eggs, and some plants.
• Hedgehogs can readily digest chitin but poorly digest cellulose. Chitin is the main source of dietary fiber in the wild.
• High-quality insectivore diets formulated specifically for pet hedgehogs are not readily available for purchase at most pet stores. As a result, most owners feed cat or dog foods, with little attention paid to fat and calorie content. Additionally, most owners are aware that hedgehogs are insectivores. The most readily available insects are mealworms. Mealworms are very high in fat, with little nutritional value. Owners tend to feed 6–10 mealworms per day, rather than the recommended 6–10 small mealworms twice weekly.
• Owners also tend to feed ad lib and consistently do not recognize obesity in these pets.

SYSTEMS AFFECTED
• Musculoskeletal—articular and locomotor problems
• Hepatobiliary—hepatic lipidosis
• Respiratory—lipid pneumonia reported in obese hedgehogs
• Integument
• Cardiovascular

GENETICS
N/A

INCIDENCE/PREVALENCE
Extremely common in pet hedgehogs

GEOGRAPHIC DISTRIBUTION
N/A

SIGNALMENT
No sex predisposition
Inactive older patients at greater risk, but can occur at any age.

SIGNS
Historical Findings
• Free choice feeding of high fat commercial foods, insects, and sugary treats.
• Weight gain may be significant but not noticeable to the owner
• Owners may report lethargy and impaired mobility.

Physical Examination Findings
• Unable to fully roll up
• Excess fat deposits, measured as a body condition score of 4–5/5, 1 = cachectic (>20% underweight), 2 = lean (10%–20% underweight), 3 = ideal, 4 = overweight/stout (20%–40% overweight), and 5 = obese (>40% overweight)
• Quills may appear sparse—widely separated due to the increased surface area of skin on dorsum.
• Moist dermatitis between skin rolls on ventral body

CAUSES
• Most commonly, excessive access to highly palatable food, often combined with insufficient activity; owners usually leave food out continuously and supplement by feeding sugary treats, excessive mealworms, and other palatable foods as part of social interaction.

RISK FACTORS
Owner lifestyle
Owner perception
Diet palatability and energy density
Inappropriate diet composition
Activity level

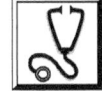

DIAGNOSIS

DIFFERENTIAL DIAGNOSIS
• Ascites
• Intraabdominal neoplasia or organomegaly
• Pregnancy

CBC/BIOCHEMISTRY/URINALYSIS
• Often normal although triglycerides and cholesterol may be elevated.
• In instances of hepatic lipidosis, liver isoenzymes may be normal or elevated.

OTHER LABORATORY TESTS
• N/A

IMAGING
• Demonstrates excess body fat.
• Hepatomegaly common due to hepatic lipidosis.

PATHOLOGIC FINDINGS
May vary depending on the presence of concurrent illnesses.
Hepatic lipidosis, lipid pneumonia commonly occurs

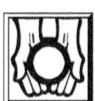

TREATMENT
• Successful treatment requires lifelong diet and activity change
• Gradual reduction in caloric intake and activity level are critical to avoid hepatic lipidosis

ACTIVITY
It is important to provide access to a gradual increase in activity level and exercise.

DIET
General principles of diet change:
• A diet change should never be made abruptly. In ill patients, wait until the patient is stable before changing to an appropriate diet.
• Weight loss should occur gradually to avoid exacerbation of hepatic lipidosis
Dietary recommendations:
• Basic requirements: 30%–50% protein (dry matter basis) and 10%–20% fat.
• The majority (>75%) of the diet should consist of a high-quality commercial insectivore diet formulated specifically for pet hedgehogs.
• If a commercial hedgehog food is not available, a premium commercial feline adult or "lite" adult cat food or high protein, low-fat ferret food may be used. Dry foods are preferred, as they help to prevent periodontal disease.
• For variety, the diet can be supplemented with 1–2 tsp of low-fat foods such as cooked lean meats/fish, eggs, fruits, dark leafy greens, and vegetables
• Calcium-rich foods are preferred, but milk products should be avoided as hedgehogs are lactose intolerant.
• Insects, including mealworms, earthworms, waxworms, crickets, and other available insects, can be fed at treats. Mealworms are high in fat and contain little nutritional value—limit to 6–10 small worms/week. Gut load crickets and dust all insects with a calcium powder before feeding.
• Do not feed ad libitum. Hedgehogs are nocturnal and feed at night.

CLIENT EDUCATION
• Education on appropriate diet is essential to treatment and prevention.
• Advise owners to weigh their hedgehog at least once weekly.
• The author recommends a wellness examination every 6 months.

CONTRAINDICATIONS
• Abrupt reduction in caloric intake.

PRECAUTIONS
N/A

OBESITY

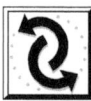

FOLLOW-UP

PATIENT MONITORING
• Regular weight checks and documentation of gradual weight loss.

PREVENTION/AVOIDANCE
• Avoid oversupplementation with highly palatable, sugary treats.
• Provide appropriate access to a large enough enclosure to allow for normal activity.
• Weigh weekly on a gram scale.

POSSIBLE COMPLICATIONS
• Difficulty breathing
• Hepatic lipidosis
• Cardiovascular disease
• Orthopedic/musculoskeletal abnormalities
• Dermatitis, pododermatitis
• Increased risk of complications/death from anesthesia
• Hypocalcemia

EXPECTED COURSE AND PROGNOSIS
The prognosis is based on the presence of concurrent illness and owner's ability to achieve weight loss.

MISCELLANEOUS

ASSOCIATED CONDITIONS
Neoplasia
Hepatic lipidosis

AGE-RELATED FACTORS
N/A

ZOONOTIC POTENTIAL
• Hedgehogs can be asymptomatic carriers of *Salmonella*. Use gloves and careful handwashing after handling.

PREGNANCY/FERTILITY/BREEDING
Reproductive failure may be more common in hedgehogs.

SYNONYMS
N/A

SEE ALSO
Neoplasia
Dyspnea and tachypnea

Suggested Reading
Dierenfeld ES. Feeding behavior and nutrition of the African pygmy hedgehog (*Atelerix albiventris*). Vet Clin North Am Exot Anim Pract 2009;12(2):335–337.

Ivey E, Carpenter J. African hedgehogs. In: Quesenberry KE, Carpenter JW, eds. Ferrets, Rabbits, and Rodents: Clinical Medicine and Surgery, 3rd ed. St Louis, MO: Saunders, 2012:411–427.

Smith AJ. Husbandry and nutrition of hedgehogs. Vet Clin North Am Exot Anim Pract;2(1):127–141.

Wissink-Argilaga N. Veterinary care of African pygmy hedgehogs. In Pract 2020;42(3):151–158.

Author Barbara Oglesbee, DVM, DABVP (Avian) and Amanda Steinagel, DVM

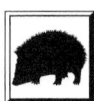

BASICS

DEFINITION
• Vomiting—a complex reflex that results in the expulsion of food or fluid from the alimentary tract through the oral cavity.
• Diarrhea—abnormal frequency, liquidity, and volume of feces

PATHOPHYSIOLOGY
Vomiting
• Vomiting can be caused by diseases of the alimentary tract or can occur secondary to toxic, neurologic, metabolic, infectious, and noninfectious causes.
• Vomiting can be stimulated by peripheral receptors located in the gastrointestinal tract or in various organs.
• Vomiting can also be initiated directly by stimulation of the receptors in the vomiting center in animals with CNS disease. Stimulation of the chemoreceptor trigger zone by metabolic or bacterial toxins, drugs, motion sickness, or vestibulitis will also trigger vomiting

Diarrhea
• Caused by an imbalance in the absorptive, secretory, and motility actions of the intestines
• Can result from a combination of factors: increased membrane permeability, hypersecretion, and malabsorption
• Death occurs from loss of electrolytes and water, acidosis, and from the effects of toxins.
• Antibiotics, stress, and/or poor diet may disrupt the commensal flora of the gut. Pathogenic bacteria, such as *Escherichia coli*, *Clostridium* spp., and *Salmonella* spp. may overgrow and lead to enterotoxemia, ileus, and gas distension.

SYSTEMS AFFECTED
• Gastrointestinal
• Endocrine/Metabolic—fluid, electrolyte, and acid–base imbalances
• Respiratory—aspiration pneumonia

GENETICS
N/A

INCIDENCE/PREVALENCE
Common—gastrointestinal tract diseases rank 3rd in the most common disorders in pet hedgehogs, behind dermatologic disorders and neoplasia.

GEOGRAPHIC DISTRIBUTION
Worldwide

SIGNALMENT
• No specific gender predilection
• Younger animals are more commonly affected by infectious causes.
• See neoplasia more commonly in middle-aged to older animals
• Diet changes can precipitate diarrhea.

SIGNS
General Comments
• Vomiting and diarrhea can occur with or without systemic illness.
• The choice of diagnostic and therapeutic measures depends on the severity of illness.
• Patients that are not systemically ill tend to have normal hydration and minimal systemic signs.
• Signs of more severe illness (e.g., anorexia, weight loss, severe dehydration, depression, and shock) should prompt more aggressive diagnostic and therapeutic measures.

Historical Findings
• Signs of nausea, such as ptyalism, licking the lips, pawing at the mouth
• Soft, formed stool to liquid diarrhea noted.
• Change in color of feces, consistency, and/or containing blood and/or mucous. Owner may note straining to defecate
• History of diet change, spoiled/rotten food
• Lethargy, anorexia may also be noted
• Changes in appetite
• Weight loss
• Recent stress—hospitalization, transportation, environmental changes, and concurrent illness

Physical Examination Findings
• Vary with the severity of disease
• Anorexia, lethargy, and depression
• Fecal staining of the perineum
• Tenesmus, hematochezia, and rectal prolapse
• Dehydration, hypothermia, hypotension, and weakness
• Fever
• Abdominal distention—due to thickened or fluid-filled bowel loops, impaction, bloat, masses, or organomegaly
• Fluid or gas may be palpable within the gastrointestinal tract
• Weight loss in chronically infected animals
• Animals may be found dead in the absence of clinical signs.

CAUSES
• Bacterial infections including *Salmonella* spp., *Escherichia coli*, *Clostridium* spp, *Klebsiella* sp., *Yersinia pseudotuberculosis*. These causes may lead to enterotoxemia.
• *Salmonella typhimurium, S tilene, and S. enteritica* have been reported in hedgehogs—may act as asymptomatic carriers.
• Parasitic causes—coccidiosis, cryptosporidium; Nematodes (*Crenosoma* sp., *Capillaria erinaceid*)
• Yeast—*Candida albicans*
• Dietary—diet change, spoiled/rotten food
• Gastrointestinal obstruction—foreign body, neoplasia, and intussusception
• Inflammatory disorders—*Eosinophilic gastroenteritis* has been reported
• Metabolic disorders—hepatic disease, renal disease
• Neoplasia—primary gastrointestinal tumor, or as a sequela to other organ involvement

RISK FACTORS
• Environmental stressors—improper temperature, poor sanitation, overcrowding, and transportation stress
• Immunosuppressors (corticosteroids, concurrent disease)
• Poor nutrition
• Unsupervised chewing (foreign bodies)

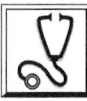

DIAGNOSIS

DIFFERENTIAL DIAGNOSIS
• Differentiate from normal behavior—anting or self-anointing—when encountering a new smell, hedgehogs will produce copious amounts of thick, foamy saliva and spread it on their quills. Direct contact with the object creating the odor is not necessary. It is believed that this is a defensive mechanism.
• Consider all causes of enteropathy, including diet change, inappropriate antibiotics, enterotoxemia, systemic or metabolic disease, as well as specific intestinal disorders
• Infectious and parasitic causes may be primary or secondary.

CBC/BIOCHEMISTRY
• Often normal with mild illness
• Moderate to severe illness should prompt a complete evaluation.
• Increased PCV and TS seen with dehydration
• Anemia may be seen with chronic gastrointestinal bleeding.
• TWBC elevation with neutrophilia may be seen with bacterial enteritis.
• Hemogram abnormalities may be consistent with sepsis and/or systemic infection.
• Hypoalbuminemia may be seen with protein loss from the intestinal tract.
• Serum biochemistry abnormalities may suggest renal or hepatic disease.
• Electrolyte abnormalities secondary to anorexia, fluid loss, and dehydration.

OTHER LABORATORY TESTS
Fecal Examination
• Fecal direct examination, fecal floatation, and zinc sulfate centrifugation may demonstrate gastrointestinal parasites or spore-forming bacteria.
• Fecal cytology—may reveal red blood cells or fecal leukocytes, which are associated with inflammation or infection of the intestines

- Fecal culture should be performed if a bacterial infection is suspected; however, interpretation may be difficult since *E. coli* may be normal inhabitants in some cases.
- Fecal occult blood testing—to confirm melena when suspected

IMAGING

- Survey abdominal radiography may indicate intestinal obstruction, organomegaly, mass, foreign body, or ascites.
- Contrast radiography may indicate mucosal irregularities, mass, ileus, foreign body, stricture, or thickening of the intestinal wall.
- Abdominal ultrasonography may demonstrate intestinal wall thickening, gastrointestinal mass, foreign body, ileus, or mesenteric lymphadenopathy. Hyperechogenicity may be seen with hepatic lipidosis or fibrosis; hypoechoic nodules are suggestive of hepatic necrosis, abscess, or neoplasia.

DIAGNOSTIC PROCEDURES

- Exploratory laparotomy and surgical biopsy—if there is evidence of obstruction or intestinal mass, and/or for definitive diagnosis of gastrointestinal inflammatory or neoplastic diseases

PATHOLOGIC FINDINGS

- Vary with cause
- Gross pathology may reveal lesions suggestive of etiology
- Histopathology is often the best method to obtain a definitive diagnosis for neoplasia, infiltrative or inflammatory conditions, and certain infections.

TREATMENT

APPROPRIATE HEALTH CARE

- Treatment must be specific to the underlying cause to be successful.
- Patients with mild vomiting or diarrhea that are otherwise bright and alert usually respond to outpatient treatment.
- Patients with moderate to severe disease usually require hospitalization and supportive care including parenteral medication, fluid therapy, and thermal support.
- Patients exhibiting signs of lethargy, depression, dehydration, and/or shock should be hospitalized
- When infectious disease is suspected, strict isolation of affected and exposed animals is indicated.

NURSING CARE

- Ensure that the patient is kept warm—between 80 and 85°F (27 and 29°C). Topor occurs when the environmental temperature falls below 65°F (18°C).
- Fluid therapy is used to correct hydration following standard protocols (5%–10% of

body weight administered in SQ boluses). Fluids should be kept warm to prevent hypothermia and can be warmed by placing the prepared syringe in a warm water bath prior to administration. Administration via a 22–25-gauge butterfly needle can reduce stress on the patient by minimizing restraint.
- For critical patients, administer fluid therapy via IV or intraosseous (IO) catheter. In addition to crystalloids, the patient may need colloids such as hetastarch at 10 mL/kg IO per day in several small boluses. Maintenance requirement is 100 mL/kg/day

ACTIVITY

Depending on the cause, activity may or may not need to be restricted. Most small mammals that do not feel well will be less active of their own accord.

DIET

- Hedgehogs rarely have intractable vomiting such that holding NPO for long periods is necessary. If holding NPO, monitor carefully for hypoglycemia.
- Once vomiting has subsided, offer a bland diet such as canned chicken baby foods.
- It is imperative that the animal receive nutritional support if it is not eating. Supplementation with a liquid diet may be required, such as Oxbow Carnivore Care (Oxbow Enterprises, Inc., Murdock, NE) or Emeraid Omnivore (Lafeber's, Cornell, IL), supplements such as Ensure (Abott Nutrition, Columbus, OH).
- A diet change should never be made abruptly. If the diet is inappropriate, wait until the patient is stable and eating again, then convert to an appropriate diet.

CLIENT EDUCATION

- If infectious disease is suspected, strict isolation and zoonotic precautions should be initiated.
- Most neoplasms are malignant, and treatment is generally palliative

SURGICAL CONSIDERATIONS

Exploratory laparotomy if intestinal obstruction or neoplasia is suspected, or to obtain biopsies for diagnosis of IBD

MEDICATIONS
DRUG(S) OF CHOICE
Antibiotic Therapy

- Indicated in patients with bacterial disorders of the gastrointestinal tract; also indicated in patients with disruption of the intestinal mucosa evidenced by blood in the feces
- Selection should be broad-spectrum antibiotics, based on the results of culture and susceptibility testing when possible.

- Some choices for empirical use while waiting for culture results include chloramphenicol (30–50 mg/kg PO q12h), or enrofloxacin (5–10 mg/kg PO, SC, IM q12h) or trimethoprim-sulfa (30 mg/kg PO q12h), or chloramphenicol (30–50 mg/kg PO q12h)
  - If *Salmonella* is suspected—enrofloxacin. ciprofloxacin (5–20 mg/kg PO q12h) or amoxicillin (15 mg/kg PO, SC, IV q12h) while waiting for culture results. Treatment for 3–4 weeks is needed.
- For anaerobic bacteria—metronidazole (20 mg/kg PO q24h × 14 days)
- For candida—ketoconazole (10 mg/kg PO q12h) or nystatin (300,000 IU/kg PO q8–12h)

Antiparasitic Agents

- Indicated based upon fecal examination for internal parasites, ova, or cysts
- For nematodes—fenbendazole (10–30 mg/kg PO q24h × 5 days, repeat in 14 days) or (25 mg/kg PO q14d × 3 treatments)
- For cestodes—praziquantel (7 mg/kg PO or SQ, repeat in 14 days)
- For coccidia—sulfadimethoxine (10–20 mg/kg PO q24h × 5 days; 5 days off, then repeat) or toltrazuril (10 mg/kg PO q24 × 2 treatments, then repeat q7d for 3 treatments)
- For protozoa—metronidazole (25 mg/kg PO q12h × 5 days)

Gastroprotectant and Antiemetic Agents

- Antisecretory agents: omeprazole (0.5–1 mg/kg PO, SC q24h), famotidine (1 mg/kg PO, SC, IV q24h), and ranitidine (2–4 mg/kg PO, SQ, IV q24h)
- Sucralfate suspension (10–25 mg/kg PO q8h) protects ulcerated tissue (cytoprotection) by binding to ulcer sites.
- Antiemetics should be reserved for patients with refractory vomiting that have not responded to treatment of the underlying disease. Options include metoclopramide (0.2–0.5 mg/kg PO, SC, IM q6–8h), ondansetron (0.5 mg/kg PO q12h), or maropitant citrate (1–2 mg/kg PO, SC q24h).

Suggested Treatment of IBD

- Treat with antiparasitic medication—fenbendazole (10–30 mg/kg PO q24h × 5 days, repeat in 14 days), followed by a novel food trial for 3–4 weeks
- If no response, an antibacterial trial for 3–4 weeks: enrofloxacin (10 mg/kg PO q12h) or amoxicillin (15 mg/kg PO, SC, IV q12h)
- If no response, immunosuppressive therapy—prednisolone (0.5–2 mg/kg PO q12h) weaning back to the lowest effective dose

For Pain Control

Meloxicam (0.2 mg/kg PO q24h), tramadol (2–5 mg/kg PO q8–12h) and/or buprenorphine (0.03–0.05 mg/kg IM, SQ, PO q6–12h).

CONTRAINDICATIONS
Corticosteroids with bacterial enteritis, especially if *Salmonella* is suspected.

PRECAUTIONS
• It is important to determine the cause of vomiting and diarrhea. A general "shotgun" approach with antibiotics may be ineffective or detrimental.
• Chloramphenicol may cause aplastic anemia in susceptible people. Clients and staff should use appropriate precautions when handling this drug.
• Metronidazole is neurotoxic if overdosed.
• Isolate affected and exposed animals when infectious disease is suspected.

POSSIBLE INTERACTIONS
N/A

ALTERNATIVE DRUGS
N/A

FOLLOW-UP

PATIENT MONITORING
• Fecal volume and character, appetite, attitude, and body weight
• If symptoms do not resolve, consider reevaluation of the diagnosis.

PREVENTION/AVOIDANCE
• Providing appropriate diet and husbandry
• Reducing stress and providing sanitary conditions
• When infectious disease is suspected, strict isolation of affected and exposed animals is indicated.

POSSIBLE COMPLICATIONS
• Aspiration pneumonia
• Dehydration due to fluid loss
• Ileal obstruction, intussusception, tenesmus, and cloacal prolapse.

Septicemia due to bacterial invasion of enteric mucosa
Shock, death from enterotoxicosis

EXPECTED COURSE AND PROGNOSIS
• Depends on cause and severity of disease
• Most neoplasms are malignant, and treatment is generally palliative

MISCELLANEOUS

ASSOCIATED CONDITIONS
• Dehydration
• Malnutrition
• Hypoproteinemia
• Anemia
• Septicemia

AGE-RELATED FACTORS
• All ages susceptible to diarrhea
• Neoplasia common in older animals

ZOONOTIC POTENTIAL
• Hedgehogs can be asymptomatic carriers of *Salmonella*. Use gloves and careful handwashing after handling.

PREGNANCY/FERTILITY/BREEDING
• Severe diarrhea and associated metabolic disturbance may reduce fertility or cause abortion.
• Some infections (e.g., *Salmonella*) can cause abortion.

SEE ALSO
Anorexia
Neoplasia

ABBREVIATIONS
IBD = inflammatory bowel disease
PCV = packed cell volume
TS = total solids
TWBC = total white blood cell count

Suggested Reading
Hoff C, Nichols M, Gollarza L, Scheftel J, Adams J, Tagg KA, Francois Watkins L, Poissant T, Stapleton GS, Morningstar-Shaw B, Signs K. Multistate outbreak of *Salmonella Typhimurium* linked to pet hedgehogs, United States, 2018–2019. Zoonoses Public Health 2022;69(3): 167–174.
Hrysyzen TM, Malmberg JL, Johnston MS. Diagnosis and clinical management of eosinophilic gastroenteritis in an African pygmy hedgehog (*Atelerix albiventris*). J Exot Pet Med 2019;30:88–91.
Johnson DH. Geriatric hedgehogs. Vet Clin Exot Anim Pract 2020;23(3):615–637.
Keeble E, Koterwas B. Salmonellosis in hedgehogs. Vet Clin Exot Anim Pract 2020;23(2):459–470.
Lennox AM. Emergency and critical care procedures in sugar gliders (*Petaurus breviceps*), African hedgehogs (*Atelerix albiventris*), and prairie dogs (*Cynomys* spp). Vet Clin North Am Exot Anim Pract 2007;10:533–555.
McLaughlin A, Strunk A. Common emergencies in small rodents, hedgehogs, and sugar gliders. Vet Clin Exot Anim Pract 2016;19(2):465–499.
Pignon C, Mayer J. Zoonoses of ferrets, hedgehogs, and sugar gliders. Vet Clin North Am Exot Anim Pract 2011;14(3):533–549.
Authors Amanda Steinagel, DVM and Barbara Oglesbee, DVM, DABVP (Avian)

HEDGEHOGS

WOBBLY HEDGEHOG SYNDROME

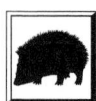

BASICS

DEFINITION
• Wobbly Hedgehog syndrome (WHS) is a progressive, fatal neurodegenerative disorder of the spinal cord and brain.

PATHOPHYSIOLOGY
• Progressive neurodegeneration as a result of spongiform changes in the white matter of the brain and spinal cord. The disease ascends from the hind limbs to the forelimbs, causing progressive ataxia, muscle degeneration, paresis, and paralysis. Eventually, tetraplegia and aphagia result in an inability to eat, progressive wasting and death. The cause is unknown.

SYSTEMS AFFECTED
• Neuromuscular

GENETICS
Due to regional disease prevalence of Wobbly Hedgehog syndrome, a genetic predisposition is suspected

INCIDENCE/PREVALENCE
10% of North American hedgehogs are affected

GEOGRAPHIC DISTRIBUTION
Wobbly Hedgehog syndrome (WHS) is seen more commonly in North America

SIGNALMENT
Most common in animals <2 years of age, but has been reported in older animals. No sex differences

SIGNS
Historical Findings
• Usually begins with an inability to roll up, progresses to rear limb ataxia, weakness, and paralysis. Ascends to front limbs over a period of 9–15 months. In later stages, weight loss despite a good appetite, followed by general debility and an inability to swallow.

Physical Examination Findings
• Initially, unable to ball up.
• Progresses to rear limb ataxia, weakness, and paralysis.
• In late stages, tetraparesis, weight loss, and general debility.

CAUSES
• Unknown, genetic predisposition suspected

RISK FACTORS
• None

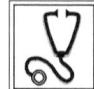

DIAGNOSIS

DIFFERENTIAL DIAGNOSIS
• Tupor—a hibernation-like state which occurs when the environmental temperature falls below 65°F (18°C).
• IVDD—more acute onset, rear legs only involved
• Spondylosis—acute or gradual onset; usually does not progress to front legs or severe debility
• Trauma to the brain, ear, or spinal cord—may have been noted in history, more acute onset
• Infectious: otitis, encephalitis, viral infections; may be a sequela to rhinitis and URI; see circling, head tilt, nystagmus
• Neoplastic—usually older animals, more rapid progression as compared to WHS
• Poisoning, including lead (rare)

CBC/BIOCHEMISTRY/URINALYSIS
Important to rule out an infectious cause or metabolic disorder

OTHER LABORATORY TESTS
None

IMAGING
• To rule out other causes of ataxia, paresis, and paralysis: Skull radiographs to identify or rule out ear pathology
• Radiographs or CT—identify IVDD, spondylosis, spinal injury, and injury that would explain lameness (versus ataxia); identify neoplasia, cardiopulmonary disease, or abdominal masses that may explain difficulty ambulating

DIAGNOSTIC PROCEDURES
• Necropsy—the diagnosis of WHS can only be made by histological examination of the nervous system.

PATHOLOGIC FINDINGS
Vacuolization of the white matter tract of the cerebrum, cerebellum, brain stem, and throughout the spinal cord.

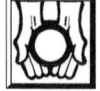

TREATMENT

APPROPRIATE HEALTH CARE
As long as the patient is eating and drinking, outpatient care is appropriate

NURSING CARE
• Ensure that the patient is kept warm—between 80 and 85°F (27–29°C). Topor occurs when the environmental temperature falls below 65°F (18°C).
• Fluid therapy is used to correct hydration following standard protocols (5%–10% of body weight administered in SQ boluses). Fluids should be kept warm to prevent hypothermia and can be warmed by placing the prepared syringe in a warm water bath prior to administration. Administration via a 22–25-gauge butterfly needle can reduce stress on the patient by minimizing restraint.
• For critical patients, administer fluid therapy via IV or intraosseous (IO) catheter. In addition to crystalloids, the patient may need colloids such as hetastarch at 10 mL/kg IO per day in several small boluses. Maintenance requirement is 100 mL/kg/day

ACTIVITY
Exercise should be restricted. Remove ramps, exercise wheels; limit to one level of the cage.

DIET
• It is imperative that the animal receive nutritional support if it is not eating. Supplementation with a liquid diet may be required, such as Oxbow Carnivore Care (Oxbow Enterprises, Inc., Murdock, NE) or Emeraid Exotic Carnivore (Lafeber's, Cornell, IL), is essential.

CLIENT EDUCATION
• WHS is uniformly fatal. The progression of the disease varies from weeks to months; will become immobile within 9–15 months following the onset of ataxia
• Supportive care, including assisted feeding, frequent bedding changes, padding, and cleanliness are important components of home nursing care.

SURGICAL CONSIDERATIONS
N/A

MEDICATIONS

DRUG(S) OF CHOICE
• For pain: meloxicam (0.2 mg/kg PO q24h), tramadol (2–5 mg/kg PO q8–12h), or buprenorphine (0.03–0.05 mg/kg IM, SQ, PO q6–12h)

CONTRAINDICATIONS
• N/A

PRECAUTIONS

POSSIBLE INTERACTIONS
N/A

ALTERNATIVE DRUGS
N/A

FOLLOW-UP

PATIENT MONITORING
• Monitor for signs of pain or worsening of neurological abnormalities

PREVENTION/AVOIDANCE
N/A

POSSIBLE COMPLICATIONS
N/A

EXPECTED COURSE AND PROGNOSIS
• WHD is progressive and fatal

 MISCELLANEOUS

ASSOCIATED CONDITIONS
Dysphagia
Weight loss

AGE-RELATED FACTORS
• Older animals—neoplasia, IVDD
• Younger animals—WHS

ZOONOTIC POTENTIAL
• Hedgehogs can be asymptomatic carriers of *Salmonella*. Use gloves.

PREGNANCY/FERTILITY/BREEDING
N/A

SYNONYMS
• Degenerative myelopathy
• Spongiform leukoencephalopathy

SEE ALSO
• Anorexia
• Ataxia

ABBREVIATIONS
CT = computed tomography
IVDD = intravertebral disc disease
WHS = Wobbly Hedgehog syndrome

INTERNET RESOURCES
www.vin.com

Suggested Reading
Berg CC, Doss GA, Guevar J. Neurologic examination of healthy adult African pygmy hedgehogs (*Atelerix albiventris*). J Am Vet Med Assoc 2021;258(9): 971–976.

Díaz-Delgado J, Whitley DB, Storts RW, Heatley JJ, Hoppes S, Porter BF. The pathology of wobbly hedgehog syndrome. Vet Pathol 2018;55(5):711–718.
Ivey E, Carpenter J. African hedgehogs. In: Quesenberry KE, Carpenter JW, eds. Ferrets, Rabbits, and Rodents: Clinical Medicine and Surgery, 3rd ed. St Louis, MO: Saunders, 2012:411–427.
Johnson DH. Geriatric hedgehogs. Vet Clin Exot Anim Pract 2020;23(3):615–637.
Keeble E, Koterwas B. Selected emerging diseases of pet hedgehogs. Vet Clin Exot Anim Pract 2020;23(2):443–458.
Lennox AM. Emergency and critical care procedures in sugar gliders (*Petaurus breviceps*), African hedgehogs (*Atelerix albiventris*), and prairie dogs (*Cynomys* spp). Vet Clin North Am Exot Anim Pract 2007;10:533–555.

Authors Amanda Steinagel, DVM and Barbara Oglesbee, DVM, DABVP (Avian)

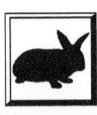

RABBITS

ABSCESSES

 BASICS

DEFINITION
An abscess is a localized collection of purulent exudate contained within a fibrous capsule. Abscesses are an extremely common finding in rabbits.

PATHOPHYSIOLOGY
• Unlike cats and dogs, abscesses in rabbits do not often rupture and drain. Rabbit abscesses are filled with a thick, caseous exudate, surrounded by a fibrous capsule. They can be either slow growing or become large very quickly and often extend aggressively into surrounding soft tissue and bone. Abscesses with bony involvement (facial, plantar, and joints) can be extremely difficult to treat, requiring surgical intervention and prolonged medical care. Prognosis is fair to poor depending on the severity and location.
• Abscesses in rabbits are usually associated with an underlying cause. Identification and correction of the underlying cause are paramount for successful treatment.
• Abscesses occur most commonly on the face and are almost always caused by dental disease; occasionally, they may be secondary to upper respiratory infections, otitis, or trauma.
• Abscesses on the trunk or extremities are usually caused by trauma, puncture, or bite wounds, abrasions, foreign bodies, furunculosis, or osteomyelitis.
• Hepatic abscessation is often secondary to corticosteroid use.
• Abscessation secondary to bacteremia may occur anywhere on the body, including internal organs; often, the original source cannot be identified.
• Affected rabbits often appear to not be painful, unless osteomyelitis or dental disease is present. However, assessment of pain in rabbits is often difficult for owners, as compared to predatory species such as dogs and cats.

SYSTEMS AFFECTED
• Skin/Exocrine—percutaneous
• Skeletal—especially skull and plantar abscesses
• Ophthalmic—periorbital tissues
• Hepatobiliary—liver parenchyma
• Respiratory—lung parenchyma, nasal turbinates, sinuses
• Reproductive—mammary gland

INCIDENCE/PREVALENCE
Extremely common in pet rabbits; most common cause of subcutaneous swelling

SIGNALMENT
• No age or sex predilection for most abscesses
• Dwarf and lop-eared rabbits are predisposed to abscesses secondary to dental disease.

SIGNS
General Comments
• Determined by organ system and/or tissue affected
• Associated with a combination of inflammation (pain, swelling, loss of function), tissue destruction, and/or organ system dysfunction caused by accumulation of exudate

Historical Findings
• Facial abscesses—history of dental disease, ptyalism, nasal or ocular discharge, exopthalmous, otitis externa, interna, or media
• Anorexia, depression—seen with dental disease, pain from skeletal abscesses. Intrathoracic or hepatic abscesses—often only clinical signs until abscess is large enough to cause space-occupying effects
• Lameness, reluctance to move—plantar or digital abscesses; pain
• Occasionally history of traumatic insult or previous infection
• Dyspnea with large intrathoracic abscesses
• A rapidly appearing, variably painful, swelling if affected area is visible

Physical Examination Findings
Determined by the organ system or tissue affected
• Mandibular, cheeks, nasal rostrum, retrobulbar—usually caused by dental disease. Palpable mass of fluctuant to firm consistency, usually attached to and involving underlying bone. Findings may include ptyalism, anorexia, nasal discharge, ocular discharge, and exophthalmia. Always perform a thorough oral exam under anesthesia, including skull radiographs. Occasionally, mass is freely movable within the subcutaneous tissues and not attached to bone—more likely caused by external trauma, better prognosis
• Anorexic rabbits—may show signs of GI hypomotility; scant, dry feces, dehydration, firm stomach or cecal contents, gas-filled intestinal loops
• Ears—mass occasionally palpable arising from ear canal; vestibular signs (torticollis, ataxia, rolling, and nystagmus) with extension into inner ear or brain
• Limbs—lameness, single or multiple palpable masses, especially on plantar or interdigital surfaces, hair loss, cellulitis (erythemia, swelling); may rupture and form scabs with caseous exudate underneath

• Superficial abscess—variable size mass; firm or fluctuant; nonpainful; freely movable unless attached to underlying tissues; occasionally large areas of necrotic skin (may slough)
• Intrathoracic abscesses—dull or absent lung sounds on thoracic auscultation; dyspnea; anorexia; depression

CAUSES
• Pyogenic bacteria—odontogenic abscesses—*Pasteurella* generally not present; common isolates from dental-related abscesses include anaerobic bacteria such as *Fusobacterium nucleatum*, *Prevotella* spp., *Peptostreptococcus micros*, *Actinomyces israelii*, and *Arcanobacterium haemolyticum*. *Streptococcus* spp. may also be cultured from odontogenic abscesses. Other abscesses—may culture *Pasteurella multocida*, *Staphylococcus aureus*, *Pseudomonas* spp., *Escherichia coli*, b-hemolytic *Streptococcus* spp., *Proteus* spp., *Bacteroides* spp.
• Dental disease—periapical or tooth root abscesses, food lodged between teeth and/or gingival mucosa; malocclusion causing sharp points on crowns that penetrate oral mucosa
• Foreign objects

RISK FACTORS
• Mandibular, cheeks—elongated cheek teeth, incisor malocclusion often caused by feeding of diets containing inadequate roughage; pulpal trauma from inappropriate trimming of teeth or blunt trauma
• Periorbital—dental disease; periapical abcesses of the maxillary cheek teeth
• Brain—otitis interna, sinusitis; often caused by chronic nasal pasteurellosis extending via eustachian tube, sinuses; may be extension of otitis externa/media
• Percutaneous—abrasions, puncture (bite) wounds, sepsis
• Plantar/digital—improper surfaces (wire cages, nonpadded surfaces), urine scald, sitting on soiled bedding material, abrasions, furunculosis, trauma, puncture wounds, foreign bodies; immobility from pain; obesity
• Liver—use of topical or systemic corticosteroids, sepsis
• Lung—sepsis, bacterial pneumonia, foreign object aspiration
• Mammary gland—mastitis
• Immunosuppression—systemic or topical corticosteroid use, immunosuppressive chemotherapy, underlying predisposing disease (e.g., diabetes mellitus, chronic renal failure)

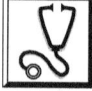 **DIAGNOSIS**

DIFFERENTIAL DIAGNOSIS
Mass lesions
• Granuloma—generally firmer without fluctuant center

- Neoplasia—variable growth; variably painful
- Cyst—lack of white caseous exudate
- Fibrous scar tissue—firm; nonpainful; does not enlarge
- Hematoma/seroma—nonencapsulated; unattached to surrounding tissues; fluctuant and fluid-filled initially but more firm with organization
- Cuterebra

CBC/BIOCHEMISTRY/URINALYSIS
- CBC—often normal; TWBC elevations generally do not occur; instead the neutrophil:lymphocyte ratio shifts to a relative neutrophilia and lymphopenia
- Urinalysis and serum chemistry profile—depend on system affected
- Liver—slight to moderate increases in liver enzymes if hepatic involvement

OTHER LABORATORY TESTS
- Serology for *Pasteurella*—usefulness is severely limited and generally not helpful in the diagnosis of pasteurellosis in pet rabbits. Positive results, even when high, only indicate prior exposure to *Pasteurella* and the development of antibodies, and do not confirm active infection. Low positive results may occur due to cross-reaction with other, nonpathogenic bacteria (false positive). False-negative results are common with immunosuppression or early infection. No evidence exists to support correlation of titers to the presence or absence of disease.

IMAGING
- Radiography—to determine the extent of bone involvement; essential in guidance of treatment plan and expected prognosis; osteomyelitis carries poorer prognosis, prolonged treatment
- Thoracic and abdominal radiographs may help identify and determine the extent of internal abscesses.
- Skull radiographs—essential to identify type and extent of dental disease in rabbits with facial abscesses; perform under general anesthesia; five views are recommended for a thorough assessment, including ventral-dorsal, lateral, two lateral obliques, and rostral-caudal.
- Ultrasonography—determine organ system affected; extent of disease
- Echocardiography—helpful for diagnosis of pericardial abscess
- CT—more accurate than radiographs for assessment of facial abscesses, bullae involvement, or brain abscess

DIAGNOSTIC PROCEDURES
- Thorough oral examination under sedation to look for dental disease is crucial in the diagnosis and treatment of all rabbits with facial abscesses.

Aspiration
- Reveals a thick, creamy to caseous, white exudate
- High nucleated cell count; primarily degenerative neutrophils with lesser numbers of macrophages and lymphocytes
- Pyogenic bacteria—may be seen in cells, higher number in wall of abscess; Gram's stain to direct antibiotic therapy

Biopsy
- To rule out neoplasia, granuloma, and other causes of masses
- Sample should contain both normal and abnormal tissue in the same specimen.
- Submit tissues for histopathologic examination and culture

Culture
- Affected tissue and/or exudate—aerobic and anaerobic bacteria; lack of growth is common, especially with anaerobic infections or fastidious bacterial infections
- If anaerobic culture is not possible, diagnosis is often presumed.
- Growth may be more likely if wall or capsule is sampled; bacteria deep within exudate are often nonviable.
- Bacterial susceptibility testing to direct antibiotic therapy

PATHOLOGIC FINDINGS
- Exudate—large numbers of neutrophils in various stages of degeneration; other inflammatory cells; necrotic tissue
- Surrounding tissue congested; fibrin; large number of neutrophils; variable number of lymphocytes; plasma cells; macrophages, fibrous connective tissue
- Causative agent variably detectable, especially with anaerobic infections

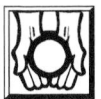

TREATMENT

APPROPRIATE HEALTH CARE
- Simple lancing, flushing, and draining are not adequate to treat rabbits' abscesses. Thick exudates do not drain well, and the abscess will recur. It is crucial to remove/correct the underlying cause for long-term success.
- Depends on location of abscess and treatment required
- Outpatient—smaller, well-demarcated subcutaneous abscesses
- Inpatient—sepsis; extensive surgical procedures; treatment requiring extended hospitalization
- Surgical removal of abscess, nidus of infection (e.g., teeth), or foreign object is necessary
- Institution of long-term antimicrobial therapy
- Correction of underlying disease or predisposing factors if possible

NURSING CARE
- Depends on location of abscess and type of surgical repair (see below).
- Use protective bandaging and/or Elizabethan collars as needed.
- Sepsis or peritonitis—aggressive fluid therapy and support

ACTIVITY
Restrict until the abscess has resolved and adequate healing of tissues has taken place.

DIET
- It is imperative that the rabbit continues to eat during and following treatment. Anorexia will often cause GI hypomotility, derangement of the gastrointestinal microflora, and overgrowth of intestinal bacterial pathogens.
- Offer a large selection of fresh, moistened greens such as cilantro, romaine lettuce, parsley, carrot tops, dandelion greens, spinach, collard greens, etc., and good-quality grass hay. Many rabbits will begin to eat these foods, even if they were previously anorectic. Also, try offering the rabbit's usual pelleted diet.
- If the patient refuses these foods, syringe-feed a gruel such as Critical Care for Herbivores (Oxbow Pet Products) or Emeraid Herbivore (Lafeber Company, Cornell, IL) 10–15 mL/kg PO q6–8h. Larger volumes and more frequent feedings are often accepted; feed as much as the rabbit will readily accept. Alternatively, pellets can be ground and mixed with fresh greens, vegetable baby foods, water, or juice to form a gruel. If sufficient volumes of food are not accepted in this manner, nasogastric intubation is indicated.
- High-carbohydrate, high-fat nutritional supplements should be avoided.

CLIENT EDUCATION
- Discuss the need to correct or prevent risk factors
- Abscesses of the head and those involving bone have a fair to guarded prognosis for complete resolution. Most will require extensive surgery, sometimes multiple surgeries and multiple follow-up visits. Recurrences, in the same or other locations, are common. Clients must be aware of the monetary and time investment.

SURGICAL CONSIDERATIONS
Superficial Abscesses (Not Involving Bone or Teeth)
- Drainage or debridement alone will not be sufficient. Exudate does not drain, and placement of Penrose or similar drains is contraindicated. Abscesses must be debrided; debridement must be followed by local treatment until no evidence of infection exists.
- En bloc excision of entire abscess, leaving wide margins (similar to excision of

ABSCESSES

malignant sarcoma in dogs or cats); exercise care not to rupture capsule
• If entire abscess cannot be removed en bloc, lance, remove exterior wall, curette all exudates, leave wound to heal via second intention. Irrigate wound with dilute antiseptic solution (chorhexidine or iodine) 2–3 times daily until healthy granulation bed forms followed by antibiotic cream until re-epithelialization occurs; long-term antibiotic therapy
• Remove any foreign objects(s), necrotic tissue, or nidus of infection.
• Place on long-term antibiotic therapy.

Facial Abscesses
• Remove, in entirety, all teeth involved in the abscess.
• Remove the abscess, abscess capsule, and affected bone, in entirety, whenever possible.
• If all affected tissues cannot be removed entirely, remove abscess at the level of the bone, curette/debride all grossly abnormal bone, teeth, and soft tissue. Flush copiously to remove exudates.
Post debridement, local treatment options include:
• Marsupialization of soft tissues, followed by daily flushing, debridement as needed, and instillation of antibiotic ointments until healing occurs via second intention
• Pack the wound with sterile, antibiotic-soaked gauze (antibiotics selected should be effective against anaerobic bacteria), then close the skin. Unpack and debride the cavity weekly until a healthy granulation bed forms, followed by primary closure.
• Fill the defect with antibiotic-impregnated polymethyl methacrylate (AIPMMA) beads, which release a high concentration of antibiotic into local tissues for several months. Selection of antibiotic is limited to those known to elute appropriately from bead to tissues and should be based on culture and susceptibility testing. Beads must be manufactured and inserted aseptically. Beads should be left in the incision site for at least 2 months but can be left in indefinitely.
• In rabbits with extensive head abscesses, aggressive debridement of bone is often indicated, and special expertise may be required. Given the expense and pain involved in these procedures, the author recommends referral to a specialist.
• Place on long-term antibiotic therapy; appropriate pain management

Abscesses Involving Joints or Feet
• As above, remove as much abscess en bloc as possible, using care not to rupture the abscess and further contaminate the incision site
• Debride, curette all visible abnormal tissue; flush copiously

• Treat as open wound—flush, debride would daily initially, followed by twice weekly to weekly debridement as healing occurs. Follow debridement with the application of soft bandages. Bandages must be changed immediately if they become wet.
• Severe osteomyelitis may require amputation.
• Correct underlying cause—provide soft bedding, improve husbandry, weight loss
• Place on long-term antibiotic therapy; appropriate pain management

Internal Abscesses
• Thoracic abscess—occasionally may be amenable to surgical excision or lobectomy via thoracotomy; if not excised, treat with supportive care, long-term antibiotics
• Abdominal abscesses—surgical removal when possible, followed by long-term antibiotic therapy

MEDICATIONS
DRUG(S) OF CHOICE
Antibiotics
• Combine with topical treatment (surgical debridement and post-debridement care).
• Antimicrobial drugs effective against the infectious agent; gain access to site of infection. Choice of antibiotic is ideally based on results of culture and susceptibility testing. Depending on the severity of infection, long-term antibiotic therapy is required (4–6 weeks minimum, to several months). Use broad-spectrum antibiotics such as enrofloxacin (10–20 mg/kg PO, SC, IM, IV q12h), marbofloxacin (5 mg/kg PO q24h), trimethoprim-sulfa (15–30 mg/kg PO q12h), or chloramphenicol (50 mg/kg PO q8h). Most facial or dental abscesses contain anaerobic bacteria; use antibiotics effective against anaerobes such as azithromycin (15–30 mg/kg PO q24h); can be used alone or combined with metronidazole (20 mg/kg PO q12h). Alternatively, use penicillin G procaine (40,000–60,000 IU/kg SC q24h). Combine with topical or surgical treatment.

Acute Pain Management
• Butorphanol (0.1–0.5 mg/kg SQ, IM, IV q4–6h); may cause profound sedation; short acting
• Buprenorphine (0.02–0.05 mg/kg SQ, IM IV q8–12h); less sedating, longer acting than butorphanol
• Hydromorphone (0.1 mg/kg SC IM q2–4h) or oxymorphone (0.05–0.2 mg/kg SC IM q8–12h); use with caution; more than 1–2 doses may cause gastrointestinal stasis
• Meloxicam (1 mg/kg PO, SC, IM q24h)
• Carprofen (2–4 mg/kg PO, SC q12–24h)

Long-Term Pain Management
• Nonsteroidal anti-inflammatories—have been used for short- or long-term therapy to reduce pain and inflammation; meloxicam (1 mg/kg PO q24h); carprofen (2–4 mg/kg PO q12–24h)
• For sedation—light sedation with midazolam (0.5–2 mg/kg IM); for deeper sedation and longer procedures the author prefers ketamine (10–20 mg/kg IM) plus midazolam (0.5–1.0 mg/kg IM) or dexmedetomidine (0.03–0.05 mg/kg IM) plus hydromorphone (0.1 mg/kg IM) and ketamine (5–15 mg/kg IM); many other sedation protocols exist

CONTRAINDICATIONS
• Oral administration of most antibiotics effective against anaerobes will cause a fatal GI dysbiosis in rabbits. Do not administer penicillins, macrolides, lincosamides, and cephalosporins by oral administration.
• The use of corticosteroids (systemic or topical in otic preparations) can severely exacerbate abscesses.
• Placement of Penrose or similar drains

PRECAUTIONS
• Chloramphenicol—avoid human contact with chloramphenicol due to potential blood dyscrasia. Advise owners of potential risks.
• Meloxicam or other NSAIDs—use with caution in rabbits with compromised renal function; monitor renal values
• Oral administration of any antibiotic may potentially cause enteric dysbiosis; discontinue use if diarrhea or anorexia occur.
• Azithromycin—use with caution due to risk of enteric dysbiosis

POSSIBLE INTERACTIONS
N/A

ALTERNATIVE DRUGS
• 50% dextrose-soaked gauze has been anecdotally used with success as a topical abscess treatment following surgical debridement. Dextrose has bactericidal properties and promotes granulation bed formation. The abscess cavity is filled with dextrose-laden gauze and replaced daily until a healthy granulation bed appears. Manduca honey has been used in a similar manner. Effectiveness varies, depending on the severity of disease and owner compliance.

FOLLOW-UP
PATIENT MONITORING
Monitor for progressive decrease in exudate, resolution of inflammation, and improvement of clinical signs.

(CONTINUED)

PREVENTION/AVOIDANCE
• Prevent progressive dental disease by selecting pets without congenital predisposition (when possible), providing high-fiber foods, good-quality hay, and periodic trimming of overgrown crowns.
• Prevent joint or feet abscess by providing clean, solid surfaces and appropriate surface substrates; prevent obesity.
• Treating otitis or upper respiratory infections in early stages may prevent otitis media and/or brain abscesses.
• Prevent fighting between rabbits.

POSSIBLE COMPLICATIONS
• Severe deformation of face with chronic facial abscesses
• Compromise of organ function
• Sepsis
• Peritonitis/pleuritis if intra-abdominal or intrathoracic abscess ruptures
• Recurrence, chronic pain, or extensive tissue destruction warranting euthanasia due to poor quality of life

EXPECTED COURSE AND PROGNOSIS
• Depend on organ system involved and amount of tissue destruction
• Superficial abscess—good to fair prognosis; recurrence locally or in other sites possible
• Facial abscesses, osteomyelitis—depend on severity of bone involvement and location. Rabbits with abscesses in the nasal passages or with exophthalmos, multiple or severe maxillary abscesses, or brain abscesses have a fair to guarded prognosis. Multiple surgeries and follow-up treatments are often required; recurrence rates are high. Euthanasia may be warranted if rabbits are painful and quality of life is unacceptable.
• Internal abscesses—fair to grave prognosis depending on location
• Without surgical treatment—many abscesses are slow growing. If surgical treatment is not elected, continue antibiotic treatment long-term. Many rabbits will live for months in comfort, even with relatively large abscesses.

MISCELLANEOUS

ASSOCIATED CONDITIONS
• Immunosuppression
• Gastrointestinal hypomotility

AGE-RELATED FACTORS
N/A

ZOONOTIC POTENTIAL
N/A

PREGNANCY/FERTILITY/BREEDING
N/A

ABBREVIATIONS
AIPPMA = antibiotic-impregnated polymethyl methacrylate
CT = computed tomography
ELISA = enzyme-linked immunosorbent assay
GI = gastrointestinal
MRI = magnetic resonance imaging
TWBC = total white blood cell count

Suggested Reading
Deeb BJ, Carpenter JW. Neurologic and musculoskeletal diseases. In: Quesenberry KE, Carpenter JW, eds. Ferrets, Rabbits, and Rodents: Clinical Medicine and Surgery, 2nd ed. St Louis: WB Saunders, 2004:203–210.
Harcourt-Brown F. Neurological and locomotor diseases. In: Harcourt-Brown F, ed. Textbook of Rabbit Medicine. Oxford, UK: Butterworth-Heinemann, 2002:307–323.
Hess L. Dermatologic diseases. In: Quesenberry KE, Carpenter JW, eds. Ferrets, Rabbits, and Rodents: Clinical Medicine and Surgery, 2nd ed. St Louis: WB Saunders, 2004:194–202.
Kapatkin A. Orthopedics in small mammals. In: Quesenberry KE, Carpenter JW, eds. Ferrets, Rabbits, and Rodents: Clinical Medicine and Surgery, 2nd ed. St Louis: WB Saunders, 2004:383–391.
Author Barbara Oglesbee, DVM, DABVP (Avian)

ALOPECIA

BASICS

DEFINITION
• A complete or partial lack of hair in areas where it is normally present
• May be associated with a multifactorial cause
• May be the primary problem or only a secondary phenomenon

PATHOPHYSIOLOGY
• Multifactorial causes
• All of the disorders represent a disruption in the growth of the hair follicle from infection, trauma, immunologic attack, mechanical "plugging," or blockage of the receptor sites for stimulation of the cycle.

SYSTEMS AFFECTED
Skin/Exocrine

SIGNALMENT
No specific age, breed, or sex predilection

SIGNS
• The pattern and degree of hair loss are important for establishing a differential diagnosis.
• Multifocal patches of alopecia—most frequently associated with folliculitis from parasitic, mycotic, or bacterial infection
• Large diffuse areas of alopecia—indicate a follicular dysplasia or metabolic component; not reported in rabbits
• May be acute in onset or slowly progressive

CAUSES
• Normal shedding pattern—some breeds, especially dwarf, miniature lop, and angora rabbits, lose hair in patches when shedding.
• Behavioral—barbering—dominant cage mates may chew or pull out hair of submissive rabbit, especially on flanks.
• Parasitic—*Cheyletiella* spp., *Leporacarus gibbus*, ear mites, fleas
• Endocrine—pregnant or pseudopregnant females will pull hair from chest and abdomen to line nest.
• Infectious—bacterial pyoderma, dermatophytosis; most often a secondary problem, especially moist dermatitis
• Neoplastic—cutaneous lymphoma, mast cell tumor
• Immunologic—contact dermatitis
• Nutrition—particularly protein deficiencies
• Trauma—foot pad alopecia

RISK FACTORS
N/A

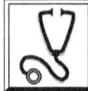

DIAGNOSIS

DIFFERENTIAL DIAGNOSIS
Differentiating Causes
Pattern and degree—important features for formulating a differential diagnosis
Symmetrical
• Barbering—hair loss along the flanks, face, nape of neck, and/or body wall. Close examination reveals broken hair. Dominant cage mate pulls/chews hairs on submissive rabbit; owners may not observe this behavior
Multifocal to focal
• *Cheyletiella* spp. (or less commonly, *Leporacarus gibbus*): Lesions are usually located in the intrascapular or tail base region and associated with copious amounts of large, white scale. Mites are readily identified in skin scrapes or acetate tape preparations under low magnification.
• Ear mites—alopecia around ear base, pinna; may extend to face, neck, abdomen, perineal region; intense pruritus; brown, beige crusty exudate in the ear canal and pinna
• Fleas—patchy alopecia; finding flea dirt will help to differentiate; secondary pyoderma sometimes seen
• Other ectoparasites—*Sarcoptes scabiei* and *Notoedres cati* rarely infest rabbits. Lesions are located around the head and neck and are intensely pruritic.
• Injection reactions—alopecia, scabs, scale, erythema, usually in the intrascapular region as this is a common site of subcutaneous injections
• Normal shedding pattern—some breeds, especially dwarf, miniature lop, and angora rabbits lose hair in patches when shedding, leaving well-demarcated alopecic areas.
• Lack of grooming—may cause alopecia and an accumulation of scale in intrascapular or tail base regions
• Contact dermatitis—alopecia with or without erythema, scale on ventral abdomen or other contact areas
• Moist dermatitis—alopecia, with or without erythema, scale, or ulceration. Facial—associated with epiphora or ptyalism; perineal/ventrum—associated with urinary disease, diarrhea, or uneaten cecotrophs
• Dermatophytosis—partial to complete alopecia with scaling; with or without erythema; not always ringlike; may begin as small papules

• *Treponema cuniculi* (rabbit syphilis)—alopecia, crusts at mucocutaneous junctions, especially nose, lips, and genitalia
• Neoplasia—cutaneous lymphoma, cutaneous epitheliotropic lymphoma (mycoses fungoides) or mast cell tumors—rare in rabbits; focal or diffuse truncal alopecia; scaling and erythema; may see plaque formation; similar lesions occur in association with thymoma in some rabbits

CBC/BIOCHEMISTRY/URINALYSIS
To identify underlying disease, especially in rabbits with perineal dermatitis or urine scald

OTHER LABORATORY TESTS
Serologic testing for *Treponema cuniculi* if consistent lesions are identified

IMAGING
Radiographs—skull/dental to identify underlying dental disease in rabbits with moist dermatitis secondary to chronic epiphora or ptyalism; whole-body radiographs may be helpful in identifying spinal/orthopedic, GI, or renal diseases contributing to perineal or ventral moist dermatitis

DIAGNOSTIC PROCEDURES
• Fungal culture
• Skin scraping; acetate tape preparation
• Cytology
• Skin biopsy

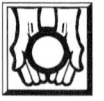

TREATMENT
• Treatment must be specific to the underlying cause to be successful.
• Moist dermatitis—identify and correct underlying cause (dental disease in facial or dewlap dermatitis, urinary, GI, or musculoskeletal disease in perineal/ventral dermatitis)
• Separate from dominant rabbits if barbering is suspected.

MEDICATIONS
DRUG(S) OF CHOICE
Varies with specific cause:
• Ear mites, *Cheyletiella* or *Leptogibbus* mites—1% ivermectin—0.4 mg/kg SC q10–14d for 2–3 doses; or selamectin-10 (Revolution, Pfizer)—12 mg/kg applied topically q30d, or Imidacloprid/moxidectin (Advantage-Multi for Cats Bayer)—10 mg/kg

RABBITS

(i) + 1 mg/kg (m) topically q30d; Treat all in-contact animals
• Fleas—imidacloprid (Advantage, Bayer) or imidacloprid/moxidectin (Advantage-Multi, Bayer)—10 mg/kg (i) + 1 mg/kg (m) topically q30d; or selamectin (Revolution, Pfizer)—12 mg/kg applied topically q30d; treat all in-contact animals
• Sarcoptic mange—ivermectin 0.4 mg/kg SC q14d for 3–4 doses; treat all in-contact animals
• Bacterial folliculitis—shampoos and antibiotic therapy, preferably based on culture and susceptibility testing; good initial choices include enrofloxacin (5–20 mg/kg PO q12–24h), trimethoprim-sulfa (30 mg/kg PO q12h)
• Dermatomycosis—lime sulfur dip q7d has been used to successfully; lime sulfur is odiferous and can stain; dipping is often difficult to perform on rabbits; clotrimazole cream (Lotrimin Cream 1%, Schering-Plough Corp.) for focal lesions; itraconazole (5–10 mg/kg PO q24h × 30days) or Terbinafine (10 mg/kg PO q24h)
• Treponema cuniculi—penicillin G, procaine 42,000–84,000 IU/kg SC q7d for 3 treatments. Treat all affected rabbits.
• Neoplasia—various chemotherapy protocols

CONTRAINDICATIONS
• Do not use fipronil (Frontline, Merial) on rabbits—Fatal toxicity reported
• Oral administration of antibiotics that select against gram-positive bacteria (penicillins, macrolides, lincosamides, and cephalosporins) can cause fatal enteric dysbiosis and enterotoxemia.
• The use of corticosteroids (systemic or topical) can severely exacerbate infectious causes of alopecia. Corticosteroid use is associated with gastrointestinal ulceration and hemorrhage, delayed wound healing, and heightened susceptibility to infection.
• Do not use flea collars on rabbits.
• Do not use organophosphate-containing products on rabbits.
• Do not use straight permethrin sprays or permethrin spot-ons on rabbits.

PRECAUTIONS
• Use extreme caution when dipping or bathing rabbits due to the high risk of skeletal fractures and excessive chilling with inexperienced owners.

• Most flea control products discussed above are off-label use. Safety and efficacy have not been evaluated in rabbits. Use with caution, especially in young or debilitated animals.
• Prevent rabbits or their cage mates from licking topical spot-on products before they are dry.
• Toxicity—if any signs are noted, the animal should be bathed thoroughly to remove any remaining chemicals and treated appropriately.
• Topical flea preparation for use in dogs and cats, such as permethrins and pyrethrins, are less effective and may be toxic to rabbits.
• Griseofulvin—bone marrow suppression reported in dogs/cats as an idiosyncratic reaction or with prolonged therapy; not yet reported in rabbits but may occur; weekly or biweekly CBC is recommended. Neurologic side effects reported in dogs and cats—monitor for this possibility in rabbits; do not use during the first two trimesters of pregnancy; it is teratogenic.
• Oral administration of any antibiotic may potentially cause enteric dysbiosis; discontinue use if diarrhea or anorexia occurs.

POSSIBLE INTERACTIONS
None

ALTERNATIVE DRUGS
Ketaconazole (10–15 mg/kg PO q24h) for dermatophytes—efficacy and safety in rabbits are unknown. Hepatopathy reported in dogs and cats can be quite severe.

 FOLLOW-UP

PATIENT MONITORING
Varies with cause

POSSIBLE COMPLICATIONS
N/A

 MISCELLANEOUS

ASSOCIATED CONDITIONS
• Dental disease
• Musculoskeletal disease
• Obesity

AGE-RELATED FACTORS
N/A

ZOONOTIC POTENTIAL
Dermatophytosis and Cheyletiella can cause skin lesions in people.

PREGNANCY/FERTILITY/BREEDING
Avoid griseofulvin and ivermectin in pregnant animals.

SYNONYMS
None

SEE ALSO
Cheyletiellosis (fur mites)
Dermatophytosis
Ear mites
Epiphora
Fleas and flea infestation
Ptyalism (slobbers)

ABBREVIATIONS
GI = gastrointestinal

Suggested Reading
d'Ovidio D, Santoro F. Leporacarus gibbus infestation in client-owned rabbits and their owners. Vet Dermatol 2014;25:46–e17.
Meredith A. Dermatoses. In: Meredith A, Lord B, eds. BSAVA Manual of Rabbit Medicine. Gloucester: British Small Animal Veterinary Association, 2014:255–263.
Palmerio BS, Roberts H. Clinical approach to dermatologic disease in exotic animals. Vet Clin North Am Exot Anim Pract 2013;16(3):523–577.
Snook TS, White SD, Hawkins MG et al. Skin diseases in pet rabbits: a retrospective study of 334 cases seen at the University of California at Davis, USA (1984–2004). Vet Dermatol 2013;24:613–618.
Varga M. Skin diseases. In: Varga M, ed. Textbook of Rabbit Medicine, 2nd ed. Elsiver, 2014:224–248.
Varga M, Patterson S. Dermatologic diseases of rabbits. In: Quesenberry KE, Carpenter JW, eds. Ferrets, Rabbits and Rodents, (4th ed.). Clinical Medicine and Surgery. 2021, St. Louis: Saunders, 2020:220–222.

Author Barbara Oglesbee, DVM, Dipl ABVP (Avian)

ANOREXIA AND PSEUDOANOREXIA

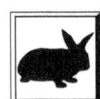 **BASICS**

DEFINITION
• The lack or loss of appetite for food; appetite is psychologic and depends on memory and associations, compared with hunger, which is physiologically aroused by the body's need for food; the existence of appetite in animals is assumed.
• Anorexia is a much more urgent presenting complaint in rabbits as compared to dogs and cats. An acute onset of refusing all food can become life threatening within 6–8 hours as this is the most common presenting complaint in rabbits with GI obstruction or liver lobe torsion. Even with a gradual onset, rabbits that have not eaten for more than 24 hours have a guarded to poor prognosis.
• The term *pseudoanorexia* is used to describe animals that have a desire for food but are unable to eat because they cannot prehend, chew, or swallow food. Pseudoanorexia due to dental disease is one of the most common causes of lack of food intake in rabbits.

PATHOPHYSIOLOGY
• In rabbits, anorexia is most often associated gastrointestinal disorders, stress, or with systemic disease but can be caused by many different mechanisms.
• Acute onset of refusing all food is the hallmark of life-threatening disorders such as intestinal obstruction, liver lobe torsion, or sepsis
• Rabbits are hind gut fermenters with a complex cecal flora. This flora must be continuously fed, or potentially pathogenic bacteria can overpopulate and cause serious diseases. Anorexia for any reason should be addressed immediately.
• Pseudoanorexia is commonly associated with oral pain or inability to chew due to dental disease.

SYSTEMS AFFECTED
All body systems are affected; breakdown of the intestinal mucosal barrier is particularly important in sick patients.

SIGNALMENT
Depends on the underlying cause

SIGNS
Historical Findings
• The history is extremely useful in assessing the cause and urgency of disease.
  ◦ An acute onset of refusing all food, even favorite treats with a corresponding acute cessation of fecal production is characteristic of urgent, potentially life-threatening disease.
  ◦ A more gradual onset of progressively declining appetite over a period of hours to days is more common and can be due to a variety of causes. With this history, fecal

pellets gradually become scant, dark in color, and small in size.
  ◦ Rabbits with GI tract hypomotility/GI stasis often initially stop eating pellets and/or hay, but continue to eat treats, followed by complete anorexia
• Signs of pain can be subtle as rabbits are prey species and instinctively hide signs of disease. The most common sign of mild to moderate discomfort is hiding or appearing less social.
• Signs of more severe pain, such as teeth grinding, a hunched posture and reluctance to move indicate more urgent and serious disease.
• Patients with disorders causing dysfunction or pain of the face, neck, oropharynx, and esophagus may display an interest in food but be unable to complete prehension and swallowing (pseudoanorexia).
• Pseudoanorectic patients commonly display weight loss, excessive drooling, difficulty in prehension and mastication of food, halitosis, dysphagia, and odynophagia (painful eating). This may be preceded by a preference for softer foods such as lettuces.

Physical Examination Findings
Abdominal palpation and gut sounds
• Abdominal palpation is an extremely valuable tool in the diagnosis of gastrointestinal disorders.
• Even in rabbits that do not have access to food or those that are anorexic, the rabbit stomach is never empty. Rabbits consume cecotrophs, formed in the cecum and consumed from the rectum, which will fill the stomach even when food is not provided. If anorexic, stomach contents do not empty, either due to the onset of GI hypmotility/stasis or due to GI obstruction.
• The normal stomach should be easily deformable, feel soft and pliable, and does not remain pitted on compression.
• A firm, noncompliant stomach, or stomach contents that remain pitted on compression, is an abnormal finding and characteristic of GI hypomotility/GI stasis.
• Fluid distention of the stomach occurs in rabbits with intestinal obstruction. The degree of distention depends on the region of intestinal obstruction and progresses with time. Rabbits cannot vomit and eventually, the stomach can become severely fluid-distended, turgid and can even rupture. A distended, fluid-filled stomach is an emergency.
• Gas distension of the intestines and/or cecum is common in rabbits with GI tract disease such as GI hypomotility/stasis or cecal disorders.
• Auscultation of gut sounds is helpful. Decreased or absent gut sounds with little or no borborygmus is consistent with GI hypomotility. Increased gut sounds can be heard in the early phases of intestinal obstruction. In the late stages of obstruction, gut sound decreases.

Other exam findings
• Signs of shock such as hypothemia (body temp <98° F), pale mucus membranes, lethargy, collapse, or stiff body posture are common with acute intestinal obstruction, and often accompany the finding of a fluid distended stomach.
• Rabbits with other causes of anorexia may have a normal physical examination
• Auscultation of the thorax may reveal an underlying cause—look for cardiac murmurs, arrhythmias, or abnormal breath sounds.
• Most underlying causes of pseudoanorexia can be identified by a thorough examination of the face, mandible, and teeth for evidence of dental disease, ulceration, traumatic lesions, masses, foreign bodies, and neuromuscular dysfunction.
• A thorough exam of the oral cavity, including the incisors, molars, and buccal and lingual mucosa is necessary to rule out dental disease. Use of an otoscope or speculum may be useful in identifying severe abnormalities; however, many problems will be missed by using this method alone. A thorough examination of the cheek teeth requires heavy sedation or general anesthesia and specialized equipment. Use a focused, directed light source and magnification (or a rigid endoscope, if available) to provide optimal visualization. Use a rodent mouth gag and cheek dilators (Jorgensen Laboratories, Inc., Loveland, CO) to open the mouth and pull buccal tissues away from teeth surfaces to allow adequate exposure. Identify cheek teeth elongation, irregular crown height, spikes, curved teeth, oral ulceration, or abscesses.
• Significant tooth root abnormalities may be present despite normal-appearing crowns. Skull films are required to identify apical disorders.

CAUSES
Anorexia
• Almost any systemic disease process
• Gastrointestinal disease is one of the most common causes—especially problems related to GI hypomotility/stasis or intestinal obstruction
• Pain—especially in rabbits with dental disease, orthopedic disorders, or urolithiasis
• Metabolic disease—especially hepatic or renal disease
• Neoplasia involving any site
• Cardiac failure
• Infectious disease
• Respiratory disease
• Neurologic disease
• Psychologic—unpalatable diets, alterations in routine or environment, stress
• Toxicosis and drugs
• Musculoskeletal disorders
• Acid–base disorders
• Miscellaneous—high environmental temperature, etc.

(CONTINUED)

Pseudoanorexia
• Diseases causing painful prehension and mastication are extremely common, especially dental disease (e.g., malocclusion, dental abscess); soft tissue inflammation (usually secondary to acquired dental disease), retrobulbar abscess, oral or glossal neoplasia (rare), musculoskeletal disorders (mandible fracture or subluxation)
• Diseases causing oropharyngeal dysphagia (uncommon); glossal disorders (neurologic, neoplastic), pharyngitis, pharyngeal neoplasia, retropharyngeal disorders (lymphadenopathy, abscess, hematoma), neuromuscular disorders (CNS lesions, botulism)
• Diseases of the esophagus (rare)—esophagitis, neoplasia, and neuromuscular disorders

RISK FACTORS
• Rabbits on a diet containing inadequate amounts of long-stem hay are at risk for developing diseases related to GI hypomotility and dental disease
• Rabbits with limited exercise or mobility (cage restriction, orthopedic disorders, and obesity) are at higher risk of developing GI motility disorders and hypercalciuria.
• Anesthesia and surgical procedures commonly cause temporary anorexia.
• Risk factors for acute intestinal obstruction are unknown

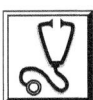

DIAGNOSIS

DIFFERENTIAL DIAGNOSIS
• Gastrointestinal hypomotility/stasis disorders are the most common causes of anorexia in rabbits, followed by acute anorexia due to intestinal obstruction. Pseudoanorexia is usually due to dental disease.
• The timeline of anorexia and corresponding fecal production and extremely helpful in differentiating GI obstruction from other causes of anorexia. Rabbits with GI obstruction have an acute onset of refusing all food while simultaneously go from producing normal feces to complete absence of fecal production.
• Obtain a minimum database (CBC, biochemistry, whole-body radiographs) to help delineate underlying medical disorders.
• Questioning about the patient's interest in food and its ability to prehend, masticate, and swallow food, along with a thorough examination of the animal's teeth, oropharynx, face, and neck, will help identify pseudoanorexia; if the owners are poor historians, the patient should be observed while eating.
• A thorough history regarding the animals' environment, diet, other animals and people in the household, and any recent changes

involving any of these help identify psychologic anorexia.
• Any abnormalities detected in the physical examination or historical evidence of illness mandate a diagnostic workup for the identified problem.

CBC/BIOCHEMISTRY/URINALYSIS
• These tests are often normal but can be used to differentiate GI hypomotility/stasis from GI obstruction. Rabbits with GI hypomotility/stasis are either normo- or mildly hyperglycemic (BG <300 mg/dl) with normal serum Na concentration, whereas those with GI obstruction are severely hyperglycemic, with BG ranging from 300–600 mg/dL and mildly hyponatremic Na <140 mEq/L)
• BUN and creatinine may be elevated due to dehydration or, in rabbits with obstruction, due to decreased renal perfusion
• PCV and TS elevation in dehydrated patients
• Serum ALT elevation in rabbits with liver disease, especially lipidosis
• May be used to identify underlying causes of GI hypomotility or anorexia

OTHER LABORATORY TESTS
Special tests may be necessary to rule out specific diseases suggested by the history, physical examination, or minimum database (See other topics on specific diseases).

IMAGING
• Due to the practice of cecotrophy, the stomach is never empty. Gastric contents are normally present and visible radiographically, even if the rabbit is not eating. The presence of ingesta in the stomach is a normal finding.
• *With GI hypomotility/Stasis*—Depending on the duration of the disease, the stomach may appear to contain normal ingesta or, as the disease progresses and fluid is pulled from the stomach, contents appear dense, the stomach appears small and may have a halo of gas around the inspissated stomach contents. If the owners have been assist-feeding, the stomach may be distended with food. Gas distension is sometimes seen throughout the intestinal tract, including the cecum in rabbits with GI hypomotility/stasis.
• *With GI obstruction*—The stomach becomes fluid distended. In addition to fluid, a gas cap may form within the stomach causing a "fried egg" appearance. The degree of distension depends on the location and time of onset of obstruction. With increasing severity, the stomach will extend caudal to the last rib and have direct contact with the ventral body wall. If the stomach distends past the caudal aspect of L2 vertebrae, the prognosis worsens. Fluid and/or gas distension occurs in the intestinal loops proximal (orad) to the obstruction. If the obstruction is in the proximal GI tract (located near the pyloric outflow), no gas or distended intestinal loops are found.

• If underlying disease is suspected but no abnormalities are revealed by the physical examination or minimum database, perform abdominal radiography and abdominal ultrasonography to identify hidden conditions such as hepatic disease, urolithiasis, orthopedic disease, or neoplasia. Consider thoracic radiography to rule out cardiac or pulmonary disease.
• Skull films are necessary to identify the presence of and extent of dental disease.
• The need for further diagnostic imaging varies with the underlying condition suspected (see other topics on specific diseases).

DIAGNOSTIC PROCEDURES
Vary with underlying condition suspected (see other topics regarding specific diseases)

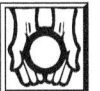

TREATMENT
Treatment is directed towards the underlying cause.

APPROPRIATE HEALTH CARE
• Rabbits with acute onset of complete anorexia and lack of fecal production generally have serious, potentially life-threatening disease such as intestinal obstruction, liver lobe torsion, and sepsis and require hospitalization.
• Rabbits with a gradual onset of anorexia and those still accepting some foods can often be treated on an outpatient basis. Those which have not eaten for more than 24 hours generally require hospitalization.

NURSING CARE
Fluid Therapy
• For patients with signs of shock or severe depression (seen with acute GI obstructions, liver lobe torsion, and sepsis) balanced crystalloid fluids are indicated IV at a rate appropriate for shock or the level of dehydration. For patients in shock, fluids should be warmed.
• Intravenous fluids are indicated in patients that are severely dehydrated or depressed. Maintenance fluid requirements are estimated at 60 mL/kg/day for large breeds, 80–100 mL/kg/day for small or dwarf breeds.
• Fluid therapy is an essential component of the medical management of all anorexic patients. Administer both oral and parenteral fluids (except when GI obstruction is suspected). Oral fluid administration in the form of commercially available assist feeding slurries (see below) will aid in the rehydration of inspissated gastric contents. Mildly affected rabbits will usually respond well to oral and subcutaneous fluid administration, treatment with analgesics, intestinal motility modifiers, and dietary modification described below.

ANOREXIA AND PSEUDOANOREXIA   (CONTINUED)

ACTIVITY
Depends on the cause of anorexia.

DIET
- Rabbits with suspected GI obstructions should not be assist or force fed. However, food should be offered free choice. Once the obstruction begins to move, affected rabbits usually begin to eat. This may serve as a prognostic indicator.
- If obstruction is ruled out, it is imperative that the rabbit begins eating as soon as possible. Continued anorexia will exacerbate GI hypomotility, causing further derangement of the gastrointestinal microflora and overgrowth of intestinal bacterial pathogens.
- Offer a large selection of fresh, moistened greens such as cilantro, romaine lettuce, parsley, carrot tops, dandelion greens, spinach, collard greens, etc. and good-quality grass hay. Many rabbits will begin to eat these foods, even if they were previously anorectic. Also offer the rabbit's usual pelleted diet, as the initial goal is to get the rabbit to eat.
- If the patient refuses these foods, syringe-feed a gruel such as Critical Care for Herbivores (Oxbow Pet Products) or Emeraid Herbivore (Lafeber Company, Cornell, IL) 10–15 mL/kg PO q6–8h. Larger volumes and more frequent feedings are often accepted; feed as much as the rabbit will readily accept. Alternatively, pellets can be ground and mixed with fresh greens, vegetable baby foods, water, or juice to form a gruel. If sufficient volumes of food are not accepted in this manner, nasogastric intubation is indicated.
- High-carbohydrate, high-fat nutritional supplements are contraindicated.
- The diet should be permanently modified to include sufficient amounts of roughage and long-stemmed hay.

CLIENT EDUCATION
- Discuss the importance of monitoring appetite in prey species such as rabbits. These species have a strong instinct to hide illness and may appear active and "normal" to owners unfamiliar with this concept. Stress the importance of seeking veterinary care any time the appetite is reduced. An acute onset of refusing all food and simultaneous lack of fecal output is an emergency.
- Discuss the importance of monitoring appetite in prey species such as rabbits. These species have a strong instinct to hide illness and may appear active and "normal" to owners unfamiliar with this concept. Stress the importance of seeking veterinary care any time the appetite is reduced. An acute onset of refusing all food and simultaneous lack of fecal output is an emergency.
- Advise owners to regularly monitor food consumption and fecal output and to seek veterinary attention with a noticeable decrease in either.
- Discuss the importance of feeding hay and high-quality pellets.

SURGICAL CONSIDERATIONS
- Depend on the underlying cause

MEDICATIONS
Use parenteral medications in animals with severely compromised intestinal motility; oral medications may not be properly absorbed. Begin oral medication when intestinal motility begins to return (fecal production, return of appetite, radiographic evidence)

DRUG(S) OF CHOICE
- Treat the underlying cause
- Analgesics such as meloxicam (1 mg/kg SC, IM q24h), hydromorphone (0.05–0.2 mg/kg IV, IM, SC q6–8h), buprenorphine (0.02–0.05 mg/kg SC, IM, IV q8–12h), or carprofen (2–4 mg/kg SC, IV q24h) are essential to treatment of rabbits with GI hypomotility. Intestinal pain, either postoperative or from gas distention and ileus, impairs mobility and decreases appetite, and may severely inhibit recovery.
- Maropitant (2 mg/kg SC q24h) is used to treat visceral pain. Combine this with one of the analgesics listed above.
- Anorexia, regardless of the cause, causes or exacerbates GI tract hypomotility. Motility modifiers such as cisapride (0.5 mg/kg PO q8–12h), metoclopramide (0.5–1.0 mg/kg PO, SC, IM q12h or 1–2 mg/kg/day IV as a constant rate infusion) are generally helpful in rabbits with GI hypomotility. These can also be used in rabbits with intraluminal intestinal obstruction as the most common GI foreign body is a compressed pellet of hair and the goal of therapy is to keep the hair pellet moving through the intestinal tract. Motility modifiers are contraindicated if an extraluminal obstruction is suspected.
- H_2-receptor antagonists may ameliorate or prevent gastric ulceration; cimetidine (5–10 mg/kg PO, SC, IM IV q6–12h); ranitidine (2 mg/kg SC, IV q24h or 2–5 mg/kg PO q12–24h)

CONTRAINDICATIONS
Assisted or force-feeding rabbits with ab suspected GI obstruction is contraindicated

FOLLOW-UP

PATIENT MONITORING
- Appetite will return with successful treatment
- Fecal production—both the size, shape, and number of fecal pellets should gradually improve

POSSIBLE COMPLICATIONS
- Dehydration, malnutrition, and cachexia are most likely; these exacerbate the underlying disease.
- Hepatic lipidosis is a common complication of anorexia, especially in obese rabbits.
- Breakdown of the intestinal mucosal barrier is a concern in debilitated patients.
- Anorexia may cause enteric dysbiosis and subsequent enterotoxemia.

MISCELLANEOUS

ASSOCIATED CONDITIONS
See causes

SYNONYMS
Inappetence

SEE ALSO
Cheek teeth (premolar and molar) malocclusion and elongation
Clostridial enteritis/enterotoxicosis
Diarrhea, chronic
Gastric dilation (bloat)
Gastrointestinal hypomotility and gastrointestinal stasis
Hypercalciuria and urolithiasis
Intestinal obstruction
Liver lobe torsion

ABBREVIATIONS
ALT = alanine aminotransferase
BG = blood glucose
BUN = blood urea nitrogen
GI = gastrointestinal
Na = sodium
PCV = packed cell volume
TS = total solids

Suggested Reading
Bays TB. Geriatric care of rabbits, guinea pigs, and chinchillas. Vet Clin Exot Anim 2020;23:567–593.
Debenham JJ, Brinchmann T, Sheen J, Vella D. Radiographic diagnosis of small intestinal obstruction in pet rabbits (*Oryctolagus cuniculus*): 63 cases. J Sm Anim Pract 2019;60:691–696.
DeCubellis J. Common emergencies in rabbits, guinea pigs, and chinchillas. Vet Clin Exot Anim 2016;19:411–429.
Hartcourt-Brown F. Digestive system disease. In: Meredith A, Lord B, eds. BSAVA Manual of Rabbit Medicine. Gloucester: British Small Animal Veterinary Association, 2014:168–190.
Oglesbee B, Lord B. Gastrointestinal diseases of rabbits. In: Quesenberry KE, Carpenter JW, eds. Ferrets, Rabbits and Rodents, (4th ed.). Clinical Medicine and Surgery. 2021, St. Louis: Saunders, 2020:174–187.
Varga M. Digestive disorders. In: Varga M, ed. Textbook of Rabbit Medicine, 2nd ed. London, UK: Elsevier, 2014:303–349.
Author Barbara Oglesbee, DVM, DABVP (Avian)

RABBITS

BASICS

DEFINITION
Inflammation of the iris and/or ciliary body

PATHOPHYSIOLOGY
• Common theme from all causes—tissue destruction secondary to breakdown of the blood-aqueous barrier
• Iridal abscesses, corneal stromal abscesses, and phacoclastic uveitis secondary to *Encephalitozoon cuniculi* and ulcerative keratitis are the most common causes in rabbits.
• Associated most commonly with cellular infiltration, iridal congestion, aqueous flare, and hypopyon; keratic precipitates and corneal edema are occasionally seen.

SYSTEMS AFFECTED
• Ophthalmic
• Others—if the cause is a systemic disease

GENETICS
N/A

INCIDENCE/PREVALENCE
• Common
• True incidence unknown

GEOGRAPHIC DISTRIBUTION
N/A

SIGNALMENT
• *Encephalitozoon cuniculi*—more common in young, dwarf breeds
• Other causes—no age, breed, or gender predilection

SIGNS

Historical Findings
• Usually owner complains of a change in the appearance of the affected eye(s).
• May have a history of respiratory disease, dental disease, abscesses, or CNS signs, depending on the underlying cause

Physical Examination Findings
• Iridal swelling, white or pink nodule on the iris—common, especially in rabbits with *E. cuniculi* or iridal bacterial abscesses. Rabbits are often presented for evaluation of an intraocular white mass, with the remainder of the eye appearing relatively quiet.
• Ocular discomfort—suggested by photophobia, blepharospasm, and epiphora. Rabbits are less likely to show discomfort, but pain is more difficult to assess in rabbits, as they are prey species and less likely to outwardly demonstrate pain.
• Conjunctival hyperemia—common; a nonspecific indication of ocular irritation
• Fibrinous exudation—severe disease; may cause fibrin clot formation within the anterior chamber

• Intraocular pressure—usually low with anterior uveitis; depends on severity and duration of disease; may be high with severe disease and secondary glaucoma
• Miosis—pupillary constriction; subtle miosis best observed in a darkened room by simultaneously examining both eyes with retroillumination
• Hypopyon (accumulation of WBCs in the anterior chamber)—develop with extreme breakdown of blood-aqueous barrier; cellular components typically settle homogeneously in the ventral anterior chamber; common finding in rabbits with iridal or corneal stromal abscesses, and with ocular *E. cuniculi* infection.
• Ciliary flush—may be observed in the limbal region; result of hyperemia of the perilimbal anterior ciliary vessels; along with conjunctival hyperemia, may contribute to red eye
• Aqueous flare—increased turbidity of aqueous humor; occasionally seen, but less common than in dogs and cats. It is not uncommon to have a large iris stromal abscess or granuloma present without seeing significant flare.
• Keratic precipitates—occasionally seen on the corneal endothelial surface; indicates active or previous disease
• Corneal edema—not as common as in dogs or cats
• Hyphema (accumulation of RBCs in the anterior chamber) is common with intraocular tumors and systemic hypertension.

CAUSES
Most common causes are bacterial iridal or corneal stromal abscesses, phacoclastic uveitis from *E. cuniculi*, or ulcerative keratitis.
• Bacterial—iridial or corneal stromal abscess most often seen; either hematogenous spread (iridial abscess) or secondary to keratitis (corneal stromal abscess); caused by any systemic bacterial disease (Pasteurella most common) or underlying dental or respiratory disease (corneal stromal abscess).
• *Encephalitozoon cuniculi*—in utero infection, vertical transmission of organism into the developing lens; replication of spores within the lens of young rabbits results in cataract formation, thin anterior portion or lens ruptures resulting in phacoclastic uveitis with focal granuloma formation at site of rupture
• Ulcerative keratitis—common cause, secondary to trauma, chronic dacryocystitis, conjunctivitis, or environmental irritants
• Other infectious agents—fungal, protozoan, or viral not well described in rabbits
• Traumatic—blunt or penetrating injuries—common

• Immune mediated—naturally occurring or spontaneous cataracts (lens-induced uveitis); lens trauma (rupture of lens capsule)
• Neoplastic (primary or secondary)—primary uncommon in rabbits- intraocular sarcoma and iridociliary tumors have been described; lymphoma and metastasis from other neoplasia (e.g., uterine adenocarcinoma) more likely
• Metabolic—not described in rabbits

RISK FACTORS
Immunosuppression—stress, poor diet, dental disease, and glucocorticoid therapy, especially rabbits with bacterial infection or *E. cuniculi*

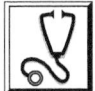

DIAGNOSIS

DIFFERENTIAL DIAGNOSIS
• Conjunctivitis—clinical signs (hyperemia, chemosis, ocular discharge, and pain) vary, depending on the duration and severity; normal intraocular pressure and intraocular examination
• Glaucoma—common sequela to intraocular *E. cuniculi* infection; pupil usually dilated; clinical signs may be identical; must measure intraocular pressure to distinguish
• Ulcerative keratitis—may be accompanied by anterior uveitis
• Horner syndrome—may have a similar appearance because the pupil is miotic and upper lid ptosis creates the impression of blepharospasm; normal intraocular pressure; no aqueous flare; conjunctiva not or only mildly injected

CBC/BIOCHEMISTRY/URINALYSIS
• CBC serum biochemistry and urinalysis—usually unremarkable; may reflect underlying systemic disease

OTHER LABORATORY TESTS
• Serologic testing for E. cuniculi—many tests are available, but usefulness is extremely limited since a positive titer indicates only exposure and does not confirm *E. cuniculi* as the cause of uveitis. *E. cuniculi* can only be definitively diagnosed by finding organisms and resultant lesions on ocular histopathology or by positive DNA probe (PCR) on the removed lens material. Antibody titers usually become positive by 2 weeks post-infection but generally do not continue to rise with active infection or decline with treatment. No correlation exists between antibody titers and shedding of organism, or the presence or severity of the disease. It is unknown if exposed rabbits eventually become seronegative. Available tests include PCR, ELISA, indirect IFA, and carbon immunoassay.

ANTERIOR UVEITIS   (CONTINUED)

• Plasma protein electrophoresis—some evidence exists that increases in gamma globulins, concurrent with high ELISA antibody titers, may be supportive of infection.

• Serology for *Pasteurella*—usefulness is severely limited and generally not helpful in the diagnosis of pasteurellosis in pet rabbits. An ELISA is available, and results reported as negative, low positive or high positive. Positive results, even when high, only indicate prior exposure to *Pasteurella* and the development of antibodies and does not confirm active infection. Low positive results may occur due to cross reaction with other, nonpathogenic bacteria (false positive). False-negative results are common with immunosuppression or early infection. No evidence exists to support the correlation of titers to the presence or absence of disease.

IMAGING

• Skull radiographs—to rule out underlying dental disease nasal, sinus, or maxillary bone lesions

• CT—superior to radiographs to identify underlying dental disease nasal, sinus, or maxillary bone lesions

• Thoracic radiographs—rule out neoplastic (and possibly fungal) diseases

• Abdominal radiographs and ultrasound—for palpable abdominal mass

• Ocular ultrasonography—for trauma; rule out penetrating wounds and foreign bodies not obviously visible; when the ocular media are too opaque to allow complete examination of the eye

DIAGNOSTIC PROCEDURES

• Aqueous humor paracentesis—seldom helpful

• Tonometry—usually reveals low intraocular pressure unless primary or secondary glaucoma is present. Normal intraocular pressure was reported as 10–20 mmHg when measured by applanation tonometry.

• Nasolacrimal duct flush—identify patients with dacryocystitis

• Fluorescein stain—rule out ulcerative keratitis; corneal epithelium usually intact with corneal stromal abscess; test for nasolacrimal function

• Thorough adnexal examination—rule out lid abnormalities, lash abnormalities, and foreign bodies in cul-de-sacs or under nictitans.

PATHOLOGIC FINDINGS

• *E. cuniculi*—phacoclastic uveitis secondary to lens rupture; leakage results in inflammation and granuloma formation, usually on the iris surrounding the rupture. Histologically, may see *E. cuniculi* organisms in lens material, or may detect using DNA probe.

• Eye—conjunctival hyperemia; ciliary flush; aqueous flare; miosis; variable vision

• Iridal abcesses—often walled off; composed of accumulations of degenerate neutrophils, lymphocytes, and plasma cells

TREATMENT

APPROPRIATE HEALTH CARE

• Inpatient—severe disease and/or high intraocular pressure; for initial diagnostic workup and medical management

• Outpatient—mild to moderate disease

NURSING CARE

N/A

ACTIVITY

No restrictions

DIET

Make sure that the rabbit continues to eat to avoid secondary gastrointestinal disorders.

CLIENT EDUCATION

• Discuss the need for early aggressive medical management and a thorough diagnostic workup to identify the cause.

• Warn client of the adverse sequelae, including blindness, cataracts, endophthalmitis, or panophthalmitis, lens luxation, phthisis bulbi, posterior synechiae with iris bombé, and secondary glaucoma.

SURGICAL CONSIDERATIONS

• Lens removal by phacoemulsification is recommended in rabbits with ocular *E. cuniculi*. Spontaneous lens regeneration occurs in rabbits; however, insertion of a prosthetic lens ± capsular tension ring (IOL ± CTR placement) may markedly decrease the degree of lens regrowth and improve postoperative visual outcome. Uveitis may recur following treatment, requiring medical treatment or enucleation.

• Enucleation may be indicated in rabbits with iridal abscess, severe phacoclastic uveitis, or panophthalmitis when medical therapy is not successful, or rabbit is painful. Enucleation can be more difficult than dogs or cats due to the presence of a large orbital venous plexus that increases the risk of hemorrhage.

MEDICATIONS

DRUG(S) OF CHOICE

Topically Applied Agents

• Frequency of treatment depends on the severity of disease

• NSAIDs—0.5% ketorolac, or 1% diclofenac; q6h daily to control inflammation

• Mydriatic-cycloplegic drugs—1% atropine q12h for acute disease; to dilate the pupil, minimize posterior synechia, paralyze the ciliary muscle (cycloplegia); reduces ocular pain. May not be effective in all rabbits, since some species of rabbits produce atropinase; the addition of 10% phenylephrine may facilitate mydriasis in these rabbits.

• Topical antibiotics, chloramphenicol, or ciprofloxacin first choice for corneal stromal abscess, dacryocystitis, keratitis; alternatively, triple antibiotic or gentocin q6–12h, depending on organism isolated and severity of infection, if cornea ulcerated

• Corticosteroids—1% prednisolone acetate; q6–12h with severe disease; use with extreme caution in rabbits (see Precautions)

Systemic Medications

• Systemic antibiotics—indicated in rabbits with iridal or corneal stromal abscess or to treat underlying bacterial disease. Choice of antibiotic is ideally based on results of culture and susceptibility testing. Use broad-spectrum antibiotics such as enrofloxacin (10–20 mg/kg PO, SC, IM q12–24h), marbofloxacin (5 mg/kg PO q24h), trimethoprim-sulfa (15–30 mg/kg PO q12h), or chloramphenicol (25 mg/kg PO q8–12h).

• Pain management—Nonsteroidal anti-inflammatories have been used for short- or long-term therapy to reduce pain and inflammation in rabbits with ocular pain; meloxicam (1.0 mg/kg PO q24h); carprofen (2–4 mg/kg PO q12h)

• *E. cuniculi*—Benzimidazole anthelmintics are effective against *E. cuniculi* in vitro and have been shown to prevent experimental infection in rabbits. However, efficacy in rabbits with clinical signs is unknown. Anecdotal reports suggest a response to treatment in rabbits with *E. cuniculi* associated phacoclastic uveitis. Published treatments include fenbendazole (20 mg/kg q24h × 28 days) as the most commonly used and anecdotally effective treatment.

CONTRAINDICATIONS

• Topical corticosteroids—never use if the cornea retains fluorescein stain (corneal ulceration), if abscesses are present, or if bacterial infection is suspected.

• Oral administration of most antibiotics effective against anaerobes will cause a fatal gastrointestinal dysbiosis in rabbits. Do not administer penicillins, macrolides, lincosamides, and cephalosporins by oral administration.

• Atropine in rabbits with glaucoma

PRECAUTIONS

• Topical corticosteroids or antibiotic-corticosteroid combinations—avoid; associated with gastrointestinal ulceration and hemorrhage, iatrogenic diabetes mellitus,

delayed wound healing, and heightened susceptibility to infection; rabbits are very sensitive to the immunosuppressive effects of both topic and systemic corticosteroids; use may exacerbate subclinical bacterial infection
• Meloxicam or other NSAIDs—use with caution in rabbits with compromised renal function; monitor renal values.
• Topical aminoglycosides—may be irritating; may impede reepithelization if used frequently or at high concentrations
• Topical solutions—are preferable to ointments if corneal perforation is possible
• Topical antibiotics—may lead to enteric dysbiosis if excessive ingestion occurs during grooming.
• Atropine—may exacerbate KCS and glaucoma
• Topical atropine—may cause salivation

POSSIBLE INTERACTIONS
N/A

ALTERNATIVE DRUGS
N/A

FOLLOW-UP

PATIENT MONITORING
• Complete ocular examination—repeated 5–7 days after initiation of treatment for severe disease
• Intraocular pressure—monitored for secondary glaucoma
• Reevaluation—every 2–3 weeks, depending on the response to treatment

PREVENTION/AVOIDANCE
N/A

POSSIBLE COMPLICATIONS
• Adverse sequelae—blindness; cataracts; endophthalmitis or panophthalmitis; iris atrophy; lens luxation; phthisis bulbi; rubeosis iridis; posterior synechiae with iris bombé; secondary glaucoma
• Secondary glaucoma—frequent complication; tends to be recalcitrant to medical treatment

EXPECTED COURSE AND PROGNOSIS
• Regardless of the initial response to treatment, treat for at least 2 months with decreasing frequency because the blood-aqueous barrier remains disrupted for about 8 weeks after an insult.
• *E. cuniculi*–associated uveitis—depends on the severity and chronicity of infection and presence of secondary bacterial infections—if cannot treat surgically, prognosis for viability of the affected eye is guarded as most will progress to glaucoma.
• Iridal abscesses—often do not respond well to medical treatment; enucleation may be necessary
• Corneal stromal abscess—good to fair prognosis when treated early and aggressively with topical and systemic antibiotics; with advanced disease and panophthalmitis—poor prognosis for the viability of affected eye; enucleation may be required
• Secondary to a systemic disease—prognosis usually determined by the systemic disease rather than by the anterior uveitis
• Prognosis for resolution of inflammation without deleterious sequelae—depends on the severity of the disease at initial examination and on the response to aggressive medical treatment

MISCELLANEOUS

ASSOCIATED CONDITIONS
N/A

AGE-RELATED FACTORS
E. cuniculi–related anterior uveitis seen most often in young <2-year-old rabbits.

ZOONOTIC POTENTIAL
E. cuniculi—unlikely, but possible in immunosuppressed humans. Mode of transmission and susceptibility in humans is unclear

PREGNANCY/FERTILITY/BREEDING
• Systemic steroids—do not use in pregnant animals if at all avoidable.
• Topical steroids—use with caution; systemic absorption occurs.

SYNONYMS
Iridocyclitis

SEE ALSO
Encephalitozoonosis
Abscesses
Red eye

ABBREVIATIONS
CNS = central nervous system
KCS = keratoconjunctivitis sicca
NSAID = nonsteroidal anti-inflammatory drug

Suggested Reading
Bedard KM. Ocular surface disease of rabbits. Vet Clin Exot Anim 2019;922:1–14.
Florin M, Rusanen E, Haessig M et al. Clinical presentation, treatment, and outcome of dacryocystitis in rabbits: a retrospective study of 28 cases (2003–2007). Vet Ophthalmol 2009;12(6):350–356.
Lennox AM, Capello V, Legendre LF. Small mammal dentistry. In: Quesenberry KE, Carpenter JW, eds. Ferrets, Rabbits and Rodents, (4th ed). Clinical Medicine and Surgery. 2021, St. Louis: Saunders, 2020:514–535.
Van der Woerdt A. Ophthalmologic diseases of small mammals. In: Quesenberry KE, Carpenter JW, eds. Ferrets, Rabbits and Rodents, (4th ed). Clinical Medicine and Surgery. 2021, St. Louis: Saunders, 2020:583–594.
Williams DL. Laboratory animal ophthalmology. In: Gelatt KN, ed. Veterinary Ophthalmology, 3rd ed. Philadelphia: Lippincott, Williams & Wilkins, 1999:151–181.

Author Georgina Newbold, DVM, Dipl. ACVO

ARTHRITIS—OSTEOARTHRITIS

BASICS

OVERVIEW
• Progressive deterioration of articular cartilage found in diarthrodial joints
• Degenerative joint disease—more appropriate term in veterinary medicine

SIGNALMENT
• No breed or gender predilection
• Actual incidence not reported
• Hereditary or developmental disorders—young animals
• Trauma/infection induced—any age

SIGNS

General Comments
Radiographic severity may not correlate with clinical severity.

Historical Findings
• Lameness or stiff gait; may be intermittent; slowly becomes more severe and frequent; may have a history of previous joint trauma (fracture, ligament injury, dislocation), osteochondral disease, or developmental disorder
• Restricted motion, inability to hop (may be intermittent)
• Signs referable to an inability to properly groom or attain a normal stance while urinating due to stiffness or pain may be seen. Affected rabbits may not be able to groom the intrascapular, perineal, or tail head region, or may be unable to consume cecotrophs from the rectum, resulting in feces or cecotrophs pasted to perineum. If unable to attain a normal stance while urinating, urine may soak the ventrum, resulting in urine scald.
• May be exacerbated by exercise, long periods of recumbency

Physical Examination Findings
• Stiffness of gait
• Lameness
• Decreased range of motion
• Crepitus
• Joint swelling and pain
• Joint instability (ligament tear, subluxation), depending on the duration of disease
• Signs referable to inability to groom, depending on which joints are involved—feces pasted to perineum, flaky skin, urine scald, and unkempt hair coat
• Obesity

CAUSES AND RISK FACTORS
• Primary—thought to be the result of long-term use combined with aging; associated with a known predisposing cause
• Secondary—results from an initiating cause: joint instability, trauma, joint incongruity

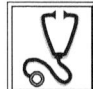

DIAGNOSIS

DIFFERENTIAL DIAGNOSIS
• Septic arthritis
• Neoplasia
• Spondylosis deformans
• Urolithiasis
• Pododermatitis

CBC/BIOCHEMISTRY/URINALYSIS
• CBC/biochemistry profile is usually normal
• Urinalysis may reflect hypercalciuria or urinary tract infection secondary to insufficient voiding

OTHER LABORATORY TESTS
N/A

IMAGING
Radiographic changes—joint capsular distension; osteophytosis; soft tissue thickening; soft tissue mineralization; narrowed joint spaces. Oblique views of the spine may be helpful in delineating spinal arthritis.

DIAGNOSTIC PROCEDURES
• Arthrocentesis and synovial fluid analysis—may support the diagnosis; slight increase in mononuclear cells; large numbers of neutrophils are likely the result of infectious arthritis
• Bacterial culture and sensitivity—synovial fluid
• Biopsy of synovial tissue—helps rule out other arthritides or neoplasia

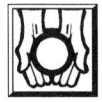

TREATMENT

APPROPRIATE HEALTH CARE
Treat as an outpatient with limited exercise and analgesic administration

NURSING CARE
• Keep perineum clean, dry, and free of fecal matter.
• Use soft bedding and keep bedding clean and dry to prevent dermatitis or bed sores
• Physical therapy—may be beneficial in enhancing limb function and general well-being; range-of-motion exercises, a combination of heat and cold therapy

ACTIVITY
Limited to a level that minimizes aggravation of clinical signs

DIET
• Weight reduction for obese patients—decreases stress placed on affected joints
• Painful rabbits often refuse food. Make sure that patients are eating normally to prevent gastrointestinal motility disorders.

CLIENT EDUCATION
• Inform the client that medical therapy is palliative and the condition is likely to progress.
• Discuss treatment options, activity level, and diet.

SURGICAL CONSIDERATIONS
N/A

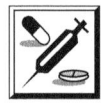

MEDICATIONS

DRUG(S) OF CHOICE
• Nonsteroidal anti-inflammatories—have been used for short- or long-term therapy to reduce pain and inflammation in rabbits with musculoskeletal disease; meloxicam (1.0 mg/kg PO q24h; carprofen (2 mg/kg PO q12h)
• Tramadol—5–15 mg/kg PO q8–12h
• Gabapentin—5–20 mg/kg PO q8–12h

CONTRAINDICATIONS
Corticosteroids—associated with gastrointestinal ulceration and hemorrhage, delayed wound healing, and heightened susceptibility to infection. Rabbits are very sensitive to the immunosuppressive effects of both topical and systemic corticosteroids; use may exacerbate subclinical bacterial infection.

PRECAUTIONS
• Meloxicam—use with caution in rabbits with compromised renal function

ALTERNATIVE DRUGS
• Chondroitin sulfate (Cosequin, Nutramax) has been used anecdotally using feline dosage protocols; polysulfated glycosaminoglycan (Adequan, Luitpold) 2.2 mg/kg SC, IM q3d × 21–28 days, then q14d
• Acupuncture may be effective for rabbits with chronic pain.

FOLLOW-UP

PATIENT MONITORING
Clinical deterioration—indicates the need to change drug selection or dosage; may indicate the need for surgical intervention

PREVENTION/AVOIDANCE
Early identification of predisposing causes and prompt treatment—help reduce progression of secondary condition

POSSIBLE COMPLICATIONS
• Gastrointestinal hypomotility or stasis
• Dermatitis, urine scald, ulcerative pododermatitis (sore hocks)
• Hypercalciuria

EXPECTED COURSE AND PROGNOSIS
• Slow progression of disease likely
• Pain control and limited exercise usually allow a good quality of life.

 MISCELLANEOUS

ASSOCIATED CONDITIONS
N/A

AGE-RELATED FACTORS
N/A

ZOONOTIC POTENTIAL
N/A

PREGNANCY/FERTILITY/BREEDING
N/A

SYNONYMS
Degenerative joint disease

Suggested Reading
Bays TB. Geriatric care of rabbits, guinea pigs, and chinchillas. Vet Clin Exot Anim 2020;23:567–593.
Fisher PG, Künzel F, Rylander H. Neurologic and musculoskeletal disease. In: Quesenberry KE, Carpenter JW, eds. Ferrets, Rabbits and Rodents, (4th ed). Clinical Medicine and Surgery. St. Louis: Saunders, 2020:583–594.
Harkness JE, Turner PV, VandeWoude S, Wheeler CL. Clinical signs and differential diagnoses: nervous and musculoskeletal conditions. In: Harkness JE, Turner PV, VandeWoude S, Wheeler CL, eds. Biology and Medicine of Rabbits and Rodents, 5th ed. Ames: Wiley-Blackwell, 2010:214–216.
Keeble E. Nervous system and musculoskeletal disorders. In: Meredith A, Lord B, eds. BSAVA Manual of Rabbit Medicine. Gloucester: British Small Animal Veterinary Association, 2014:233–248.
Varga M. Neurological and locomotive disorders. In: Varga M, ed. Textbook of Rabbit Medicine, 2nd ed. London, UK: Elsevier, 2014:367–389.
Author Barbara Oglesbee, DVM, DABVP (Avian)

ARTHRITIS—SEPTIC

BASICS

OVERVIEW
• Definition—pathogenic microorganisms within the closed space of one or more synovial joints
• Usually caused by the hematogenous spread of microorganisms from a distant septic focus, contamination associated with traumatic injury (e.g., a direct penetrating injury such as bite wounds or cage injury), the extension of a primary osteomyelitis (especially on the plantar/palmar surfaces of the feet), or a contaminated surgery
• Sources of infection—abscesses; dental disease; upper respiratory infection; skin; wounds; sometimes not identified

SIGNALMENT
No age, breed, or gender predilection

SIGNS
General Comments
Consider the diagnosis in patients with lameness associated with soft tissue swelling, heat, and pain.

Historical Findings
• Lameness
• Lethargy, anorexia
• History of upper respiratory infection, dental disease, abscess
• May report previous trauma—bite wound, penetrating injury

Physical Examination Findings
• Joint pain and swelling
• Localized joint heat
• Decreased range of motion
• Signs of concurrent infection—URI, dental disease, ulcerative pododermatitis, abscess

CAUSES AND RISK FACTORS
• Pyogenic bacteria—especially staphylo-cocci, pasteurella, and anaerobic bacteria
• Predisposing factors—immunosuppression, chronic bacterial infection, and penetrating trauma to the joint

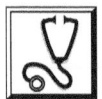

DIAGNOSIS

DIFFERENTIAL DIAGNOSIS
• Lameness affecting one limb—fracture, soft tissue injury, abscess, ulcerative pododermati-tis, and neoplasia
• Lameness affecting multiple limbs—spinal trauma, spondylosis, disc disease, and encephalitozoonosis

CBC/BIOCHEMISTRY/URINALYSIS
• Hemogram—normal or lymphopenia; inflammatory left shift not usually seen in rabbits; may see mild anemia
• Other results normal

OTHER LABORATORY TESTS
• Serology for pasteurella—usefulness is severely limited, and generally not helpful in the diagnosis of pasteurellosis in pet rabbits. An ELISA is available; however, positive results, even when high, only indicate prior exposure to pasteurella and the development of antibodies, and do not confirm active infection. Low positive results may occur due to cross-reaction with other, nonpathogenic bacteria (false positive). False-negative results are common with immunosuppression or early infection. No evidence exists to support the correlation of titers to the presence or absence of disease.

IMAGING
Radiography—similar to lesions found in dogs and cats—may reveal thickened periarticular tissues; evidence of synovial effusion; bone destruction, osteolysis, irregular joint space, erosions, and periarticular osteophytosis

DIAGNOSTIC PROCEDURES
Synovial Fluid Analysis
• Increased volume
• Turbid fluid
• Elevated WBC count—predominate neutrophils
• Bacteria in the synovial fluid or within neutrophils

Synovial Fluid Culture
• Must be collected aseptically; requires heavy sedation or general anesthesia
• Submit fluid samples for aerobic and anaerobic culture; bacterial susceptibility testing to direct antibiotic therapy

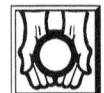

TREATMENT

APPROPRIATE HEALTH CARE
• It is essential to remove/correct the underlying cause for long-term success
• Inpatient—for initial stabilization or surgical debridement
• Outpatient—for long-term management

NURSING CARE
• Depends on severity of disease
• Bandage changes postarthrotomy
• Anorectic rabbits require assistance feeding
• Soft bedding, daily bedding changes

ACTIVITY
Restricted until resolution of symptoms

DIET
• It is imperative that the rabbit continues to eat during and following treatment. This condition is often painful, resulting in anorexia. Anorexia will often cause GI hypomotility, derangement of the GI microflora, and overgrowth of intestinal bacterial pathogens.
• If the patient refuses food, syringe-feed a gruel such as Critical Care for Herbivores (Oxbow Pet Products) or Emeraid Herbivore (Lafeber Company, Cornell, IL) 10–15 mL/kg PO q6–8h. Larger volumes and more frequent feedings are often accepted; feed as much as the rabbit will accept. Alternatively, pellets can be ground and mixed with fresh greens, vegetable baby foods, water, or juice to form a gruel. If sufficient volumes of food are not accepted in this manner, nasogastric intubation is indicated.
• High-carbohydrate, high-fat nutritional supplements are contraindicated.

CLIENT EDUCATION
• Warn client about the need for long-term antibiotics, repeated treatments and the likelihood of residual degenerative joint disease.
• Severe disease, especially with multiple joint involvement, carries a guarded to poor prognosis for complete resolution. Most will require surgical debridement, sometimes multiple surgeries, and multiple follow-up visits. Recurrences are common, especially if the underlying cause cannot be corrected. Clients must be aware of the monetary and time investment.

SURGICAL CONSIDERATIONS
• Open arthrotomy with debridement of the synovium; debride all visibly necrotic tissue
• Simple lancing and draining are not adequate. In rabbits, septic joints usually contain thick exudates that do not drain well. Instead of draining, curette all visible exudates and flush copiously with warmed physiologic saline.
• Given the expense and pain involved in these procedures, the author recommends referral to a specialist with surgical expertise.
• Place on long-term systemic antibiotic therapy; appropriate pain management
• Severe infection that is not responsive to therapy may require amputation. Most rabbits tolerate amputation of a single front or hind limb well.

(CONTINUED)

MEDICATIONS

DRUG(S) OF CHOICE
• Antimicrobial drugs are effective against the infectious agent; gain access to site of infection. Choice of antibiotic is ideally based on the results of culture and susceptibility testing. Depending on the severity of infection, long-term antibiotic therapy is required (4–6 weeks minimum, to several months). Use broad-spectrum antibiotics such as enrofloxacin (10–20 mg/kg PO, SC, IM, IV q12h), marbofloxacin (5 mg/kg PO q24h), trimethoprim-sulfa (15–30 mg/kg PO q12h), or chloramphenicol (50 mg/kg PO q8h). For anaerobic bacteria: azithromycin (15–30 mg/kg PO q24h); can be used alone or combined with metronidazole (20 mg/kg PO q12h). Alternatively, use penicillin G procaine (40,000–60,000 IU/kg SC q24h).
• Combine with the surgical treatment listed above.

Acute Pain Management
• Butorphanol (0.1–0.5 mg/kg SQ, IM, IV q4–6h); may cause profound sedation; short acting
• Buprenorphine (0.02–0.05 mg/kg SQ, IM IV q8–12h); less sedating, longer acting than butorphanol
• Hydromorphone (0.1 mg/kg SC IM q2–4h) or oxymorphone (0.05–0.2 mg/kg SC IM q8–12h)
• Meloxicam (1 mg/kg PO, SC, IM q24h)
• Carprofen (2–4 mg/kg PO, SC q12–24h)

Long-Term Pain Management
• Nonsteroidal anti-inflammatories—have been used for short- or long-term therapy to reduce pain and inflammation in rabbits with musculoskeletal disease; meloxicam (1.0 mg/kg PO q24h; carprofen (2 mg/kg PO q12h)
• Tramadol—5–15 mg/kg PO q8–12h
• Gabapentin—5–20 mg/kg PO q8–12h

CONTRAINDICATIONS
• Oral administration of antibiotics that select against gram-positive bacteria (penicillins, macrolides, lincosamides, and cephalosporins) can cause fatal enteric dysbiosis and enterotoxemia.
• The use of corticosteroids (systemic or topical preparations) can severely exacerbate septic arthritis.

PRECAUTIONS
• Meloxicam and other NSAIDs—use with caution in patients with renal compromise; monitor renal values
• Failure to respond to conventional antibiotic therapy—may indicate anaerobic disease or other unusual causes (fungal, spirochete)
• Oral administration of any antibiotic can potentially cause intestinal dysbiosis. Discontinue use if anorexia or diarrhea occurs.

POSSIBLE INTERACTIONS
N/A

ALTERNATIVE DRUGS
N/A

FOLLOW-UP

PATIENT MONITORING
• Duration of antibiotic therapy—4–8 weeks or longer; depends on clinical signs and pathogenic organism
• Monitor for progressive decrease in swelling, resolution of inflammation, and improvement of clinical signs.

PREVENTION/AVOIDANCE
N/A

POSSIBLE COMPLICATIONS
• Chronic disease—severe degenerative joint disease
• Recurrence of infection
• Limited joint range of motion
• Generalized sepsis
• Osteomyelitis

EXPECTED COURSE AND PROGNOSIS
• Acutely diagnosed disease—good to fair prognosis with aggressive treatment
• Advanced disease, multiple joint involvement, or resistant or highly virulent organisms—guarded to poor prognosis

MISCELLANEOUS

ASSOCIATED CONDITIONS
• Immunosuppression
• Dental disease

• Rhinitis/sinusitis
• Hypercalciuria
• Ulcerative pododermatitis
• Moist pyoderma

AGE-RELATED FACTORS
N/A

ZOONOTIC POTENTIAL
N/A

PREGNANCY/FERTILITY/BREEDING
N/A

SYNONYMS
Infectious arthritis

SEE ALSO
Abscesses
Ulcerative pododermatitis (sore hocks)

ABBREVIATIONS
ELISA = enzyme-linked immunosorbent assay
GI = gastrointestinal
NSAID = nonsteroidal anti-inflammatory drug

Suggested Reading
Bays TB. Geriatric care of rabbits, guinea pigs, and chinchillas. Vet Clin Exot Anim 2020;23:567–593.
Fisher PG, Künzel F, Rylander H. Neurologic and musculoskeletal disease. In: Quesenberry KE, Carpenter JW, eds. Ferrets, Rabbits and Rodents, (4th ed). St. Louis: Saunders, 2020:583–594.
Harkness JE, Turner PV, VandeWoude S, Wheeler CL. Clinical signs and differential diagnoses: nervous and musculoskeletal conditions. In: Harkness JE, Turner PV, VandeWoude S, Wheeler CL, eds. Biology and Medicine of Rabbits and Rodents, 5th ed. Ames: Wiley-Blackwell, 2010: 214–216.
Keeble E. Nervous system and musculoskeletal disorders. In: Meredith A, Lord B, eds. BSAVA Manual of Rabbit Medicine. Gloucester: British Small Animal Veterinary Association, 2014:233–248.
Varga M. Neurological and locomotive disorders. In: Varga M, ed. Textbook of Rabbit Medicine, 2nd ed. London, UK: Elsevier, 2014:367–389.
Author Barbara Oglesbee, DVM, DABVP (Avian)

ATAXIA

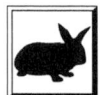

BASICS

DEFINITION
• A sign of sensory dysfunction that produces incoordination of the limbs, head, and/or trunk
• Three clinical types—sensory (proprioceptive), vestibular, and cerebellar; all produce changes in limb coordination, but vestibular and cerebellar ataxia also produce changes in head and neck movement.

PATHOPHYSIOLOGY

Sensory
• Proprioceptive pathways in the spinal cord relay limb and trunk position to the brain.
• When the spinal cord is slowly compressed, proprioceptive deficits are usually the first signs observed because these pathways are located more superficially in the white matter and their larger-sized axons are more susceptible to compression than other tracts.
• Generally accompanied by weakness owing to early concomitant upper motor neuron involvement, weakness is not always obvious early in the course of the disease

Vestibular
• Changes in head and neck position are relayed through the vestibulocochlear nerve to the brain stem.
• Diseases that affect the vestibular receptors, the nerve in the inner ear, or the nuclei in the brain stem cause various degrees of disequilibrium with ensuing vestibular ataxia.
• Affected animal leans, tips, falls, or rolls toward the side of the lesion; accompanied by head tilt

Cerebellar
• The cerebellum regulates, coordinates, and smooths motor activity.
• Proprioception is normal because the ascending proprioceptive pathways to the cortex are intact; weakness does not occur because the upper motor neurons are intact.
• Inadequacy in the performance of motor activity; strength preservation; no proprioceptive deficits

SYSTEMS AFFECTED
Nervous—spinal cord (and brain stem); cerebellum; vestibular system

SIGNALMENT
Any age, breed, or sex

SIGNS
• Important to define the type of ataxia to localize the problem
• Only one limb involved—consider a lameness problem

• Only hind limbs affected—likely a spinal cord disorder
• All or both ipsilateral limbs affected—cerebellar
• Head tilt—vestibular
• Nasal/ocular discharge—likely vestibular; spread of upper respiratory infection to inner/middle ear
• Urine scald, perineal dermatitis, alopecia in the intrascapular region—seen in rabbits with spinal disease due to inability to maintain normal stance while urinating or inability to properly groom

CAUSES

Neurologic
Cerebellar and CNS vestibular
• Infectious—bacterial most common, especially central erosion caused by otitis media and interna; encephalitis due to *Pasteurella* spp. or other bacteria; listeriosis (rare); *Encephalitozoon cuniculi*, reportedly common; aberrant *Baylisascariasis* migration (unusual cause); rabies virus and herpes virus (rare)
• Toxin ingestion—lead most common
• Degenerative and anomalous—not yet described in rabbits
• Neoplastic—any tumor of the CNS (primary or secondary) localized to the cerebellum
• Inflammatory, idiopathic, immune-mediated—granulomatous meningoencephalomyelitis, common postmortem finding in rabbits both with and without antemortem neurologic signs; has been attributed to *E. cuniculi* infection, but organisms generally not found; similar lesions can be found on postmortem examination of rabbits in the absence of clinical signs
Vestibular—PNS
• Infectious—otitis media interna the most common cause; Pasteurella multocida, Staphylococcus aureus, Pseudomonas aeruginosa, E. coli, and Listeria monocytogenes most often cultured
• Idiopathic—not well described in rabbits; however, a definitive diagnosis is often not found, and many rabbits with vestibular signs improve with supportive care
• Neoplastic—not well described in rabbits
Spinal cord
• Traumatic—fracture or luxation, very common in pet rabbits; intervertebral disc herniation—anecdotally reported
• Degenerative—spondylosis, common in older rabbits
• Anomalous—kyphosis, lordosis, hemivertebrae
• Infectious—*E. cuniculi*, spinal cord, and nerve route lesions anecdotally reported
• Vascular and neoplastic diseases—uncommon, not well described in rabbits

Metabolic
• Anemia
• Electrolyte disturbances—hypokalemia and hypoglycemia

Miscellaneous
• Respiratory compromise
• Cardiac compromise

RISK FACTORS
• Otitis media/interna—chronic upper respiratory infection, immunosuppression (stress, corticosteroid use, concurrent disease)
• Spinal fractures, luxations, or intervertebral disk disease—improper restraint, possibly disuse atrophy from confinement
• *Encephalitozoon cuniculi*—immunosuppression (stress, corticosteroid use, concurrent disease)
• *Baylisascariasis*—outdoor housing, exposure to raccoon feces
• Spondylosis—unknown, possibly related to small caging, lack of exercise, aging change

DIAGNOSIS

DIFFERENTIAL DIAGNOSIS
• Differentiate the types of ataxia
• Differentiate from other disease processes that can affect gait—musculoskeletal; metabolic; cardiovascular; respiratory
• Musculoskeletal disorders—typically produce lameness and a reluctance to move
• Systemic illness, cardiovascular, and metabolic disorders—can cause intermittent ataxia, especially of the pelvic limbs; fever, weight loss, murmurs, arrhythmias, or collapse with exercise suspect a non-neurologic cause; obtain minimum data from hemogram, biochemistry analysis, and urinalysis
• Head tilt or nystagmus—likely vestibular
• Intention tremors of the head or hypermetria—likely cerebellar
• Only limbs affected—likely spinal cord dysfunction; all four limbs are affected: lesion is in the cervical area or is multifocal to diffuse; only pelvic limbs affected: lesion is anywhere below the second thoracic vertebra
• Upper respiratory disease—likely vestibular; spread of infection to inner/middle ear or brain stem

CBC/BIOCHEMISTRY/URINALYSIS
Normal unless metabolic cause (e.g., hypoglycemia, electrolyte imbalance, and anemia)

OTHER LABORATORY TESTS
• Electrolyte imbalance—correct the problem; see if ataxia resolves
• Serologic testing for *E. cuniculi*—many tests are available, but usefulness is limited since a positive titer indicates only exposure

and does not confirm *E. cuniculi* as the cause of neurologic signs. *E. cuniculi* can only be definitively diagnosed by finding organisms and resultant lesions on histopathologic examination in areas that anatomically correlate with observed clinical signs. A combination of IgM, IgG, and C-reactive protein appears to be most reliable.
• Serology for pasteurella—usefulness is severely limited and generally not helpful in the diagnosis of pasteurellosis in pet rabbits. An ELISA is available, and positive results, even when high, only indicate prior exposure to *Pasteurella* and the development of antibodies but do not confirm active infection. Low positive results may occur due to cross-reaction with other, nonpathogenic bacteria (false positive). False-negative results are common with immunosuppression or early infection. No evidence exists to support the correlation of titers to the presence or absence of disease.
• Bacterial culture and sensitivity testing—from ear exudate or nasal discharge

IMAGING
• Spinal radiographs—if spinal cord dysfunction is suspected; referral for myelogram may be indicated
• Bullae radiographs—if peripheral vestibular disease is suspected; CT scans are superior; many rabbits with bullae disease have normal-appearing radiographs
• Thoracic radiographs—identify heart disease, neoplasia
• CT—if cerebellar disease is suspected; evaluate potential brain disease
• Abdominal ultrasonography—if underlying metabolic disease (renal, hepatic) is suspected

DIAGNOSTIC PROCEDURES
• Otoscopic examination—in rabbits with otitis externa, thick, white, creamy exudate may be found in the horizontal and/or vertical canals. Otitis interna/media often occurs in the absence of otitis externa via extension through the eustachian tube. Most rabbits with otitis interna have no visible otoscopic abnormalities.
• CSF—may aid in confirming nervous system causes; may see increased protein, lymphocyte and monocytes with *E. cuniculi* infection. Studies were unable to find organisms or evidence of organisms utilizing PCR testing on CSF.

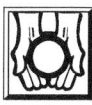

TREATMENT
Usually outpatient, depending on the severity and acuteness of clinical signs

ACTIVITY
• Exercise—decrease or restrict if spinal cord disease suspected; if vestibular signs—restrict (e.g., avoid stairs and slippery surfaces)

according to the degree of disequilibrium; encourage a return to activity as soon as safely possible; activity may enhance recovery of vestibular function
• The client should monitor gait for increasing dysfunction or weakness; if paresis worsens or paralysis develops, other testing is warranted.

DIET
• It is important that the rabbit continue to eat. Although rabbits cannot vomit, many with vestibular disorders appear to be nauseated and will not eat. Anorexia will cause GI hypomotility or GI stasis, derangement of the GI microflora, and overgrowth of intestinal bacterial pathogens.
• Bring the food to the rabbit if non-ambulatory, or offer food by hand.
• If the patient refuses these foods, syringe feed a gruel such as Critical Care for Herbivores (Oxbow Pet Products) or Emeraid Herbivore (Lafeber Company, Cornell, IL) 10–15 mL/kg PO q6–8h. Larger volumes and more frequent feedings are often accepted; feed as much as the rabbit will readily accept. Alternatively, pellets can be ground and mixed with fresh greens, vegetable baby foods, water, or juice to form a gruel.
• High-carbohydrate, high-fat nutritional supplements are contraindicated.
• Encourage oral fluid intake by offering fresh water, wetting leafy vegetables, or flavoring water with vegetable juices.

MEDICATIONS
DRUG(S) OF CHOICE
Not recommended until the source or cause of the problem is identified

CONTRAINDICATIONS
• Oral administration of antibiotics that select against gram-positive bacteria (penicillins, macrolides, lincosamides, and cephalosporins) can cause fatal enteric dysbiosis and enterotoxemia.
• Topical and systemic corticosteroids—rabbits are very sensitive to the immunosuppressive effects of corticosteroids; use may exacerbate subclinical bacterial infection. Use is contraindicated unless intervertebral disc disease is demonstrated by myelography.

FOLLOW-UP
PATIENT MONITORING
Periodic neurologic examinations to assess condition

POSSIBLE COMPLICATIONS
• Spinal cord or neuromuscular disease—progression to weakness and possibly paralysis
• Cerebellar disease—head tremors, severe torticollis, rolling, and anorexia

MISCELLANEOUS
SEE ALSO
See specific diseases
Head tilt (vestibular disease)
Paresis and paralysis

ABBREVIATIONS
CSF = cerebrospinal fluid
CT = computed tomography
ELISA = enzyme-linked immunosorbent assay
IFA = indirect immunofluorescence assay
PCR = polymerase chain reaction
PNS = peripheral nervous system

Suggested Reading
Bays TB. Geriatric care of rabbits, guinea pigs, and chinchillas. Vet Clin Exot Anim 2020;23:567–593.
DeCubellis J. Common emergencies in rabbits, guinea pigs, and chinchillas. Vet Clin Exot Anim 2016;19:411–429.
Fisher PG, Künzel F, Rylander H. Neurologic and musculoskeletal disease. In: Quesenberry KE, Carpenter JW, eds. Ferrets, Rabbits and Rodents, Clinical Medicine and Surgery, 4th ed. St. Louis: Saunders, 2020:583–594.
Harkness JE, Turner PV, VandeWoude S, Wheeler CL. Clinical signs and differential diagnoses: nervous and musculoskeletal conditions. In: Harkness JE, Turner PV, VandeWoude S, Wheeler CL, eds. Biology and Medicine of Rabbits and Rodents, 5th ed. Ames: Wiley-Blackwell, 2010:214–216.
Keeble E. Nervous system and musculoskeletal disorders. In: Meredith A, Lord B, eds. BSAVA Manual of Rabbit Medicine. Gloucester: British Small Animal Veterinary Association, 2014:233–248.
Lennox AM, Gladden JN. Emergency and critical care of small mammals. In: Quesenberry KE, Carpenter JW, eds. Ferrets, Rabbits and Rodents, (4th ed). Clinical Medicine and Surgery. 2021, St. Louis: Saunders, 2020:595–608.
Varga M. Neurological and locomotive disorders. In: Varga M, ed. Textbook of Rabbit Medicine, 2nd ed. London, UK: Elsevier, 2014:367–389.
Author Barbara Oglesbee, DVM, DABVP (Avian)

RABBITS

CATARACTS

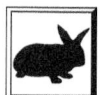

BASICS

OVERVIEW
- Opacification of the lens
- The term *cataract* may refer to an entire lens that is opaque or to an opacity within the lens; does not imply cause
- Most common causes—*Encephalitozoon cuniculi* in utero infection with vertical transmission of organism into the developing lens; replication of spores within the lens of young rabbits results in cataract formation, thin anterior portion, or rupture of lens, resulting in phacoclastic uveitis with focal granuloma formation at the site of rupture. Congenital and naturally occurring, spontaneous cataracts also reported.
- Other causes (nutritional deficiency; elevated blood glucose; toxins; altered composition of the aqueous humor caused by uveitis) not well described in rabbits
- Traditional terminology—immature (only part of the lens is involved); mature (entire lens is opaque); hypermature (lens liquefaction has occurred); implies progressive condition

SIGNALMENT
- *E. cuniculi*—most common in dwarf breeds <2 years old, but can occur in any age or breed
- Spontaneous juvenile cataracts—one study demonstrated an incidence of 4.3% in laboratory New Zealand white rabbits
- No breed predilection described for congenital cataracts

SIGNS
- Opacification of lens
- Liquefied lens material leaking from the lens—seen most often with *E. cuniculi*
- Iridal swelling, white nodule on the iris—common in rabbits with *E. cuniculi*; consists of granulomatous reaction to leakage of lens material. Rabbits are often presented for evaluation of an intraocular white mass, with the remainder of the eye appearing relatively quiet.
- Associated with uveitis—typically see hypopyon and low intraocular pressure

Choroid Reflection
- Easiest method of detection
- Obstruction of light by lenticular opacities (retroillumination)
- Appear as black or gray spots
- Cloudiness owing to sclerosis—will not detect discrete foci of obstruction; fundic examination possible through lenticular sclerosis

CAUSES AND RISK FACTORS
- Congenital
- In utero infection with *E. cuniculi*
- Spontaneous—unknown cause; senile or degenerative cataracts have not been well described
- Uveitis—secondary to synechia formation or altered aqueous humor composition
- Diabetes mellitus—not reported in rabbits

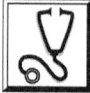

DIAGNOSIS

DIFFERENTIAL DIAGNOSIS
- For white mass protruding from iris—iridal abscess (common); neoplasia

CBC/BIOCHEMISTRY/URINALYSIS
- Routine hematology and blood chemistry profiles—screen for infectious diseases when associated with uveitis

OTHER LABORATORY TESTS
- Serologic testing for *E. cuniculi*—many tests are available, but usefulness is limited since a positive titer indicates only exposure and does not confirm *E. cuniculi* as the cause of uveitis. Can only be definitively diagnosed by finding an organism on ocular histopathology or positive DNA probe (PCR) on removed lens material. Antibody titers usually become positive by 2 weeks post-infection but may not continue to rise with active infection or decline with treatment. No correlation exists between antibody titers and the shedding of organism or severity of disease.

IMAGING
Ocular ultrasound may detect posterior or equatorial lens capsule rupture secondary to cataract ± *E. cuniculi*

DIAGNOSTIC PROCEDURES
N/A

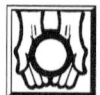

TREATMENT

APPROPRIATE HEALTH CARE
Rabbits undergoing surgery—inpatient

NURSING CARE
N/A

ACTIVITY
N/A

DIET
Make certain that the rabbit continues to eat to avoid secondary gastrointestinal disorders.

CLIENT EDUCATION
- Inform the client that surgery can be performed on congenital or spontaneous cataract that is causing or is anticipated to cause vision loss if no other ocular pathology is present. Spontaneous regeneration of the lens following phacoemulsification has been reported in rabbits; however, recent studies have shown that insertion of a prosthetic lens ± capsular tension ring (IOL ± CTR placement) may markedly decrease the degree of lens regrowth and improve postoperative visual outcome
- Warn client that the prognosis for surgery is better if it is done early in the course of cataract development, before hypermaturity, lens-induced uveitis, and retinal detachment occur.
- Phacoemulsification may offer the best prognosis for cataracts caused by *E. cuniculi*.

SURGICAL CONSIDERATIONS
- Phacoemulsification—ultrasonic lens fragmentation; procedure of choice.
- *E. cuniculi*—may recur following surgery, requiring medical treatment or enucleation.

MEDICATIONS

DRUG(S) OF CHOICE
- Topical NSAIDs—0.5% ketorolac, or 1% diclofenac; q6h daily to control inflammation
- 1% prednisolone acetate—has been used q6h to prevent and control lens-induced uveitis; use with extreme caution in rabbits (see Precautions).
- *E. cuniculi*—Benzimidazole anthelmintics are effective against *E. cuniculi* in vitro and have been shown to prevent experimental infection in rabbits. However, efficacy in rabbits with clinical signs is unknown. Anecdotal reports suggest a response to treatment in rabbits with *E. cuniculi*-associated phacoclastic uveitis. Published treatments include fenbendazole (20 mg/kg q24h × 5–28 days) as the most commonly used and anecdotally effective treatment.

CONTRAINDICATIONS
Topical corticosteroids—never use if the cornea retains fluorescein stain (corneal ulceration)

PRECAUTIONS
- Topical corticosteroids or antibiotic-corticosteroid combinations—avoid; associated with gastrointestinal ulceration and hemorrhage, delayed wound healing, and heightened susceptibility to infection; rabbits are very sensitive to the

immunosuppressive effects of both topic and systemic corticosteroids; use may exacerbate subclinical bacterial infection
• Albendazole has been associated with bone marrow toxicity in rabbits. Several anecdotal reports of pancytopenia leading to death in rabbits exist.

POSSIBLE INTERACTIONS
N/A

ALTERNATIVE DRUGS
N/A

FOLLOW-UP

PATIENT MONITORING
• All patients—monitored carefully for progression
• Intraocular pressure—monitored for secondary glaucoma in rabbits with *E. cuniculi*; normal intraocular pressure reported as 10–20 mmHg when measured by applanation tonometry

POSSIBLE COMPLICATIONS
• Complete cataracts—potential to cause lens-induced uveitis, secondary glaucoma, and retinal detachment

EXPECTED COURSE AND PROGNOSIS
• Congenital or spontaneous cataracts—insufficient data available on prognosis following phacoemulsification or progression to uveitis.

• *E. cuniculi*–associated uveitis—depends on the severity and chronicity of infection and the presence of secondary bacterial infections. If cannot treat surgically, the prognosis for viability of the affected eye is guarded, as most will progress to glaucoma; enucleation may be indicated.

MISCELLANEOUS

ASSOCIATED CONDITIONS
N/A

AGE-RELATED FACTORS
E. cuniculi-related anterior uveitis is seen most often in young (<2 years old) rabbits.

ZOONOTIC POTENTIAL
E. cuniculi—unlikely, but possible in immunosuppressed humans. Mode of transmission and susceptibility in humans are unclear.

PREGNANCY/FERTILITY/ BREEDING
• Systemic steroids—do not use in pregnant animals if at all avoidable
• Topical steroids—use with caution; systemic absorption occurs

SYNONYMS
N/A

SEE ALSO
Encephalitozoonosis
Red eye

ABBREVIATIONS
ELISA = enzyme-linked immunosorbent assay
IFA = indirect immunofluorescence assay
NSAID = nonsteroidal anti-inflammatory

Suggested Reading
Bedard KM. Ocular surface disease of rabbits. Vet Clin Exot Anim 2019;922:1–14.
Florin M, Rusanen E, Haessig M et al. Clinical presentation, treatment, and outcome of dacryocystitis in rabbits: a retrospective study of 28 cases (2003–2007). Vet Ophthalmol 2009;12(6):350–356.
Lennox AM, Capello V, Legendre LF. Small mammal dentistry. In: Quesenberry KE, Carpenter JW, eds. Ferrets, Rabbits and Rodents, (4th ed.). Clinical Medicine and Surgery. 2021, St. Louis: Saunders, 2020:514–535.
Van der Woerdt A. Ophthalmologic diseases of small mammals. In: Quesenberry KE, Carpenter JW, eds. Ferrets, Rabbits and Rodents, (4th ed.). Clinical Medicine and Surgery. 2021, St. Louis: Saunders, 2020:583–594.
Williams DL. Laboratory animal ophthalmology. In: Gelatt KN, ed. Veterinary Ophthalmology, 3rd ed. Philadelphia: Lippincott, Williams & Wilkins, 1999:151–181.
Author Georgina Newbold, DVM, Dipl. ACVO

CHEYLETIELLOSIS AND *L. GIBBUS* (FUR MITES)

BASICS

OVERVIEW
• A highly contagious parasitic skin disease of rabbits, dogs, and cats caused by infestation with *Cheyletiella* spp. mites
• Nonburrowing mite lives on the epidermal keratin layer
• Life cycle is approximately 35 days; the entire cycle is spent on the host
• Most rabbits are asymptomatic—disease occurs in young animals, debilitated animals, or those with underlying diseases that prohibit adequate grooming
• Signs of scaling and pruritus can mimic other diseases.
• With *Cheyletiella* and Leporacaurs infestation, human (zoonotic) lesions can occur.
• Lesions may less commonly be caused by the fur mite *Leporacarus gibbus*

SIGNALMENT
• Seen in any age rabbit
• Most common in young animals, debilitated animals, or those with underlying diseases that prohibit adequate grooming to remove keratin and mites
• May be more common in long-haired rabbits

SIGNS
Historical Findings
• Pruritus—none to severe, depending on the individual's response to infestation
• Alopecia; focal, most commonly in the intrascapular region
• May have a history of dental disease, obesity, or underlying musculoskeletal disease

Physical Examination Findings
• Scaling—important clinical sign. Copious amounts of large, white flakes of scale can sometimes be seen. Most often focal, beginning in intrascapular region; most severe in chronically infested and debilitated animals
• Lesions—dorsal location, either between the scapulae or at the tail base most common. Some rabbits are unable to adequately groom these regions, especially obese animals or those with dental or musculoskeletal disease. Lesions are most commonly found in these regions, where lack of grooming allows the proliferation of mites.
• Underlying skin irritation may be minimal. With chronic infestation, the underlying skin may become thickened.
• Alopecia occurs often with excessive scaling. Alopecia is generally located centrally within the lesion.

• A thorough oral examination is indicated to rule out underlying dental disease.
• Ataxia, proprioceptive deficits, paresis; pain on palpation or manipulation of the spine in rabbits may be found in rabbits with underlying musculoskeletal disease.
• Facial or perineal dermatitis may be seen in rabbits with underlying skeletal disease due to an inability to groom these areas or inability to maintain a normal posture while urinating.
• Obesity—often an underlying cause; obese rabbits have difficulty reaching key areas while grooming

CAUSES AND RISK FACTORS
• Healthy rabbits with normal grooming habits usually remain asymptomatic.
• Disease is seen in young animals and those with underlying diseases that prohibit adequate grooming.
• Inability to adequately reach the intrascapular or tail base regions for grooming contributes to the formation of lesions in these areas.
• Common sources of initial infestation—pet stores, animal shelters, breeders

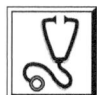

DIAGNOSIS

DIFFERENTIAL DIAGNOSIS
• *Cheyletiella* sp. or *Leporacarus gibbus* should be considered in every animal that has scaling, with or without pruritus.
• Also consider ear mite (*Psoroptes cuniculi*) infestation, *Sarcoptes scabiei* and *Notoedres cati* (rare), flea hypersensitivity dermatitis, dermatophytes, and bacterial dermatitis.
• In some rabbits, lack of grooming alone may cause an accumulation of scale, without the presence of mites.
• Injection reactions—The intrascapular region is a common site of subcutaneous injections (including fluids); reaction to irritating substances (especially enrofloxacin) in this region may mimic Cheyletiellosis.
• Sebaceous adenitis—very similar appearance; usually begins around the head and neck; often associated with thymoma or thymic lymphoma. Differentiate by skin biopsy and histologic examination.

CBC/BIOCHEMISTRY/URINALYSIS
N/A

OTHER LABORATORY TESTS
N/A

IMAGING
Spinal or dental radiographs to rule out underlying dental or musculoskeletal disease

DIAGNOSTIC PROCEDURES
• Examination of epidermal debris—very effective in diagnosing infestation
• Collection of debris—flea combing (most effective), skin scraping, and acetate tape preparation
• *Cheyletiella* sp. and *Leporacarus gibbus* mites are large—scales and hair may be examined under low magnification; staining is not necessary.
• A thorough physical examination, including oral, orthopedic, and neurologic, is indicated to rule out the underlying cause.
• Skin biopsy with histological examination to rule out sebaceous adenitis

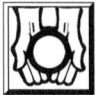

TREATMENT
• Identification and correction of any underlying disease that may prohibit normal grooming behavior are essential to ensure complete resolution.
• Treat all animals in the household, including cats and dogs.
• Comb daily with a fine-toothed comb to remove the scale.
• Bathing is also effective in removing scale, but is often difficult to perform on rabbits. Bathing can be dangerous in nervous rabbits and inexperienced owners and can result in spinal fractures and excessive chilling.
• Environmental treatment—adult mites can live up to 10 days off of the host.
• Combs, brushes, and grooming utensils—discard or thoroughly disinfect before reuse
• Zoonotic lesions (*Cheyletiella* sp.)—self-limiting after eradication of the mites from household animals

MEDICATIONS
DRUG(S) OF CHOICE
Treat all affected animals.
• Ivermectin—usually effective—0.2–0.4 mg/kg SC q8–14d for 2–3 doses
• Selamectin (Revolution, Pfizer)—(12 mg/kg) applied topically q30d)
• Imidacloprid/moxidectin (Advantage-Multi, Bayer)—10 mg/kg (i) + 1 mg/kg (m) topically q30d; one treatment is usually effective.

ALTERNATIVE DRUGS
• Carbaryl powder (5%) is applied topically once weekly; may also be used to treat the environment

(CONTINUED) CHEYLETIELLOSIS AND *L. GIBBUS* (FUR MITES)

CONTRAINDICATIONS/POSSIBLE INTERACTIONS
• Do not use fipronil fipronil (Frontline, Merial) on rabbits—fatal toxicity reported
• Do not use flea collars on rabbits.
• Do not use organophosphate-containing products on rabbits.
• Do not use straight permethrin sprays or spot-ons on rabbits.
• Topical flea preparation for use in dogs and cats, such as permethrins and pyrethrins, is less effective and may be toxic to rabbits.
• Use extreme caution when dipping or bathing rabbits due to the high risk of skeletal fractures and excessive chilling with inexperienced owners.
• Topical medications may be accidentally ingested during self-grooming or grooming by cage mates.

FOLLOW-UP
• Treatment failure necessitates reevaluation for other causes of pruritus and scaling.
• Reinfestation may indicate contact with an asymptomatic carrier or the presence of an unidentified source of mites (e.g., untreated bedding).

MISCELLANEOUS

ZOONOTIC POTENTIAL
A pruritic papular rash may develop in areas of contact with the pet. This rash is self-limiting with the removal of the mite from pets and the environment.

SYNONYMS
Fur mites
Walking dandruff

SEE ALSO
Dermatophytosis
Ear mites
Fleas and flea infestation
Pruritus

ABBREVIATIONS
N/A

Suggested Reading
d'Ovidio D, Santoro F. *Leporacarus gibbus* infestation in client-owned rabbits and their owners. Vet Dermatol 2014;25:46–e17.
Hansen O, Gall Y, Pfister K et al. Efficacy of a formulation containing imidacloprid and moxidectin against naturally acquired ear mite infestations (*Psoroptes cuniculi*) in Rabbits. Intern J Appl Res Vet Med 2005;3(4):281–286.

Meredith A. Dermatoses. In: Meredith A, Lord B, eds. BSAVA Manual of Rabbit Medicine. Gloucester: British Small Animal Veterinary Association, 2014:255–263.
Palmerio BS, Roberts H. Clinical approach to dermatologic disease in exotic animals. Vet Clin North Am Exot Anim Pract 2013;16(3):523–577.
Rosen LB. Dermatologic manifestations of zoonotic diseases in exotic animals. J Exotic Pet Med 2011;20:9–13.
Snook TS, White SD, Hawkins MG et al. Skin diseases in pet rabbits: a retrospective study of 334 cases seen at the University of California at Davis, USA (1984–2004). Vet Dermatol 2013;24:613–618.
Varga M. Skin diseases. In: Varga M, ed. Textbook of Rabbit Medicine, 2nd ed. Elsiver, 2014:224–248.
Varga M, Patterson S. Dermatologic diseases of rabbits. In: Quesenberry KE, Carpenter JW, eds. Ferrets, Rabbits and Rodents, (4th ed.). Clinical Medicine and Surgery. 2021, St. Louis: Saunders, 2020:220–222.

Author Barbara Oglesbee, DVM, Dipl ABVP (Avian)

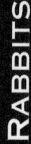

CHEEK TEETH (PREMOLAR AND MOLAR) MALOCCLUSION

BASICS

DEFINITION
• Cheek teeth elongation—occurs when normal occlusion and wear does not occur

ANATOMY AND PHYSIOLOGY
• Normal dentition: 6 incisor teeth, including 4 large primary (mandibular and maxillary) incisors and 2 smaller secondary maxillary incisors (or "peg teeth") located lingual to the primary maxillary incisors. Lack of canine teeth, with the presence of a large diastema between the incisor and the cheek teeth. Since the premolars and molars are anatomically similar and are aligned as one functional unit, they are referred to as cheek teeth. Cheek teeth consist of 3 maxillary premolars, 3 maxillary molars, 2 mandibular premolars, and 3 mandibular molars on each side, for a total of 22 cheek teeth and a total of 28 teeth.
• All teeth are elodont (open-rooted) and grow continuously throughout life, with growth originating from the germinal bud located at the apex of the tooth.
• The rate of normal wear should equal the rate of eruption. Normal wear requires proper occlusion with the opposing set of teeth, and a highly abrasive, fresh food diet to encourage proper movement of the mandible and grind coronal surfaces.

PATHOPHYSIOLOGY
• Malocclusion of the cheek teeth—can be due to congenital prognathism of the mandible/brachygnathim of the maxilla or acquired tooth elongation and malocclusion secondary to improper diet
• The cause of acquired cheek teeth elongation (acquired dental disease) is likely multifactorial and not completely known. The most significant contributing or exacerbating factor is diets that contain inadequate amounts of the coarse roughage material required to properly grind coronal surfaces. Malocclusion may also be an inherited or congenital defect.
• When erupted crowns (clinical crowns) are at a normal length, they will contact the opposing set of cheek teeth at an angle such that the teeth will wear normally. If normal wear does not occur and teeth overgrow, sharp spikes or spurs will often form, angling toward the tongue on the mandibular set and toward buccal mucosa on the maxillary set.
• Spikes on the cheek teeth can become very long and sharp—may penetrate into adjacent soft tissues. Secondary bacterial infections are common.
• Other common sequelae of excessive coronal elongation include longitudinal fractures, marked differences in coronal

length of adjacent teeth (step mouth), or an irregular occlusal plane (wave mouth).
• Cheek teeth that do not occlude normally will continue to elongate into the oral cavity until normal jaw tone arrests upward growth. At this point, pressure from the opposing set of cheek teeth will cause the reserve crowns of cheek teeth to grow in an apical direction (ventrally into the mandible, or upward into the maxilla) such that the apices intrude into cortical bone.
• Poor skull mineralization due to metabolic bone disease can also be a contributing factor, more or less predominant depending on individual patients.

SYSTEMS AFFECTED
• Oral cavity
• Ocular—involvement of the nasolacrimal duct (obstruction or dacyocystitis)
• Gastrointestinal—secondary functional stasis and related complications.
• Respiratory—chronic rhinitis following advanced dental disease of maxillary cheek teeth
• Musculoskeletal—weight loss, muscle wasting

GENETICS
More common in dwarf breeds due to flattened facial features

INCIDENCE/PREVALENCE
One of the most common presenting complaints in pet rabbits

GEOGRAPHIC DISTRIBUTION
N/A

SIGNALMENT
• Usually seen in middle-aged or older rabbits—acquired cheek tooth elongation
• Young animals—congenital malocclusion
• Dwarf and lop breeds—congenital malocclusion
• No breed or gender predilection for the acquired dental disease of the cheek teeth

SIGNS

General Comments
• Always perform a thorough oral examination under sedation or general anesthesia to examine the cheek teeth. Rabbits have a long, narrow mouth; the use of a directed light source, cheek dilators, mouth gag, or endoscope is needed to thoroughly examine the teeth. Significant cheek teeth apical abnormalities may be present despite normal-appearing crowns. Skull radiographs are required to identify apical (root) disorders.
• Owners sometimes notice incisor overgrowth first, as these teeth are readily visible. In many cases, rabbits with incisor overgrowth also have cheek teeth elongation and generalized dental disease.

Historical Findings
• A history of feeding diets deficient in coarse fiber hay; diets primarily consisting of pellets

• Preference for soft foods
• Anorexia or decreased appetite; often show an interest in food, but unable to eat; may be anorectic from pain with advanced disease
• Weight loss
• Ptyalism and moist dermatitis on the chin and dewlap
• Tooth grinding
• Epiphora
• Nasal discharge
• Facial asymmetry or exophthalmos in rabbits with periapical infections and abscesses
• Signs of pain—reluctance to move, depression, lethargy, hiding, hunched posture
• Unkempt hair coat, lack of grooming

Physical Examination Findings
Oral examination
• A thorough examination of the cheek teeth requires heavy sedation or general anesthesia and specialized equipment. A cursory examination using an otoscope for illumination and visualization is insufficient for rabbits with dental disease.
• A focused, directed light source and magnification will provide optimal visualization.
• Use a rabbit mouth gag and cheek dilators (Jorgensen Laboratories, Inc., Loveland, CO) to open the mouth and pull buccal tissues away from cheek teeth to allow adequate exposure. Use a cotton swab or tongue depressor to retract the tongue from lingual surfaces.
• Normal cheek teeth—coronal surfaces have small cusp
• Identify cheek teeth abnormalities—elongation, irregular coronal height, spikes, curved teeth, discolored teeth, longitudinal fractures, missing teeth, purulent exudate, odor, impacted food, oral ulceration, or abscesses
• Identify concurrent incisor abnormalities—overgrown incisors, horizontal ridges or grooves, malformation, discoloration, fractures, increased or decreased curvature, loose teeth
• Buccal or lingual mucosa and lip margins—ulceration, abrasions, secondary bacterial infection, or abscess formation if incisors or cheek teeth spikes have damaged soft tissues
• Significant cheek teeth apical abnormalities may be present despite normal-appearing crowns. Skull radiographs or advanced diagnostic imaging are required to identify apical and reserve crowns disorders.
Other findings
• Ptyalism causing secondary moist pyoderma and alopecia around the mouth, neck, and dewlap areas
• A scalloped edge or single bony protrusions may be palpable on the ventral rim of the mandible in rabbits in which the cheek teeth have intruded into and distorted surrounding bone.

(CONTINUED) CHEEK TEETH (PREMOLAR AND MOLAR) MALOCCLUSION

• Soft tissue swelling and abscesses most commonly located on the mandible or below the eye.
• Exophthalmos in rabbits with retrobulbar abscesses from periapical abscess arising from most caudal maxillary cheek teeth.
• Weight loss, emaciation
• Nasal discharge—chronic rhinitis following advanced dental disease of maxillary cheek teeth
• Ocular discharge—obstruction of the nasolacrimal duct; pressure on the eye from retrobulbar abscess or overgrown tooth roots
• Signs of gastrointestinal hypomotility—scant feces, intestinal pain, and soft stools

CAUSES
• Congenital skeletal malocclusion—most likely in dwarf or lop-eared breeds
• Acquired dental disease—multiple etiologies; inadequate fibrous, tough foods or foods containing silicates (grasses) to encourage proper mandibular motion and properly grind coronal surfaces; metabolic bone disease may play a role
• Trauma—longitudinal fractures of the cheek teeth, usually mandibular premolars

RISK FACTORS
• Feeding pelleted and mixed diets and simple carbohydrate treats
• Breeding rabbits with congenital malocclusion

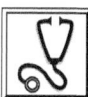

DIAGNOSIS
DIFFERENTIAL DIAGNOSIS
• For epiphora—upper respiratory tract disease, blocked nasolacrimal duct (exudate, stricture), primary ocular disease
• For ptyalism—wet dewlap from water bowls, oral trauma or non-odontogenic abscess, oral neoplasia (rare), swallowing disorders (rare)

CBC/BIOCHEMISTRY/URINALYSIS
Usually normal even when oral or facial abscess occur; may see abnormalities in liver enzymes in rabbits with hepatic lipidosis secondary to anorexia.

OTHER LABORATORY TESTS
N/A

IMAGING
Skull Radiographs
• Mandatory to identify the type and extent of dental disease, to plan treatment strategies, and to monitor progression of treatment.
• Perform under general anesthesia
• A standard set of five extraoral views are recommended for thorough assessment: lateral, ventro-dorsal, two lateral obliques, and rostro-caudal. Additional extraoral

oblique projections, as well as additional intraoral views may also be used.
• Early stage of dental disease—elongation of the reserve crowns and apices, apical deformities, loss of normal coronal occlusal pattern, mild radiolucency around reserve crowns, bone lysis
• Moderate to severe disease—curved teeth, widening of the interdental space, apical radiolucency and bony lysis, protrusion or penetration of the apices into surrounding cortical bone
• Periapical *abscess* infection—severe lysis of cortical bone; bony proliferation
• CT—superior to radiographs to evaluate the extent of dental disease and bony destruction

DIAGNOSTIC PROCEDURES
• Bacterial culture and sensitivity testing of affected tissue and/or exudate—aerobic and anaerobic bacteria. Growth more likely if wall or capsule is sampled; bacteria deep within exudate are often nonviable, culture results often yield no growth with anaerobic infections. Anaerobic infection is often presumed based on evidence derived from previous studies of odontogenic abscess in rabbits.
• Rabbits with epiphora—instill fluorescein stain into the affected eye to determine patency of the nasolacrimal duct or perform nasolacrimal duct irrigation.

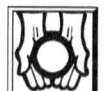

TREATMENT
APPROPRIATE HEALTH CARE
• Outpatient—patients with mild to moderate dental disease requiring coronal reduction
• Inpatient—patients with periapical or facial abscess, patients requiring extraction or debilitated patients

NURSING CARE
Keep fur around face clean and dry and shave where needed.

ACTIVITY
N/A

DIET
• It is absolutely imperative that the rabbit continues to eat during and following treatment. Many rabbits with dental disease will become anorexic. Rabbits may be reluctant to eat solid food following coronal reduction, extractions, or surgical treatment of abscesses. Anorexia will cause or exacerbate GI hypomotility, derangement of the gastrointestinal microflora, and overgrowth of intestinal bacterial pathogens.
• Syringe feed a gruel such as Critical Care for Herbivores (Oxbow Pet Products) or Emeraid Herbivore (Lafeber Company,

Cornell, IL), 10–15 mL/kg PO q8–12h. Larger volumes and more frequent feedings are often accepted; feed as much as the rabbit will readily accept. Alternatively, pellets can be ground and mixed with fresh greens, vegetable baby foods, water, or juice to form a gruel.
• High-carbohydrate, high-fat nutritional supplements are contraindicated.
• Return the rabbit to a solid food diet as soon as possible to encourage normal occlusion and wear. Increase the amount of tough, fibrous foods and foods containing abrasive silicates such as hay and wild grasses; avoid pelleted food and soft fruits or vegetables.
• Encourage oral fluid intake by offering fresh water or wetting leafy vegetables.

CLIENT EDUCATION
• Early tooth elongation may sometimes be corrected by sequential coronal reduction and diet change.
• By the time severe signs of cheek teeth elongation are noted, the disease is usually advanced. Lifelong treatment, consisting of periodic coronal reduction (teeth trimming), may be required, usually every 3–12 months.
• Rabbits with severe dental disease (apical abscesses and severe bony destruction) have a guarded prognosis for complete resolution. Most will require surgery (sometimes multiple surgeries) and multiple follow-up visits. Recurrences in other locations are common. Clients must be aware of the monetary and time investment.
• With severe disease, euthanasia may be the most humane option, especially in rabbits with intractable pain or those that cannot eat.

SURGICAL CONSIDERATIONS
Coronal Reduction of Cheek Teeth (Trimming)
• Trimming of spurs and sharp points alone will be of little benefit for most rabbits; in most cases, the crowns all of the cheek teeth are elongated and will need to be reduced to normal length.
• Always perform under general anesthesia.
• Use a focused, directed light source and magnification (e.g., lighted magnification loops).
• Adequate exposure of the teeth and protection of soft tissues are crucial. Use a rabbit mouth gag or the rabbit and rodent table retractor/restrainer (Veterinary Instrumentations, UK) and cheek dilators (Jorgensen Laboratories, Inc., Loveland, CO) to open the mouth and pull buccal tissues away from cheek teeth to allow adequate exposure. Protect soft tissues by using dental spatulas to protect the tongue and buccal tissues and a bur guard while trimming the teeth.

CHEEK TEETH (PREMOLAR AND MOLAR) MALOCCLUSION   (CONTINUED)

RABBITS

• Trim using a straight dental handpiece with an appropriate bur and bur guard to protect soft tissues. Burs with long shanks made specifically for use in rabbits are available. Alternatively, a dremel tool with a diamond bit or X-long Dental Bits (Veterinary Specialty Products, Inc, Shawnee, KS) can be used.

• Do not "float" the teeth with a rasp or file. These procedures can traumatize the teeth and gums and are generally insufficient for coronal reduction.

• Reducing the crowns to a normal length, combined with dietary correction, may realign occlusal surfaces, preventing or slowing elongation in some cases. However, owner compliance is essential.

Extraction of Cheek Teeth
• Indicated in rabbits with loose, fractured, significantly misdirected teeth, or apical abscesses.

• Because rabbits have very long, deeply embedded, and slightly curved reserve crown, extraction per os can be extremely time consuming and labor intensive compared with that of dogs and cats. If the germinal bud is not completely removed, the teeth may regrow. If the practitioner is not experienced with tooth extraction in rabbits, the author recommends referral to a veterinarian with special expertise whenever feasible.

MEDICATIONS
DRUG(S) OF CHOICE
Antibiotics
• Indicated in rabbits with periapical abscesses, after appropriate dental procedures. The choice of antibiotic is ideally based on results of culture and sensitivity testing. Most facial or dental abscesses are caused by anaerobic bacteria; use antibiotics effective against anaerobes such as azithromycin (15–30 mg/kg PO q24h); can be used alone or combined with metronidazole (20 mg/kg PO q12h). Alternatively, use penicillin G procaine (40,000–60,000 IU/kg SC q24h). Combine with topical or surgical treatment

• If aerobic bacteria are present, use broad-spectrum antibiotics such as enrofloxacin (10–20 mg/kg PO, SC, IM, IV q12h), marbofloxacin (5 mg/kg PO q24h), trimethoprim-sulfa (15–30 mg/kg PO q12h), or chloramphenicol (50 mg/kg PO q8h)

Acute Pain Management
• Buprenorphine (0.02–0.05 mg/kg PO, SQ, IM IV q8–12h); use preoperatively for extractions, coronal reduction, or surgical abscess treatment

• Butorphanol (0.1–0.5 mg/kg SQ, IM, IV q4–6h); may cause profound sedation at higher dosage; short acting

• Hydromorphone (0.1 mg/kg SC IM q2–4h) or oxymorphone (0.05–0.2 mg/kg SC IM q8–12h); use with caution; more than 1–2 doses may cause gastrointestinal stasis

• Meloxicam (1 mg/kg PO, SC, IM q24h)

• Carprofen (2–4 mg/kg PO, SC q12–24h)

Long-Term Pain Management
Nonsteroidal anti-inflammatories have been used for short- or long-term therapy to reduce pain and inflammation; meloxicam (1 mg/kg PO q24h); carprofen (2–4 mg/kg PO q12h)

CONTRAINDICATIONS
• Oral administration of most antibiotics effective against anaerobes will cause a fatal gastrointestinal dysbiosis in rabbits. Do not administer penicillins, macrolides, lincosamides, and cephalosporins by oral administration.

• Corticosteroids—associated with gastrointestinal ulceration and hemorrhage, delayed wound healing, and heightened susceptibility to infection; rabbits are very sensitive to the immunosuppressive effects of both topical and systemic corticosteroids; use may exacerbate subclinical bacterial infection

PRECAUTIONS
• Chloramphenicol—avoid human contact with chloramphenicol due to potential blood dyscrasia. Advise owners of potential risks.

• Meloxicam—use with caution in rabbits with compromised renal function

• Azithromycin—use with caution due to risk of enteric dysbiosis

POSSIBLE INTERACTIONS
N/A

ALTERNATIVE DRUGS
N/A

FOLLOW-UP
PATIENT MONITORING
• Reevaluate, and trim as needed, every 3–12 months, depending on the severity of the disease. Evaluate the entire oral cavity with each recheck and repeat skull radiographs periodically to monitor progression.

• Monitor for signs of apical abscess or invasion of the tooth roots into surrounding bone (epiphora, nasal discharge, facial swelling).

PREVENTION/AVOIDANCE
• In rabbits with acquired dental disease of cheek teeth, prevention is not possible once clinical signs of malocclusion are

present. With periodic coronal reduction and appropriate diet, progression of disease may be arrested, but treatment is often lifelong.

• To help prevent acquired dental disease, discontinue or limit the feeding of pellets and avoid soft fruits or vegetables; provide adequate tough, fibrous foods such as hay and grasses to encourage normal wear of teeth.

• Do not breed rabbits with congenital malocclusion.

POSSIBLE COMPLICATIONS
• Periapical abscesses, recurrence, chronic pain, or extensive tissue destruction warranting euthanasia due to poor quality of life

• Hepatic lipidosis with prolonged anorexia

• Chronic epiphora with nasolacrimal duct occlusion

EXPECTED COURSE AND PROGNOSIS
• Mild to moderate disease—good prognosis with regular trimming and appropriate diet change, depending on severity of disease; lifelong trimming may be required

• Periapical or facial abscesses, osteomyelitis—depend on the severity of bone involvement and location. Rabbits with multiple or severe apical abscesses have a guarded prognosis. Euthanasia may be warranted with severe or advanced disease, especially in rabbits that are painful or cannot eat.

MISCELLANEOUS
ASSOCIATED CONDITIONS
N/A

AGE-RELATED FACTORS
N/A

ZOONOTIC POTENTIAL
N/A

PREGNANCY/FERTILITY/BREEDING
N/A

SYNONYMS
N/A

SEE ALSO
Abscessation
Epiphora
Incisor malocclusion and overgrowth

Suggested Reading
Capello V. Dental diseases. In: Capello V, Lennox AM, eds. Rabbit and Rodent Dentistry Handbook. Lake Worth: Zoological Education Network, 2005:113–138.

(CONTINUED) CHEEK TEETH (PREMOLAR AND MOLAR) MALOCCLUSION

Capello V. Intraoral treatment of dental disease in pet rabbits. Vet Clin Exot Anim 2016;19(3):783–798.

Easson W. Tooth extraction. In: Harcourt-Brown F, Chitty J, eds. BSAVA Manual of Rabbit Surgery, Dentistry, and Imaging. Gloucester, UK: BSAVA, 2013:370–381.

Harcourt-Brown F. Treatment of dental problems: principles and options. In: Harcourt-Brown F, Chitty J, eds. BSAVA Manual of Rabbit Surgery, Dentistry, and Imaging. Gloucester, UK: BSAVA, 2013:349–369.

Lennox AM, Capello V, Legendre LF. Small mammal dentistry. In: Quesenberry KE, Carpenter JW, eds. Ferrets, Rabbits and Rodents, (4th ed). Clinical Medicine and Surgery. 2021, St. Louis: Saunders, 2020:514–535.

Varga M. Dental Disease. Textbook of Rabbit Medicine, 2nd ed. London, UK: Elsevier, 2014:203–248.

Authors Barbara Oglesbee, DVM, and Vittorio Capello, DVM

CLOSTRIDIAL ENTERITIS/ENTEROTOXICOSIS

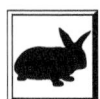

BASICS

OVERVIEW
• Clostridial enteritis and enterotoxicosis are common in rabbits. In weanlings or severely affected adults, acute diarrhea and death due to enterotoxin production by *Clostridium spiroforme* are most common. In adult rabbits, cecal dysbiosis characterized by anorexia, gut pain, and ± cecal diarrhea is more common.
• Young, weanling-aged rabbits (5–8 weeks old) are more susceptible to acute enteric colonization *by C. spiroforme*. This is often due to incomplete enteric colonization by commensal bacteria, allowing rapid colonization by *C. spiroforme* from the environment. This may cause either a profuse, watery diarrhea, or mucoid diarrhea (mucoid enteritis) with cecal colonization. Disease is acute and severe, usually causing death in 1–3 days.
• Older rabbits require one or more predisposing factors to allow enteric colonization of clostridial species. These include stress, inappropriate diet, and inappropriate antibiotic use. Colonization may cause acute, often fatal disease as seen in neonates, or a milder form of disease that is more amenable to treatment.
• In any aged rabbit, diets containing high-carbohydrate concentrations provide excessive fermentable products that can lead to an overgrowth of intestinal clostridia organisms.
• In any aged rabbit, antibiotic usage can cause severe, acute, often fatal diarrhea due to alteration of normal gut flora. Diarrhea follows the oral administration of antibiotics that are effective against gram-positive bacteria and some gram-negative anaerobes, such as lincomycin, clindamycin, erythromycin, ampicillin, amoxicillin, cephalosporins, and penicillins. These antibiotics should not be orally administered to rabbits.

SIGNALMENT
• Post-weaning-age rabbits (2–4 months old)—acute, often fatal diarrhea
• Adult rabbits—variable severity of disease, generally cecal dysbiosis

SIGNS
General Comments
Two clinical syndromes are seen, depending on the age of the rabbit and severity of infection. Both syndromes are potentially life-threatening due to enterotoxemia

In weanlings and severely affected adults: acute, watery or mucoid diarrhea, dehydration, and death

In adults: Cecal dysbiosis with gas distention of cecum, GI stasis, or cecal diarrhea

Historical Findings
• In young weanling rabbits: most common—acute onset of watery or mucoid diarrhea. Initially, most appear bright and alert; Depression, anorexia, and listlessness typically begin 1–2 days post onset of diarrhea.
• In adults—with severe infection (carbohydrate overload, inappropriate antibiotic use)—acute onset of mucoid or watery diarrhea, anorexia, listlessness, abdominal pain, and cecal distention
• In adults with mild/moderate cecal dysbiosis—diarrhea, often intermixed with normal, formed fecal pellets. The "diarrhea" is actually abnormal cecotrophs often described as soft and sticky with foul odor
• In adults—history of diets low in roughage and long-stemmed hay, diets high in simple carbohydrates (pellets, excessive fruits, or sugary vegetables, cereal "treats," grain or bread products, sugars; infrequent feeding of good-quality long-stemmed hay and fresh leafy greens)
• In adults—history of recent stress or fearful stimuli (surgery, hospitalization, illness, diet change, and environmental change)
• History of antibiotic use—especially those with a gram-positive spectrum (clindamycin, lincomycin, penicillin, ampicillin, and amoxicillin)

Physical Examination Findings
Cecal dysbiosis (adults)
• Abdominal discomfort and gas- or fluid-filled cecum may be detected on palpation.
• May be evidence of fecal staining of perineum
• Abdominal pain characterized by a hunched posture, reluctance to move, or bruxism palpation
• May have cecal diarrhea (soft, odiferous, intermixed with formed fecal pellets) or lack of fecal production with concurrent GI stasis
Acute, severe diarrhea; enterotoxic shock
• Dehydration and depression
• Abdominal distension; tympanic abdomen
• Tachycardia or bradycardia
• Tachypnea
• Signs of hypovolemic shock (e.g., pale mucous membranes, decreased capillary refill time, and weak pulses)
• Hypothermia

CAUSES AND RISK FACTORS
• Low-fiber, high-carbohydrate diet
• Improper antibiotic use
• Stress
• Dirty environment

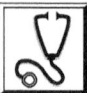

DIAGNOSIS

DIFFERENTIAL DIAGNOSIS
• Diarrhea should be differentiated from normal cecotrophs (or night feces). Cecotrophs are formed in the cecum, are rich in nutrients, and are usually eliminated once daily. Normally, cecotrophs are not observed because rabbits will ingest them directly from the rectum. Occasionally rabbits are unable to consume the cecotroph, which may be mistaken for diarrhea. Cecotrophs are dark in color, have a soft consistency and strong odor, tend to clump together, and are covered with mucous.
• Weaning-aged rabbits—coccidia, other bacterial pathogens (*E. coli*, *Salmonella*), *Clostridium pilforme* (Tyzzer's disease), rotavirus, coronavirus
• Adult rabbits—other bacterial pathogens (*E. coli*, *Salmonella*, and *Campylobacter*), intussusception, partial GI tract obstruction; chronic disease can sometimes present as acute diarrhea; systemic illness may also result in diarrhea as a secondary event

CBC/BIOCHEMISTRY/URINALYSIS
• With mild/moderate diarrhea—usually normal
• With acute severe diarrhea, expect hemogram abnormalities consistent with acute inflammation and hemoconcentration/shock; electrolyte abnormalities and acid–base alterations may be seen.

OTHER LABORATORY TESTS
• Fecal direct examination and fecal flotation to rule out coccidia in young or debilitated patients

Microbiology
• Anaerobic fecal cultures may demonstrate clostridia organisms, but usually are negative due to the fastidious nature of the organism.

Fecal Cytology
• Large numbers of large, gram-positive, endospore-producing bacteria can sometimes be found in the feces in a patient with diarrhea.
• Gram's stain—preferred stain; allows identification of concurrent overgrowth of gram-negative bacteria.
• Must differentiate from normal enteric yeast (Saccharomyces spp. or Cyniclomyces guttulatus)—much larger than enteric bacteria

IMAGING
• Gas-filled intestines, colon, and cecum common in rabbits with acute diarrhea and clostridial enterotoxicosis
• In adult rabbits with cecal dybiosis—stomach contains ingesta, and cecum is distended with varying amounts of gas

PATHOLOGIC FINDINGS

With cecal dysbiosis—grossly dilated, thin-walled cecum ± intestines with erythemia and serosal petechia; diffuse congestion of lungs and liver is common in those dying from enterotoxemia

With acute diarrhea—fluid, gas, and/or mucus-filled intestines and colon; diffuse necrosis of mucosa on histologic examination

TREATMENT

APPROPRIATE HEALTH CARE

• Most adult rabbits with mild, intermittent cecal diarrhea that are otherwise bright and alert can be treated as outpatients. These patients can usually be successfully treated with oral or subcutaneous fluid therapy, dietary modification, and metronidazole.
• Hospitalize rabbits with signs of anorexia, lethargy, depression, dehydration, or shock, even if diarrhea is mild or absent.
• Hospitalize when diarrhea is profuse, resulting in dehydration and electrolyte imbalance.
• Hospitalize rabbits under 5 months of age, regardless of the severity of diarrhea.

NURSING CARE

• Fluid therapy and correction of electrolyte imbalances are the mainstay of treatment in most cases.
• Can give crystalloid fluid therapy subcutaneously or intravenously, as required
• Aim to return the patient to proper hydration status (over 12–24 hours) and replace any ongoing losses. Maintenance fluid requirements are estimated at 60 mL/kg/day for large breeds, 80–100 mL/kg/day for small or dwarf breeds
• Severe volume depletion can occur with acute diarrhea; aggressive shock fluid therapy may be necessary.
• Fluid choice for intravenous or subcutaneous use should take into consideration the electrolyte and hydration status.

DIET

• It is imperative that the rabbit continues to eat during and following treatment. Continued anorexia will exacerbate GI motility disorders, cause further derangement of the gastrointestinal microflora, and cause overgrowth of intestinal bacterial pathogens.
• Offer a good-quality grass hay and high-quality commercial pellets.
• Withhold greens, vegetables, fruits, and treats as these foods are higher in carbohydrates and can exacerbate clostridial overgrowth.

• If the patient refuses these foods, syringe-feed a gruel such as Critical Care for Herbivores (Oxbow Pet Products) or Emerald Herbivore (Lafeber Company, Cornell, IL) 10–15 mL/kg PO q6–8h. Larger volumes and more frequent feedings are often accepted; feed as much as the rabbit will readily accept.
• The diet should be permanently modified to include sufficient amounts of long-stemmed hay. Offer high-quality, fresh hay (grass or timothy preferred; commercially available hay cubes are not sufficient) and an assortment of washed, fresh leafy greens. These foods should always constitute the bulk of the diet. Pellets should be limited (¼ cup pellets per 5 lbs body weight), and foods high in simple carbohydrates prohibited or limited to the occasional treat.

CLIENT EDUCATION

• Warn owners of rabbits with acute, severe diarrhea that death may occur despite treatment. Young rabbits (<6 months old) and rabbits showing signs of depression and shock also have a guarded to grave prognosis with treatment, even when diarrhea is mild.
• Emphasize the importance of permanent dietary modification (described above) in surviving rabbits.

MEDICATIONS

DRUG(S) OF CHOICE

• Antibiotics for *Clostridium* spp.—metronidazole (20 mg/kg PO, 5–20 mg/kg IV q12h); rabbits that are anorexic and/or those with watery diarrhea should receive this IV
• Cholestyramine (Questran, Bristol Laboratories) is an ion exchange resin that binds clostridial iota toxins. A dose of 2 g in 20 mL of water q24h for up to 18–21 days has been reported to be effective in preventing death in rabbits with acute clostridia enterotoxemia.
• Analgesics such as meloxicam (1 mg/kg SC, IM q24h), hydromorphone (0.05–0.2 mg/kg IV, IM, SC q6–8h), buprenorphine (0.02–0.05 mg/kg SC, IM, IV q8–12h), or carprofen (2–4 mg/kg SC, IV q24h) are essential to treatment of rabbits with GI hypomotility. Intestinal pain, either postoperative or from gas distention and ileus, impairs mobility and decreases appetite, and may severely inhibit recovery.
• Maropitant (2 mg/kg SC q24h) is used to treat visceral pain. Combine this with one of the analgesics listed above.

CONTRAINDICATIONS

• Antibiotics that are generally effective against clostridia in other species, such as clindamycin or penicillins, are contraindicated in rabbits. Do not administer

lincomycin, clindamycin, erythromycin, ampicillin, amoxicillin cephalosporins, or penicillins orally to rabbits.
• Do not use corticosteroids in the treatment of shock in rabbits.

PRECAUTIONS

Meloxicam or other NSAIDs—use with caution in rabbits with compromised renal function; monitor renal values

FOLLOW-UP

PATIENT MONITORING

• Response to therapy supports the diagnosis; repeat diagnostics are rarely necessary.
• Monitor body temperature, appetite, hydration, fecal production, and serial fecal gram stain for a positive response to therapy.

PREVENTION/AVOIDANCE

• Feed a diet consisting of good-quality grass hay, fresh leafy greens, and minimal pellets. Avoid fruit, vegetable, or cereal-based treats.
• Do not administer oral antibiotics that are primarily gram positive in spectrum (penicillins, cephalosporins, macrolides, and lincosamides)
• Infection in weaning-aged rabbits is associated with environmental contamination; disinfection is difficult.

POSSIBLE COMPLICATIONS

Death due to continued diarrhea, dehydration, electrolyte imbalances, or enterotoxic shock

EXPECTED COURSE AND PROGNOSIS

• Most animals with mild to moderate disease respond well to therapy.
• The prognosis is fair to grave in rabbits with acute, severe watery diarrhea, depending on the extent of infection and time elapsed to treatment.
• The prognosis is poor to grave in rabbits demonstrating signs of shock (hypothermia, bradycardia, and lethargy) and in young rabbits (<6 months old), even with treatment.

MISCELLANEOUS

ASSOCIATED CONDITIONS

Frequently other enteric disease

AGE-RELATED FACTORS

• Young, weaning-aged rabbits develop acute, watery diarrhea, or mucoid diarrhea; prognosis is poorer.
• Adult rabbits require predisposing factors (poor diet, stress, and antibiotic usage) and usually carry a better prognosis.

CLOSTRIDIAL ENTERITIS/ENTEROTOXICOSIS (CONTINUED)

ZOONOTIC POTENTIAL
Unknown

SYNONYMS
Enterotoxemia
Mucoid enteritis

SEE ALSO
Diarrhea, acute
Gastrointestinal hypomotility and gastrointestinal stasis

ABBREVIATIONS
GI = gastrointestinal
NSAID = nonsteroidal anti-inflammatory drug

Suggested Reading
Bays TB. Geriatric care of rabbits, guinea pigs, and chinchillas. Vet Clin Exot Anim 2020;23:567–593.
DeCubellis J. Common emergencies in rabbits, guinea pigs, and chinchillas. Vet Clin Exot Anim 2016;19: 411–429.
Hartcourt-Brown F. Digestive system disease. In: Meredith A, Lord B eds. BSAVA Manual of Rabbit Medicine. Gloucester: British Small Animal Veterinary Association, 2014. pp 168–190
Oglesbee B, Lord B. Gastrointestinal diseases of rabbits. In: Quesenberry KE, Carpenter JW, eds. Ferrets, Rabbits and Rodents, (4th ed). Clinical Medicine and Surgery. 2021, St. Louis: Saunders, 2020:174–187.
Varga M. Digestive disorders. In: Varga M, ed. Textbook of Rabbit Medicine, 2nd ed. London, UK: Elsevier, 2014:303–349.
Author Barbara Oglesbee, DVM

BASICS

OVERVIEW
- An enteric or hepatic infection, associated with *Eimeria* spp.
- Twelve different species of coccidia have been reported to infect the rabbit intestinal tract. Many rabbits that are clinically ill have more than one species of coccidia.
- Only one species, *E. stiedae*, infects the liver.
- Strictly host specific (i.e., no cross-transmission)
- Asexual multiplication occurs in intestinal epithelial cells, causing cellular damage and disease.
- Following asexual multiplication, sexual reproduction results in shedding of oocysts in the feces.
- Oocysts become infective 1–4 days after shedding in the feces.
- Immunity naturally develops against each *Eimeria* species following exposure; however, no cross-protection exists. Therefore, young or adult rabbits can become clinically ill following exposure to a species that they have not developed immunity to.
- Disease severity depends on the species of *Eimeria*, the immune status of the rabbit (including age and environmental stressors), and the number of oocysts ingested.
- Infection may predispose to bacterial enteritis

SIGNALMENT
- Usually a disease of young and recently weaned rabbits, 4–16 weeks of age
- Rarely causes clinical disease in adult rabbits. Clinical disease is possible with adults that are debilitated or exposed to large numbers of oocyst.

SIGNS
- Often asymptomatic, especially in adults
- Watery-to-mucoid, sometimes blood-tinged, diarrhea with intestinal form
- Tenesmus with intestinal form
- Weakness, lethargy, dehydration, and weight loss with heavy infection in young rabbits.
- May cause intussusception and death
- With hepatic involvement—Jaundice and abdominal distention in a 4–16-week-old rabbit is nearly pathognomonic

CAUSES AND RISK FACTORS
- Infected rabbits contaminating environment with oocysts of *Eimeria* spp. Screen rabbits for shedding of oocysts and separate those shedding from young rabbits.
- Poor sanitation—Sanitation is critical for control, especially within rabbit colonies or

multirabbit homes. Routinely disinfect food bowls, water bottles, and cages.
- Stress, debility, and concurrent disease may predispose older animals to infection.

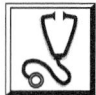

DIAGNOSIS

DIFFERENTIAL DIAGNOSIS
- Blood and mucus in stool is also seen with bacterial dysbiosis, especially overgrowth of clostridia or *E. coli*; differentiate by fecal cytology
- Fluid, blood-tinged or mucous-covered diarrhea—usually associated with coccidia or bacterial enteritis in young rabbits; in older rabbits—associated with bacterial enteritis following antibiotic use, severe systemic illness, or intestinal obstruction/intussusception; less often coccidia
- Anorexia, hepatomegaly, and jaundice—consider other causes of hepatitis, hepatic lipidosis, or neoplasia

CBC/BIOCHEMISTRY/URINALYSIS
- Usually normal; may be hemoconcentrated if dehydrated
- Increased liver enzymes (even mild increases can be significant) or bilirubin with hepatic involvement

OTHER LABORATORY TESTS
N/A

IMAGING
- Hepatomegaly or ascites may be seen in rabbits with hepatic coccidiosis; often unremarkable in rabbits with intestinal coccidiosis

DIAGNOSTIC PROCEDURES
- Fecal examination for oocysts using routine fecal floatation or fecal wet mount
- Oocysts range in size from 15 to 40 μm
- Organisms can be identified from intestinal mucosal scrapings on necropsy, or on histologic examination of intestinal specimens.

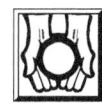

TREATMENT
- Usually treated as an outpatient
- Patients with moderate to severe disease usually require hospitalization and 24-hour care for parenteral medication and fluid therapy.

NURSING CARE
- Fluid therapy and correction of electrolyte imbalances are the mainstay of treatment in most cases.
- Can give crystalloid fluid therapy subcutaneously or intravenously, as required

- Aim to return the patient to proper hydration status (over 12–24 hours) and replace any ongoing losses. Maintenance fluid requirements are estimated at 60 mL/kg/day for large breeds, 80–100 mL/kg/day for small or dwarf breeds.
- Severe volume depletion can occur with acute diarrhea; aggressive shock fluid therapy may be necessary.
- Fluid choice for intravenous or subcutaneous use should take into consideration the electrolyte and hydration status.

DIET
- It is imperative that the rabbit continues to eat during and following treatment. Continued anorexia will exacerbate gastrointestinal motility disorders, causing further derangement of the gastrointestinal microflora and overgrowth of intestinal bacterial pathogens.
- Offer a large selection of fresh, moistened greens such as cilantro, romaine lettuce, parsley, carrot tops, dandelion greens, spinach, collard greens, and good-quality grass hay. Many rabbits will begin to eat these foods, even if they were previously anorectic. Also, offer the rabbit's normal pelleted diet.
- If the patient refuses these foods, syringe-feed a gruel such as Critical Care for Herbivores (Oxbow Pet Products) or Emeraid Herbivore (Lafeber Company, Cornell, IL) 10–15 mL/kg PO q6–8h. Larger volumes and more frequent feedings are often accepted; feed as much as the rabbit will accept.
- The diet should be permanently modified to include sufficient amounts of indigestible fiber. Pellets should be limited to ¼ cup per 5 lbs body weight per day.

MEDICATIONS

DRUG(S) OF CHOICE
- Coccidiostats—only slow multiplication of organisms until host immunity develops. Adult animals with subclinical infections will develop natural immunity and may not require medication.
- Sulfadimethoxine—50 mg/kg PO first dose, then 25 mg/kg q24h for 10–20 days
- Trimethoprim/sulfamethoxazole—30 mg/kg PO q12h for 10 days
- Toltrazuril (25 mg/kg daily for 2 days PO, then repeat after 5 days)
- Antibiotics—if secondary gastrointestinal bacterial infection is present. If indicated, use only broad-spectrum antibiotics such as trimethoprim sulfa (30 mg/kg PO q12h) or enrofloxacin (10–20 mg/kg PO, SC, IM q12–24h). For *Clostridium* spp.—metronidazole (5–20 mg/kg PO, IV q12h)

CONTRAINDICATIONS

The use of antibiotics that are primarily gram-positive in spectrum is contraindicated in rabbits. Use of these antibiotics will suppress the growth of commensal flora, allowing overgrowth of enteric pathogens, and often a fatal enterotoxemia. Do not orally administer lincomycin, clindamycin, erythromycin, ampicillin, amoxicillin cephalosporins, or penicillins.

ALTERNATE DRUGS

• Coccidia—amprolium 9.6% in drinking water (0.5 mL per 500 mL); not consistently effective as water consumption is variable
• Ponazuril has been anecdotally used (20–50 mg/kg PO q24h). Safety and efficacy are unknown.

FOLLOW-UP

Fecal examination for oocysts 1–2 weeks following treatment

EXPECTED COURSE AND PROGNOSIS

• Intestinal coccidiosis—variable, depending on severity of infection, dehydration, age, and immunocompetency of the rabbit
• Hepatic coccidiosis—guarded to poor in rabbits with heavy infestation and signs of hepatic failure on presentation

MISCELLANEOUS

AGE-RELATED FACTORS

Disease usually in young patients 4–16 weeks old

SEE ALSO

Clostridial enteritis/enterotoxicosis
Diarrhea, acute

ABBREVIATIONS

N/A

Suggested Reading

Bays TB. Geriatric care of rabbits, guinea pigs, and chinchillas. Vet Clin Exot Anim 2020;23:567–593.

DeCubellis J. Common emergencies in rabbits, guinea pigs, and chinchillas. Vet Clin Exot Anim 2016;19:411–429.

Hartcourt-Brown F. Digestive system disease. In: Meredith A, Lord B, eds. BSAVA Manual of Rabbit Medicine. Gloucester: British Small Animal Veterinary Association, 2014:168–190.

Oglesbee B, Lord B. Gastrointestinal diseases of rabbits. In: Quesenberry KE, Carpenter JW, eds. Ferrets, Rabbits and Rodents, (4th ed). Clinical Medicine and Surgery. 2021, St. Louis: Saunders, 2020:174–187.

Varga M. Digestive disorders. In: Varga M, ed. Textbook of Rabbit Medicine, 2nd ed. London, UK: Elsevier, 2014:303–349.

Author Barbara Oglesbee, DVM, DABVP (Avian)

CONGESTIVE HEART FAILURE

BASICS

DEFINITION
• Left-sided congestive heart failure (L-CHF)—failure of the left side of the heart to advance blood at a sufficient rate to meet the metabolic needs of the patient or to prevent blood from pooling within the pulmonary venous circulation
• Right-sided congestive heart failure (R-CHF)—failure of the right side of the heart to advance blood at a sufficient rate to meet the metabolic needs of the patient or to prevent blood from pooling within the systemic venous circulation

PATHOPHYSIOLOGY
• CHF in rabbits may be due to cardiomyopathy, tricuspid or mitral insufficiency, and less commonly, congenital heart disease.
• Rabbits have limited collateral myocardial circulation and may therefore be more prone to myocardial ischemia.
• L-CHF—low cardiac output may cause lethargy, exercise intolerance, or syncope. High hydrostatic pressure causes leakage of fluid from pulmonary venous circulation into pulmonary interstitium and alveoli resulting in pulmonary edema.
• R-CHF—high hydrostatic pressure leads to leakage of fluid from venous circulation into the pleural and peritoneal space and interstitium of peripheral tissue. When fluid leakage exceeds the ability of lymphatics to drain the affected areas, pleural effusion, ascites, and peripheral edema develop.

SYSTEMS AFFECTED
All organ systems can be affected by either poor delivery of blood or the effects of passive congestion from backup of venous blood.

INCIDENCE/PREVALENCE
Although anecdotally reported as common, only a few published case reports exist. True incidence is unknown.

SIGNALMENT
• Little information available
• Dilated cardiomyopathy may be more common in giant breeds.
• Atherosclerosis is reported most often in New Zealand White—often bred for research purposes.
• CHF in pet rabbits—published case reports in smaller breeds (<2 kg)
• Incidence increases with age

SIGNS
Historical Findings
• Weakness, lethargy, exercise intolerance

• Anorexia or inappetence, weight loss
• Dyspnea or tachypnea
• Syncope or episodes of collapse
• Abdominal distension with ascites

Physical Examination Findings
L-CHF
• Inspiratory and expiratory dyspnea when the animal has pulmonary edema
• Pulmonary crackles and wheezes
• Prolonged capillary refill time
• Possible murmur
• Possible arrhythmia (normal heart rate is 180–330 beats/min)
• Weak, irregular pulses
R-CHF
• Hepatomegaly
• Ascites rarely seen
• Possible murmur
• Muffled heart sounds if the animal has pleural or pericardial effusion
• Rapid, shallow respiration if the animal has pleural effusion

CAUSES AND RISK FACTORS
• Idiopathic cardiomyopathy—most commonly reported cause
• Myocarditis secondary to *Pasteurella multocida*, *Salmonella* sp., coronavirus, or *Encephalitozoon cuniculi*
• Mitral valve insufficiency secondary to endocardiosis reported
• Aortic insufficiency
• Ventricular septal defect anecdotally reported, other congenital defects have not been reported

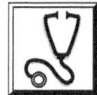

DIAGNOSIS

DIFFERENTIAL DIAGNOSIS
• Must differentiate from other causes of dyspnea and weakness; requires a complete diagnostic workup, including CBC, biochemistry profile, thoracocentesis or abdominocentesis with fluid analysis, and thoracic and abdominal ultrasound
• Dyspnea—rhinitis/sinusitis (rabbits are obligate nasal breathers), primary pulmonary disease (abscess, pneumonia), and thymoma (most common); other neoplasia (primary lung tumors, metastatic neoplasia); trauma resulting in diaphragmatic hernia, pulmonary hemorrhage, pneumothorax; airway obstruction due to foreign body or laryngeal edema
• Pleural effusion—thymoma or lymphoma, other neoplasia, abscess
• Ascites—consider end-stage liver disease, ruptured bladder, peritonitis, abdominal neoplasia, and abdominal hemorrhage

CBC/BIOCHEMISTRY/URINALYSIS
• CBC usually normal
• Mild to moderately high alanine transaminase, aspartate transaminase, and serum alkaline phosphatase with R-CHF
• Prerenal azotemia in some animals

OTHER LABORATORY TESTS
• Cytologic examination of pleural fluid

IMAGING
Radiographic Findings
• Generalized cardiomegaly—bear in mind that the thoracic cavity is smaller in rabbits compared with other mammals, and the heart may be large relative to thoracic cage.
• Soft tissue density cranial to heart—normal and often indistinguishable from the cranial border of the heart due to thymus (does not regress in rabbits) and intrathoracic fat
• Pulmonary edema (L-CHF) or pleural effusion or both in some animals
• Hepatomegaly may be seen in R-CHF.

Echocardiography
• Echocardiography is the diagnostic modality of choice to differentiate forms of cardiomyopathy, cardiac masses, pericardial effusion, and valvular insufficiency

DIAGNOSTIC PROCEDURES
Electrocardiographic Findings
• Respiratory sinus arrhythmias are not normal findings in rabbits.
• The ECG of normal rabbits differs from the feline ECG in that p, R, and T waves are shorter in lead II.
• Both ventricular and supraventricular arrhythmias can be seen.
• May show atrial or ventricular enlargement patterns.

Pleural Effusion Analysis
• Pleural effusion typically is a modified transudate with total protein less than 4.0 g/dL and nucleated cell counts of less than 2500/mL (these values have been extrapolated from other mammalian species to be used as a guideline). Analysis of the pleural effusion is important to rule out other causes of pleural effusion; can be both diagnostic and therapeutic

PATHOLOGIC FINDINGS
Cardiac findings vary with disease.

TREATMENT

APPROPRIATE HEALTH CARE
• Severely dyspneic, weak, or anorectic rabbits in congestive heart failure should be treated as inpatients.

CONGESTIVE HEART FAILURE　　(CONTINUED)

• Mildly affected animals can be treated as outpatients.

NURSING CARE
• Supplemental oxygen therapy is extremely important for dyspneic rabbits. Face mask delivery of oxygen can be very stressful to rabbits; oxygen cage should be used if available.
• Minimize handling of critically dyspneic animals. Stress can kill!
• Thoracocentesis is both therapeutic and diagnostic. If there is significant pleural effusion, drain each hemithorax with a 20-gauge butterfly catheter after the rabbit is stable enough to be handled. Sedation is necessary.
• If hypothermic, external heat (incubator or heating pad) is recommended. Monitor temperature carefully, as rabbits are extremely sensitive to heat stress.

ACTIVITY
Restrict activity

DIET
• If the patient refuses food, syringe-feed a gruel such as Critical Care for Herbivores (Oxbow Pet Products) or Emeraid Herbivore (Lafeber Company, Cornell, IL) 10–15 mL/kg PO q6–8h. Alternatively, pellets can be ground and mixed with fresh greens, vegetable baby foods, water, or juice to form a gruel.
• Encourage oral fluid intake by offering fresh water from multiple sources, wetting leafy vegetables

CLIENT EDUCATION
CHF is not curable and will progress.

SURGICAL CONSIDERATIONS
N/A

MEDICATIONS
DRUG(S) OF CHOICE
Diuretics
• Furosemide is recommended at the lowest effective dose to eliminate pulmonary edema and pleural effusion. If the rabbit is in fulminant cardiac failure, administer furosemide at 1–4 mg/kg q8–12h IM or IV. Initially, furosemide should be administered parenterally. Long-term therapy should be continued at a dose of 1–4 mg/kg q8–12h PO.
• Predisposes the patient to dehydration, prerenal azotemia, and electrolyte disturbances

ACE Inhibitors
• Benazepril (0.25–0.5 mg/kg PO q24h) or Enalapril (0.25–0.5 mg/kg PO q24h)

Positive Inotropes
Pimobendan (0.1–0.3 mg/kg PO q12h–24h) sensitizes calcium channels, resulting in arterial dilation and increased myocardial contractility and increasing afterload.

Digoxin
• Digoxin is used in animals with dilated cardiomyopathy or mitral or tricuspid regurgitation at a dose of 0.005–0.01 mg/kg PO q24–48h. Use the low end of dosage range initially and increased gradually. Monitor for signs of digoxin toxicity (anorexia); monitor serum digoxin concentrations.

Venodilators
• Nitroglycerin (2% ointment) 1/16–1/8 inch applied topically to the inner pinna can be used in conjunction with diuretics in the acute management of congestive heart failure to further reduce preload. Nitroglycerin may lower the dose of furosemide and is particularly useful in patients with hypothermia or dehydration.

Other Medications
Beta-blockers may be beneficial in patients with hypertropic cardiomyopathy; doses have not been reported in rabbits; extrapolate from cat or ferret doses. Beneficial effects may include slowing of sinus rate, correcting atrial, and ventricular arrhythmias. Role in asymptomatic patients unresolved

CONTRAINDICATIONS
Positive inotropic drugs should be avoided in patients with HCM.

PRECAUTIONS
• Anecdotal reports of anorexia with enalapril administration. If anorexia occurs, decrease the dosage and/or frequency of administration.
• ACE inhibitors and digoxin must be used cautiously in patients with renal disease.
• Overzealous diuretic therapy may cause dehydration and hypokalemia.

POSSIBLE INTERACTIONS
• The use of a calcium channel blocker in combination with a beta-blocker should be avoided as clinically significant bradyarrhythmias can develop in other small animals and are likely to also occur in rabbits.
• Combination of high-dose diuretics and ACE inhibitor may alter renal perfusion and cause azotemia.

ALTERNATIVE DRUGS
• Other vasodilators, including hydralazine, may be used instead of or in addition to an ACE inhibitor. Dosages have been anecdotally extrapolated from feline dosages; however, their use is not widespread, and

efficacy and safety are unknown (beware of hypotension).
• Other beta-blockers, such as atenolol, carvedilol, or metoprolol, can be used instead of propranolol to help control ventricular response rate in atrial fibrillation. Dosages have been anecdotally extrapolated from feline dosages; however, their use is not widespread, and efficacy and safety are unknown.

FOLLOW-UP
PATIENT MONITORING
• Monitor radiographs, echocardiography, renal status, electrolytes, hydration, respiratory rate and effort, heart rate, body weight, and abdominal girth.
• If azotemia develops, reduce the dosage of diuretic. If azotemia persists and the animal is also on an ACE inhibitor, reduce or discontinue the ACE inhibitor. Use digoxin with caution if azotemia develops.
• Monitor ECG if arrhythmias are suspected.
• Check digoxin concentration periodically. The therapeutic range (as extrapolated from dogs and cats) is between 1 and 2 ng/dL 8–12 hours postpill.

PREVENTION/AVOIDANCE
Minimize stress and exercise in patients with heart disease.

POSSIBLE COMPLICATIONS
• Sudden death due to arrhythmias
• Iatrogenic problems associated with medical management (see above)

EXPECTED COURSE AND PROGNOSIS
Prognosis varies with underlying cause; little data exist for rabbits

MISCELLANEOUS
ASSOCIATED CONDITIONS
N/A

AGE-RELATED FACTORS
Degenerative heart conditions are generally seen in middle-aged to old animals

ZOONOTIC POTENTIAL
N/A

PREGNANCY/FERTILITY/BREEDING
N/A

SYNONYMS
N/A

RABBITS

SEE ALSO

Dyspnea and tachypnea

ABBREVIATIONS

ACE = angiotensin-converting enzyme
HCM = hypertrophic cardiomyopathy
L-CHF = left-sided congestive heart failure
R-CHF = right-sided congestive heart failure

Suggested Reading

Capello V, Lennox AM. Diagnostic imaging of the respiratory system in exotic companion mammals. Vet Clin Exot Anim 2011;14:369–389.

Fitzgerald BC, Dias S, Martorell J. Cardiovascular drugs in avian, small mammal, and reptile medicine. Vet Clin Exot Anim 2018;21:399–442.

Lennox AM, Gladden JN. Emergency and critical care of small mammals. In: Quesenberry KE, Carpenter JW, eds. Ferrets, Rabbits and Rodents, (4th ed). Clinical Medicine and Surgery. 2021, St. Louis: Saunders, 2020:595–608.

Orcutt CJ, Malakoff RJ. Cardiovascular disorders. In: Quesenberry KE, Carpenter JW, eds. Ferrets, Rabbits and Rodents, (4th ed). Clinical Medicine and Surgery. St. Louis: Saunders, 2020:250–256.

Author Barbara Oglesbee, DVM, DABVP (Avian)

CONJUNCTIVITIS

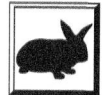

BASICS

DEFINITION
Inflammation of the conjunctiva, the vascularized mucous membrane that covers the anterior portion of the globe (bulbar portion) and lines the lids and third eyelid (palpebral portion)

PATHOPHYSIOLOGY
• Primary—infectious; environmental; KCS
• Secondary to an underlying ocular or systemic disease—tooth root disorders; glaucoma; uveitis; neoplasia

SYSTEMS AFFECTED
• Ophthalmic—ocular with occasional lid involvement (e.g., blepharoconjunctivitis)
• Respiratory
• Oral cavity

GENETICS
N/A

INCIDENCE/PREVALENCE
Common

GEOGRAPHIC DISTRIBUTION
N/A

SIGNALMENT
• Acquired cheek tooth elongation causing blockage of nasolacrimal duct or intrusion into the retrobulbar space—usually seen in middle-aged rabbits
• Young animals—congenital tooth malocclusion, congenital eyelid deformities
• Dwarf and lop breeds—congenital tooth malocclusion
• Dwarf and Himalayan breeds—glaucoma more common
• Rex and New Zealand White breeds—entropion and trichiasis more common

Mean Age and Range
N/A

Predominant Sex
N/A

SIGNS

Historical Signs
• History of previous treatment for dental disease
• History of nasal discharge or previous upper respiratory infection
• Facial asymmetry, masses, or exophthalmos in rabbits with tooth root abscesses
• Signs of pain—reluctance to move, depression, lethargy, hiding, hunched posture in rabbits with painful ocular conditions or underlying dental disease
• Unilateral or bilateral alopecia, crusts, matted fur in periocular area, cheeks, and/or nasal rostrum

Physical Examination Findings
• Blepharospasm
• Conjunctival hyperemia
• Ocular discharge—serous, mucoid, or mucopurulent
• Thick white exudate accumulation in medial canthus in rabbits with dacryocystitis
• Corneal ulcers associated with dacryocystitis are usually superficial and ventrally located; ulcers secondary to exposure keratitis are usually central and may be superficial or deep.
• Chemosis
• Excessive conjunctival tissue—may partially or completely occlude the cornea
• Facial pyoderma—alopecia, erythema, matted fur in periocular area, cheeks, and/or nasal rostrum; due to constant moisture in rabbits with epiphora
• A thorough examination of the oral cavity is indicated in every rabbit with epiphora to rule out dental disease. Use of an otoscope or speculum may be useful in identifying severe abnormalities; however, many problems will be missed by using this method alone. A thorough examination of the cheek teeth requires heavy sedation or general anesthesia and specialized equipment. Use a focused, directed light source and magnification (or a rigid endoscope, if available) to provide optimal visualization. Use a rodent mouth gag and cheek dilators (Jorgensen Laboratories, Inc., Loveland, CO) to open the mouth and pull buccal tissues away from teeth surfaces to allow adequate exposure. Use a cotton swab or tongue depressor to retract tongue from lingual surfaces.
• Identify cheek teeth elongation, irregular crown height, spikes, curved teeth, tooth discoloration, tooth mobility, missing teeth, purulent exudate, oral ulceration, or abscesses.
• Incisors—may see overgrowth, horizontal ridges or grooves, malformation, discoloration, fractures, malocclusion, increased or decreased curvature
• Significant tooth root abnormalities may be present despite normal-appearing crowns. Skull radiographs are required to identify apical disorders.

CAUSES AND RISK FACTORS

Bacterial
• Primary condition (i.e., not secondary to another condition such as dacryocystitis or KCS)—rare
• Secondary infection—*Staphylococcus* spp., *Pseudomonas* spp., *Moraxella* spp., *Pasteurella multocida*, *Niesseria* spp., and *Bordetella* spp. frequently cultured. Usually secondary to URI or dental disease.

Secondary to Adnexal Disease
• Secondary to obstruction of the outflow of the nasolacrimal duct or dacryocystitis—one of the most common causes—obstruction usually secondary to tooth root elongation or tooth root abscesses blocking outflow; or due to the presence of thick exudates, scarring, or inflammation of the duct from chronic upper respiratory tract infection.
• Secondary to maxillary tooth root elongation—irritation to the globe due to impingement of overgrown tooth roots or abscesses into the retrobulbar space
• Lid diseases (e.g., entropion, ectropion, and blepharitis) and lash diseases (e.g., distichiasis, ectopic cilia) or trichiasis from periocular fur—may lead to clinical signs of conjunctivitis
• Aqueous tear film deficiency (KCS); often secondary to facial nerve paralysis

Secondary to Trauma or Environmental Causes
• Conjunctival foreign body—hay or other bedding material common offenders
• Irritation—dust, chemicals, or ophthalmic medications

Secondary to Other Ocular Diseases
• Ulcerative keratitis—trauma most common; exposure keratitis following anesthesia, facial nerve paralysis; corneal abrasion in rabbits with torticollis
• Anterior uveitis—most commonly bacterial or encephalitozoon cuniculi
• Glaucoma

Viral Causes
Myxomatosis—unusual

Neoplastic Causes
Tumors involving conjunctiva—rare

Aberrant Conjunctival Overgrowth
• Cause not completely understood; may occur as congenital disorder, idiopathic or secondary to trauma or inflammation. Conjunctiva grows from the limbus, is nonadherent to the cornea, and may completely cover the cornea; does not appear to be painful, may not be associated with significant inflammation in patients with congenital or idiopathic disease

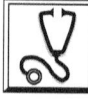

DIAGNOSIS

DIFFERENTIAL DIAGNOSIS
• Primary—must distinguish from condition that is secondary to other ocular diseases
• Differentiate between conjunctival vessels (freely mobile and will blanch with sympathomimetic) and episcleral (deep) vessels (immobile and do not blanch with

sympathomimetics) because episcleral congestion indicates intraocular disease, whereas conjunctival hyperemia may be a sign of primary conjunctivitis or intraocular disease.
• Unilateral condition with ocular pain (blepharospasm)—usually indicates a tooth root disorder, foreign body, or corneal injury
• Chronic, bilateral condition—usually due to chronic upper respiratory tract infection (scarring, inflammation of duct), can indicate a congenital problem; bilateral tooth root disorders also seen
• Acute, bilateral condition with severe eyelid edema—consider myxomatosis
• Facial pain, swelling, nasal discharge, or sneezing—seen with tooth root elongation or abscess; may indicate nasal or sinus infection; may indicate obstruction from neoplasm
• White discharge confined to the medial canthus—usually indicates dacryocystitis

CBC/BIOCHEMISTRY/URINALYSIS
Normal, except with systemic disease

OTHER LABORATORY TESTS
N/A

IMAGING
• Skull radiographs are mandatory to identify dental disease, nasal, sinus, or maxillary bone lesions and, if present, to plan treatment strategies and to monitor progression of treatment.
• Perform under general anesthesia
• Five views are recommended for thorough assessment, including ventral-dorsal, lateral, two lateral obliques, and rostral-caudal.
• CT or MRI—superior to radiographs to localize nasolacrimal duct obstruction and characterize associated lesions
• Orbital ultrasonography—helpful in defining retrobulbar abscess or neoplasia and extent of the lesion
• Dacryocystorhinography—radiopaque contrast material to help localize nasolacrimal duct obstruction

DIAGNOSTIC PROCEDURES
• Complete ophthalmic examination
• Schirmer tear test—rule out KCS. Average values reported as 5 mm/min; however, even lower values can be seen in normal rabbits. KCS defined as lower than the normal STT value in conjunction with keratoconjunctivitis
• Fluorescein stain—rule out ulcerative keratitis; test for nasolacrimal function and patency, dye flows through the nasolacrimal system and reaches the external nares in approximately 10 seconds in normal rabbits.
• Intraocular pressures—rule out glaucoma (normal values 10–20 mmHg with applanation tonometry)

• Examine for signs of anterior uveitis (e.g., hypotony, aqueous flare, and miosis).
• Thorough adnexal examination—rule out lid abnormalities, lash abnormalities, and foreign bodies in cul-de-sacs or under nictitans.
• Perform a nasolacrimal flush—rule out nasolacrimal disease; may dislodge foreign material. Topical administration of an ophthalmic anesthetic is generally sufficient for this procedure; nervous rabbits may require mild sedation. Rabbits have only a single nasolacrimal punctum located in the ventral eyelid at the medial canthus. A 23-gauge lacrimal cannula or a 24-gauge Teflon intravenous catheter can be used to flush the duct. Irrigation will generally produce a thick white exudate from the nasal meatus.
• Aerobic bacterial culture and sensitivity—consider with mucopurulent discharge; ideally specimens taken before anything is placed in the eye (e.g., topical anesthetic, fluorescein, and flush) to prevent inhibition or dilution of bacterial growth; not routinely indicated for KCS and a mucopurulent discharge (secondary bacterial overgrowth almost certain). Often, only normal organisms are isolated (*Bacillus subtilis*, *Staphylococcus aureus*, and *Bordetella* spp.).
• Conjunctival cytology—may reveal a cause (rare); may see degenerate neutrophils and intracytoplasmic bacteria, which indicate bacterial infection
• Conjunctival biopsy—may be useful with mass lesions and immune-mediated disease; may help with chronic disease for which a definitive diagnosis has not been made
• Rhinoscopy—with or without biopsy or bacterial culture; may be indicated if previous tests suggest a nasal or sinus lesion

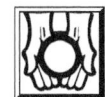

TREATMENT
APPROPRIATE HEALTH CARE
Primary—often outpatient
　Secondary to other diseases (e.g., tooth root elongation or abscess)—may require hospitalization while the underlying problem is diagnosed and treated
　Nasolacrimal duct irrigation—as described above if obstruction is diagnosed; if blocked or inflamed, irrigation of the duct often needs to be repeated, either daily for 2–3 consecutive days, or once every 3–4 days until irrigation produces a clear fluid. Failure to keep ducts patent may result in scarring or permanent obstruction.
　Keep fur around face clean and dry.

DIET
• Make sure that the rabbit continues to eat to avoid secondary gastrointestinal disorders.
• Rabbits with underlying dental disease—encourage normal occlusion and wear by increasing the amount of tough, fibrous foods and foods containing abrasive silicates such as hay and wild grasses; avoid pelleted food and soft fruits or vegetables.

CLIENT EDUCATION
• If copious discharge is noted, instruct the client to clean the eyes before giving topical treatments.
• If solutions and ointments are both prescribed, instruct the client to use the solution(s) before the ointment(s).
• If several solutions are prescribed, instruct the client to wait several minutes between treatments.
• Instruct the client to call for instructions if the condition worsens, which indicates that the condition may not be responsive or may be progressing or that the animal may be having an adverse reaction to a prescribed medication.
• Inform client that an Elizabethan collar should be placed on the patient if self-trauma occurs.

SURGICAL CONSIDERATIONS
• Irritation of the globe or blocked nasolacrimal duct due to elongation of cheek tooth roots—trimming of cheek teeth (coronal deduction) may correct or control progression of root elongation
• Tooth extraction—Because rabbits have very long, deeply embedded and curved tooth roots, extraction per os can be extremely time consuming and labor intensive compared with that of dogs and cats. If practitioner is not experienced with tooth extraction in rabbits, the author recommends referral to a veterinarian with special expertise whenever feasible.
• In rabbits with extensive tooth root abscesses, aggressive debridement is indicated, and special expertise may be required. Maxillary and retrobulbar abscesses can be particularly challenging. If practitioner is not experienced with facial abscesses in rabbits, the author recommends referral to a veterinarian with special expertise whenever feasible.
• Aberrant conjunctival overgrowth—surgical excision of the excessive conjunctiva; often only palliative, may reform; to minimize recurrence, the cut edge may be sutured to the limbus. Immunomodulating agents may prevent reformation.
• Chronic corneal ulcers not responsive to medical treatment—may require debridement of loose epithelium; punctate or grid keratotomy, or diamond burr

RABBITS

debridement, followed by collagen shield placement or conjunctival flap. Procedures are similar to those performed in cats and dogs.

MEDICATIONS

DRUG(S) OF CHOICE

Bacterial
- Based on bacterial culture and sensitivity results
- Initial treatment—broad-spectrum topical antibiotic or based on results of cytologic examination while waiting culture results; may try empirical treatment, performing a culture only if patient is refractory to treatment
- Topical triple antibiotic, chloramphenicol, gentamicin, ofloxacin, or ciprofloxacin—q6–12h, depending on severity
- Systemic antibiotics—indicated in rabbits with tooth root abscess or upper respiratory infection as the cause of conjunctivitis
- Topical nonsteroidal anti-inflammatory agents—0.5% ketorolac or 1% diclofenac may help reduce inflammation and irritation associated with nasolacrimal duct flushes.
- Artificial tears and lubricant ointments—for alleviation of keratoconjunctivitis sicca; must be applied frequently; only transiently relieve dryness
- Cyclosporine A has also been used in rabbits to increase tear production (0.2% ointment instilled q12h). Use with discretion—information on use in rabbits is limited; be aware that Schirmer tear test results can be very low in normal rabbits.

CONTRAINDICATIONS
- Topical corticosteroids—never use if the cornea retains fluorescein stain. Never use in the face of evidence of local or systemic bacterial infection.
- Oral administration of most antibiotics effective against anaerobes will cause a fatal gastrointestinal dysbiosis in rabbits. Do not administer penicillins, macrolides, lincosamides, and cephalosporins by oral administration.

PRECAUTIONS
- Topical corticosteroids or antibiotic-corticosteroid combinations—avoid; associated with gastrointestinal ulceration and hemorrhage, delayed wound healing, and heightened susceptibility to infection; rabbits are very sensitive to the immunosuppressive effects of both topical and systemic corticosteroids; use may exacerbate subclinical bacterial infection
- Aggressive flushing of the nasolacrimal duct may cause temporary swelling of the

periocular tissues. Swelling usually resolves within 12–48 hours.
- Topical aminoglycosides—may be irritating
- Topical antibiotics—may lead to enteric dysbiosis if excessive ingestion occurs during grooming.

POSSIBLE INTERACTIONS
N/A

ALTERNATIVE DRUGS
N/A

FOLLOW-UP

PATIENT MONITORING
Recheck shortly after beginning treatment (i.e., 5–7 days); then recheck as needed.

PREVENTION/AVOIDANCE
Treat any underlying disease that may be causing or exacerbating the condition (e.g., dental disease, eyelid disorders, and KCS) and assess husbandry for potential changes in bedding material, etc.

POSSIBLE COMPLICATIONS
N/A

EXPECTED COURSE AND PROGNOSIS
- Warn client that recurrence is common in patients with nasolacrimal obstruction. The nasolacrimal duct may become completely obliterated in rabbits with severe infection or tooth root disease (abscesses, elongation, neoplasia). Epiphora may be lifelong. Home management, including keeping the face clean and dry, is crucial to prevent secondary pyoderma. In many cases, acquisition of a second rabbit can beneficial if the second rabbit grooms discharges from the face.
- Rabbits with aberrant conjunctival overgrowth—recurrence is common; more than one surgery may be required
- Mild conjunctivitis as part of upper respiratory tract infection—prognosis is good, although recurrence is common
- Rabbits with cheek tooth root elongation—by the time clinical signs are noted, disease is usually advanced. Lifelong treatment consisting of periodic coronal reduction (teeth trimming) is required, usually every 1–3 months. Incisor extraction may be necessary if causing nasolacrimal duct blockage.
- Severe dental disease, especially those with tooth root abscesses and severe bony destruction, carry a guarded to poor prognosis for complete resolution. Most will require extensive surgery, sometimes multiple surgeries and multiple follow-up visits. Recurrences in the same or other locations are common. Clients must be aware of the monetary and time investment.

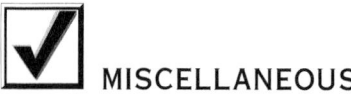

MISCELLANEOUS

ASSOCIATED CONDITIONS
- Moist dermatitis ventral to the medial canthus
- Nasal discharge
- Dental disease

AGE-RELATED FACTORS
N/A

ZOONOTIC POTENTIAL
N/A

PREGNANCY/FERTILITY/BREEDING
- Use systemic antibiotics and corticosteroids with caution, if at all, in pregnant animals.
- Consider absorption of topically applied medications; weigh benefits of treatment against possible complications.

SEE ALSO
Cheek teeth malocclusion
Incisor malocclusion
Abscesses
Red eye

ABBREVIATIONS
KCS = keratoconjunctivitis sicca
URI = upper respiratory infection

Suggested Reading
Bedard KM. Ocular surface disease of rabbits. Vet Clin Exot Anim 2019;922:1–14.
Florin M, Rusanen E, Haessig M et al. Clinical presentation, treatment, and outcome of dacryocystitis in rabbits: a retrospective study of 28 cases (2003–2007). Vet Ophthalmol 2009;12(6):350–356.
Lennox AM, Capello V, Legendre LF. Small mammal dentistry. In: Quesenberry KE, Carpenter JW, eds. Ferrets, Rabbits and Rodents, (4th ed). Clinical Medicine and Surgery. 2021, St. Louis: Saunders, 2020:514–535.
Van der Woerdt A. Ophthalmologic diseases of small mammals. In: Quesenberry KE, Carpenter JW, eds. Ferrets, Rabbits and Rodents, (4th ed). Clinical Medicine and Surgery. 2021, St. Louis: Saunders, 2020:583–594.
Williams DL. Laboratory animal ophthalmology. In: Gelatt KN, ed. Veterinary Ophthalmology, 3rd ed. Philadelphia: Lippincott, Williams & Wilkins, 1999:151–181.

Author Georgina Newbold, DVM, Dipl. ACVO

RABBITS

CONSTIPATION (LACK OF FECAL PRODUCTION)

BASICS

DEFINITION
• Constipation—infrequent, incomplete, or difficult defecation with passage of scant, small, hard, or dry fecal pellets
• Constipation and obstipation, in which the colon is filled with large amounts of hard, dry feces, generally does not occur in rabbits. The exception to this is a very distal colonic outflow obstruction (neoplasia, abscess, and stricture).
• Scant fecal production or lack of fecal production is usually the result of anorexia and/or gastrointestinal motility dysfunction (GI hypomotility/stasis).
• A sudden, complete lack of fecal output corresponding with sudden anorexia is seen in rabbits with acute, life-threatening disorders such as intestinal obstruction, liver lobe torsion, or sepsis.

PATHOPHYSIOLOGY
• Rabbits are hind-gut fermenters and are extremely sensitive to alterations in diet.
• Proper hind-gut fermentation and gastrointestinal tract motility are dependent on the ingestion of large amounts of roughage and long-stemmed hay. If adequate amounts of roughage are ingested and GI tract motility is normal, fur ingested as a result of normal grooming behavior will pass through the gastrointestinal tract with the ingesta.
• Diets that contain inadequate amounts of long-stemmed, coarse fiber (such as the feeding of only commercial pelleted food without hay or grasses) cause cecocolonic hypomotility that may lead to accumulation of ingesta in the stomach and lack of fecal production.
• Affected rabbits suddenly or gradually refuse food; as motility slows, ingesta accumulates proximal to the colon (stomach, cecum); fecal pellets become small and scant; water is removed from fecal pellets in the colon, making the fecal pellets drier than normal.
• Anorexia due to infectious or metabolic disease, pain, stress, or starvation may cause or exacerbate GI hypomotility.

SYSTEMS AFFECTED
Gastrointestinal

INCIDENCE/PREVALENCE
• GI hypomotility/stasis resulting in scant amounts of small, misshapen fecal pellets, or a lack of feces is one of the most common clinical problems seen in the rabbit.
• Sudden onset of complete lack of fecal production in a rabbit that was producing normal feces is equally common and seen in rabbits with an acute onset of life-threatening disorders.
• Other causes of constipation are uncommon.

SIGNALMENT
• Can occur in any aged rabbit
• No breed or gender predilections

SIGNS
Historical Findings
• The history is extremely useful in assessing the cause and urgency of disease.
  ○ An acute onset of cessation of fecal production and concurrent refusal all food, even favorite treats is characteristic of urgent, potentially life-threatening disease.
  ○ A more gradual onset of fecal pellets gradually become scant, dark in color, and small in size along with a progressively declining appetite over a period of hours to days is characteristic of GI hypomotility/stasis and can be due to a variety of causes
• Signs of pain can be subtle as rabbits are prey species and instinctively hide signs of disease. The most common sign of mild to moderate discomfort is hiding or appearing less social.
• Signs of more severe pain, such as teeth grinding, a hunched posture, and reluctance to move indicate more urgent and serious disease.

Physical Examination Findings
Abdominal Palpation and Gut Sounds
• Abdominal palpation is an extremely valuable tool in the diagnosis of gastrointestinal disorders.
• Even in rabbits that do not have access to food or those that are anorexic, the rabbit's stomach is never empty. Rabbits consume cecotrophs, formed in the cecum, and consumed from the rectum, which will fill the stomach even when food is not provided. If anorexic, stomach contents do not empty, either due to the onset of GI hypomotility/stasis or due to GI obstruction.
• The normal stomach should be easily deformable, feel soft and pliable, and does not remain pitted on compression.
• A firm, noncompliant stomach, or stomach contents that remain pitted on compression, is an abnormal finding and characteristic of GI hypomotility/GI stasis. In these rabbits, the colon is relatively empty or contains small, scant feces that may be difficult to detect on palpation.
• Fluid distension of the stomach occurs in rabbits with intestinal obstruction. The degree of distention depends on the region of intestinal obstruction and progresses with time. Rabbits cannot vomit, and eventually, the stomach can become severely fluid distended, turgid, and can even rupture. A distended, fluid-filled stomach is an emergency. In these rabbits, fecal production abruptly stops, and normal, round fecal pellets are palpable in the colon.
• Gas distension of the intestines and/or cecum is common in rabbits with GI tract disease such as GI hypomotility/stasis or cecal disorders.
• Occasionally, large amounts of hard, dry feces are palpable in the distal colon, similar to constipation or obstipation in dogs and cats. This may be caused by a very distal colonic outflow obstruction (neoplasia, abscess, stricture, or anal atresia).
• Auscultation of gut sounds is helpful. Decreased or absent gut sounds with little or no borborygmus is consistent with GI hypomotility. Increased gut sounds can be heard in the early phases of intestinal obstruction. In late stages of obstruction, gut sound decrease.
Other Exam Findings
• Signs of shock such as hypothemia (body temp <98° F), pale mucus membranes, lethargy, collapse, or stiff body posture are common with acute intestinal obstruction, and often accompany the finding of a fluid-distended stomach.
• Rabbits with other causes of anorexia may have a normal physical examination
• Auscultation of the thorax may reveal an underlying cause—look for cardiac murmurs, arrhythmias, or abnormal breath sounds.
• Other physical examination findings depend on the underlying cause; perform a complete physical examination, including a thorough oral exam.

CAUSES
Dietary and Environmental Causes
• GI hypomotility—may be caused by feeding diets with insufficient roughage such as grasses and long-stemmed hay and/or excessive simple carbohydrate content. Examples of improper diets include a diet consisting primarily of commercial pellets, especially those containing seeds, oats, or other high-carbohydrate treats; feeding of cereal products (bread, crackers, and breakfast cereals); feeding large amounts of fruits containing simple carbohydrates. Proper hind-gut fermentation and GI motility rely on large quantities of indigestible coarse fiber, as found in long-stemmed hay and grasses. Most commercial pelleted diets contain inadequate roughage, coarse fiber, and excessive calories. This high caloric content often contributes to obesity and hepatic lipidosis, both of which may exacerbate intestinal disease.
• Stress is a major cause of GI stasis/hypomotility. Stress may be the result of pain

such as trauma, surgery, or dental disease or from underlying metabolic disease. Even minor changes such as changes in the daily schedule, new animals or people in the household, or changes in environment such as hospitalization or boarding can cause GI hypomotility/stasis.
• Lack of exercise (cage confinement, obesity)—often a significant contributing factor
• Foreign material—ingestion of cloth (towels, carpeting, etc.) may cause GI tract obstruction; scoopable cat litters can cause severe cecal impaction.
• Change of environment—hospitalization, boarding; can cause significant stress and contribute to GI hypomotility

Drugs
• Anesthetic agents may cause or exacerbate GI hypomotility
• Anticholinergics
• Opioids
• Barium sulfate, kaopectolin, or sucralfate
• Diuretics

Mechanical Obstruction
• Intestinal foreign body—extremely common cause of sudden lack of fecal production. Most foreign bodies consist of a firm pellet of hair. This hair pellet is formed in the cecum and consumed inadvertently during normal cecotrophy. If the pellet is small, it may move through the GI tract causing few or no signs of discomfort. Larger pellets move slowly or not at all, leading to potentially life-threatening blockage of the intestinal tract (see bloat, intestinal obstruction). Occasionally, other foreign materials such as cloth or hard foods can become GI foreign bodies.
• Extraluminal—intra-abdominal adhesions (commonly develop post ovariohysterectomy), intra-abdominal abscess, and intrapelvic neoplasia,
• Colonic Disorders—intraluminal and intramural—colonic intussusception, colonic or rectal neoplasia or polyp, rectal stricture, rectal foreign body, and rectal prolapse.

Neuromuscular Disease
• Central nervous system—paraplegia, spinal trauma, intervertebral disk disease, and cerebral disease (lead toxicity, *Baylisascaris*, abscess, *Encephalitozoon cuniculi*)
• Peripheral nervous system—sacral nerve trauma

Painful Defecation
• Anorectal disease—abscess, perineal moist dermatitis, myiasis, anal stricture, rectal foreign body, and rectal prolapse
• Trauma—fractured pelvis, fractured limb, dislocated hip, perianal bite wound or laceration, and perineal abscess

Metabolic and Dental Disease
• Conditions that result in inappetence or anorexia may also cause GI hypomotility/stasis. Common causes of anorexia include dental disease (malocclusion, molar elongation, and tooth root abscesses), metabolic disease (renal disease, liver disease), pain (oral, trauma, postoperative pain, and adhesions), neoplasia (gastrointestinal, uterine), and toxins.
• Debility—general muscle weakness, dehydration, neoplasia

RISK FACTORS
• Diets with inadequate indigestible coarse fiber content
• Inactivity due to pain, obesity, and cage confinement
• Anesthesia and surgical procedures
• Unsupervised chewing behavior
• Underlying dental, gastrointestinal tract, or metabolic disease

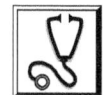

DIAGNOSIS
DIFFERENTIAL DIAGNOSIS
• Dyschezia and tenesmus—seen rarely and only in patients with colonic outflow obstruction (intussecption, strictures, and extraluminal compression)—may be mistaken for constipation by owners; associated with increased frequency of attempts to defecate, and frequent production of small amounts of feces containing blood and/or mucus
• Stranguria (e.g., caused by hypercalciuria)—may be mistaken for constipation by owners; can be associated with hematuria and abnormal findings on urinalysis; rabbits with calciuria may produce thick, sandlike urine that can be mistaken for feces

CBC/BIOCHEMISTRY/URINALYSIS
• These tests are often normal but can be used to differentiate GI hypomotility/stasis from GI obstruction. Rabbits with GI hypomotility/stasis are either normo- or mildly hyperglycemic (BG <300 mg/dL) with normal serum Na concentration, whereas those with GI obstruction are severely hyperglycemic, with BG ranging from 300 to 600 mg/dL and mildly hyponatremic Na <140 mEq/L)
• BUN and creatinine may be elevated due to dehydration or, in rabbits with obstruction, due to decreased renal perfusion
• PCV and TS elevation in dehydrated patients
• Serum ALT elevation in rabbits with liver disease, especially lipidosis
• May be used to identify underlying causes of GI hypomotility or anorexia

OTHER LABORATORY TESTS
N/A
IMAGING
• Due to the practice of cecotrophy, the stomach is never empty. Gastric contents are normally present and visible radiographically, even if the rabbit is not eating. The presence of ingesta in the stomach is a normal finding.
• Depending on the duration of disease, the stomach may appear to contain normal ingesta or, as disease progresses and fluid is pulled from the stomach, contents appear dense, and the stomach appears small and may have a halo of gas around the inspissated stomach contents. If the owners have been assist feeding, the stomach may be distended with food. Few or no feces are visible in the colon.
• This contrasts with the appearance of the stomach in rabbits with GI obstruction, where the stomach becomes fluid filled. Normal, round fecal pellets can be seen throughout the colon. Normal fecal pellets are spherical and consist of hay and air, so may be mistaken for air bubbles within the colon.
• Gas distension is sometimes seen throughout the intestinal tract, including the cecum in rabbits with GI hypomotility/stasis.
• Ultrasound can be helpful to identify foreign bodies, masses, or intussusception. However, use is often limited due to large volumes of intestinal gas.

DIAGNOSTIC PROCEDURES
• Contrast enema—in patients with suspected colonic disorders such as entrapment by postoperative adhesions, strictures, abscess, tumor, or intussusception. Barium can be administered via a soft red rubber catheter.

TREATMENT
APPROPRIATE HEALTH CARE
• Rabbits with acute onset of complete anorexia and lack of fecal production generally have serious, potentially life-threatening disease uch as intestinal obstruction, liver lobe torsion, and sepsis and require hospitalization.
• Rabbits with a gradual onset of anorexia and those still accepting some foods can often be treated on an outpatient basis. Those who have not eaten for more than 24 hours generally require hospitalization.

NURSING CARE
Fluid Therapy
• For patients with signs of shock or severe depression (seen with acute GI obstructions,

liver lobe torsion, and sepsis) balanced crystalloid fluids are indicated IV at a rate appropriate for shock or the level of dehydration. For patients in shock, fluids should be warmed.
• Intravenous fluids are indicated in patients that are severely dehydrated or depressed. Maintenance fluid requirements are estimated at 60 mL/kg/day for large breeds, 80–100 mL/kg/day for small or dwarf breeds.
• Fluid therapy is an essential component of the medical management of all anorexic patients. Administer both oral and parenteral fluids (except when GI obstruction is suspected). Oral fluid administration in the form of commercially available assist feeding slurries (see below) will aid in the rehydration of inspissated gastric contents. Mildly affected rabbits will usually respond well to oral and subcutaneous fluid administration, treatment with analgesics, intestinal motility modifiers, and dietary modification described below.

ACTIVITY
Depends on the cause of lack of fecal production

DIET
• Rabbits with suspected GI obstructions should not be assist or force fed. However, food should be offered free choice. Once the obstruction begins to move, affected rabbits usually begin to eat. This may serve as a prognostic indicator.
• If obstruction is ruled out, it is imperative that the rabbit begins eating as soon as possible. Continued anorexia will exacerbate GI hypomotility, causing further derangement of the gastrointestinal microflora and overgrowth of intestinal bacterial pathogens.
• Offer a large selection of fresh, moistened greens such as cilantro, romaine lettuce, parsley, carrot tops, dandelion greens, spinach, and collard greens and good-quality grass hay. Many rabbits will begin to eat these foods, even if they were previously anorectic. Also offer the rabbit's usual pelleted diet, as the initial goal is to get the rabbit to eat.
• If the patient refuses these foods, syringe feed a gruel such as Critical Care for Herbivores (Oxbow Pet Products) or Emeraid Herbivore (Lafeber Company, Cornell, IL) 10–15 mL/kg PO q6–8h. Larger volumes and more frequent feedings are often accepted; feed as much as the rabbit will readily accept. Alternatively, pellets can be ground and mixed with fresh greens, vegetable baby foods, water, or juice to form a gruel. If sufficient volumes of food are not accepted in this manner, nasogastric intubation is indicated.

• High-carbohydrate, high-fat nutritional supplements are contraindicated.
• The diet should be permanently modified to include sufficient amounts of roughage and long-stemmed hay.

CLIENT EDUCATION
• Discuss the importance of monitoring appetite in prey species such as rabbits. These species have a strong instinct to hide illness and may appear active and "normal" to owners unfamiliar with this concept. Stress the importance of seeking veterinary care any time the appetite is reduced. An acute onset of refusing all food and simultaneous lack of fecal output is an emergency.
• Discuss the importance of monitoring appetite in prey species such as rabbits. These species have a strong instinct to hide illness and may appear active and "normal" to owners unfamiliar with this concept. Stress the importance of seeking veterinary care any time the appetite is reduced. An acute onset of refusing all food and simultaneous lack of fecal output is an emergency.
• Advise owners to regularly monitor food consumption and fecal output and to seek veterinary attention with a noticeable decrease in either.
• Discuss the importance of feeding hay and high-quality pellets.

SURGICAL CONSIDERATIONS
Depend on the underlying cause

MEDICATIONS
Use parenteral medications in animals with severely compromised intestinal motility; oral medications may not be properly absorbed; begin oral medication when intestinal motility begins to return (fecal production, return of appetite, and radiographic evidence)

DRUG(S) OF CHOICE
• Treat the underlying cause
• Analgesics such as meloxicam (1 mg/kg SC, IM q24h), hydromorphone (0.05–0.2 mg/kg IV, IM, SC q6–8h), buprenorphine (0.02–0.05 mg/kg SC, IM, IV q8–12h), or carprofen (2–4 mg/kg SC, IV q24h) are essential to treatment of rabbits with GI hypomotility. Intestinal pain, either postoperative or from gas distention and ileus, impairs mobility and decreases appetite, and may severely inhibit recovery.
• Maropitant (2 mg/kg SC q24h) is used to treat visceral pain. Combine this with one of the analgesics listed above.
• Anorexia, regardless of the cause, causes or exacerbates GI tract hypomotility. Motility modifiers such as cisapride (0.5 mg/kg PO q8–12h), metoclopramide (0.5–1.0 mg/kg

PO, SC, IM q12h or 1–2 mg/kg/day IV as a constant rate infusion) are generally helpful in rabbits with GI hypomotility. These can also be used in rabbits with intraluminal intestinal obstruction as the most common GI foreign body is a compressed pellet of hair and the goal of therapy is to keep the hair pellet moving through the intestinal tract. Motility modifiers are contraindicated if an extraluminal obstruction is suspected.
• H$_2$-receptor antagonists may ameliorate or prevent gastric ulceration; cimetidine (5–10 mg/kg PO, SC, IM IV q6–12h); ranitidine (2 mg/kg SC, IV q24h or 2–5 mg/kg PO q12–24h).

CONTRAINDICATIONS
Assisted or force-feeding rabbits with ab suspected GI obstruction is contraindicated
• The use of gastrointestinal motility enhancers is contraindicated in rabbits with complete GI tract obstruction, due to the possibility of intestinal rupture.

PRECAUTIONS
• Meloxicam—use with caution in rabbits with compromised renal function
• Oral administration of any antibiotic may potentially cause enteric dysbiosis; discontinue use if diarrhea or anorexia occurs.

POSSIBLE INTERACTIONS
N/A

FOLLOW-UP
PATIENT MONITORING
• Monitor the appetite and production of fecal pellets. Rabbits that are successfully treated will regain a normal appetite and begin to produce normal volumes of feces. Initially, the fecal pellets are sometimes expelled and bound together with hair. Both the size/shape and number of fecal pellets should gradually improve.

PREVENTION/AVOIDANCE
• Strict feeding of diets containing adequate amounts of indigestible coarse fiber (long-stemmed hay) and low simple carbohydrate content along with access to fresh water will often prevent episodes.
• Be certain that postoperative patients are eating and passing feces prior to release.

POSSIBLE COMPLICATIONS
• Death due to gastric rupture or hypovolemic or endotoxic shock
• Postoperative GI stasis
• Overgrowth of bacterial pathogens

EXPECTED COURSE AND PROGNOSIS
• Varies with cause

CONSTIPATION (LACK OF FECAL PRODUCTION)   (CONTINUED)

MISCELLANEOUS

ASSOCIATED CONDITIONS
- See causes

AGE-RELATED FACTORS
Older rabbits on a poor diet are more likely to develop GI hypomotility.

ZOONOTIC POTENTIAL
N/A

PREGNANCY/FERTILITY/BREEDING
N/A

SYNONYMS
N/A

SEE ALSO
Cheek teeth (premolar and molar) malocclusion and elongation
Clostridial enteritis/enterotoxicosis

Diarrhea, chronic
Gastric dilation (bloat)
Gastrointestinal hypomotility and gastrointestinal stasis
Hypercalciuria and urolithiasis
Intestinal obstruction
Liver lobe torsion

ABBREVIATIONS
ALP = alkaline phosphatase
ALT = alanine aminotransferase
GI = gastrointestinal
PCV = packed cell volume
TS = total solids

Suggested Reading
Bays TB. Geriatric care of rabbits, guinea pigs, and chinchillas. Vet Clin Exot Anim 2020;23:567–593.
Debenham JJ, Brinchmann T, Sheen J, Vella D. Radiographic diagnosis of small intestinal obstruction in pet rabbits (*Oryctolagus cuniculus*): 63 cases. J Sm Anim Pract 2019;60:691–696.
DeCubellis J. Common emergencies in rabbits, guinea pigs, and chinchillas. Vet Clin Exot Anim 2016;19:411–429.
Hartcourt-Brown F. Digestive system disease. In: Meredith A, Lord B, eds. BSAVA Manual of Rabbit Medicine. Gloucester: British Small Animal Veterinary Association, 2014:168–190.
Oglesbee B, Lord B. Gastrointestinal diseases of rabbits. In: Quesenberry KE, Carpenter JW, eds. Ferrets, Rabbits and Rodents, (4th ed). Clinical Medicine and Surgery. 2021, St. Louis: Saunders, 2020:174–187.
Varga M. Digestive disorders. In: Varga M, ed. Textbook of Rabbit Medicine, 2nd ed. London, UK: Elsevier, 2014:303–349.

Author Barbara Oglesbee, DVM, DABVP (Avian)

BASICS

OVERVIEW
• A cutaneous fungal infection affecting the cornified regions of hair, nails, and occasionally the superficial layers of the skin
• Isolated organisms most commonly include Trichophyton mentagrophytes, *Microsporum canis*, and *M. gypseum*.
• Exposure to or contact with a dermatophyte does not necessarily result in an infection.
• Dermatophytes—grow in the keratinized layers of hair, nail, and skin; do not thrive in living tissue or persist in the presence of severe inflammation
• Rabbits can be asymptomatic carriers.

SIGNALMENT
• Uncommon disease of rabbits
• More common in young or debilitated animals

SIGNS

Historical Findings
• Lesions often begin as alopecia and dry, scaly skin.
• A history of previously confirmed infection or exposure to an infected animal or environment is a useful but not consistent finding.
• Variable pruritus

Physical Examination Findings
• Often begins as focal areas of alopecia
• Classic circular alopecia may be seen
• Scales, crust, erythema—variable, usually in more advanced cases
• Lesions most commonly begin on the face, head, and feet but may occur anywhere on the body.
• Variable pruritus

CAUSES AND RISK FACTORS
• Exposure to affected animals, including other rabbits, cats, and dogs
• Poor management practices—overcrowding, poor ventilation, dirty environment, and poor nutrition
• As in other species, immunocompromising diseases or immunosuppressive medications may predispose to infection, but this has not been clearly demonstrated in rabbits.

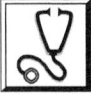

DIAGNOSIS

DIFFERENTIAL DIAGNOSIS
• Fur mites—*Cheyletiella* spp., *Leporacarus gibbus.* May be concurrent with dermatophyte infection. Fur mite lesions are usually located in the intrascapular or tail base region and associated with copious amounts of large white scale. Mites are readily identified in skin scrapes or acetate tape preparations under low magnification.
• Ear mites (*Psoroptes cuniculi*)—usually intensely pruritic; lesions typically localized to areas inside pinnae, surrounding ears, face, and neck. Skin thickening and exudative crusts form with chronic infestation. Mites can be seen with unaided eye or with microscopic examination under low power.
• Other ectoparasites—*Sarcoptes scabiei* and *Notoedres cati* rarely infest rabbits. Lesions are located around the head and neck and are intensely pruritic.
• Fleas—patchy alopecia usually appears in other areas in addition to head and feet; finding flea dirt will help to differentiate
• Demodicosis—extremely rare, may occur in association with corticosteriod use; mites will be present on skin scrape
• Contact dermatitis—usually ventral distribution of lesions; acute onset
• Barbering—by cagemates or self-inflicted—causes hair loss alone without pruritus, scale, or skin lesions
• Lack of grooming due to obesity or underlying dental or musculoskeletal disease may cause an accumulation of scale, especially in the intrascapular region.
• Injection site reactions, especially with irritating substances such as enrofloxacin, may cause alopecia and crusting

CBC/BIOCHEMISTRY/URINALYSIS
Not useful for diagnosis

OTHER LABORATORY TESTS
For the most common dermatophyte, *T. mentagrophytes,* an enzyme-linked immunosorbent assay (ELISA) is available

IMAGING
N/A

DIAGNOSTIC PROCEDURES

Fungal Culture
• Best means of confirming diagnosis
• Hair that exhibit a positive apple-green florescence under Wood's lamp examination are considered ideal candidates for culture (*M. canis* only).
• Pluck hair from the periphery of an alopecic area and do not use a random pattern.
• Test media—change to red when they becomes alkaline; dermatophytes typically produce this color during the early growing phase of their culture; saprophytes, which also produce this color, do so in the late growing phase; thus, it is important to examine DTM daily.
• Positive culture—indicates existence of a dermatophyte; however, it may have been there only transiently, as may occur when the culture is obtained from the feet, which are likely to come in contact with a geophilic dermatophyte.

Wood's Lamp Examination
• Not a very useful screening tool; many pathogenic dermatophytes do not fluoresce
• Skin Biopsy
• Can be helpful in confirming true invasion and infection
• Can be helpful to rule out other causes of alopecia

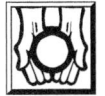

TREATMENT

APPROPRIATE HEALTH CARE
• May resolve spontaneously with no treatment
• Management of dermatophytosis must be directed at eradication of infectious material from affected animals, in-contact animals, and the environment.
• Environmental treatment is mandatory. Dilute bleach out (1:10) is a practical and relatively effective means of environmental decontamination. Gloves should be worn during cleaning.

NURSING CARE
Gloves should be worn when handling animals with this disease due to the zoonotic nature of the organism.

ACTIVITY
Isolate patient and in-contact animals during treatment as dermatophytosis is very infective and zoonotic.

CLIENT EDUCATION
• Dermatophytosis is zoonotic to humans and other household pets.
• Wear gloves when handling animal or in-contact animals and when cleaning environment.
• Clean the environment of the animal, including all living areas, clothing of the owners, toys, etc., using 10% bleach. Discard wooden cage materials and toys as they cannot be disinfected adequately.

SURGICAL CONSIDERATIONS
When obtaining biopsy specimens, care should be taken to avoid transfer of organisms to other noninfected sites via contaminated surgical instruments.

MEDICATIONS

DRUG(S) OF CHOICE
Regardless of therapy chosen, treatment should continue until two negative cultures 4 weeks apart are obtained. In general,

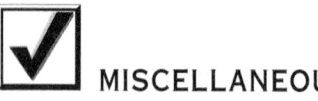

combination topical therapy with systemic antifungals is required for successful treatment of severe infections.

Topical Therapy

• Prior to topical therapy, the affected areas should be gently clipped to expose the affected skin, realizing that organisms might be moved to another location with the clipping. Thoroughly cleanse clipper blades after use. Always wear gloves when handling the patient.

• 2% chlorhexidine/2% miconazole shampoo—shown to have moderate success in cats and dogs; anecdotally used in rabbits, but efficacy and toxicity are unknown.

• Clotrimazole, ketoconazole, or miconazole creams or ointments may not be as effective, as they are not formulated to penetrate infected hair shafts and follicles.

Systemic Therapy

• Itraconazole (5–10 mg/kg PO q24h) for 30 days
• Terbinafine (10 mg/kg PO q24h)
• Fluconazole (5 mg/kg PO q24h)
• Griseofulvin (12.5–25 mg/kg PO q24h or divided q12h) for 4–6 weeks (or until negative cultures) for refractory or severe cases; less effective than itraconazole

CONTRAINDICATION

The use of corticosteroids (systemic or topical) can severely exacerbate dermatophytosis.

PRECAUTIONS

Griseofulvin

• Bone marrow suppression (anemia, pancytopenia, and neutropenia) reported in dogs/cats as an idiosyncratic reaction or with prolonged therapy; not yet reported in rabbits but may occur; weekly or biweekly CBC is recommended
• Neurologic side effects reported in dogs and cats—monitor for this possibility in rabbits
• Do not use during the first two trimesters of pregnancy; it is teratogenic.

Ketaconazole and Fluconazole

Can be hepatotoxic; monitor hepatic enzymes during therapy

Bathing, Dipping

Use extreme caution when dipping or bathing rabbits due to the high risk of skeletal fractures and excessive chilling with inexperienced owners.

POSSIBLE INTERACTIONS

The imidazole antifungal medications (especially ketaconazole) can induce hepatotoxicity, which could interfere with metabolism of other drugs metabolized by the liver.

ALTERNATIVE DRUGS

• Lime sulfur dip (1:16 in water) is safe and efficacious q3–7d. The animal should not be rinsed but should be towel dried. Avoid contact with the eyes and ears as it can be irritating. It is odiferous and can stain. Dipping is often difficult to perform on rabbits. Dipping and bathing can be dangerous with nervous rabbits and inexperienced owners and can result in serious consequences such as spinal fractures or excessive chilling.

• Ketoconazole (10–40 mg/kg PO q24h)— efficacy and safety in rabbits are unknown. Hepatopathy reported in dogs and cats can be quite severe.

FOLLOW-UP

PATIENT MONITORING

Repeat fungal cultures toward the end of the treatment regimen and continue treatment until at least one culture result is negative.

PREVENTION/AVOIDANCE

• Initiate a quarantine period and obtain dermatophyte cultures of all animals entering the household to prevent reinfection from other animals.
• Avoid infective soil, if a geophilic dermatophyte is involved.

POSSIBLE COMPLICATIONS

False-negative dermatophyte cultures

EXPECTED COURSE AND PROGNOSIS

• Infection will recur if the environment and all in-contact animals are not treated.
• Many animals will "self-clear" a dermatophyte infection over a period of a few months, but recontamination can occur, and it is most prudent to treat affected animals.
• Treatment periods can be long; continue treatment until two negative cultures are obtained if possible.

✓ MISCELLANEOUS

ASSOCIATED CONDITIONS
N/A

AGE-RELATED FACTORS
N/A

ZOONOTIC POTENTIAL
Dermatophytosis is zoonotic.

PREGNANCY/FERTILITY/BREEDING

• Griseofulvin is teratogenic and should not be used in pregnant animals.
• Ketoconazole can affect steroidal hormone synthesis, especially testosterone.

SYNONYMS
Ringworm

SEE ALSO
Cheyletiellosis (fur mites)
Ear mites
Fleas and flea infestation
Pruritus

ABBREVIATIONS
DTM = dermatophyte test media
GI = gastrointestinal

Suggested Reading
Kraemer A, Mueller RS, Werckenthin C et al. Dermatophytes in pet guinea pigs and rabbits. Vet Microbiol 2012;157(1–2):208–213.
Meredith A. Dermatoses. In: Meredith A, Lord B, eds. BSAVA Manual of Rabbit Medicine. Gloucester: British Small Animal Veterinary Association, 2014:255–263.
Palmerio BS, Roberts H. Clinical approach to dermatologic disease in exotic animals. Vet Clin North Am Exot Anim Pract 2013;16(3):523–577.
Snook TS, White SD, Hawkins MG et al. Skin diseases in pet rabbits: a retrospective study of 334 cases seen at the University of California at Davis, USA (1984–2004). Vet Dermatol 2013;24:613–618.
Varga M. Skin diseases. In: Varga M, ed. Textbook of Rabbit Medicine, 2nd ed. Elsiver, 2014:224–248.
Varga M, Patterson S. Dermatologic diseases of rabbits. In: Quesenberry KE, Carpenter JW, eds. Ferrets, Rabbits and Rodents, 4th ed. Clinical Medicine and Surgery. 2021. St. Louis: Saunders, 2020:220–222.
Author Barbara Oglesbee, DVM, DABVP (Avian)

BASICS

DEFINITION
Abrupt or recent onset of abnormally frequent, soft or fluid fecal matter. True diarrhea is uncommon in adult rabbits.

PATHOPHYSIOLOGY
• Caused by imbalance in the absorptive, secretory, and motility actions of the intestines
• Normally, the intestinal epithelium secretes fluid and electrolytes to aid in the digestion, absorption, and propulsion of food. In rabbits with enteric dysbiosis, this secretion can overwhelm the absorptive activity and produce a secretory diarrhea.
• Rabbits are hind-gut fermenters and are extremely sensitive to alterations in diet. Proper hind-gut fermentation is dependent on the ingestion of large amounts of roughage and long-stemmed hay. Diets that contain inadequate amounts of coarse fiber (such as the feeding of only commercial pelleted food without hay or grasses) cause cecocolonic hypomotility and produce diarrhea due to motility changes and secondary decreases in absorption.
• A common predisposing cause of diarrhea in rabbits is disruption of enteric commensal flora. Flora may be altered by antibiotic usage, stress, or poor nutrition. Cecocolonic hypomotility can cause alterations in cecal fermentation, pH, and substrate production, which alter enteric microflora populations. Diets low in coarse fiber typically contain high simple carbohydrate concentrations, which provide a ready source of fermentable products and promote the growth of bacterial pathogens such as *E. coli* and *Clostridium* spp. Bacterial dysbiosis can cause acute diarrhea and/or enterotoxemia.
• Antibiotic usage can cause severe, acute, often fatal diarrhea due to alteration of normal gut flora. Diarrhea follows the oral administration of antibiotics that are effective against gram-positive bacteria and some gram-negative anaerobes, such as lincomycin, clindamycin, erythromycin, ampicillin, amoxicillin cephalosporins, and penicillins. These antibiotics should not be orally administered to rabbits.

SYSTEMS AFFECTED
• Gastrointestinal
• Endocrine/Metabolic—fluid, electrolyte, and acid-base imbalances

SIGNALMENT
No specific age or gender predilection

SIGNS
General Comments
• Rabbits with acute diarrhea usually quickly develop signs of severe illness (e.g., anorexia, abdominal pain, watery diarrhea, severe dehydration, depression, and shock), generally considered an emergency.

Historical Findings
• Most common—acute onset of watery diarrhea, depression, anorexia, and listlessness; owners may describe a foul-smelling diarrhea
• Mucoid enteritis—acute onset of mucoid diarrhea, depression, anorexia in weaning-aged rabbits
• Diarrhea may be described as soft and sticky, mucus covered, or watery in adults
• In adults—history of diets low in roughage and long-stemmed hay, diets high in simple carbohydrates (pellets, excessive fruits, or sugary vegetables, cereal treats, grain or bread products, sugars; infrequent feeding of good-quality long-stemmed hay and fresh leafy greens)
• In adults—history of recent stress or fearful stimuli (surgery, hospitalization, illness, diet change, and environmental change)
• History of antibiotic use—especially those with a gram-positive spectrum (clindamycin, lincomycin, penicillin, ampicillin, and amoxicillin)

Physical Examination Findings
Mild to moderate diarrhea
• Abdominal discomfort and gas- or fluid-filled intestines or cecum may be detected on palpation.
• May be evidence of fecal staining of perineum
• Abdominal pain characterized by a hunched posture, reluctance to move, or bruxism palpation
Acute, severe diarrhea; enterotoxic shock
• Dehydration and depression
• Abdominal distension; tympanic abdomen
• Tachycardia or bradycardia
• Tachypnea
• Signs of hypovolemic shock (e.g., pale mucous membranes, decreased capillary refill time, and weak pulses)
• Hypothermia—body temperature is usually low in rabbits that are in shock. Incomplete insertion of the thermometer into the rectum is a common cause of falsely low body temperature measurement. Be certain that the thermometer is completely inserted into the rectum (approximately 3 cm) to register an accurate body temperature.

CAUSES
• Dietary—high simple carbohydrate, low coarse fiber diets, diet changes—most common cause

• Bacterial dysbiosis/enterotoxemia—*Escherica coli, Clostridium spiroforme, Clostridium piliforme* (Tyzzer's disease), *Salmonella* spp., *Pseudomonas* spp., *Campylobacter* spp.
• Obstruction—neoplasia, abscess, and intussusception
• Drugs and toxins—oral administration of lincomycin, clindamycin, erythromycin, ampicillin, amoxicillin cephalosporins, and penicillins; plant toxins
• Viral infection—coronavirus (3–10-week-old rabbits), rotavirus (usually a copathogen with coronavirus); seen in neonates
• Parasitic causes—coccidia (*Eimeria* spp., hepatic or intestinal)

RISK FACTORS
• Diets with inadequate indigestible coarse fiber content and high simple carbohydrate content
• Improper antibiotic usage
• Stress
• Weaning

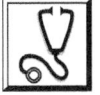

DIAGNOSIS

DIFFERENTIAL DIAGNOSIS
Differentiating Similar Signs
• Diarrhea should be differentiated from uneaten cecotrophs (or night feces). Cecotrophs are formed in the cecum, are rich in nutrients, and are usually eliminated during the early morning hours. Normally, cecotrophs are not observed because rabbits will ingest them directly from the anus. If rabbits are unable to consume cecotrophs (due to orthopedic or neuromuscular disorders, obesity, dental disease or application of Elizabethan collars), uneaten cecotrophs are often mistaken for diarrhea. Cecotrophs are dark in color, have a soft consistency, tend to clump together, are covered with mucus and have a strong, unpleasant odor.
• Fluid, blood-tinged diarrhea—usually associated with coccidia or bacterial enteritis in young rabbits; in older rabbits—associated with bacterial enteritis (esp. *Clostridia* spp., *E. coli*, or *Salmonella* spp.) or intestinal obstruction/intussusception
• Severe depression, lethargy, hypothermia, and signs of shock—usually associated with clostridial enterotoxicosis
• Soft stool, sticky or pasty consistency—usually associated with inappropriate diet or diet changes

CBC/BIOCHEMISTRY
• Increased hematocrit and serum protein concentration seen with dehydration

• TWBC elevation may be seen with bacterial enteritis, but rarely occurs
• Electrolytes may be abnormal because of intestinal losses (hypokalemia, hypochloremia, hyponatremia).
• Altered protein levels because of intestinal loss (decreased) or dehydration (increased)
• Altered renal values with dehydration or gastrointestinal hemorrhage (prerenal azotemia) or with renal disease
• Liver enzymes can be elevated with disease in these organ systems.

OTHER LABORATORY TESTS
• Fecal direct examination, fecal flotation to rule out coccidia in young or debilitated patients
• Anaerobic fecal cultures may demonstrate clostridia organisms but often are negative due to the fastidious nature of the organism.

IMAGING
Radiographic Findings
• Gas-filled cecum and intestines are a common finding in rabbits with acute diarrhea and enterotoxicosis
• May be helpful to rule out other causes of diarrhea (mesenteric torsion, neoplasia, and intussusception)

OTHER DIAGNOSTIC PROCEDURES
N/A

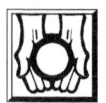

TREATMENT

APPROPRIATE HEALTH CARE
• Treatment must be specific to the underlying cause to be successful.
• Most adult rabbits with mild diarrhea that are otherwise bright and alert can be treated as outpatients.
• Hospitalize rabbits with signs of lethargy, depression, dehydration, or shock, even if diarrhea is mild or absent.
• Hospitalize when diarrhea is profuse, resulting in dehydration and electrolyte imbalance.
• Hospitalize rabbits under 5 months of age, regardless of the severity of diarrhea.
• Rabbits with mild, intermittent diarrhea, characterized by the production of soft, pasty stool and lack of other clinical signs, may respond to dietary correction alone. These rabbits will have a few soft stools each day, with the remainder of the feces normal, formed pellets. See "Diarrhea, Chronic Intermittent" for details.

NURSING CARE
• Fluid therapy and correction of electrolyte imbalances is the mainstay of treatment in most cases.

• Can give crystalloid fluid therapy orally, subcutaneously, or intravenously, as required
• Aim to return the patient to proper hydration status (over 12–24 hours) and replace any ongoing losses. Maintenance fluid requirements are estimated at 60 mL/kg/day for large breeds, 80–100 mL/kg/day for small or dwarf breeds.
• Severe volume depletion can occur with acute diarrhea; aggressive shock fluid therapy may be necessary.
• Fluid choice for intravenous or subcutaneous use should take into consideration the electrolyte and hydration status.

DIET
• It is imperative that the rabbit continue to eat during and following treatment. Continued anorexia will exacerbate GI motility disorders, cause further derangement of the gastrointestinal microflora, and cause overgrowth of intestinal bacterial pathogens.
• Offer a good-quality grass hay and high-quality commercial pellets.
• Withhold greens, vegetables, fruits, and treats as these foods are higher in carbohydrates and can exacerbate clostridial overgrowth
• If the patient refuses these foods, syringe-feed a gruel such as Critical Care for Herbivores (Oxbow Pet Products) or Emeraid Herbivore (Lafeber Company, Cornell, IL) 10–15 mL/kg PO q6–8h. Larger volumes and more frequent feedings are often accepted; feed as much as the rabbit will readily accept.
• High-carbohydrate, high-fat nutritional supplements are contraindicated.
• The diet should be permanently modified to include sufficient amounts of roughage and long-stemmed hay. Offer high-quality fresh hay (grass or timothy preferred; commercially available hay cubes are not sufficient) and an assortment of washed, fresh leafy greens. These foods should always constitute the bulk of the diet. Pellets should be limited (1/4 cup pellets per 5 lbs body weight) and foods high in simple carbohydrate prohibited or limited to the occasional treat.

CLIENT EDUCATION
• Warn owners of rabbits with acute, severe diarrhea that death may occur despite treatment. Young rabbits (<6 months old) and rabbits showing signs of depression and shock also have a guarded to grave prognosis with treatment, even when diarrhea is mild.
• Emphasize the importance of permanent dietary modification (described above) in surviving rabbits.

MEDICATIONS
DRUG(S) OF CHOICE
• Antibiotics for *Clostridium* spp.— metronidazole (20 mg/kg PO; 5–20 mg/kg IV q12h); for other bacterial infections, use broad-spectrum antibiotics such as trimethoprim sulfa (30 mg/kg PO q12h) or enrofloxacin (10–20 mg/kg PO, SC, IV q12–24h)
• Coccidia—sulfadimethoxine—50 mg/kg PO first dose, then 25 mg/kg q24h for 10–20 days, trimethoprim sulfa (30 mg/kg PO q12h × 10 days) or toltrazuril (25 mg/kg daily for 2 days PO, then repeat after 5 days)
• Cholestyramine (Questran, Bristol Laboratories) is an ion exchange resin that binds clostridial iota toxins. A dose of 2 g in 20 mL of water administered by gavage q24h for up to 18–21 days has been reported to be effective in preventing death in rabbits with acute clostridia enterotoxemia.
• Analgesics such as meloxicam (1 mg/kg SC, IM q24h), hydromorphone (0.05–0.2 mg/kg IV, IM, SC q6–8h), buprenorphine (0.02–0.05 mg/kg SC, IM, IV q8–12h), or carprofen (2–4 mg/kg SC, IV q24h) are essential to treatment of rabbits with GI hypomotility. Intestinal pain, either postoperative or from gas distention and ileus, impairs mobility and decreases appetite and may severely inhibit recovery.
• Maropitant (2 mg/kg SC q24h) is used to treat visceral pain. Combine this with one of the analgesics listed above.

CONTRAINDICATIONS
• The use of antibiotics that are primarily gram positive in spectrum is contraindicated in rabbits. Use of these antibiotics will suppress the growth of commensal flora, allowing overgrowth of enteric pathogens, and often a fatal enterotoxemia. Do not orally administer lincomycin, clindamycin, erythromycin, ampicillin, amoxicillin cephalosporins, or penicillins.
• Administration of corticosteriods may cause immunosuppression and should not be used in rabbits with infectious causes of diarrhea. Corticosteroid use is associated with gastrointestinal ulceration and hemorrhage, delayed wound healing, and heightened susceptibility to infection.

PRECAUTIONS
• Meloxicam—use with caution in rabbits with compromised renal function
• Oral administration of any antibiotic may potentially cause enteric dysbiosis; discontinue use if diarrhea or anorexia occurs.

POSSIBLE INTERACTIONS
N/A

ALTERNATE DRUGS
Coccidia—amprolium 9.6% in drinking water (0.5 mL per 500 mL)

FOLLOW-UP

PATIENT MONITORING
• Fecal volume and character, fecal cytology, appetite, attitude, and body weight
• If diarrhea does not resolve, consider reevaluation of the diagnosis.

POSSIBLE COMPLICATIONS
• Septicemia due to bacterial invasion of enteric mucosal
• Dehydration due to fluid loss
• Shock, death from clostridial enterotoxicosis

EXPECTED COURSE AND PROGNOSIS
• Most animals with mild to moderate diarrhea respond well to therapy.
• The prognosis is fair to grave in rabbits with acute, severe, watery diarrhea, depending on the extent of infection and time elapsed to treatment.

• The prognosis is poor to grave in rabbits demonstrating signs of shock (hypothermia, bradycardia, lethargy) and in young rabbits (<6 months old), even with treatment.

MISCELLANEOUS

ASSOCIATED CONDITIONS
• Gastrointestinal hypomotility
• Hypercalciuria

AGE-RELATED FACTORS
• *E. coli*, *Clostridia* spp., coccidia, and viral-related diarrhea more severe in neonates
• Young, weaning-aged rabbits develop acute, watery diarrhea or mucoid diarrhea; prognosis is poorer.
• Adult rabbits require predisposing factors (poor diet, stress, and antibiotic usage) and usually carry a better prognosis.

ZOONOTIC POTENTIAL
Salmonella

PREGNANCY/FERTILITY/BREEDING
N/A

SEE ALSO
Clostridial enteritis/enterotoxicosis
Diarrhea, chronic
Gastrointestinal hypomotility and gastrointestinal stasis

ABBREVIATIONS
GI = gastrointestinal
TWBC = total white blood cell count

Suggested Reading
Bays TB. Geriatric care of rabbits, guinea pigs, and chinchillas. Vet Clin Exot Anim 2020;23:567–593.
DeCubellis J. Common emergencies in rabbits, guinea pigs, and chinchillas. Vet Clin Exot Anim 2016;19:411–429.
Hartcourt-Brown F. Digestive system disease. In: Meredith A, Lord B, eds. BSAVA Manual of Rabbit Medicine. Gloucester: British Small Animal Veterinary Association, 2014:168–190.
Oglesbee B, Lord B. Gastrointestinal diseases of rabbits. In: Quesenberry KE, Carpenter JW, eds. Ferrets, Rabbits and Rodents, 4th ed. Clinical Medicine and Surgery. 2021. St. Louis: Saunders;2020:174–187.
Varga M. Digestive disorders. In: Varga M, ed. Textbook of Rabbit Medicine, 2nd ed. London, UK: Elsevier, 2014:303–349.
Author Barbara Oglesbee, DVM, DABVP (Avian)

DIARRHEA—CHRONIC, INTERMITTENT

BASICS

DEFINITION
• True diarrhea is rare in adult rabbits. The most common cause of what owners perceive to be chronic, intermittent diarrhea is uneaten cecotrophs. This is characterized by the passage of soft, pasty, odiferous stool, concurrent with the passage of normal, firm fecal pellets.

PATHOPHYSIOLOGY
• Cecotrophs (aka, "cecals" or "night feces") are formed by cecal fermentation of indigestible fiber (hay, grasses) in the cecum and constitute up to 60% of a rabbits daily caloric needs. They are rich in protein, vitamins, and other essential nutrients.
• A separate, distinct contraction of the cecum occurs, filling the colon with cecotrophs. The rabbit perceives this contraction and instinctively consumes them directly from the anus as they are passed. They are ingested quickly and swallowed whole, so owners usually do not recognize cecotrophy and perceive this as grooming behavior.
• It is normal for a rabbit to miss, or not eat an occasional normal cecotroph. These can be distinguished from normal feces by their appearance. Cecotrophs appear as clusters of soft, dark brown/black, shiny spheres resembling a large blackberry. They have a characteristic strong, unpleasant odor. When uneaten, they often stick to the fur around the perineum or are stepped on, losing their characteristic shape. This, combined with the texture and strong odor cause their misidentification as diarrhea.
• The cause of uneaten cecotrophs fall into 2 categories: (1) difficulty or inability to reach the anus to ingest normal cecotrophs or (2) abnormal cecotrophs (texture, odor) due to cecal dysbiosis.

SYSTEMS AFFECTED
Gastrointestinal
Neurologic
Musculoskeletal
Dental

INCIDENCE/PREVALANCE
Extremely common reason for presentation in pet rabbits

SIGNALMENT
For uneaten normal cecotrophs: Middle aged to older rabbits
For cecal dysbiosis: No specific age or gender predilection

SIGNS

Historical Findings
The key historical finding is the passage of "diarrheic" feces interspersed with normal, firm, round feces. If the rabbit is passing normal feces through the "diarrhea" episode, the soft feces are uneaten cecotrophs.
For uneaten, normal cecotrophs:
• Owners describe soft, pasty stools that stick together; these will often stick to the fur around the perineum or become stepped on, losing their characteristic shape
• Frequency of "abnormal" stools may vary from several times a day to weekly or monthly
• History of dental disease
• History of orthopedic, musculoskeletal, or neurologic disorders
• Obesity
For cecal dysbiosis:
• History of diet change or diets containing inadequate amounts of long-stemmed hay or grasses and excessive simple carbohydrates (e.g., feeding only pellets, excessive fruits, sugary vegetables, sweets, or grain products)
• Antibiotic usage—the use of antibiotics that are primarily gram-positive in spectrum will suppress the growth of commensal flora, allowing overgrowth of enteric pathogens
• Stress—hospitalization, environmental changes, and concurrent illness may contribute to alterations in intestinal commensal flora.

Physical Examination Findings
• Fecal staining of the perineum
• Secondary perineal dermatitis
For uneaten, normal cecotrophs:
• Unkempt haircoat—retained shed, cheyletiella, or leptogibbus mite infestation due to inability to groom
• Signs of dental disease—ptyalism, moist dermatitis around the mouth and chin. Perform a thorough oral examination
• Obesity
• Signs of musculoskeletal disease—back pain—can often be identified by applying pressure to each interverterbral space, weakness, and muscle wasting
• Neurologic signs—vestibular signs, generalized weakness
For cecal dysbiosis:
• Cecal dysbiosis often occurs without signs of systemic illness.
• Fluid or gas is often palpable within the cecum.
• Severe, acute dysbiosis—abdominal pain characterized by a hunched posture, reluctance to move, or pain on palpation. Signs of GI stasis

CAUSES
For uneaten, normal cecotrophs:
• Dental disease—overgrown incisors or oral pain make it difficult to consume cecotrophs
• Obesity—inability to bend and reach the anus
• Musculoskeletal disease—pain when reaching toward the anus
• Neurologic disease—vestibular disorders, generalized weakness
For cecal dysbiosis:
• Dietary—the most common cause in patients that appear otherwise normal is inappropriate diet. Diets that are high in simple carbohydrates (yogurt drops or other sweets, sugary fruits and vegetables, bread, and grain products) and low in coarse, indigestible fiber such as long-stemmed hay cause disruption of normal cecal flora and function.
• Bacterial infection/enterotoxemia—*Escherica coli*, *Clostridium spiroforme*, *Salmonella* sp., *Pseudomonas* sp., and *Campylobacter* sp. Seen with inappropriate antibiotic use or in patients fed a diet consisting of commercial pellets only, especially pellet mixes containing dehydrated fruits, vegetables, nuts, and grains; fed excessive treats: sugary fruits and vegetables, grains, or bread products.

RISK FACTORS
• Inactivity due to pain, cage confinement
• Obesity
• Diets with inadequate indigestible coarse fiber content and high simple carbohydrate content—most prominent risk factor
• Stress
• Dietary changes

DIAGNOSIS

DIFFERENTIAL DIAGNOSIS
• If only soft or liquid feces are passed (no normal, round firm fecal balls are seen) this is true diarrhea or cecal diarrhea
• Anorexia, hunched posture: intestinal obstruction, GI stasis.

CBC/BIOCHEMISTRY
• Usually normal
• Useful in identifying underlying metabolic disorders, when present

IMAGING
Radiographic Findings
• Often no gastrointestinal abnormalities are noted in rabbits with uneaten, normal cecotrophs or mild cecal dysbiosis

- Look for spinal abnormalities, especially spondylosis deformans
- In rabbits that are obese—large intraabdominal fat pads
- Skull films indicated with suspected dental disease/malocclusion
- Rabbits with more severe cecal dysbiosis may have gas and/or fluid cecal distension

OTHER DIAGNOSTIC PROCEDURES

Fecal cytology or culture—generally not helpful; clostridial overgrowth may occasionally be identified rabbits with moderate-to-severe cecal dysbiosis

TREATMENT

For uneaten, normal cecotrophs:
- Dental disease—trim or extract overgrown incisors, trim cheek teeth as needed
- Obesity—caloric restriction (increased hay, decrease pellets and treats)
- Musculoskeletal disease—pain control
- Neurologic disease—treatment varies with cause

For cecal dysbiosis:
- Most rabbits with intermittent cecal diarrhea lack other clinical signs and will respond to dietary correction alone (see Diet, below). Often these rabbits will have a few soft stools each day, with the remainder of the feces being normally formed pellets.
- Patients with moderate to severe disease (anorexia, lack or normal fecal production) may require hospitalization and 24-hour care for parenteral medication and fluid therapy. Correct electrolyte and acid–base disturbances.

DIET

For Cecal Dysbiois
Dietary modification is the mainstay of treatment. It may take days to weeks for these dietary recommendations to change intestinal flora. Allow sufficient time on strict dietary modification for diarrhea to resolve. Warn clients not to give up if a change is not noted immediately; sometimes soft stools may worsen slightly before improving. Strict client compliance is essential to successful treatment.
- First eliminate *all* fruits, vegetable, greens and treats
- Offer only high-quality, fresh, long-stemmed hay (grass or timothy preferred; commercially available hay cubes are not sufficient) until soft stool production

is no longer noted. This may occur within days or may require weeks of diet change.
- Gradually return pellets to the diet. Offer only a limited amount (¼ cup pellets per 5 lbs body weight) of high-quality, timothy-based pellet
- Gradually introduce greens. Start with a small amount such as 1–2 leaves of high fiber greens. If no soft feces are noted, gradually increase the volume and diversity.
- A few rabbits cannot tolerate fresh leafy greens, fruits, vegetables, or treats in the diet. Intermittent soft stools may return with the reintroduction any or, in some cases, only certain foods. Instruct owners to keep a log of which foods trigger these episodes.

DRUG(S) OF CHOICE
- Antibiotic therapy—not indicated in rabbits that are otherwise asymptomatic. Treatment is with diet change alone, and antibiotics are generally contraindicated as all oral antibiotics can potentially alter normal cecal flora.
- For uneaten cecotrophs due to pain: Analgesics such as meloxicam (1 mg/kg SC, IM q24h), or carprofen (2–4 mg/kg SC, IV q24h), can combine with gabapentin (5–20 mg/kg PO q8–12h) for orthopedic or nerve pain.

CONTRAINDICATIONS
- The use of antibiotics that are primarily gram-positive in spectrum is contraindicated in rabbits. Use of these antibiotics will suppress the growth of commensal flora, allowing overgrowth of enteric pathogens and often a fatal enterotoxemia.
- Administration of corticosteriods may cause immunosuppression and should not be used in rabbits with infectious causes of diarrhea. Corticosteroids use is associated with gastrointestinal ulceration and hemorrhage, delayed wound healing, and heightened susceptibility to infection.

PRECAUTIONS
- Oral administration of any antibiotic may potentially cause enteric dysbiosis; discontinue use if diarrhea or anorexia occurs.
- Meloxicam—use with caution in rabbits with compromised renal function.

FOLLOW-UP
PATIENT MONITORING
- It often takes days to weeks for dietary modification for resolution of diarrhea. Owners must be diligent in feeding only the recommended diet.

- Monitor fecal volume and character, appetite, attitude, and body weight.
- If intermittent soft stools persist, consider reevaluation of the diagnosis.

POSSIBLE COMPLICATIONS
- Perineal dermatitis
- Myiasis

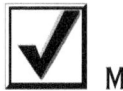

MISCELLANEOUS
ASSOCIATED CONDITIONS
- Dental disease
- Dermatitis
- Pododermatitis (sore hocks)
- Hypercalciuria (bladder sludge)

AGE-RELATED FACTORS
Obesity, orthopedic pain, and dental disorders are usually seen in middle aged to older rabbits.

SEE ALSO
Clostridial enteritis/enterotoxicosis
Diarrhea, acute
Dental disease
Obesity
Arthritis

ABBREVIATIONS
GI = gastrointestinal

Suggested Reading
Bays TB. Geriatric care of rabbits, guinea pigs, and chinchillas. Vet Clin Exot Anim 2020;23:567–593.
DeCubellis J. Common emergencies in rabbits, guinea pigs, and chinchillas. Vet Clin Exot Anim 2016;19:411–429.
Hartcourt-Brown F. Digestive system disease. In: Meredith A, Lord B, eds. BSAVA Manual of Rabbit Medicine. Gloucester: British Small Animal Veterinary Association, 2014:168–190.
Oglesbee B, Lord B. Gastrointestinal diseases of rabbits. In: Quesenberry KE, Carpenter JW, eds. Ferrets, Rabbits and Rodents, (4th ed). Clinical Medicine and Surgery. 2021, St. Louis: Saunders, 2020:174–187.
Varga M. Digestive disorders. In: Varga M, ed. Textbook of Rabbit Medicine, 2nd ed. London, UK: Elsevier, 2014:303–349.
Author Barbara Oglesbee, DVM, DABVP (Avian)

RABBITS

DYSPNEA AND TACHYPNEA

BASICS

DEFINITION
• Dyspnea is difficult or labored breathing; tachypnea is rapid breathing (not necessarily labored), and hyperpnea is deep breathing. In animals, the term *dyspnea* often is applied to labored breathing that appears to be uncomfortable.
• Rabbits are obligate nasal breathers. The rim of the epiglottis is normally situated dorsal to the elongated soft palate to allow air passage from the nose to the trachea during normal respiration. With complete obstruction of the nasal passages, rabbits may attempt open mouth breathing, which is an extremely poor prognostic indicator.

PATHOPHYSIOLOGY
• Dyspnea and/or tachypnea are common symptoms of respiratory or cardiovascular system disorders.
• Primary respiratory diseases may be divided into upper and lower respiratory tract problems.
• Nonrespiratory causes of dyspnea may include abnormalities in pulmonary vascular tone (CNS disease, shock), pulmonary circulation, (congestive heart failure), oxygenation (anemia), or ventilation (heat stress, obesity, ascites, abdominal organomegaly, and musculoskeletal disease).

SYSTEMS AFFECTED
• Respiratory
• Cardiovascular
• Nervous (secondary to hypoxia)

SIGNALMENT
Any

SIGNS

Historical Findings
• Orthopnea (recumbent dyspnea), restlessness, and poor sleeping may occur in rabbits with pleural space disease (effusions, abscesses) or CHF.
• Exercise intolerance may occur with upper respiratory tract disease (rabbits are obligatory nasal breathers), lower respiratory tract disease, or CHF.
• Sneezing or naso-ocular discharge, facial abscess, and dental disease, ptyalism may be seen with upper respiratory infections.
• Anorexia and lethargy often only historical complaint in rabbits with pneumonia
• Coughing is unusual in this species.

Physical Examination Findings
• Upper airway/nasal obstruction—stridor, stertor
• Serous or mucopurulent nasal discharge, ocular discharge, facial abscess, dental disease, ptyalism with URT disease

• Pneumonia—harsh inspiratory and expiratory bronchovesicular sounds sometimes auscultated
• Pulmonary abscesses—absent lung sounds over site of abscess
• Pleural effusion—absent lung sounds ventrally, harsh lung sounds dorsally
• Pulmonary edema—fine inspiratory crackles
• Pyrexia (viral or bacterial infections)
• Weight loss and poor hair coat in rabbits with chronic respiratory disease
• Anorexic rabbits—may show signs of GI hypomotility; scant, dry feces, dehydration, firm stomach or cecal contents, and gas-filled intestinal loops

CAUSES

Nonrespiratory Causes
• Pain, fever, heat stroke, obesity, anxiety
• Neuromuscular disease—severe CNS disease (trauma, abscess, neoplasia, and inflammation), spinal disease (trauma, *E. cuniculi*)
• Hematologic—anemia
• Metabolic disease—(acidosis, uremia)
• Cardiac disease—CHF, cardiogenic shock
• Abdominal distension—organomegaly, ascites, pregnancy, and gastric dilation

Respiratory Causes
Upper respiratory tract (URT)
• Nasal obstruction—rhinitis/sinusitis (bacterial is extremely common), dental disease (periapical abscess, elongated maxillary tooth roots are extremely common), foreign body (hay most common), neoplasia
• Laryngotracheal obstruction—choke/ aspiration of food is most common; laryngeal edema following traumatic intubation also common; abscess or neoplasia are rare
• Traumatic airway rupture—rare
• Extraluminal tracheal compression— abscess, neoplasia
Lower respiratory tract (LRT)
• Extraluminal tracheal compression— abscess, mediastinal mass (thymoma, thymic lymphoma)
• Pneumonia (bacterial is common), pulmonary contusion (trauma), neoplasia (primary, metastatic), pulmonary edema (cardiogenic and noncardiac)
Plural space disease
• Mediastinal masses (thymoma most common)
• Pneumothorax, hemothorax, pleural effusion caused by trauma, cardiac, or pericardial disease
• Diaphragmatic hernia (rare)

RISK FACTORS
• Dental disease—periapical or tooth root abscesses, malocclusion

• Dysphagia, aspiration
• Trauma, bite wounds
• Poor husbandry—dirty, urine-soaked bedding (high ammonia concentrations); poor ventilation, dusty hay or litter; diets too low in fiber content may predispose to dental disease
• Bleach, smoke, or other inhaled irritants
• Stress
• Immunosuppression, concurrent disease, and corticosteroid use

DIAGNOSIS

DIFFERENTIAL DIAGNOSIS
• Tachypnea without dyspnea may be a physiologic response to fear, physical exertion, anxiety, fever, pain, or acidosis. The respiratory rate in normal rabbits is generally very high (100–200 bpm) during veterinary visits.
• With dyspnea, nasal flare with or without increased abdominal effort is noted.
• Pneumonia usually presents with signs of systemic disease (emaciation, anorexia, and depression).
• URT dyspnea is often more pronounced on inspiration; nasal discharge, facial abscesses, or signs of dental disease usually present
• Primary cardiac disease often presents with a constellation of other signs (e.g., heart murmur, arrhythmias). Respiratory rate generally slows with increased effort (nasal flare, abdominal effort)
• Tracheal foreign body (choke)—acute onset of severe dyspnea with nasal flare, abdominal effort. Owner may have witnessed event. If food becomes lodged in the nasopharynx, copious mucoid (sometimes green) nasal discharge may be seen.
• Pleural space disease often presents as exaggerated thoracic excursions that generate only minimal airflow at the mouth or nose.
• Trauma—history and physical examination findings consistent with trauma

CBC/BIOCHEMISTRY/URINALYSIS
• Hemogram—TWBC elevations are usually not seen with bacterial diseases. A relative neutrophilia and/or lymphopenia are more common
• Biochemistry panel—may help to define underlying cause with metabolic diseases; increased liver enzyme activity or bile acids (liver disease), increased CK (muscle wasting, heart disease), uremia

OTHER LABORATORY TESTS
• Culture and sensitivity testing
• Serology for *Pasteurella*—ELISA—high IG G results may corelate with active infection. Low positive results may occur due to

cross-reaction with other, nonpathogenic bacteria (false positive). False-negative results are common with immunosuppression or early infection. Titers may not correlate well to the presence or absence of disease. Test may be useful to monitor SPF colonies.
• *Pasteurella* PCR assay may also be performed on samples taken from deep nasal swabs. PCR may be more sensitive in detecting the presence of *Pasteurella*; however, it should be combined with anaerobic and aerobic culture to identify other bacterial primary or copathogens.

IMAGING

Radiography
• Skull—nasal obstructions, sinusitis, bone destruction from tooth root abscesses, neoplasia, mycotic, or severe bacterial infections. CT scans are much more useful in the diagnosis of URT disease
• Thoracic—pulmonary diseases (small airway disease, pulmonary edema, and pneumonia) and pleural space disease (effusions, mediastinal mass, and pneumothorax)
• Cardiac shadow—cardiomegaly, lifting of the trachea
• Abdominal—gas-filled stomach due to aerophagia, organomegaly, and ascites

Ultrasonography
• Echocardiography to evaluate pericardial effusion, cardiomyopathy, congenital defects, and valvular disease
• Thoracic ultrasound is useful to identify thymoma
• Abdominal ultrasound may be used to evaluate masses or organomegaly.

DIAGNOSTIC PROCEDURES
• Microbiologic and cytologic examinations—LRT samples—transtracheal washing and bronchoalveolar lavage are difficult procedures in rabbits due to the location of glottis—collect airway washings via transoral (endotracheal) wash or during bronchoscopy
• Fine-needle lung aspiration can be performed under ultrasound guidance.
• URT samples—nasal swab or flush for cytologic examination and culture
• Cultures—may be difficult to interpret, since commonly isolated bacteria (e.g., *Bordetella* sp.) often represent only commensal organisms or opportunistic pathogens. A heavy growth of a single organism is usually significant. Deep cultures obtained by inserting a mini-tipped culturette 2–4 cm into each nostril are sometimes reliable; sedation is required for this procedure.
• A lack of growth does not rule out infection, since the organism may be in an inaccessible, deep area of the nasal cavity or

sinuses. *Pasteurella* sp. are often difficult to grow on culture
• Rhinoscopy is valuable to visualize nasal abnormalities, retrieve foreign bodies, or obtain biopsy samples.
• Laryngopharygnoscopy—to evaluate for laryngeal trauma, foreign bodies, or neoplasia
• Biopsy of the nasal cavity is indicated in any animal with chronic nasal discharge in which neoplasia is suspected.
• Thoracocentesis—fluid analysis and culture

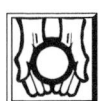

TREATMENT

APPROPRIATE HEALTH CARE
• Severe dyspnea requires hospitalization for supplemental oxygen administration and supportive care; supply O_2 enrichment (O_2 cage or induction chamber) in a quiet environment.
• Gentle suction with a bulb syringe or pediatric aspirator to clear nasal discharges in rabbits with URT disease or acute aspiration (choke)
• Maintain normal systemic hydration—important to aid mucociliary clearance and secretion mobilization; use a balanced multielectrolyte solution
• Nebulization with normal saline or hypertonic saline—may contribute to a more rapid resolution if used in conjunction with antibiotics
• Chest tap—may be both diagnostic and therapeutic in animals with pleural space disease (rare in rabbit). In acutely dyspneic animals, perform tap prior to radiography. A negative tap for air or fluid suggests solid pleural space (mass, abscess or hernia), primary pulmonary disease, or cardiac disease.

DIET
• If the patient refuses food, syringe-feed a gruel such as Critical Care for Herbivores (Oxbow Pet Products) or Emerald Herbivore (Lafeber Company, Cornell, IL) 10–15 mL/kg PO q6–8h. Alternatively, pellets can be ground and mixed with fresh greens, vegetable baby foods, water, or juice to form a gruel.
• Encourage oral fluid intake by offering fresh water from multiple sources, wetting leafy vegetables

SURGICAL CONSIDERATIONS
Surgery may be necessary to remove foreign bodies, obtain samples for biopsy, or to debulk tumors, abscesses, or granulomas; however, maintaining adequate ventilation can be challenging.

MEDICATIONS

DRUG(S) OF CHOICE
• Oxygen is the single most useful drug in the treatment of acute severe dyspnea.
• See primary disorder for definitive therapy.

CONTRAINDICATIONS
• Oral administration of antibiotics that select against gram-positive bacteria (penicillins, macrolides, lincosamides, and cephalosporins) can cause fatal enteric dysbiosis and enterotoxemia.
• The use of corticosteroids (systemic or topical in otic preparations) can severely exacerbate bacterial infection; use is almost never indicated in rabbits.
• In animals with CHF and blunt chest trauma, iatrogenic fluid overload and pulmonary edema is a potential problem. Intravenous administration of crystalloids should be used judiciously.
• Respiratory rate and effort should be monitored carefully and frequently in these patients.

FOLLOW-UP

PATIENT MONITORING
• Repeat any abnormal tests
• Radiographs—monitor response to therapy in animals with pulmonary disease. Pulmonary edema should be visibly improved within 12 hours of therapy, if effective therapy is used. Monitor the recurrence of pleural effusion, based upon how quickly effusion accumulates. Pneumonia—radiographic lesions improve more slowly than the clinical appearance; may not improve with pulmonary abscesses
• Cardiac ultrasound—3–12 weeks, depending on the condition

POSSIBLE COMPLICATIONS
• Depends on the underlying disease
• Relapse, progression of disease, and death are common.

MISCELLANEOUS

ASSOCIATED CONDITIONS
• Dental disease
• Gastrointestinal hypomotility

SEE ALSO
Cheek teeth malocclusion
Congestive heart failure
Pneumonia
Rhinitis and sinusitis

ABBREVIATIONS

CHF = congestive heart failure
CNS = central nervous system
CT = computed tomography
ELISA = enzyme-linked immunosorbent assay
GI = gastrointestinal
LRT = lower respiratory tract
PCR = polymerase chain reaction
URT = upper respiratory tract

Suggested Reading
Capello V, Lennox AM. Diagnostic imaging of the respiratory system in exotic companion mammals. Vet Clin Exot Anim 2011;14:369–389.
DeCubellis J. Common emergencies in rabbits, guinea pigs, and chinchillas. Vet Clin Exot Anim 2016;19:411–429.
Hedley J. Respiratory disease. In: Meredith A, Lord B, eds. BSAVA Manual of Rabbit Medicine. Gloucester: British Small Animal Veterinary Association, 2014:160–167.
Lennox AM, Gladden JN. Emergency and critical care of small mammals. In: Quesenberry KE, Carpenter JW, eds. Ferrets, Rabbits and Rodents, (4th ed). Clinical Medicine and Surgery. 2021, St. Louis: Saunders, 2020:595–608.
Lennox AM, Mancinelli E. Respiratory disorders. In: Quesenberry KE, Carpenter JW, eds. Ferrets, Rabbits and Rodents, (4th ed). Clinical Medicine and Surgery. St. Louis: Saunders, 2020:188–200.
Orcutt CJ, Malakoff RJ. Cardiovascular disorders. In: Quesenberry KE, Carpenter JW, eds. Ferrets, Rabbits and Rodents, (4th ed). Clinical Medicine and Surgery. St. Louis: Saunders, 2020:250–256.

Author Barbara Oglesbee, DVM, DABVP (Avian)

BASICS

DEFINITION
• Dysuria—difficult or painful urination
• Pollakiuria—voiding small quantities of urine with increased frequency

PATHOPHYSIOLOGY
Inflammatory and noninflammatory disorders of the lower urinary tract may decrease bladder compliance and storage capacity by damaging structural components of the bladder wall or by stimulating sensory nerve endings located in the bladder or urethra. Sensations of bladder fullness, urgency, and pain stimulate premature micturition and reduce functional bladder capacity. Dysuria and pollakiuria are caused by lesions of the urinary bladder and/or urethra and provide evidence of lower urinary tract disease; these clinical signs do not exclude concurrent involvement of the upper urinary tract or disorders of other body systems.

SYSTEMS AFFECTED
Renal/Urologic—bladder, urethra

SIGNS

Historical Findings
• Frequent trips to the litter box, urination outside of the litter box
• Urinating when picked up by owners
• Thick white- or tan-appearing urine
• Urine staining in the perineum
• Recurrent GI stasis
• Anorexia, weight loss, lethargy, tooth grinding, tenesmus, and a hunched posture in rabbits with chronic or obstructive lower urinary tract disease

Physical Examination Findings
• May be normal
• Abdominal palpation may demonstrate urocystoliths; failure to palpate uroliths does not exclude them from consideration.
• In rabbits with crystalluria (bladder sludge), the bladder may palpates as a soft, doughy mass.
• An extremely large, often soft urinary bladder may be palpable in rabbits with chronic bladder sludge due to stretching and loss of tone
• A large, turgid urinary bladder may be palpable in patients with partial or complete urethral obstruction.
• Manual expression of the bladder may reveal thick beige- to brown-colored urine. Manual expression of the bladder may expel thick brown urine even in rabbits that have normal-appearing voided urine.

CAUSES

Urinary Bladder
• Hypercalciuria (bladder sludge)—most common cause
• Urinary tract infection—bacterial; sometimes accompanies hypercalciuria
• Urolithiasis—may occur with or without accompanying hypercalciuria (bladder sludge)
• Neoplasia
• Trauma
• Iatrogenic—e.g., catheterization, overdistension of the bladder during contrast radiography, and surgery

Urethra
• Urinary tract infection
• Urethrolithiasis—occasionally seen with hypercalciuria
• Urethral plugs—consisting of calcium precipitates
• Trauma—especially bite wounds
• Neoplasia (rare)

Reproductive
• Endometrial hyperplasia
• Uterine adenoma or adenocarcinoma

Other Organ Systems
• Neurological/Musculoskeletal—any disease that inhibits normal posturing for urination (e.g., pododermatitis, arthritis) can lead to these signs. Contributes to formation of bladder sludge (hypercalciuria) as pain or neurologic disorders lead to retention of urine and accumulation of sludge in the bladder
• Other abdominal organomegaly may put undue pressure on the urinary system, causing straining

RISK FACTORS
• Inadequate water intake—dirty water bowls, unpalatable water, inadequate water provision, changing water sources predisposes to hypercalciuria (bladder sludge)
• Feeding diets high in bioavailable calcium such as alfalfa pellets and alfalfa hay alone may predispose to hypercalciuria (bladder sludge) and cystic calculi.
• Obese, sedentary rabbits are prone to hypercalciuria (bladder sludge)
• Urine retention—underlying bladder pathology, neuromuscular disease, painful conditions causing a reluctance to ambulate (pododermatitis, arthritis)
• Intact females likely to develop uterine disease
• Diseases, diagnostic procedures, or treatments that (1) alter normal host urinary tract defenses and predispose to infection, (2) predispose to formation of uroliths, or

(3) damage the urothelium or other tissues of the lower urinary tract
• Mural or extramural diseases that compress the bladder or urethral lumen

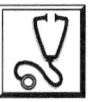

DIAGNOSIS

DIFFERENTIAL DIAGNOSIS

Differentiating from Other Abnormal Patterns of Micturition
• Rule out polyuria—increased frequency and volume of urine
• Rule out urethral obstruction—stranguria, anuria, overdistended urinary bladder, signs of postrenal uremia

Differentiate Causes of Dysuria and Pollakiuria
• Rule out uterine disease—female rabbits; rabbits with uterine disease often strain and expel blood when urinating. Blood may mix with urine and be mistaken for hematuria.
• Rule out urinary tract infection—hematuria; malodorous or cloudy urine; painful, thickened bladder
• Rule out hypercalciuria (bladder sludge)—thick beige urine; radiopaque bladder
• Rule out urolithiasis—palpable uroliths in bladder; radiopaque bladder
• Rule out neoplasia—hematuria; palpable masses in urethra or bladder possible; radiographs and ultrasound may differentiate
• Rule out neurogenic disorders—flaccid bladder wall; residual urine and calcium sludge in bladder lumen after micturition; other neurologic deficits to hind legs, tail, perineum, and anal sphincter
• Rule out iatrogenic disorders—history of catheterization, reverse flushing, contrast radiography, or surgery

CBC/BIOCHEMISTRY/URINALYSIS
• Results may be normal
• Elevated serum calcium concentration seen in both rabbits with hypercalciuria and normal rabbit
• Lower urinary tract disease complicated by urethral obstruction may be associated with azotemia.
• Patients with concurrent pyelonephritis may have impaired urine-concentrating capacity, leukocytosis, and azotemia.
• Disorders of the urinary bladder are best evaluated with a urine specimen collected by cystocentesis.
• Pyuria (normal value 0–1 WBC/hpf), hematuria (normal value 0–1 RBC/hpf), and proteinuria (normal value 0–33 mg/dL) indicate urinary tract inflammation, but these are nonspecific findings that may result from

infectious and noninfectious causes of lower urinary tract disease.
• Urine pH: normal rabbit urine is alkaline; pH >8 suggestive of bacterial cystitis due to urease-producing bacteria
• Identification of bacteria in urine sediment suggests that urinary tract infection is causing or complicating lower urinary tract disease.
• Identification of neoplastic cells in urine sediment indicates urinary tract neoplasia (rare).
• Normal rabbits have numerous crystals in the urine. The most common types are calcium oxalate and calcium carbonate.

OTHER LABORATORY TESTS
Quantitative urine culture—the most definitive means of identifying and characterizing bacterial urinary tract infection; negative urine culture results suggest a noninfectious cause

IMAGING
• Survey abdominal radiography, contrast cystography, urinary tract, and uterine ultrasonography are important means of identifying and localizing causes of dysuria and pollakiuria.
• Urinary sludge and calculi in rabbits are radiopaque, allowing for ease of identification using survey radiography. The majority of urinary calculi are located in the bladder but may also be found in the kidneys, ureters, or urethra.
• Ultrasound may be useful to identify uroliths mixed with sludge in the urinary bladder.

TREATMENT
• Patients with nonobstructive lower urinary tract diseases are typically managed as outpatients; diagnostic evaluation may require brief hospitalization.
• Dysuria and pollakiuria associated with systemic signs of illness (e.g., pyrexia, depression, anorexia, and dehydration) or laboratory findings of azotemia or leukocytosis warrant aggressive diagnostic evaluation and initiation of supportive and symptomatic treatment.
• Treatment depends on the underlying cause and specific sites involved. See specific chapters describing diseases listed in section on causes.

NURSING CARE
• Fluid therapy—rabbits with large amounts of bladder sludge often benefit from SC fluids 2–3 times weekly to dilute urine and keep calcium in solution
• Bladder sludge/sediment can often be manually expressed. This is painful and

requires sedation or anesthesia. Sedation with benzodiazepines may help to relax the urethral sphincter—Midazolam 0.5–1.0 mg/kg IM, IV combined with an opioid for pain control is often sufficient. Repeated expression, usually weekly along with SC fluid therapy at home, may be needed until all sludge is removed.
• Urinary catheterization to flush the bladder with warm saline may be needed to remove residual sludge
• Keep fur clean and dry.

ACTIVITY
• Long-term—increase activity level by providing large exercise areas to encourage voiding and prevent recurrence.
• Activity should be reduced during the time of tissue repair if surgery is required for urinary obstruction.

DIET
• Many affected rabbits are anorectic or have a decreased appetite. It is an absolute requirement that the patient continue to eat during and following treatments. Anorexia may cause or exacerbate gastrointestinal hypomotility and cause derangement of the gastrointestinal microflora and overgrowth of intestinal bacterial pathogens. If the patient refuses these foods, syringe-feed Critical Care for Herbivores (Oxbow Animal Health, Murdock, NE) or Emerald Herbivore (Lafeber Company, Cornell, IL) diet at approximately 10–15 mL/kg PO q6–8h. Larger volumes and more frequent feedings are often accepted; feed as much as the patient will readily accept. Alternatively, pellets can be ground and mixed with fresh greens, vegetable baby foods, water, or sugar-free juice to form a gruel
• Encourage oral fluid intake by offering fresh water, wetting leafy vegetables, or flavoring water with vegetable juices.
• If calcium uroliths or bladder sludge is present, decrease the amount of bioavailable calcium in the diet: Offer only low calcium grass hays; avoid vegetables that are high in calcium content such as kale, spinach, dandelion greens, and watercress.
• Encourage weight loss in overweight patients

CLIENT EDUCATION
• Limiting risk factors such as obesity, sedentary life, and inappropriate diet combined with increasing water consumption is necessary to minimize or delay recurrence of lower urinary tract disease. Even with these changes, however, recurrence may occur.
• Surgical removal of urinary tract calculi does not alter the causes responsible for their formation; limiting risk factors such as high calcium diets is necessary to minimize or delay recurrence. Even with these changes, however, recurrence is likely.

MEDICATIONS
DRUG(S) OF CHOICE
• Depend on the underlying cause
• If bacterial cystitis is demonstrated, begin treatment with a broad-spectrum antibiotic such as enrofloxacin (10–20 mg/kg PO, SC, IM, IV q12h), marbofloxacin (5 mg/kg PO q24h), trimethoprim-sulfa (15–30 mg/kg PO q12h), or chloramphenicol (50 mg/kg PO q8h).
• Modify antibacterial treatment based on results of urine culture and susceptibility testing.
• Pain Management: Symptomatic rabbits with hypercalciuria are sometimes painful and therefore reluctant to urinate. Pain management may aid in urination and promote appetite and water consumption.
   ◦ NSAIDs (meloxicam, carprofen) reduce pain and may decrease inflammation in the bladder; meloxicam (1.0 mg/kg PO q24h); carprofen (2 mg/kg PO q12h)
   ◦ Tramadol—5–15 mg/kg PO q8–12h
   ◦ Gabapentin—5–20 mg/kg PO q8–12h
• Consider diuretic therapy for patients with bladder sludge or uroliths. Give a calcium-sparing thiazide diuretic such as hydrochlorothiazide 0.5–2 mg/kg PO q12h
• Potassium citrate 33 mg/kg PO q8h may help to prevent formation of calcium crystals in urine

CONTRAINDICATIONS
• Glucocorticoids or other immunosuppressive agents
• Oral administration of antibiotics that select against gram-positive bacteria (penicillins, macrolides, lincosamides, and cephalosporins) can cause fatal enteric dysbiosis and enterotoxemia
• Potentially nephrotoxic drugs (e.g., aminoglycosides, NSAIDs) in patients that are febrile, dehydrated, or azotemic or that are suspected of having pyelonephritis, septicemia, or preexisting renal disease

PRECAUTIONS
Meloxicam or other NSAIDs: Use caution in patients with compromised renal function; monitor renal values.

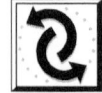

FOLLOW-UP
PATIENT MONITORING
• Response to treatment by clinical signs, serial physical examinations, laboratory testing, and radiographic and ultrasonic

evaluations appropriate for each specific cause
• Refer to specific chapters describing diseases listed in section on causes.

PREVENTION/AVOIDANCE
• Prevention is based upon the specific underlying cause. Limiting risk factors such as obesity, sedentary life, and inappropriate diet combined with increasing water consumption is necessary to minimize or delay recurrence of urinary tract diseases. Even with these changes, however, recurrence may occur.
• For animals with hypercalciuria or urolithiasis, water is the cornerstone to any prevention protocol. Prevention is targeted at increasing water intake and reducing (but not eliminating) dietary calcium. Avoid alfalfa-based diets. Diets containing a high percentage of timothy, oat, or grass hays, a lower overall percentage pellets, and a wider variety of vegetables and fruits may decrease the risk of hypercalciuria or urolithiaisis.

POSSIBLE COMPLICATIONS
• Urine scald
• Refer to specific chapters describing diseases listed in section on causes.

 MISCELLANEOUS

ASSOCIATED CONDITIONS
• Obesity
• Gastrointestinal hypomotility
• Pyoderma (urine scald)

SEE ALSO
Hypercalciuria and urolithiasis
Lower urinary tract infection
Urinary tract obstruction

Suggested Reading
Di Girolamo N, Selleri P. Disorders of the urinary and reproductive system. In: Quesenberry KE, Carpenter JW, eds. Ferrets, Rabbits and Rodents, (4th ed). Clinical Medicine and Surgery. St. Louis: Saunders, 2020:201–220.
Hallman RM, Brandão J. Diagnostic imaging of the renal system in exotic companion mammals. Vet Clin Exot Anim 2020;23:195–214.
Mancinelli E, Lord B. Urogenital and reproductive disease. In: Meredith A, Lord B, eds. BSAVA Manual of Rabbit Medicine. Gloucester: British Small Animal Veterinary Association, 2014:191–204.
Reavill DR, Lennox AM. Disease overview of the urinary tract in exotic companion mammals and tips on clinical management. Vet Clin Exot Anim 2020;23(1):169–193.
Author Barbara Oglesbee, DVM

RABBITS

EAR MITES

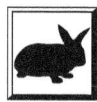

BASICS

OVERVIEW
• *Psoroptes cuniculi* is the rabbit ear mite. Most affected rabbits are intensely pruritic and painful, with thick crust accumulation within the ear canal and pinnae, although early infestations may be asymptomatic or only mildly pruritic.
• Mites are spread to other areas of the body during grooming. Lesions may be seen around the head, abdomen, and perineal regions.
• *Psoroptes cuniculi* are nonburrowing mites and spend their entire 3-week life cycle on the host; eggs hatch within 4 days.

SIGNALMENT
Can be seen in any aged rabbit; no gender predilection

SIGNS
• Intense pruritus (most common) primarily located around the ears, head, and neck; occasionally generalized. Affected areas may become extremely painful.
• Thick brown to beige crusty exudate in the ear canal, eventually spreading to cover the pinna. As infestation becomes more severe, the thick crust layer develops a foliated appearance that is pathognomonic for ear mites in rabbits.
• Alopecia and excoriations around the pinnae may occur, owing to the intense pruritus.
• Mites and lesions may extend to the face, neck, abdomen, perineal region, and even feet via grooming.
• In early infestation—mild to moderate pruritus around the pinna, head, and neck
• Signs of otitis interna/media such as head tilt and vestibular signs may occur with secondary infections and chronic disease.

CAUSES AND RISK FACTORS
• Exposure to affected rabbits—pet stores, shelters, and multiple rabbit households
• Exposure to fomites—hay, grass, straw, or wood chip bedding

DIAGNOSIS

DIFFERENTIAL DIAGNOSIS
Exudate in the Ear Canal
• Normal wax—most rabbits normally have a light yellow-beige, waxy exudate in the ear canal. Exudate normally does not extend onto the pinnae, as seen in ear mite infestations.

• Bacterial or mycotic otitis externa—more common than ear mite infestation in rabbits; exudate is usually thick, white, creamy, and limited to the external canal; differentiate by microscopic examination of exudate

Pruritus/Alopecia
• Fur mites—*Cheyletiella* sp., or less commonly, *Leporacarus gibbus*. May be concurrent with ear mite infestation. Fur mite lesions are usually located in the intrascapular or tail base region and associated with copious amounts of large white scale. Mites are readily identified in skin scrapes or acetate tape preparations under low magnification. No exudate in ear canals
• Other ectoparasites—*Sarcoptes scabiei* and *Notoedres cati* rarely infest rabbits. Lesions are located around the head and neck and are intensely pruritic. Exudate in ear canals is not seen.
• Fleas—patchy alopecia usually appears in other areas in addition to head; finding flea dirt will help to differentiate

CBC/BIOCHEMISTRY/URINALYSIS
Normal

OTHER LABORATORY TESTS
N/A

IMAGING
N/A

DIAGNOSTIC PROCEDURES
• Ear swabs placed in mineral oil and examined under low magnification—usually a very effective means of identification
• Skin scrapings—identify mites, if signs are generalized
• Otoscopic examination—to visualize mites
• Mites are also visible to the unaided eye.

TREATMENT
• Contagious; important to treat all in-contact rabbits
• Thoroughly clean and treat the environment. Extremely important for eliminating infestation; mites can live on exfoliated crusts in the environment up to 21 days, depending on conditions. Remove and discard all organic material from cage (wood or paper products, bedding); replace bedding with shredded paper bedding that can be discarded, and the cage thoroughly cleaned every day during the treatment period.
• Combs, brushes, and grooming utensils—discard or thoroughly disinfect before reuse
• Do not clean crusts from the ear canal or pinnae. Cleaning not enhance treatment, can

be very painful, and can traumatize the ear canal. Treat first with ivermectin or selamectin. Most crusts and lesions will resolve rapidly without the need for manually removing crusts.

MEDICATIONS

DRUG(S) OF CHOICE
• Selamectin (Revolution, Pfizer)—12 mg/kg applied topically q30d; one treatment is usually effective
• Imidacloprid/moxidectin (Advantage-Multi, Bayer)—10 mg/kg (i) + 1 mg/kg (m) topically q30d; one treatment is usually effective
• Topical otic antibiotic or antifungal medications are usually not required. Secondary bacterial and/or yeast otitis is usually the result of overzealous cleaning of the pinnae and/or ear canals.

CONTRAINDICATIONS
• Avoid cleaning of the ear canal; do not attempt to manually remove crusts as this is extremely painful, does not hasten resolution of infection and may cause secondary infections. The crusts will be removed by the rabbit with normal grooming after the mites are killed.
• Ivermectin—do not use in pregnant animals
• Do not use topical and parenteral ivermectin concurrently.
• Do not use fipronil on rabbits.
• Do not use organophosphate-containing products on rabbits.
• Do not use straight permethrin sprays or permethrin spot-ons on rabbits.

PRECAUTIONS
• Topical otic medications containing corticosteriods should be avoided in rabbits.
• Prevent rabbits or their cagemates from licking topical spot-on products before they are dry.

ALTERNATIVE DRUGS
• Ivermectin 1%—0.4 mg/kg SC q10–14d for 2–3 doses. The eggs are not killed, so repeated dosing and thorough environmental cleaning are needed
• Moxidectin (Advocate, Bayer) 0.2 mg/kg q10 days for two doses

FOLLOW-UP
• An ear swab and physical examination should be done 1 month after therapy commences.

(CONTINUED)

- For most patients, prognosis is excellent.
- Infestation is more likely to recur or fail to respond to treatment with ivermectin or moxidectin if the environment is not thoroughly cleaned

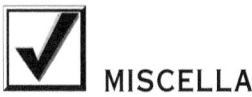 **MISCELLANEOUS**

ZOONOTIC POTENTIAL
N/A

SEE ALSO
Cheyletiellosis (fur mites)
Dermatophytosis
Fleas and flea infestation
Pruritus

Suggested Reading
Hansen O, Gall Y, Pfister K et al. Efficacy of a formulation containing imidacloprid and moxidectin against naturally acquired ear mite infestations (*Psoroptes cuniculi*) in rabbits. Int J Appl Res Vet Med 2005; 3(4):281–286.
Meredith A. Dermatoses. In: Meredith A, Lord B, eds. BSAVA Manual of Rabbit Medicine. Gloucester: British Small Animal Veterinary Association, 2014:255–263.
Palmerio BS, Roberts H. Clinical approach to dermatologic disease in exotic animals. Vet Clin North Am Exot Anim Pract 2013; 16(3):523–577.
Rosen LB. Dermatologic manifestations of zoonotic diseases in exotic animals. J Exotic Pet Med 2011;20:9–13.
Snook TS, White SD, Hawkins MG et al. Skin diseases in pet rabbits: a retrospective study of 334 cases seen at the University of California at Davis, USA (1984–2004). Vet Dermatol 2013;24:613–618.
Varga M. Skin diseases. In: Varga M, ed. Textbook of Rabbit Medicine, 2nd ed. Elsiver, 2014:224–248.
Varga M, Patterson S. Dermatologic diseases of rabbits. In: Quesenberry KE, Carpenter JW, eds. Ferrets, Rabbits and Rodents, (4th ed). Clinical Medicine and Surgery. 2021, St. Louis: Saunders, 2020:220–222.

Author Barbara Oglesbee, DVM, DABVP (Avian)

ENCEPHALITOZOONOSIS

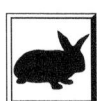

BASICS

DEFINITION
Encephalitozoon cuniculi—an obligate intracellular microsporidian parasite that infects rabbits, mice, guinea pigs, hamsters, dogs, cats, primates, and humans

PATHOPHYSIOLOGY
• Infection—ingestion of spores in urine-contaminated food or water; spores spread to extraintestinal organs via reticuloendothial system; rupture of intracellular spore-filled vacuoles results in granulomatous inflammation
• In normal life cycle—localizes in renal tubular epithelial cells, resulting in spores shed in urine 6 weeks after infection, shedding peaks 2 months postinfection and ends 3 months postinfection
• In utero infection—vertical transmission of organism into the developing lens; replication of spores within the lens of young rabbits results in cataract formation, lens rupture, uveitis, and glaucoma
• The prevalence of *E. cuniculi* as a cause of CNS disease is controversial since definitive antemortem diagnosis is not possible, and postmortem lesions do not correlate with clinical disease.
• Severity and manifestation—depend on location and degree of tissue injury; most infections are asymptomatic or remain asymptomatic unless the rabbit becomes immunocompromised (stress, debility, and age); symptomatic rabbits generally display nervous system, ocular, or renal disease
• Myocarditis, vasculitis, pneumonitis, hepatitis, splenitis, and spinal nerve root inflammation have also been reported.
• Clinical disease—most likely occurs in older or immunosuppressed animals

SYSTEMS AFFECTED
• CNS—granulomatous encephalitis, spinal nerve root inflammation
• Ophthalmic—cataract formation and phacoclastic uveitis from in utero infections
• Renal—lesions typically incidental finding; may cause renal compromise if severe

GENETICS
N/A

INCIDENCE/PREVALENCE
• Many rabbits (at least 52% of those tested) in US and Europe are serologically positive for *E. cuniculi*.
• Most animals asymptomatic
• The true incidence of clinical disease is unknown.

GEOGRAPHIC DISTRIBUTION
Worldwide

SIGNALMENT
• No sex predilection
• Phacoclastic uveitis seen in young animals, dwarf breeds more commonly affected
• CNS disease anecdotally more likely in older animals

SIGNS

General Comments
• Determined mainly by site and extent of tissue damage; ocular and CNS signs most commonly reported
• Most infections are asymptomatic.
• The extent to which *E. cuniculi* causes neurologic disease in rabbits is controversial. Many rabbits with CNS signs demonstrate postmortem histologic CNS lesions compatible with *E. cuniculi*, but the organism itself is often not identified in tissues. On the other hand, many rabbits have similar postmortem lesions (and sometimes, organism identified) in the absence of neurologic signs.

Historical Findings
• Ocular—hypopyon, intraocular granuloma, cataract; usually unilateral
• Neurologic—vestibular signs (with head tilt, nystagmus, anorexia, ataxia, and rolling) predominate; seizures; tremors; paresis/paralysis also reported anecdotally
• Renal compromise (unusual)—nonspecific signs of lethargy, depression, anorexia, and weight loss

Physical Examination Findings
• Neurologic—vestibular signs predominate (ataxia, head tilt, nystagmus, and torticollis); tremors, paresis, paralysis, seizures, stiff rear limb gait and incontinence also reported
• Ocular signs—often unilateral, iridal abscess, cataract, lens rupture, uveitis (aqueous flare, hyphema, and mydriasis); hypopyon
• Renal disease—irregular, pitted kidneys (usually incidental finding); if renal compromise (unusual)—depression, dehydration, cachexia, and evidence of GI hypomotility
• Cardiac or hepatic involvement—occurs; usually not clinically apparent

CAUSES
Encephalitazoon cuniculi

RISK FACTORS
Immunosuppression—predisposes to clinical disease: stress, poor diet, concurrent disease, and glucocorticoid or antitumor chemotherapy. Asymptomatic rabbits with subclinical infections often demonstrate clinical signs following one or more of these events.

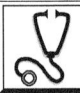

DIAGNOSIS
Antemortem diagnosis is usually presumed based on clinical signs, exclusion of other diagnoses, positive antibody titers, and possibly, response to treatment. Definitive antemortem diagnosis is problematic, since a positive antibody titer indicates exposure only, rabbits often respond minimally or not at all to treatment, and many rabbits will improve with no treatment at all. Definitive diagnosis requires identification of organisms and characteristic inflammation in affected tissues, generally acquired at postmortem examination. However, multiple studies have failed to demonstrate a correlation between the severity of CNS lesions and clinical signs.

DIFFERENTIAL DIAGNOSIS
• Neurologic—vestibular signs due otitis interna/media are identical to those seen in rabbit with encephalitozoonosis. Many rabbits with otitis interna/media lack exudate in external canal or other signs of otitis externa. Bulla disease is not always visible on skull radiographs, and may require CT to diagnose. Every attempt should be made to rule out otic disease prior to assuming *E. cuniculi* infection. Other causes—CNS abscess, neoplasia, trauma; parasitic (toxoplasmosis, aberrant migration of *Baylisascaris* sp). Rear limb weakness/ataxia—spinal disease, lead toxicosis, generalized weakness from metabolic disease, orthopedic disease
• Intraocular disease (anterior uveitis)—bacterial; trauma; lens-induced; corneal ulceration with reflex uveitis

CBC/BIOCHEMISTRY/URINALYSIS
• CBC usually unremarkable; increased PCV with dehydration possible secondary to renal disease or anorexia
• Biochemistry—increased BUN and creatinine with renal disease (rare)

OTHER LABORATORY TESTS
Serologic testing
• The usefulness of serum antibody testing is limited in pet rabbits since a positive titer indicates only exposure and does not confirm *E. cuniculi* as the cause of clinical signs. *E. cuniculi* can only be definitively diagnosed by finding organisms and resultant lesions on histopathologic examination in areas that anatomically correlate with observed clinical signs.
• IgG titers usually become positive by 2 weeks post infection. A rising titer after 4 weeks may confirm infection, but titers do not always continue to rise with active

infection. IgG levels can decline after 8 weeks in some rabbits, in others may persist for life. No correlation exits between antibody titers and shedding of organism or severity of disease. Available tests include ELISA and IFA.

• IgM titers may indicate a more recent, active infection. Titers become positive shortly after infection and appear to persist for up to 18 weeks.

• C-reactive protein, an inflammatory marker, appears to be elevated in rabbits with active infection. Although this marker is nonspecific, concurrent elevation with IgG and IgM supports active infection.

• A negative test may rule out infection; however, false negatives can be seen in early infections, before titers have a chance to rise.

• Cerebrospinal fluid analysis—may see increased protein, lymphocyte, and monocytes. In recent studies, the organism was only detected in 10% of known positives with PCR testing on CSF.

• PCR testing—Conventional PCR appears to be reliable in diagnosing E. cuniculi on liquefied lens material from rabbits with uveitis. Can be used to detect organism in urine if actively shedding.

IMAGING
• Radiographs—skull films to rule out otitis interna/media; spinal films to rule out spinal disease/trauma; may see small, malformed kidneys with severe renal involvement
• CT—to rule out bulla disease, CNS neoplasia, abscess

DIAGNOSTIC PROCEDURES
• Urine sedimentation—gram's stain may demonstrate spores, oval $2.5 \times 1.5\,\mu m$, in diameter. Spores are only passed for up to 4 weeks following infection, and generally are not present in urine when neurologic, ophthalmologic, or renal signs are present.

PATHOLOGIC FINDINGS
• CNS—multifocal nonsuppurative granulomatous meningoencephalomyelitis; astrogliosis; perivascular lymphocytic infiltration; lymphocytic meningitis. Spores $(1.5 \times 2.5\,mm)$ stain positive with gram and carbol fuchsin stains. The cerebrum is most commonly infected, followed by the brain stem, spinal cord, and to a much lesser extent, the cerebellum. Several studies have demonstrated that there is no evident correlation between the severity, presence, or absence of CNS lesions and clinical signs of CNS disease.
• Kidneys—gross: multifocal, depressed areas of fibrosis pitting the surface of the kidney—usually an incidental finding; histologic with active disease—lymphohistiocytic

tubulointerstitial nephritis, interstitial nephrosis, renal tubular necrosis. Protozoa may be identified with Gram's stain.
• Ocular—lens capsule rupture with anterior uveitis; organisms may be identified on histologic examination of the liquefied lens; iridal abscesses or hypopyon with secondary bacterial infection

TREATMENT
APPROPRIATE HEALTH CARE
• Outpatient if eating and able to maintain posture
• Inpatient—severe disease; patient cannot maintain adequate nutrition, hydration or posture

NURSING CARE
• Dehydration—intravenous fluids or subcutaneous fluids
• Assist-feed anorexic animals
• Support posture, prevent rolling in rabbits with severe vestibular signs. House in a quiet space with dim lighting.

ACTIVITY
• Restrict or confine patients with neurologic signs; provide padded cages for rabbits that are severely ataxic, seizuring, or rolling.
• Encourage return to activity as soon as safely possible; activity may enhance recovery of vestibular function

DIET
• It is imperative that the rabbit continue to eat. Although rabbits cannot vomit, many appear to experience nausea with vestibular disorders, and become anorexic. Anorexia will cause GI hypomotility or GI stasis, derangement of the gastrointestinal microflora, and overgrowth of intestinal bacterial pathogens.
• Make sure that food and water are within reach; may need to bring food to patient.
• If the patient refuses food, syringe-feed a gruel such as Critical Care for Herbivores (Oxbow Pet Products) or Emeraid Herbivore (Lafeber Company, Cornell, IL) 10–15 mL/kg PO q6–8h. Larger volumes and more frequent feedings are often accepted; feed as much as the rabbit will accept. Alternatively, pellets can be ground and mixed with fresh greens, vegetable baby foods, water, or juice to form a gruel. Caution: be aware of aspiration secondary to abnormal body posture in patients with severe head tilt and vestibular disequilibrium or brainstem dysfunction.
• High-carbohydrate, high-fat nutritional supplements are contraindicated.

CLIENT EDUCATION
• Prognosis is guarded in symptomatic patients; response to therapy inconsistent
• Long-term home nursing care (assist-feed, padded bedding in recumbent animals) may be required; residual neurologic signs common in rabbits that partially recover; a waxing and waning course of progression is seen in some rabbits; some rabbits take weeks to months to recover.
• Head tilt may be permanent but does not appear to affect quality of life in most recovered patients.

SURGICAL CONSIDERATIONS
Phacoclastic uveitis—phacoemulsification has been successfully performed. Rabbits with glaucoma secondary to E. cuniculi require enucleation.

MEDICATIONS
DRUG(S) OF CHOICE
• Fenbendazole (20 mg/kg q24h × 28 days) is the most common treatment and has been shown to reduce clinical signs and increase survival rates in symptomatic patients. Benzimidazole anthelmintics are effective against E. cuniculi in vitro and have been shown to prevent experimental infection in rabbits. However, efficacy in rabbits with clinical signs is unknown. Long-term treatment has been recommended, as treatment only prevents replication, rather than kills the parasite.
• Severe vestibular signs (rolling, torticollis) or seizures—diazepam (0.5–2.0 mg/kg SC, IM, IV) or midazolam (0.5–2.0 mg/kg SC, IM, IV)
• If anorexic, maropitant (2 mg/kg SC, PO q24h) or metoclopramide (0.5–1.0 mg/kg PO, SC, IV q12h)
• Vestibular signs—meclizine 2–12 mg/kg PO q24h may reduce clinical signs, control nausea, and induce mild sedation

CONTRAINDICATIONS
N/A

PRECAUTIONS
• Benzimidazole anthelmintics have been associated with fatal bone marrow toxicity in rabbits. Although this is rare with use of fenbendazole, periodic monitoring of CBC is recommended.
• Topical and systemic corticosteroids—topical corticosteroids have been used to decrease ocular inflammation, progression of uveitis, and development of glaucoma. However, the use of either topical or systemic corticosteroids in rabbits with E. cuniculi is

RABBITS

controversial. Rabbits are very sensitive to the immunosuppressive effects of corticosteroids; use may exacerbate signs of *E. cuniculi* or subclinical bacterial infection.

POSSIBLE INTERACTIONS
None

ALTERNATIVE DRUGS
• Systemic corticosteroids have been advocated by some practitioners for treatment of *E. cuniculi*-induced CNS granulomatous inflammation. Most recommend a single dose of a short-acting corticosteroid at immunosuppressive doses, followed by anti-inflammatory doses only if necessary. Use of corticosteroids is controversial. Rabbits are very sensitive to the immunosuppressive effects of corticosteroids; immunosuppression may exacerbate subclinical bacterial or *E. cuniculi* infection.
• Ponazuril has been anecdotally used to treat *E. cuniculi* (20–50 mg/kg PO q24h × 30 days). Safety and efficacy are unknown.

FOLLOW-UP

PATIENT MONITORING
• Uveitis—monitor for progression of uveitis and development of glaucoma
• Monitor for progression of neurologic signs

PREVENTION/AVOIDANCE
• Most infections occur when rabbits are young
• Rabbits with CNS, ocular, or renal signs are no longer shedding spores.
• Clean environment daily; spores are inactivated by most common disinfectants. Select serologically negative rabbits for breeding, when possible.
• Some practitioners advocate serologic testing prior to purchase or addition of a new rabbit and excluding seropositive rabbits. Antibody titers may be helpful in the development of SPF colonies: testing every

2 weeks for 2 months and removing all positive rabbits.

POSSIBLE COMPLICATIONS
N/A

EXPECTED COURSE AND PROGNOSIS
• Prognosis—guarded; varied response to drug treatment; many rabbits improve with supportive care alone
• Acute, severe neurologic signs or renal insufficiency—guarded to poor prognosis; some improve with supportive care
• Residual deficits (especially neurologic) cannot be predicted until after a course of therapy
• Ocular disease—variable response to medical therapy; removal of the lens by phacoemulsion necessary to prevent progression to glaucoma; ocular disease is not expected to progress to CNS or renal disease
• Severe muscular or neurologic disease—usually chronic debility

MISCELLANEOUS

ASSOCIATED CONDITIONS
• Hypercalciuria
• Gastrointestinal hypomotility/stasis
• Dermatitis

AGE-RELATED FACTORS
N/A

ZOONOTIC POTENTIAL
Unlikely, but possible in immunosuppressed humans. All confirmed human cases have been in severely immunocompromised patients and not correlated with *E. cuniculi*-positive rabbits. Mode of transmission and susceptibility in humans are unclear

PREGNANCY/FERTILITY/BREEDING
Placental transmission possible

ABBREVIATIONS
BUN = blood urea nitrogen
CNS = central nervous system
CT = computed tomography
ELISA = enzyme-linked immunosorbent assay
GI = gastrointestinal
IFA = immunofluorescence assay
PCV = packed cell volume
SPF = specific pathogen free

Suggested Reading
Bays TB. Geriatric care of rabbits, guinea pigs, and chinchillas. Vet Clin Exot Anim 2020;23:567–593.
DeCubellis J. Common emergencies in rabbits, guinea pigs, and chinchillas. Vet Clin Exot Anim 2016;19:411–429.
Fisher PG, Künzel F, Rylander H. Neurologic and musculoskeletal disease. In: Quesenberry KE, Carpenter JW, eds. Ferrets, Rabbits and Rodents, (4th ed.) Clinical Medicine and Surgery. St. Louis: Saunders, 2020:583–594.
Harkness JE, Turner PV, VandeWoude S, Wheeler CL. Clinical signs and differential diagnoses: nervous and musculoskeletal conditions. In: Harkness JE, Turner PV, VandeWoude S, Wheeler CL, eds. Biology and Medicine of Rabbits and Rodents, 5th ed. Ames: Wiley-Blackwell, 2010:214–216.
Keeble E. Nervous system and musculoskeletal disorders. In: Meredith A, Lord B, eds. BSAVA Manual of Rabbit Medicine. Gloucester: British Small Animal Veterinary Association, 2014:233–248.
Lennox AM, Gladden JN. Emergency and critical care of small mammals. In: Quesenberry KE, Carpenter JW, eds. Ferrets, Rabbits and Rodents, (4th ed.) Clinical Medicine and Surgery. 2021, St. Louis: Saunders, 2020:595–608.
Varga M. Neurological and locomotive disorders. In: Varga M, ed. Textbook of Rabbit Medicine, 2nd ed. London, UK: Elsevier, 2014:367–389.
Author Barbara Oglesbee, DVM, DABVP (Avian)

ENCEPHALITIS AND MENINGOENCEPHALITIS

BASICS

DEFINITION
• Encephalitis—inflammation of the brain that may be accompanied by spinal cord and/or meningeal involvement
• Meningoencephalitis—inflammation of the meninges and brain

PATHOPHYSIOLOGY
• Inflammation—caused by an infectious agent (bacterial, viral, or parasitic) or by the patient's own immune system
• Bacterial infection of the CNS by extension of an infected extraneural site, especially ears or sinuses (most common) or by hematogenous route
• Immune-mediated—cause of immune system derangement generally unknown; not reported in rabbits

SYSTEMS AFFECTED
• Nervous
• Multisystemic signs—may be noted in patients with infectious diseases

INCIDENCE/PREVALENCE
Unknown

GEOGRAPHIC DISTRIBUTION
Varies with the cause or agent implicated

SIGNALMENT
• Lop-eared rabbits may be more likely to show signs of otitis with subsequent meningeal/brain involvement.
• Dwarf breeds, older and immunosuppressed rabbits may be more predisposed to signs due to infectious causes.

SIGNS

Historical Findings
• Usually a peracute to acute onset of clinical signs
• History of upper respiratory infection, dental disease, otitis externa/interna in rabbits with bacterial meningoencephalitis or brain abscesses
• History of grazing outdoors consistent with parasitic encephalitis (*Baylisascariasis*, *Toxoplasmosis*)

Physical Examination Findings
• Head tilt accompanied by other vestibular signs often seen in rabbits with brain abscess or encephalitozoonosis
• In rabbits with otitis externa, thick, white, creamy exudate may be found in the horizontal and/or vertical canals. Otitis interna/media may occur in the absence of otitis externa via extension through the eustachian tube; may see bulging tympanum. Most rabbits with otitis interna have no visible otoscopic abnormalities.

Neurologic Examination Findings
• Determined by the portion of the brain most affected
• Forebrain—seizures, personality change, decreasing level of responsiveness
• Brainstem—depression, head tilt, rolling, abnormal nystagmus, facial paresis/paralysis, and incoordination

CAUSES
• Protozoal—*Encephalitozoon cuniculi*: very common. How often *E. cuniculi* is truly the cause of neurologic signs is controversial, since antemortem definitive diagnosis is not possible and postmortem changes do not correlate well with clinical disease; toxoplasmosis: sporadic cause
• Bacterial—common, especially secondary to local extension from infection of the ears, eyes, sinuses, nasal passages caused by *Pasteurella* spp. or other bacteria
• Inflammatory, idiopathic, immune-mediated—granulomatous meningoencephalomyelitis, common postmortem finding in rabbits both with and without antemortem neurologic signs; has been attributed to *E. cuniculi* infection, but organisms not always found
• Parasite migration—sporadic; *Baylisascaris* (raccoon roundworm)
• Viral—rare; rabies virus and herpes reported
• Mycotic—not yet reported in rabbits

RISK FACTORS
• Bacterial—otitis interna/media, dental disease, chronic upper respiratory infection, immunosuppression (stress, corticosteroid use, concurrent disease)
• *Encephalitozoon cuniculi*—immunosuppression (stress, corticosteroid use, concurrent disease)
• *Toxoplasma* sp., *Baylisascaris* sp.—grazing outdoors, exposure to feed contaminated with cat or raccoon feces
• Injury involving the CNS or adjacent structures

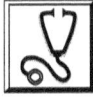

DIAGNOSIS

DIFFERENTIAL DIAGNOSIS
• Bacterial diseases—usually proceeded by history of, or accompanied by, signs of upper respiratory disease, dental disease, or otitis. Not all rabbits with otitis interna/media have signs of otitis externa since bacterial extension from the eustachian tube is common.
• Encephalitozoonosis—diagnosis of exclusion; rule out other causes of encephalitis, especially bacterial
• Primary CNS neoplasia—rare in rabbits; signs may be similar to encephalitis

• Metabolic or toxic encephalopathy—bilateral, symmetrical neurologic abnormalities that relate to the cerebrum
• Trauma—history and physical evidence of injury

CBC/BIOCHEMISTRY/URINALYSIS
• Hemogram—frequently normal
• Serum chemistry—to rule out metabolic disease

OTHER LABORATORY TESTS
• Serologic testing for *E. cuniculi*
  ○ The usefulness of serum antibody testing is limited in pet rabbits since a positive titer indicates only exposure and does not confirm *E. cuniculi* as the cause of clinical signs. *E. cuniculi* can only be definitively diagnosed by finding organisms and resultant lesions on histopathologic examination in areas that anatomically correlate with observed clinical signs.
  ○ IgG titers usually become positive by 2 weeks post infection. A rising titer after 4 weeks may confirm infection, but titers do not always continue to rise with active infection. IgG levels can decline after 8 weeks in some rabbits, in others may persist for life. No correlation exits between antibody titers and shedding of organism or severity of disease. Available tests include ELISA and IFA.
  ○ IgM titers may indicate a more recent, active infection. Titers become positive shortly after infection and appear to persist for up to 18 weeks.
  ○ C-reactive protein, an inflammatory marker, appears to be elevated in rabbits with active infection. Although this marker is nonspecific, concurrent elevation with IgG and IgM supports active infection.
  ○ A negative test may rule out infection; however, false negatives can be seen in early infections, before titers have a chance to rise.
• Serologic testing for toxoplasmosis—ELISA testing for IgM and IgG is commercially available. The overall seroprevalence is low and most seropositive rabbits are asymptomatic.
• Serologic testing for *Pasteurella*—usefulness is severely limited and generally not helpful in the diagnosis of pasteurellosis in pet rabbits. An ELISA is available, and positive results, even when high, only indicate prior exposure to *Pasteurella* and the development of antibodies and does not confirm active infection. Low positive results may occur due to cross-reaction with other, nonpathogenic bacteria (false positive). False negative results are common with immunosuppression or early infection. No evidence exists to support correlation of titers to the presence or absence of disease.

ENCEPHALITIS AND MENINGOENCEPHALITIS

• Serologic testing for toxoplasmosis—anecdotal reports exist of using serum antibody titers available for testing in dogs and cats to diagnose infection in rabbits.

IMAGING
• Tympanic bullae and skull radiography—may help rule out otitis interna/media; however, normal radiographs do not rule out bulla disease.
• CT—valuable for confirming bulla lesions and CNS extension from otitis; or to document localized tumor, granuloma, and extent of inflammation

DIAGNOSITIC PROCEDURES
• Bacterial culture and sensitivity testing in rabbits with concurrent otitis—sample from myringotomy or surgical drainage of tympanic bulla is most accurate
• Culture of the nasal cavity—may be helpful to direct antibiotic therapy in rabbits with intact tympanum and evidence of concurrent respiratory infection if extension of URI is suspected. To obtain a sample, a mini-tip culturette is inserted 1–4 cm inside the nares near the nasal septum. Sedation and appropriate restraint are required to obtain a deep, meaningful sample. The nasal cavity is extremely sensitive, and rabbits that appear sedated may jump or kick when the nasal mucosa is touched. Inadequate sedation or restraint may result in serious spinal or other musculoskeletal injury.
• CSF analysis—sample from the cerebellomedullary cistern; may be valuable for evaluating central disease; detect inflammatory process; sample collection may put the patient at risk for herniation if there is a mass or high intracranial pressure.

PATHOLOGIC FINDINGS
The lesions are a function of the brain response to the infectious agent or other cause. Nonsuppurative granulomatous meningoencephalomyelitis is common on postmortem examination of rabbits suspected of encephalitazoonosis. However, there is often no direct correlation between the severity, presence, or absence of CNS lesions and clinical signs of CNS disease.

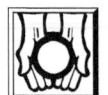

TREATMENT

APPROPRIATE HEALTH CARE
Inpatient—diagnosis and initial therapy

NURSING CARE
Supportive fluids—replacement or maintenance fluids (depend on clinical state); may be required in the acute phase when disorientation and nausea preclude oral intake

ACTIVITY
Restrict (e.g., avoid stairs and slippery surfaces) according to the degree of disequilibrium; encourage return to activity as soon as safely possible; activity may enhance recovery of vestibular function

DIET
• It is important that the rabbit continue to eat during and following treatment. Many rabbits with encephalitis, especially those with vestibular signs, will not eat. Anorexia will cause GI hypomotility or GI stasis, derangement of the gastrointestinal microflora, and overgrowth of intestinal bacterial pathogens.
• Make sure that food and water are within reach; may need to bring food to patient.
• If the rabbit refuses food, syringe-feed a gruel such as Critical Care for Herbivores (Oxbow Pet Products) or Emeraid Herbivore (Lafeber Company, Cornell, IL) 10–15 mL/kg PO q6–8h. Larger volumes and more frequent feedings are often accepted; feed as much as the rabbit will accept. Alternatively, pellets can be ground and mixed with fresh greens, vegetable baby foods, water, or juice to form a gruel.
• High-carbohydrate, high-fat nutritional supplements are contraindicated.
• Encourage oral fluid intake by offering fresh water, wetting leafy vegetables, or flavoring water with vegetable juices.

CLIENT EDUCATION
• Inform client that the condition can be life threatening
• Emphasize the importance of the diagnostic workup.
• Prognosis is guarded; response to therapy inconsistent
• Long-term home nursing care (assist-feed, padded bedding in recumbent animals) may be required; residual neurologic signs common in rabbits that partially recover; a waxing and waning course of progression is seen in some rabbits; some rabbits take weeks to months to recover
• Head tilt may be permanent but may not affect quality of life in most recovered patients.

MEDICATIONS

DRUG(S) OF CHOICE
• Apply specific therapy once diagnosis is reached or highly suspected.
• Seizures—control may be erratic unless the encephalitis can be treated; diazepam—1–5 mg/kg IV, IM; begin with 0.5–1.0 mg/kg IV bolus; may repeat if gross

seizure activity has not stopped within 5 minutes; can be administered rectally if IV access cannot be obtained; may diminish or stop the gross motor seizure activity to allow IV catheter placement; constant rate infusion protocols used in dogs and cats have been anecdotally used
• Severe vestibular signs (continuous rolling, torticollis)—diazepam 1–2 mg/kg IM or midazolam 0.5–2.0 mg/kg IM; meclizine 2–12 mg/kg PO q24h may reduce clinical signs, control nausea, and induce mild sedation
• If anorexic, maropitant (2 mg/kg SC, PO q24h) or metoclopramide (0.5–1.0 mg/kg PO, SC, IV q12h)
• Vestibular signs—meclizine 2–12 mg/kg PO q24h may reduce clinical signs, control nausea, and induce mild sedation
• Bacterial meningoencephalitis; abscess—antibiotics; choice is ideally based on results of culture and susceptibility testing when possible (otitis, extension from sinuses). Long-term antibiotic therapy is generally required (4–6 weeks minimum, to several months). Use broad-spectrum antibiotics such as enrofloxacin (10–20 mg/kg PO, SC, IM, IV q12h), marbofloxacin (5 mg/kg PO q24h), trimethoprim-sulfa (15–30 mg/kg PO q12h), or chloramphenicol (50 mg/kg PO q8h). Most facial or dental abscesses contain anaerobic bacteria; use antibiotics effective against anaerobes such as azithromycin (15–30 mg/kg PO q24h); can be used alone or combined with metronidazole (20 mg/kg PO q12h). Alternatively, use penicillin G procaine (40,000–60,000 IU/kg SC q24h).
• Encephalitozoonosis—Fenbendazole (20 mg/kg q24h × 28 days) is the most common treatment and has been shown to reduce clinical signs and increase survival rates in symptomatic patients. Benzimidazole anthelmintics are effective against *E. cuniculi* in vitro and have been shown to prevent experimental infection in rabbits. However, efficacy in rabbits with clinical signs is unknown. Long-term treatment has been recommended, as treatment only prevents replication, rather than kills the parasite.
• Toxoplasmosis—trimethoprim-sulfa 15–30 mg/kg PO q12h; sulfadiazine in combination with pyrimethamine for 2 weeks has also been recommended

CONTRAINDICATIONS
• Dexamethasone—contraindicated in patients with infectious diseases, but may help decrease brain edema when impending brain herniation or life-threatening edema is suspected
• Oral administration of antibiotics that select against gram-positive bacteria (penicillins, macrolides, lincosamides, and

cephalosporins) can cause fatal enteric dysbiosis and enterotoxemia.

PRECAUTIONS
• Topical and systemic corticosteroids—rabbits are very sensitive to the immunosuppressive effects of corticosteroids; use may exacerbate subclinical bacterial or *E. cuniculi* infection.
• Albendazole has been associated with bone marrow toxicity in rabbits. Many anecdotal reports of pancytopenia leading to death in rabbits exist.

POSSIBLE INTERACTIONS
N/A

ALTERNATIVE DRUGS
• Systemic corticosteroids have been advocated by some practitioners for treatment of *E. cuniculi*–induced CNS granulomatous inflammation. Use of corticosteroids is controversial. Although clinical improvement has been anecdotally reported, rabbits are very sensitive to the immunosuppressive effects of corticosteroids; immunosuppression may exacerbate subclinical bacterial or *E. cuniculi* infection.
• Ponazuril has been anecdotally used to treat *E. cuniculi* (20–50 mg/kg PO q24h × 30 days). Safety and efficacy are unknown.

FOLLOW-UP

PATIENT MONITORING
• Repeat the neurologic examination at a frequency dictated by the underlying cause.
• Head tilt or other neurologic signs may persist.

POSSIBLE COMPLICATIONS
• Progression of disease with deterioration of mental status
• CSF collection or natural course of the disease—tentorial herniation and death

EXPECTED COURSE AND PROGNOSIS
• Resolution of signs—generally gradual (2–16 weeks)

• Prognosis—guarded depending on underlying cause; viral, parasitic migration—almost always progress to death; protozoal—course varies greatly, response to treatment erratic; many improve with supportive care; bacterial—depends on extent of infection, may improve with long-term antibiotic care
• Following acute episodes of vestibular signs, head tilt often persists. Most rabbits adapt well to this, will ambulate, eat well, and appear to live comfortable lives. Recurrence of acute episodes may occur.
• Residual neurologic deficits cannot be predicted.

MISCELLANEOUS

ASSOCIATED CONDITIONS
• Dental disease
• Upper respiratory infections
• Facial abscesses
• Gastrointestinal hypomotility

AGE-RELATED FACTORS
Encephalitozoonosis and bacterial disease may be more common in older, especially immunosuppressed, animals.

ZOONOTIC POTENTIAL
• Rabies—consider in endemic areas if the patient is an outdoor animal that has rapidly progressive encephalitis
• Encephalitozoonosis—unlikely, but possible in immunosuppressed humans; mode of transmission and susceptibility in humans is unclear

PREGNANCY/FERTILITY/BREEDING
N/A

SYNONYMS
N/A

SEE ALSO
Ataxia
Head tilt (vestibular disease)
Seizures

ABBREVIATIONS
CNS = central nervous system
CSF = cerebrospinal fluid

CT = computed tomography
ELISA = enzyme-linked immunosorbent assay
IFA = immunofluorescence assay
PCR = polymerase chain reaction
URI = upper respiratory infection

Suggested Reading

Bays TB. Geriatric care of rabbits, guinea pigs, and chinchillas. Vet Clin Exot Anim 2020;23:567–593.
DeCubellis J. Common emergencies in rabbits, guinea pigs, and chinchillas. Vet Clin Exot Anim 2016;19:411–429.
Fisher PG, Künzel F, Rylander H. Neurologic and musculoskeletal disease. In: Quesenberry KE, Carpenter JW, eds. Ferrets, Rabbits and Rodents, (4th ed). Clinical Medicine and Surgery. St. Louis: Saunders, 2020:583–594.
Harkness JE, Turner PV, VandeWoude S, Wheeler CL. Clinical signs and differential diagnoses: nervous and musculoskeletal conditions. In: Harkness JE, Turner PV, VandeWoude S, Wheeler CL, eds. Biology and Medicine of Rabbits and Rodents, 5th ed. Ames: Wiley-Blackwell, 2010: 214–216.
Keeble E. Nervous system and musculoskeletal disorders. In: Meredith A, Lord B, eds. BSAVA Manual of Rabbit Medicine. Gloucester: British Small Animal Veterinary Association, 2014:233–248.
Lennox AM, Gladden JN. Emergency and critical care of small mammals. In: Quesenberry KE, Carpenter JW, eds. Ferrets, Rabbits and Rodents, (4th ed). Clinical Medicine and Surgery. 2021, St. Louis: Saunders, 2020:595–608.
Varga M. Neurological and locomotive disorders. In: Varga M, ed. Textbook of Rabbit Medicine, 2nd ed. London, UK: Elsevier, 2014:367–389.
Author Barbara Oglesbee, DVM, DABVP (Avian)

EPIPHORA

BASICS

DEFINITION
Abnormal overflow of the aqueous portion of the precorneal tear film

PATHOPHYSIOLOGY
• Caused by blockage of the nasolacrimal drainage system, overproduction of the aqueous portion of tears (usually in response to ocular irritation), or poor eyelid function secondary to malformation or deformity
• In rabbits, epiphora is most often caused by blockage of the nasolacrimal duct either due to dental disease (most commonly incisor malocclusion) or blockage by dried exudate.
• Rabbits have only one nasolacrimal punctum, with a nasolacrimal duct that runs in close association with the roots of the cheek teeth (premolars and molars) and upper incisors. Elongation of the tooth roots is an extremely common disorder in pet rabbits. Root elongation and tooth root abscesses can impinge on or erode into the nasolacrimal duct, resulting in blockage and/or dacryocystitis. In most cases, the blocked duct fills with inflammatory cells, oil, and debris; however, secondary bacterial infections can occur.
• Also commonly caused by blockage of the nasolacrimal duct with inspissated exudate or scarring secondary to chronic upper respiratory infections.

SYSTEMS AFFECTED
Ophthalmic
Dermatologic (secondary moist pyoderma)

SIGNALMENT
• Acquired cheek tooth elongation causing blockage of nasolacrimal duct or intrusion into the retrobulbar space—usually seen in middle-aged rabbits
• Young animals—congenital tooth malocclusion, congenital eyelid deformities
• Dwarf and lop breeds—congenital tooth malocclusion
• Dwarf and Himalayan breeds—glaucoma more common
• Rex and New Zealand White breeds—entropion and trichiasis more common
• Blockage of the nasolacrimal duct due to dried exudate can be seen in any age rabbit

SIGNS

Historical Signs
• History of previous treatment for dental disease
• History of incisor overgrowth
• History of nasal discharge or previous upper respiratory infection

• Facial asymmetry, masses, or exophthalmos in rabbits with tooth root abscesses or facial nerve paralysis
• Unilateral or bilateral alopecia, crusts, matted fur in periocular area, cheeks, and/or nasal rostrum
• History of red or painful eyes in rabbits with primary ocular disease

Physical Examination Findings
• Facial pyoderma—alopecia, erythema, matted fur, in periocular are cheeks and/or nasal rostrum; due to constant moisture from epiphora
• Thick white exudate accumulation in medial canthus in rabbits with dacryocystitis
• Corneal ulcers associated with dacryocystitis are usually superficial and ventrally located; ulcers secondary to exposure keratitis are usually central and may be superficial or deep.
• Depending on the underlying cause, may see blepharospasm, conjunctival hyperemia, exophthalmia, entropion, or corneal disease. Perform a complete ocular examination including pupillary light reflex, Schirmer tear test, tonometry; examination of the orbit, cornea, anterior chamber, iris, fundus, conjunctiva, nictitating membrane, and eyelids
Oral examination
• A thorough examination of the oral cavity is indicated in every rabbit with epiphora. A thorough examination includes the incisors, molars, and buccal and lingual mucosa to rule out dental disease. Use of an otoscope or speculum may be useful in identifying severe abnormalities; however, many problems will be missed by using this method alone. Complete exam requires heavy sedation or general anesthesia and specialized equipment.
• A focused, directed light source and magnification (or a rigid endoscope) will provide optimal visualization.
• Use a rodent mouth gag and cheek dilators (Jorgensen Laboratories, Inc., Loveland, CO) to open the mouth and pull buccal tissues away from teeth surfaces to allow adequate exposure. Use a cotton swab or tongue depressor to retract tongue from lingual surfaces.
• Identify cheek teeth elongation, irregular crown height, spikes, curved teeth, tooth discoloration, tooth mobility, missing teeth, purulent exudate, oral ulceration, or abscesses.
• Significant tooth root abnormalities may be present despite normal-appearing crowns. Skull films are required to identify apical disorders.
• Incisors—may see overgrowth, horizontal ridges or grooves, malformation,

discoloration, fractures, increased or decreased curvature

CAUSES AND RISK FACTORS

Obstruction of the Nasolacrimal Drainage System (Most Common Cause)
Acquired
• Dacryocystitis—inflammation of the canaliculi, lacrimal sac, or nasolacrimal ducts. Can extend from primary rhinitis or conjunctivitis. If bacterial infection is present (primary or secondary), *Staphylococcus* spp., *Pseudomonas* spp., *Moraxella* spp., *Pasteurella multocida*, *Niesseria* spp., and *Bordetella* spp. frequently cultured
• Cheek tooth or incisor elongation—common cause; the nasolacrimal duct is normally very closely associated with the roots of the incisors and cheek teeth; elongation or abscessation of the tooth roots (most commonly the second upper premolar) impinges or invades into the nasolacrimal duct
• Rhinitis or sinusitis—causes swelling adjacent to the nasolacrimal duct
• Trauma or fractures of the lacrimal or maxillary bones
• Neoplasia—conjunctiva, medial eyelids, nasal cavity, maxillary bone, or periocular sinuses
Congenital
• Imperforate nasolacrimal puncta, ectopic nasolacrimal openings, and nasolacrimal atresia—not yet documented in rabbits

Overproduction of Tears Secondary to Ocular Irritants
Congenital
• Distichiasis or trichiasis
• Entropion
Acquired
• Corneal or conjunctival foreign bodies (especially hay, litter, or bedding)
• Corneal stromal abscess
• Conjunctivitis—often associated with upper respiratory infections, environmental irritants, or rarely, blepharoconjuntivitis due to mxyomatosis
• Ulcerative keratitis—trauma most common; exposure keratitis following anesthesia, facial nerve paralysis; corneal abrasion in rabbits with torticollis
• Anterior uveitis—most commonly bacterial or *Encephalitozoon cuniculi*
• Glaucoma
• Eyelid neoplasms
• Blepharitis

Eyelid Abnormalities or Poor Eyelid Function
Tears never reach the nasolacrimal puncta but instead spill over the eyelid margin.

Congenital
• Entropion
Acquired
• Posttraumatic eyelid scarring
• Facial nerve paralysis

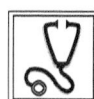

DIAGNOSIS

DIFFERENTIAL DIAGNOSIS
• Other ocular discharges (e.g., mucus or purulent)—epiphora is a watery, serous discharge.
• Eye—often red when caused by overproduction of tears; quiet when secondary to impaired outflow; however, chronic blockage of the nasolacrimal duct and dacryocystitis can lead to corneal ulceration or secondary conjunctivitis
• Unilateral condition with ocular pain (blepharospasm)—usually indicates a tooth root disorder, foreign body, or corneal injury
• Chronic, bilateral condition—usually due to chronic upper respiratory tract infection (scarring, inflammation of duct); can indicate a congenital problem; bilateral tooth root disorders also seen
• Acute, bilateral condition with severe eyelid edema—consider myxomatosis
• Facial pain, swelling, nasal discharge, or sneezing—seen with tooth root elongation or abscess; may indicate nasal or sinus infection; and may indicate obstruction from neoplasm
• White discharge confined to the medial canthus—usually indicates dacryocystitis

CBC/BIOCHEMISTRY/URINALYSIS
N/A

OTHER LABORATORY TESTS
N/A

IMAGING
• Skull radiographs are needed to identify dental disease, nasal, sinus, or maxillary bone lesions and, if present, to plan treatment strategies and to monitor progression of treatment.
• Perform under general anesthesia
• Five views are recommended for thorough assessment: ventral-dorsal, lateral, two lateral obliques, and rostral-caudal.
• CT—superior to radiographs to localize obstruction and characterize associated lesions
• Dacryocystorhinography—radiopaque contrast material to help localize obstruction

DIAGNOSTIC PROCEDURES
• Bacterial culture and sensitivity testing and cytologic examination of the material—with purulent material at the medial canthus (e.g., dacryocystitis); performed before instilling any substance into the eye. Often, only normal organisms are isolated (*Bacillus subtilis*, *Staphylococcus aureus*, and *Bordetella* sp.)
• Topical fluorescein dye application to the eye—most physiologic test for nasolacrimal function; should be performed first; dye flows through the nasolacrimal system and reaches the external nares in approximately 10 seconds in normal rabbits.
• Rhinoscopy—with or without biopsy or bacterial culture; may be indicated if previous tests suggest a nasal or sinus lesion

Nasolacrimal Flush
• Confirms obstruction
• May dislodge foreign material
• Topical administration of an ophthalmic anesthetic is generally sufficient for this procedure; nervous rabbits may require mild sedation.
• Rabbits have only a single nasolacrimal punctum located in the ventral eyelid at the medial canthus. A 23-gauge lacrimal cannula or a 24-gauge Teflon intravenous catheter can be used to flush the duct. Irrigation will generally produce a thick white exudate from the nasal meatus.

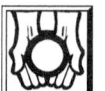

TREATMENT
• Remove cause of ocular irritation—removal of a conjunctival or corneal foreign body; treatment of the primary ocular disease (e.g., conjunctivitis, ulcerative keratitis, and uveitis); entropion correction
• Treat primary obstructing lesion (e.g., dental disease, nasal or sinus mass, and infection)—can be frustrating with advanced underlying dental disease
• Nasolacrimal duct irrigation—as described above
• Irrigation of the duct often needs to be repeated, either daily for 2–3 consecutive days, or once every 3–4 days until irrigation produces a clear fluid.
• Instill an ophthalmic antibiotic solution such as ciprofloxacin or chloramphenicol 4–6 times a day for 14–21 days following nasolacrimal duct irrigation.
• Keep fur around face clean and dry.

CLIENT EDUCATION
• Warn client that recurrence is common in patients with nasolacrimal obstruction.
• Inform client that early detection and intervention provides a better long-term prognosis.
• The nasolacrimal duct may become completely obliterated in rabbits with severe tooth root disease, abscesses involving the duct, or scarring due to chronic infection. Epiphora may be lifelong. Home management, including keeping the face clean and dry, is crucial to prevent secondary pyoderma. In many cases, acquisition of a second rabbit can beneficial if the second rabbit grooms discharges from the face.
• Rabbits with cheek tooth root elongation—by the time clinical signs are noted, disease is usually advanced. Lifelong treatment, consisting of periodic coronal reduction (teeth trimming), is required, usually every 3–12 months.
• Severe dental disease, especially those with tooth root abscesses and severe bony destruction, carries a guarded to poor prognosis for complete resolution. Most will require extensive surgery, sometimes multiple surgeries and multiple follow-up visits. Recurrences in the same or other locations are common. Clients must be aware of the monetary and time investment.

SURGICAL CONSIDERATIONS
• Trimming of cheek teeth (coronal reduction)—may control progression of root elongation
• Tooth extraction—indicated in rabbits with congenital incisor malocclusion or teeth that are severely diseased; extracting teeth may not improve tear duct patency if extraluminal compression cannot be relieved.
• In rabbits with extensive tooth root abscesses, aggressive debridement is indicated, and special expertise may be required. Maxillary and retrobulbar abscesses can be particularly challenging. If practitioner is not experienced with facial abscesses in rabbits, the author recommends referral to a veterinarian with special expertise whenever feasible.

MEDICATIONS
DRUG(S) OF CHOICE
• Topical broad-spectrum antibiotic ophthalmic solutions—use following nasolacrimal duct irrigation and while waiting for results of diagnostic tests (e.g., bacterial culture and sensitivity testing; diagnostic radiographs); q4–6h; may try triple antibiotic solution, ciprofloxacin, ofloxacin, gentocin, or ophthalmic chloramphenicol solution
• Dacryocystitis—based on bacterial culture and sensitivity test results; continued for at least 21 days
• Systemic antibiotics—indicated in rabbits with tooth root abscess as cause of conjunctivitis
• Topical nonsteroidal anti-inflammatory agents—0.03% flurbiprofen or 1% diclofenac may help reduce inflammation and irritation associated with flushes.

EPIPHORA

CONTRAINDICATIONS
• Topical corticosteroids or antibiotic-corticosteroid combinations—avoid; associated with gastrointestinal ulceration and hemorrhage, delayed wound healing, and heightened susceptibility to infection; rabbits are very sensitive to the immunosuppressive effects of both topical and systemic corticosteroids; use may exacerbate subclinical bacterial infection
• Topical corticosteroids—never use if the cornea retains fluorescein stain

PRECAUTIONS
Aggressive flushing of the nasolacrimal duct may cause temporary swelling of the periocular tissues. Swelling usually resolves within 12–48 hours.

POSSIBLE INTERACTIONS
N/A

ALTERNATIVE DRUGS
N/A

FOLLOW-UP

PATIENT MONITORING
Dacryocystitis
• Reevaluate every 3–4 days until the condition is resolved.
• Problem persists more than 7–10 days with treatment or recurs soon after cessation of treatment—indicates a nidus of persistent infection or obstruction; requires further diagnostics (e.g., skull films, dacryostorhinography)

POSSIBLE COMPLICATIONS
• Recurrence—most common complication; caused by nonresolution of underlying dental disease, recurrence of ocular irritation (e.g., corneal ulceration, distichiasis, and entropion), or chronic URI
• In rabbits with chronic dental disease, lifelong treatment is required.
• Permanent blockage of the nasolacrimal duct may occur due to scarring from chronic URI, abscess, or neoplasia

MISCELLANEOUS

ASSOCIATED CONDITIONS
• Immunosuppression
• Recurrent eye "infections"
• Moist dermatitis ventral to the medial canthus
• Nasal discharge

AGE-RELATED FACTORS
N/A

ZOONOTIC POTENTIAL
N/A

PREGNANCY/FERTILITY/BREEDING
N/A

SEE ALSO
Cheek teeth (premolar and molar) malocclusion and elongation
Conjunctivitis
Incisor malocclusion and overgrowth
Abscesses (periapical infections and osteomyelitis)
Pyoderma

ABBREVIATIONS
URI = upper respiratory infection

Suggested Reading
Harcourt-Brown F. Treatment of dental problems: principles and options. In: Harcourt-Brown F, Chitty J, eds. BSAVA Manual of Rabbit Surgery, Dentistry, and Imaging. Gloucester, UK: BSAVA, 2013:349–369.
Lennox AM, Capello V, Legendre LF. Small mammal dentistry. In: Quesenberry KE, Carpenter JW, eds. Ferrets, Rabbits and Rodents, (4th ed). Clinical Medicine and Surgery. 2021, St. Louis: Saunders, 2020:514–535.
Varga M. Dental Disease. Textbook of Rabbit Medicine, 2nd ed. London, UK: Elsevier, 2014:203–248.
Van der Woerdt A. Ophthalmologic diseases of small mammals. In: Quesenberry KE, Carpenter JW, eds. Ferrets, Rabbits and Rodents, (4th ed). Clinical Medicine and Surgery. 2021, St. Louis: Saunders, 2020:583–594.

Author Barbara Oglesbee, DVM, DABVP (Avian)

FACIAL NERVE PARESIS/PARALYSIS

BASICS

DEFINITION
Dysfunction of the facial nerve (seventh cranial nerve), causing paralysis or weakness of the muscles of the ears, eyelids, lips, and nostrils

PATHOPHYSIOLOGY
Weakness or paralysis caused by impairment of the facial nerve or the neuromuscular junction peripherally or the facial nucleus in the brain stem

SYSTEMS AFFECTED
• Nervous—facial nerve peripherally or its nucleus in the brain stem
• Ophthalmic—if parasympathetic preganglionic neurons that supply the lacrimal glands and course with the facial nerve are involved, keratoconjunctivitis sicca develops because of lack of tear secretion.

GENETICS
N/A

INCIDENCE/PREVALENCE
Common sequela to otic and dental disease in rabbits

GEOGRAPHIC DISTRIBUTION
N/A

SIGNALMENT
• Lop-eared rabbits may be more likely to develop otitis externa, dental disease, and subsequent facial nerve paralysis.
• Dwarf breeds are more likely to have dental disease and subsequent facial nerve paralysis.
• No age or sex predilection

SIGNS

General Comments
• Assess strength of the palpebral closure; there should be full eyelid closure when a finger is gently passed over both eyelids simultaneously.
• Bilateral nerve involvement is rare in rabbits—consider systemic disease or bilateral otitis.
• Unilateral paresis or paralysis—may accompany other clinical signs; may indicate focal or systemic disease

Historical Findings
• History of otitis externa, interna, or media
• History of vestibular disease
• Head tilt
• Holding one ear down
• Excessive drooling
• Facial asymmetry
• Eye—inability to close; rubbing; discharge; cloudy cornea, redness

Physical Examination Findings
Findings associated with facial nerve disorder:
• Ipsilateral ear and lip drooping
• Excessive drooling
• Food falling from the side of mouth
• Collapse of the nostril
• Inability to close the eyelids
• Wide palpebral fissure
• Palpebral reflex decreased or absent
• Chronic—patient may have deviation of the face toward the affected side
• Nasal discharge, facial abscesses
Findings associated with ear disease:
• Many rabbits with otitis interna/media have normal-appearing external canals, since infection often spreads from upper respiratory tract via the eustachian tube
• Evidence of aural erythema, white creamy discharge, and thick and stenotic canals support otitis externa
• White, dull, opaque, and bulging tympanic membrane on otoscopic examination sometimes visible when middle ear exudate is present
• Abscess at the base of the ear common finding
• Pain—may be detected upon opening the mouth or bulla palpation
Other findings:
• Mucopurulent discharge from the affected eye and exposure conjunctivitis or keratitis—may be noted
• When secondary to brain stem disease—altered mentation (e.g., depression or stupor); other cranial nerve and gait abnormalities may be noted

CAUSES

Unilateral Peripheral
• Inflammatory—otitis media or interna
• Trauma—fracture of the petrous temporal bone; injury to the facial nerve external to the stylomastoid foramen or secondary to surgical ablation of external ear canal
• Neoplasia
• Idiopathic vestibular disease
• Metabolic causes not reported in rabbits, but should be considered

Bilateral Peripheral
• Bilateral ear disease
• Idiopathic, metabolic, inflammatory, and immune-mediated—not reported in rabbits
• Toxic—botulism

CNS
• Most unilateral
• Inflammatory—infectious (bacterial abscess as extension from ear or dental disease), protozoal (*Encephalitozoon cuniculi*), fungal (not well described in rabbits), and noninfectious (granulomatous meningoencephalomyelitis)
• Neoplastic—primary brain tumor; metastatic tumor

RISK FACTORS
Chronic ear disease

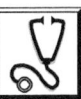

DIAGNOSIS

DIFFERENTIAL DIAGNOSIS
• Differentiate unilateral from bilateral
• Look for other neurologic deficits
• Be sure that abnormal head posture is not due to holding one ear down due to pain, as may occur in otitis externa alone, and not associated with neurologic pathology.
• *Encephalitozoon cuniculi*—this is a diagnosis of exclusion. Every attempt should be made to rule out otic disease prior to assuming *E. cuniculi* infection. Antemortem diagnosis of *E. cuniculi* is usually presumed based on clinical signs, exclusion of other diagnoses, positive antibody titers, and sometimes, response to treatment. Definitive antemortem diagnosis is problematic, since a positive antibody titer indicates exposure only, some rabbits respond minimally or not at all to anthelmintic treatment, and many rabbits will improve spontaneously with supportive care alone. Definitive diagnosis requires identification of organisms and characteristic inflammation in tissues anatomically correlated with clinical signs, generally acquired at postmortem examination. Results of several studies demonstrate a poor or no correlation between the severity of CNS lesions on postmortem and clinical signs.
• Central vestibular diseases—difficult to differentiate in rabbits; may see lethargy, somnolence, stupor, and other brain stem signs
• Neoplasia—uncommon causes of refractory and relapsing otitis media and interna; diagnosed by imaging of the head
• Trauma—history and physical evidence of injury
• Idiopathic—consider if patient has no historical or physical signs of ear disease and no other neurologic deficits

CBC/BIOCHEMISTRY/URINALYSIS
Usually normal

OTHER LABORATORY TESTS
• Serologic testing for *E. cuniculi*—many tests are available, but usefulness is extremely limited since a positive titer only indicates exposure and does not confirm *E. cuniculi* as the cause of neurologic signs. *E. cuniculi* can only be definitively diagnosed by finding organisms and resultant lesions on histopathologic examination in areas that anatomically correlate with observed clinical signs. A combination of IgM, IgG, and C-reactive protein appears to be most reliable.
• Serology for *Pasteurella*—has been used to attempt to rule out pasteurellosis as a cause of

FACIAL NERVE PARESIS/PARALYSIS (CONTINUED)

underlying disease. However, the usefulness of antibody titers is severely limited and generally not helpful in the diagnosis of pasteurellosis in pet rabbits. An ELISA is available; however, positive results, even when high, only indicate prior exposure to *Pasteurella* and the development of antibodies, and do not confirm active infection. Low positive results may occur due to cross-reaction with other, nonpathogenic bacteria (false positive). False-negative results are common with immunosuppression or early infection. No evidence exists to support correlation of titers to the presence or absence of disease.

IMAGING
• Bullae radiographs—tympanic bullae may appear cloudy if exudate is present; may see thickening of the bullae and petrous temporal bone with chronic disease; may see lysis of the bone with severe cases of osteomyelitis; may be normal in some rabbits, even with severe otitis interna and/or bullae disease; normal-appearing radiographs does not rule out bullae disease.
• CT—superior to radiographs to diagnose bullae disease. Detailed evidence of fluid and soft tissue density within the middle ear and the extent of involvement of the adjacent structures; defines brain stem disease

DIAGNOSTIC PROCEDURES
• Schirmer tear test—evaluate tear production. Average values reported as 5 mm/min; however, even lower values can be seen in normal rabbits.
• CSF examination—may be helpful in detecting brain stem disease
• Bacterial culture and sensitivity testing—sample from myringotomy or surgical removal of exudate from the tympanic bulla is most accurate

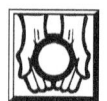

TREATMENT

APPROPRIATE HEALTH CARE
• Outpatient—otherwise healthy rabbits
• Inpatient—initial medical workup and management of systemic or CNS disease

NURSING CARE
• Concurrent otitis externa—culture and clean the ear; use warm normal saline if the tympanum is ruptured; if a cleaning solution is used, follow with a thorough flush with normal saline; dry the ear canal with a cotton swab and low vacuum suction; sedation or general anesthesia may be necessary in rabbits with painful ears

• Keep fur around face clean and dry
• Instill artificial tears if indicated

ACTIVITY
N/A

DIET
• Make sure that the patient continues to eat to prevent GI motility disorders.

CLIENT EDUCATION
• Advise client that the clinical signs are usually permanent, as muscle fibrosis develops.
• Inform client that the other side can become affected.
• Discuss eye care: the cornea on the affected side may need lubrication; must regularly check for corneal ulcers
• Inform client that most animals tolerate this nerve deficit well.

SURGICAL CONSIDERATIONS
Bulla osteotomy—may be indicated in patients with disorders of the middle ear to alleviate discomfort and prevent spread of infection into the brain; nerve paralysis will persist following surgery

MEDICATIONS

DRUG(S) OF CHOICE
• Treat specific disease if possible
• Tear replacement—if Schirmer tear test value low; with ectropion or exophthalmic globes

CONTRAINDICATIONS
• Corticosteroids—no evidence of improvement with use; will exacerbate infectious disease
• Oral administration of antibiotics that select against gram-positive bacteria (penicillins, macrolides, lincosamides, and cephalosporins) can cause fatal enteric dysbiosis and enterotoxemia.

PRECAUTIONS
N/A

POSSIBLE INTERACTIONS
N/A

ALTERNATIVE DRUGS
N/A

FOLLOW-UP

PATIENT MONITORING
• Reevaluate early for evidence of corneal ulcers.

• Assess monthly for palpebral reflexes, and lip and ear movements to evaluate return of function and condition of affected eye, although damage is often permanent.

PREVENTION/AVOIDANCE
Treating otitis or upper respiratory infections in early stages may prevent otitis media/interna and/or brain abscesses.

POSSIBLE COMPLICATIONS
• Keratoconjunctivitis sicca
• Corneal ulcers
• Severe contracture on side of lesion
• Progression of underlying disease

EXPECTED COURSE AND PROGNOSIS
• Depend on cause
• Improvement may take weeks or months or may never occur.
• Lip contracture sometimes develops.

MISCELLANEOUS

ASSOCIATED CONDITIONS
N/A

AGE-RELATED FACTORS
N/A

ZOONOTIC POTENTIAL
N/A

PREGNANCY/FERTILITY/BREEDING
N/A

SYNONYMS
Idiopathic facial paresis and paralysis

SEE ALSO
Conjunctivitis
Encephalitozoonosis
Head tilt (vestibular disease)
Otitis media and interna

ABBREVIATIONS
CNS = central nervous system
CSF = cerebrospinal fluid
CT = computed tomography
ELISA = enzyme-linked immunosorbent assay
GI = gastrointestinal
IFA = immunofluorescence assay

Suggested Reading
Csomos R, Bosscher G, Mans C, Hardie R. Surgical management of ear diseases in rabbits. Vet Clin Exot Anim 2016;19: 189–204.
Fisher PG, Künzel F, Rylander H. Neurologic and musculoskeletal disease. In: Quesenberry KE, Carpenter JW, eds.

RABBITS

Ferrets, Rabbits and Rodents, (4th ed). Clinical Medicine and Surgery. St. Louis: Saunders, 2020:583–594.

Keeble E. Nervous system and musculoskeletal disorders. In: Meredith A, Lord B, eds. BSAVA Manual of Rabbit Medicine. Gloucester: British Small Animal Veterinary Association, 2014:233–248.

Mancinelli E, Lennox AM. Management of otitis in rabbits. J Exot Pet Med 2017; 26:63–67.

Varga M. Neurological and locomotive disorders. In: Varga M, ed. Textbook of Rabbit Medicine, 2nd ed. London, UK: Elsevier, 2014:367–389.

Author Barbara Oglesbee, DVM, DABVP (Avian)

FLEAS AND FLEA INFESTATION

BASICS

OVERVIEW
• Flea infestation—the presence of fleas and flea dirt; *Ctenocephalides canis* or *C. felis* most commonly found on rabbits
• Heavy infestations may cause anemia, especially in young rabbits.
• Fleabite hypersensitivity has not been documented in rabbits; however, some rabbits appear to be significantly more pruritic than others, suggesting that a hypersensitivity reaction may exist in these animals.

SIGNALMENT
• Incidence varies with climatic conditions and flea population
• No age or sex predilection
• Clinical signs vary with individual animals
• Young animals more likely to develop anemia

SIGNS
Historical Findings
• History of flea infestation in other pets, including dogs and cats
• Some animals asymptomatic
• Biting, chewing, scratching, or excessive licking
• Signs of fleas and flea dirt

Physical Examination Findings
• Depends on the severity of the reaction and the degree of exposure to fleas (i.e., seasonal vs. year-round)
• Finding fleas and flea dirt
• Papules, alopecia, excoriations, and scaling may appear anywhere on the body.
• Secondary bacterial infections sometimes seen
• Pale mucous membranes, tachycardia in anemic animals

CAUSES AND RISK FACTORS
Exposure to other flea-infested animals within the household; keeping animals outdoors in hutches

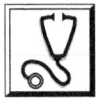

DIAGNOSIS

DIFFERENTIAL DIAGNOSIS
• Fur mites—*Cheyletiella* spp., or less commonly, *Leporacarus gibbus*. May be concurrent with flea infestation. Fur mite lesions are usually located in the intrascapular or tail base region and associated with copious amounts of large white scale. Mites are readily identified in skin scrapes or acetate tape preparations under low magnification.
• Ear mites (*Psoroptes cuniculi*)—usually intensely pruritic; lesions typically localized to areas inside of pinnae, surrounding ears, face, and neck. Skin thickening and exudative crusts form with chronic infestation. Mites can be seen with unaided eye or with microscopic examination under low power.
• Other ectoparasites—*Sarcoptes scabiei* and *Notoedres cati* rarely infest rabbits. Lesions are located around the head and neck and are intensely pruritic.
• Contact dermatitis—usually ventral distribution of lesions; acute onset
• Sebaceous adenitis—often profuse amounts of white scale and flakes, alopecia; diagnose by skin biopsy
• Barbering—by cagemates or self-inflicted—causes hair loss alone without pruritus, scale, or skin lesions
• Lack of grooming due to obesity or underlying dental or musculoskeletal disease may cause an accumulation of scale.
• Injection site reactions—especially with irritating substances such as enrofloxacin—may cause alopecia and crusting

CBC/BIOCHEMISTRY/URINALYSIS
Usually normal; hypereosinophilia inconsistently detected and not well documented

OTHER LABORATORY TESTS
• Skin scrapings—negative
• Flea combings—fleas or flea dirt usually found in affected rabbits
• Cytology of ear exudate—no mites seen

IMAGING
N/A

DIAGNOSTIC PROCEDURES
• Diagnosis usually based on historical information and ruling out other causes of dermatitis
• Fleas or flea dirt is supportive but may be difficult to find
• The most accurate test may be response to appropriate treatment.

PATHOLOGIC FINDINGS
• Superficial dermatitis
• Histopathologic lesions not well described

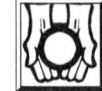

TREATMENT

CLIENT EDUCATION
• Inform owners that controlling exposure to fleas is currently the only means of therapy.
• Treat all animals in the household.

MEDICATIONS

DRUG(S) OF CHOICE
• Selamectin (Revolution, Pfizer)—12 mg/kg applied topically q30d
• Imidacloprid (Advantage, Bayer)1—0–16 mg/kg topically or imidacloprid/moxidectin (Advantage-Multi for Cats, Bayer)—monthly spot treatment for cats; 10 mg/kg (i) + 1 mg/kg (m) topically q30d
• Sprays and powders—usually contain pyrethrins and pyrethroids (synthetic pyrethrins) or carbaryl with an insect growth regulator or synergist; products labeled for use in kittens and puppies are anecdotally considered safe and generally effective, advantages are low toxicity, and repellent activity; disadvantages are frequent applications and expense
• Antibiotics—may be necessary to treat secondary pyoderma, if severe

CONTRAINDICATIONS
• Do not use fipronil (Frontline, Merial) on rabbits—fatal toxicity reported
• Do not use flea collars on rabbits.
• Do not use organophosphate-containing products on rabbits.
• Do not use straight permethrin sprays or permethrin spot-ons on rabbits
• Oral administration of antibiotics that select against gram-positive bacteria (penicillins, macrolides, lincosamides, and cephalosporins) can cause fatal enteric dysbiosis and enterotoxemia.
• Do not use corticosteroids (systemic or topical) to treat pruritic dermatitis in rabbits with fleas. Corticosteroid use is associated with gastrointestinal ulceration and hemorrhage, delayed wound healing, hepatopathy/hepatic abscess formation, and heightened susceptibility to infection.

PRECAUTIONS
• Use extreme caution when dipping or bathing rabbits due to the high risk of skeletal fractures and excessive chilling with inexperienced owners.
• Prevent rabbits or their cagemates from licking topical spot-on products before they are dry.
• Pyrethrin-/pyrethroid-type flea products—adverse reactions include depression, hypersalivation, muscle tremors, vomiting, ataxia, dyspnea, and anorexia
• Toxicity—if any signs are noted, the animal should be bathed thoroughly to remove any remaining chemicals and treated appropriately.

(CONTINUED)

POSSIBLE INTERACTIONS
• Do not use more than one flea treatment at a time.

ALTERNATIVE DRUGS
N/A

FOLLOW-UP

PATIENT MONITORING
• Pruritus and alopecia—should decrease with effective flea control; if signs persist evaluate for other causes
• Fleas and flea dirt—should decrease with effective flea control; however, absence is not always a reliable indicator of successful treatment in very sensitive animals

PREVENTION/AVOIDANCE
• Flea control for all other pets in the household, especially dogs and cats
• See medications
• Year-round warm climates—may require year-round flea control
• Seasonally warm climates—usually begin flea control in May or June

POSSIBLE COMPLICATIONS
• Secondary bacterial infections
• Adverse reaction to flea control products
• Anemia

EXPECTED COURSE AND PROGNOSIS
Prognosis is good if strict flea control is instituted.

MISCELLANEOUS

ASSOCIATED CONDITIONS
N/A

AGE-RELATED FACTORS
Use caution with flea control products in young animals; remove fleas with a flea comb instead and treat other pets in the household.

ZOONOTIC POTENTIAL
In areas of moderate-to-severe flea infestation, people can be bitten by fleas; usually papular lesions are located on the wrists and ankles.

PREGNANCY/FERTILITY/BREEDING
Carefully follow the label directions of each individual product to estimate its safety; however, bear in mind that these products have not been used extensively in pregnant rabbits, and safety is unknown.

SYNONYMS
N/A

SEE ALSO
Cheyletiellosis (fur mites)
Dermatophytosis
Ear mites

Suggested Reading
Hansen O, Gall Y, Pfister K et al. Efficacy of a formulation containing imidacloprid and moxidectin against naturally acquired ear mite infestations (*Psoroptes cuniculi*) in rabbits. Int J Appl Res Vet Med 2005;3(4): 281–286.

Meredith A. Dermatoses. In: Meredith A, Lord B, eds. BSAVA Manual of Rabbit Medicine. Gloucester: British Small Animal Veterinary Association, 2014:255–263.
Palmerio BS, Roberts H. Clinical approach to dermatologic disease in exotic animals. Vet Clin North Am Exot Anim Pract 2013; 16(3):523–577.
Rosen LB. Dermatologic manifestations of zoonotic diseases in exotic animals. J Exotic Pet Med 2011;20:9–13.
Snook TS, White SD, Hawkins MG et al. Skin diseases in pet rabbits: a retrospective study of 334 cases seen at the University of California at Davis, USA (1984–2004). Vet Dermatol 2013;24:613–618.
Varga M. Skin diseases. In: Varga M, ed. Textbook of Rabbit Medicine, 2nd ed. Elsiver, 2014:224–248.
Varga M, Patterson S. Dermatologic diseases of rabbits. In: Quesenberry KE, Carpenter JW, editors. Ferrets, Rabbits and Rodents (4th ed). Clinical Medicine and Surgery. 2021, St. Louis: Saunders; 2020. p.220-222

Author Barbara Oglesbee, DVM, Dipl ABVP (Avian)

GASTRIC DILATION (BLOAT)

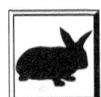

BASICS

DEFINITION
An acute, life-threatening disorder of rabbits caused by intra or extraluminal intestinal obstruction. Untreated, the stomach fills with fluid or fluid and gas, resulting in hypovolemic shock and/or necrosis of distended stomach and intestinal loops. Depending on the proximity of the obstruction to the stomach, death can occur within 6–8 hours.

PATHOPHYSIOLOGY
• Rabbits cannot vomit, due to a well-developed cardiac sphincter.
• When outflow from the stomach is obstructed, sodium and chloride are actively pumped into the intestines orad (proximal) to the obstruction, followed by water. The volume and rapidity of fluid accumulation depend on the distance of the obstruction from the stomach. With obstruction in the proximal duodenum, over 500 ml of fluid can be pumped into the stomach within 6–8 hours, resulting in hypovolemic shock. Untreated, death results from shock or stomach rupture.
• The further the obstruction location is from the stomach, the longer it takes for fluid to accumulate. With distal obstructions (jejunum, ileo-cecal-colonic junction), signs of shock and intestinal dilation may take 12–24 hours.
• Due to changes in gastric pH with fluid accumulation, fermentation of gastric contents can cause a characteristic bubble of gas within the stomach. This can be seen radiographically as a "fried egg" appearance of the stomach.
• Acute, intraluminal foreign body (FB) obstructions cause increased motility of intestinal loops proximal (orad) to the obstruction, in an attempt to move the obstruction through the intestines. In many cases, this is successful, and smaller FB's may progress to the cecum with transient clinical signs. Larger FB's either do not move or move slowly. Eventually, either pain and stress or dilation of intestinal loops with resultant pressure necrosis causes GI hypomotility, and the FB stops moving.
• Dilation of the stomach results in compression of intraabdominal vessels, reducing venous return and compromising renal perfusion. Pressure on the diaphragm reduces lung volume, cardiac efficiency, and activates sympathetic nervous system. Sequestration of bicarbonate in the stomach leads to progressively worsening acidosis

• In most cases, the FB is a pellet of compressed fur. It is believed that these pellets are formed in the cecum and inadvertently swallowed during normal cecotrophy. Occasionally, other materials can act as a FB.
• Extraluminal causes of intestinal obstruction, include abscesses, neoplasia, postoperative adhesions, mesenteric torsion, intussusception, or entrapment of intestines by hernia.

SYSTEMS AFFECTED
• Gastrointestinal—gastric ischemia and necrosis; ileus
• Cardiovascular—decreased in venous return to the heart; hypovolemic shock
• Renal—decreased renal perfusion; acute renal failure

INCIDENCE/PREVALANCE
Extremely common disorder in pet rabbits

SIGNALMENT
No age, breed, or sex predilections

SIGNS

Historical Findings
• The history is extremely useful in differentiating intestinal obstruction from other causes of anorexia and GI hypomotility/stasis.
  ◦ An acute onset of refusing all food, even favorite treats with a corresponding acute cessation of fecal production is the hallmark of rabbits with intestinal obstruction. Affected rabbits suddenly go from a normal appetite and normal round fecal pellets to refusing all food and producing no fecal pellets.
  ◦ A more gradual onset of progressively declining appetite over a period of hours to days is seen in rabbits with GI hypomotility/stasis. Patients often initially stop eating pellets and/or hay, but continue to eat treats, followed by complete anorexia. With this history, fecal pellets gradually become scant, dark in color and small in size.
• Signs of pain can be subtle as rabbits are prey species and instinctively hide signs of disease. The most common sign of mild to moderate discomfort is hiding or appearing less social.
• Signs of more severe pain, such as teeth grinding, a hunched posture and reluctance to move indicate more urgent and serious disease.
• Rabbits with acute FB obstruction in the proximal duodenum are often found dead when owners return after a 6–8 hour period. Owners typically report that the rabbit appeared normal when they left home.

Physical Examination Findings
Abdominal Palpation and Gut Sounds
  Abdominal palpation is an extremely valuable tool in the diagnosis of gastrointestinal disorders.
• *Intestinal obstruction:* Fluid distention of the stomach. The degree of distention depends on the region of intestinal obstruction and progresses with time. Rabbits cannot vomit and eventually, the stomach can become severely fluid distended, and turgid and can even rupture. In rabbits with intestinal obstruction, fecal production abruptly stops, and normal, round fecal pellets are palpable in the colon.
• *Normal findings:* Even in rabbits that do not have access to food or those that are anorexic, the rabbit stomach is never empty. Rabbits consume cecotrophs, formed in the cecum and consumed from the rectum, which will fill the stomach even when food is not provided. If anorexic, stomach contents do not empty, either due to the onset of GI hypmotility/stasis or due to GI obstruction. The normal stomach should be easily deformable, feel soft, and pliable and does not remain pitted on compression.
• *GI hypomotility/stasis:* Depending on the duration of disease, the stomach may contain normal ingesta or, as disease progresses and fluid is pulled from the stomach, contents feel firm, dense, and remain pitted on compression. If the owners have been assist-feeding, the stomach may be distended with food.
• Auscultation of gut sounds is helpful. Decreased or absent gut sounds with little or no borborygmus is consistent with GI hypomotility. Increased gut sounds can be heard in the early phases of intestinal obstruction. In late stages of obstruction, gut sound decrease.
Other Exam Findings
• Signs of shock such as hypothemia (body temp <98°F), pale mucus membranes, lethargy, collapse, or stiff body posture are common with acute intestinal obstruction, depending on the location of obstruction and time to presentation.

CAUSES AND RISK FACTORS
• Most acute duodenal obstructions are caused by ingested pellets of compacted hair. These pellets are likely formed in the cecum and ingested whole with other cecotrophs. Other intestinal foreign bodies include carpet or other cloth, locust beans, plastic, or rubber.
• Peritoneal adhesions, neoplasia, or intraabdominal abscesses occasionally cause pyloric outflow obstruction; presentation is usually more chronic (preceded by signs of gastrointestinal hypomotility).

RABBITS

- Intestinal intussusception and torsion at the mesenteric root are rare causes of gastric dilation.
- Rarely, the stomach dilates and fills with fluid and gas, in the absence of an obstructing foreign body. The cause of this is unknown; functional pyloric outflow obstruction, gastric myoelectric abnormalities, dynamic movement of the stomach following ingestion of food or water, aerophagia, and severe ileus or stress may play a role.

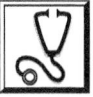

DIAGNOSIS

DIFFERENTIAL DIAGNOSIS
- Gastrointestinal hypomotility—onset is more gradual; usually present for anorexia, lack of fecal production; patients generally bright and alert or only mild to moderately depressed; abdominal palpation reveals a large, doughy or firm mass within the stomach (vs. air or fluid-filled stomach with gastric dilation); radiographs demonstrate stomach full of ingesta; sometimes surrounded by a halo of air; and air is often also visible in the remainder of the intestinal tract as well.
- Overgrowth of gas-producing *Clostridia* spp.—similar presentation, as patients also are often in shock on presentation. With clostridial overgrowth, gas is usually palpable throughout the intestinal tract and visible radiographically; history of inappropriate antibiotic use, gastric stasis, or feeding of foods high in simple carbohydrates. Overgrowth may occur simultaneously with mechanical causes of gastric dilation.
- Aerophagia—rabbits with severe dyspnea; history of respiratory tract disease
- Liver lobe torsion—also acute in onset and can have similar presentation and history; however, the stomach is not fluid-filled on physical examination or radiographically.
- Differentiate nongastric dilation conditions via examination and imaging; rabbits with gastric dilation are extremely painful; often present in shock or moribund; tympanic, fluid-filled stomach is palpable; and borborygmus is often increased on abdominal auscultation, radiographs demonstrate dilated, gas- and/or fluid-filled stomach

CBC/BIOCHEMISTRY/URINALYSIS
- Blood glucose concentration—extremely useful to differentiate GI hypomotility/stasis from GI obstruction and to assess the severity of disease. Rabbits with GI hypomotility/stasis are either normo- or have a mild stress hyperglycemia (BG <300 mg/dL). Rabbits regulate serum osmolaity via changes in

glucose. With loss of Na, Cl, and water into the stomach, BG proportionally increases. Rabbits with GI are severely hyperglycemic, with BG ranging from 300 to 600 mg/dL.
- Serum sodium concentration—rabbits with GI obstruction are typically mildly hyponatremic (Na <140 mEq/L)
- BUN and creatinine may be elevated due to decreased renal perfusion
- PCV and TS elevation due to fluid loss into the intestinal tract

IMAGING
- *With GI obstruction*—the stomach becomes fluid distended. In addition to fluid, a gas cap may form within the stomach causing a "fried egg" appearance. The degree of distension depends on the location and time of onset of obstruction. With increasing severity, the stomach will extend caudal to the last rib and have direct contact with the ventral body wall. If the stomach distends past the caudal aspect of L2 vertebrae, the prognosis worsens. Fluid and/or gas distension occurs in the intestinal loops proximal (orad) to the obstruction. If the obstruction is in the proximal GI tract (located near the pyloric outflow), no gas or distended intestinal loops are found.
- Normal, round fecal pellets can be seen throughout the colon. Normal fecal pellets are spherical and consist of hay and air, so may be mistaken for air bubbles within the colon.
- This contrast with patients with GI hypomotility/stasis. Depending on the duration of disease, the stomach may appear to contain normal ingesta or, as disease progresses and fluid is pulled from the stomach, contents appear dense, and the stomach appears small and may have a halo of gas around the inspissated stomach contents. If the owners have been assist-feeding, the stomach may be distended with food. Gas distension is sometimes seen throughout the intestinal tract, including the cecum.

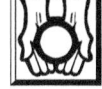

TREATMENT

APPROPRIATE HEALTH CARE
This disorder is an emergency. Patients require immediate medical therapy with special attention to establishing improved cardiovascular function and gastric decompression.

NURSING CARE
Provide Warmth
Patients are usually hypothermic (body temp <99° F) and shock treatment will not be effective until the patient is warmed.

Fluid Therapy
- For patients with signs of shock or severe depression balanced crystalloid fluids are indicated IV at a rate appropriate for shock (60–90 mg/kg/hr IV, IO over 20–60 min) followed by maintenance rate. For patients in shock, fluids should be warmed.
- Supportive fluids on the basis of hydration status are recommended for animals not in shock.

Orogastric Decompression
- Indicated only in patients with signs of shock and severe gastric dilation. Guidelines for the need to manually decompress the stomach include: body temperature <98° F; fluid distension of stomach—radiographically, the stomach extends past the caudal aspect of L2 vertebrae, comes in contact with the ventral body wall, and contents are a fluid density (often with a round gas cap, giving the "fried egg" sign); blood glucose—BG >300 mg/dL (typically will be 400–600 mg/dL)
- Perform gastric decompression by orogastric intubation; sedation or general anesthesia with isoflurane or sevoflurane is required unless the animal is severely depressed. Depending on the degree of depression, use midazolam (0.5–2 mg/kg IV, IM) ± ketamine (2–10 mg/kg IV, IM) or Alfaxalone (1–2 mg/kg IV give slowly over 1 minute to effect; 0.5–1 mg/kg IM when combined with midazolam, opioids, and ketamine). Rabbits are obligatory nasal breathers, so gas anesthesia, if needed, can be administered via nosecone, leaving access to the mouth.
- Use an appropriately sized flexible red-rubber or other rubber tube. If open-ended, be certain that the end of the tube is blunt and smooth to prevent perforation. If a red-rubber catheter is used, it is helpful to cut the holes in the side of the tube to extend the diameter of the openings. Lubricate well. Measure to the caudal aspect of the last rib and mark the tube.
- Place the rabbit in ventral recumbency with the head over the edge of the exam table. Ventroflex the head to direct the orogastric tube into the esophagus. A large-diameter otoscope is useful as a mouth gag through which the tube can be directed into the esophagus.
- Fluid and/or gas will move via gravity out of the tube.
- Clumps of hay, hair, and other ingesta may repeatedly block the orogastric tube. If this occurs, a catheter tip syringe can sometimes be used to push the obstruction out of the tube followed by repositioning the tube until fluid is again encountered. If the tube obstruction cannot be dislodged, remove and replace the tube.

• The character of the fluid obtained from the stomach has prognostic value. The fluid should be green or pale brown in color. Fetid, blood tinged, dark brown fluid is suggestive of avascular necrosis of the stomach lining and carries a poor prognosis.

• After successful decompensation, hospitalize and monitor closely for recurrent dilation. This can occur if the FB does not begin to move or pass with medical treatment or if the obstruction is caused by extraluminal compression of the intestine. If dilation returns, an additional orogastric decompression may be needed. If the patient does not improve after initial decompression or after 2 decompressions within 12 hours, exploratory laparotomy is recommended.

• Decompression by other techniques such as trocarization is contraindicated in rabbits, as gastric rupture is a likely consequence.

ACTIVITY

Surgical patients may resume normal activity after the foreign body passes or is removed.

DIET

• Offer, but do not assist or force feed. Rabbits with intestinal obstruction will not voluntarily eat. If the patient begins eating, the obstruction is moving. This can be used an indication of successful treatment.

• If orogastric decompression was performed, patients may eat a small amount if the stomach was successfully decompressed. Continuing to offer food, but not assist feed and monitor. If the obstruction does not begin to move, appetite will again cease.

CLIENT EDUCATION

• Most rabbits with gastric dilation present in critical condition. Prognosis is guarded, even with immediate decompression, treatment for shock, and/or surgery.

• Discuss the importance of monitoring appetite in prey species such as rabbits. These species have a strong instinct to hide illness and may appear active and "normal" to owners unfamiliar with this concept. Stress the importance of seeking veterinary care any time the appetite is reduced. An acute onset of refusing all food and simultaneous lack of fecal output is an emergency.

• Advise owners to regularly monitor food consumption and fecal output and to seek veterinary attention with a noticeable decrease in either.

• Discuss the importance of feeding hay and high-quality pellets.

SURGICAL CONSIDERATIONS

• Gastric dilation is most commonly caused by a hair pellet FB and will respond to medical treatment.

• Indications for exploratory laparotomy include diagnosis of extraluminal compression of the intestine, inability to alleviate gastric dilation by means of orogastric decompression, inability to closely monitor patients during hospitalization, recurrence of gastric dilation, or worsening signs with treatment.

• Prolonged delay may result in death of the patient.

• Most FB obstructions are found in the proximal duodenum 1–4 inches from the pylorus. The second most common location is mid-jejunum, followed by the ileoceco-colonic junction.

• If a hair pellet FB is located and the intestine appears healthy, milk the pellet into the cecum. The pellet will generally pass from the cecum uneventfully.

• If the pellet cannot be milked into the cecum or another foreign object is encountered, manipulate the object into the stomach and perform a gastrotomy rather than an enterotomy. Gastrotomy is generally better tolerated, and there is less chance of postoperative complications such as stricture or leakage.

• Intestinal necrosis at the site of the obstruction may necessitate resection and anastomosis.

• If no foreign body is seen, examine the intestinal tract for masses, adhesions, or abscess or other causes of extraluminal obstruction.

• Examine the stomach and/or dilated intestinal loops for evidence of necrosis secondary to distention; euthanasia may be indicated depending on the area or extent of necrosis.

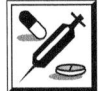

MEDICATIONS

DRUG(S) OF CHOICE

• Lidocaine administered as a CRI (loading dose 2 mg/kg then 50 mcg/kg/min) alleviates intestinal pain, is anti-inflammatory, and may help to prevent ileus.

• Analgesics such as hydromorphone (0.05–0.2 mg/kg IV, IM, SC q6–8h), buprenorphine (0.02–0.05 mg/kg SC, IM, IV q8–12h), or carprofen (2–4 mg/kg SC, IV q24h) are essential to treatment. Intestinal pain, either postoperative or from GI distention impairs mobility, decreases appetite and may severely inhibit recovery.

• Maropitant (2 mg/kg SC q24h) is used to treat visceral pain. Combine this with one of the analgesics listed above.

• Motility modifiers such as metoclopramide (0.5–1.0 mg/kg IV, SC, IM q12h or, ideally, 1–2 mg/kg/day IV as a constant rate infusion)

can be used in rabbits with intraluminal intestinal obstruction as the most common GI foreign body is a compressed pellet of hair and the goal of therapy is to keep the hair pellet moving through the intestinal tract. Motility modifiers are contraindicated if an extraluminal obstruction is suspected.

• H_2-receptor antagonists may ameliorate or prevent gastric ulceration; cimetidine (5–10 mg/kg PO, SC, IM IV q6–12h) and ranitidine (2 mg/kg SC, IV q24h or 2–5 mg/kg PO q12–24h).

CONTRAINDICATIONS

• Trocarization of the stomach will result in gastric rupture.

• Avoid NSAIDs and other drugs that may lead to renal compromise, in patients with signs of shock or dehydration.

PRECAUTIONS

Meloxicam and other NSAIDs—use with caution in patients with renal compromise; monitor renal values

FOLLOW-UP

PATIENT MONITORING

• Monitor for recurrence of gastric dilation after initiation of medical treatment. Patients are hospitalized and monitored until eating and passing feces. Palpate the stomach every 2–3 hours until then. If recurrence of dilation is suspected, frequent repeat abdominal radiographs.

• With successful treatment, see return of appetite, normal feces produced. In many cases, a larger, mucus covered fecal pellet is passed. If broken open and examined, the hair pellet is often contained within.

PREVENTION/AVOIDANCE

This syndrome is not related to diet or husbandry; no known prevention

POSSIBLE COMPLICATIONS

• Death due to gastric rupture
• Acute renal failure
• Postoperative GI stasis and subsequent overgrowth of bacterial pathogens
• Stricture formation at the site of removal
• Gastric dilation may recur.

EXPECTED COURSE AND PROGNOSIS

• If the patient presents in shock, the prognosis is guarded, even with immediate decompression, treatment for shock, and/or surgical removal of obstruction.

• Patients that begin eating and passing feces within 24 hours of treatment have a good prognosis for complete recovery.

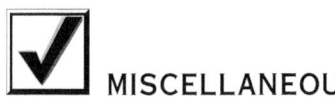 MISCELLANEOUS

SYNONYMS
Acute gastrointestinal obstruction
Bloat
Gastric stasis and dilation syndrome
Intestinal obstruction

SEE ALSO
Gastrointestinal foreign bodies
Gastrointestinal hypomotility and
gastrointestinal stasis
Constipation
Anorexia

ABBREVIATIONS
ALP = alkaline phosphatase
ALT = alanine aminotransferase
GI = gastrointestinal
LRS = lactated Ringer's solution
NSAID = nonsteroidal anti-inflammatory
drugs
PCV = packed cell volume
TS = total solids

Suggested Reading
Debenham JJ, Brinchmann T, Sheen J, Vella
D. Radiographic diagnosis of small
intestinal obstruction in pet rabbits
(*Oryctolagus cuniculus*): 63 cases. J Sm
Anim Pract 2019;60:691–696.

DeCubellis J. Common emergencies in
rabbits, guinea pigs, and chinchillas. Vet
Clin Exot Anim 2016;19:411–429.
Hartcourt-Brown F. Digestive system disease.
In: Meredith A, Lord B, eds. BSAVA
Manual of Rabbit Medicine. Gloucester:
British Small Animal Veterinary
Association, 2014:168–190.
Oglesbee B, Lord B. Gastrointestinal diseases
of rabbits. In: Quesenberry KE, Carpenter
JW, eds. Ferrets, Rabbits and Rodents,
(4th ed). Clinical Medicine and Surgery.
2021, St. Louis: Saunders, 2020:174–187.
Varga M. Digestive disorders. In: Varga M,
ed. Textbook of Rabbit Medicine, 2nd ed.
London, UK: Elsevier, 2014:303–349.

Author Barbara Oglesbee, DVM, DABVP
(Avian)

GASTROINTESTINAL HYPOMOTILITY, AND GASTROINTESTINAL STASIS

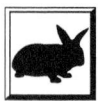

BASICS

DEFINITION
• Gastrointestinal hypomotility—delayed gastrointestinal transit time characterized by decreased frequency of ceocolonic segmental contractions
• Gastrointestinal (GI) stasis—severe ileus with little to no caudal movement of ingesta
• "GI Stasis" or "Stasis" are terms commonly used as a catch-all phrases for colic in rabbits, characterized by decreased or absent appetite and fecal production. However, it is important to distinguish true GI hypomotility disorders from other causes of colic, such as intestinal obstruction, liver lobe torsion, or cecal disorders.

PATHOPHYSIOLOGY
• Rabbits are hind-gut fermenters and are extremely sensitive to alterations in diet.
• Proper hind-gut fermentation and gastrointestinal tract motility are dependent on the ingestion of large amounts of roughage and long-stemmed hay. Diets that contain inadequate amounts of long-stemmed, coarse fiber (such as the feeding of only commercial pelleted food without hay or grasses) can cause gastrointestinal tract hypomotility.
• The presence of hair balls or trichobezoars in the stomach is not a disease but a symptom or consequence of GI hypomotility or stasis. Rabbits normally ingest hair during grooming. Healthy rabbits will always have some amount of hair and ingesta in the stomach. These stomach contents are both palpable and visible radiographically in the normal, healthy rabbit.
• With proper nutrition and GI tract motility, fur ingested as a result of normal grooming behavior, as well as some small or easily deformed foreign bodies, will pass through the gastrointestinal tract with the ingesta uneventfully.
• When gastrointestinal motility slows or stops, ingesta, including fur and other material, accumulates in the stomach. Rabbits cannot vomit to expel nonfood contents from the stomach.
• Over time, fluid is actively pulled from the stomach, eventually resulting in dehydration of stomach contents in rabbits with GI stasis.
• Affected rabbits suddenly or gradually refuse food; as motility slows, ingesta accumulates proximal to the colon (stomach, cecum); fecal pellets become small and scant; water is removed from fecal pellets in the colon, making the fecal pellets drier than normal

• Cecocolonic hypomotility also causes alterations in cecal fermentation, pH, and substrate production, resulting in alteration of enteric microflora populations. Diets low in coarse fiber typically contain high simple carbohydrate concentrations, which provide a ready source of fermentable products and promote the growth of bacterial pathogens such as *E. coli* and *Clostridium* spp. Bacterial dysbiosis can cause acute diarrhea, enterotoxemia, ileus, or chronic intermittent diarrhea.
• Anorexia due to infectious or metabolic disease, pain, stress, or starvation may cause or exacerbate GI hypomotility.
• The process is often self-perpetuating; GI hypomotility and dehydration promote anorexia and exacerbation of stasis.

SYSTEMS AFFECTED
• Gastrointestinal
• Hepatic—lipidosis secondary to anorexia

INCIDENCE/PREVALENCE
• GI hypomotility resulting in scant or lack of feces, chronic intermittent diarrhea, abdominal pain, and ill-thrift is one of the most common clinical problems seen in the rabbit.

SIGNALMENT
• More commonly seen in middle-aged to older rabbits on inappropriate diets, but can occur in any aged rabbit
• No breed or gender predilections

SIGNS

Historical Findings
• History of progressive inappetence or anorexia over a period of hours to days. Rabbits often initially stop eating pellets but continue to eat treats, followed by complete anorexia.
• History of reduced fecal output. Fecal pellets progressively become more scant, dark, misshaped and small in size, eventually no fecal pellets produced with complete GI stasis
• History of signs of pain such as hiding, appearing less social. Rabbits are prey species and instinctively hide signs of illness, so signs of pain can be subtle.
• History of inappropriate diet (e.g., cereals, grains, commercial pellets only, sweets, large quantities of fruits, and lack of feeding long-stemmed hay)
• Recent history of illness or stressful event
• History of decreased activity—cage confinement, orthopedic, or neuromuscular disease
• Weight loss in rabbits with underlying or chronic disease
• Obesity in rabbits on diets consisting of mainly commercial pellets

Physical Examination Findings
• Small, misshaped, hard fecal pellets or absence of fecal pellets palpable in the colon; examine feces in cage or carrier—appear small, dark, firm, irregularly shaped, and scant with GI hypomotility/stasis
• Cecum may palpate as gas-filled, fluid-filled, or firm, depending on the underlying cause.
• Palpation of the stomach is an extremely valuable tool in the diagnosis. Ingesta normally should be palpable in the stomach of a healthy rabbit. The normal stomach should be easily deformable, feel soft, and pliable and not remain pitted on compression. Rabbits with early GI hypomotility will have a firm, often enlarged stomach that remains pitted when compressed. With complete GI stasis, severe dehydration, or prolonged hypomotility, the stomach contents may become hard and nondeformable.
• The presence of firm ingesta in the stomach of a rabbit that has been anorectic for 1–3 days is compatible with the diagnosis of GI hypomotility.
• Decreased or absent gut sounds—little or no borborygmus is heard on abdominal auscultation in rabbits with GI hypomotility.
• Other physical examination findings depend on the underlying cause; perform a complete physical examination, including a thorough oral exam.

CAUSES AND RISK FACTORS

Dietary and Environmental Causes
• GI hypomotility may be caused by feeding diets with insufficient roughage such as grasses and long-stemmed hay and/or excessive simple carbohydrate content. Examples of improper diets include a diet consisting primarily of commercial pellets, especially those containing seeds, oats, or other high-carbohydrate treats; feeding of cereal products (bread, crackers, and breakfast cereals); feeding large amounts of fruits containing simple carbohydrates. Proper hind-gut fermentation and GI motility rely on large quantities of indigestible coarse fiber, as found in long-stemmed hay and grasses. Most commercial pelleted diets contain inadequate roughage, coarse fiber, and excessive calories. This high caloric content often contributes to obesity and hepatic lipidosis, both of which may exacerbate intestinal disease.
• Stress is a major cause of GI stasis/ hypomotility. Stress may be the result of pain such a trauma, surgery, or dental disease or from underlying metabolic disease. Even minor changes such as changes in the daily schedule, new animals or people in the

household, or changes in environment such as hospitalization or boarding can cause GI hypomotility/stasis
• Lack of exercise (cage confinement, obesity)—often a significant contributing factor

Drugs
• Anesthetic agents may cause or exacerbate GI hypomotility.
• Anticholinergics
• Opioids

Anorexia or Inappetence
• Conditions that result in inappetence or anorexia may also cause GI hypomotility. Common causes of anorexia include dental disease (malocclusion, molar elongation, and tooth root abscesses), metabolic disease (renal disease, liver disease), pain (oral, trauma, postoperative pain, and adhesions), neoplasia (gastrointestinal, uterine), toxins, changes in the environment, or accidental starvation.

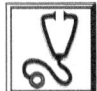

DIAGNOSIS
DIFFERENTIAL DIAGNOSIS
• GI obstruction—it is important to differentiate acute small intestinal obstruction (bloat) from GI hypomotility/stasis, as acute intestinal obstruction is a life-threatening emergency. Signs and history with acute GI obstruction include—acute onset of complete anorexia coinciding with abrupt cessation of fecal production, abdominal pain, reluctance to move, progression to lateral recumbency, and signs of hypovolemic shock (e.g., pale mucous membranes, decreased capillary refill time, weak pulses, and hypothermic). Stomach is severely distended, tympanic, and full of gas and/or fluid. Patients can often in shock and require emergency treatment. Monitor rectal temperature; rabbits that become hypothermic are critically ill.
• For palpable mass in the cranial abdomen: neoplasia, abscess, hepatomegaly, and normal gastric contents
• For anorexia: liver lobe torsion, dental disease, metabolic disease, pain, neoplasia, cardiac disease, and toxin
• For decreased fecal output: anorexia, GI obstruction, liver lobe torsion, intussusception, and intestinal neoplasia

CBC/BIOCHEMISTRY/URINALYSIS
• These tests are often normal but can be used to differentiate GI hypomotility/stasis from GI obstruction. Rabbits with GI hypomotility/stasis are either normo- or mildly hyperglycemic (BG <300 mg/dL) with normal serum Na concentration, whereas those with GI obstruction are severely

hyperglycemic, with BG ranging from 300 to 600 mg/dL and mildly hyponatremic Na <140 mEq/L)
• BUN and creatinine may be elevated due to dehydration or, in rabbits with obstruction, due to decreased renal perfusion
• PCV and TS elevation in dehydrated patients
• Serum ALT elevation in rabbits with liver disease, especially lipidosis
• May be used to identify underlying causes of GI hypomotility or anorexia

OTHER LABORATORY TESTS
N/A

IMAGING
Radiography
• Due to the practice of cecotrophy, the stomach is never empty. Gastric contents are normally present and visible radiographically, even if the rabbit is not eating. The presence of ingesta in the stomach is a normal finding.
• Depending on the duration of disease, the stomach may appear to contain normal ingesta or, as disease progresses and fluid is pulled from the stomach, contents appear dense, the stomach appears small, and may have a halo of gas around the inspissated stomach contents. If the owners have been assist-feeding, the stomach may be distended with food.
• This contrasts with the appearance of the stomach in rabbits with GI obstruction, where the stomach becomes fluid filled.
• Gas distension is sometimes seen throughout the intestinal tract, including the cecum in rabbits with GI hypomotility/stasis.
• Small fecal balls or the absence of fecal balls in the colon are highly suggestive.

OTHER DIAGNOSTIC PROCEDURES
N/A

PATHOLOGIC FINDINGS
N/A

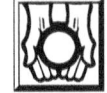

TREATMENT
APPROPRIATE HEALTH CARE
• Remove or ameliorate any underlying cause if possible.
• Rabbits that have not produced feces or have been anorectic for over 24 hours should be treated as soon as possible; emergency evaluation should be recommended in all cases of anorexia to rule out acute intestinal obstruction (bloat).
• Rabbits that are stable should be treated on an outpatient basis when possible. Hospitalization increases stress and may exacerbate GI stasis.

• Rabbits that are severely dehydrated, weak, or demonstrating signs of shock (often indicative of acute intestinal obstruction) require hospitalization.

NURSING CARE
Fluid Therapy
• Fluid therapy is an essential component of the medical management of all patients with GI hypomotility. Administer both oral and parenteral fluids. Oral fluid administration in the form of commercially available assist feeding slurries (see below) will aid in the rehydration of inspissated gastric contents. Mildly affected rabbits will usually respond well to oral and subcutaneous fluid administration, treatment with analgesics, intestinal motility modifiers, and dietary modification described below.
• Intravenous fluids are indicated in patients that are severely dehydrated or depressed. Maintenance fluid requirements are estimated at 60 mL/kg/day for large breeds and 80–100 mL/kg/day for small or dwarf breeds.
• Rehydration is essential to treatment success in severely ill rabbits. Initially, a balanced fluid (e.g., lactated Ringer's solution) may be used.
• A warm, quiet environment should be provided.

ACTIVITY
If patient is not debilitated, encourage exercise (hopping) for at least 10–15 minutes every 6–8 hours as activity promotes gastric motility; provide supervised freedom from the cage or access to a safe grazing area.

DIET
• Diet is the keystone of successful treatment of GI hypomotility/stasis.
• It is imperative that the rabbit continue to eat during and following treatment. Continued anorexia will exacerbate GI hypomotility, cause further derangement of the gastrointestinal microflora, and cause overgrowth of intestinal bacterial pathogens.
• Offer high-quality rabbit pellets and grass or timothy hays. If greens have been a part of the patient's diet, offer these as well.
• If the patient refuses these foods, syringe-feed a gruel such as Critical Care for Herbivores (Oxbow Pet Products) or Emeraid Herbivore (Lafeber Company, Cornell, IL) 10–15 mL/kg PO q6–8h. Larger volumes and more frequent feedings are often accepted; feed as much as the rabbit will readily accept. Alternatively, pellets can be ground and mixed with fresh greens, vegetable baby foods, or water to form a gruel.
• Do not assist feed rabbits with confirmed or suspected GI obstructive disorders.

GASTROINTESTINAL HYPOMOTILITY, AND GASTROINTESTINAL STASIS

• High-carbohydrate, high-fat nutritional supplements are contraindicated.
• Encourage oral fluid intake by offering many sources of fresh water and/or wetting leafy vegetables.
• The diet should be permanently modified to include sufficient amounts of indigestible, coarse fiber. Offer long-stemmed grass or timothy hay (commercially available hay cubes are not sufficient) and an assortment of washed, fresh leafy greens. These foods should always constitute the bulk of the diet. Pellets should be limited to ¼ cup/5 lb body weight and foods high in simple carbohydrate prohibited or limited to the occasional treat.

CLIENT EDUCATION
• Discuss the importance of monitoring appetite in prey species such as rabbits. These species have a strong instinct to hide illness and may appear active and "normal" to owners unfamiliar with this concept. Stress the importance of seeking veterinary care any time the appetite is reduced. An acute onset of refusing all food and simultaneous lack of fecal output is an emergency.
• Advise owners to regularly monitor food consumption and fecal output and to seek veterinary attention with a noticeable decrease in either.
• Discuss the importance of feeding hay and high-quality pellets.

SURGICAL CONSIDERATIONS
• Gastrointestinal hypomotility—accumulation of inspissated gastric contents (including ingested hair) will usually pass with medical treatment alone; surgery is generally contraindicated in rabbits with GI hypomotility. Surgical manipulation of the intestinal tract, hypothermia, anesthetic agents, and pain all exacerbate GI hypomotility; GI stasis is often worse postoperatively. The combination of these factors results in a significantly worsened prognosis with surgical treatment.

MEDICATIONS
• Use parenteral medications in animals with severely compromised intestinal motility; oral medications may not be properly absorbed. Begin oral medication when intestinal motility begins to return (fecal production, return of appetite, and radiographic evidence).

DRUG(S) OF CHOICE
• Analgesics such as meloxicam (1 mg/kg SC, IM q24h), hydromorphone (0.05–0.2 mg/kg IV, IM, SC q6–8h), buprenorphine (0.02–0.05 mg/kg SC, IM, IV q8–12h), or

carprofen (2–4 mg/kg SC, IV q24h) are essential to treatment of rabbits with GI hypomotility. Intestinal pain, either postoperative or from gas distention and ileus, impairs mobility and decreases appetite and may severely inhibit recovery.
• Maropitant (2 mg/kg SC q24h) is used to treat visceral pain. Combine this with one of the analgesics listed above.
• Motility modifiers such as cisapride (0.5 mg/kg PO q8–12h) and metoclopramide (0.5–1.0 mg/kg PO, SC, IM q12h or 1–2 mg/kg/day IV as a constant rate infusion) are generally helpful in rabbits with GI hypomotility.
• H_2-receptor antagonists may ameliorate or prevent gastric ulceration; cimetidine (5–10 mg/kg PO, SC, IM IV q6–12h); ranitidine (2 mg/kg SC, IV q24h or 2–5 mg/kg PO q12–24h)
• Antibiotic therapy—generally not indicated in patients with GI hypomotility/stasis.

Other Treatment
• Simethicone 65–130 mg/rabbit q1h for 2–3 treatments may be helpful in alleviating painful intestinal gas.

CONTRAINDICATIONS
• The use of antibiotics that are primarily gram positive in spectrum is contraindicated in rabbits. Use of these antibiotics will suppress the growth of commensal flora, allowing overgrowth of enteric pathogens. Do not orally administer lincomycin, clindamycin, erythromycin, ampicillin, amoxicillin cephalosporins, or penicillins.
• Enzymatic digestion of trichobezoars with fresh pineapple juice, papaya extract, or pancreatic enzymes have been advocated. However, these substances should not be fed as they may exacerbate gastric mucosal ulceration/erosions and may contribute to gastric rupture. Additionally, these substances do nothing to treat the underlying cause of trichobezoars and GI hypomotility.
• Assist feeding is contraindicated in rabbits with intestinal obstruction.

PRECAUTIONS
• NSAIDs—use with caution in rabbits with compromised renal function or if gastric ulceration is suspected
• Oral administration of any antibiotic may potentially cause enteric dysbiosis; discontinue use if diarrhea or anorexia occur.

POSSIBLE INTERATIONS
N/A

ALTERNATIVE DRUGS
• Intestinal lubricants such as cat laxatives are unlikely to aid in the passage of trichobezoars as they simply lubricate the intestinal

contents and do nothing to treat the underlying motility disorder.

FOLLOW-UP
PATIENT MONITORING
• Monitor hydration, appetite, and production of fecal pellets. Rabbits that are successfully treated will regain a normal appetite and begin to produce normal volumes of feces. Initially, the fecal pellets are sometimes expelled bound together with hair.
• Appetite and fecal production should improve daily. The average course of GI hypomotility/stasis is 3–5 days.

PREVENTION/AVOIDANCE
• Strict feeding of diets containing adequate amounts of indigestible coarse fiber (long-stemmed hay) and low simple carbohydrate content along with access to fresh water will often prevent episodes.
• Allow sufficient daily exercise.
• Prevent obesity.
• Be certain that all postoperative patients are eating and passing feces prior to release.

POSSIBLE COMPLICATIONS
• Continued ileus leading to hepatic lipidosis, other metabolic derangements and death
• Death due to gastric rupture
• Overgrowth of bacterial pathogens; clostridial enterotoxicosis

EXPECTED COURSE AND PROGNOSIS
• Depends on the underlying cause
• Early medical management of animals with GI hypomotility/stasis carries a good to excellent prognosis.
• May recur if underlying disease cannot be addressed.

MISCELLANEOUS
ASSOCIATED CONDITIONS
• Dental disease
• Hypercalciuria
• Hepatic lipidosis
• Bacterial dysbiosis
• Bacterial endotoxemia

AGE-RELATED FACTORS
Middle-aged to older rabbits on a poor diet are more likely to GI hypomotility.

ZOONOTIC POTENTIAL
N/A

(CONTINUED)

PREGNANCY/FERTILITY/BREEDING
N/A

SYNONYMS
Rabbit gastrointestinal syndrome (RGIS)
Stasis
Wool block

SEE ALSO
Anorexia and pseudoanorexia
Clostridial enteritis/enterotoxicosis
Diarrhea, chronic
Gastric dilation (bloat)

ABBREVIATIONS
ALT = alanine aminotransferase
BG = blood glucose
BUN = blood urea nitrogen
GI = gastrointestinal
Na = sodium
PCV = packed cell volume
TS = total solids

Suggested Reading
Debenham JJ, Brinchmann T, Sheen J, Vella D. Radiographic diagnosis of small intestinal obstruction in pet rabbits (*Oryctolagus cuniculus*): 63 cases. J Sm Anim Pract 2019;60:691–696.
Hartcourt-Brown F. Digestive system disease. In: Meredith A, Lord B, eds. BSAVA Manual of Rabbit Medicine. Gloucester: British Small Animal Veterinary Association, 2014:168–190.

Oglesbee B, Lord B. Gastrointestinal diseases of rabbits. In: Quesenberry KE, Carpenter JW, eds. Ferrets, Rabbits and Rodents, (4th ed). Clinical Medicine and Surgery. 2021, St. Louis: Saunders, 2020:174–187.
Varga M. Digestive disorders. In: Varga M, ed. Textbook of Rabbit Medicine, 2nd ed. London, UK: Elsevier, 2014:303–349.
Author Barbara Oglesbee, DVM, DABVP (Avian)

HEAD TILT (VESTIBULAR DISEASE)

BASICS

DEFINITION
Tilting of the head away from its normal orientation with the trunk and limbs; associated with disorders of the vestibular system

PATHOPHYSIOLOGY
• Vestibular system—coordinates position and movement of the head with that of the eyes, trunk, and limbs by detecting linear acceleration and rotational movements of the head; includes vestibular nuclei in the rostral medulla of the brainstem, vestibular portion of the vestibulocochlear nerve (cranial nerve VIII), and receptors in the semicircular canals of the inner ear
• Head tilt—most consistent sign of diseases affecting the vestibular system and its projections to the cerebellum, spinal cord, cerebral cortex, reticular formation, and extraocular eye muscles
• In rabbits, vestibular disease is most commonly caused by bacterial otitis interna/media, *Encephalitozoon cuniculi* infection, trauma, or idiopathic vestibular disease.

SYSTEMS AFFECTED
Nervous—peripheral or CNS
Gastrointestinal—associated inappetence leading to GI stasis

SIGNALMENT
• Lop-eared rabbits may be more likely to show signs of otitis externa.
• Dwarf breeds, older and immunosuppressed rabbits may be more predisposed to signs due to infection with *E. cuniculi.*

SIGNS
• Often acute presentation regardless of the cause
• Often severe initially—see rolling, torticollis, lateral recumbency, unable or unwilling to lift head from the ground
• Head tilt usually accompanied by other vestibular signs; nystagmus (resting, positional); ataxia and disequilibrium with a tendency to fall, lean, or roll toward the side of the tilt; often acute in onset
• Peripheral deficits—spontaneous nystagmus: may be horizontal or rotatory with fast phase in the direction opposite the head tilt; however, type and direction of nystagmus may not correlate well with location of the deficit (CNS vs. PNS); patient may have Horner's syndrome or concomitant ipsilateral facial nerve paresis or paralysis
• Central deficits—positional nystagmus: vertical, horizontal, or rotatory; sometimes

changes with the position of the head; altered mentation possible; proprioceptive deficits common; ipsilateral paresis, general weakness, ataxia, or wide-based stance possible; other signs related to the cerebellum such as intention tremors possible
• Rolling common with both peripheral and central disease
• Anorexia, inappetence due to nausea
• Nasal/ocular discharge—historical or present on physical examination; spread of upper respiratory infection to inner/middle ear via Eustachian tube is common
• In rabbits with otitis externa, thick, white, creamy exudate may be found in the horizontal and/or vertical canals.
• In rabbits with otitis media only, the external canal usually has a normal appearance on otoscopic examination; the tympanum sometimes bulges out into the external canal.

CAUSES
Peripheral Disease
• Inflammatory—otitis media and interna most common cause; primarily bacterial but occasionally related to parasitic (e.g., *Psoroptes cuniculi*) and fungal origins. *Pasteurella multocida, Staphylococcus aureus, Pseudomonas aeruginosa, E. coli,* and *Listeria monocytogenes* most often cultured in otitis media/interna; foreign body (rare)
• Idiopathic vestibular disease—not well described in rabbits; however, a definitive diagnosis is often not found, and many rabbits improve with supportive care
• Traumatic—tympanic bulla or petrosal bone fracture; aggressive ear flush
• Neoplastic—neoplasia of the bone and surrounding tissue (rare)
• Toxic—lead; aminoglycosides
• Metabolic and immune mediated—not described in rabbits

Central Disease
Inflammatory, infectious
• Protozoal—*Encephalitozoon cuniculi* infections are believed to be a very common cause of vestibular disease in rabbits; however, the prevalence of *E. cuniculi* as a cause of CNS disease is controversial since definitive antemortem diagnosis is not possible, and postmortem lesions do not correlate well with clinical disease; toxoplasmosis (rare)
• Bacterial—very common cause; otitis media and interna; encephalitis due to *Pasteurella* spp. or other bacteria
• Aberrant larval migrans—*Baylisascaris* sp. (raccoon roundworm)
• Viral—rabies extremely rare, but should be considered in any rabbit with neurologic disease; herpesvirus also described

• Fungal (e.g., cryptococcosis, blastomycosis, and histoplasmosis)—not yet described in rabbits
Inflammatory, noninfectious
• Granulomatous meningoencephalomyelitis—common postmortem finding in rabbits both with and without antemortem signs of vestibular disease; has been attributed to *E. cuniculi* infection, but organisms not always found
Degenerative
Demyelinating disease; vascular event; incidence unknown
Trauma
Bone fracture with brain stem injury
Neoplastic
Nervous system neoplasia rarely reported in rabbits; skull tumor (e.g., osteosarcoma); metastasis (e.g., hemangiosarcoma and melanoma)
Nutritional—hypovitaminosis A (rare)
Toxic—lead; metronidazole (rare)

RISK FACTORS
• Immunosuppression, especially for *E. cuniculi* or bacterial infection—predisposes to clinical disease: stress, poor diet, concurrent disease, and glucocorticoid or antitumor chemotherapy
• For otitis interna/media—previous URI, since most infections spread from the respiratory tract via eustachian tube; abnormal or breed-related conformation of the external canal (e.g., stenosis, lop-eared breeds); excessive moisture (e.g., from frequent cleanings with improper solutions) can lead to infection

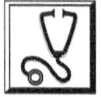

DIAGNOSIS

GENERAL COMMENTS
Every attempt should be made to rule out otic disease prior to assuming *E. cuniculi* infection. Antemortem diagnosis of *E. cuniculi* is presumed based on clinical signs, exclusion of other diagnoses, positive antibody titers, and sometimes response to treatment. Definitive antemortem diagnosis is problematic, since a positive antibody titer indicates exposure only, some rabbits respond minimally or not at all to anthelmintic treatment, and many rabbits will improve spontaneously with supportive care alone. Definitive diagnosis requires identification of organisms and characteristic inflammation in affected tissues that anatomically correlate with clinical signs; generally acquired at postmortem examination. Results of several studies demonstrate a poor or no correlation between the severity of CNS lesions on postmortem and clinical signs.

DIFFERENTIAL DIAGNOSIS

NonVestibular Head Tilt and Head Posture

• Be sure that abnormal head posture is not due to holding one ear down due to pain, as may occur in otitis externa/media alone, and not associated with vestibular pathology.
• Rabbits with vestibular dysfunction demonstrate nystagmus, torticollis, ataxia, and/or tremors in addition to head tilt.

CBC/BIOCHEMISTRY/URINALYSIS

• Usually normal
• May reflect underlying disorder in stressed immunosuppressed rabbits

OTHER LABORATORY TESTS

• Serologic Testing for *E. cuniculi*
  ◦ The usefulness of serum antibody testing is limited in pet rabbits since a positive titer indicates only exposure and does not confirm *E. cuniculi* as the cause of clinical signs. *E. cuniculi* can only be definitively diagnosed by finding organisms and resultant lesions on histopathologic examination in areas that anatomically correlate with observed clinical signs.
  ◦ IgG titers usually become positive by 2 weeks post infection. A rising titer after 4 weeks may confirm infection, but titers do not always continue to rise with active infection. IgG levels can decline after 8 weeks in some rabbits, in others may persist for life. No correlation exits between antibody titers and shedding of organism or severity of disease. Available tests include ELISA and IFA.
  ◦ IgM titers may indicate a more recent, active infection. Titers become positive shortly after infection and appear to persist for up to 18 weeks.
  ◦ C-reactive protein, an inflammatory marker, appears to be elevated in rabbits with active infection. Although this marker is nonspecific, concurrent elevation with IgG and IgM supports active infection.
  ◦ A negative test may rule out infection; however, false negatives can be seen in early infections, before titers have a chance to rise.
• Serologic testing for toxoplasmosis—ELISA testing for IgM and IgG are commercially available. The overall seroprevalence is low, and most seropositive rabbits are asymptomatic.
• Serology for *Pasteurella*—usefulness is severely limited and generally not helpful in the diagnosis of pasteurellosis in pet rabbits. An ELISA is available; however, positive results, even when high, only indicate prior exposure to *Pasteurella* and the development of antibodies, and does not confirm active infection. Low positive results may occur due to cross-reaction with other, nonpathogenic bacteria (false positive). False negative results are common with immunosuppression or early infection. No evidence exists to support correlation of titers to the presence or absence of disease.
• Bacterial culture and sensitivity testing—sample from external ear canal in rabbits with otitis externa, or from myringotomy or surgical drainage of tympanic bulla if otitis media or interna is suspected
• Microscopic examination of ear swab

IMAGING

• Tympanic bullae and skull radiography—may help rule out otitis interna/media; however, normal radiographs do not rule out bulla disease.
• CT—more reliable for confirming bulla lesions and CNS extension from otitis; or to document localized tumor, granuloma, and extent of inflammation

DIAGNOSTIC PROCEDURES

• Otoscopic examination—in rabbits with otitis externa, thick, white, creamy exudate may be found in the horizontal and/or vertical canals. Otitis interna/media often occurs in the absence of otitis externa via extension through the eustachian tube; may see bulging tympanum. Many rabbits with otitis interna have no visible otoscopic abnormalities.
• CSF analysis—sample from the cerebellomedullary cistern; may be valuable for evaluating central vestibular disease; detect inflammatory process; sample collection may put the patient at risk for herniation if there is a mass or high intracranial pressure. May see increased protein, lymphocyte, and monocytes with *E. cuniculi* infection. Studies were unable to find organism or evidence of organism utilizing PCR testing on CSF.
• Biopsy—when a tumor or osteomyelitis is suspected

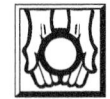

TREATMENT

APPROPRIATE HEALTH CARE

• Inpatient vs. outpatient—depends on severity of the signs (especially vestibular ataxia and need for supportive care). If the rabbit can eat and drink a normal amount, home nursing care is usually appropriate. Instruct clients to place food and water in reach of non-ambulatory patients, or to assist-feed gruel if not eating.
• Many rabbits improve with supportive care alone.

NURSING CARE

• Supportive fluids—replacement or maintenance fluids (depend on clinical state); usually required in the acute phase when disorientation and nausea preclude oral intake
• Trauma—supportive care (e.g., anti-inflammatory drugs, antibiotics, and intravenous fluid administration); specific fracture repair or hematoma removal is difficult, considering the location.

ACTIVITY

• Restrict (e.g., avoid stairs and slippery surfaces) according to the degree of disequilibrium; encourage return to activity as soon as safely possible; activity may enhance recovery of vestibular function

DIET

• It is important that the rabbit continue to eat. Although rabbits cannot vomit, many rabbits with vestibular disorders become anorexic, suggesting nausea. Anorexia will cause GI hypomotility or GI stasis, derangement of the gastrointestinal microflora, and overgrowth of intestinal bacterial pathogens.
• Bring the food to the rabbit if non-ambulatory, or offer food by hand.
• If the patient refuses these foods, syringe-feed a gruel such as Critical Care for Herbivores (Oxbow Pet Products) or Emeraid Herbivore (Lafeber Company, Cornell, IL) 10–15 mL/kg PO q6–8h. Larger volumes and more frequent feedings are often accepted; feed as much as the rabbit will readily accept. Alternatively, pellets can be ground and mixed with fresh greens, vegetable baby foods, water, or juice to form a gruel.
• High-carbohydrate, high-fat nutritional supplements are contraindicated.
• Encourage oral fluid intake by offering fresh water, wetting leafy vegetables, or flavoring water with vegetable juices.

CLIENT EDUCATION

• Advise client that the prognosis for central vestibular disorders is usually poorer than that for peripheral disorders.
• Long-term home nursing care (assist-feed, padded bedding in recumbent animals) may be required; residual neurologic signs common in rabbits that partially recover; a waxing and waning course of progression is seen in some rabbits; and some rabbits take weeks to months to recover
• Head tilt may be permanent but often does not appear to affect quality of life in recovered patients.

SURGICAL CONSIDERATIONS

• Total ear canal ablation and or bullae osteotomy may be required in patients with bulla disease and otitis media or interna to

HEAD TILT (VESTIBULAR DISEASE)

alleviate discomfort and prevent extension into the brain; however, vestibular signs persist following surgery.
• Surgical resection of abscess or tumor may be indicated, if accessible.

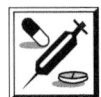

MEDICATIONS

DRUG(S) OF CHOICE
• If anorexic, Maropitant (2 mg/kg SC, PO q24h) or Metoclopramide (0.5–1.0 mg/kg PO, SC, IV q12h)
• Otitis media or interna, bacterial encephalitis—antibiotics; choice is ideally based on results of culture and susceptibility testing, if possible. Depending on the severity of infection, long-term antibiotic therapy is required (4–6 weeks minimum, to several months). Use broad-spectrum antibiotics such as enrofloxacin (10–20 mg/kg PO, SC, IM, IV q12h), marbofloxacin (5 mg/kg PO q24h), trimethoprim-sulfa (15–30 mg/kg PO q12h), or chloramphenicol (50 mg/kg PO q8h). Most facial or dental abscesses contain anaerobic bacteria; use antibiotics effective against anaerobes such as azithromycin (15–30 mg/kg PO q24h); can be used alone or combined with metronidazole (20 mg/kg PO q12h). Alternatively, use penicillin G procaine (40,000–60,000 IU/kg SC q24h).
• Encephalitozoonosis—fenbendazole (20 mg/kg q24h × 28 days) is the most common treatment and has been shown to reduce clinical signs and increase survival rates in symptomatic patients. Benzimidazole anthelmintics are effective against E. cuniculi in vitro and have been shown to prevent experimental infection in rabbits. However, efficacy in rabbits with clinical signs is unknown. Long-term treatment has been recommended, as treatment only prevents replication, rather than kills the parasite.
• Severe vestibular signs (continuous rolling, torticollis) or seizures—diazepam (1–2 mg/kg IM) or midazolam (0.5–2 mg/kg IM)
• Meclizine (12.5–25 mg/kg PO q8–12h) may reduce clinical signs, control nausea, and induce mild sedation.

CONTRAINDICATIONS
• Oral administration of antibiotics that select against gram-positive bacteria (penicillins, macrolides, lincosamides, and cephalosporins) can cause fatal enteric dysbiosis and enterotoxemia.
• Drugs potentially toxic to the vestibular system—aminoglycoside antibiotics; prolonged high-dose metronidazole

PRECAUTIONS
• Albendazole has been associated with in rabbits. Several anecdotal reports exist of pancytopenia leading to death in rabbits.
• Topical and systemic corticosteroids—rabbits are very sensitive to the immunosuppressive effects of corticosteroids; use may exacerbate subclinical bacterial infection. The use of corticosteroids (systemic or topical in otic preparations) can severely exacerbate otitis.
• Avoid topical otic preparations if the tympanic membrane is ruptured.

POSSIBLE INTERACTIONS
Several topical otic medications may induce contact irritation or allergic response; reevaluate all worsening cases.

ALTERNATIVE DRUGS
• Systemic corticosteroids have been advocated by practitioners for treatment of E. cuniculi-induced CNS granulomatous inflammation. Use of corticosteroids is controversial. Although clinical improvement has been anecdotally reported, rabbits are very sensitive to the immunosuppressive effects of corticosteroids; immunosuppression may exacerbate subclinical bacterial or E. cuniculi infection.
• Ponazuril has been anecdotally used to treat E. cuniculi (20–50 mg/kg PO q24h × 30 days). Safety and efficacy are unknown.

FOLLOW-UP

PATIENT MONITORING
• Monitor for corneal ulceration—secondary to facial nerve paralysis or abrasion during vestibular episodes
• Repeat the neurologic examination at a frequency dictated by the underlying cause.
• Head tilt may persist.

POSSIBLE COMPLICATIONS
• Progression of disease with deterioration of mental status
• Corneal ulceration

EXPECTED COURSE AND PROGNOSIS
• Most rabbits improve slowly with supportive care; advise owners that nursing care may be required for weeks to months.
• Following acute episode, head tilt often persists. Most rabbits adapt well to this, will ambulate, eat well, and appear to live comfortable lives. Recurrence of acute episodes may occur.
• Prognosis—guarded depending on underlying cause; varied response to drug treatment; many rabbits improve with

antibiotic therapy and/or supportive care alone
• Residual deficits (especially neurologic) cannot be predicted until after a course of therapy; long-term quality of life is good for the majority of rabbits with mild to moderate residual head tilt or facial nerve paralysis.

MISCELLANEOUS

ASSOCIATED CONDITIONS
• Dental disease
• Facial abscesses
• Upper respiratory infections
• Gastrointestinal hypomotility

AGE-RELATED FACTORS
E. cuniculi and bacterial otitis interna/media may be more common in older, especially immunosuppressed animals

ZOONOTIC POTENTIAL
• Rabies—consider in endemic areas if the patient is an outdoor animal that has rapidly progressive encephalitis
• E. cuniculi—unlikely but possible in immunosuppressed humans. Mode of transmission and susceptibility in humans are unclear.

PREGNANCY/FERTILITY/BREEDING
N/A

SYNONYMS
N/A

SEE ALSO
Encephalitozoonosis
Otitis media and interna
Pasteurellosis

ABBREVIATIONS
CNS = central nervous system
CSF = cerebrospinal fluid
CT = computed tomography
ELISA = enzyme-linked immunosorbent assay
GI = gastrointestinal
IFA = immunofluorescence assay
PCR = polymerase chain reaction
PNS = peripheral nervous system

Suggested Reading
Bays TB. Geriatric care of rabbits, guinea pigs, and chinchillas. Vet Clin Exot Anim 2020;23:567–593.
DeCubellis J. Common emergencies in rabbits, guinea pigs, and chinchillas. Vet Clin Exot Anim 2016;19:411–429.
Fisher PG, Künzel F, Rylander H. Neurologic and musculoskeletal disease. In: Quesenberry KE, Carpenter JW, eds. Ferrets, Rabbits and Rodents, (4th ed). Clinical Medicine and Surgery. St. Louis: Saunders, 2020:583–594.

RABBITS

Harkness JE, Turner PV, VandeWoude S, Wheeler CL. Clinical signs and differential diagnoses: nervous and musculoskeletal conditions. In: Harkness JE, Turner PV, VandeWoude S, Wheeler CL, eds. Biology and Medicine of Rabbits and Rodents, 5th ed. Ames: Wiley-Blackwell, 2010:214–216.

Keeble E. Nervous system and musculoskeletal disorders. In: Meredith A, Lord B, eds. BSAVA Manual of Rabbit Medicine. Gloucester: British Small Animal Veterinary Association, 2014:233–248.

Lennox AM, Gladden JN. Emergency and critical care of small mammals. In: Quesenberry KE, Carpenter JW, eds. Ferrets, Rabbits and Rodents, (4th ed). Clinical Medicine and Surgery. 2021, St. Louis: Saunders, 2020:595–608.

Varga M. Neurological and locomotive disorders. In: Varga M, ed. Textbook of Rabbit Medicine, 2nd ed. London, UK: Elsevier, 2014:367–389.

Author Barbara Oglesbee, DVM, DABVP (Avian)

HEATSTROKE AND HEAT STRESS

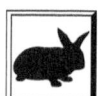

BASICS
- Rabbits are very sensitive to heatstroke and heat stress, especially in humid conditions
- Rabbits are obligate nasal breathers and cannot pant to dissipate heat. They rely primarily on distribution of blood flow to the large surface area of the pinnae for evaporative cooling.

PATHOPHYSIOLOGY
- The primary pathophysiologic processes of heatstroke are related to thermal damage that can lead to cellular necrosis, hypoxemia, and protein denaturalization.

SYSTEMS AFFECTED
- Nervous—neuronal damage, parenchymal hemorrhage, and cerebral edema
- Cardiovascular—hypovolemia, cardiac arrhythmias, myocardial ischemia, and necrosis
- Gastrointestinal—mucosal ischemia and ulceration, bacterial translocation, and endotoxemia
- Hepatobiliary—hepatocellular necrosis
- Renal/Urologic—acute renal failure
- Hemic/Lymph/Immune— hemoconcentration, thrombocytopenia, and disseminated intravascular coagulopathy
- Musculoskeletal—rhabdomyolysis

GENETICS
N/A

GEOGRAPHIC DISTRIBUTION
May be seen in any climate but more common in warm and or humid environments

SIGNALMENT
No breed, age, or sex predilection

SIGNS

Historical Findings
- Identifiable underlying cause—hot day, outdoor rabbits in the sun, ambient temperature >85°F, lack of shade, lack of ventilation, lack of drinking water, and excessive exercise
- Predisposing underlying disease— cardiovascular disease, neuromuscular disease, obesity, and previous history of heat-related disease

Physical Examination Findings
- Weakness, depression, ataxia early findings
- Seizures
- Coma
- Hyperthermia
- Hyperemic mucous membranes
- Tachycardia
- Cardiac arrhythmias
- Respiratory distress
- Muscle tremors
- Hematochezia
- Melena
- Petechiation
- Shock
- Oliguria/anuria
- Respiratory arrest
- Cardiopulmonary arrest

CAUSES AND RISK FACTORS
- Excessive environmental heat and humidity—may be due to weather conditions or accidents such as enclosed in unventilated room or car, or housed outdoors with a lack of shade and ventilation
- Exercise
- Age extremes
- Obesity
- Underlying cardiopulmonary disease
- Thick hair coat
- Dehydration

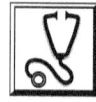

DIAGNOSIS

DIFFERENTIAL DIAGNOSIS
- If temperatures exceed 105°F without evidence of inflammation, consider heatstroke.
- Early clinical signs are nonspecific (lethargy, ataxia) and may resemble many other diseases. History is the most helpful factor in differentiating cause. However, many owners do not realize that the environment may have been too warm or ventilation inadequate for a pet rabbit. Always carefully question owners if heat stress is suspected.

CBC/BIOCHEMISTRY/URINALYSIS
- May help identify underlying disease process
- May help identify sequelae to hyperthermia
- CBC abnormalities may include anemia, thrombocytopenia, or hemoconcentration.
- Biochemistry profile may show azotemia, hyperalbuminemia, high ALT, high AST, high CK, and electrolyte abnormalities.

OTHER LABORATORY TESTS
N/A

IMAGING
Thoracic and abdominal radiographs may help identify underlying cardiopulmonary disease or predisposing factors.

DIAGNOSTIC PROCEDURES
Frequent body temperature monitoring

TREATMENT

APPROPRIATE HEALTH CARE
- Hospitalize patients until temperature is stabilized; intensive care for several days likely

needed; however, many rabbits do not survive.

NURSING CARE
- Immediate correction of hyperthermia
  ° Wet rabbit by spraying with water or soaking with cool, wet clothes before transporting to veterinary facility, if possible
  ° Wet rabbit in veterinary hospital by above means, or by immersing body in cool water
  ° Convection cooling with fans
  ° Evaporative cooling (e.g., alcohol on ears, foot pads, axilla, and groin)
- Stop cooling procedures when temperature reaches 103°F, to avoid hypothermia.
- Supplement oxygen via oxygen cage, mask, or nasal catheter.
- Give ventilatory support if required.
- Give fluid support with shock doses of crystalloids.
- Treat complications such as renal failure, cerebral edema.
- Treat underlying disease or correct predisposing factors.

ACTIVITY
Restricted

DIET
Be certain that the rabbit continues to eat to prevent secondary GI stasis.

CLIENT EDUCATION
- Be aware of clinical signs.
- Know how to cool animals.
- An episode of heatstroke may predispose pets to additional episodes.

SURGICAL CONSIDERATIONS
N/A

MEDICATIONS

DRUG(S) OF CHOICE
- No specific drugs are required for hyperthermia or heatstroke; therapy depends on clinical presentation.
- Fluid therapy for hypovolemic shock—LRS or other crystalloid (60–90 mg/kg/hr IV, IO over 20–60 minutes; followed by maintenance rate) or crystalloid bolus (30 mL/kg) plus hetastarch bolus (5 mL/kg initially) followed by crystalloids at a maintenance rate and hetastarch at 20 mL/kg divided over 24 hours.
- Cerebral edema—mannitol using canine/ feline protocols
- Ventricular arrhythmia—lidocaine bolus (1–2 mg/kg IV or 2–4 mg/kg IT) followed by continuous-rate intravenous infusion using feline dosage if necessary

- Metabolic acidosis—sodium bicarbonate (2 mEq/kg IV)
- Hemorrhagic diarrhea—broad-spectrum antibiotics
- Seizures—diazepam (1–2 mg/kg IV to effect)

CONTRAINDICATIONS
- Oral administration of antibiotics that select against gram-positive bacteria (penicillins, macrolides, lincosamides, and cephalosporins) can cause fatal enteric dysbiosis and enterotoxemia.
- Nonsteroidal anti-inflammatory agents not indicated in nonpyrogenic hyperthermia because the hypothalamic set point is not altered
- Corticosteroids—not demonstrated to be of benefit. Rabbits are extremely sensitive to the immunosuppressive effects
- Cooling with ice—may lead to peripheral vasoconstriction and poor heat dissipation

PRECAUTIONS
N/A

POSSIBLE INTERACTIONS
N/A

ALTERNATIVE DRUGS
N/A

 **FOLLOW-UP**

PATIENT MONITORING
- Monitor closely during cooling-down period and for a minimum of 24 hours post episode; most need several days, depending on clinical presentation and sequelae.

Perform a thorough physical examination daily; also consider monitoring the following:
- Body temperature
- Body weight
- Blood pressure
- ECG
- Thoracic auscultation
- Urinalysis and urine output
- PCV, TP
- CBC, biochemical profile

PREVENTION/AVOIDANCE
Avoid risk factors.

POSSIBLE COMPLICATIONS
- Cardiac arrhythmias
- Hemorrhagic diarrhea
- Organ failure
- Coma
- Seizures
- Acute renal failure
- Pulmonary edema—acute respiratory distress
- Hepatocellular necrosis
- Disseminated intravascular coagulation
- Respiratory arrest
- Cardiopulmonary arrest

EXPECTED COURSE AND PROGNOSIS
- Guarded—depending on complications and duration of episode
- May predispose to further episodes due to damage to thermoregulatory center

 MISCELLANEOUS

ASSOCIATED CONDITIONS
N/A

AGE-RELATED FACTORS
N/A

ZOONOTIC POTENTIAL
N/A

PREGNANCY/FERTILITY/BREEDING
N/A

SYNONYMS
Heat exhaustion
Heat prostration
Heat-related disease

ABBREVIATIONS
ALT = alanine aminotransferase
AST = aspartate aminotransferase
CK = creatine kinase
ECG = electrocardiogram
LRS = lactated Ringer's solution
PCV = packed cell volume
TP = total protein

Suggested Reading
DeCubellis J. Common emergencies in rabbits, guinea pigs, and chinchillas. Vet Clin Exot Anim 2016;19:411–429.
Lennox AM, Gladden JN. Emergency and critical care of small mammals. In: Quesenberry KE, Carpenter JW, eds. Ferrets, Rabbits and Rodents, 4th Ed). Clinical Medicine and Surgery. 2021 ed. St. Louis: Saunders, 2020:595–608.
Varga M. Cardiorespiratory diseases. In: Varga M, ed. Textbook of Rabbit Medicine, 2nd ed. London, UK: Elsevier, 2014:390–405.

Author Barbara Oglesbee, DVM, DABVP (Avian)

HEMATURIA

BASICS

DEFINITION
The presence of blood in the urine. Important to differentiate from red or red/brown colored urine caused by the excretion of dietary pigments in urine or from blood originating from the reproductive tract in females.

PATHOPHYSIOLOGY
• Must distinguish from blood originating from the reproductive tract in female rabbits. Blood expressed from the uterus or vaginal vault during micturition is a much more common cause of perceived hematuria than actual urinary tract bleeding.
• Secondary to loss of endothelial integrity in the urinary tract.
• Clotting factor deficiency or thrombocytopenia possible but not commonly reported

SYSTEMS AFFECTED
• Renal/Urologic
• Reproductive

SIGNALMENT
N/A

SIGNS
Historical Findings
• Red-tinged urine with or without pollakiuria
• Blood clots expelled during micturition

Physical Examination Findings
• May be normal
• Palpable mass in patients with uterine or cystic neoplasia
• Turgid, painful bladder on abdominal palpation in rabbits with hypercalciuria/bladder sludge, uroliths, or cystitis
• Detect urocystoliths by abdominal palpation; failure to palpate uroliths does not exclude them from consideration. Often one single, large calculus is palpated within the urinary bladder. Surprisingly, large calculi can be palpated in the distal urethra of both males and females, often causing hematuria and/or stranguria but not complete obstruction.
• In rabbits with crystalluria, the bladder sometimes palpates as a soft, doughy mass.
• With chronic disease, the bladder may markedly increase in size and may even fill most of the abdomen.
• Petechia or ecchymoses in patients with coagulopathies

CAUSES
Genitalia (Most Common Cause of Hematuria in Females)
• Uterine neoplasia, endometrial hyperplasia, or endometrial venous aneurysm—female

rabbits with uterine disease often expel blood when urinating. Blood may mix with urine and be mistaken for hematuria.
• Pyometra

Lower Urinary Tract (Most Common)
• Hypercalciuria, urolithiasis—calculi most commonly found in bladder or distal urethra
• Infectious—bacterial cystitis—relatively uncommon in rabbits
• Neoplasia
• Trauma

Systemic
• Coagulopathy (anticoagulant rodenticides)
• Thromboctyopenia

RISK FACTORS
• Sedentary, obese rabbits on diets consisting mainly of commercial pellets or high alfalfa hay content are at high risk for hypercalciuria and urolithiasis.
• Middle-aged to older intact females at risk for uterine neoplasia or pyometra.

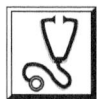

DIAGNOSIS

DIFFERENTIAL DIAGNOSIS
• Rule out physiologic red-brown colored urine—this is an extremely common cause of perceived hematuria and occurs much more commonly than true hematuria. Normal rabbits may have brown to red colored urine. This color change may be intermittent and is caused by the excretion of plant pigments. Differentiate blood from pigment excretion by cytologic examination or urine dipstick for blood; pigments may also fluoresce using an ultraviolet light (black light).
• Rule out blood originating from uterus in intact females—perform urinalysis, collect sample via ultrasound-guided cystocentesis to differentiate true hematuria from uterine bleeding
• Rule out other causes of discolored urine (myoglobinuria, hemoglobinuria)

CBC/BIOCHEMISTRY/URINALYSIS
• Elevated serum calcium concentration (normal range 12–16 mg/dL) in rabbits with hypercalciuria; the significance of this is unclear since many normal rabbits have high serum calcium concentration and never develop hypercalciuria.
• Azotemia in some patients with bilateral renal disease or urinary tract obstruction
• Thrombocytopenia, anemia with bleeding disorders
• Anemia with uterine adenocarcinoma
• Urinary sediment evaluation usually reveals calcium oxalate or calcium carbonate crystals; however, this is a normal finding in rabbits, and the presence of large amounts of crystals

in the urine does not necessarily indicate disease. Disease occurs only when the concentration of crystals is excessive, forming thick, white to brown, sand-like urine, and subsequent inflammatory cystitis or partial to complete blockage of the urethra.
• Pyuria (normal value 0–1 WBC/hpf), hematuria (normal value 0–1 RBC/hpf), and proteinuria (normal value 0–33 mg/dL) indicate urinary tract inflammation, but these are nonspecific findings that may result from infectious and noninfectious causes of lower urinary tract disease.
• Identification of neoplastic cells in urine sediment indicates urinary tract neoplasia.

OTHER LABORATORY TESTS
Bacterial culture of urine to identify urinary tract infection

IMAGING
Ultrasonography, radiography, and possibly contract radiographs may be useful in obtaining a diagnosis.

DIAGNOSTIC PROCEDURES
• Cystoscopy
• Biopsy of mass lesions

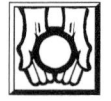

TREATMENT
• Hematuria may indicate a serious disease process.
• Hypercalciuria requires diet and husbandry modification. Diuresis and mechanical removal of urine "sludge" often necessary.
• Uroliths require surgical removal.
• Uterine disease requires surgical intervention.

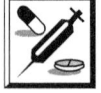

MEDICATIONS

DRUG(S) OF CHOICE
• Blood transfusion may be necessary if patient is severely anemic
• Fluids to treat dehydration
• Symptomatic rabbits with hypercalciuria or urinary calculi are sometimes painful and therefore reluctant to urinate. Pain management may aid in urination and promote appetite and water consumption. NSAIDs (meloxicam, carprofen) reduce pain and may decrease inflammation in the bladder.

CONTRAINDTICATIONS
• Glucocorticoids or other immunosuppressive agents
• Oral administration of antibiotics that select against gram-positive bacteria (penicillins, macrolides, lincosamides, and

(CONTINUED)

cephalosporins) can cause fatal enteric dysbiosis and enterotoxemia.

PRECAUTIONS
N/A

ALTERNATIVE DRUGS
N/A

FOLLOW-UP

PATIENT MONITORING
• Response to treatment by clinical signs, serial physical examinations, laboratory testing, and radiographic and ultrasonic evaluations appropriate for each specific cause
• Refer to specific chapters describing diseases listed in section on causes.

POSSIBLE COMPLICATIONS
• Anemia
• Urinary tract obstruction with urolithiasis or hypercalciuria
• Renal failure with urolithiasis or hypercalciuria
• Metastases with uterine adenocarcinoma

MISCELLANEOUS

ASSOCIATED CONDITIONS
• Obesity
• Gastrointestinal hypomotility
• Musculoskeletal disorders

AGE-RELATED FACTORS
• Neoplasia tends to occur in middle-aged to older rabbits
• Hypercalciuria tends to occur in middle-aged to older rabbits

ZOONOTIC POTENTIAL
N/A

PREGNANCY/FERTILITY/BREEDING
N/A

SYNONYMS
N/A

SEE ALSO
• Hypercalciuria and urolithiasis
• Pyometra and nonneoplastic uterine disorders
• Uterine neoplasia
• Vaginal discharge

Suggested Reading
Di Girolamo N, Selleri P. Disorders of the urinary and reproductive system. In: Quesenberry KE, Carpenter JW, eds. Ferrets, Rabbits and Rodents, 4th Ed). Clinical Medicine and Surgery ed. St. Louis: Saunders, 2020:201–220.
Hallman RM, Brandão J. Diagnostic imaging of the renal system in exotic companion mammals. Vet Clin Exot Anim 2020;23: 195–214.
Mancinelli E, Lord B. Urogenital and reproductive disease. In: Meredith A, Lord B, eds. BSAVA Manual of Rabbit Medicine. Gloucester: British Small Animal Veterinary Association, 2014:191–204.
Reavill DR, Lennox AM. Disease overview of the urinary tract in exotic companion mammals and tips on clinical management. Vet Clin Exot Anim 2020;23(1):169–193.

Author Barbara Oglesbee, DVM, DABVP (Avian)

HERPES SIMPLEX

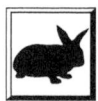

BASICS

DEFINITION
Human herpesvirus-1 (HHV-1) can be transmitted from humans with cold sores to rabbits. The virus is strongly neurotropic with a 67% of human <50 years of age infected worldwide. Mammals of the superorder Euarchontoglires—primates, rabbits, and rodents are susceptible to the virus. Rabbits are particularly susceptible and are used for research of HHV-1. In research rabbits, the virus is exclusively neurotropic and infection is almost always fatal. Although spontaneous transmission is rare, this represents another differential when considering causes of neurologic disease with and without concurrent conjunctivitis in rabbits.

PATHOPHYSIOLOGY
Transmission from infected, shedding human to rabbit via oral-oral, oral-ocular, or oronasal routes. Rabbit to rabbit transmission is also possible. Neurotropic in rabbits, likely ascending infection to brain/spinal cord via olfactory, optical, or trigeminal nerves

SYSTEMS AFFECTED
Neurologic
Ophthalmic

INCIDENCE/PREVALENCE
Rare in rabbits

SIGNALMENT

Species
Rabbits, rodents, nonhuman primates, humans

Breed Predilection
None known

Mean Age and Range
Assume all ages

Predominant Sex
None

SIGNS

Historical Findings
Owner has HHV-1 and recent, active cold sores leading to shedding of virus, along with close interactions with rabbit.

Physical Examination Findings
• Bilateral epiphora and conjunctivitis, uveitis, and keratitis may be noted.
• Ptyalism, bruxism
• Severe signs of CNS dysfunction such as incoordination, muscle tremors, intermittent myoclonic seizures, and opisthotonus.

CAUSES
HHV-1

RISK FACTORS
Owner with HHV-1 with recent a flare-up, close contact of affected area of infected human with mucous membranes of the rabbit

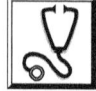

DIAGNOSIS

DIFFERENTIAL DIAGNOSIS
Neurologic disorders such as head trauma, brain abscess or tumor, infection with *E. cuniculi* or *T. gondii*, migration of *Baylisascaris* spp. larvae, uremia, hepatoencephalic syndrome, rabies, arteriosclerosis, and intoxication

CBC/BIOCHEMISTRY/URINALYSIS
Lymphopenia, a relative monocytosis, and an increase in creatine phosphokinase and serum concentration of total protein was reported in a single case.

OTHER LABORATORY TESTS
N/A

IMAGING
Ultrasound-guided atlanto-occipital CSF collection

DIAGNOSTIC PROCEDURES
• Corneal/subconjunctival swab testing for HHV1 by PCR amplification
• HHV-1-specific PCR and immunohistochemical staining (poly- and monoclonal) analysis of brain tissue.

PATHOLOGIC FINDINGS
• Gross—mild, focal, erosive keratitis of the eye. No gross abnormalities in the brain, spinal cord, or musculoskeletal system unless concurrent disease.
• Histopathologic—severe, diffuse, nonsuppurative meningoencephalitis with severe, acute, multifocal neuronal degeneration and necrosis and degeneration in the cerebrum, cerebellum, and brain stem. Large, eosinophilic, intranuclear inclusion bodies multifocally distributed in neurons and glial cells of the cerebrum. Giemsa and periodic acid-Schiff staining of sections of brain tissue fail to reveal the presence of *E. cuniculi* and *T. gondii*; however, their presence does not preclude dual infection.

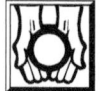

TREATMENT

NURSING CARE
General supportive care as clinical signs warrant, such as antibiotics, anti-inflammtories, fluids, and supportive nutrition
    Isolate from other rabbits and people

ACTIVITY
Limit until neurologic signs resolve

DIET
Ensure that the rabbit is eating to prevent gastrointestinal motility disorders.

CLIENT EDUCATION
Reverse zoonotic, proper hygiene/interaction with pet, especially during an HHV-1 outbreak

SURGICAL INDICATIONS
N/A

MEDICATIONS

DRUG(S) OF CHOICE
None reported, as most cases result in acute death, but if not, could consider:
Acyclovir 5 mg/kg PO q12h
L-lysine—12.5 mg/kg PO daily

CONTRAINDICATIONS/POSSIBLE INTERATIONS
N/A

PRECAUTIONS
N/A

ALTERNATIVE DRUGS
N/A

FOLLOW-UP

PATIENT MONITORING
N/A

PREVENTION/AVOIDANCE
Limit close human contact with rabbits during active HHV-1 outbreak.

POSSIBLE COMPLICATIONS
If survives, possible recrudenscence

EXPECTED COURSE AND PROGNOSIS
All reported cases have been fatal.

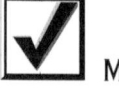

MISCELLANEOUS

ASSOCIATED CONDITIONS
None known

AGE-RELATED FACTORS
N/A

ZOONOTIC POTENTIAL
Reverse zoonoses, possible normal zoonotic to naïve humans

PREGNANCY/FERTILITY/BREEDING
Unknown

RABBITS

(CONTINUED)

SYNONYMS
Herpes simplex virus

SEE ALSO
Encephalitis

ABBREVIATIONS
CSF = cerebrospinal fluid
HHV-1 = human herpesvirus 1

Suggested Reading
Anselmi C, Dias S, Martorell J et al. Ultrasonographic anatomy of the atlanto-occipital region and ultrasound-guided cerebrospinal fluid collection in rabbits (*Oryctolagus cuniculus*). Vet Radiol Ultrasound 2018;59(2):188–197.
Bauer K, Steeil J, Adkins E et al. Management of ocular human herpesvirus 1 infection in a white-faced saki monkey (*Pithecia pithecia*). Comp Med 2018;68(4):319–323.
De Matos R, Russell D, Alstine W, Miller A. Spontaneous fatal human herpesvirus 1 encephalitis in two domestic rabbits (*Oryctolagus cuniculus*). J Vet Diagn Investig. 2014;26(5):689–694.
Meredith A, Richardson J. Neurological diseases of rabbits and rodents. J Exot Pet Med 2015;24(1):21–33.

Author Eric Klaphake, DVM, Dipl. ABVP, Dipl. ACZM

RABBITS

HYPERCALCIURIA (BLADDER SLUDGE) AND UROLITHIASIS

BASICS

DEFINITION
Formation of crystals or uroliths composed of calcium salts (usually calcium oxalate and calcium carbonate) within the urinary tract and associated clinical conditions. Excessive crystal formation and retention in the bladder results in thick sand- or paste-like urine ("sludge") and inflammation of the bladder wall. Crystals can condense to form uroliths in the bladder, urethra, ureters, or renal pelvis.

PATHOPHYSIOLOGY
In rabbits, nearly all calcium in the diet is absorbed. Calcium excretion occurs primarily through the kidneys (vs. the gall bladder in other mammals); the fractional urinary excretion is 45%–60% in rabbits compared to less than 2% in other mammals.
• Rabbits normally eat a diet high in calcium; however, not all rabbits develop hypercalciuria.
• The factors leading to hypercalciuria and urolith formation in rabbits are unclear; however, the disease is seen more commonly in obese, sedentary rabbits fed a diet composed primarily of commercial alfalfa-based pellets.
• Inadequate water intake leading to a more concentrated urine, and factors that impair complete evacuation of the bladder, such as lack of exercise, obesity, cystitis, neoplasia, or neuromuscular disease are the primary cause of hypercalciuria. Without frequent urination and dilute urine, calcium crystals may precipitate out of solution within the bladder. Precipitated crystals form a thick sand or sludge within the bladder that does not mix normally with urine and is not eliminated during voiding.
• Most commercial diets contain excessive amounts of calcium. The dietary requirement of calcium for rabbits is only 0.22 g of calcium/100 g food, but most commercial diets contain up to 0.9–1.6 g of calcium/100 g of food. It is unlikely that high dietary calcium content alone is the cause of hypercalciuria, but it may exacerbate urinary sludge formation when combined with other factors leading to urine retention.

SYSTEMS AFFECTED
• Renal/Urologic
• Skin—urine scald, perineal, and ventral dermatitis

GENETICS
Unknown—but may play a role in determining which rabbits develop hypercalciuria

INCIDENCE/PREVALENCE
Clinical conditions related to hypercalciuria and urolith formation are extremely common in pet rabbits.

GEOGRAPHIC DISTRIBUTION
Ubiquitous

SIGNALMENT
Breed Predilections
All breeds are equally affected

Mean Age and Range
Seen most often in middle-aged rabbits 3–5 years old.

Predominant Sex
N/A

SIGNS
General Comments
• Some animals remain asymptomatic, despite large amounts of calcium sludge accumulation in the bladder.
• Depend on location, size, and amount of material in the bladder

Historical Findings
• Pollakiuria, dysuria, hematuria, and urine staining in the perineum in rabbits with urocystoliths, ureteroliths, or large amounts of crystalline sludge in the bladder
• Urinating outside of the litter box
• Urinating when picked up by owners
• Owners may report thick, pasty, beige- to brown-colored urine; sometimes this urine so thick that it is mistaken for diarrhea.
• Abnormal-appearing urine is not always reported. Some rabbits void clear urine while sludge remains in the bladder; sometimes cloudy urine is reported.
• Hunched posture, ataxia, or difficulty ambulating in rabbits with neurologic or orthopedic disorders leading to urine retention
• Anorexia, weight loss, lethargy, tooth grinding, tenesmus, and a hunched posture in rabbits with large urocystoliths, large amounts of sludge in the bladder, or complete or partial obstruction of the ureters or urethra

Physical Examination Findings
• Detect urocystoliths by abdominal palpation; failure to palpate uroliths does not exclude them from consideration. Most often one single, large calculus is palpated. In rabbits with crystalluria (urine sludge), the bladder may palpate as a soft, doughy mass.
• With chronic disease, the bladder loses tone, may markedly increase in size, and may even fill most of the abdomen.
• A large urinary bladder may also be palpable in patients with partial or complete urethral obstruction.
• Manual expression of the bladder may reveal thick beige- to brown-colored urine.

Manual expression of the bladder may expel thick brown urine even in rabbits that have normal-appearing voided urine.
• A large kidney may be palpated in rabbits with ureteroliths and subsequent hydronephrosis (rare).

CAUSES
See pathophysiology

RISK FACTORS
• Inadequate water intake (dirty water bowls, unpalatable water, changing water sources, and inadequate water provision)
• Urine retention (underlying bladder pathology, neuromuscular disease)
• Inadequate cleaning of litter box or cage may cause some rabbits to avoid urinating for abnormally long periods.
• Obesity
• Pain and a reluctance to ambulate
• Lack of exercise
• Feeding of exclusively commercial pelleted diets
• Renal disease
• Calcium or vitamin/mineral supplements added to the diet

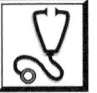

DIAGNOSIS

DIFFERENTIAL DIAGNOSIS
• Other, less common causes of hematuria, dysuria, and pollakiuria, with or without urethral obstruction, include urinary tract infection and lower urinary tract neoplasia.
• Female rabbits with pyometra or uterine neoplasia may expel blood or a thick, often blood-tinged vaginal discharge when urinating. This discharge may mix with urine and mimic hypercalciuria.

CBC/BIOCHEMISTRY/URINALYSIS
• Most affected rabbits are hypercalcemic (normal range 12–16 mg/dL); however, the significance of this is unclear since many normal rabbits have high serum calcium concentration and never develop hypercalciuria.
• Complete urinary outflow obstruction can cause postrenal azotemia (e.g., high BUN, creatinine).
• Urinary sediment evaluation reveals calcium oxalate or calcium carbonate crystals; however, this is a normal finding in rabbits, and the presence of large amounts of crystals in the urine does not necessarily indicate disease. Disease occurs only when the concentration of crystals is excessive, forming thick, white to brown, sandlike urine, and subsequent inflammatory cystitis or partial to complete blockage of the urethra.
• Pyuria (normal value 0–1 WBC/hpf), hematuria (normal value 0–1 RBC/hpf), and

(CONTINUED) HYPERCALCIURIA (BLADDER SLUDGE) AND UROLITHIASIS

proteinuria (normal value 0–33 mg/dL) indicate urinary tract inflammation, but these are nonspecific findings that may result from infectious and noninfectious causes of lower urinary tract disease.
• Urine pH: normal rabbit urine is alkaline; pH >8 suggestive of bacterial cystitis due to urease-producing bacteria

OTHER LABORATORY TESTS
• Prior to antibiotic use, culture the urine or bladder wall if high numbers of red or white blood cells, bacteria, or a combination of these are present on sediment examination. Collect urine via cystocentesis, as free-catch samples are commonly contaminated.
• If surgery is necessary to relieve obstruction from urolithiasis, collect and submit the calculi for analysis and culture and sensitivity, and submit the bladder wall for culture and sensitivity.

IMAGING
• Calcium oxalate uroliths are radiopaque and may be detected by survey radiography. Uroliths must be differentiated from calcium "sand" or sludge in the bladder, which resembles a bladder full of contrast material. Ultrasonic examination of the bladder and palpation can be helpful to distinguish solitary calculi from amorphous sand.
• A small amount of sand or sludge in the bladder can be normal and is frequently discovered serendipitously in rabbits undergoing radiographs for other causes.
• Nephroliths and/or ureteroliths may also been seen. Renal calcification can resemble renoliths on abdominal radiographs. Renal calcification can be differentiated from renoliths on ultrasound.
• Occasionally, relatively large uroliths can be found in the urethra, sometimes causing only partial obstruction.

DIAGNOSTIC PROCEDURES
• Perform a urine culture—occasionally, rabbits with hypercalciuria have concurrent bacterial cystitis.

PATHOLOGIC FINDINGS
N/A

TREATMENT

APPROPRIATE HEALTH CARE
• Look for and treat any underlying medical problem that may cause a reluctance or inability to urinate.
• Retrograde urohydropropulsion to flush urethral stones back into the urinary bladder or voiding urohydropropulsion to eliminate

bladder "sand" can be performed on an outpatient basis. Voiding urohydropropulsion is contraindicated in patients with urethral obstruction.
• Surgery requires a short period of hospitalization.

NURSING CARE
• Unobstructed rabbits diagnosed with hypercalciuria usually respond to diuresis via subcutaneous fluid administration, increasing water consumption, dietary modification, weight loss, and increase in exercise alone.
• Severely affected rabbits with large amounts of calcium precipitate (sand or sludge) in the urinary bladder may require medical treatment with fluid therapy and voiding urohydropropulsion. Manually express the bladder to remove as much precipitated calcium sand as possible. Gentle ballottement or agitation of the bladder may help to mobilize sludge. Administer fluid therapy SC daily for 2–4 days to increase the amount of urine in the bladder. If precipitated calcium sand is detected in the bladder (via palpation or imaging) after this time, continue fluid therapy and manually express the bladder, gently forcing the non-voided sludge out the urethra. This is a painful procedure and requires sedation or anesthesia. Sedation with benzodiazepines may help to relax the urethral sphincter—Midazolam 0.5–1.0 mg/kg IM, IV combined with an opioid for pain control is often sufficient.
• If large amounts of precipitate are present and manual expression does not remove the accumulated sludge, flushing the bladder with warm saline via urethral catheterization may be effective.
• Fortunately, ureteroliths are relatively rare. However, when present can be surprisingly large and may only cause partial obstruction. Retrograde urohydropropulsion can sometimes be used to push small stones back into the bladder to be removed via cystotomy. Catheterization should be attempted under heavy sedation or general anesthesia.

ACTIVITY
• Reduce during the period of tissue repair after surgery
• Increase activity level by providing large exercise areas to encourage voiding and prevent recurrence—important part of treatment and prevention

DIET
• Many affected rabbits are anorectic or have a decreased appetite. It is an absolute requirement that the patient continue to eat during and following treatments. Anorexia may cause or exacerbate gastrointestinal

hypomotility and cause derangement of the gastrointestinal microflora and overgrowth of intestinal bacterial pathogens. If the patient refuses these foods, syringe-feed Critical Care for Herbivores (Oxbow Animal Health, Murdock, NE) or Emeraid Herbivore (Lafeber Company, Cornell, IL) diet at approximately 10–15 mL/kg PO q6–8h. Larger volumes and more frequent feedings are often accepted; feed as much as the patient will readily accept. Alternatively, pellets can be ground and mixed with fresh greens, vegetable baby foods, water, or sugar-free juice to form a gruel
• Encourage oral fluid intake by offering fresh water, wetting leafy vegetables, or flavoring water with vegetable juices.
• Increasing water consumption is essential to prevention and treatment of hypercalciuria. Provide multiple sources of fresh water. Automatic, continuously pouring water fountains available for cats entice some rabbits to drink. Flavoring the water with fruit or vegetable juices (with no added sugars) may be helpful. Provide a variety of clean, fresh, leafy vegetables sprayed, or soaked with water.
• No reports of dissolution of calcium oxalate uroliths with special diets
• Following treatment, reduction in the amount of calcium in the diet may help to prevent or delay recurrence. Eliminate feeding of alfalfa pellets and switch to a high-fiber timothy-based pellet (Oxbow Pet Products, Murdock, NE). Feed timothy and grass hay instead of alfalfa hay and offer large volumes of fresh, green, leafy vegetables with lower calcium content

CLIENT EDUCATION
Urolith removal or removal of calcium sand does not alter the factors responsible for their formation; eliminating risk factors such as obesity, sedentary life, and poor diet combined with increasing water consumption is necessary to minimize or delay recurrence. Even with these changes, however, recurrence is likely.

SURGICAL CONSIDERATIONS
• Uroliths within the bladder, ureters, or renal pelvis must be removed surgically. The procedures are similar to those performed on dogs or cats.
• Large urethral calculi may require surgical removal. In males, distal urethral calculi are common and can be surprisingly large. Remove stones via urethrotomy, leaving the incision open to heal by second intention.
• Calcium sludge in the bladder that does not respond to medical therapy may require cystotomy for removal.

HYPERCALCIURIA (BLADDER SLUDGE) AND UROLITHIASIS   (CONTINUED)

MEDICATIONS

DRUG(S) OF CHOICE

• No available drugs effectively dissolve calcium oxalate uroliths.
• Some rabbits with large amounts of calcium precipitate or uroliths have an underlying chronic bacterial cystitis. Treat with antibiotics, based on culture and susceptibility testing, when possible.
• Pain management is essential during and following surgery, urohydropropulsion, urinary catheterization, or if pain is causing reduced frequency of voiding. Perioperative choices include butorphanol (0.1–0.5 mg/kg SQ, IM, IV q4–6h, buprenorphine (0.02–0.05 mg/kg SQ, IM IV q8–12h), Hydromorphone (0.1 mg/kg SC IM q2–4h) or oxymorphone (0.05–0.2 mg/kg SC IM q8–12h). To manage long-term pain: meloxicam (1.0 mg/kg PO q24h), carprofen (2 mg/kg PO q12h), tramadol (5–15 mg/kg PO q8–12h), and/or gabapentin (5–20 mg/kg PO q8–12h)
• Consider diuretic therapy for patients with bladder sludge or uroliths. Give a calcium-sparing thiazide diuretic such as hydrochlorothiazide 0.5–2 mg/kg PO q12h
• Potassium citrate 33 mg/kg POq8h may help to prevent formation of calcium crystals in urine
• For a bladder that is chronically distended and will not empty completely during micturition, bethanechol chloride has been anecdotally used at feline dosages (2.5–5 mg/kg q8–12h).

CONTRAINDICATIONS

• Oral administration of antibiotics that select against gram-positive bacteria (penicillins, macrolides, lincosamides, and cephalosporins) can cause fatal enteric dysbiosis and enterotoxemia.

PRECAUTIONS

NSAIDs—use with caution in patients with renal disease

POSSIBLE INTERACTIONS

N/A

ALTERNATIVE DRUGS

N/A

FOLLOW-UP

PATIENT MONITORING

• Radiographs are essential following surgery or urohydropropulsion to verify complete removal
• Repeat radiographs to monitor for recurrence every 1–3 months

PREVENTION/AVOIDANCE

• Increase water consumption for the remainder of the rabbit's life.
• Avoid alfalfa-based diets. Diets containing a high percentage of timothy, oat, or grass hays, a lower overall percentage pellets, and a wider variety of vegetables and fruits decrease the risk of urolith development.
• Diruetics such as furosemide (1–2 mg/kg PO q12–24h) or hydrochlorothiazide (0.5–2 mg/kg PO q12h) have been anecdotally used in rabbits with recurrent urolithiasis to increase water intake and urination when husbandry changes alone were not successful in preventing recurrence.

POSSIBLE COMPLICATIONS

• Renal failure, urinary tract obstruction, hydronephrosis, and bladder atony
• Urine scald

EXPECTED COURSE AND PROGNOSIS

• The prognosis following surgical removal of uroliths or urohydropropulsion for the removal of calcium sand is fair to good. Although husbandry changes and dietary management may decrease the likelihood of recurrence, many rabbits will develop clinical disease again within 1–2 years.

MISCELLANEOUS

ASSOCIATED CONDITIONS

• Obesity
• Gastrointestinal hypomotility
• Urine scald

AGE-RELATED FACTORS

Rare in young animals

ZOONOTIC POTENTIAL

None

PREGNANCY/FERTILITY/BREEDING

N/A

SYNONYMS

Calcium oxalate urolithiasis
Bladder sludge

SEE ALSO

Dysuria and pollakiuria
Lower urinary tract infection
Urinary tract obstruction

ABBREVIATIONS

BUN = blood urea nitrogen
GI = gastrointestinal
NSAID = nonsteroidal anti-inflammatory drug

Suggested Reading
Di Girolamo N, Selleri P. Disorders of the urinary and reproductive system. In: Quesenberry KE, Carpenter JW, eds. Ferrets, Rabbits and Rodents, 4th Ed). Clinical Medicine and Surgery ed. St. Louis: Saunders, 2020:201–220.
Hallman RM, Brandão J. Diagnostic imaging of the renal system in exotic companion mammals. Vet Clin Exot Anim 2020;23: 195–214.
Mancinelli E, Lord B. Urogenital and reproductive disease. In: Meredith A, Lord B, eds. BSAVA Manual of Rabbit Medicine. Gloucester: British Small Animal Veterinary Association, 2014:191–204.
Reavill DR, Lennox AM. Disease overview of the urinary tract in exotic companion mammals and tips on clinical management. Vet Clin Exot Anim 2020;23(1):169–193.

Author Barbara Oglesbee, DVM, DABVP (Avian)

INCISOR MALOCCLUSION AND OVERGROWTH

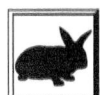

BASICS

DEFINITION
• Incisor overgrowth—occurs when occlusion is not normal. Rabbit teeth are elodont (open-rooted) and grow continuously throughout life. Normal rabbit incisors are very long and curved (considering both the clinical and the reserve crown) and rely on proper contact of the mandibular incisors between the primary and secondary maxillary incisors during chewing, to create a chisel-shaped occlusal plane.
• Malocclusion of the incisors—can occasionally be caused by congenital skeletal malocclusion, trauma, or secondary to malocclusion of the cheek teeth.

ANATOMY AND PHYSIOLOGY
• Normal dentition: 6 incisor teeth, including 4 large primary (mandibulary and maxillary) incisors and 2 smaller secondary maxillary incisors (or "peg teeth") located lingual to the primary maxillary incisors. Lack of canine teeth with the presence of a large diastema between the incisor and the cheek teeth. Since the premolars and molars are anatomically similar and are aligned as one functional unit, they are referred to as cheek teeth. Cheek teeth consist of 3 maxillary premolars, 3 maxillary molars, 2 mandibular premolars, and 3 mandibular molars on each side, for a total of 22 cheek teeth and a total of 28 teeth.
• All teeth are elodont (open-rooted) and grow continuously at a rate of approximately 2–2.5 mm per week, with growth originating from the germinal bud located at the apex of the tooth, the rate of tooth growth, and eruption matches the rate of wear.
• The rate of normal wear should match the rate of growth and eruption. Normal wear requires proper occlusion with the opposing set of teeth. When at rest, the mandibular incisors should rest between the primary and secondary (peg teeth) bmaxillary incisors.

PATHOPHYSIOLOGY
• Incisor malocclusion can be caused by trauma (falling, being dropped, or chewing on cage bars), congenital malocclusion, or may be secondary to malocclusion and overgrowth of the cheek teeth (acquired dental disease). Metabolic bone disease may also be an underlying or concurrent factor. Cheek teeth malocclusion eventually leads to a prognathic position of the mandible and subsequent incisor malocclusion.
• Incisors may grow into or damage adjacent soft tissues; secondary bacterial infections may occur.

SYSTEMS AFFECTED
• Oral cavity
• Ocular—involvement of the nasolacrimal duct (obstruction or dacyocystitis)
• Gastrointestinal—secondary functional stasis and related complications.
• Musculoskeletal—weight loss, muscle wasting

GENETICS
Unknown

INCIDENCE/PREVALENCE
• One of the most common presenting complaints in pet rabbits

GEOGRAPHIC DISTRIBUTION
N/A

SIGNALMENT
• Young animals—congenital malocclusion (prognathism of the mandible and/or brachygnathism of the maxilla)
• Middle-aged to older rabbits—incisor overgrowth secondary to acquired dental disease or congenital malocclusion
• Dwarf and lop breeds—congenital malocclusion

SIGNS

General Comments
• Owners generally notice incisor overgrowth first, as these teeth are readily visible when abnormal. In many cases, incisor overgrowth is a sign of generalized dental disease.
• Always perform a thorough oral examination under sedation or general anesthesia to examine the cheek teeth. Rabbits have a long, narrow mouth; the use of a directed light source, cheek dilators, mouth gag, or endoscope are needed to thoroughly examine the teeth. Significant cheek teeth apical abnormalities may be present despite normal-appearing crowns. Skull radiographs are required to identify apical (root) disorders.

Historical Findings
• Incisor overgrowth may be the only clinical sign in rabbits with congenital incisor malocclusion.
• Inability to prehend food
• Epiphora if nasolacrimal duct is secondarily affected because of compression by the abnormal apices of primary maxillary incisor teeth.
If generalized dental disease is present:
• Anorexia or reduced food intake
• Weight loss
• Excessive drooling and moist dermatitis on the chin and dewlap
• Nasal discharge
• Tooth grinding
• Facial asymmetry or exophthalmos in rabbits with periapical infections and abscesses

• Signs of pain—reluctance to move, depression, lethargy, hiding, and hunched posture
• Unkempt hair coat, lack of grooming

Physical Examination Findings
• Incisors—coronal elongation, horizontal ridges or grooves, malocclusion, discoloration, fractures, increased or decreased curvature, and loose teeth

Oral Examination
• Always thoroughly examine the cheek teeth to look for generalized dental disease. This requires heavy sedation or general anesthesia and specialized equipment. A cursory examination using an otoscope for illumination and visualization is insufficient for rabbits with dental disease.
• A focused, directed light source and magnification will provide optimal visualization.
• Use a rabbit mouth gag and cheek dilators (Jorgensen Laboratories, Inc., Loveland, CO) to open the mouth and pull buccal tissues away from cheek teeth to allow adequate exposure. Use a cotton swab or tongue depressor to retract the tongue from lingual surfaces.
• Normal cheek teeth—coronal surfaces have small cusps)
• Identify cheek teeth abnormalities—elongation, irregular coronal height, spikes, curved teeth, longitudinal fractures, missing teeth, purulent exudate, odor, impacted food, oral ulceration, or abscesses
• Buccal or lingual mucosa and lip margins—ulceration, abrasions, secondary bacterial infection, or abscess formation if incisors or cheek teeth spikes have damaged soft tissues
Other findings in rabbits with generalized dental disease:
• Ptyalism, secondary moist pyoderma around the mouth, neck, and dewlap areas
• A scalloped edge or single bony protrusions may be palpable on the ventral rim of the mandible in some rabbits with apical cheek teeth disorders.
• Soft tissue swelling, abscess most commonly located on the mandible or below the eye
• Exophthalmos in rabbits with retrobulbar abscesses from periapical infection arising from most caudal maxillary cheek teeth.
• Weight loss, emaciation
• Nasal discharge
• Ocular discharge—obstruction of the nasolacrimal duct; pressure on the eye from retrobulbar abscess or overgrown tooth roots
• Signs of gastrointestinal hypomotility—scant feces, intestinal pain, soft stools

INCISOR MALOCCLUSION AND OVERGROWTH

CAUSES
• Congenital skeletal malocclusion—common cause; most common in dwarf or lop-eared breeds
• Trauma—traumatic fracture of the incisors from falls, chewing cage bars or other objects; iatrogenic damage from inappropriate teeth trimming
• Elongated cheek teeth (acquired dental disease)—likely multiple etiologies; inadequate hay or tough foods to properly grind teeth so that coronal surfaces cannot wear normally; metabolic bone disease may play a role

RISK FACTORS
• Feeding pelleted and mixed diets (without supplementing long-stem hay and grasses)—these diets lack sufficient fiber to encourage proper mandibular motion and properly grind coronal surfaces
• Breeding rabbits with congenital malocclusion
• Broken incisors—improper restraint or inappropriate trimming of the incisors

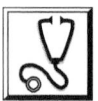

DIAGNOSIS
DIFFERENTIAL DIAGNOSIS
• Overgrowth due to trauma—may have history of trauma (jumping, falling, and being dropped), history of chewing on cage bars or other hard objects, or history of having the teeth "clipped." May see fractured incisors, discoloration secondary to pulpitis.
• Rule out cheek teeth elongation by performing thorough oral examination under anesthesia and skull radiographs.
• Congenital malocclusion—seen in young animals. Diagnosis of exclusion if cheek teeth elongation has been ruled out by performing thorough oral examination under anesthesia and mandatory skull radiographs.

CBC/BIOCHEMISTRY/URINALYSIS
Usually normal; may see abnormalities in liver enzymes in rabbits with hepatic lipidosis secondary to anorexia.

OTHER LABORATORY TESTS
N/A

IMAGING
Skull Radiographs
• Mandatory to identify type and extent of dental disease, to plan treatment strategies, and to monitor progression of treatment
• Perform under general anesthesia
• A standard set of five extraoral views are recommended for thorough assessment: lateral, ventrodorsal, two lateral obliques, and rostro-caudal. Additional extraoral oblique

projections, as well as additional intraoral views, may also be used.
• Common incisor abnormalities—incisors may appear elongated or excessively curved; abnormal occlusal plane, mandibular incisors will often lose their normal curvature and protrude rostrally from the mandible; the apex of the mandibular incisors may superimpose on the reserve crowns of the first of the mandibular premolars; increased curvature of the primary maxillary incisors and apical elongation is usually seen
• With cheek teeth elongation and malocclusion—elongation of the reserve crowns and apices, apical deformities, loss of normal coronal occlusal pattern, mild radiolucency around reserve crowns, curved teeth, widening of the interdental space, apical radiolucency and bony lysis, protrusion or penetration of the apices into surrounding cortical bone
• CT—superior to radiographs to evaluate the extent of dental disease and bony destruction

DIAGNOSTIC PROCEDURES
• Fine-needle aspiration of facial swelling—may be helpful to identify abscess
• Bacterial culture and sensitivity testing of abscess or nasal discharge, if present—aerobic and anaerobic bacteria

TREATMENT
APPROPRIATE HEALTH CARE
• Outpatient—patients with mild to moderate dental disease requiring coronal reduction
• Inpatient—patients with periapical or facial abscess, patients requiring extraction, or debilitated patients

NURSING CARE
Keep fur around face clean and dry, shave where needed.

ACTIVITY
N/A

DIET
• It is absolutely imperative that the rabbit continue to eat during and following treatment. Most rabbits with congenital malocclusion of the incisors alone continue to eat until the teeth are very long. Many rabbits with generalized dental disease will become anorexic. Anorexia will cause or exacerbate GI hypomotility, derangement of the gastrointestinal microflora, and overgrowth of intestinal bacterial pathogens.
• Syringe-feed a gruel such as Critical Care for Herbivores (Oxbow Pet Products) or Emeraid Herbivore (Lafeber Company,

Cornell, IL), 10–15 mL/kg PO q6–8h. Larger volumes and more frequent feedings are often accepted; feed as much as the rabbit will readily accept. Alternatively, pellets can be ground and mixed with fresh greens, vegetable baby foods, water, or juice to form a gruel.
• High-carbohydrate, high-fat nutritional supplements are contraindicated.
• Return the rabbit to a solid food diet as soon as possible to encourage normal occlusion and wear. Increase the amount of tough, fibrous foods such as hay and wild grasses; avoid pelleted food and soft fruits or vegetables.
• Encourage oral fluid intake by offering fresh water or wetting leafy vegetables.

CLIENT EDUCATION
• Extraction of the incisor teeth is indicated in most cases. Extraction of the incisors will not impede the rabbit's ability to prehend food with lips.
• Many incisor malocclusions are acquired secondary to cheek teeth elongation. By the time clinical signs are noted, disease is usually advanced. Lifelong treatment, consisting of periodic coronal reduction of cheek teeth, may be required, usually every 3–12 months.
• Severe generalized dental disease, especially those with tooth root abscesses and severe bony destruction, carry a guarded prognosis for complete resolution. Most will require extensive surgery, sometimes multiple surgeries and multiple follow-up visits. Recurrences in other locations are common. Clients must be aware of the monetary and time investment.
• Teach owners how to recognize signs of oral discomfort and pain.

SURGICAL CONSIDERATIONS
Incisor Extraction
• Is the preferred option, since incisors will need to be trimmed every 4–8 weeks, often for life. Each trimming can be stressful to the rabbit, expensive and time consuming for the client, and carries the risk of pulp exposure or trauma to teeth during trimming.
• Incisor extraction will not limit food prehension.
• Regular examination of the cheek teeth to monitor for overgrowth is still required in rabbits with generalized dental disease.
• Because incisor teeth have very long, deeply embedded and curved reserve crowns, extraction can be challenging. If the germinal bud is not completely removed, the reserve crown may regrowth, with or without eruption of the clinical crown. If practitioner is not experienced with tooth extraction in rabbits, the author recommends referral to a veterinarian with special expertise whenever feasible.

Trimming of Incisors (Coronal Reduction)

• Coronal reduction will rarely correct malocclusion. It is painful and stressful to the rabbit when performed without sedation or anesthesia, requires frequent visits to the veterinarian, is generally more expensive in the long term, and carries the risk of significant damage to the pulp.
• In selected cases where extraction of the incisors is not an option, coronal reduction is usually necessary every 4–8 weeks.
• Sedation or general anesthesia is indicated to trim the incisors.
• Never clip the teeth with nail trimmers, rongeurs, or any other clipping device—clipping may cause longitudinal fractures of the teeth, leading to pulpitis and subsequent periapical abscessation, or damage periapical tissues.
• Trim incisors with dremel tool using a diamond cutting blade or a high-speed thin-cutting dental bur.
• Protect soft tissues from the cutting blade.
• Avoid cutting through the pulp—the pulp grows beyond the level of gingiva with overgrown teeth and is visible as a pink coloration. Cutting the pulp is painful and may cause pulpitis, pulp necrosis, and periapical abscess formation.
• If the pulp is accidentally cut, indicated by bleeding at the cut surface of the tooth, perform a partial pulpectomy and cap the pulp with calcium hydroxide cement. Do not use conventional filling materials as these prevent normal tooth wear.

MEDICATIONS

DRUG(S) OF CHOICE

• Buprenorphine (0.02–0.05 mg/kg PO, SQ, IM IV q8–12h); use preoperatively for extractions, coronal reduction, or surgical abscess treatment
• Butorphanol (0.1–0.5 mg/kg SQ, IM, IV q4–6h); may cause profound sedation at higher dosage; short acting
• Hydromorphone (0.1 mg/kg SC IM q2–4h) or oxymorphone (0.05–0.2 mg/kg SC IM q8–12h); use with caution; more than 1–2 doses may cause gastrointestinal stasis
• Meloxicam (1 mg/kg PO, SC, IM q24h)
• Carprofen (2–4 mg/kg PO, SC q12–24h)

CONTRAINDICATIONS

• Trimming of the incisors with nail trimmers, rongeurs, or other clipping devices
• Oral administration of most antibiotics effective against anaerobes will cause a fatal

gastrointestinal dysbiosis in rabbits. Do not administer penicillins, macrolides, lincosamides, and cephalosporins by oral administration.
• Corticosteroids—associated with gastrointestinal ulceration and hemorrhage, delayed wound healing, and heightened susceptibility to infection; rabbits are very sensitive to the immunosuppressive effects of both topical and systemic corticosteroids; use may exacerbate subclinical bacterial infection

PRECAUTIONS

• Meloxicam—use with caution in rabbits with compromised renal function

POSSIBLE INTERACTIONS
N/A

ALTERNATIVE DRUGS
N/A

FOLLOW-UP

PATIENT MONITORING

• Not usually necessary after incisor extraction
• If incisor extraction is declined, reevaluate and trim as needed every 4–8 weeks. Evaluate the entire oral cavity with each recheck.

PREVENTION/AVOIDANCE

• Avoid breeding rabbits with congenital malocclusion.
• In rabbits with acquired generalized dental disease, prevention is not possible once clinical signs of malocclusion are present. With periodic coronal reduction and appropriate diet, progression of disease may be arrested, but treatment is lifelong.
• Provide adequate tough, fibrous foods such as hay and grasses to encourage normal wear of teeth.

POSSIBLE COMPLICATIONS

• Complications are rare with incisor extraction. Periapical infection and abscess in case of septic complication during the dental procedure.
• With periodic coronal reduction—pulp trauma and necrosis, periapical abscesses, recurrence, trauma to soft tissues
• Chronic epiphora with nasolacrimal duct occlusion

EXPECTED COURSE AND PROGNOSIS

• Incisor overgrowth only (congenital malocclusion or trauma)—excellent prognosis with incisor extraction

• Incisor overgrowth due to cheek teeth elongation and generalized dental disease—fair to poor prognosis, depending on severity of disease; lifelong treatment is required.

MISCELLANEOUS

ASSOCIATED CONDITIONS
N/A

AGE-RELATED FACTORS
N/A

ZOONOTIC POTENTIAL
N/A

PREGNANCY/FERTILITY/BREEDING
N/A

SYNONYMS
N/A

SEE ALSO
Abscessation
Cheek teeth (premolar and molar teeth) malocclusion and elongation
Epiphora

ABBREVIATIONS
N/A

Suggested Reading
Capello V. Dental diseases. In: Capello V, Lennox AM, eds. Rabbit and Rodent Dentistry Handbook. Lake Worth: Zoological Education Network, 2005:113–138.
Capello V. Intraoral treatment of dental disease in pet rabbits. Vet Clin Exot Anim 2016;19(3):783–798.
Easson W. Tooth extraction. In: Harcourt-Brown F, Chitty J, eds. BSAVA Manual of Rabbit Surgery, Dentistry, and Imaging. Gloucester, UK: BSAVA, 2013:370–381.
Harcourt-Brown F. Treatment of dental problems: principles and options. In: Harcourt-Brown F, Chitty J, eds. BSAVA Manual of Rabbit Surgery, Dentistry, and Imaging. Gloucester, UK: BSAVA, 2013:349–369.
Lennox AM, Capello V, Legendre LF. Small mammal dentistry. In: Quesenberry KE, Carpenter JW, eds. Ferrets, Rabbits and Rodents, 4th Ed). Clinical Medicine and Surgery. 2021 ed. St. Louis: Saunders, 2020:514–535.
Varga M. Dental Disease. Textbook of Rabbit Medicine, 2nd ed. London, UK: Elsevier, 2014:203–248.
Authors Barbara Oglesbee, DVM, and Vittorio Capello, DVM

INCONTINENCE, URINARY

BASICS

DEFINITION
Loss of voluntary control of micturition, usually observed as involuntary urine leakage

PATHOPHYSIOLOGY
Usually, a disorder of the storage phase of micturition. Urine storage failure is caused by failure of urinary bladder accommodation, failure of urethral continence mechanisms, or anatomic bypass of urinary storage structures. Partial outlet obstruction and other causes of urinary bladder overdistension may result in paradoxical, or overflow, urinary incontinence.

SYSTEMS AFFECTED
• Renal/Urologic
• Nervous
• Skin—urine scald, perineal, and ventral dermatitis

SIGNALMENT
Most common in middle-aged rabbits 3–5 years old

SIGNS

Historical Findings
• Owners often observe urine scald or report dribbling of urine when the rabbit is picked up.
• Trauma, rear limb paresis, or paralysis in rabbits with spinal disease
• Other CNS signs in rabbits with CNS abscess or *Encephalitozoon cuniculi*
• Cloudy or thick, beige- to brown-colored urine in rabbits with hypercalciuria
• May be only historical finding in rabbits with hypercalciuria or urinary calculi

Physical Examination Findings
• Rear limb paresis or paralysis
• Urine scald in perineal region
• Detect urocystoliths by abdominal palpation; failure to palpate uroliths does not exclude them from consideration. Sometimes, relatively large uroliths can be palpated in the distal urethra of both males and females.
• In rabbits with crystalluria, the bladder sometimes palpates as a soft, doughy mass.
• With chronic disease, the bladder may markedly increase in size and may even fill most of the abdomen.
• Manual expression of the bladder may reveal thick, beige- to brown-colored urine in rabbits with hypercalciuria. Manual expression of the bladder may expel thick, brown urine even in rabbits that have normal-appearing voided urine.

CAUSES

Neurologic
• Disruption of local neuroreceptors, peripheral nerves, spinal pathways, or higher centers involved in the control of micturition can disrupt urine storage.
• Lesion of the sacral spinal cord, such as traumatic fractures or dislocation (common), disk disease, or spinal neoplasia, can result in a flaccid, overdistended urinary bladder with weak outlet resistance. Urine retention and overflow incontinence develop.
• Lesions of the cerebellum or cerebral micturition center (e.g., *Pasteurella* abscess or *E. cuniculi*) affect inhibition and voluntary control of voiding.

Urinary Bladder Storage Dysfunction
• Hypercalciuria/urinary calculi, urinary tract infection, infiltrative neoplastic lesion, external compression, and chronic partial outlet obstruction.

Urethral Disorders
• Acquired urethral incompetence— estrogen-responsive urinary incontinence in ovariohysterectomized females has been reported.
• Urinary tract infection or inflammation from hypercalciuria

Anatomic
• Developmental or acquired anatomic abnormalities that divert urine from normal storage mechanisms or interfere with urinary bladder or urethral function
• Ectopic ureters—the only congenital abnormality reported in the literature

RISK FACTORS
• For hypercalciuria/urinary calculi— inadequate water intake (dirty water bowls, unpalatable water, changing water sources, inadequate water provision), inadequate cleaning of litter box or cage may cause some rabbits to avoid urinating for abnormally long periods; obesity; lack of exercise; feeding of exclusively alfalfa-based pelleted diets; renal disease; and adding calcium or vitamin/mineral supplements to the diet
• For neurologic causes—improper restraint (fracture/luxation); debility, stress, or immunosuppression (bacterial infection and *E. cuniculi*)

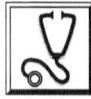

DIAGNOSIS

DIFFERENTIAL DIAGNOSIS

Differentiating Similar Signs
• Voluntary but inappropriate urination

• Inability to maintain proper stance for micturition due to musculoskeletal disease or obesity—rabbits normally lift their hindquarters and spray urine caudally; an inability to maintain this posture causes urine to soak the perineal region and ventrum and may mimic incontinence
• Urine spraying—territorial marking in intact animals

Differentiating Causes
• Polyuria—may precipitate or exacerbate urinary incontinence or lead to nocturia and inappropriate urination
• Hypercalciuria/Bladder sludge—urinary incontinence occasionally the only clinical sign; urine scald in perineum or ventrum; doughy consistency to bladder on palpation; manual expression of the bladder may reveal thick, beige- to brown-colored urine in rabbits with hypercalciuria
• Other neurologic signs are usually present in rabbits with CNS disease or spinal disorders.
• A large, distended urinary bladder may be seen in rabbits with neurologic causes of incontinence or chronic, severe hypercalciuria.

CBC/BIOCHEMISTRY/URINALYSIS
• Hematologic and biochemical analyses may be helpful in identifying causes or polyuric disorders.
• Hypercalciuria/Bladder sludge—urinary sediment evaluation reveals calcium oxalate or calcium carbonate crystals; however, this is a normal finding in rabbits, and the presence of large amounts of crystals in the urine does not necessarily indicate disease. Disease occurs only when the concentration of crystals is excessive, forming thick, white to brown, paste- or sand-like urine, and subsequent inflammatory cystitis or partial to complete blockage of the urethra
• Pyuria (normal value 0–1 WBC/hpf), hematuria (normal value 0–1 RBC/hpf), and proteinuria (normal value 0–33 mg/dL) indicate urinary tract inflammation, but these are nonspecific findings that may result from infectious and noninfectious causes of lower urinary tract disease
• Urine pH: normal rabbit urine is alkaline; pH >8 suggestive of bacterial cystitis due to urease-producing bacteria

OTHER LABORATORY TESTS
• Serologic testing for *E. cuniculi*—the usefulness of serum antibody testing is limited in pet rabbits since a positive titer indicates only exposure and does not confirm *E. cuniculi* as the cause of clinical signs.

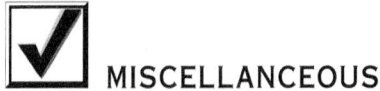

A combination of IgM, IgG, and C-reactive protein appears to be most reliable.

IMAGING

Radiographic Finding
• Calcium oxalate uroliths are radiopaque and may be detected by survey radiography. Uroliths must be differentiated from calcium "sand" or "sludge" in the bladder, which resembles a bladder full of contrast material. With chronic disease, the bladder may enlarge significantly.
• Radiographs may demonstrate spondylosis or other orthopedic abnormalities that prohibit normal posture during micturition.

Ultrasonographic Findings
Can evaluate the kidneys and urinary bladder to identify uroliths, hypercalciuria, masses, hydroureter, or evidence of pyelonephritis

DIAGNOSTIC PROCEDURES
• Neurologic examination—examination of anal tone, tail tone, and perineal sensation provide a brief assessment of caudal spinal and peripheral nerve function
• Urethral catheterization may be required to assess patency of the urethra if urine retention is observed.

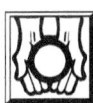 **TREATMENT**

• Usually outpatient
• Address primary neurologic disorders specifically, if possible.
• Identify urinary tract infection and treat appropriately.
• Urolithiasis may be surgically corrected.
• Symptomatic rabbits with calcium precipitate (sand or sludge) in the urinary bladder often respond to medical treatment with fluid therapy and periodic bladder expression or bladder flushing.
• Treat secondary urine scald; keep area clean and dry.

 MEDICATIONS

DRUG(S) OF CHOICE
• Pain management is essential during and following surgery, urohydropropulsion, urinary catheterization, or if pain is causing reduced frequency of voiding. Perioperative choices include butorphanol (0.1–0.5 mg/kg SQ, IM, IV q4–6h, buprenorphine (0.02–0.05 mg/kg SQ, IM IV q8–12h), hydromorphone (0.1 mg/kg SC IM q2–4h), or oxymorphone (0.05–0.2 mg/kg SC IM

q8–12h). To manage long-term pain: meloxicam (1.0 mg/kg PO q24h; carprofen (2 mg/kg PO q12h), tramadol (5–15 mg/kg PO q8–12h), and/or gabapentin (5–20 mg/kg PO q8–12h)
• Consider diuretic therapy for patients with bladder sludge or uroliths. Give a calcium-sparing thiazide diuretic such as hydrochlorothiazide 0.5–2 mg/kg PO q12h
• Potassium citrate 33 mg/kg PO q8h may help to prevent formation of calcium crystals in urine
• For a bladder that is chronically distended and will not empty completely during micturition, bethanechol chloride has been anecdotally used at feline dosages (2.5–5 mg/kg q8–12h).
• Some rabbits with large amounts of calcium precipitate or uroliths have an underlying chronic bacterial cystitis. Treat with antibiotics, based on culture and susceptibility testing when possible.
• Urethral incompetence in ovariohysterectomized rabbits may respond to diethystilbestrol (0.5 mg PO 1–2 times per week)

CONTRAINDICATIONS
Oral administration of antibiotics that select against gram-positive bacteria (penicillins, macrolides, lincosamides, and cephalosporins) can cause fatal enteric dysbiosis and enterotoxemia.

PRECAUTIONS
NSAIDs—use with caution in patients with renal disease

POSSIBLE INTERACTIONS
N/A

ALTERNATIVE DRUGS
N/A

 **FOLLOW-UP**

PATIENT MONITORING
• Radiographs are essential following treatment of hypercalciuria to verify complete removal of calcium precipitate or uroliths.
• Periodic urinalysis
• Rabbits with incontinence caused by neurologic disease carry a poor prognosis.

POSSIBLE COMPLICATIONS
• Recurrent and ascending urinary tract infection
• Urine scald with perineal and ventral dermatitis, myiasis, and pododermatitis
• Refractory and unmanageable incontinence

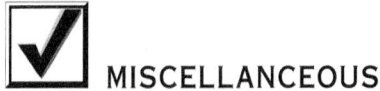 **MISCELLANEOUS**

ASSOCIATED CONDITIONS
Gastrointestinal hypomotility
Pyoderma

AGE-RELATED FACTORS
N/A

ZOONOTIC POTENTIAL
Possible with *E. cuniculi*

PREGNANCY/FERTILITY/BREEDING
N/A

SEE ALSO
Encephalitis and meningoencephalitis
Hypercalciuria and urolithiasis
Polyuria and polydipsia

ABBREVIATIONS
BUN = blood urea nitrogen
GI = gastrointestinal
NSAID = nonsteroidal anti-inflammatory drug

Suggested Reading
Bays TB. Geriatric care of rabbits, guinea pigs, and chinchillas. Vet Clin Exot Anim 2020;23:567–593.
DeCubellis J. Common emergencies in rabbits, guinea pigs, and chinchillas. Vet Clin Exot Anim 2016;19:411–429.
Di Girolamo N, Selleri P. Disorders of the urinary and reproductive system. In: Quesenberry KE, Carpenter JW, eds. Ferrets, Rabbits and Rodents, 4th Ed). Clinical Medicine and Surgery ed. St. Louis: Saunders, 2020:201–220.
Fisher PG, Künzel F, Rylander H. Neurologic and musculoskeletal disease. In: Quesenberry KE, Carpenter JW, eds. Ferrets, Rabbits and Rodents, 4th Ed). Clinical Medicine and Surgery ed. St. Louis: Saunders, 2020:583–594.
Hallman RM, Brandão J. Diagnostic imaging of the renal system in exotic companion mammals. Vet Clin Exot Anim 2020;23: 195–214.
Mancinelli E, Lord B. Urogenital and reproductive disease. In: Meredith A, Lord B, eds. BSAVA Manual of Rabbit Medicine. Gloucester: British Small Animal Veterinary Association, 2014:191–204.
Reavill DR, Lennox AM. Disease overview of the urinary tract in exotic companion mammals and tips on clinical management. Vet Clin Exot Anim 2020;23(1):169–193.
Author Barbara Oglesbee, DVM, DABVP (Avian)

LAMENESS

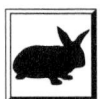

BASICS

DEFINITION
A disturbance in gait and locomotion in response to pain or injury

PATHOPHYSIOLOGY
• Severe, sharp pain—when moving, patient carries or puts no weight on the affected limb.
• Milder, dull, or aching pain—when moving, patient limps or bears little weight on the affected limb; at rest, the patient bears less weight on the affected limb.
• Many rabbits are reluctant to move at all with mild to moderate limb pain.
• Pain produced only during certain phases of movement—patient adjusts its motion and gait to minimize discomfort

SYSTEMS AFFECTED
• Musculoskeletal
• Nervous
• Dermatologic—secondary disorders (urine scald, dermatitis)

SIGNALMENT
• Age, breed, and sex predilection—depend on specific disease

SIGNS

General Comments
• Always assess the patient's neurologic status, especially with a suspected proximal lesion.

Historical Findings
• Complete history—signalment; identification of affected limb(s); known trauma; changes with exercise or rest; responsiveness to previous treatments
• Determine onset of lameness—acute or chronic
• Determine progression—static; slow; rapid
• Signs of pain—depression, lethargy, hunched posture while sitting, reluctance to move, hiding, teeth grinding, grunting, decreased appetite, lack of grooming

Physical Examination Findings
• Use secure restraint when examining painful rabbits
• Perform a complete routine examination.
• Observe gait—hopping, climbing
• Palpate—asymmetry of muscle mass; bony prominences; swelling over joints
• Manipulate bones and joints, beginning distally and working proximally.
• Assess—instability; luxation or subluxation; pain; abnormal range of motion; and abnormal sounds
• Examine suspected area of involvement last—by starting with normal limbs, patient

may relax, allowing assessment of normal reaction to maneuvers.
• Urine scald in the perineal region; dermatitis or alopecia due to inappropriate grooming; pododermatitis

CAUSES

General Comments
The causes listed below are the most common causes of lameness in rabbits, with most common listed first. Also consider other causes common to dogs and cats; these may also occur in rabbits but have not been described.

Forelimb
• Trauma—soft tissue; bone; joint
• Infection—abscess, septic arthritis, and pododermatitis
• Degenerative joint disease
• Soft tissue or bone neoplasia—primary; metastatic
• Shoulder luxation or subluxation
• Elbow luxation or subluxation
• Congenital anomalies

Hind Limb
• Trauma—soft tissue; bone; and joint
• Infection—ulcerative pododermatitis (sore hocks), abscess, and septic arthritis
• Degenerative joint disease
• Patella luxation
• Congenital anomalies
• Hip luxation or subluxation
• Soft tissue or bone neoplasia—primary; metastatic

Spinal Disease
• Spondylosis, spinal arthritis
• Fractures, luxation
• Intervertebral disc disease

RISK FACTORS
• Trauma, dislocations—improper restraint, trauma in caged rabbits suddenly startled, possibly disuse atrophy from confinement
• Ulcerative pododermatitis (sore hocks)—excoriation, friction, or constant moisture on the skin and soft tissues of the plantar aspect of the hock. Caused by lack of protective fur covering and/or feces and urine coating the feet
• Abscesses, infection—immunosuppression (stress, corticosteroid use, concurrent disease); poor husbandry
• Obesity, lack of exercise

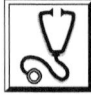

DIAGNOSIS

DIFFERENTIAL DIAGNOSIS
• Must differentiate musculoskeletal from neurogenic causes
• Lameness affecting one limb—fracture, soft tissue injury, abscess, ulcerative pododermatitis, and neoplasia

• Lameness affecting multiple limbs—spinal trauma, spondylosis, disc disease, and septic arthritis

CBC/BIOCHEMISTRY/URINALYSIS
Usually normal; relative heterophilia and/or lymphopenia sometimes seen with bacterial diseases.

OTHER LABORATORY TESTS
Depend on suspected cause

IMAGING
• Radiographs—recommended for all suspected musculoskeletal causes
• CT—more accurate to identify and delineate causative lesions

DIAGNOSTIC PROCEDURES
• Cytologic examination of joint fluid—identify and differentiate intra-articular disease
• EMG—differentiate neuromuscular from musculoskeletal disease
• Muscle and/or nerve biopsy—reveal and identify neuromuscular disease

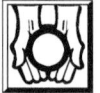

TREATMENT
Depends on underlying cause

NURSING CARE
• Depends on severity of disease
• Bandage or splint care
• Anorectic rabbits require assist feeding
• Soft bedding; daily bedding changes
• Remove soiled bedding; keep fur clean and dry.

ACTIVITY
Restricted until resolution of symptoms

DIET
• It is imperative that the rabbit continue to eat during and following treatment. This condition is often painful, resulting in anorexia. Anorexia will often cause GI hypomotility, derangement of the gastrointestinal microflora, and overgrowth of intestinal bacterial pathogens.
• If the patient refuses food, syringe-feed a gruel such as Critical Care for Herbivores (Oxbow Pet Products) or Emeraid Herbivore (Lafeber Company, Cornell, IL) 10–15 mL/kg PO q6–8h. Larger volumes and more frequent feedings are often accepted; feed as much as the rabbit will readily accept. Alternatively, pellets can be ground and mixed with fresh greens, vegetable baby foods, water, or juice to form a gruel. If sufficient volumes of food are not accepted in this manner, nasogastric intubation is indicated.
• High-carbohydrate, high-fat nutritional supplements are contraindicated.

SURGICAL CONSIDERATIONS
- Abscesses, osteomyelitis, and septic joints require aggressive surgical management.
- Simple, closed fractures distal to the elbow may respond to external coaptation; most other fractures require open reduction.
- Joint injuries—closed reduction of coxofemoral luxation is difficult due to powerful hind limb musculature, most require FHO; most elbow luxations require internal fixation as the shoulder is difficult to incorporate in a bandage

MEDICATIONS
DRUG(S) OF CHOICE
Acute Pain Management
- Butorphanol (0.1–0.5 mg/kg SQ, IM, IV q4–6h); may cause profound sedation; short acting
- Buprenorphine (0.02–0.05 mg/kg SQ, IM IV q8–12h); less sedating, longer acting than butorphanol
- Hydromorphone (0.1 mg/kg SC IM q2–4h) or oxymorphone (0.05–0.2 mg/kg SC IM q8–12h)
- Meloxicam (1 mg/kg PO, SC, IM q24h)
- Carprofen (2–4 mg/kg PO, SC q12–24h)

Long-Term Pain Management
- Nonsteroidal anti-inflammatories—have been used for short- or long-term therapy to reduce pain and inflammation in rabbits with musculoskeletal disease; meloxicam (1.0 mg/kg PO q24h; carprofen (2 mg/kg PO q12h)
- Tramadol—5–15 mg/kg PO q8–12h
- Gabapentin—5–20 mg/kg PO q8–12h

Bacterial Infection
- Antimicrobial drugs effective against the infectious agent; gain access to site of infection. Choice of antibiotic is ideally based on results of culture and susceptibility testing. Depending on the severity of infection, long-term antibiotic therapy is required (4–6 weeks minimum, to several months). Use broad-spectrum antibiotics such as enrofloxacin (10–20 mg/kg PO, SC, IM, IV q12h), marbofloxacin (5 mg/kg PO q24h), trimethoprim-sulfa (15–30 mg/kg PO q12h), or chloramphenicol (50 mg/kg PO q8h). For anaerobic bacteria: azithromycin (15–30 mg/kg PO q24h), and it can be used alone or combined with metronidazole (20 mg/kg PO q12h). Alternatively, use penicillin G procaine (40,000–60,000 IU/kg SC q24h).

CONTRAINDICATIONS
- Corticosteroids—associated with gastrointestinal ulceration and hemorrhage, delayed wound healing, and heightened susceptibility to infection; rabbits are very sensitive to the immunosuppressive effects of both topical and systemic corticosteroids; use may exacerbate subclinical bacterial infection

PRECAUTIONS
- Meloxicam and other NSAIDs—use with caution in rabbits with compromised renal function

POSSIBLE INTERACTIONS
N/A

ALTERNATIVE DRUGS
- Chondroprotective agents, nutraceuticals (oral glycosaminoglycans, cosequin)—use not well described in rabbits; have been anecdotally used at feline dosages in addition to analgesics
- Acupuncture may be effective for rabbits with chronic pain.

FOLLOW-UP
PATIENT MONITORING
- Depends on underlying cause
- Monitor for complications arising secondary to chronic pain and immobility such as urine scald, hypercalciuria, obesity, sore hocks, and GI hypomotility.

POSSIBLE COMPLICATIONS
- Secondary to chronic pain and immobility—urine scald, hypercalciuria, obesity, sore hocks, gastrointestinal hypomotility; ankylosis common with severe joint disorders

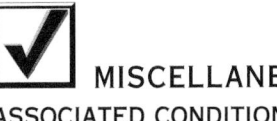

MISCELLANEOUS
ASSOCIATED CONDITIONS
N/A

AGE-RELATED FACTORS
N/A

ZOONOTIC POTENTIAL
N/A

PREGNANCY/FERTILITY/BREEDING
N/A

SEE ALSO
Abscesses
Ulcerative pododermatitis (sore hocks)
Vertebral fracture or luxation

ABBREVIATIONS
CT = computed tomography
EMG = electromyogram
FHO = femoral head ostectomy
GI = gastrointestinal
NSAID = nonsteroidal anti-inflammatory drug

Suggested Reading
Bays TB. Geriatric care of rabbits, guinea pigs, and chinchillas. Vet Clin Exot Anim 2020;23:567–593.
Fisher PG, Künzel F, Rylander H. Neurologic and musculoskeletal disease. In: Quesenberry KE, Carpenter JW, eds. Ferrets, Rabbits and Rodents, 4th Ed). Clinical Medicine and Surgery ed. St. Louis: Saunders, 2020:583–594.
Harkness JE, Turner PV, VandeWoude S, Wheeler CL. Clinical signs and differential diagnoses: nervous and musculoskeletal conditions. In: Harkness JE, Turner PV, VandeWoude S, Wheeler CL, eds. Biology and Medicine of Rabbits and Rodents, 5th ed. Ames: Wiley-Blackwell, 2010: 214–216.
Keeble E. Nervous system and musculoskeletal disorders. In: Meredith A, Lord B, eds. BSAVA Manual of Rabbit Medicine. Gloucester: British Small Animal Veterinary Association, 2014:233–248.
Varga M. Neurological and locomotive disorders. In: Varga M, ed. Textbook of Rabbit Medicine, 2nd ed. London, UK: Elsevier, 2014:367–389.
Author Barbara Oglesbee, DVM, DABVP (Avian)

RABBITS

LEAD TOXICITY

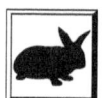

BASICS

OVERVIEW
- Intoxication (blood lead concentrations >10 µg/dL) owing to acute or chronic exposure to some form of lead
- Many rabbits chew or lick lead containing household substances, especially painted surfaces; occasionally metallic objects
- Lead—interferes with numerous enzymes, including those involved in heme synthesis; causes fragility and decreased survival of RBCs
- Damage to CNS capillaries—may account for brain lesions

SYSTEMS AFFECTED
- Hemic/Lymph/Immune—interference with hemoglobin synthesis
- Gastrointestinal—unknown mechanism
- Nervous—capillary damage; possible direct toxic affect
- Renal/Urologic—damage to proximal tubule cells

SIGNALMENT
- Incidence unknown; more common in rabbits living in older homes and rabbits that roam free in the house
- No age, breed, or gender predisposition

SIGNS
- Nonspecific signs such as weight loss, anorexia, depression, and lethargy predominate.
- Gastrointestinal—decreased appetite, anorexia, gastrointestinal hypomotility, or stasis; rarely diarrhea
- CNS—blindness, weakness, lethargy, ataxia, and seizures

CAUSES
- Ingestion of some form of lead—paint and paint residues or dust from sanding; linoleum; solder; plumbing materials and supplies; lubricating compounds; putty; tar paper; lead foil; and lead objects
- Use of improperly glazed ceramic food or water bowl
- Lead paint or solder on cages

RISK FACTORS
- Living in economically depressed areas or old housing that is being renovated
- Unsupervised chewing
- Lead-containing cages or cage contents

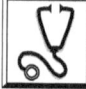

DIAGNOSIS

DIFFERENTIAL DIAGNOSIS
For CNS Signs
- Other, more common causes of encephalopathy—infectious: *Encephalitozoon cuniculi*, bacterial (brain abscess, extension from otitis interna/media, meningoencephalitis); parasitic migration (*Baylisascaris*—raccoon roundworm), fungal rare in rabbits; brain tumor; trauma
- Heat stroke—acute onset, supportive history
- Physical examination findings helpful in diagnosing more common problems: nasal/ocular discharge—either historical or currently present—common finding with spread of upper respiratory infection to inner/middle ear; otitis externa—thick, white, creamy exudate may be found in the horizontal and/or vertical canals; otitis interna/media may occur in the absence of otitis externa via extension through the eustachian tube; may see bulging tympanum. Some rabbits with otitis interna have no visible otoscopic abnormalities.

For Anorexia, Depression, Weight Loss
- Almost any systemic disease process
- Gastrointestinal disease is one of the most common causes—especially problems related to GI hypomotility or stasis
- Pain
- Dental disease

CBC/BIOCHEMISTRY/URINALYSIS
- Anemia common finding; may be only abnormality found in rabbit that is otherwise clinically normal or exhibiting vague, nonspecific signs
- Nucleated erythrocytes, hypochromasia, poikilocytosis, and cytoplasmic basophilic stippling of RBCs sometimes seen

OTHER LABORATORY TESTS
Lead Concentration
- Submit whole, unclotted blood; lithium heparin tube or check with diagnostic laboratory for anticoagulant preference
- Toxic—antemortem whole blood lead concentrations >10 µg/dL
- Lower values—must be interpreted in conjunction with history and clinical signs
- Blood levels—may not correlate with occurrence or severity of clinical signs

IMAGING
- May note radiopaque material in gastrointestinal tract; not diagnostic. Radiopaque densities often not present with ingestion of paint

DIAGNOSTIC PROCEDURES
N/A

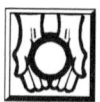

TREATMENT

APPROPRIATE HEALTH CARE
- Inpatient—first course of chelation, depending on severity of clinical signs; for rabbits that are actively seizuring, debilitated, or anorectic and require supportive care
- Outpatient—rabbits that are stable and eating, if owner can administer injections

NURSING CARE
- Balanced electrolyte fluids—replacement of hydration deficit
- Treat GI stasis if present (see GI stasis)

ACTIVITY
N/A

DIET
- It is imperative that the rabbit continue to eat during and following treatment. Anorexia will often cause GI hypomotility, derangement of the gastrointestinal microflora, and overgrowth of intestinal bacterial pathogens.
- Offer a large selection of fresh, moistened greens such as cilantro, romaine lettuce, parsley, carrot tops, dandelion greens, spinach, collard greens, and good-quality grass hay. Many rabbits will begin to eat these foods, even if they were previously anorectic.
- If the patient refuses these foods, syringe-feed a gruel such as Critical Care for Herbivores (Oxbow Pet Products, Murdock NJ) or Emeraid Herbivore (Lafeber Company, Cornell, IL) 10–15 mL/kg PO q6–8h. Larger volumes and more frequent feedings are often accepted; feed as much as the rabbit will readily accept. Alternatively, pellets can be ground and mixed with fresh greens, vegetable baby foods, water, or juice to form a gruel.
- High-carbohydrate, high-fat nutritional supplements are contraindicated.
- Encourage oral fluid intake by offering fresh water, wetting leafy vegetables, or flavoring water with vegetable juices.

CLIENT EDUCATION
- Inform client of the potential of adverse human health effects of lead.
- Notify public health officials.
- Determine the source of the lead.

SURGICAL CONSIDERATIONS
Removal of lead objects from the gastrointestinal tract

RABBITS

(CONTINUED)

MEDICATIONS

DRUG(S) OF CHOICE
• Control of seizures—diazepam (1–5 mg/kg IV, IM) or midazolam (0.5–2 mg/kg IV, IM) begin with 0.5–1.0 mg/kg IV bolus; may repeat if gross seizure activity has not stopped within 5 minutes; can be administered rectally if IV access cannot be obtained; may diminish or stop the gross motor seizure activity to allow IV catheter placement. Constant rate infusion protocols used in dogs and cats have been anecdotally used.
• Reduction of lead body burden—CaEDTA (25 mg/kg SC q6h for 5 days); dilute to 1% solution with D5W before administration; may need multiple treatments; allow a 5-day rest period between treatments.

CONTRAINDICATIONS
EDTA—do not administer to patients with renal impairment or anuria; establish urine flow before administration.

PRECAUTIONS
CaEDTA—safety in pregnancy not established

POSSIBLE INTERACTIONS
N/A

ALTERNATIVE DRUGS
Alternatives to CaEDTA—D-penicillamine or succimer—use not reported in rabbits

FOLLOW-UP

PATIENT MONITORING
Blood lead—assess 10–14 days after cessation of chelation therapy and again 2–3 months later

PREVENTION/AVOIDANCE
Determine source of lead and remove it from the patient's environment.

POSSIBLE COMPLICATIONS
• Permanent neurologic signs (e.g., blindness) occasionally
• Derangement of the gastrointestinal microflora and overgrowth of intestinal bacterial pathogens secondary to GI hypomotility or stasis

EXPECTED COURSE AND PROGNOSIS
• Signs should dramatically improve within 24–48 hours after initiating chelation therapy.
• Prognosis—favorable with treatment
• Uncontrolled seizures—guarded prognosis

MISCELLANEOUS

ASSOCIATED CONDITIONS
N/A

AGE-RELATED FACTORS
N/A

ZOONOTIC POTENTIAL
None, however, humans in the same environment may be at risk for exposure

PREGNANCY
• Transplacental passage—may cause neonatal poisoning
• Lactation—lead mobilized from bones unlikely to poison nursing animals

SYNONYMS
Plumbism

SEE ALSO
Gastrointestinal hypomotility and gastrointestinal stasis
Seizures

ABBREVIATIONS
CaEDTA = calcium ethylenediaminetetraacetic acid
D5W = dextrose 5% in water
GI = gastrointestinal
HSV = herpes simplex virus
RBC = red blood cell

Suggested Reading
DeCubellis J. Common emergencies in rabbits, guinea pigs, and chinchillas. Vet Clin Exot Anim 2016;19:411–429.
Fisher PG, Künzel F, Rylander H. Neurologic and musculoskeletal disease. In: Quesenberry KE, Carpenter JW, eds. Ferrets, Rabbits and Rodents, 4th Ed). Clinical Medicine and Surgery ed. St. Louis: Saunders, 2020:583–594.
Hung M, Boyeaux A. Assessment and care of the critically ill rabbit. Vet Clin North Am Exot Anim Pract 2016;19:379–409.
Lennox AM, Gladden JN. Emergency and critical care of small mammals. In: Quesenberry KE, Carpenter JW, eds. Ferrets, Rabbits and Rodents, 4th Ed). Clinical Medicine and Surgery. 2021 ed. St. Louis: Saunders, 2020:595–608.
Murphy LA. Environmental toxicology: considerations for exotic pets. J Exotic Pet Medicine 2015;24(4):390–397.
Swartout MS, Gerken DF. Lead-induced toxicosis in two domestic rabbits. J Am Vet Med Assoc 1987;191:717–719.
Varga M. Neurological and locomotive disorders. In: Varga M, ed. Textbook of Rabbit Medicine, 2nd ed. London, UK: Elsevier, 2014:367–389.

Author Barbara Oglesbee, DVM, DABVP (Avian)

LIVER LOBE TORSION

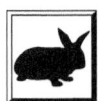

BASICS

DEFINITION
An acute, life-threatening disorder of rabbits in which one lobe of the liver (most commonly the caudate lobe) twists at the base, resulting in venous congestion and diffuse necrosis of the lobe. In most cases, hemorrhage occurs at the origin, resulting in acute hemoabdomen.

PATHOPHYSIOLOGY
- The cause of liver lobe torsion is unknown.
- Torsion of caudate lobe has been reported in over 60% of cases, possibly because of its narrow attachment to the dorsal hilar region of the liver.
- Torsion of the right lobe, quadrate lobe, and the posterior lobule of the left hepatic lobe have also been reported
- Lobe torsion results in venous obstruction leading to arterial and venous thrombosis, followed by tissue necrosis
- Acute pain and tissue necrosis lead to signs similar to those seen with GI stasis: anorexia, decreased fecal output, and signs of abdominal pain.
- In the majority of cases, hemorrhage occurs at the point of torsion, resulting in acute hemoabdomen and death without surgical intervention.
- If hemorrhage does not occur, rabbits can survive without surgical treatment, although supportive care for pain and secondary GI stasis are needed. In some cases, GI stasis episodes become recurrent for months to years. The affected lobe eventually becomes cirrhotic and may be an incidental finding at necropsy.

SYSTEMS AFFECTED
- Gastrointestinal—hepatic necrosis, secondary GI stasis
- Hemodynamic—hemorrhage, sepsis

INCIDENCE/PREVALANCE
Unusually common, often under-recognized disorder in pet rabbits as signs resemble GI stasis. Although overall incidence has not been reported, approximately 1 case/month is seen in the author's practice.

SIGNALMENT
- Seen most commonly in middle-aged rabbits
- No sex or breed predilection reported

SIGNS

Historical Findings
- Acute onset of anorexia. Often, all food is refused, similar to anorexia seen rabbits with intestinal obstruction, although some will continue to accept small amounts of treats or favorite foods. This differs from rabbits with other causes of GI hypomotility/stasis where a more gradual onset of progressively declining appetite over a period of hours to days is seen.
- Acute onset of lack of or decrease stool production occurring simultaneously with the onset of anorexia. Feces produced are often normal or soft in appearance.
- Acute onset of pain. Signs of pain can be subtle as rabbits are prey species and instinctively hide signs of disease. The most common sign of mild to moderate discomfort is hiding or appearing less social.
- With onset of hemorrhage, weakness, tachypnea, signs of shock, or sudden death.

Physical Examination Findings
- Pain is often elicited on palpation of the cranial abdomen is common. Occasionally, a mass effect may be palpable in the region of the affected lobe, but his finding should not be relied on.
- Initially, the stomach is usually full of normal ingesta; normal feces can usually be palpated in the colon. With the onset of GI stasis, stomach contents may become firm, intestinal gas is often palpable.
- Auscultation of gut sounds may be normal initially, progressing to decreased or absent gut sounds.
- Tachypnea, tachycardia, pale mucus membranes, lethargy, and collapse with the onset of hemorrhage and hemoabdomen.

CAUSES AND RISK FACTORS
- Although the cause is unknown, affected rabbits often have a history of one or more prior episodes of GI stasis or small intestinal obstruction (bloat). It is possible that the left triangular ligament becomes stretched following gastric dilation and may predispose to torsion.

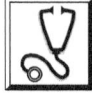

DIAGNOSIS

DIFFERENTIAL DIAGNOSIS

Small Intestinal Obstruction (Bloat)
- Onset of anorexia and absence of fecal production may be similar. Rabbits with intestinal obstruction abruptly refuse *all* food (even treats), simultaneous with an abrupt cessation of fecal production. Most rabbits with liver lobe torsion will accept some favorite foods and pass small amounts of feces.
- With intestinal obstruction, the stomach is dilated with fluid—the volume of fluid depends on the time of onset and location of obstruction. Normal or firm ingesta is palpable in rabbits with liver lobe torsion

GI Stasis/Hypomotility
- Onset of anorexia is usually more gradual, progressing over a period of hours to days; abdominal palpation reveals a large, doughy, or firm mass within the stomach (vs. fluid-filled stomach with gastric dilation); feces become progressively small, dark, and dry.

CBC/BIOCHEMISTRY/URINALYSIS
- Elevation of ALT, ALP, and AST most common. These values may be normal initially, but typically increase by a factor of 5–10x normal within 24 hours of onset. GGT and total bilirubin elevations are also common.
- With onset of hemorrhage—decreased PCV, TS

IMAGING

Radiographs
- Abnormalities of the affected lobe are rarely visible on radiographs, but radiographs are helpful in differentiating liver lobe torsion from intestinal obstruction.
- The stomach typically contains normal ingesta initially, with normal, round fecal pellets throughout the colon. With the onset of GI stasis, dehydrated stomach contents, small amounts of gas in the stomach may be seen; gas may be seen in intestinal loops and cecum. Rabbits with intestinal obstruction have a fluid filled stomach.
- With hemorrhage, decreased abdominal detail

Ultrasound
- Often very useful in diagnosis of liver lobe torsion and to monitor for hemoabdomen
- Affected liver lobe usually appears mildly enlarged with rounded margins with decreased or mixed parenchymal echogenicity. Color flow Doppler demonstrates decreased or absent blood flow to the affected lobe.
- Free abdominal fluid with hemorrhage and hemoabdomen. Perform ultrasound-guided abdominocentesis to confirm.

TREATMENT

APPROPRIATE HEALTH CARE
This disorder is an emergency. Immediate exploratory celiotomy and removal of the affected lobe are the treatment of choice. Hospitalization for supportive care is necessary.

NURSING CARE

Fluid Therapy
- Supportive fluids on the basis of hydration status are recommended for animals not in shock.

(CONTINUED)

• For patients with signs of shock or severe depression balanced crystalloid fluids are indicated IV at a rate appropriate for shock (60–90 mg/kg/hr IV, IO over 20–60 min) followed by maintenance rate. For patients in shock, fluids should be warmed.

DIET
• Offer the normal diet
• If the patient refuses food, syringe-feed a gruel such as Critical Care for Herbivores (Oxbow Pet Products) or Emeraid Herbivore (Lafeber Company, Cornell, IL) 10–15 mL/kg PO q6–8h. Larger volumes and more frequent feedings are often accepted; feed as much as the rabbit will readily accept.

CLIENT EDUCATION
• Prompt surgical treatment provides the best prognosis. Although a small percentage of patients do not develop hemoadomen and may recover with supportive care alone, this is unusual.
• Even with surgical treatment, the prognosis is guarded. If hemorrhage is significant prior to surgery, the prognosis is poor.
• Discuss the importance of monitoring appetite in prey species such as rabbits. These species have a strong instinct to hide illness and may appear active and "normal" to owners unfamiliar with this concept. Stress the importance of seeking veterinary care any time the appetite is reduced. An acute onset of refusing all food and simultaneous lack of fecal output is an emergency.

SURGICAL CONSIDERATIONS
• Liver lobe torsion is a surgical emergency. Hemorrhage will often occur at the base of the affected lobe within 8–72 hours of onset of torsion. Prolonged delay may result in death of the patient.
• The affected lobe should be completely removed. Ligate the vessels at the base of the lobe using monofilament absorbable suture, vascular clips, surgical stapling, or sealing devices.

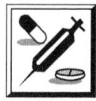 **MEDICATIONS**

DRUG(S) OF CHOICE
• Lidocaine administered as a CRI (loading dose 2 mg/kg then 50 mcg/kg/min) alleviates intestinal pain, is anti-inflammatory, and may help to prevent ileus.
• Analgesics such as hydromorphone (0.05–0.2 mg/kg IV, IM, SC q6–8h),

buprenorphine (0.02–0.05 mg/kg SC, IM, IV q8–12h), or carprofen (2–4 mg/kg SC, IV q24h) are essential to treatment. Intestinal pain, either postoperative or from GI distention impairs mobility, decreases appetite, and may severely inhibit recovery.
• Maropitant (2 mg/kg SC q24h) is used to treat visceral pain. Combine this with one of the analgesics listed above.
• Motility modifiers such as metoclopramide (0.5–1.0 mg/kg IV, SC, IM q12h or, ideally, 1–2 mg/kg/day IV as a constant rate infusion) can be used in rabbits with intraluminal intestinal obstruction. As the most common GI foreign body is a compressed pellet of hair and the goal of therapy is to keep the hair pellet moving through the intestinal tract. Motility modifiers are contraindicated if an extraluminal obstruction is suspected.
• H_2-receptor antagonists may ameliorate or prevent gastric ulceration; cimetidine (5–10 mg/kg PO, SC, IM IV q6–12h); ranitidine (2 mg/kg SC, IV q24h or 2–5 mg/kg PO q12–24h)

CONTRAINDICATIONS
• Avoid NSAIDs and other drugs that may lead to renal compromise, in patients with signs of shock or dehydration

PRECAUTIONS
Meloxicam and other NSAIDs—use with caution in patients with renal compromise; monitor renal values

 FOLLOW-UP

PATIENT MONITORING
• Monitor for evidence of hemorrhage in patients treated with supportive care alone and for 24 hours postoperatively.
• Monitor appetite and fecal production. GI stasis is common immediately postoperatively and in the following weeks to months.

PREVENTION/AVOIDANCE
This syndrome is not related to diet or husbandry, no known prevention

POSSIBLE COMPLICATIONS
• Death due to blood loss or sepsis
• Postoperative GI stasis

EXPECTED COURSE AND PROGNOSIS
• Good with successful surgical removal.

• Once hemorrhage begins, the prognosis is guarded, even with immediate surgical removal of the affected lobe.
• Guarded to poor with medical treatment alone.

 MISCELLANEOUS

SYNONYMS
Hepatic torsion

SEE ALSO
Small intestinal obstruction
Gastrointestinal hypomotility and gastrointestinal stasis
Anorexia

ABBREVIATIONS
ALP = alkaline phosphatase
ALT = alanine aminotransferase
GGT = gamma-glutamyl transferase
GI = gastrointestinal
LRS = lactated Ringer's solution
NSAID = nonsteroidal anti-inflammatory drugs
PCV = packed cell volume
TS = total solids

Suggested Reading
DeCubellis J. Common emergencies in rabbits, guinea pigs, and chinchillas. Vet Clin Exot Anim 2016;19:411–429.
Graham J, Basseches J. Liver lobe torsion in pet rabbits: clinical consequences, diagnosis, and treatment. Vet Clin Exot Anim 2014;17:195–202.
Hartcourt-Brown F. Digestive system disease. In: Meredith A, Lord B, eds. BSAVA Manual of Rabbit Medicine. Gloucester: British Small Animal Veterinary Association, 2014:168–190.
Oglesbee B, Lord B. Gastrointestinal diseases of rabbits. In: Quesenberry KE, Carpenter JW, eds. Ferrets, Rabbits and Rodents, 4th Ed). Clinical Medicine and Surgery. 2021 ed. St. Louis: Saunders, 2020:174–187.
Szabo Z, Bradley K, Cahalane AK. Rabbit soft tissue surgery. Vet Clin Exot Anim 2016;19:159–188.
Author Barbara Oglesbee, DVM, DABVP (Avian)

RABBITS

MASTITIS, CYSTIC, AND SEPTIC

BASICS

OVERVIEW

Septic Mastitis
- Bacterial infection of one or more lactating glands; result of ascending infection, trauma to the gland, or hematogenous spread
- Potentially life-threatening infection may lead to septic shock
- Mammary gland abscesses—may occur in nonlactating does due to trauma or hematogenous spread

Cystic Mastitis
- Sterile, fluid-filled cysts arising from mammary papillary ducts; usually single, but may be multiple, coalesce, and involve several glands
- Associated with endometrial cystic hyperplasia or uterine adenocarcinoma; hormonally mediated, resolves with ovariohysterectomy.
- May progress to mammary adenocarcinoma if untreated

SIGNALMENT
- Septic mastitis—postpartum lactating does or pseudopregnant does; no age predilection
- Cystic mastitis—highest incidence in does >3–4 years old, as this is the age range in which associated endometrial disorders occur; all breeds at risk; occurrence rate independent of breeding status

SIGNS

Historical Findings
Septic mastitis
- Anorexia, lethargy, and depression
- Polydipsia/polyuria
- May have had signs of pseudopregnancy—pulling hair, nest building
- Illness or death in suckling young
Cystic mastitis
- Usually bright, alert, nonpainful
- May have history of hematuria—due to associated endometrial disorder. Not true hematuria since blood originates from the uterus but is expelled during micturition. Hematuria is often reported as intermittent or cyclic; usually occurs at the end of micturition

Physical Examination Findings
Septic mastitis
- Firm, swollen, warm, erythematous (possibly deep purple to cyanotic) and painful mammary gland(s) from which purulent or hemorrhagic fluid can be expressed
- May involve single or multiple glands
- Fever, dehydration—with systemic involvement
- Abscessation of gland(s)

Cystic mastitis
- Swelling around nipple(s) or within mammary gland; filled with clear or serosanguinous fluid; no signs of inflammation (heat, pain, induration)
- May see signs of associated uterine disorder—palpably enlarged uterus; fresh blood or serosanguinous vaginal discharge; usually expelled during urination, but can appear independent of micturition; may see discharge adhered to fur

CAUSES AND RISK FACTORS

Septic Mastitis
- Trauma
- Poor hygiene
- Systemic infection originating elsewhere (e.g., metritis)
- *Staphylococcus aureus*, *Streptococcus* sp., and *Pasteurella* sp. most common isolates

Cystic Mastitis
- Intact reproductive status
- Endometrial disorders—endometrial hyperplasia, endometriosis, endometritis, and pyometra
- Uterine adenocarcinoma

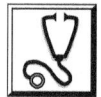

DIAGNOSIS

DIFFERENTIAL DIAGNOSIS
- Mammary gland hyperplasia—with pregnancy, common in rabbits with ovarian or uterine disorders, has been reported secondary to pituitary tumors
- Inflammatory mammary adenocarcinoma—differentiated by biopsy; may have simultaneous mammary abscess or neoplasia
- Subcutaneous abscess—may or may not involve mammary gland

CBC/BIOCHEMISTRY/URINALYSIS
- CBC—usually normal or lymphopenia; neutrophilia and left shift not common
- Azotemia, increases in ALT, electrolyte disturbances—all can be abnormal in rabbits with septicemia or severe dehydration, depending on clinical course
- Urinalysis—in rabbits with associated vaginal bleeding; sample collected by ultrasound-guided cystocentesis to differentiate true hematuria from uterine bleeding

IMAGING
- Abdominal radiography—in rabbits with cystic mastitis or mammary hyperplasia—may detect a large uterus with uterine adenocarcinoma or other endometrial disorder

- Thoracic radiographs—if mammary or uterine neoplasia is suspected; assess for metastasis

ULTRASONOGRAPHY
Assess size of uterus and nature of uterine contents.

OTHER LABORATORY TESTS
- Fine-needle aspiration of firm masses—may be helpful in differentiating mammary neoplasia from abscess; can be misleading if necrotic, septic foci are present within tumor
- Fine-needle aspiration of fluid—usually serosanguinous fluid with atypical epithelial cells in does with cystic mastitis
- Fine-needle aspiration of regional lymph node—to identify metastases if adenocarcinoma is suspected
- Excisional biopsy—may be required to identify adenocarcinoma
- Bacterial culture and susceptibility testing—from wall of abscess or expressed fluid/milk

DIAGNOSTIC PROCEDURES
Express milk or fluid from teats—if septic may see degenerative neutrophils with intracellular bacteria or macrophages; obtain bacterial culture to identify the organism; serosanguinous fluid with atypical epithelial cells seen with cystic mastitis

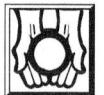

TREATMENT

SEPTIC MASTITIS
- Inpatient until stable
- Neonates—do not foster to surrogate doe as may transmit infection to surrogate
- Dehydration or sepsis—intravenous fluid therapy
- Apply warm compress and milk out affected gland(s) several times daily.
- Abscessed or necrotic glands—require surgical debridement
- Assist-feed any rabbit that is anorexic to avoid secondary gastrointestinal disorders.
- Clean and disinfect the environment.

CYSTIC MASTITIS
Usually resolves with ovariohysterectomy, no other treatment indicated

MAMMARY NEOPLASIA
Mastectomy and ovariohysterectomy

MEDICATIONS

DRUG(S) OF CHOICE

Septic Mastitis
- Combine with topical treatment (surgical debridement and post-debridement care).

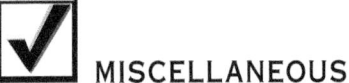

• Antimicrobial drugs effective against the infectious agent; gain access to site of infection. Choice of antibiotic is ideally based on results of culture and susceptibility testing. Use broad-spectrum antibiotics such as enrofloxacin (10–20 mg/kg PO, SC, IM, IV q12h), marbofloxacin (5 mg/kg PO q24h), trimethoprim-sulfa (15–30 mg/kg PO q12h), or chloramphenicol (50 mg/kg PO q8h). Penicillin G procaine (40,000–60,000 IU/kg SC q24h). Combine with topical or surgical treatment.

Acute Pain Management
• Butorphanol (0.1–0.5 mg/kg SQ, IM, IV q4–6h); may cause profound sedation; short acting
• Buprenorphine (0.02–0.05 mg/kg SQ, IM IV q8–12h); less sedating, longer acting than butorphanol
• Hydromorphone (0.1 mg/kg SC IM q2–4h) or oxymorphone (0.05–0.2 mg/kg SC IM q8–12h); use with caution; more than 1–2 doses may cause gastrointestinal stasis
• Meloxicam (1 mg/kg PO, SC, IM q24h)
• Carprofen (2–4 mg/kg PO, SC q12–24h)

Long-Term Pain Management
• Nonsteroidal anti-inflammatories—have been used for short- or long-term therapy to reduce pain and inflammation; meloxicam (1 mg/kg PO q24h); carprofen (2–4 mg/kg PO q12–24h)

CONTRAINDICATIONS
• Oral administration of most antibiotics effective against anaerobes will cause a fatal gastrointestinal dysbiosis in rabbits. Do not administer penicillins, macrolides, lincosamides, and cephalosporins by oral administration.
• Corticosteroids—associated with gastrointestinal ulceration and hemorrhage, delayed wound healing, and heightened susceptibility to infection; rabbits are very sensitive to the immunosuppressive effects of both topical and systemic corticosteroids; use may exacerbate subclinical bacterial infection

PRECAUTIONS
• Chloramphenicol—avoid human contact with chloramphenicol due to potential blood dyscrasia. Advise owners of potential risks.

• Meloxicam or other NSAIDs—use with caution in rabbits with compromised renal function.
• Oral administration of any antibiotic may potentially cause enteric dysbiosis; discontinue use if diarrhea or anorexia occurs.

FOLLOW-UP

PATIENT MONITORING
Physical examination; monitor for development of neoplasia in intact females

PREVENTION/AVOIDANCE
• Septic mastitis—clean environment
• Cystic mastitis—ovariohysterectomy for all nonbreeding rabbits; usually performed between 6 months and 2 years of age. Breeding rabbits—recommend stop breeding and spay after 4 years of age, as this is when most endometrial disorders (including adenocarcinoma) occur.

POSSIBLE COMPLICATIONS
• Abscessation may cause loss of gland(s), septicemia, death, and death of suckling neonates
• Cystic mastitis—progression to mammary adenocarcinoma with metastasis to lymph nodes and lungs if owner elects not to spay; hemorrhage, possible death in rabbits with associated bleeding uterine disorders

EXPECTED COURSE AND PROGNOSIS
• Septic mastitis—prognosis is fair to guarded with treatment, depending on severity
• Cystic mastitis—prognosis is good if ovariohysterectomy is performed; affected glands usually return to normal within 3–4 weeks.
• Mammary neoplasia—frequently metastasizes to region lymph nodes and lungs; survival times not reported

✔️ MISCELLANEOUS

ASSOCIATED CONDITIONS
• Mammary neoplasia
• Endometrial disorders
• Uterine adenocarcinoma
• Ovarian neoplasia
• Ovarian abscess

AGE-RELATED FACTORS
• Uterine neoplasia—rare in rabbits under 2 years of age; risk increases with age; seen in up to 60% of does over 3 years old

SEE ALSO
Abscesses
Pyometra and nonneoplastic endometrial disorders
Uterine adenocarcinoma

ABBREVIATIONS
ALT = alanine aminotransferase
NSAID = nonsteroidal anti-inflammatory drug

Suggested Reading
Di Girolamo N, Selleri P. Disorders of the urinary and reproductive system. In: Quesenberry KE, Carpenter JW, eds. Ferrets, Rabbits and Rodents, 4th Ed). Clinical Medicine and Surgery ed. St. Louis: Saunders, 2020:201–220.
Hallman RM, Brandão J. Diagnostic imaging of the renal system in exotic companion mammals. Vet Clin Exot Anim 2020;23: 195–214.
Mancinelli E, Lord B. Urogenital and reproductive disease. In: Meredith A, Lord B, eds. BSAVA Manual of Rabbit Medicine. Gloucester: British Small Animal Veterinary Association, 2014:191–204.
Reavill DR, Lennox AM. Disease overview of the urinary tract in exotic companion mammals and tips on clinical management. Vet Clin Exot Anim 2020;23(1):169–193.
Author Barbara Oglesbee, DVM

MAMMARY TUMORS

BASICS

DEFINITION
Malignant and benign tumors involving the mammary gland tissue

PATHOPHYSIOLOGY
Prolactin favors the multiplication of the tumor cells and inhibits their apoptosis.
• Seen in intact females, most often with underlying uterine or ovarian disease (especially endometrial hyperplasia or uterine adenocarcinoma)
• Can arise spontaneously, but often begins as cystic mastitis; progresses to adenoma then adenocarcinoma if ovariohysterectomy is not performed
• Mixed adenoma, adenocarcinoma, and mammary papilloma have been reported

SYSTEMS AFFECTED
• Reproductive
• Metastasis sites—lungs, lymph nodes, other system

INCIDENCE/PREVALENCE
Mammary tumors are nearly always seen in intact does with underlying uterine or ovarian disease. Exact incidence is not reported.

GEOGRAPHIC DISTRIBUTION
Worldwide

SIGNALMENT
Breed Predilections
Most often reported in New Zealand White and New Zealand White mixed breeds but can occur in any intact female.

Predominant Sex
Females; not reported in males.

Age
Intact females over 3 years of age

SIGNS
Historical Findings
• Intact female >2 years of age
• Owners often note signs of uterine disease—hematuria (blood arising from uterus, expelled during micturition), increased aggression, and sexual behavior
• Owner may palpate mass

Physical Examination Findings
• Can begin as cystic mastitis—swelling around nipple(s) or within mammary gland; filled with clear or serosanguinous fluid; no signs of inflammation (heat, pain, induration)
• Single or multiple coalescing subcutaneous nodules surrounding nipples; may have clear, milky, or serosanguinous discharge

• Concurrent reproductive tract signs predominate. May find vaginal discharge, hematuria (due to blood expelled from the uterus during micturition), or palpable uterine enlargement

CAUSES
• Usually due to underlying hyperestrogenism from ovarian and uterine disease; can be secondary to prolactin-secreting pituitary adenomas

RISK FACTORS
• Intact reproductive status
• Endometrial disorders—endometrial hyperplasia, endometriosis, endometritis, and pyometra
• Uterine adenocarcinoma
• Age—more common in does >2 years old

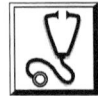

DIAGNOSIS

DIFFERENTIAL DIAGNOSIS
• Subcutaneous abscess—secondary to trauma
• Cystic Mastitis—swelling around nipple(s) or within mammary gland; filled with clear or serosanguinous fluid; no signs of inflammation (heat, pain, induration)
• Septic Mastitis—firm, swollen, warm, erythematous (possibly deep purple to cyanotic) and painful mammary gland(s) from which purulent or hemorrhagic fluid can be expressed
• Mammary gland hyperplasia—with pregnancy, common in rabbits with ovarian or uterine disorders, has been reported secondary to pituitary tumors

CBC/BIOCHEMISTRY/URINALYSIS
Nonspecific findings, usually normal

OTHER LABORATORY TESTS
• Fine-needle aspiration of the mass—may be helpful in differentiating benign, malignant tumor, mastitis
• Fine-needle aspiration of the regional lymph node—to identify metastasis if adenocarcinoma suspected

IMAGING
Thoracic radiography—to detect metastasis if malignant tumor suspected.

Whole-body radiographs or ultrasound to identify concurrent reproductive disease (uterine, ovarian).

DIAGNOSTIC PROCEDURES
Excisional biopsy—histologic evaluation for definitive diagnosis

PATHOLOGIC FINDINGS
• Gross—most tumors are well-circumscribed, multilobular, and easily separated from surrounding tissues. Malignant tumors sometimes invade into skin and underlying musculature.
• Histopathology—adenoma, fibroadenoma, papilloma, or adenocarcinoma most common

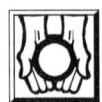

TREATMENT

APPROPRIATE HEALTH CARE
• Most are treated as outpatients following ovariohysterectomy and surgical excision.

NURSING CARE
Assist-feeding and fluid therapy to prevent secondary GI stasis if the patient is not eating.

ACTIVITY
Decrease activity level following surgical removal by confining to cage.

DIET
• Many affected rabbits are anorectic or have a decreased appetite. It is an absolute requirement that the patient continues to eat during and following treatments. Anorexia may cause or exacerbate gastrointestinal hypomotility and cause derangement of the gastrointestinal microflora and overgrowth of intestinal bacterial pathogens. If the patient refuses these foods, syringe-feed Critical Care for Herbivores (Oxbow Animal Health, Murdock, NE) or Emeraid Herbivore (Lafeber Company, Cornell, IL) diet at approximately 10–15 mL/kg PO q6–8h. Larger volumes and more frequent feedings are often accepted; feed as much as the patient will readily accept. Alternatively, pellets can be ground and mixed with fresh greens, vegetable baby foods, or water to form a gruel

CLIENT EDUCATION
• Advice clients of the benefits of ovariohysterectomy prior to 2 years of age.

SURGICAL CONSIDERATIONS
• Ovairohysterectomy is always indicated. Most uterine disorders carry risk of hemorrhage into the uterus; can become life threatening; can progress; all are at risk for developing uterine adenocarcinoma; reproductive performance is reduced in does with endometrial disorders
• With benign small masses, removal can be achieved via a simple incision in the overlying skin, shelling out the underlying mass.
• With ulcerated large masses, or suspected malignant masses, remove via an elliptical incision with wide margins.

(CONTINUED)

MAMMARY TUMORS

MEDICATIONS

DRUG(S) OF CHOICE

Pain Management
- Butorphanol (0.1–0.5 mg/kg SQ, IM, IV q4–6h); may cause profound sedation; short acting
- Buprenorphine (0.02–0.05 mg/kg SQ, IM IV q8–12h); less sedating, longer acting than butorphanol
- Hydromorphone (0.1 mg/kg SC IM q2–4h) or oxymorphone (0.05–0.2 mg/kg SC IM q8–12h)
- Meloxicam (1 mg/kg PO, SC, IM q24h)
- Carprofen (2–4 mg/kg PO, SC q12–24h)

Antibiotics
Indicated in large masses with ulceration. Use broad-spectrum antibiotics such as enrofloxacin (10–20 mg/kg PO, SC, IM, IV q12h), marbofloxacin (5 mg/kg PO q24h), trimethoprim-sulfa (15–30 mg/kg PO q12h), or chloramphenicol (50 mg/kg PO q8h).

Chemotherapy
Success in metastatic disease has not been reported in rabbits.

CONTRAINDICATIONS
- Oral administration of most antibiotics effective against anaerobes will cause a fatal gastrointestinal dysbiosis in rabbits. Do not administer penicillins, macrolides, lincosamides, and cephalosporins by oral administration.
- Corticosteroids—associated with gastrointestinal ulceration and hemorrhage, delayed wound healing, and heightened susceptibility to infection; rabbits are very sensitive to the immunosuppressive effects of both topical and systemic corticosteroids; use may exacerbate subclinical bacterial infection

PRECAUTIONS
- Chloramphenicol—avoid human contact with chloramphenicol due to potential blood dyscrasia. Advise owners of potential risks.

- Meloxicam or other NSAIDs—use with caution in rabbits with compromised renal function
- Oral administration of any antibiotic may potentially cause enteric dysbiosis; discontinue use if diarrhea or anorexia occurs

FOLLOW-UP

PATIENT MONITORING
- Postoperatively, monitor the suture line. Rabbits are extremely likely to chew sutures and open the wound. An Elizabethan collar is generally needed.
- Monitor for postoperative GI stasis (appetite, fecal production).
- Consider thoracic and abdominal radiographs every 3 months for the first 6–12 months post ovariohysterectomy. Not all metastases are grossly visible at the time of surgery.

PREVENTION/AVOIDANCE
Ovariohysterectomy for all nonbreeding rabbits; usually performed between 6 months and 2 years of age. For breeding rabbits—recommend stop breeding and spay before 4 years of age, as this is when most tumors occur.

POSSIBLE COMPLICATIONS
- Suture line dehiscence
- Self-mutilation
- Regrowth of the mass if the margins are not clean

EXPECTED COURSE AND PROGNOSIS
- Excellent (cure) if ovariohysterectomy prior to metastasis or mammary neoplasia; poor to grave if metastasis has occurred (5 month to 2 years to metastasize); after chemotherapy, unknown
- Without ovariohysterectomy—metastasis, death in 12–24 months
- Associated cystic mastitis will resolve with ovariohysterectomy alone unless secondary infection has developed.

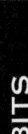

MISCELLANEOUS

ASSOCIATED CONDITIONS
Uterine and ovarian disorders

AGE-RELATED FACTORS
Rare in does under 2 years of age.

ZOONOTIC POTENTIAL
N/A

PREGNANCY/FERTILITY/BREEDING
Tumors grow more rapidly in pregnant animals due to high levels of prolactin secretion.

SYNONYMS
N/A

SEE ALSO
Hematuria
Mastitis, cystic, and septic
Pyometra and nonneoplastic endometrial disorders

Suggested Reading
Di Girolamo N, Selleri P. Disorders of the urinary and reproductive system. In: Quesenberry KE, Carpenter JW, eds. Ferrets, Rabbits and Rodents, 4th Ed). Clinical Medicine and Surgery ed. St. Louis: Saunders, 2020:201–220.
Hallman RM, Brandão J. Diagnostic imaging of the renal system in exotic companion mammals. Vet Clin Exot Anim 2020;23: 195–214.
Mancinelli E, Lord B. Urogenital and reproductive disease. In: Meredith A, Lord B, eds. BSAVA Manual of Rabbit Medicine. Gloucester: British Small Animal Veterinary Association, 2014:191–204.
Reavill DR, Lennox AM. Disease overview of the urinary tract in exotic companion mammals and tips on clinical management. Vet Clin Exot Anim 2020;23(1):169–193.
Author Barbara Oglesbee, DVM, DABVP (Avian)

MYXOMATOSIS

BASICS

OVERVIEW
• A systemic, usually fatal disease in domestic and wild European rabbits and hares caused by a myxomavirus in the poxvirus family
• Disease in wild rabbits is less severe due to the development of genetic resistance to the virus.
• Virus was originally intentionally introduced into Australia and Europe in an effort to control wild rabbit populations; resistance has since developed.
• Several strains of mxyoma viruses exist, and pathogenicity varies with strain and host immunity.
• Virus is spread primarily through insect bites (mosquitos, flies, fur mites, and fleas), but can also be transmitted by mechanical vectors (nonbiting insects, thorns, bedding, and food)
• Wild rabbits often only show mild disease, with the development of firm cutaneous nodules at the site of transmitting bites.
• Clinical signs in pet rabbit depend on how long the rabbit survives; most pet rabbits will die within 2 weeks.

GEOGRAPHIC DISTRIBUTION
• Europe, South America, North America, and Australia
• In the United States, seen primarily in California. The California strain is extremely virulent, with mortality rates exceeding 99%.

SIGNALMENT
• Domestic, pet rabbits (*Oryctolagus cuniculus*) more susceptible to disease than wild cottontail rabbits (*Sylviagus* spp.) and other North American species of rabbits.
• Outdoor rabbits may be at greater risk due to mode of viral transmission.
• Seen primarily in rabbits living in California; ease of transportation of pet rabbits raises concern over spread to other parts of the country

SIGNS
California Strain in Pet (Domestic) Rabbits
• Incubation period is usually 1–3 days
• Peracute—death with few premonitory signs; lethargy; eyelid edema; pyrexia; death within 7 days
• Acute form—eyelid edema usually develops first; perioral and perineal swelling and edema; cutaneous hemorrhage; lethargy; anorexia; dyspnea; seizures or other CNS signs (excitement, opisthotonus); death within 1–2 weeks
• Chronic form—few rabbits live long enough to develop this form; see blepharoconjunctivitis, swelling, edema around base of ears, generalized cutaneous tumors; lethargy; anorexia; dyspnea; high fever; death within 2 weeks

Wild Rabbits
• Cutaneous nodules at the site of transmission (insect bite, scratch)—firm fibroma-like swellings may be only clinical signs
• Young wild or feral rabbits may develop disease similar to pet rabbits

CAUSES AND RISK FACTORS
• Myxoma virus, a strain of Leporipoxvirus
• Outbreaks may be more likely when mosquitos are numerous (summer, fall)

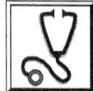

DIAGNOSIS

DIFFERENTIAL DIAGNOSIS
• For periocular, perioral, and perineal rash—*Treponema cuniculi* (rabbit syphilis); usually not associated with edema or fever; usually otherwise healthy
• For neurologic signs—meningitis, otitis interna/media, rabies; usually not associated with dermatologic signs

CBC/BIOCHEMISTRY/URINALYSIS
N/A

OTHER LABORATORY TESTS
Serologic testing—various serologic tests are available for research purposes, may not be commercially available in North America

IMAGING
N/A

DIAGNOSTIC PROCEDURES
Virus isolation

PATHOLOGIC FINDINGS
Gross
• Cutaneous nodules—characteristic lesions fibrous nodule with mucinous material in the center
• Hepatic necrosis, splenomegaly, infarcts, or hemorrhage in lungs, trachea, and thymus
• Subcutaneous ecchymoses; ecchymoses in serosal surfaces of the gastrointestinal tract
• May be no gross lesions in peracute cases

Histopathologic
• Undifferentiated mesenchymal cells, inflammatory cells, mucin, and edema.
• Necrotizing lesions—may be seen in fetal placentas

TREATMENT
• None effective
• Supportive care—generally unsuccessful

MEDICATIONS

DRUG(S) OF CHOICE
N/A

CONTRADINDICATIONS/POSSIBLE INTERACTIONS
N/A

FOLLOW-UP

PREVENTION/AVOIDANCE
• Control of vectors—screening to keep out insects; flea control; keep indoors
• Disinfection—10% bleach, 10% NaOH, 1%–1.4% formalin
• Quarantine new rabbits; do not house wild rabbits with domestic pet rabbits.
• Vaccination with an attenuated myxoma virus vaccine may provide temporary protection; not available in the United States; vaccination may cause atypical myomatosis

MISCELLANEOUS

ZOONOTIC POTENTIAL
None

Suggested Reading
Farrella S, Noble PJ, Pinchbeck GL et al. Seasonality and risk factors for myxomatosis in pet rabbits in Great Britain. Prev Vet Med 2020;176.
Harcourt-Brown F. Infectious diseases of domestic rabbits. In: Harcourt-Brown F, ed. Textbook of Rabbit Medicine. Oxford, UK: Butterworth-Heinemann, 2002:361–385.
Kerar PJ. Myxomatosis in Australia and Europe: a model for emerging infectious diseases. Antiviral Res 2012;93:387–415.
Author Barbara Oglesbee, DVM, DABVP (Avian)

NASAL DISCHARGE AND SNEEZING

BASICS

DEFINITION
• Nasal discharges may be serous, mucoid, mucopurulent, purulent, blood tinged, or frank blood (epistaxis).
• Sneezing is the reflexive expulsion of air through the nasal cavity and is commonly associated with nasal discharge.

PATHOPHYSIOLOGY
• Secretions are produced by mucous cells of the epithelium and glands. Irritation of the nasal mucosa (by mechanical, chemical, or inflammatory stimulation) increases nasal secretion production.
• The most common cause of nasal discharge and sneezing in rabbits is bacterial infection. Infection usually begins in the nasal cavity and may spread via the eustachian tubes to the inner or middle ears, into the sinuses and bones of the face, via the nasolacrimal duct to the eye, via the trachea to the lower respiratory tract and hematogenously to joints, bones, and other organ systems.
• Dental disease or abscesses can cause destruction and/or chronic infection of the nasal turbinates or facial bones (osteomyelitis), which may result in refractory or recurrent infections.
• Choke, or aspiration of food, can cause an acute onset of nasal discharge and dyspnea. Rabbits are obligate nasal breathers. The rim of the epiglottis is normally situated dorsal to the elongated soft palate to allow air passage from the nose to the trachea during normal respiration. With complete obstruction of the nasal passages, rabbits may attempt open mouth breathing, which is an extremely poor prognostic indicator. After aspirating food, the foreign material can flip up into the nasopharynx and cause copious discharge.

Types of Nasal Discharge and Common Associations
• Serous—mild irritation, allergies, acute phase of inflammation, early bacterial infection
• Copious, acute, mucoid (often green tinged)—foreign body/food aspiration (choke).
• Mucoid—allergies or contact irritation, acute inflammation or infection, early neoplastic conditions
• Purulent (or mucopurulent, generally thick and white)—bacterial infections, nasal foreign bodies, rarely mycotic in rabbits
• Serosanguinous—destructive processes (bacterial pathogens, primary nasal tumors), associated with coagulopathies

SYSTEMS AFFECTED
• Respiratory—mucosa of the upper respiratory tract, including the nasal cavities, sinuses, and nasopharynx
• Ophthalmic—extension to the eyes via nasolacrimal duct
• Musculoskeletal—extension of infection into bones of the skull
• Neurologic—extension of infection via eustachian tube causing vestibular signs from otitis interna/media
• Hemic/Lymphatic/Immune—systemic diseases may cause blood-tinged nasal discharge or epistaxis due to hemostasis disorders.

SIGNALMENT
• Young animals—bacterial infections
• Middle-aged to older animals—nasal tumors, dental disease, and bacterial infections

SIGNS

Historical Findings
• Nasal discharge and sneezing may be reported as concurrent problems. Information concerning both the initial and present character of the discharge and whether it was originally unilateral or bilateral are important historical findings.
• The response to previous antibiotic therapy may be helpful in determining secondary bacterial involvement. Bacterial infections, dental disease, or foreign body will often respond initially to antibiotic therapy but commonly relapse after treatment. Nasal tumors typically show little response.
• Acute onset of copious discharge with dyspnea is characteristic of food aspiration (choke). Owners may have witnessed event; may have history of previous choking events.
• History of ocular discharge; ptyalism with tooth involvement; head tilt, vestibular signs, scratching at ears with extension into the ears
• History of feeding poor diets, such as commercial pelleted foods without the addition of long-stemmed hay or grasses, is common in rabbits with dental disease.

Physical Examination Findings
• Secretions or dried discharges on the hair around the nose and front limbs
• Concurrent dental disease, especially tooth root impaction, malocclusion, and incisor overgrowth. Findings may include ptyalism, anorexia, nasal discharge, ocular discharge, and exophthalmia. Always perform a thorough oral exam.
• Ocular discharge—may be serous with nasolacrimal duct occlusion or mucopurulent; conjunctivitis secondary to nasolacrimal duct obstruction or extension of upper respiratory infection; exophthalmos with retrobulbar abscess

• Bony involvement (tooth root abscess, tumor, pasteurellosis, or other bacteria) may cause facial swelling or pain.
• Lethargy, anorexia, or depression with pain, extension to lower respiratory tract or hematogenous spread
• Dyspnea, stridor—especially with exertion with extension to lower respiratory tract or complete nasal occlusion (rabbits are obligate nasal breathers)

CAUSES
• Pyogenic bacteria—Pasteurella multocida; Staphylococcus aureus, Bordetella bronchiseptica, Moraxella catarrhalis, Pseudomonas aeruginosa, Mycobacterium sp., and various anaerobes have also been implicated.
• Odontogenic abscesses—Pasteurella not causative; common isolates from these sites include anaerobic bacteria such as Fusobacterium nucleatum, Prevotella spp., Peptostreptococcus micros, Actinomyces israelii, and Arcanobacterium haemolyticum. Aerobic bacteria—Streptococcus sp. most common isolate
• Dental disease—periapical or tooth root abscesses, elongated maxillary tooth roots penetrating into nasal passages
• Foreign objects, especially hay, straw, or other bedding material
• Aspiration of food
• Allergies or irritants—dust (often from hay), cat litter, bedding, and plant material
• Neoplasia
• Unilateral discharge often is associated with nonsystemic processes—dental-related disease, nasal tumors, or foreign bodies
• Discharge may be unilateral or bilateral with bacterial respiratory tract infections, allergies, nasal tumors, dental disease, or foreign bodies.

RISK FACTORS
• Dental disease
• Immunosuppression
• Stress
• Corticosteroid use
• Poor husbandry—inappropriate diet; urine-soaked bedding

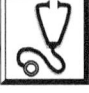

DIAGNOSIS

DIFFERENTIAL DIAGNOSIS
Allergic, irritant, neoplastic, infectious, inflammatory, and traumatic disorders

CBC/BIOCHEMISTRY
• TWBC elevations are usually not seen with bacterial diseases. A relative neutrophilia and/or lymphopenia are more common.
• Although not specific for any particular cause of nasal discharge, a chemistry profile

NASAL DISCHARGE AND SNEEZING   (CONTINUED)

may be valuable for detecting concurrent problems and as part of a thorough evaluation prior to any procedure requiring anesthesia.

OTHER LABORATORY TESTS
• Serology for *Pasteurella*—usefulness is severely limited and generally not helpful in the diagnosis of pasteurellosis in pet rabbits. An ELISA is available; however, positive results, even when high, only indicate prior exposure to *Pasteurella* and the development of antibodies, but do not confirm active infection. Low positive results may occur due to cross-reaction with other, nonpathogenic bacteria (false positive). False negative results are common with immunosuppression or early infection. No evidence exists to support correlation of titers to the presence or absence of disease.

IMAGING
Radiographic Findings
• Radiography of the nasal cavities can be helpful in cases of chronic nasal discharge, especially to rule out bacterial rhinitis/ sinusitis, neoplasia, foreign body, or associated dental disease. Because of difficulties with overlying structures, the patient should be anesthetized and carefully positioned.
• The lateral view is useful in detecting any periosteal reaction over the nasal bones, for gross changes in the maxillary teeth, nasal cavity, and frontal sinus and for evaluating the air column of the nasopharynx.
• The ventrodorsal view useful for evaluating the nasal cavities and turbinates; disease may be localized to the affected side.
• The lateral oblique views are best for detecting maxillary teeth abnormalities.
• The rostrocaudal view is used to evaluate each frontal sinus (e.g., periosteal reaction, filling).
• CT or MRI: provides better imaging quality and may be more diagnostic than skull radiographs especially if nasal detail is obscured by nasal discharge; can help to determine whether the cause of disease is nasal, sinus, or dental disease. CT specifically is excellent for providing bony detail, and the procedure time is relatively short.

OTHER DIAGNOSTIC PROCEDURES
• Cultures—may be difficult to interpret, since commonly isolated bacteria (e.g., *Bordetella* sp.) often represent only commensal organisms or opportunistic pathogens. A heavy growth of a single organism is usually significant. Deep cultures obtained by inserting a mini-tipped culturette 2–4 cm into each nostril are sometimes reliable. However, samples taken from the nostrils should not be overinterpreted, since the causative agent may be located only deep within the sinuses, and not present at the rostral portion of the nostrils, where samples are readily accessible.
• A lack of growth does not rule out bacterial disease, since the infection may be in an inaccessible, deep area of the nasal cavity or sinuses, and many organisms (especially anaerobes and *Pasteurella* sp.) can be difficult to grow on culture.
• PCR assay for pasteurellosis may also be performed on samples taken from deep nasal swabs. Positive results should not be overinterpreted. Pasteurella is often a copathogen with other bacteria; presence of organism alone does not confirm pasteurella as the sole causative agent.
• Nasal cytology—nonspecific inflammation is most commonly found
• Biopsy of the nasal cavity is indicated in any animal in which neoplasia is suspected. Specimens may be obtained by direct endoscopic biopsy or rhinotomy. Multiple samples may be necessary to ensure adequate representation of the disease process.
• Rhinoscopy can be extremely valuable to visualize nasal abnormalities, retrieve foreign bodies, or obtain biopsy samples; sometimes, the only method of identifying foreign bodies

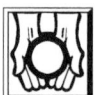

TREATMENT
• Provide oxygen supplementation if patient appears to be dyspneic; rabbits are obligate nasal breathers; nasal discharge can cause severe dyspnea. Keep nostrils clear of discharge.
• Outpatient treatment is acceptable unless surgery is required or the patient is exhibiting signs of systemic illness in addition to nasal discharge.
• Symptomatic treatment and nursing care are important in the treatment of rabbits with sneezing and nasal discharge. Patient hydration, nutrition, warmth, and hygiene (keeping nostrils clean) are important.
• Surgery may be necessary to remove foreign bodies, obtain samples for biopsy, or to debulk abscesses, tumors, or granulomas.
• Treat associated dental disease— extractions, complete debridement of abscesses
• If epiphora or ocular discharge is present, always flush the nasolacrimal duct.
• Remove environmental allergens/irritants (dusty litters, moldy hay, or betting); provide clean airspace.

DIET
• Rabbits with nasal discharge are often inappetent. It is absolutely imperative that the rabbit continue to eat during and following treatment. Anorexia will often cause GI hypomotility, derangement of the gastrointestinal microflora, and overgrowth of intestinal bacterial pathogens.
• Offer a large selection of fresh, moistened greens such as cilantro, romaine lettuce, parsley, carrot tops, dandelion greens, spinach, collard greens, etc., and good-quality grass hay. Many rabbits will begin to eat these foods, even if they were previously anorectic.
• If the patient refuses these foods, syringe-feed a gruel such as Critical Care for Herbivores (Oxbow Pet Products) or Emeraid Herbivore (Lafeber Company, Cornell, IL) 10–15 mL/kg PO q6–8h. Alternatively, pellets can be ground and mixed with fresh greens, vegetable baby foods, water, or juice to form a gruel.
• High-carbohydrate, high-fat nutritional supplements are contraindicated.
• Encourage oral fluid intake by offering fresh water, wetting leafy vegetables, or flavoring water with vegetable juices.

CLIENT EDUCATION
• Discuss need to correct or prevent risk factors.
• Warn clients that signs may recur following discontinuation of antibiotic therapy. Rabbits with chronic nasal discharge and turbinate destruction are unlikely to be cured; the goal of medication is to control more severe signs, and lifelong therapy may be required.

MEDICATIONS
DRUG(S) OF CHOICE
• Nasal secretions clear more easily if the patient is well hydrated; fluid therapy should be considered if hydration is marginal.
• Antimicrobial drugs effective against the infectious agent; gain access to site of infection. Choice of antibiotic is ideally based on results of culture and susceptibility testing. Depending on the severity of infection, long-term antibiotic therapy is required (2 weeks minimum, to several months or intermittently for years in cases of chronic, recurrent bacterial rhinitis/sinusitis).
• Use broad-spectrum antibiotic such as enrofloxacin (10–20 mg/kg PO, SC, IM, IV q12h), marbofloxacin (5 mg/kg PO q24h), trimethoprim-sulfa (15–30 mg/kg PO q12h), chloramphenicol (50 mg/kg PO q8h), or penicillin G procaine (40,000–60,000 IU/kg SC q24h).
• Nebulization—used in conjunction with systemic treatment. Nebulize for 15 minutes 1–3 times daily. Choices include enrofloxacin 100 mg in 10 mL saline; doxycycline 200 mg in 15 mL saline; gentamicin 50 mg I 10 mL saline; and amikacin 50 mg in 10 mL saline

(CONTINUED)

• Antihistamines have been used rabbits with allergic rhinitis and symptomatically in rabbits with infectious rhinitis. Use is anecdotal and dosages have been extrapolated from feline dosages. Hydroxyzine (2 mg/kg PO q8–12h); diphenhydramine (2.0 mg/kg PO, SC q8–12h)
• Topical ophthalmic preparations, such as those containing quinolones, to treat associated conjunctivitis

CONTRAINDICATIONS
• Topical nasal decongestants containing phenylephrine can exacerbate nasal inflammation and cause nasal ulceration and purulent rhinitis.
• Oral administration of antibiotics that select against gram-positive bacteria (penicillins, macrolides, lincosamides, and cephalosporins) can cause fatal enteric dysbiosis and enterotoxemia.
• The use of corticosteroids (systemic or topical in ophthalmic preparations) can severely exacerbate bacterial infection.

PRECAUTIONS
• Chloramphenicol—avoid human contact with chloramphenicol due to potential blood dyscrasia. Advise owners of potential risks.
• Nebulization or oral administration of any antibiotic may potentially cause enteric dysbiosis; discontinue use if diarrhea or anorexia occurs.

POSSIBLE INTERACTIONS
N/A

ALTERNATIVE DRUGS
• Topical (intranasal) administration of ciprofloxacin ophthalmic drops may be used in conjunction with systemic antibiotic therapy. Rabbits do not like having things placed in their nose and should be restrained appropriately before intranasal treatment administration.

• Nebulization with saline or antibiotic solutions may be helpful in chronic cases.

FOLLOW-UP
PATIENT MONITORING
Clinical assessment and monitoring for relapse of clinical signs

PREVENTION/AVOIDANCE
• Improve husbandry (good ventilation and appropriate substrate) and diet.
• Avoid stressful situations and corticosteroid use.
• Prevent dental disease by providing high-fiber foods, especially good-quality hay. Yearly veterinary exams with periodic trimming of overgrown teeth as needed.

POSSIBLE COMPLICATIONS
• Loss of appetite
• Extension of primary disease into mouth, eyes, ears, lungs, or brain
• Dyspnea as a result of nasal obstruction

MISCELLANEOUS
ASSOCIATED CONDITIONS
• Cheek teeth malocclusion and elongation
• Gastrointestinal hypomotility
• Abscessation

AGE-RELATED FACTORS
N/A

ZOONOTIC POTENTIAL
N/A

PREGNANCY/FERTILITY/BREEDING
N/A

SYNONYMS
Snuffles

SEE ALSO
Abscessation
Cheek teeth (premolar and molar) malocclusion and elongation
Pasteurellosis
Rhinitis and sinusitis

ABBREVIATIONS
CT = computed tomography
ELISA = enzyme-linked immunosorbent assay
GI = gastrointestinal
PCR = polymerase chain reaction

Suggested Reading
Capello V, Lennox AM. Diagnostic imaging of the respiratory system in exotic companion mammals. Vet Clin Exot Anim 2011;14:369–389.
DeCubellis J. Common emergencies in rabbits, guinea pigs, and chinchillas. Vet Clin Exot Anim 2016;19:411–429.
Hedley J. Respiratory disease. In: Meredith A, Lord B, eds. BSAVA Manual of Rabbit Medicine. Gloucester: British Small Animal Veterinary Association, 2014:160–167.
Jekl V. Respiratory disorders in rabbits. Vet Clin Exot Anim 2021;24:459–482.
Lennox AM, Mancinelli E. Respiratory diseases. In: Quesenberry KE, Carpenter JW, eds. Ferrets, Rabbits and Rodents, 4th Ed). Clinical Medicine and Surgery ed. St. Louis: Saunders, 2020:188–201.
Varga M. Cardiorespiratory diseases. In: Varga M, ed. Textbook of Rabbit Medicine, 2nd ed. London, UK: Elsevier, 2014:390–405.

Author Barbara Oglesbee, DVM, DABVP-Avian

NECK AND BACK PAIN

BASICS

DEFINITION
Discomfort along the spinal column

PATHOPHYSIOLOGY
Pain may originate in the epaxial muscle, vertebrae and associated structures, spinal nerves, nerve roots or dorsal root ganglia, and meninges.

SYSTEMS AFFECTED
- Nervous
- Musculoskeletal

SIGNALMENT
No age, breed, or sex predilection

SIGNS
Historical Findings
- Owner may describe an abnormal gait; the rabbit may be unable to hop or be reluctant to jump or climb; rabbit may have difficulty getting in and out of litter box, climbing stairs, hopping onto furniture; may drag the affected limbs or may be unable get up
- Sudden onset of paresis/paralysis is common with traumatic vertebral fractures or luxation
- History of improper restraint—inexperienced handlers or owners; restraint for mask induction of anesthesia; very nervous animals escaping from appropriate restraint
- Trauma may not have been witnessed. A rabbit can fracture or luxate vertebrae by suddenly jumping while in their cages. History may include startling event such as a loud thunderstorm, fireworks, or unfamiliar people or pets in the house.
- Ataxia, rear limb weakness
- Perineal dermatitis, urine scald
- Flaking, alopecia in intrascapular region or tail head
- Feces or cecotrophs pasted to perineum
- Teeth grinding or reluctance to move due to pain

PHYSICAL EXAMINATION FINDINGS
- Pain on epaxial palpation
- Neurologic deficits referable to the spinal cord or nerve root compression
- Ataxia, rear limb weakness
- Perineal dermatitis—matted fur, urine-soaked perineum or ventrum, feces pasted to perineum, alopecia, erythema, ulceration, myiasis; seen secondary to inability to groom and in rabbits with fecal or urinary incontinence
- Pododermatitis (sore hocks) due to inactivity

- Alopecia, flaking, *Cheyletiella* mites in intrascapular or tail head region due to inadequate grooming
- Accumulation of wax in ear canals from inadequate grooming
- Hypercalciuria secondary to insufficient voiding in chronically painful rabbits or rabbits with loss of bladder control
- Obesity

CAUSES (LISTED IN ORDER OF FREQUENCY)
Epaxial Muscle
- Traumatic myositis
- Abscess, cellulitis

Vertebrae and Associated Structures
- Spondylosis/spinal arthritis
- Fracture
- Luxation and subluxation
- Malformation and malarticulation
- Vertebral osteomyelitis
- Vertebral neoplasia

Spinal Nerves
- Compression or inflammation of dorsal root ganglion
- Traumatic entrapment, tearing, or laceration
- Meningitis—bacterial, protozoal
- Neoplasia—primary or metastatic
- Entrapment by disk herniation (rare)

RISK FACTORS
- Trauma
- Spinal fractures, luxations, or intervertebral disk disease—improper restraint, trauma in caged rabbits suddenly startled, possibly disuse atrophy from confinement
- Age—with spondylosis/spinal arthritis

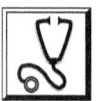

DIAGNOSIS

DIFFERENTIAL DIAGNOSIS
- Diseases involving thoracic structures—pleura, cardiovascular system, and lungs
- Diseases involving abdominal structures—uterine neoplasia, hypercalciuria or urolithiasis, and abdominal abscesses
- Rule out limb musculoskeletal pain, especially coxofemoral degenerative joint disease (DJD)
- *Encephalitozoon cuniculi*—nonpainful disease of the spinal cord

CBC/BIOCHEMISTRY/URINALYSIS
- Creatine kinase—can be high with any diseases affecting the muscle
- CBC—TWBC elevations are usually not seen with bacterial diseases. A relative heterophilia and/or lymphopenia are more common.

IMAGING
- Survey radiographs—identify spondylosis/spinal arthritis, hypercalciuria, other causes of pain or reluctance to move
- Spinal radiographs—lesion localized to the spinal cord; may reveal fracture or luxation, spondylosis, diskospondylitis, bony tumor, congenital vertebral malformation
- Thoracic radiography—detect metastasis
- CT—more accurate for evaluation of spine, underlying causes of pain
- Abdominal ultrasonography—if underlying metabolic disease is suspected

DIAGNOSTIC PROCEDURES
Epaxial Muscle
- Bone biopsy—helps confirm vertebral neoplasia and infection
- Cytology and culture—from the affected intervertebral space; may help identify cause
- CSF analysis—sample from the cerebellomedullary cistern; may be valuable for evaluating central disease; detect inflammatory process; sample collection may put the patient at risk for herniation if there is a mass or high intracranial pressure.

TREATMENT
- Varies widely according to the nature and extent of the tissues involved
- Inpatient vs. outpatient—depends on severity of disease

NURSING CARE
- Keep perineum clean, dry, and free of fecal matter
- Use soft bedding, keep bedding clean and dry to prevent dermatitis or bed sores
- Manual expression of the bladder if unable to urinate
- Comb frequently to remove matted hair and scale from areas in which the rabbit cannot groom.
- Clean ears to remove buildup of wax

ACTIVITY
Restrict until spinal trauma can be ruled out.

DIET
- It is imperative that the rabbit continues to eat during and following treatment. Painful animals are often anorectic. Anorexia will often cause GI hypomotility, derangement of the gastrointestinal microflora, and overgrowth of intestinal bacterial pathogens.
- If the patient refuses food, syringe-feed a gruel such as Critical Care for Herbivores (Oxbow Pet Products) or Emeraid Herbivore (Lafeber Company, Cornell, IL) 10–15 mL/kg PO q6–8h. Alternatively, pellets can be

RABBITS

ground and mixed with fresh greens, vegetable baby foods, water, or juice to form a gruel.

MEDICATIONS

DRUG(S) OF CHOICE

Acute Pain Management
• Butorphanol (0.1–0.5 mg/kg SQ, IM, IV q4–6h); may cause profound sedation; short acting
• Buprenorphine (0.02–0.05 mg/kg SQ, IM IV q8–12h); less sedating, longer acting than butorphanol
• Hydromorphone (0.1 mg/kg SC IM q2–4h) or oxymorphone (0.05–0.2 mg/kg SC IM q8–12h)
• Meloxicam (1 mg/kg PO, SC, IM q24h)
• Carprofen (2–4 mg/kg PO, SC q12–24h)

Long-term Pain Management
• Nonsteroidal anti-inflammatories—have been used for short- or long-term therapy to reduce pain and inflammation in rabbits with musculoskeletal disease; meloxicam (1.0 mg/kg PO q24h); carprofen (2 mg/kg PO q12h)
• Tramadol—5–15 mg/kg PO q8–12h
• Gabapentin—5–20 mg/kg PO q8–12h
• Antimicrobial therapy—for infection; depends on the causative agent
• Chemotherapy and radiotherapy—depends on tumor type

CONTRAINDICATIONS
• Oral administration of antibiotics that select against gram-positive bacteria (penicillins, macrolides, lincosamides, and cephalosporins) can cause fatal enteric dysbiosis and enterotoxemia.
• Corticosteroids—do not use for routine treatment of inflammatory or painful musculoskeletal disorders; associated with gastrointestinal ulceration and hemorrhage, delayed wound healing, and heightened susceptibility to infection; rabbits are very sensitive to the immunosuppressive effects of both topical and systemic corticosteroids; use may exacerbate subclinical bacterial infection

PRECAUTIONS
• Corticosteroids—use with caution, only in acute spinal trauma;

• Meloxicam—use with caution in rabbits with compromised renal function

POSSIBLE INTERACTIONS
N/A

ALTERNATIVE DRUGS
• Chondroitin sulfate (Cosequin, Nutramax) has been used anecdotally using feline dosage protocols; Polysulfated glycosaminoglycan (Adequan, Luitpold) 2.2 mg/kg SC, IM q3d × 21–28 days, then q14d.
• Acupuncture may be effective for rabbits with chronic pain.

FOLLOW-UP

PATIENT MONITORING
• Monitor response to treatment closely and make adjustments as necessary.
• Instruct client to watch for signs of gastrointestinal hypomotility, pyoderma, and urinary tract disease.

POSSIBLE COMPLICATIONS
• Fibrous replacement of muscle fibers, causing chronic pain and immobility
• Permanent paralysis or dysfunction
• Urinary tract infection, bladder atony, urine scalding and pyoderma, fecal incontinence, decubital ulcer formation, and myiasis
• Exacerbation of bacterial infections (possibly life threatening), gastric ulceration with corticosteroid usage
• Chronic pain

MISCELLANEOUS

ASSOCIATED CONDITIONS
• Gastrointestinal hypomotility
• Hypercalciuria
• Ulcerative pododermatitis (sore hocks)
• Dermatitis

AGE-RELATED FACTORS
• Anomalous conditions—usually seen in younger animals
• Spondylosis/spinal arthritis—seen in middle-aged to older animals
• Neoplastic conditions—more often seen in middle-aged to older animals

ZOONOTIC POTENTIAL
N/A

PREGNANCY/FERTILITY/BREEDING
Use of corticosteroids is contraindicated

SEE ALSO
See Causes

ABBREVIATIONS
CSF = cerebrospinal fluid
CT = computed tomography
DJD = degenerative joint disease
NSAID = nonsteroidal anti-inflammatory drug

Suggested Reading
Bays TB. Geriatric care of rabbits, guinea pigs, and chinchillas. Vet Clin Exot Anim 2020;23:567–593.
Fisher PG, Künzel F, Rylander H. Neurologic and musculoskeletal disease. In: Quesenberry KE, Carpenter JW, eds. Ferrets, Rabbits and Rodents, 4th Ed). Clinical Medicine and Surgery ed. St. Louis: Saunders, 2020:583–594.
Harkness JE, Turner PV, VandeWoude S, Wheeler CL. Clinical signs and differential diagnoses: nervous and musculoskeletal conditions. In: Harkness JE, Turner PV, VandeWoude S, Wheeler CL, eds. Biology and Medicine of Rabbits and Rodents, 5th ed. Ames: Wiley-Blackwell, 2010:214–216.
Keeble E. Nervous system and musculoskeletal disorders. In: Meredith A, Lord B, eds. BSAVA Manual of Rabbit Medicine. Gloucester: British Small Animal Veterinary Association, 2014:233–248.
Varga M. Neurological and locomotive disorders. In: Varga M, ed. Textbook of Rabbit Medicine, 2nd ed. London, UK: Elsevier, 2014:367–389.

Author Barbara Oglesbee, DVM, DABVP (Avian)

OBESITY

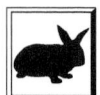

BASICS

DEFINITION
The presence of body fat in sufficient excess to compromise normal physiologic function or predispose to metabolic, surgical, and/or mechanical problems. Obesity has become an extremely common and often debilitating problem in pet rabbits.

PATHOPHYSIOLOGY
• Caging—inactivity is an important risk factor since many pet rabbits are kept in small cages for long periods of time. Most cages sold commercially are inadequate in size. Access to exercise areas is often limited.
• Dietary factors—most commercial pelleted diets are very nutrient dense. Free choice feeding of pellets is one of the primary causes of obesity in rabbits. Most pelleted diets are low in fiber and high in protein, calories, and carbohydrates. The feeding of commercially marketed rabbit treats such as honey sticks, yogurt drops, and pellets containing seed or grains contribute to obesity. Additionally, the high simple carbohydrate content of these treats can cause or exacerbate serious disorders such as gastrointestinal hypomotility and dysbiosis.
• Feeding management—some rabbits will overeat and become obese if pelleted food is left in the cage all day, due to boredom and lack of exercise.
• Animal factors—some rabbits refuse to eat hay or other foods high in coarse, indigestible fiber (this behavior contributes not only to obesity but also to dental disease, hypercalciuria, and GI hypomotility as well). Rabbits with orthopedic, musculoskeletal, or painful disorders may be unwilling or unable to ambulate; inactivity contributes to obesity. Increasing age may also contribute.
• Owner factors—rabbits tend to prefer sweet-tasting treats; overfeeding of these treats contributes to obesity in pet rabbits. Rabbits are often treated as family members, and owners have difficulty denying them these treats.

SYSTEMS AFFECTED
• Musculoskeletal—articular and locomotor problems
• Hepatobiliary—hepatic lipidosis
• Cardiovascular
• Gastrointestinal—GI hypomotility and stasis; dysbiosis associated with inappropriate diets
• Urogenital—hypercalciuria common in obese, sedentary rabbits
• Dermatologic—poor grooming; fecal pasting of perineum; moist dermatitis; pododermatitis; myiasis

SIGNALMENT
• Caged, inactive, middle-aged animals of either gender are at increased risk.
• Dwarf and lop breeds may be predisposed to obesity.

SIGNS
• Excess amounts of body fat for body size, often measured as body condition score of 4 on a 1–5 scale in which 1 = cachectic (>20% underweight), 2 = lean (10%–20% underweight), 3 = moderate, 4 = stout (20%–40% overweight), and 5 = obese (>40% overweight)
• Sites of adipose tissue to evaluate during physical examination include the rib cage, intrabdominal, axilla, and dewlap.
• In some overweight rabbits, fat accumulation in the axillary region is multilobulated and may resemble neoplasia.
• In a normal, nonobese rabbit, the ribs should be palpable without an overlying layer of fat; no rolls of fat should extend over the rear limbs or hindquarters.
• Lethargy, weakness
• Perineal pyoderma, feces, or cecotrophs pasted to perineal region due to inability to groom or consume cecotrophs
• Flaky dermatitis in intrascapular region due to inability to groom
• Moist dermatitis of dewlap in females

CAUSES
• Most commonly, excessive access to pelleted diets and treats, often combined with insufficient activity

RISK FACTORS
• Owner lifestyle
• Diet palatability and energy density
• Cage confinement

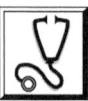

DIAGNOSIS

DIFFERENTIAL DIAGNOSIS
• Intra-abdominal neoplasia or organomegaly
• Similar problems/diseases should be differentiated via history, physical examination, laboratory evaluation, and imaging.

CBC/BIOCHEMISTRY/URINALYSIS
Normal

OTHER LABORATORY TESTS
Normal

IMAGING
Many obese rabbits have a large, radiographically visible, intra-abdominal fat pad located in the retroperitoneal space, surrounding the kidneys and displacing the gastrointestinal tract ventrally.

DIAGNOSTIC PROCEDURES
N/A

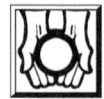

TREATMENT
Success is lifelong amelioration of the problem.

NURSING CARE
• Keep perineum clean, dry, and free of fecal matter.
• Remove matted hair. Be extremely cautious when clipping hair or pulling on mats since rabbit skin is extremely fragile and will easily tear. Sedation may be required.
• Treat secondary dermatitis.
• Provide soft, clean flooring to help prevent secondary pododermatitis.

ACTIVITY
Increase activity level by providing access to exercise areas.

DIET
• Either eliminate or reduce the volume of pelleted foods. A maximum volume of ¼ cup pellets per 5 lbs body weight has been recommended. Switch to a high-fiber, timothy-based pelleted diet.
• Do not feed alfalfa-based pelleted foods or pellet mixes containing seeds and/or dried fruits and vegetables.
• Do not feed commercial rabbit treats or dried fruits as these are more calorie dense.
• Offer a large selection of fresh, moistened greens such as cilantro, romaine lettuce, parsley, carrot tops, dandelion greens, collard greens, broccoli leaves and tops, endive, basil, escarole, kale, swiss chard, chicory, and mustard greens.
• Feed high-quality timothy or grass hay ad lib in addition to fresh greens daily.
• Limit fresh fruits and nonleafy vegetable treats to 2–3 tsp/5 lbs of body weight daily.
• Strictly prohibit simple sugars (such as yogurt drops, candies, or cookies), high starch foods (such as bread products, grains, nuts, cereals, oats, corn, and peas), and legumes.

CLIENT EDUCATION
• Most important part of obesity therapy: must be tailored to each particular circumstance
• In addition to obesity, advise clients that feeding high-calorie, high-carbohydrate, low-fiber diets can lead to gastrointestinal hypomotility, chronic soft stools, hypercalciuria, dental disease, and hepatic lipidosis, all of which can be life threatening.
• Therapeutic suggestions include reasonable, functional weight loss goals, rather than recommending achieving a poorly defined "optimal adult weight" for esthetic reasons.

Keeping a food record that identifies all food sources may help some clients appreciate how many the pet consumes. Suggest that snacks replace regular food rather than supplement it and that the snacks consist of a portion of the regularly allotted food.
• The amount fed should be tailored to the specific needs of individual pets. Caloric requirements reported for rabbits: 2,500 kCal/kg feed for growing, pregnant, or lactating rabbits; 2,100 kCal/kg feed for adult maintenance.

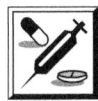

MEDICATIONS
N/A

FOLLOW-UP
PATIENT MONITORING
• Lifelong follow-up and support are essential to maintain the reduced weight.
• At the initial visit, instruct clients to recognize moderate body condition score and to feed the quantity of food necessary to maintain this condition during the changing physiologic and environmental conditions of the pet's life; remind them at checkups.

POSSIBLE COMPLICATIONS
• Never fast rabbits
• Do not make sudden, drastic reductions in available food; may predispose to hepatic lipidosis or GI hypomotility
• Hypercalciuria
• Increased anesthetic risk
• Cardiovascular disease
• Orthopedic disease
• Hepatic lipidosis
• Moist dermatitis, pododermatitis; myiasis

MISCELLANEOUS
ASSOCIATED CONDITIONS
• Orthopedic problems
• Skin problems
• Hypercalciuria
• Respiratory problems
• Hepatic lipidosis

AGE-RELATED FACTORS
N/A

ZOONOTIC POTENTIAL
N/A

PREGNANCY/FERTILITY/BREEDING
Obesity may increase risk of dystocia, but because of potential risk to fetus, do not treat pregnant animals.

SYNONYMS
N/A

SEE ALSO
Diarrhea, chronic, intermittent
Gastrointestinal hypomotility and gastrointestinal stasis
Hypercalciuria and urolithiasis
Pyoderma

ABBREVIATIONS
N/A

Suggested Reading
Bays TB. Geriatric care of rabbits, guinea pigs, and chinchillas. Vet Clin Exot Anim 2020;23:567–593.
Oglesbee B, Lord B. Gastrointestinal diseases of rabbits. In: Quesenberry KE, Carpenter JW, editors. Ferrets, Rabbits and Rodents (4th Ed). Clinical Medicine and Surgery. 2021, St. Louis: Saunders; (2020) 174-187
Varga M. Digestive disorders. In: Varga M, ed. Textbook of Rabbit Medicine, 2nd ed. London, UK: Elsevier, 2014:303–349.
Author Barbara Oglesbee, DVM, DABVP (Avian)

OTITIS EXTERNA AND MEDIA

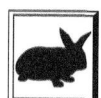

BASICS

OVERVIEW
• Inflammation of the external ear canal—not a diagnosis but descriptions of clinical signs.
• Otitis media may occur as an extension of otitis externa through a ruptured tympanum.
• Otitis media may occur as an extension of upper respiratory infection (rhinitis, sinusitis) via the eustachian tube. In this case, the tympanum may be intact.
• A thorough otic examination, including visualization of the tympanum, should be part of routine physical examination. The normal rabbit ear has a small amount of yellow/beige wax, which may need to be removed with a small curette in order to visualize the tympanum. Dwarf and lop-eared breeds tend to form more wax than other breeds.
• Lop-eared rabbits tend to have stenotic external canals, predisposing to otitis externa
• Rabbits with otitis externa/media have thick, white exudate in the horizontal or vertical canal. Often, this exudate is located deep within the horizontal canal, near the tympanum, and may not be associated with signs of inflammation. A thorough otic examination is required to detect this exudate.
• Some rabbits are asymptomatic—otitis is detected on otic exam
• Exudate is generally extremely caseous, does not drain, and is difficult to flush. Successful removal of all exudate from the horizontal canal can be challenging, requires consistent owner compliance, and frequently involves multiple office visits.
• With chronic infections, an abscess may form at the base of the ear canal.

SIGNALMENT
• Lop-eared rabbits may be more likely to show signs of otitis externa.
• No age or sex predilection

SIGNS

Historical Findings
• Pain—may be manifested by anorexia, holding the ear down, depression, or repeated digging at the floor
• Head shaking
• Scratching at the pinnae
• Malodorous ears (uncommon)

Physical Examination Findings
• Thick, white, creamy exudate in the horizontal and/or vertical canals

• In rabbits with otitis media only, the external canal may have a normal appearance on otoscopic examination; the tympanum may bulge out into the external canal, and a white, creamy exudate may be seen behind the tympanum.
• In some cases, the otic examination appears normal, despite significant otitis media.
• Redness and swelling of the external canal, leading to stenosis
• Swelling of the base of the canal with abscess formation
• Exudate caused by ear mites often forms distinctive, large, tan foliated crusts that may entirely fill the pinna.
• Excessive wax production
• Scaling and exudation—may result in canal obstruction
• Holding the pinna down or tilting the head due to pain
• Alopecia, excoriations at the base of the ear
• Vestibular signs (with head tilt, nystagmus, anorexia, ataxia, and rolling) indicate development of otitis interna/media.

CAUSES
• Parasitic—*Psoroptes cuniculi* (ear mites)
• Bacterial infections—common; *Pasteurella multocida* and Staphylococcus aureus most often cultured from the horizontal canal in otitis externa; *Pasteurella multocida*, *Staphylococcus aureus*, *Pseudomonas aeruginosa*, *E. coli*, and *Listeria monocytogenes* most often cultured in otitis media/interna
• Yeast infections—bacterial infections can be mixed with, or entirely the result of, Malassezia sp. or other yeast species
• Hypersensitivities—rabbits often develop hypersensitivity reactions to many of the topical ear cleaning solutions or medications commonly used in other mammalian species.
• Obstruction—neoplasia, excessive cerumen production, foreign bodies
• Progressive changes—canal hypertrophy, fibrosis, and cartilage calcification
• Otitis media—can produce symptoms on its own; can act as a reservoir for organisms, causing recurrent condition

RISK FACTORS
• Abnormal or breed-related conformation of the external canal (e.g., stenosis, pendulous pinnae) restricts proper air flow into the canal.
• Excessive moisture (e.g., from frequent cleanings with improper solutions) can lead to infection.
• Topical drug reaction and irritation and trauma from abrasive cleaning techniques

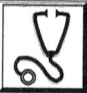

DIAGNOSIS

DIFFERENTIAL DIAGNOSIS

Exudate in the Ear Canal
• Normal wax—most rabbits normally have a light yellow-beige, waxy exudate in the ear canal. Exudate from bacterial otitis is typically creamy white to beige in color. However, white exudate may turn yellow-brown on the surface after drying out and may be mistaken for wax. To differentiate, remove a small amount of dried exudate to reveal white, creamy exudate below.
• Ear mites—intense pruritus primarily located around the ears, head, and neck; occasionally generalized. Thick, brown, beige crusty exudate in the ear canal and extending onto the pinna. With severe infestations, crust layer may be very thick.

Head Tilt
• Rabbits with otitis externa/media may hold the ear down or tilt the head due to pain. This must be differentiated from a head tilt caused by lesions affecting the vestibular apparatus. Rabbits with vestibular dysfunction demonstrate nystagmus, torticollis, ataxia, and/or tremors in addition to head tilt.
• Progression of otitis interna/media may lead to lesions of the vestibular apparatus, so that clinical signs of both may be seen concurrently.

CBC/BIOCHEMISTRY/URINALYSIS
May indicate a primary underlying disease

OTHER LABORATORY TESTS
• Serology for *Pasteurella*—usefulness is severely limited and generally not helpful in the diagnosis of pasteurellosis in pet rabbits. An ELISA is available; however, positive results, even when high, only indicate prior exposure to *Pasteurella* and the development of antibodies, and do not confirm active infection. Low positive results may occur due to cross-reaction with other, nonpathogenic bacteria (false positive). False-negative results are common with immunosuppression or early infection. No evidence exists to support correlation of titers to the presence or absence of disease.

IMAGING
• Bullae radiographs—may demonstrate otitis media; increased soft tissue density in the bullae, bony lysis, or periosteal proliferation. Normal appearance of bullae radiographs does not rule out otitis media. Occasionally, rabbits with severely affected

bullae have normal-appearing radiographs. The bullae are best evaluated using CT scans when available; in many cases, severe abnormalities are found on CT scan even when bullae radiographs appeared normal.

DIAGNOSTIC PROCEDURES
• Gross appearance of the exudate—bacterial infections commonly produce a thick, creamy white exudate; yeast infections commonly produce a yellow-tan thick exudate; however, appearance does not allow an accurate diagnosis of the type of infection; microscopic examination necessary. Ear mites produce a characteristic profuse, tan foliated crusting on the pinnae.
• Microscopic examination of aural exudate—extremely important diagnostic tool. Make preparations from both canals (the contents of the canals may not be the same); spread samples thinly on a glass microscope slide; findings—type(s) of bacteria or yeast—assist in the choice of therapy; WBCs within the exudate—active infection
• Culture of exudate—perform both aerobic and anaerobic culture to identify bacterial pathogens and base antibiotic selection
• Culture of the nasal cavity—to direct antibiotic therapy in rabbits with intact tympanum and evidence of concurrent respiratory infection. In these rabbits, otitis media is assumed to be the result of extension of upper respiratory infections. To obtain a sample, a mini-tip culturette is inserted 1–4 cm inside the nares near the nasal septum. Sedation and appropriate restraint are required to obtain a deep, meaningful sample. The nasal cavity is extremely sensitive, and rabbits that appear sedated may jump or kick when the nasal mucosa is touched. Inadequate sedation or restraint may result in serious spinal or other musculoskeletal injury.
• Skin scrapings from the pinnae—parasites
• Skin biopsy—neoplasia

PATHOLOGIC FINDINGS
N/A

TREATMENT
APPROPRIATE HEALTH CARE
General Comments
• Occasionally, rabbits have thick white exudate in the horizontal canal, preventing visualization of the tympanum, but no signs of inflammation of the ear canal are present. Many of these rabbits are asymptomatic and may remain so lifelong. One study demonstrated that 32% of asymptomatic

rabbits had exudate in the horizontal canal and/or otitis media on necropsy. The decision as to how aggressively one should treat asymptomatic rabbits, or whether to treat at all, is multifactorial; age of the animal, concurrent diseases, owner compliance, and financial issues should be considered. Exudate is generally extremely caseous, does not drain, and can be difficult to flush. Successful removal of all exudate from the horizontal canal can be challenging, requires consistent owner compliance, and frequently involves multiple office visits for cleaning under anesthesia. Occasionally, aggressive cleaning and medication of the ear canal will irritate the lining of the ear canal and/or may cause rupture of the tympanum, resulting in clinical signs of otitis externa and/or interna in a previously asymptomatic rabbit. However, when possible, treatment of asymptomatic animals is recommended, since many of these rabbits are painful (even if that pain is not recognized by the owner), and the ear may serve as a nidus for infection. Early intervention in asymptomatic rabbits may prevent severe disease such as otitis interna or brain abscess from occurring.
• Treatment is indicated in all rabbits showing clinical signs of otitis externa/media.
• Outpatient, unless severe vestibular signs are noted

NURSING CARE
• Ear cleaning under sedation may be helpful in rabbits with large amounts of exudate in the horizontal canal or otitis media. Warmed, physiologic saline is recommended, especially if the tympanum is not intact. Even if the tympanum is intact, use caution with commercial otic cleaning solutions. Rabbits often develop hypersensitivity reactions to many of the topical ear cleaning solutions or medications commonly used in other mammalian species.
• Rabbits with ear mites—do not attempt to clean the ears; not necessary since crusts will fall off following treatment with ivermectin; cleaning can cause painful ulceration and worsening of otitis.

ACTIVITY
No restrictions

DIET
Make sure that the patient continues to eat during treatment to prevent gastrointestinal motility disorders or derangement of enteric flora.

CLIENT EDUCATION
• Chronic otitis can be extremely frustrating to treat, especially once otitis media develops. Successful outcome requires long-term therapy, consistent client compliance, and possibly, surgical intervention.

• Teach clients, by demonstration, the proper method for medicating ears. Proper restraint is critical—severe injury to the back may occur if proper restraint is not employed.

SURGICAL CONSIDERATIONS
• Indicated when the canal is severely stenotic, when medical treatment fails, or when neoplasia is diagnosed
• Medical treatment failure is common. A total ear canal ablation is indicated with aural abscesses or with severe or long-standing disease, especially when aural pain diminishes the quality of life. In most rabbits with disease severe enough to warrant surgery, otitis media is also present, requiring concurrent bullae osteotomy. The two procedures are similar to those performed in dogs and cats. However, careful pain management and the use of antibiotic-impregnated polymethyl methacrylate (AIPMMA) beads are necessary for a successful outcome. Complete excision of all abnormal tissue, followed by filling the defect with long lasting topical anibiotic preparations are needed to prevent postsurgical abscess formation. Unlike dogs and cats, bullae and ear canals in affected rabbits are filled with a thick, caseous exudate, surrounded by a fibrous capsule, and often extend aggressively into surrounding soft tissue and bone. Given the expense and pain involved in these procedures, referral to a specialist may be indicated.

MEDICATIONS
DRUG(S) OF CHOICE
Systemic
• Antibiotics—necessary in most cases of bacterial otitis externa; mandatory when the tympanum has ruptured. Choice of antibiotic is ideally based on results of culture and susceptibility testing. Depending on the severity of infection, long-term antibiotic therapy is required (4–6 weeks minimum, to several months). Use broad-spectrum antibiotics such as enrofloxacin (10–20 mg/kg PO, SC, IM, IV q12h), marbofloxacin (5 mg/kg PO q24h), trimethoprim-sulfa (15–30 mg/kg PO q12h), or chloramphenicol (50 mg/kg PO q8h). Most facial or dental abscesses contain anaerobic bacteria; use antibiotics effective against anaerobes such as azithromycin (15–30 mg/kg PO q24h); can be used alone or combined with metronidazole (20 mg/kg PO q12h). Alternatively, use penicillin G procaine (40,000–60,000 IU/kg SC q24h).

Pain Management
- Butorphanol (0.1–0.5 mg/kg SQ, IM, IV q4–6h); may cause profound sedation; short acting
- Buprenorphine (0.01–0.05 mg/kg SQ, IM IV q8–12h); less sedating, longer acting than butorphanol
- Hydromorphone (0.1 mg/kg SC IM q2–4h) or oxymorphone (0.05–0.2 mg/kg SC IM q8–12h); use with caution; more than 1–2 doses may cause gastrointestinal stasis
- Meloxicam (0.2–0.3 mg/kg SC, IM q24h)
- Carprofen (2–4 mg/kg SC q24h)
- For long-term pain management—meloxicam (0.2–0.5 mg/kg PO, SC, IM q12–24h) or carprofen (1.5 mg/kg PO q12h)
- For sedation—light sedation with midazolam (0.5–2 mg/kg IM) or diazepam (1–2 mg/kg IM); for deeper sedation and longer procedures, the author prefers ketamine (10–20 mg/kg IM) plus midazolam (0.5 mg/kg IM); many other sedation protocols exist

Topical
- For ear mites: Selamectin (Revolution, Pfizer)—12 mg/kg applied topically q30d or Imidacloprid/moxidectin (Advantage-Multi, Bayer)—10 mg/kg (i) + 1 mg/kg (m) topically q30d; one treatment is usually effective
- Bacterial—topical antibiotics (e.g., enrofloxacin, gentocin) or antiyeast drops (miconazole), without corticosteroids; treatment duration is generally longer than in cats and dogs.
- Commercial ear cleansers with cerumenolytics, antiseptics, and astringents available for dogs and cats should be used with caution as some rabbits will develop contact irritation or an allergic response. Routine use of these products at home is not recommended; liquids tend to accumulate in rabbit's deep ear canals.

CONTRAINDICATIONS
- Oral administration of antibiotics that select against gram-positive bacteria (penicillins, macrolides, lincosamides, and cephalosporins) can cause fatal enteric dysbiosis and enterotoxemia.
- Ruptured tympanum—use caution with topical cleansers and medications other than sterile saline or dilute acetic acid; potential for ototoxicity is a concern; controversial
- The use of corticosteroids (systemic or topical in otic preparations) can severely exacerbate otitis.

PRECAUTIONS
- Proper restraint is critical when examining, cleaning, or medicating the ears—severe injury to the back may occur if proper restraint is not employed.
- Postflushing vestibular complications are common, sometimes temporary, but can be permanent if otitis media is present; warn clients of possible complications and residual effects.
- Meloxicam or other NSAIDs—use with caution in rabbits with compromised renal function; monitor renal values
- Oral administration of any antibiotic may potentially cause enteric dysbiosis; discontinue use if diarrhea or anorexia occur.

POSSIBLE INTERACTIONS
Several topical medications may induce contact irritation or allergic response; reevaluate all worsening cases.

ALTERNATIVE DRUGS
N/A

 **FOLLOW-UP**

PATIENT MONITORING
Repeat exudate examinations can assist in monitoring infection.

PREVENTION/AVOIDANCE
Control of underlying diseases

POSSIBLE COMPLICATIONS
- Uncontrolled otitis externa can lead to otitis media, deafness, vestibular disease, cellulitis, facial nerve paralysis, progression to otitis interna, and rarely meningoencephalitis.
- Pain may contribute to GI hypomotility or stasis.

EXPECTED COURSE AND PROGNOSIS
- Otitis externa—often recurs; goal is management rather than cure.
- Otitis media—may take months of systemic antibiotic therapy; most will improve, but many are nonresponsive to medical treatment; guarded to good prognosis with proper surgical treatment

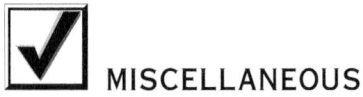 **MISCELLANEOUS**

ASSOCIATED CONDITIONS
Upper respiratory infections
Dental disease
Abscesses
Epiphora

AGE-RELATED FACTORS
N/A

ZOONOTIC POTENTIAL
N/A

PREGNANCY/FERTILITY/BREEDING
N/A

SYNONYMS
N/A

ABBREVIATIONS
CT = computed tomography
ELISA = enzyme-linked immunosorbent assay
GI = gastrointestinal
NSAID = nonsteroidal anti-inflammatory

Suggested Reading
Csomos R, Bosscher G, Mans C, Hardie R. Surgical management of ear diseases in rabbits. Vet Clin Exot Anim 2016;19:189–204.
Fisher PG, Künzel F, Rylander H. Neurologic and musculoskeletal disease. In: Quesenberry KE, Carpenter JW, eds. Ferrets, Rabbits and Rodents, 4th Ed). Clinical Medicine and Surgery ed. St. Louis: Saunders, 2020:583–594.
Keeble E. Nervous system and musculoskeletal disorders. In: Meredith A, Lord B, eds. BSAVA Manual of Rabbit Medicine. Gloucester: British Small Animal Veterinary Association, 2014:233–248.
Mancinelli E, Lennox AM. Management of otitis in rabbits. J Exot Pet Med 2017;26:63–67.
Varga M. Neurological and locomotive disorders. In: Varga M, ed. Textbook of Rabbit Medicine, 2nd ed. London, UK: Elsevier, 2014:367–389.
Author Barbara Oglesbee, DVM, DABVP (Avian)

RABBITS

BASICS

DEFINITION
Inflammation of the middle (otitis media) and inner (otitis interna) ears most commonly caused by bacterial infection

PATHOPHYSIOLOGY
• Most commonly arises from extension of infection from the oral and nasopharyngeal cavities via the eustachian tube (most common) or from extension of external ear infection through the tympanic membrane
• Interna—may also result from hematogenous spread of a systemic infection

SYSTEMS AFFECTED
• Nervous—vestibulocochlear receptors in the inner ear and the facial nerve in the middle ear (peripheral) with possible extension of infection intracranially (central)
• Ophthalmic—cornea and conjunctiva; from exposure and/or lack of tear production after nerve damage
• Gastrointestinal—hypomotility secondary to anorexia from nausea in the acute phase

INCIDENCE/PREVALENCE
One of the most common disorders seen in pet rabbits

GEOGRAPHIC DISTRIBUTION
N/A

SIGNALMENT
• Lop-eared rabbits may be more likely to show signs of otitis externa.
• No age or sex predilection

SIGNS

General Comments
Related to the severity and extent of the infection; may range from none to those related to bulla discomfort and nervous system involvement

Historical Findings
• Most commonly an acute onset of vestibular signs; often severe initially
• Torticollis; can be severe; affected rabbit often unwilling or unable to lift its head off the ground
• Head tilt
• Patient may lean, veer, or roll toward the side affected with peripheral vestibulitis.
• Owners often mistake severe episodes of rolling for seizures.
• Anorexia due to nausea—may occur during the acute phase; rabbits cannot vomit
• Pain manifested as reluctance to chew; shaking the head; pawing at the affected ear; holding the affected ear down; inappetence; reluctance to move; digging at the cage floor
• Facial nerve damage—facial asymmetry; an inability to blink; ocular discharge

Neurologic Examination Findings
• Damage to the associated neurologic structures depends on the severity and location.
• Vestibular portion of cranial nerve VIII—when vestibular portion is affected, there is an ipsilateral head tilt.
• Nystagmus—resting or positional (more common); rotatory or horizontal may be seen; does not appear to aid in differentiating central from peripheral
• Vestibular strabismus—ipsilateral ventral deviation of eyeball with neck extension; may be noted
• Ipsilateral leaning, veering, falling, or rolling
• Facial nerve damage—ipsilateral paresis/paralysis of the ear, eyelids, lips, and nares; may be reduced tear production; with chronic facial nerve paralysis, contracture of the affected side of the face caused by fibrosis of the denervated muscles; deficits can be bilateral

Other Findings
• Evidence of aural erythema, white creamy discharge, and thick and stenotic canals support otitis externa (not always present; extension from eustachian tube more common source of infection)
• White, dull, opaque, and bulging tympanic membrane on otoscopic examination indicates a middle ear exudate.
• In some cases, the otic examination appears normal, despite significant otitis interna/media.
• Nasal discharge, facial abscesses—may be associated
• Abscess at the base of the ear common finding
• Pain—upon opening the mouth or bulla palpation may be detected
• Corneal ulcer—may be caused by inability to blink or a dry eye

CASES
• Bacteria—most common; primary agents include *Pasteurella multocida, Staphylococcus aureus, Pseudomonas aeruginosa, E. coli, Listeria monocytogenes*, and various anaerobes
• Yeast (*Malassezia* sp., *Candida* sp.)—agents to consider
• Mites—*Psoroptes cuniculi* infestation infrequently leads to secondary bacterial infections
• Unilateral disease—usually bacterial; look for foreign bodies, trauma, and tumor

RISK FACTORS
• Immunosuppression (stress, corticosteroid use, concurrent disease, and debility) increases susceptibility to and extension of bacterial infections, especially pasteurellosis.
• Abnormal or breed-related conformation of the external canal (e.g., stenosis, pendulous pinnae) restricts proper air flow into the canal.
• Vigorous ear flush
• Ear cleaning solutions—may be irritating to the middle and inner ear; avoid if the tympanum is ruptured

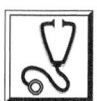

DIAGNOSIS

DIFFERENTIAL DIAGNOSIS
• Be sure that abnormal head posture is not due to holding one ear down due to pain, as may occur in otitis externa alone, and not associated with vestibular pathology; rabbits with vestibular dysfunction demonstrate nystagmus, torticollis, ataxia, and/or tremors in addition to head tilt.
• *Encephalitozoon cuniculi*—this is a diagnosis of exclusion. Every attempt should be made to rule out otic disease prior to assuming *E. cuniculi* infection. Antemortem diagnosis of *E. cuniculi* is usually presumed based on clinical signs, exclusion of other diagnoses, and possibly response to treatment. Definitive antemortem diagnosis is problematic, since a positive antibody titer indicates exposure only, some rabbits respond minimally or not at all to anthelmintic treatment, and many rabbits will improve spontaneously with supportive care alone. Definitive diagnosis requires identification of organisms and characteristic inflammation in tissues that correspond anatomically to observed clinical signs, generally acquired at postmortem examination. Results of several studies demonstrate a poor or no correlation between the severity of CNS lesions on postmortem and clinical signs.
• Idiopathic vestibular disease—not well described in rabbits; however, many rabbits with vestibular signs demonstrate no evidence of concurrent or previous respiratory or otic disease and recover with supportive care alone
• Central vestibular diseases—abscess most common; difficult to differentiate in rabbits; may see lethargy, somnolence, stupor, and other brainstem signs
• Neoplasia—uncommon causes of refractory and relapsing otitis media and interna; diagnosed by imaging of the head
• Trauma—history and physical evidence of injury

CBC/BIOCHEMISTRY/URINALYSIS
• Usually normal; abnormalities may suggest concurrent disease resulting in immunosuppression
• Hemogram—TWBC elevations are usually not seen with bacterial diseases. A relative heterophilia and/or lymphopenia are more common.

OTITIS MEDIA AND INTERNA

OTHER LABORATORY TESTS
• Serologic testing for *E. cuniculi*—many tests are available, but usefulness is extremely limited since a positive titer only indicates exposure and does not confirm *E. cuniculi* as the cause of neurologic signs. *E. cuniculi* can only be definitively diagnosed by finding organisms and resultant lesions on histopathologic examination in areas that anatomically correlate with observed clinical signs. A combination of IgM, IgG, and C-reactive protein appears to be most reliable.
• Serology for *Pasteurella*—usefulness is severely limited and generally not helpful in the diagnosis of pasteurellosis in pet rabbits. An ELISA is available; however, positive results, even when high, only indicate prior exposure to *Pasteurella*, and the development of antibodies, and does not confirm active infection. Low positive results may occur due to cross-reaction with other, nonpathogenic bacteria (false positive). False-negative results are common with immunosuppression or early infection. No evidence exists to support correlation of titers to the presence or absence of disease.

IMAGING
• Bullae radiographs—tympanic bullae may appear cloudy if exudate is present; may see thickening of the bullae and petrous temporal bone with chronic disease; may see lysis of the bone with severe cases of osteomyelitis; may be normal in some rabbits, even with severe otitis interna and/or bullae disease; normal-appearing radiographs do not rule out bullae disease
• CT—superior to radiographs to diagnose bullae disease. Detailed evidence of fluid and soft tissue density within the middle ear and the extent of involvement of the adjacent structures.

DIAGNOSTIC PROCEDURES
• Bacterial culture and sensitivity testing—sample from myringotomy or surgical debridement of tympanic bulla is most accurate
• Culture of the nasal cavity—to direct antibiotic therapy in rabbits with intact tympanum and evidence of concurrent respiratory infection. In these rabbits, otitis media is assumed to be the result of extension of upper respiratory infections. To obtain a sample, a mini-tip culturette is inserted 1–4 cm inside the nares near the nasal septum. Sedation and appropriate restraint are required to obtain a deep, meaningful sample. The nasal cavity is extremely sensitive, and rabbits that appear sedated may jump or kick when the nasal mucosa is touched. Inadequate sedation or restraint

may result in serious spinal or other musculoskeletal injury.
• Microscopic examination of ear swab if otitis externa is also present
• Biopsy—when a tumor or osteomyelitis is suspected

PATHOLOGIC FINDINGS
Purulent exudate within the middle ear cavity surrounded by a thickened bullae and microscopic evidence of degenerative neutrophils with intracellular bacteria; variable degree of osteomyelitis

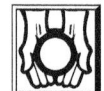

TREATMENT
APPROPRIATE HEALTH CARE
• Inpatient—severe debilitating infection; neurologic signs
• Outpatient—if patient is capable of eating and drinking alone or with assistance, and home nursing care is feasible

NURSING CARE
• Fluid therapy—if unable to eat or drink owing to nausea and disorientation and for rabbits with secondary GI stasis
• Concurrent otitis externa—culture and clean the ear; use warm normal saline if the tympanum is ruptured; if a cleaning solution is used, follow with a thorough flush with normal saline; dry the ear canal with a cotton swab and low vacuum suction; sedation or general anesthesia may be necessary in rabbits with painful ears

ACTIVITY
• Restrict with substantial vestibular signs to avoid injury.
• Encourage return to activity as soon as safely possible; activity may enhance recovery of vestibular function.

DIET
• It is important that the rabbit continue to eat during and following treatment. Many rabbits with vestibular signs will become anorexic. Anorexia will cause GI hypomotility or GI stasis, derangement of the gastrointestinal microflora, and overgrowth of intestinal bacterial pathogens.
• Bring to food to recumbent animals or hand feed.
• If the patient refuses these foods, syringe-feed a gruel such as Critical Care for Herbivores (Oxbow Pet Products) or Emerald Herbivore (Lafeber Company, Cornell, IL) 10–15 mL/kg PO q6–8h. Some rabbits will accept greater volumes more frequently; feed as much as the rabbit will readily accept. Alternatively, pellets can be ground and mixed with fresh greens, vegetable baby foods, water, or juice to form a gruel.

• High-carbohydrate, high-fat nutritional supplements are contraindicated.
• Encourage oral fluid intake by offering fresh water, wetting leafy vegetables.

CLIENT EDUCATION
• Inform client that otitis interna/media can be extremely frustrating to treat, especially in chronic cases. Successful outcome requires long-term therapy, consistent client compliance, and occasionally, surgical intervention.
• Warn client that neurologic signs, especially head tilt and facial nerve paralysis, may persist. Although most rabbits improve and seem to maintain a good quality of life despite residual neurologic deficits, some rabbits improve minimally or not at all, even with aggressive therapy.

SURGICAL CONSIDERATIONS
• Indicated when the canal is severely stenotic, when evidence of middle ear exudate or osteomyelitis refractory is present and refractory to medical management, or when neoplasia is diagnosed.
• Bullae osteotomy—allows drainage of the middle ear cavity; may alleviate discomfort and prevent extension of infection into the brain
• Total ear canal ablation—indicated when otitis media is associated with recurrent otitis externa or neoplasia, especially when aural pain diminishes the quality of life.
• Bullae osteotomy and total ear canal ablation—procedures are similar to those performed in dogs and cats. However, complete excision of all abnormal tissue, careful pain management, and the use a long-acting local antibiotic preparation are necessary for a successful outcome. Unlike dogs and cats, bullae in affected rabbits are filled with a thick, caseous exudate, surrounded by a fibrous capsule, and often extend aggressively into surrounding soft tissue and bone. Given the expense and pain involved in these procedures, refer to a specialist if possible.
• Cytologic examination, both aerobic and anaerobic culture/susceptibility testing of middle ear exudate and histopathologic evaluation of samples of abnormal tissue—perform at the time of surgery

MEDICATIONS
DRUG(S) OF CHOICE
• Systemic antibiotics—choice is ideally based on results of culture and susceptibility testing. Depending on the severity of infection, long-term antibiotic therapy is required (4–6 weeks minimum, to several

months or lifelong treatment in some cases). Use broad-spectrum antibiotics such as enrofloxacin (10–20 mg/kg PO, SC, IM, IV q12h), marbofloxacin (5 mg/kg PO q24h), trimethoprim-sulfa (15–30 mg/kg PO q12h), or chloramphenicol (50 mg/kg PO q8h). Most facial or dental abscesses contain anaerobic bacteria; use antibiotics effective against anaerobes such as azithromycin (15–30 mg/kg PO q24h); can be used alone or combined with metronidazole (20 mg/kg PO q12h). Alternatively, use penicillin G procaine (40,000–60,000 IU/kg SC q24h).
• Topical antibiotics—for treatment of concurrent otitis externa; use antibacterial (e.g., enrofloxacin, gentocin) or antiyeast drops (miconazole) without corticosteroids
• If anorexic, maropitant (2 mg/kg SC, PO q24h) or metoclopramide (0.5–1.0 mg/kg PO, SC, IV q12h)
• Severe vestibular signs (continuous rolling, torticollis) or seizures—diazepam 1–2 mg/kg IM or midazolam 1–2 mg/kg IM during acute phase
• Meclizine 2–12 mg/kg PO q24h may reduce clinical signs, control nausea, and induce mild sedation.

Acute Pain Management
• Butorphanol (0.1–0.5 mg/kg SQ, IM, IV q4–6h); may cause profound sedation; short acting
• Buprenorphine (0.02–0.05 mg/kg SQ, IM IV q8–12h); less sedating, longer acting than butorphanol
• Hydromorphone (0.1 mg/kg SC IM q2–4h) or oxymorphone (0.05–0.2 mg/kg SC IM q8–12h)
• Meloxicam (1 mg/kg PO, SC, IM q24h)
• Carprofen (2–4 mg/kg PO, SC q12–24h)

Long-Term Pain Management
• Nonsteroidal anti-inflammatories—have been used for short- or long-term therapy to reduce pain and inflammation in rabbits with musculoskeletal disease; meloxicam (1.0 mg/kg PO q24h; carprofen (2 mg/kg PO q12h)
• Tramadol—5–15 mg/kg PO q8–12h
• Gabapentin—5–20 mg/kg PO q8–12h

CONTRAINDICATIONS
• Oral administration of antibiotics that select against gram-positive bacteria (penicillins, macrolides, lincosamides, and cephalosporins) can cause fatal enteric dysbiosis and enterotoxemia.
• Topical and systemic corticosteroids— rabbits are very sensitive to the immunosuppressive effects of corticosteroids; use will exacerbate otitis
• Ruptured tympanum or associated neurologic deficits—avoid oil-based or irritating external ear preparations (e.g., chlorhexidine) and aminoglycosides, which are toxic to inner ear structures.

PRECAUTIONS
Avoid rigorously flushing the external ear; this may result in or exacerbate signs of otitis media or interna.

POSSIBLE INTERACTIONS
Several topical otic medications may induce contact irritation or allergic response; reevaluate all worsening cases.

ALTERNATIVE DRUGS
N/A

FOLLOW-UP
PATIENT MONITORING
• Monitor for corneal ulceration—secondary to facial nerve paralysis or abrasion during vestibular episodes
• Evaluate for resolution of signs after 10–14 days or sooner if the patient is deteriorating.

PREVENTION/AVOIDANCE
• Treating otitis or upper respiratory infections in early stages may prevent otitis media/interna and/or brain abscesses

POSSIBLE COMPLICATIONS
• Corneal ulcers
• Signs associated with vestibular and facial nerve damage may persist.
• Severe infections—may spread to the brain stem
• Osteomyelitis of the petrous temporal bone and middle ear cavity effusion—common sequela to severe, chronic infections
• Bulla osteotomy—postoperative complications include facial paralysis, postoperative abscess formation, and onset or exacerbation of vestibular dysfunction.

EXPECTED COURSE AND PROGNOSIS
• Otitis media and interna— may take months of systemic antibiotic therapy; most will improve, but some are nonresponsive to medical treatment
• When medical management is ineffective, a surgical evaluation should be explored.
• Vestibular signs generally do not improve after surgery; surgical treatment is to alleviate discomfort and prevent progression of infection.
• Residual deficits (especially neurologic) cannot be predicted until after a course of therapy; long-term quality of life is good for the majority of rabbits with mild to moderate residual head tilt or facial nerve paralysis.

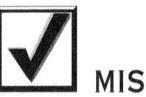

MISCELLANEOUS
ASSOCIATED CONDITIONS
• Upper respiratory infection
• Apical abscesses
• Otitis externa
• GI hypomotility

AGE-RELATED FACTORS
N/A

ZOONOTIC POTENTIAL
N/A

PREGNANCY/FERTILITY/BREEDING
N/A

SYNONYMS
Middle and inner ear infections

SEE ALSO
Encephalitozoonosis
Head tilt (vestibular disease)
Otitis externa and media

ABBREVIATIONS
CT = computed tomography
ELISA = enzyme-linked immunosorbent assay
GI = gastrointestinal
IFA = immunofluorescence assay

Suggested Reading
Csomos R, Bosscher G, Mans C, Hardie R. Surgical management of ear diseases in rabbits. Vet Clin Exot Anim 2016;19:189–204.
Fisher PG, Künzel F, Rylander H. Neurologic and musculoskeletal disease. In: Quesenberry KE, Carpenter JW, editors. Ferrets, Rabbits and Rodents (4th Ed). Clinical Medicine and Surgery. St. Louis: Saunders; 2020. p. 583–594
Keeble E. Nervous system and musculoskeletal disorders. In: Meredith A, Lord B, eds. BSAVA Manual of Rabbit Medicine. Gloucester: British Small Animal Veterinary Association, 2014:233–248.
Mancinelli E, Lennox AM. Management of otitis in rabbits. J Exot Pet Med 2017;26: 63–67.
Varga M. Neurological and locomotive disorders. In: Varga M, ed. Textbook of Rabbit Medicine, 2nd ed. London, UK: Elsevier, 2014:367–389.
Author Barbara Oglesbee, DVM, DABVP (Avian)

PARESIS AND PARALYSIS

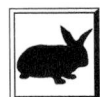

BASICS

DEFINITION
- Paresis—weakness of voluntary movement
- Paralysis—lack of voluntary movement
- Quadriparesis (tetraparesis)—weakness of voluntary movements in all limbs
- Quadriplegia (tetraplegia)—absence of all voluntary limb movement
- Paraparesis—weakness of voluntary movements in pelvic limbs
- Paraplegia—absence of all voluntary pelvic limb movement

PATHOPHYSIOLOGY
- Weakness—may be caused by lesions in the upper or lower motor neuron system. In rabbits, weakness, especially paraparesis, can be due to the effects of systemic or metabolic disease, obesity, or due to structural damage to the CNS or PNS.
- Evaluation of limb reflexes—determine which system (upper or lower motor neuron) is involved
- Upper motor neurons and their axons—inhibitory influence on the large motor neurons of the lower motor neuron system; maintain normal muscle tone and normal spinal reflexes; if injured, spinal reflexes are no longer inhibited or controlled and reflexes become exaggerated or hyperreflexic
- Lower motor neurons or their processes (peripheral nerves)—if injured, spinal reflexes cannot be elicited (areflexic) or are reduced (hyporeflexic)

SYSTEMS AFFECTED
Nervous

SIGNALMENT
No specific age, breed, or gender predisposition

SIGNS

General Comments
Limb weakness—may be acute or gradual onset; most present acutely

Historical Findings
- Owner may describe an abnormal gait; the rabbit may be unable to hop, may walk only, may drag the affected limbs, or may be unable get up.
- Sudden onset of paresis/paralysis is common with traumatic vertebral fractures or luxation and has been described in rabbits with encephalitozoonosis
- Trauma may not have been witnessed. Rabbits can fracture or luxate vertebrae by suddenly jumping while in their cages. History may include startling event such as a loud thunderstorm, fireworks, or unfamiliar people or pets in the house.

- Focal compressive spinal cord diseases often begin with ataxia and progress to weakness and finally to paralysis.
- Urinary incontinence or urine scalding in the perineal region is common in rabbits with paraparesis. Rabbits must be able to assume a normal stance during micturition. Rear limb paresis, paralysis, or pain prevents normal stance, resulting in urine soaking of the perineum and ventrum.
- Alopecia, flaking over the shoulders and tail head—due to inability to properly groom
- Severe obesity may cause locomotor difficulty.

Physical Examination Findings
- Patient usually alert
- If in pain, patient may resent handling and manipulation during the examination.
- Urine scald in the perineal region; dermatitis or alopecia due to inappropriate grooming
- Ulcerative pododermatitis—alopecia, erythema, scabs, or abscesses on the plantar aspect of the feet may occur with chronic rear limb weakness.
- With systemic or metabolic disease—weight loss, depression, or dehydration may be seen

Neurologic Examination Findings
- Confirm that the problem is weakness or paralysis
- Localize problem to either lower or upper motor neuron system
- Paraplegia—bladder may also be paralyzed in rabbits with spinal cord damage, negating voluntary urination

CAUSES

Generalized Quadriplegia
- Cervical spinal cord or multifocal cord diseases: trauma, disk herniation, *Encephalitozoon cuniculi*; neoplasia, malformations, spondylosis, and diskospondylitis

Paraplegia
Front limb paresis with normal rear limbs
- Trauma—bilateral brachial plexus or nerve root injury
- Cord lesion (vascular, *E. cuniculi*, neoplasia, and abscess) at C6–T2 affecting gray matter only
Rear limb paresis
- Trauma (lumbosacral fracture or luxation at L6–L7 most common); disk herniation; *E. cuniculi*; spondylosis; diskospondylitis; degenerative myelopathy (anecdotally reported in rabbits)
- Weakness due to systemic or metabolic disease, dental disease, and severe obesity
  Generalized Quadriplegia with Cranial Nerve Deficits, Seizures, or Stupor
  Diseases of the brain: encephalitis (bacterial, *E. cuniculi*, toxoplasmosis, rabies);

neoplasia; trauma; vascular accidents; congenital or inherited disorders

RISK FACTORS
- Spinal fractures, luxations, or intervertebral disk disease—improper restraint, trauma in caged rabbits suddenly startled, possibly disuse atrophy from confinement
- *Encephalitozoon cuniculi*—immunosuppression (stress, corticosteroid use, and concurrent disease)
- Spondylosis—unknown, possibly related to small cage, lack of exercise, or aging

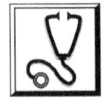

DIAGNOSIS

DIFFERENTIAL DIAGNOSIS

Weak Pelvic Limbs
- Pain or hyperesthesia elicited at site of spinal cord damage usually seen with trauma, IVD disease, discospondylitis, and rarely, bone tumors
- Lack of pain along spinal column—consider *E. cuniculi*, CNS lesions, systemic or metabolic disease; vascular disease (rare), degenerative myelopathy, and neoplasia
- Acute onset—most common with spinal cord trauma, but has been anecdotally reported with *E. cuniculi*
- Gradual onset or intermittent weakness—usually systemic or metabolic disease, spondylosis, occasionally seen with IVD extrusion, if extrusion is gradual
- Other clinical signs—lethargy, weight loss, signs referable to a specific system seen in rabbits with metabolic disease causing weakness; severe obesity
- Spinal reflexes—localize weakness to the cervical, thoracolumbar, or lower lumbar cord segments
- Musculoskeletal disorders—typically produce lameness and a reluctance to move
- Urolithiasis—affected rabbits are painful; postural changes may mimic weakness

CBC/BIOCHEMISTRY/URINALYSIS
Usually normal, unless systemic or metabolic diseases involved (e.g., electrolyte imbalance, and anemia)

OTHER LABORATORY TESTS
- Electrolyte imbalance—correct the problem; see if paresis resolves
- Serologic testing for *E. cuniculi*—many tests are available, but usefulness is extremely limited since a positive titer only indicates exposure and does not confirm *E. cuniculi* as the cause of neurologic signs. *E. cuniculi* can only be definitively diagnosed by finding organisms and resultant lesions on histopathologic examination in areas that anatomically correlate with observed clinical

signs. A combination of IgM, IgG, and C-reactive protein appears to be most reliable.

IMAGING
• Spinal radiographs—lesion localized to the spinal cord; may reveal fracture or luxation, calcified disc, narrowed disc spaces, spondylosis, diskospondylitis, bony tumor, and congenital vertebral malformation
• Skull films—identify dental disease (cause of weakness, chronic debility); severe bullae disease with extension into brain
• Whole body radiographs—identify heart disease, neoplasia, urolithiasis, and orthopedic disorders
• CT—more accurate for evaluation of spine, underlying causes of pain
• Abdominal ultrasonography—if underlying metabolic disease (renal, hepatic) is suspected

DIAGNOSTIC PROCEDURES
• CSF analysis—sample from the cerebellomedullary cistern; may be valuable for evaluating central disease; detect inflammatory process; sample collection may put the patient at risk for herniation if there is a mass or high intracranial pressure. May see increased protein, lymphocyte, and monocytes with *E. cuniculi* infection. Studies were unable to find organism or evidence of organism utilizing PCR testing on CSF.
• Muscle and nerve biopsy—to evaluate patients with generalized lower motor neuron weakness

TREATMENT
APPROPRIATE HEALTH CARE
Inpatient—with severe weakness/paralysis or until bladder function can be ascertained

NURSING CARE
• Bedding—move paralyzed, paretic, or painful rabbits away from soiled bedding, check and clean frequently to prevent urine scalding and moist pyoderma; use padded bedding to help prevent decubital ulcer formation.
• Keep fur clean and dry.
• Turn recumbent patients from side to side four to eight times daily; prevent hypostatic lung congestion and decubital ulcer formation
• Manual expression of the bladder if unable to urinate
• Carts available for small breed dogs can sometimes be fitted for larger rabbits and may be tolerated for limited periods.

ACTIVITY
Restrict until spinal trauma and disk herniation can be ruled out

DIET
• It is imperative that the rabbit continues to eat during and following treatment. Painful animals are often anorectic. Anorexia will often cause GI hypomotility, derangement of the gastrointestinal microflora, and overgrowth of intestinal bacterial pathogens.
• If the patient refuses food, syringe-feed a gruel such as Critical Care for Herbivores (Oxbow Pet Products) or Emeraid Herbivore (Lafeber Company, Cornell, IL) 10–15 mL/kg PO q6–8h. Alternatively, pellets can be ground and mixed with fresh greens, vegetable baby foods, water, or juice to form a gruel.
• High-carbohydrate, high-fat nutritional supplements are contraindicated.
• Encourage oral fluid intake by offering fresh water and by wetting leafy vegetables. Place water bottles or dishes within reach of recumbent rabbits.

MEDICATIONS
DRUG(S) OF CHOICE
• Nonsteroidal anti-inflammatories—have been used for short- or long-term therapy to reduce pain and inflammation in rabbits with musculoskeletal disease; meloxicam (1.0 mg/kg PO q24h; carprofen (2 mg/kg PO q12h)
• Tramadol—5–15 mg/kg PO q8–12h
• Gabapentin—5–20 mg/kg PO q8–12h
• Corticosteroids have been used in rabbits with disc extrusion or spinal cord trauma with some success. Although clinical improvement has been anecdotally reported, rabbits are very sensitive to the immunosuppressive and gastrointestinal side effects of corticosteroids; immunosuppression may exacerbate subclinical bacterial infections or *E. cuniculi*.
• With acute spinal trauma (fracture/luxation) or disk herniation only—Methylprednisolone sodium succinate administered IV may be of benefit. Reported canine dose—30 mg/kg IV followed by 15 mg/kg 2 and 6 hours later; doses for rabbits not reported.

CONTRAINDICATIONS
• Oral administration of antibiotics that select against gram-positive bacteria (penicillins, macrolides, lincosamides, and cephalosporins) can cause fatal enteric dysbiosis and enterotoxemia.
• Corticosteroids—do not use with diskospondylitis or other infectious diseases

PRECAUTIONS
• Corticosteroids—use with caution, only in acute spinal trauma; associated with gastrointestinal ulceration and hemorrhage,

delayed wound healing, and heightened susceptibility to infection; rabbits are very sensitive to the immunosuppressive effects of both topical and systemic corticosteroids; use may exacerbate subclinical bacterial infection

ALTERNATIVE DRUGS
• Chondroitin sulfate (Cosequin, Nutramax) has been used anecdotally using feline dosage protocols; polysulfated glycosaminoglycan (Adequan, Luitpold) 2.2 mg/kg SC, IM q3d × 21–28 days, then q14d.
• Acupuncture may be effective for rabbits with chronic pain.
• For acute spinal trauma—prednisolone (0.25 mg/kg q12h × 5d); dexamethasone (0.5–2 mg/kg IV, IM); use with caution

FOLLOW-UP
PATIENT MONITORING
• Neurologic examinations—daily to monitor status
• Bladder—evacuate (via manual expression or catheterization) three to four times a day to prevent overdistension and subsequent bladder atony; once bladder function has returned, patient can be managed at home.
• Monitor for uremia secondary to urine retention.

POSSIBLE COMPLICATIONS
• Urinary tract infection, bladder atony, urine scalding and pyoderma, constipation, decubital ulcer formation; myiasis
• Exacerbation of bacterial infections (possibly life threatening), hepatic abscesses, and gastric ulceration with corticosteroid usage
• Myelomalacia—with severe spinal cord trauma or disk herniations
• Permanent paralysis

EXPECTED COURSE AND PROGNOSIS
• Depends on the cause
• Insufficient information exists on the prognosis following surgery for intervertebral disc disease in rabbits.
• Rabbits with rear limb paresis or paralysis due to mild to moderate spinal disease may regain partial or full function with exercise restriction, supportive care, and long-term administration of NSAIDs, depending on the cause.
• Most paralyzed rabbits with severe spinal trauma (fracture, luxation) do not regain mobility; euthanasia may be warranted; rate of complicating conditions (bladder, cutaneous) is very high; quality of life often poor

RABBITS

• Wheeled carts manufactured for small dogs have been used successfully in a limited number of rabbits.

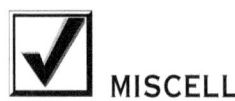 **MISCELLANEOUS**

ASSOCIATED CONDITIONS
• Gastrointestinal hypomotility
• Hypercalciuria
• Ulcerative pododermatitis (sore hocks)
• Dermatitis

ZOONOTIC POTENTIAL
N/A

ABBREVIATIONS
CNS = central nervous system
CSF = cerebrospinal fluid
CT = computed tomography
GI = gastrointestinal
IVD = intervertebral disc
NSAID = nonsteroidal anti-inflammatory drug
PNS = peripheral nervous system

Suggested Reading
Bays TB. Geriatric care of rabbits, guinea pigs, and chinchillas. Vet Clin Exot Anim 2020;23:567–593.
Fisher PG, Künzel F, Rylander H. Neurologic and musculoskeletal disease. In: Quesenberry KE, Carpenter JW, eds. Ferrets, Rabbits and Rodents, 4th Ed). Clinical Medicine and Surgery ed. St. Louis: Saunders, 2020:583–594.
Harkness JE, Turner PV, VandeWoude S, Wheeler CL. Clinical signs and differential diagnoses: nervous and musculoskeletal conditions. In: Harkness JE, Turner PV,

VandeWoude S, Wheeler CL, eds. Biology and Medicine of Rabbits and Rodents, 5th ed. Ames: Wiley-Blackwell, 2010:214–216.
Keeble E. Nervous system and musculoskeletal disorders. In: Meredith A, Lord B, eds. BSAVA Manual of Rabbit Medicine. Gloucester: British Small Animal Veterinary Association, 2014:233–248.
Varga M. Neurological and locomotive disorders. In: Varga M, ed. Textbook of Rabbit Medicine, 2nd ed. London, UK: Elsevier, 2014:367–389.

Author Barbara Oglesbee, DVM, DABVP (Avian)

BASICS

DEFINITION
• A bacterial disease that can be a cause of rhinitis, sinusitis, otitis, conjunctivitis, dacryocystitis, pleuropneumonia, bacteremia, and abscesses in subcutaneous tissues, bone, joints, or internal organs in rabbits; caused by many different serotypes of *Pasteurella*.
• Often a copathogen with other bacterial causes of rhinitis or sinusitis

PATHOPHYSIOLOGY
• *Pasteurella multocida*—a gram-negative, nonmotile cocobacillus; aerobic and facultatively anaerobic
• Transmission may be by direct contact, aerosol, or fomites; most rabbits are infected at birth from does with vaginal infection, or shortly after birth.
• Colonizes the nasal cavity and upper respiratory tract; can remain subclinical or eliminated if host's defenses are intact
• May cause rhinitis initially; may spread into the sinuses and bones of the face and/or spread via the eustachian tubes to the ears, via the nasolacrimal duct to the eye, via the trachea to the lower respiratory tract, and hematogenously to joints, bones, and other organ systems
• Not all infected rabbits become clinically ill. Outcome of infection depends on virulence of serotype and host's defenses. More virulent serotypes produce toxins that may cause nasal turbinate atrophy; purified toxin may produce pleuritis, pneumonia, and osteoclastic bone resorption; endotoxin in plasma may cause fever, depression, and shock.
• Often a coinfection with other bacteria: *Staphylococcus aureus*, *Bordetella bronchiseptica*, *Moraxella catarrhalis*, *Pseudomonas aeruginosa*, *Mycobacterium* spp., and various anaerobes are all as common.
• Several outcomes possible, including (1) elimination of infection, (2) chronic subclinical infection, (3) development of clinical signs that improve with antibiotic therapy and recur following discontinuation of therapy, and (4) chronic, progressive disease

SYSTEMS AFFECTED
• Respiratory—mucosa of the upper respiratory tract, including the nasal cavities, sinuses, and nasopharynx
• Ophthalmic—extension to the eyes via nasolacrimal duct
• Musculoskeletal—extension of infection into bones of the skull
• Neurologic—extension of infection through eustachian tube causing vestibular signs from otitis interna/media; extension into CNS; extension into joints/bones
• Potential cause of abscess formation in any organ system via hematogenous spread

GENETICS
Genetic susceptibility not well known

INCIDENCE/PREVALENCE
• True incidence in pet population unknown
• Many infections are subclinical

GEOGRAPHIC DISTRIBUTION
Worldwide

SIGNALMENT
No breed, age, or gender predilections

SIGNS

General Comments
Disease severity has a wide range—subclinical to mild, moderate, and severe clinical disease, especially in stressed rabbits

Historical Findings
• Usually begins with rhinitis: sneezing, nasal discharge, staining of the front paws
• Ptyalism, facial swelling, anorexia with sinusitis
• Epiphora, ocular discharge with extension into the eyes via nasolacrimal duct or blockage of the nasolacrimal duct
• Head tilt, rolling, nystagmus, and other vestibular signs with extension into the ears via eustachian tubes or CNS
• Dyspnea with severe rhinitis (rabbits are obligate nasal breathers), pneumonia, or large intrathoracic abscesses
• Anorexia, depression, pain from skeletal abscesses; often only clinical sign intrathoracic or hepatic abscesses until abscess is large enough to cause space-occupying effects
• Lameness, reluctance to move with plantar or digital abscesses
• Subcutaneous swelling with mammary abscess

Physical Examination Findings
• No clinical signs in rabbits with subclinical disease
• Depend on area of body involved
• Sneezing
• Serous to purulent nasal discharge
• Epiphora, purulent ocular discharge, exophthalmia, intraocular abscess
• Facial swelling, ptyalism
• Fever, malaise, depression, anorexia
• Head tilt, torticollis, nystagmus, scratching at ears
• Dyspnea, tachypnea
• Lameness, reluctance to move, single to multiple swellings with limb abscesses

CAUSES
Any one of many serotypes of *Pasteurella*

RISK FACTORS

Disease Agent Factors
Pasteurella serotype—virulence factors, infectious dose

Host Factors that Increase Susceptibility
• Age—neonatal/young rabbits; immature immune system
• Overall health status—debilitated animals: other concurrent disease (especially other respiratory bacterial pathogens)
• Stress is an important determining factor in outcome of disease.
• Corticosteroid use can severely exacerbate disease; activation of subclinical infection; hepatic abscesses common

Environmental Factors
• Poor husbandry—dirty bedding (increased ammonia concentrations) and poor nutrition contribute to stress
• Overcrowding
• Grooming habits may result in contaminated hair coat, environment, and feed and water dishes.

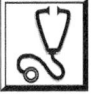

DIAGNOSIS

DIFFERENTIAL DIAGNOSIS
• Head or facial abscesses—nearly all are the result of dental disease; tooth root abscesses are caused by anaerobic bacterial and/or *Streptococcus* spp.; *Pasteurella* usually not a contributing pathogen
• Nasal discharge—other bacterial infection (*Staphylococcus aureus*, *Bordetella bronchiseptica*, *Moraxella catarrhalis*, *Pseudomonas aeruginosa*, *Mycobacterium* spp., and various anaerobes all are common causes of URI; may be copathogen with *Pasteurella*); dental disease; periapical or tooth root abscesses; elongated maxillary tooth roots penetrating into nasal passages with secondary bacterial infection; foreign body (mostly inhaled grass and seeds); allergic or irritant (inhaled pollen, moldy bedding, dusty litter, bleach or cigarette smoke); mycotic infection (rare)
• Dyspnea—laryngeal swelling from traumatic intubation, other upper airway obstruction, thoracic neoplasia, and cardiovascular disease
• Facial swelling—primary dental disease, abscess from other bacteria, neoplasia, mycoses (rare)
• Epiphora—incisor root impaction or abscess blocking the nasolacrimal duct, primary conjunctivitis, irritation
• Head tilt, vestibular signs—other causes of otitis interna/media; neoplasia, *Encephalitozoon cuniculi*

RABBITS

• Lameness, reluctance to move—orthopedic injury, spinal cord disease, pain

CBC/BIOCHEMISTRY/URINALYSIS
Hemogram—TWBC elevations are usually not seen with bacterial diseases. A relative neutrophilia and/or lymphopenia are more common.

OTHER LABORATORY TESTS
• Serology for *Pasteurella*—ELISA—high IG G results may corelate with active infection. Low positive results may occur due to cross-reaction with other, nonpathogenic bacteria (false positive). False-negative results are common with immunosuppression or early infection. Titers may not correlate well to the presence or absence of disease. Test may be useful to monitor SPF colonies.
• *Pasteurella* PCR assay may also be performed on samples taken from deep nasal swabs. PCR may be more sensitive in detecting the presence of *Pasteurella*; however, it should be combined with anaerobic and aerobic culture to identify other bacterial primary or copathogens.

IMAGING
• Thoracic radiographs are indicated in rabbits with bacterial rhinitis. Subclinical pneumonia is common; often detected only radiographically. Lung abscesses are also common and can be seen radiographically.
• Skull radiographs—must be taken under heavy sedation. Useful to rule out dental disease; may see turbinate atrophy, bone destruction in severe cases
  ○ Bony lysis or proliferation of the turbinate and facial bones important radiographic finding, consistent with chronic bacterial or neoplastic invasion
  ○ Assess the apical roots of all teeth.
• CT scans are extremely helpful in detecting the extent of bony changes associated with pasteurellosis and to rule out other causes of nasal discharge.

DIAGNOSTIC PROCEDURES
• Cytology—nasal swab or flush rarely yields diagnostic sample; nonspecific inflammation is most commonly found
• Cultures—may be difficult to interpret, since commonly isolated bacteria (e.g., *Bordetella*) often represent only commensal organisms or opportunistic pathogens. Deep cultures obtained by inserting a mini-tipped culturette 2–4 cm into each nostril are sometimes reliable. However, samples taken from the nares should not be overinterpreted, since the causative agent may be located only deep within the sinuses, and not present at the rostral portion of the nostrils, where samples are readily accessible.
• A lack of growth does not rule out *Pasteurella*, since the infection may be in an inaccessible, deep area of the nasal cavity or sinuses, and *Pasteurella* is sometimes difficult to grow on culture.

PATHOLOGIC FINDINGS
Nasal turbinate atrophy, bony lysis, abscess formation

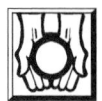

TREATMENT
APPROPRIATE HEALTH CARE
Outpatient treatment is acceptable unless surgery is required or the patient is exhibiting signs of systemic illness in addition to nasal discharge.

NURSING CARE
• Varies according to severity and location of disease
• Symptomatic treatment and nursing care are important in the treatment of rabbits with sneezing and nasal discharge. Patient hydration, nutrition, warmth, and hygiene (keeping nares clean) are important.
• Humidification of environment often helps mobilize nasal discharge; enhances patient comfort
• Saline (hypertonic or normal) nebulization may be helpful to humidify airways in rabbits with chronic rhinitis or sinusitis.
• Oxygen supplementation, low-stress environment important in rabbits with dyspnea
• If epiphora or ocular discharge is present, always cannulate and flush the nasolacrimal duct. Topical administration of an ophthalmic anesthetic is generally sufficient for this procedure.
• Postoperative wound care, bandaging necessary in rabbits treated for abscesses

ACTIVITY
Restricted in dyspneic and postsurgical patients

DIET
• If the patient refuses food, syringe-feed a gruel such as Critical Care for Herbivores (Oxbow Pet Products) or Emeraid Herbivore (Lafeber Company, Cornell, IL) 10–15 mL/kg PO q6–8h. Alternatively, pellets can be ground and mixed with fresh greens, vegetable baby foods, water, or juice to form a gruel.
• Encourage oral fluid intake by offering fresh water from multiple sources, wetting leafy vegetables

CLIENT EDUCATION
• If disease is chronic, warn client that a cure is unlikely. The goal of treatment is to control the more severe clinical signs with medication and that treatment may be lifelong.

• Abscesses of the head, and those involving bone, have a guarded to poor prognosis for complete resolution. Most will require extensive surgery, sometimes multiple surgeries and multiple follow-up visits. Recurrences in the same or other locations are common. Clients must be aware of the monetary and time investment.

SURGICAL CONSIDERATIONS
• Unlike in cats and dogs, simple lancing, flushing, and draining are not adequate to treat rabbit abscesses. Rabbit abscesses are filled with a thick, caseous exudate, surrounded by a fibrous capsule and often extending aggressively into surrounding soft tissue and bone. Abscesses with bony involvement (facial, plantar, joints) can be extremely difficult to treat, requiring surgical intervention and prolonged medical care.
• Abscesses—en bloc excision of entire abscess, leaving wide margins; exercise care not to rupture capsule; debridement must be followed by local treatment until no evidence of infection exists.
• Placement of penrose or similar drains is contraindicated.

MEDICATIONS
DRUG(S) OF CHOICE
• Choice of antibiotic is ideally based on results of culture and susceptibility testing. Depending on the severity of infection, long-term antibiotic therapy is required (4–6 weeks minimum to several months or intermittent, to lifelong in severe, refractory cases)
• Antibiotics effective against *Pasteurella* include enrofloxacin (10–20 mg/kg PO, SC, IM, IV q12h), marbofloxacin (5 mg/kg PO q24h), trimethoprim-sulfa (15–30 mg/kg PO q12h), chloramphenicol (50 mg/kg PO q8h), or penicillin G procaine (40,000–60,000 IU/kg SC q24h).
• Nebulization—used in conjunction with systemic treatment. Nebulize for 15 minutes 1–3 times daily. Choices include: enrofloxacin 100 mg in 10 mL saline; doxycycline 200 mg in 15 mL saline; gentamicin 50 mg I 10 mL saline; and amikacin 50 mg in 10 mL saline

CONTRAINDICATIONS
• Oral administration of antibiotics that select against gram-positive bacteria (penicillins, macrolides, lincosamides, and cephalosporins) can cause fatal enteric dysbiosis and enterotoxemia.
• The use of corticosteroids (systemic or topical in otic preparations) can severely exacerbate bacterial infection.

RABBITS

(CONTINUED)

• Topical nasal decongestants containing phenylephrine can exacerbate nasal inflammation and cause nasal ulceration and purulent rhinitis.

PRECAUTIONS
• Chloramphenicol—avoid human contact with chloramphenicol due to potential blood dyscrasia. Advise owners of potential risks.
• Nebulization or oral administration of any antibiotic may potentially cause enteric dysbiosis; discontinue use if diarrhea or anorexia occurs.

POSSIBLE INTERACTIONS
N/A

ALTERNATIVE DRUGS
N/A

FOLLOW-UP

PATIENT MONITORING
Clinical assessment and monitoring for relapse of clinical signs

PREVENTION/AVOIDANCE
Avoid stressful conditions, corticosteroid use; provide excellent diet and husbandry

POSSIBLE COMPLICATIONS
• Extension of infection into the brain, mouth, eyes, ears, or lungs
• Loss of appetite
• Dyspnea as a result of nasal obstruction

EXPECTED COURSE AND PROGNOSIS
• Prognosis depends on chronicity, strain of bacteria, and host factors

• Chronic infection prognosis guarded to poor for complete resolution of clinical signs, depending on invasiveness (e.g., poor with extensive turbinate destruction, CNS signs). Many will remain comfortable on lifelong antibiotic therapy.
• Thoracic abscess—usually not amenable to surgical treatment; treat with supportive care, long-term antibiotics; and fair to grave prognosis depending on location
• Recovered animals may shed *Pasteurella* intermittently.

MISCELLANEOUS

ASSOCIATED CONDITIONS
N/A

AGE-RELATED FACTORS
N/A

ZOONOTIC POTENTIAL
Pasteurella can infect humans, but there are no reports of disease in humans as a result of rabbit transmission

PREGNANCY/FERTILITY/BREEDING
• May complicate disease
• Abortion may be a sequela to infection
• Kits can be infected in the womb or when nursing

SYNONYMS
Snuffles

ABBREVIATIONS
CT = computed tomography
ELISA = enzyme-linked immunosorbent assay
GI = gastrointestinal
PCR = polymerase chain reaction
SPF = specific pathogen free
URI = upper respiratory infection

Suggested Reading
Capello V, Lennox AM. Diagnostic imaging of the respiratory system in exotic companion mammals. Vet Clin Exot Anim 2011;14:369–389.
DeCubellis J. Common emergencies in rabbits, guinea pigs, and chinchillas. Vet Clin Exot Anim 2016;19:411–429.
Hedley J. Respiratory disease. In: Meredith A, Lord B, eds. BSAVA Manual of Rabbit Medicine. Gloucester: British Small Animal Veterinary Association, 2014:160–167.
Jekl V. Respiratory disorders in rabbits. Vet Clin Exot Anim 2021;24:459–482.
Lennox AM, Mancinelli E. Respiratory diseases. In: Quesenberry KE, Carpenter JW, eds. Ferrets, Rabbits and Rodents, 4th Ed). Clinical Medicine and Surgery ed. St. Louis: Saunders, 2020:188–201.
Varga M. Cardiorespiratory diseases. In: Varga M, ed. Textbook of Rabbit Medicine, 2nd ed. London, UK: Elsevier, 2014:390–405.

Author Barbara Oglesbee, DVM, DABVP-Avian

PINWORMS (OXYURIDS)

BASICS

OVERVIEW
• Pinworms in rabbits—caused by the oxyurid *Passalurus ambiguus*
• These small worms can inhabit the cecum, small intestine, and colon.
• Pinworms are generally considered to be nonpathogenic, rarely cause clinical signs, and may be an incidental finding at necropsy.
• Transmission is fecal-oral; eggs are passed in the feces and ingested by the same or other rabbits in the environment.
• The rabbit pinworm is host specific.

SIGNALMENT
No age, gender, or breed predilection

SIGNS
Historical Findings
• Usually asymptomatic
• May cause moderate to severe perianal pruritus
• Poor reproductive performance in breeding colonies

Physical Examination Findings
• Perianal dermatitis possible
• Poor hair coat, weight loss, or rectal prolapse possible (rare) with heavy infestation
• May be an incidental finding during abdominal surgery or necropsy

CAUSES AND RISK FACTORS
• *Passalurus ambiguus*
• Infected rabbits in the environment
• Food or environment contaminated with feces

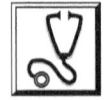

DIAGNOSIS

DIFFERENTIAL DIAGNOSIS
For perineal pruritus/dermatitis—urine scald, fleas, contact dermatitis; all are more common causes

CBC/BIOCHEMISTRY/URINALYSIS
Usually normal

OTHER LABORATORY TESTS
N/A

IMAGING
N/A

DIAGNOSTIC PROCEDURES
• Ova or adult worms can be identified in fecal float or fecal direct smear (not usually found on fur around anus)
• See adult worms around anus or incidentally found in cecum or colon during abdominal surgery or necropsy
• Worms are sexually dimorphic; male pinworms are 300 μm in diameter, 4.1 mm long, and have a single curved spicule; females are slightly longer (6.6 mm) and have a long tail.

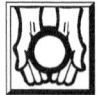

TREATMENT

• Usually asymptomatic—no treatment is indicated if found incidentally (e.g., at surgery)
• Treat if symptomatic, or if owners see worms around anus.
• Clean adult pinworms from perineal area
• Treat secondary perianal pyoderma, if present
• Recurrence is common, even in rabbits housed alone, since rabbits ingest their own feces and continue to reinfect themselves.

MEDICATIONS

DRUG(S) OF CHOICE
Adulticide/Larvicide Anthelmintics
• Fenbendazole (10–20 mg/kg once, repeat in 10–14 days)
• Thiabendazole (50 mg/kg PO once, repeat in 10–14 days)
• Retreatment may be required.
• Treat all rabbits in the environment.

CONTRAINDICATIONS
Ivermectin is not effective.

FOLLOW-UP

Monitor fecal egg counts posttreatment.

MISCELLANEOUS

ZOONOTIC POTENTIAL
Host-specific parasite; not transmissible to humans

Suggested Reading
Debenham JJ, Brinchmann T, Sheen J, Vella D. Radiographic diagnosis of small intestinal obstruction in pet rabbits (*Oryctolagus cuniculus*): 63 cases. J Sm Anim Pract 2019;60:691–696.
DeCubellis J. Common emergencies in rabbits, guinea pigs, and chinchillas. Vet Clin Exot Anim 2016;19:411–429.
Hartcourt-Brown F. Digestive system disease. In: Meredith A, Lord B, eds. BSAVA Manual of Rabbit Medicine. Gloucester: British Small Animal Veterinary Association, 2014:168–190.
Oglesbee B, Lord B. Gastrointestinal diseases of rabbits. In: Quesenberry KE, Carpenter JW, eds. Ferrets, Rabbits and Rodents, 4th Ed). Clinical Medicine and Surgery. 2021 ed. St. Louis: Saunders, 2020:174–187.
Varga M. Digestive disorders. In: Varga M, ed. Textbook of Rabbit Medicine, 2nd ed. London, UK: Elsevier, 2014:303–349.
Author Barbara Oglesbee, DVM, DABVP (Avian)

PNEUMONIA (LOWER RESPIRATORY TRACT INFECTION)

BASICS

DEFINITION
Bronchitis, pneumonia, and pulmonary abscesses are common sequalae to bacterial upper respiratory infections. Mycotic infection or inhaled foreign material in lung parenchyma may also occur.

PATHOPHYSISOLOGY
• Bacteria most common cause—enter the lower respiratory tract primarily by inhalation, aspiration, or hematogenous routes; infections incite an overt inflammatory reaction.
• Oropharyngeal bacteria—frequently aspirated; may be present for an unknown interval in the normal tracheobronchial tree and lung; have the potential to cause or complicate respiratory infection
• Respiratory infection—development depends on the complex interplay of many factors: size, inoculation site, number of organisms and their virulence, and resistance of the host
• Leukocytes infiltrate the airways and alveoli; consolidation, ischemia, tissue necrosis, and atelectasis owing to bronchial occlusion, obstructive bronchiolitis, and impaired collateral ventilation
• Abscess formation in lung parenchyma and/or pleural space is common; rabbits' abscesses are filled with a thick, caseous exudate, surrounded by a fibrous capsule. They can be either slow growing or become large very quickly and often extend aggressively into surrounding soft tissue and bone.
• Mortality—associated with severe hypoxemia (low arterial oxygen concentration) and sepsis

SYSTEMS AFFECTED
Respiratory—primary or secondary infection

GEOGRAPHIC DISTRIBUTION
Widespread

SIGNALMENT
No breed, age, or gender predilection

SIGNS

Historical Findings
• History of previous upper respiratory disease—nasal discharge, ocular discharge, sneezing, facial abscess, and ptyalism
• Anorexia, weight loss, and/or lethargy often only complaint
• Exercise intolerance—difficult to recognize in caged rabbits
• Labored breathing—usually late in the course of disease
• Coughing not seen in rabbits

Physical Examination Findings
• Lethargy
• Weight loss
• Fever
• Dehydration
• Dyspnea
• Abnormal breath sounds on auscultation—increased intensity or bronchial breath sounds, crackles, and wheezes; decreased or absent breath sounds with pulmonary abscesses. In rabbits with concurrent upper respiratory disease, referred sounds can make thoracic auscultation difficult; obtain thoracic radiographs if pneumonia is suspected
• Serous or mucopurulent nasal discharge, ocular discharge, facial abscess, dental disease, and ptyalism
• Anorexic rabbits—may show signs of GI hypomotility; scant dry feces, dehydration, firm stomach or cecal contents, gas-filled intestinal loops

CAUSES
• Bacterial—*Staphylococcus aureus, Bordetella bronchiseptica, Moraxella catarrhalis, Pseudomonas aeruginosa, Mycobacterium* spp., *Pasteurella multocida*, and various anaerobes have been implicated
• Mycotic—*Aspergillus* spp. and *Cryptococcus* spp. have been anecdotally reported; appears to be very rare, but should be considered
• Aspiration pneumonia—common cause secondary to choking episode. Rabbits do not vomit.

RISK FACTORS

Disease Agent Factors
Bacterial serotype, virulence factors, infectious dose

Host Factors that Increase Susceptibility
• Age—neonatal/young rabbits; immature immune system
• Overall health status—debilitated animals: other concurrent disease, stress, and corticosteroid use
• Dental disease—periapical or tooth root abscesses, fractured teeth; malocclusion causing sharp points on crowns penetrate oral mucosal; provide entry route for bacteria
• Dysphagia, aspiration
• Reduced level of consciousness—stupor, coma, and anesthesia

Environmental Factors
• Grooming habits may result in bacteria-contaminated hair coat, which contaminates environment and feed and water dishes
• Close contact may spread bacterial infection
• Poor husbandry—dirty, molding bedding; poor nutrition
• Inhaled irritants—ammonia buildup from urine-soaked bedding, dusty hay, bleach or other disinfectants, smoke

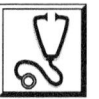

DIAGNOSIS

DIFFERENTIAL DIAGNOSIS
• Bacterial rhinitis or foreign body—rabbits are obligate nasal breathers and may become dyspneic with severe upper respiratory disease.
• Chronic sinusitis
• Thymoma or thymic lymphoma
• Congestive heart failure
• Heat stroke
• Electrocution
• Fluid overload
• Dyspnea from abdominal distension
• Tachypnea from pain, fear, heat stroke, or metabolic disease

CBC/BIOCHEMISTRY/URINALYSIS
• Hemogram—TWBC elevations are usually not seen with bacterial diseases. A relative neurtrophilia and/or lymphopenia are more common.

OTHER LABORATORY TESTS
• Serology for *Pasteurella*—ELISA—high IG G results may corelate with active infection. Low positive results may occur due to cross-reaction with other, nonpathogenic bacteria (false positive). False-negative results are common with immunosuppression or early infection. Titers may not correlate well to the presence or absence of disease. Test may be useful to monitor SPF colonies.
• *Pasteurella* PCR assay may also be performed on samples taken from deep nasal swabs. PCR may be more sensitive in detecting the presence of *Pasteurella*; however, it should be combined with anaerobic and aerobic culture to identify other bacterial primary or copathogens.

IMAGING

Thoracic Radiography
• Alveolar pattern characterized by increased pulmonary densities; air bronchograms, pulmonary abscesses; lobar consolidation; pleural fluid
• Obese rabbits often have intrathoracic fat that should not be misinterpreted as pulmonary abscess or pneumonia.

Ultrasound, CT
Distinguish pulmonary abscess from neoplasia, obtain fluid samples with effusion

DIAGNOSTIC PROCEDURES
• Microbiologic and cytologic examinations—LRT samples—transtracheal washing and bronchoalveolar lavage

PNEUMONIA (LOWER RESPIRATORY TRACT INFECTION)   (CONTINUED)

• Fine-needle lung aspiration can be performed under ultrasound guidance.
• Thoracentesis—fluid analysis with effusions

PATHOLOGIC FINDINGS

Gross
• Irregular consolidation of lung parenchyma
• Multifocal white nodules of caseous exudates of varying size within lung parenchyma
• Palpable firmness of the tissue

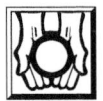

TREATMENT

APPROPRIATE HEALTH CARE
Inpatient—recommended with multisystemic signs (e.g., anorexia, fever, weight loss, and lethargy)

NURSING CARE
• Maintain normal systemic hydration—important to aid mucociliary clearance and secretion mobilization; use a balanced multielectrolyte solution
• Nebulization with normal saline—may contribute to a more rapid resolution if used in conjunction with antibiotics
• Oxygen therapy—for respiratory distress

ACTIVITY
Restrict during treatment (inpatient or outpatient)

DIET
• If the patient refuses food, syringe-feed a gruel such as Critical Care for Herbivores (Oxbow Pet Products) or Emeraid Herbivore (Lafeber Company, Cornell, IL) 10–15 mL/kg PO q6–8h. Alternatively, pellets can be ground and mixed with fresh greens, vegetable baby foods, water, or juice to form a gruel.
• Encourage oral fluid intake by offering fresh water from multiple sources, wetting leafy vegetable

CLIENT EDUCATION
Warn client that morbidity and mortality are associated with severe hypoxemia, thoracic abscesses, and sepsis.

SURGICAL CONSIDERATIONS
Surgery (lung lobectomy)—may be indicated with pulmonary abscessation or bronchopulmonary foreign body with secondary pneumonia

MEDICATIONS

DRUG(S) OF CHOICE
• Antimicrobial drugs effective against the infectious agent; gain access to site of

infection. Choice of antibiotic is ideally based on results of culture and susceptibility testing. Depending on the severity of infection, long-term antibiotic therapy is required (4–6 weeks minimum, to several months or years).
• Choose broad-spectrum antibiotics such as enrofloxacin (10–20 mg/kg PO, SC, IM, IV q12h), marbofloxacin (5 mg/kg PO q24h), trimethoprim-sulfa (15–30 mg/kg PO q12h), chloramphenicol (50 mg/kg PO q8h), or penicillin G procaine (40,000–60,000 IU/kg SC q24h).
• Nebulization—used in conjunction with systemic treatment. Nebulize for 15 minutes 1–3 times daily. Choices include: enrofloxacin 100 mg in 10 mL saline; doxycycline 200 mg in 15 mL saline; gentamicin 50 mg I 10 mL saline; amikacin 50 mg in 10 mL saline

CONTRAINDICATIONS
• Oral administration of antibiotics that select against gram-positive bacteria (penicillins, macrolides, lincosamides, and cephalosporins) can cause fatal enteric dysbiosis and enterotoxemia.
• The use of corticosteroids (systemic or topical preparations) can severely exacerbate bacterial infection.
• Anticholinergics and antihistamines—may thicken secretions and inhibit mucokinesis and exudate removal from airways

PRECAUTIONS
• Chloramphenicol—avoid human contact with chloramphenicol due to potential blood dyscrasia. Advise owners of potential risks.
• Nebulization or oral administration of any antibiotic may potentially cause enteric dysbiosis; discontinue use if diarrhea or anorexia occurs.
• Azithromycin—use with caution due to risk of enteric dysbiosis

FOLLOW-UP

PATIENT MONITORING
• Clinical assessment and monitoring for relapse of clinical signs
• Thoracic radiographs—improve more slowly than the clinical appearance

PREVENTION/AVOIDANCE
• Avoid stressful conditions, corticosteroid use; provide excellent diet and husbandry
• Treating upper respiratory infections in early stages may prevent spread to the lungs

EXPECTED COURSE AND PROGNOSIS
• Prognosis depends on chronicity and severity

• Early, mild disease—prognosis is good with aggressive antibacterial and supportive therapy; more guarded in young animals and patients that are debilitated, immunocompromised, or have severe underlying disease
• Chronic infection with widespread lung involvement—prognosis guarded to grave
• Thoracic abscess—often not amenable to surgical treatment; treat with supportive care, long-term antibiotics; fair to grave prognosis depending on location

MISCELLANEOUS

ASSOCIATED CONDITIONS
• Pasteurellosis
• GI hypomotility

AGE-RELATED FACTORS
Young rabbits may have a poorer prognosis.

PREGNANCY/FERTILITY/BREEDING
Rabbits infected with pasteurella—may transmit infection to neonates

SEE ALSO
Dyspnea and tachypnea
Rhinitis and sinusitis
Thymoma and thymic lymphoma

ABBREVIATIONS
ELISA = enzyme-linked immunosorbent assay
GI = gastrointestinal
LRT = lower respiratory tract
SPF = specific pathogen free

Suggested Reading
Capello V, Lennox AM. Diagnostic imaging of the respiratory system in exotic companion mammals. Vet Clin Exot Anim 2011;14:369–389.
DeCubellis J. Common emergencies in rabbits, guinea pigs, and chinchillas. Vet Clin Exot Anim 2016;19:411–429.
Hedley J. Respiratory disease. In: Meredith A, Lord B, eds. BSAVA Manual of Rabbit Medicine. Gloucester: British Small Animal Veterinary Association, 2014:160–167.
Jekl V. Respiratory disorders in rabbits. Vet Clin Exot Anim 2021;24:459–482.
Lennox AM, Mancinelli E. Respiratory diseases. In: Quesenberry KE, Carpenter JW, eds. Ferrets, Rabbits and Rodents, 4th Ed). Clinical Medicine and Surgery ed. St. Louis: Saunders, 2020:188–201.
Varga M. Cardiorespiratory diseases. In: Varga M, ed. Textbook of Rabbit Medicine, 2nd ed. London, UK: Elsevier, 2014:390–405.
Author Barbara Oglesbee, DVM, DABVP-Avian

POISONING (INTOXICATION)

BASICS

OVERVIEW

- Rabbits frequently ingest poisonous plants, rodent poisons, and lead.
- Many antibiotics commonly administered to other mammals can be fatal to rabbits.
- Rabbits frequently have severe adverse reactions to many topical products (cosmetic soaps, shampoos, and sprays) that are usually benign in other mammals.
- Acutely ill patients are often diagnosed as poisoned when no other diagnosis is obvious.
- Make the diagnosis after determining preexisting conditions and initially controlling clinical signs.
- Goals of treatment—providing emergency intervention; preventing further exposure; preventing further absorption; applying specific antidotes; hastening elimination; providing supportive measures; and offering client education
- Suspected intoxication—suspected toxic materials and specimens may be valuable from a medicolegal aspect; maintain a proper chain of physical evidence; and keep good medical records.

CAUSES AND RISK FACTORS

Ingested Toxins

- Poisonous plants—especially rabbits grazing outdoors; some indoor houseplants
- Lead chewing or licking lead-containing household substances, especially painted surfaces; occasionally metallic objects
- Anticoagulant rodenticides

Oral Drug Administration/Overdosage

- Antibiotics that select against gram-positive bacteria (penicillins, macrolides, lincosamides, and cephalosporins)—cause fatal enteric dysbiosis and enterotoxemia
- Nonsteroidal anti-inflammatory drugs

Topically Applied Products

- Fipronil
- Flea collars
- Organophosphate-containing products
- Permethrin sprays or permethrin spot-on products—when applied in high concentrations
- D-limolene
- Environmental insecticides/herbicides— many lawn care products; avoid contact for 3–7 days following application; consult manufacturer for specific recommendations
- Some heavily scented shampoos and soaps manufactured for human use have anecdotally caused depression, lethargy, and anorexia when used on rabbits.

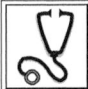

DIAGNOSIS

- Usually presumed, based on history of exposure, clinical signs, and exclusion of other diagnoses
- Resources for emergencies—National Poison Control Center; state diagnostic laboratories; local poison control centers; great value for cases of suspected intoxication, especially when labels or containers are available. PDR often has LD50 for rabbits used in pharmacologic research.
- Confirmation of diagnosis—by chemical analysis (may occur after the fact); accurate diagnosis and detailed records may help with future patients affected by the same intoxicant and are invaluable in medicolegal proceedings.

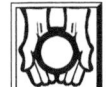

TREATMENT

NURSING CARE

Supportive

- Control of body temperature—normal rabbit rectal temperature is 101.3–104.0°F. Warm chilled rabbits using a circulating hot water blanket, hot water bottles, a circulating hot air blanket, or by placing in a warmed incubator. Gradually warm over a 20-p to 30-minute period. Cool overheated rabbits by spraying with water or soaking with cool, wet cloths; convection cool with fans or evaporative cool (e.g., alcohol on foot pads, axilla, and groin). Stop cooling procedures when temperature reaches 103°F, to avoid hypothermia.
- Supplement oxygen if necessary, via oxygen cage, mask, or nasal catheter.
- Control seizures

Emergency

- Establishment of a patent airway—intubate using a 2.0-mm endotracheal tube in small rabbits, 2.5–3.5 mm in large rabbits. Rabbits may be difficult to intubate; the glottis often cannot be directly visualized due to an elongated, curved oral cavity and small mouth opening. Place rabbit in sternal recumbency, extending head and neck forward and slightly upward. Use a laryngoscope to depress the tongue and apply pressure to the base of the tongue to expose the epiglottis; apply a topical anesthetic to the larynx to prevent laryngospasm prior to introducing the endotracheal tube. When available, a rigid endoscope can be used to visualize the trachea to guide intubation.

If intubation is not readily accomplished, administer oxygen via a face mask securely fitted over the mouth and nose an insufflating the lungs via the nostrils.
- Artificial respiration
- Cardiac massage
- Correct any cardiac abnormalities
- After stabilization—may proceed with more specific therapeutic measures

Prevent Absorption

- Major treatment factor
- Available measures—washing; use of adsorbents and cathartics
  Washing skin
- External toxicants
- Bathe with a mild liquid detergent or shampoo to remove the noxious agent. Use extreme caution when bathing rabbits due to the high risk of stress, skeletal fractures, and excessive chilling. Dry the rabbit immediately, monitor body temperature, and house in a warm, quiet cage to decrease stress.
- Avoid contamination of the people handling the patient.
  Emetics
- Cannot be used in rabbits
  Activated charcoal
- Does not detoxify but prevents absorption if properly used
- Highly absorptive of many toxicants— organic poisons, bacterial toxins, organophosphate insecticides; other insecticides; rodenticides; mercuric chloride; strychnine; other alkaloids (e.g., morphine and atropine); barbiturates; ethylene glycol
- Ineffective against cyanide, heavy metals, arsenic, or caustic materials
- Dosage—1–3 g/kg body weight in a concentration of 1 g charcoal/5–10 mL water. Dosage may need to be repeated.
- Administer via syringe (when possible) or via orogastric tube.
- Monitor rabbit for signs of GI hypomotility and treat accordingly for several days after treatment.
- Cathartic—the use of sodium sulfate or sorbitol has not been described in rabbits and is likely contraindicated due to their unique GI physiology. Use with caution, if at all.

Enhance Elimination

- Absorbed toxicants—generally excreted by the kidneys; may be excreted by other routes (e.g., bile, feces, lungs, and other body secretions)
- Apply an Elizabethan collar to prevent cecotrophy and reingestion of ingested toxins.
- Renal and urinary excretion—may be enhanced using diuretics; requires maintenance of adequate renal function

POISONING (INTOXICATION)

• Diuresis is also beneficial in rabbits with exposure to potential nephrotoxins (e.g., NSAID overdose).
• Fluid diuresis—0.9% NaCl, LRS, or other balanced crystalloid solution. Maintenance is 50–100 mL/kg/day. Attempt diuresis by IV administration of 2–3 times hourly maintenance volumes. Carefully monitor patients undergoing fluid diuresis for overhydration by monitoring urine output, weight, thoracic auscultation, and electrolytes.
• For additional diuresis—furosemide (1–4 mg/kg IV, SC, IM q4–6h)

DIET
Encourage food intake once rabbit is completely stabilized. Offer a good-quality grass hay; a large selection of fresh, moistened greens. If the patient refuses these foods, syringe-feed a gruel such as Critical Care for Herbivores (Oxbow Pet Products) or Emeraid Herbivore (Lafeber Company, Cornell, IL) 10–15 mL/kg PO q6–8h. Alternatively, pellets can be ground and mixed with fresh greens, vegetable baby foods, water, or juice to form a gruel. Fiber in the diet will promote GI motility and elimination of ingested toxins.

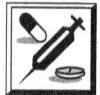

MEDICATIONS
DRUG(S) OF CHOICE
• Specific antidotes or procedures may be available for the more common toxicants. Contact national or local poison control; information may need to be extrapolated from canine/feline treatments when specific treatments for rabbits is lacking
• Control of seizures—diazepam—1–5 mg/kg IV, IM; begin with 0.5–1.0 mg/kg IV bolus; may repeat if gross seizure activity has not stopped within 5 minutes; can be administered rectally if IV access cannot be obtained
• Anticoagulant rodenticide intoxication—plasma or whole blood transfusion for acute bleeding. Perform in-house crossmatch prior to administration; blood types not described for rabbits. Vitamin K1—2.5 mg/kg PO q24h for 10–30 days (depending on the specific product); the injectable form may be administered orally; bioavailability enhanced by the concurrent feeding of a small amount of fat; has also been administered IM (2–10 mg/kg PRN); however, anaphylactic reactions have been reported anecdotally with IV or SC administration. Administer for

1 (warfarin) to 4 (longer-acting formulations) weeks.
• For antibiotic-induced enteric dysbiosis—metronidazole (20 mg/kg PO, IV q12h); cholestyramine (Questran, Bristol Laboratories) is an ion exchange resin that binds clostridial iota toxins. A dose of 2 g in 20 mL of water administered by gavage has been reported to be effective in preventing death in rabbits with acute Clostridia enterotoxemia.
• For lead intoxication—CaEDTA (25 mg/kg SC q6h for 5 days); dilute to 1% solution with D5W before administration; may need multiple treatments; allow a 5-day rest period between treatments.
• Hemorrhagic diarrhea—broad-spectrum antibiotics such as enrofloxacin (10–20 mg/kg PO, IM, SC q12h), trimethoprim-sulfa (15–30 mg/kg PO q12h)
• Gastric irritation/ulceration following NSAID intoxication—famotidine 0.5–1 mg/kg PO, SC, IV, IM q12–24h
• For gastrointestinal hypomotility—metoclopramide (0.2–1.0 mg/kg PO, SC q6–8h) or cisapride (0.5 mg/kg PO q8–12h) is usually helpful in regaining normal motility; cisapride is available through many compounding pharmacies.
• Analgesics such as buprenorphine (0.02–0.05 mg/kg SC, IM q6–12h), meloxicam (1 mg/kg PO, SC, IM q24h), or carprofen (2–4 mg/kg PO, SC, IV q12–24h) are indicated to alleviate intestinal pain. Intestinal pain from gas distention and ileus impairs mobility and decreases appetite and may severely inhibit recovery.
• Glycopyrrolate and 2-PAM have been anecdotally used at feline dosages to treat organophosphate toxicosis.

CONTRAINDICATIONS
Do not administer lincomycin, clindamycin, erythromycin, ampicillin, amoxicillin cephalosporins, or penicillins orally to rabbits.

FOLLOW-UP
• Specific monitoring depends on the toxicant, clinical signs, and laboratory abnormalities.
• Observe for improvement in the rabbit's general demeanor.
• Regularly assess the cardiopulmonary status.

• Carefully monitor for signs of overhydration in rabbits undergoing fluid diuresis.
• Observe for and treat signs of GI hypomotility following successful treatment of any type of poisoning in rabbits.

MISCELLANEOUS
ABBREVIATIONS
LD50 = median lethal dose
LRS = lactated Ringer's solution
NSAID = nonsteroidal anti-inflammatory drug
PDR = physician's desk reference

Suggested Reading
DeCubellis J. Common emergencies in rabbits, guinea pigs, and chinchillas. Vet Clin Exot Anim 2016;19:411–429.
Fisher PG, Künzel F, Rylander H. Neurologic and musculoskeletal disease. In: Quesenberry KE, Carpenter JW, eds. Ferrets, Rabbits and Rodents, 4th Ed). Clinical Medicine and Surgery ed. St. Louis: Saunders, 2020:583–594.
Hung M, Boyeaux A. Assessment and care of the critically ill rabbit. Vet Clin North Am Exot Anim Pract. 2016;19:379–409.
Lennox AM, Gladden JN. Emergency and critical care of small mammals. In: Quesenberry KE, Carpenter JW, eds. Ferrets, Rabbits and Rodents, 4th Ed). Clinical Medicine and Surgery. 2021 ed. St. Louis: Saunders, 2020:595–608.
Murphy LA. Environmental toxicology: considerations for exotic pets. J Exotic Pet Medicine 2015;24(4):390–397.
Varga M. Neurological and locomotive disorders. In: Varga M, ed. Textbook of Rabbit Medicine, 2nd ed. London, UK: Elsevier, 2014:367–389.
Author Barbara Oglesbee, DVM, DABVP (Avian)

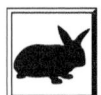 BASICS

DEFINITION
Polyuria is defined as greater than normal urine production, and polydipsia as greater than normal water consumption. Average normal water intake may vary from 50 to 150 mL/kg of body weight daily. Rabbits fed large amounts of water-containing foods, such as leafy vegetables, will drink less water than those on a dry diet of hay and pellets. Urine production has been reported as between 120 and 130 mL/kg of body weight per day.

PATHOPHYSIOLOGY
• Urine production and water consumption (thirst) are controlled by interactions between the kidneys, pituitary gland, and hypothalamus.
• Usually, polydipsia occurs as a compensatory response to polyuria to maintain hydration. The patient's plasma becomes relatively hypertonic and activates thirst mechanisms. Occasionally, polydipsia may be the primary process and polyuria is the compensatory response. Then, the patient's plasma becomes relatively hypotonic because of excessive water intake, and ADH secretion is reduced, resulting in polyuria.

SYSTEMS AFFECTED
• Renal/urologic—kidneys
• Cardiovascular—alterations in "effective" circulating volume

SIGNALMENT
• More likely to be seen in middle-aged to older rabbits
• No sex predilection

SIGNS
N/A

CAUSES
• Primary polyuria due to impaired renal response to ADH—renal failure, pyelonephritis, pyometra, hepatic failure, hypokalemia, and drugs
• Primary polyuria caused by osmotic diuresis—diabetes mellitus (rare), postobstructive diuresis, some diuretics (e.g., mannitol and furosemide), ingestion or administration of large quantities of solute (e.g., sodium chloride or glucose)
• Primary polydipsia—such as behavioral problems (especially boredom), pyrexia, or pain. Organic disease of the anterior hypothalamic thirst center of neoplastic, traumatic, or inflammatory origin has not reported in rabbits but should be considered.

RISK FACTORS
• Renal disease or liver disease
• Administration of diuretics and anticonvulsants

 DIAGNOSIS

DIFFERENTIAL DIAGNOSIS
Differentiating Similar Signs
• Differentiate polyuria from an abnormal increase in the frequency of urination (pollakiuria). Pollakiuria is often associated with dysuria, stranguria, or hematuria. Patients with polyuria void large quantities of urine; patients with pollakiuria typically void small quantities of urine.
• Measuring urinary specific gravity may provide evidence of adequate urine-concentrating ability (<1.020).

Differentiating Causes
• If associated with progressive weight loss—consider renal failure, hepatic failure, pyometra, neoplasia, pyelonephritis, and possibly diabetes mellitus
• If associated with hypercalciuria/bladder sludge—consider renal failure, nephrolithiasis
• If associated with polyphagia—consider diabetes mellitus (rare)
• If associated with recent estrus in an intact female—consider pyometra
• If associated with abdominal distention—consider hepatic failure, neoplasia

CBC/BIOCHEMISTRY/URINALYSIS
• BUN elevation (normal 9.1–22.7 mg/dL) and creatinine elevation (normal 0.5–2.0 mg/dL) are consistent with renal causes for polyuria/ polydipsia but may also indicate dehydration resulting from inadequate compensatory polydipsia
• High hepatic enzyme activities are consistent with hepatic disease.
• Hypercalcemia—rabbits have a high normal serum calcium concentration (12–15 mg/dL) that varies with dietary intake. Hypercalcemia can be a potential cause of renal failure, rather than the result of renal failure in the rabbit.
• Hypoalbuminemia supports renal or hepatic causes of polyuria/polydipsia.
• Heterophilia may suggest infectious or inflammatory disease.
• White blood cell casts and/or bacteriuria should prompt consideration of pyelonephritis.
• Urinary sediment evaluation often reveals calcium oxalate or calcium carbonate crystals; however, this is a normal finding in rabbits, and the presence of large amounts of crystals in the urine does not necessarily indicate disease. Disease occurs only when the concentration of crystals is excessive, forming thick, white to brown, sandlike urine and subsequent inflammatory cystitis or partial to complete blockage of the urethra.

• Pyuria (normal value 0–1 WBC/hpf), hematuria (normal value 0–1 RBC/hpf), and proteinuria (normal value 0–33mg/dL) indicate urinary tract inflammation, but these are nonspecific findings that may result from infectious and noninfectious causes of lower urinary tract disease.
• Urine pH: normal rabbit urine is alkaline; pH >8 suggestive of bacterial cystitis due to urease-producing bacteria

OTHER LABORATORY TESTS
Urine culture—chronic pyelonephritis cannot be conclusively ruled out by absence of pyuria or bacteriuria.

IMAGING
Abdominal survey radiography and ultrasonography may provide additional evidence of renal (e.g., primary renal diseases and hypercalciuria) and hepatic or uterine (e.g., pyometra) disorders that can contribute to polyuria/polydipsia.

DIAGNOSTIC PROCEDURES
N/A

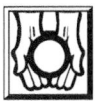 TREATMENT

APPROPRIATE HEALTH CARE
• Serious medical consequence for the patient is rare if patient has free access to water and is willing and able to drink. Until the mechanism of polyuria is understood, discourage owners from limiting access to water. Direct treatment at the underlying cause.
• Diseases associated with systemic signs of illness (e.g., pyrexia, depression, anorexia, and dehydration) or laboratory findings of azotemia and or leukocytosis warrant an aggressive diagnostic evaluation and initiation of supportive and symptomatic treatment.

NURSING CARE
• Provide polyuric patients with free access to water. Also provide fluids parenterally when other conditions limit oral intake or dehydration persists despite polydipsia.
• Base fluid selection on knowledge of the underlying cause for fluid loss. In most patients, lactated Ringer's solution is an acceptable replacement fluid.

DIET
• Many rabbits with PU/PD develop inappetence. Be certain that the rabbit continues to eat to prevent the development or exacerbation of GI hypomotility.
• Increasing water consumption is essential to prevention and treatment of hypercalciuria. Provide multiple sources of fresh water. Flavoring the water with fruit juices (with no added sugars) is usually

helpful. Provide a variety of clean, fresh, leafy vegetables sprayed or soaked with water.
• No reports of dissolution of calcium oxalate uroliths with special diets
• Following treatment, reduction in the amount of calcium in the diet may help to prevent or delay recurrence of hypercalciuria. Eliminate feeding of alfalfa pellets and switch to a high-fiber timothy-based pellet (Oxbow Pet Products, Murdock, NE). Feed timothy and grass hay instead of alfalfa hay and offer large volumes of fresh, green, leafy vegetables.

MEDICATIONS

DRUG(S) OF CHOICE
Vary with underlying cause

CONTRAINDICATIONS
• Oral administration of antibiotics that select against gram-positive bacteria (penicillins, cephalosporins, macrolides, and lincosamides) can cause fatal enteric dysbiosis and enterotoxemia.
• Potentially nephrotoxic drugs (e.g., aminoglycosides, NSAIDs) should be avoided in patients that are febrile, dehydrated, or azotemic, or that are suspected of having pyelonephritis, septicemia, or preexisting renal disease.
• Glucocorticoids or other immunosuppressive agents

PRECAUTIONS
Until renal and hepatic failure have been excluded as potential causes for polyuria/polydipsia, use caution in administering any drug eliminated via these pathways.

POSSIBLE INTERACTIONS
N/A

ALTERNATIVE DRUGS
N/A

FOLLOW-UP

PATIENT MONITORING
• Hydration status by clinical assessment of hydration and serial evaluation of body weight
• Fluid intake and urine output—provide a useful baseline for assessing adequacy of hydration therapy

POSSIBLE COMPLICATIONS
• Gastrointestinal hypomotility
• Dehydration
• Urine scald, pododermatitis, myiasis

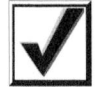

MISCELLANEOUS

ASSOCIATED CONDITIONS
• Bacterial urinary tract infection
• Hypercalciuria

AGE-RELATED FACTORS
N/A

ZOONOTIC POTENTIAL
N/A

PREGNANCY/FERTILITY/BREEDING
N/A

SYNONYMS
N/A

SEE ALSO
Dysuria and pollakiuria
Gastrointestinal hypomotility and gastrointestinal stasis
Hematuria
Hypercalciuria and urolithiasis
Pyometra and nonneoplastic endometrial disorders
Renal failure

ABBREVIATIONS
ADH = antidiuretic hormone
BUN = blood urea nitrogen
GI = gastrointestinal
NSAID = nonsteroidal anti-inflammatory drug

Suggested Reading
Di Girolamo N, Selleri P. Disorders of the urinary and reproductive system. In: Quesenberry KE, Carpenter JW, eds. Ferrets, Rabbits and Rodents, 4th Ed). Clinical Medicine and Surgery ed. St. Louis: Saunders, 2020:201–220.
Hallman RM, Brandão J. Diagnostic imaging of the renal system in exotic companion mammals. Vet Clin Exot Anim 2020;23:195–214.
Mancinelli E, Lord B. Urogenital and reproductive disease. In: Meredith A, Lord B, eds. BSAVA Manual of Rabbit Medicine. Gloucester: British Small Animal Veterinary Association, 2014:191–204.
Reavill DR, Lennox AM. Disease overview of the urinary tract in exotic companion mammals and tips on clinical management. Vet Clin Exot Anim 2020;23(1):169–193.
Author Barbara Oglesbee, DVM, DABVP (Avian)

BASICS

DEFINITION
• The sensation that provokes the desire to scratch, rub, chew, or lick; often an indicator of inflamed skin
• Pruritus, or itching, is a primary cutaneous sensation that may be elicited from the epidermis, dermis, or mucous membranes.
• Pruritus stimulates various kinds of self-trauma, including scratching, which in turn, relieves some of the sensation of itching. Self-trauma may perpetuate pruritus by contributing to skin inflammation.
• Other factors such as boredom, anxiety, and stress may exacerbate pruritus.
• Summation of effects occurs when the pruritic stimuli add up to reach the pruritus threshold.

SYSTEMS AFFECTED
• Skin/Exocrine

SIGNALMENT
Variable; depends on the underlying cause

SIGNS
• The act of scratching, licking, biting, or chewing
• Other rabbits, pets, or owners may have cutaneous signs associated with contagious dermatologic diseases.
• Behavioral changes may occur: anorexia, lethargy, lack of tolerance, vocalization, weight loss, and hiding.
• Evidence of self-trauma and cutaneous inflammation is often present.
• Alopecia may be seen.

CAUSES
• Parasitic—*Psoroptes cuniculi* (ear mites) extremely pruritic; fleas—usually pruritic; cheyletiellosis (fur mites)—can be severely pruritic; *Passalurus ambiguus* (rabbit pinworm)—severe perianal pruritus sometimes seen; *Sarcoptes scabiei* and *Notoedres cati*—rarely infest rabbits, but can be intensely pruritic; *Haemodipsus ventricosus* (rabbit louse)—very rare in pet house rabbits, may be pruritic
• Neoplastic—cutaneous lymphosarcoma; other primary or metastatic neoplasia
• Bacterial/fungal—pyoderma, moist dermatitis, and dermatomycosis
• Immunologic—contact dermatitis has been anecdotally reported in rabbits. Cutaneous lesions resembling urticaria or histologic lesions characteristic of allergic reactions in other species have also been anecdotally reported; however, there are no confirmed cases of atopy, food allergy, or other allergic dermatitis in rabbits.
• Injection reactions
• Irritants—soaps, shampoos, bedding, or harsh cleaning solutions

RISK FACTORS
N/A

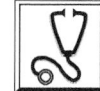

DIAGNOSIS

DIFFERENTIAL DIAGNOSIS
• Alopecia—focal: in most cases, a clear history of pruritus is noted; some animals may excessively lick themselves or may be barbered by a dominant rabbit without the owner's knowledge; ear mites, fleas, *Cheyletiella*, dermatomycosis, bacterial pyoderma, and some cutaneous neoplasms may all cause alopecia with varying degrees of inflammation and pruritus.
• Alopecia—barbering; may be associated with craving for fiber in rabbits fed diets deficient in hay or due to nesting behavior in reproductively active females; may mimic pruritus

Distribution of Lesions
• *Cheyletiella* and *Leporacarus gibbus* lesions are usually located in the intrascapular or tail base region and associated with copious amounts of large white scale. Mites are readily identified in skin scrapes or acetate tape preparations under low magnification.
• Ear mites—alopecia around ear base, pinna; may extend to face, neck, abdomen, perineal region; intense pruritus; brown, beige crusty exudate in the ear canal and pinna
• Fleas—patchy alopecia and pruritus; finding flea dirt will help to differentiate; secondary pyoderma sometimes seen
• Other ectoparasites—*Sarcoptes scabiei* and *Notoedres cati* rarely infest rabbits. Lesions are located around the head and neck and are intensely pruritic.
• Pinworms—heavy infections of intestinal pinworms sometimes cause intense perianal dermatitis and self-mutilation. Ova or adult worms can be identified in fecal float or fecal direct smear.
• Injection reactions—alopecia, scabs, scale, erythema, usually in the intrascapular region as this is a common site of subcutaneous injections
• Contact dermatitis—alopecia with or without erythema, scale on ventral abdomen or other contact areas
• Moist dermatitis—alopecia, with or without erythema, scale, or ulceration. Facial—associated with epiphora or ptyalism; perineal/ventrum—associated with urinary disease, diarrhea, or uneaten cecotrophs
• Dermatophytosis—partial to complete alopecia with scaling; with or without erythema; not always ringlike; may begin as small papules
• Sebaceous adenitis—excessive scale, alopecia; usually not pruritic

CBC/BIOCHEMISTRY/URINALYSIS
To identify underlying disease, especially in rabbits with perineal dermatitis or urine scald

OTHER LABORATORY TESTS
N/A

IMAGING
Radiographs—skull/dental to identify underlying dental disease in rabbits with moist dermatitis secondary to chronic epiphora or ptyalism; whole-body radiographs may be helpful in identifying hypercalciuria, spinal, orthopedic, renal, or gastrointestinal diseases contributing to perineal or ventral moist dermatitis.

DIAGNOSTIC PROCEDURES
• Skin scrapes, acetate tape preparations, epidermal cytology, and dermatophyte cultures (with microscopic identification)—identify primary or coexisting diseases caused by parasites or other microorganisms
• Microscopic examination of ear crust placed in mineral oil—usually a very effective means of identifying ear mites; mites may also be visualized with an otoscope
• Wood's lamp—do not use as the sole means of diagnosing or excluding dermatomycosis, owing to false negatives and misinterpretations of florescence
• Coat brushing—for fleas and *Cheyletiella parasitivorax*
• Skin biopsy—useful to diagnose cutaneous neoplasms

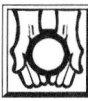

TREATMENT
• More than one disease may be contributing to the itching; if treatment for an identified condition does not result in improvement, consider other causes.
• Moist dermatitis—identify and correct underlying cause (dental disease in facial dermatitis, urinary, GI, or musculoskeletal disease in perineal/ventral dermatitis); keep the area clean and dry; apply zinc oxide + menthol powder (Gold Bond, Martin Himmel, Inc.) to clean skin q24h
• All in-contact animals should be treated in case of ectoparasites infestation. The environment will also need to be thoroughly cleaned.

RABBITS

MEDICATIONS

DRUG(S) OF CHOICE

Symptomatic Therapy
- Antihistamines—chlorpheniramine maleate (0.2–0.4 mg/kg PO q12h); hydroxyzine (2 mg/kg PO q8–12h); diphenhydramine (2 mg/kg PO, SC q8–12h)
- Topical sprays, lotions, creams, and shampoos used in dogs and cats have not been evaluated in rabbits. Use with caution as rabbits are fastidious groomers and may ingest topical medications.

Systemic/Topical Therapy
Varies with specific cause
- Ear mites, *Cheyletiella* or *Leptogibbus* sp. mites—1% ivermectin—0.4 mg/kg SC q10–14d for 2–3 doses; or selamectin-10 (Revolution, Pfizer)—12 mg/kg applied topically q30d, or imidacloprid/moxidectin (Advantage-Multi for Cats Bayer)—10 mg/kg (i) + 1 mg/kg (m) topically q30d; Treat all in-contact animals
- Fleas—imidacloprid (Advantage, Bayer) or imidacloprid/moxidectin (Advantage-Multi, Bayer)—10 mg/kg (i) + 1 mg/kg (m) topically q30d; or selamectin (Revolution, Pfizer)—12 mg/kg applied topically q30d; treat all in-contact animals
- Sarcoptic mange—ivermectin 0.4 mg/kg SC q14d for 3–4 doses; treat all in-contact animals
- Bacterial folliculitis—shampoos and antibiotic therapy, preferably based on culture and susceptibility testing; good initial choices include enrofloxacin (5–20 mg/kg PO q12–24h) and trimethoprim-sulfa (30 mg/kg PO q12h)
- Dermatomycosis—lime sulfur dip q7d has been used to successfully; lime sulfur is odiferous and can stain; dipping is often difficult to perform on rabbits; clotrimazole cream (Lotrimin Cream 1%, Schering-Plough Corp.) for focal lesions; itraconazole (5–10 mg/kg PO q24h x 30days) or terbinafine (10 mg/kg PO q24h)
- Intestinal pinworms—fendendazole (20 mg/kg PO q10–14d for 2 treatments); treat all in-contact animals

CONTRAINDICATIONS
- Do not use fipronil (Frontline, Merial) on rabbits—fatal toxicity reported
- Corticosteroids, topical or systemic—associated with gastrointestinal ulceration and hemorrhage, delayed wound healing, and heightened susceptibility to infection; rabbits

are very sensitive to the immunosuppressive effects of both topical and systemic corticosteroids; use may exacerbate subclinical bacterial infection
- Oral administration of antibiotics that select against gram-positive bacteria (penicillins, macrolides, lincosamides, and cephalosporins) can cause fatal enteric dysbiosis and enterotoxemia.
- Do not use flea collars on rabbits.
- Do not use organophosphate-containing products on rabbits.
- Do not use straight permethrin sprays or permethrin spot-ons on rabbits.

PRECAUTIONS
- Use extreme caution when dipping or bathing rabbits due to the high risk of stress, skeletal fractures, and excessive chilling with inexperienced owners.
- All flea control products discussed above are off-label use. Safety and efficacy have not been evaluated in rabbits. Use with caution, especially in young or debilitated animals.
- Prevent rabbits or their cagemates from licking topical spot-on products before they are dry.
- Toxicity—if any signs are noted, the animal should be bathed thoroughly to remove any remaining chemicals and treated appropriately.
- Topical flea preparation for use in dogs and cats, such as permethrins and pyrethrins, is less effective and may be toxic to rabbits.
- Griseofulvin—bone marrow suppression reported in dogs/cats as an idiosyncratic reaction or with prolonged therapy; not yet reported in rabbits but may occur; weekly or biweekly CBC is recommended. Neurologic side effects reported in dogs and cats—monitor for this possibility in rabbits; do not use during the first two trimesters of pregnancy; it is teratogenic.
- Sometimes the application of anything topically, including water, soap products, and products containing alcohol, iodine, and benzoyl peroxide, can exacerbate itching; cool water may be soothing.

POSSIBLE INTERACTIONS
N/A

ALTERNATIVE DRUGS
N/A

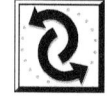

FOLLOW-UP

PATIENT MONITORING
Monitor for alleviation of itching and hair regrowth.

POSSIBLE COMPLICATIONS
Secondary pyoderma

MISCELLANEOUS

ASSOCIATED CONDITIONS
- Dental disease
- Musculoskeletal disease
- Obesity

AGE-RELATED FACTORS
N/A

ZOONOTIC POTENTIAL
Dermatophytosis and *Cheyletiella* can cause skin lesions in people.

PREGNANCY/FERTILITY/BREEDING
Avoid griseofulvin and ivermectin in pregnant animals.

SEE ALSO
Cheyletiellosis (fur mites)
Dermatophytosis
Ear mites
Fleas and flea infestation

Suggested Reading
Meredith A. Dermatoses. In: Meredith A, Lord B, eds. BSAVA Manual of Rabbit Medicine. Gloucester: British Small Animal Veterinary Association, 2014:255–263.
Palmerio BS, Roberts H. Clinical approach to dermatologic disease in exotic animals. Vet Clin North Am Exot Anim Pract 2013;16(3):523–577.
Rosen LB. Dermatologic manifestations of zoonotic diseases in exotic animals. J Exotic Pet Med 2011;20:9–13.
Snook TS, White SD, Hawkins MG et al. Skin diseases in pet rabbits: a retrospective study of 334 cases seen at the University of California at Davis, USA (1984–2004). Vet Dermatol 2013;24:613–618.
Varga M. Skin diseases. In: Varga M, ed. Textbook of Rabbit Medicine, 2nd ed. Elsiver, 2014:224–248.
Varga M, Patterson S. Dermatologic diseases of rabbits. In: Quesenberry KE, Carpenter JW, eds. Ferrets, Rabbits and Rodents, 4th Ed). Clinical Medicine and Surgery. 2021 ed. St. Louis: Saunders, 2020:220–222.
Author Barbara Oglesbee, DVM, Dipl ABVP (Avian)

BASICS

DEFINITION
• Excessive production of saliva
• *Slobbers* is the layman's term for moist dermatitis around the face or dewlap, usually caused by ptyalism and dental disease.

PATHOPHYSIOLOGY
• Saliva is constantly produced and secreted into the oral cavity from the salivary glands (parotid, sublingual, mandibular, zygomatic, and buccal).
• In rabbits, the most common cause is oral lesions secondary to dental disease or oral mucosal pain

SYSTEMS AFFECTED
• Oral cavity
• Dermatologic—moist dermatitis

SIGNALMENT
• Underlying dental disease—can be seen in any age, gender, or breed
• Dwarf and lop breeds—congenital malocclusion of teeth

SIGNS

Historical Findings
• Facial, chin, and neck alopecia and wet fur are sometimes the only signs noted by the owner.
• Reduced food intake or anorexia—often seen in patients with oral lesions, gastrointestinal disease, and systemic disease
• May have a history of dental disease
Other signs of underlying dental disease may be present, including:
• A history of an inability to prehend food, dropping food out of the mouth, or preference for soft foods
• Weight loss
• Nasal or ocular discharge
• Tooth grinding
• Facial asymmetry or exophthalmos in rabbits with apical abscesses
• Signs of pain—reluctance to move, depression, lethargy, hiding, and hunched posture
• Unkempt hair coat, lack of grooming

Physical Examination Findings
• Facial, chin, neck, or dewlap dermatitis—alopecia, erythema, matted fur, enlarged, thickened skin folds, variable crusts. Due to constant moisture from ptyalism as a symptom of dental disease.
• Always perform a thorough oral examination in rabbits with ptyalism. Complete exam requires heavy sedation or general anesthesia and specialized equipment. Use of an otoscope or speculum may be

useful in identifying severe abnormalities; however, many problems may be missed by using this method alone.
• A focused, directed light source and magnification will provide optimal visualization.
• Use a rabbit mouth gag or rodent tabletop retractor/gag (Veterinary Instrumentations, UK) and cheek dilators (Jorgensen Laboratories, Inc., Loveland, CO) to open the mouth and pull buccal tissues away from teeth surfaces to allow adequate exposure. Use a cotton swab or tongue depressor to retract the tongue and examine lingual surfaces.
• Identify cheek teeth elongation, spikes, curved teeth, ulceration, longitudinal fractures, loose or discolored teeth, halitosis, or purulent discharge.
• Abnormalities of the reserve crowns (roots) may be present despite normal-appearing clinical crowns. Skull films are required to identify apical disorders.
• Incisors—may see overgrowth, horizontal ridges or grooves, malformation, discoloration, fractures, increased or decreased curvature or malocclusion
• Stomatitis—ulceration and inflammation of many different causes are associated with ptyalism
• Lesions of the tongue—inflammation, ulceration, mass, and foreign body
• Halitosis—occasionally seen with apical abscesses
• Cranial nerve deficits—trigeminal nerve (CN V) lesions can cause drooling due to inability to close the mouth.

CAUSES

Oral Disease
• Cheek teeth elongation caused by improper wear—most common cause; from oral pain; spikes on occlusal surfaces may cause inflammation, laceration, or ulceration of soft tissues; secondary bacterial infections may occur
• Periapical abscesses and associated osteomyelitis
• Gingivitis or stomatitis—may also be secondary to ingestion of a caustic agent, poisonous plant, burns (e.g., those from biting on an electrical cord), or uremia
• Foreign body, especially hay imbedded into soft tissues
• Neoplasm (rare)
• Metabolic, esophageal, gastrointestinal disorders or nausea—do not cause ptyalism in rabbits

Neurologic Disorders
• Disorders that cause dysphagia
• Disorders that cause facial nerve palsy—especially otitis interna and media

• Disorders that cause seizures—during a seizure, ptyalism may occur because of autonomic discharge or reduced swallowing of saliva and may be exacerbated by chomping of the jaws

Drugs and Toxins
• Those that are caustic (e.g., household cleaning products and some common house plants)
• Those with a disagreeable taste—many antibiotics and anthelminthics
• Those that induce hypersalivation, including organophosphate compounds, cholinergic drugs, insecticides containing boric acid, pyrethrin, and pyrethroid insecticides, and illicit drugs such as amphetamines, cocaine, and opiates

RISK FACTORS
• Cheek teeth elongation—likely multiple etiologies; feeding pelleted foods containing inadequate fibrous, tough foods needed for normal wear of occlusal surfaces; elongation in geriatric rabbits; metabolic bone disease may also play a role
• Tooth root abscess—usually secondary to acquired or congenital malocclusion, trauma to the pulp
• Unsupervised roaming in the house—increased risk for electric cord shock; ingestion of caustic agents

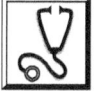

DIAGNOSIS

DIFFERENTIAL DIAGNOSIS
• Differentiate from moist dewlap pyoderma caused by sloppy drinking from a water bowl; change rabbit to sipper bottle.
• Differentiating causes of ptyalism requires a thorough history, including current medications and possible toxin exposure.
• Complete physical examination (with special attention to the oral cavity) and neurologic examination are critical; wear examination gloves when rabies exposure is possible.

CBC/BIOCHEMISTRY/URINALYSIS
• CBC—often normal
• Biochemical analysis—usually normal except in patients with renal disease or hepatic lipidosis secondary to anorexia

OTHER LABORATORY TESTS
N/A

IMAGING
• Skull radiographs are mandatory to identify dental disease and, if present, to plan treatment strategies and to monitor progression of treatment.
• Perform under general anesthesia

• Five views are recommended for thorough assessment: ventro-dorsal, lateral, two lateral obliques, and rostro-caudal.
• CT—superior to radiographs to evaluate the extent of dental disease and bony destruction

DIAGNOSTIC PROCEDURES
• Cytologic examination of oral lesions or fine-needle aspiration of oral mass
• Biopsy and histopathology of oral lesion or mass if dental disease has been ruled out

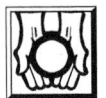

TREATMENT
Treat the underlying cause.

NURSING CARE
• Keep fur around face clean and dry.
• Clip fur and clean skin if matted fur is present and secondary dermatitis
• Supportive care in debilitated or anorexic patients; assist-feeding; subcutaneous or intravenous fluid therapy
• Symptomatic treatment to reduce the flow of saliva—generally unnecessary, may be of little value to the patient, and may mask other signs of the underlying cause

ACTIVITY
N/A

DIET
• It is absolutely imperative that the rabbit continue to eat during and following treatment. Many rabbits with dental disease will become anorexic.
• If anorectic, syringe-feed a gruel such as Critical Care for Herbivores (Oxbow Pet Products) or Emeraid Herbivore (Lafeber Company, Cornell, IL) 10–15 mL/kg PO q6–8h. Larger volumes and more frequent feedings are often accepted; feed as much as the rabbit will readily accept. Alternatively, pellets can be ground and mixed with fresh greens, vegetable baby foods, water, or juice to form a gruel.
• High-carbohydrate, high-fat nutritional supplements are contraindicated.
• Following treatment, return the rabbit to a solid food diet as soon as possible to encourage normal occlusion and wear. Increase the amount of tough, fibrous foods and foods containing abrasive silicates such as hay and wild grasses; avoid pelleted food and soft fruits or vegetables.
• Encourage oral fluid intake by offering fresh water or wetting leafy vegetables.

CLIENT EDUCATION
• Inform owner that resolution requires correction of underlying cause. The most common cause, chronic dental disease, requires a long time and financial commitment. Diet change and lifelong treatment, consisting of periodic coronal reduction (teeth trimming), are required, with reduction often being necessary every 3–12 months.
• Discuss need to correct or prevent risk factors

SURGICAL CONSIDERATIONS
• Trimming of cheek teeth (coronal reduction)—trimming of spurs and sharp points alone will be of little benefit for most rabbits; in most cases, the crowns all of the cheek teeth are elongated and maloccluded and will need to be reduced.
• Tooth extraction—because rabbits have very long, deeply embedded, and curved reserve crown (roots), intraoral extraction can be extremely time consuming and labor intensive compared with that of dogs and cats. If the reserve crown or apex is not completely removed, the tooth may regrow, or a new abscess may form. If practitioner is not experienced with tooth extraction in rabbits, the author recommends referral to a veterinarian with special expertise whenever feasible.
• In rabbits with extensive apical abscesses, aggressive debridement is indicated, and special expertise may be required. Maxillary and retrobulbar abscesses can be particularly challenging. If practitioner is not experienced with facial abscesses in rabbits, the author recommends referral to a veterinarian with special expertise whenever feasible.

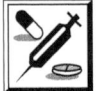

MEDICATIONS
DRUG(S) OF CHOICE
Antibiotics
• Moist pyoderma—often responds to correction of dental disease and topical treatment alone. If systemic antibiotics are needed, initially choose broad-spectrum antibiotics such as enrofloxacin (5–20 mg/kg PO, SC, IM, IV q12–24h), trimethoprim-sulfa (30 mg/kg PO q12h); for recurrent, resistant, or deep pyoderma base antibiotic therapy on culture and sensitivity testing
• Superficial, moist dermatitis—apply zinc oxide + menthol powder (Gold Bond, Martin Himmel, Inc) to clean, clipped skin q24h
• Tooth root abscess—choice of antibiotic is ideally based on results of culture and susceptibility testing. Most facial or dental abscesses are caused by anaerobic bacteria; use antibiotics effective against anaerobes such as azithromycin (15–30 mg/kg PO q24h); can be used alone or combined with metronidazole (20 mg/kg PO q12h). Alternatively, use penicillin G procaine (40,000–60,000 IU/kg SC q24h). Usually only effective when combined with topical treatment (surgical debridement, marsupialization, antibiotic-impregnated acrylic beads).

Long-Term Pain Management
• Most rabbits with dental disease are painful. Nonsteroidal anti-inflammatories have been used for short- or long-term therapy to reduce pain and inflammation; meloxicam (1 mg/kg PO q24h); carprofen (2–4 mg/kg PO q12h)

CONTRAINDICATIONS
• Oral administration of antibiotics that select against gram-positive bacteria (penicillins, macrolides, lincosamides, and cephalosporins) can cause fatal enteric dysbiosis and enterotoxemia.
• Corticosteroids—associated with gastrointestinal ulceration and hemorrhage, delayed wound healing, and heightened susceptibility to infection; rabbits are very sensitive to the immunosuppressive effects of both topical and systemic corticosteroids; use may exacerbate subclinical bacterial infection.

PRECAUTIONS
• Chloramphenicol—avoid human contact with chloramphenicol due to potential blood dyscrasia. Advise owners of potential risks.
• Meloxicam—use with caution in rabbits with compromised renal function
• Azithromycin—use with caution due to risk of enteric dysbiosis

POSSIBLE INTERACTIONS
N/A

ALTERNATIVE DRUGS
N/A

FOLLOW-UP
PATIENT MONITORING
• Depends on the underlying cause (see Causes)
• Continually monitor hydration and nutritional status in anorexic animals.

PREVENTION/AVOIDANCE
• Do not use clippers to trim incisors.
• Prevent progressive dental disease by selecting pets without congenital predisposition (when possible), providing high-fiber foods and good-quality hay, discontinuing or limiting the feeding of pellets and soft fruits or vegetables, and periodically trimming overgrown crowns.
• Do not allow unsupervised roaming or chewing; remove all potential risks from the rabbit's environment.

POSSIBLE COMPLICATIONS
• Moist pyoderma; myiasis
• Bacteremia and septicemia
• Hepatic lipidosis with prolonged anorexia
• With underlying dental disease—recurrence, chronic pain, or extensive tissue destruction

EXPECTED COURSE AND PROGNOSIS
• Depends on the underlying cause.
• In rabbits with chronic dental disease, lifelong treatment is required.

MISCELLANEOUS

ASSOCIATED CONDITIONS
• Immunosuppression
• Gastrointestinal hypomotility

AGE-RELATED FACTORS
• Congenital malocclusion in young rabbits
• Acquired tooth elongation in middle-aged to older rabbits

ZOONOTIC POTENTIAL
Rabies

PREGNANCY/FERTILITY/BREEDING
N/A

SYNONYMS
Drooling
Hypersalivation
Sialorrhea

SEE ALSO
Abscessation
Cheek teeth (premolar and molar) malocclusion and elongation
Incisor malocclusion and overgrowth
Pyoderma

ABBREVIATIONS
AIPPMA = antibiotic-impregnated polymethyl methacrylate
CN = cranial nerve
CNS = central nervous system
CT = computed tomography
GI = gastrointestinal
MRI = magnetic resonance imaging

Suggested Reading
Capello V. Dental diseases. In: Capello V, Lennox AM, eds. Rabbit and Rodent Dentistry Handbook. Lake Worth: Zoological Education Network, 2005:113–138.

Capello V. Intraoral treatment of dental disease in pet rabbits. Vet Clin Exot Anim. 2016;19(3):783–798.
Easson W. Tooth extraction. In: Harcourt-Brown F, Chitty J, eds. BSAVA Manual of Rabbit Surgery, Dentistry, and Imaging. Gloucester, UK: BSAVA, 2013:370–381.
Harcourt-Brown F. Treatment of dental problems: principles and options. In: Harcourt-Brown F, Chitty J, eds. BSAVA Manual of Rabbit Surgery, Dentistry, and Imaging. Gloucester, UK: BSAVA, 2013:349–369.
Lennox AM, Capello V, Legendre LF. Small mammal dentistry. In: Quesenberry KE, Carpenter JW, eds. Ferrets, Rabbits and Rodents, 4th Ed). Clinical Medicine and Surgery. 2021 ed. St. Louis: Saunders, 2020:514–535.
Varga M. Dental Disease: Textbook of Rabbit Medicine, 2nd ed. London, UK: Elsevier, 2014:203–248.

Authors Barbara Oglesbee, DVM, and Vittorio Capello, DVM

PYODERMA

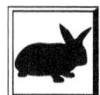 **BASICS**

DEFINITION
Bacterial infection of the skin

PATHOPHYSIOLOGY
• Skin infections occur when the surface integrity of the skin has been broken, the skin has become macerated by chronic exposure to moisture, normal bacterial flora have been altered, circulation has been impaired, or immunocompetency has been compromised.
• Pyoderma in rabbits is usually secondary to an underlying condition that prevents normal grooming or causes chronic exposure to moisture and/or contact with excrement. Identification and correction of the underlying cause(s) are essential for successful treatment.

SYSTEMS AFFECTED
Skin/Exocrine

INCIDENCE/PREVALENCE
Pyoderma is an extremely common problem in pet rabbits.

SIGNALMENT
Breed Predilections
• Breeds with dense fur or long coats such as dwarf, miniature lops, and angoras are more prone to perineal dermatitis.
• Any breed with underlying dental, musculoskeletal, gastrointestinal, or urinary disease may develop secondary pyoderma.

Mean Age and Range
Age of onset usually related to underlying cause

Predominant Sex
Female rabbits are somewhat more prone to perineal and dewlap pyodermas.

SIGNS
General Comments
• Determined by underlying cause. The location of pyoderma is important for establishing a differential diagnosis and determining the underlying cause.
• Three locations are most common: facial, chin/dewlap, and perineal.
• Pododermatitis is also a common problem; this topic is discussed in another section.
• Multifocal pyoderma or pyoderma localized to regions other than the face, dewlap, or perineal region are less common, and most frequently secondary to ectoparasites or trauma.

Historical Findings
• Facial pyoderma—history of dental disease, epiphora, nasal or ocular discharge, and exophthalmia
• Chin, neck, or dewlap dermatitis—history of dental disease, ptyalism, anorexia, and nasal or ocular discharge

• Perineal dermatitis—history of obesity, intermittent diarrhea, uneaten cecotrophs, lameness, reluctance to move, polydypsia/polyuria, lower urinary tract disease or poor sanitation
• Multifocal or focal pyoderma—history of trauma or ectoparasites

Physical Examination Findings
Determined by the underlying disease or area affected:
• Facial pyoderma—unilateral or bilateral alopecia, crusts, matted fur in periocular area, cheeks, and/or nasal rostrum. Pyoderma is secondary to chronic ocular discharge or epiphora. Most common cause of ocular discharge/epiphora is blockage of the nasolacrimal duct, usually by the elongated tooth roots or chronic upper respiratory infection. Findings may include ptyalism, anorexia, nasal discharge, ocular discharge, or exophthalmia. Always perform a thorough oral exam.
• Perineal dermatitis—alopecia or matted fur may extend from perineal region to inner thighs and abdomen; fur may be urine soaked or matted with feces/cecotrophs; underlying skin may appear ulcerated, erythemic; purulent exudate and necrotic debris may be present, especially in animals with deep perineal skin folds; may lead to myiasis (fly strike). Depending on the underlying cause, may find palpable sand within the urinary bladder, obesity, and musculoskeletal pain.
• Chin, neck, and dewlap pyoderma—alopecia, erythema, matted fur, enlarged and thickened skin folds, variable crusts. Most commonly caused by constant moisture from ptyalism as a symptom of dental disease. May see fractured teeth, food lodged between teeth and/or gingival mucosal; malocclusion causing sharp points on crowns, which penetrate oral mucosal. Always perform a thorough oral examination.

CAUSES
• *Staphylococcus aureus, Pseudomonas aeruginosa*, or *Pasteurella multocida* most frequent.
• Matting of fur—from an inability to properly groom. Matted fur traps moisture, feces, and bacteria near the skin. Inability to groom may be due to dental disease, musculoskeletal disease, obesity, or pain with severe pyoderma.
• Chronic exposure to moisture:
  ◦ Epiphora (facial) or ptyalism (dewlap); both are most commonly caused by dental disease or chronic upper respiratory infection.
  ◦ Urine scald (perineal, ventral)—due to underlying urinary tract disease, polyuria, or conditions that do not allow the rabbit to maintain a normal posture while

urinating (musculoskeletal disease, obesity). Rabbits normally lift their hindquarters and spray urine caudally; an inability to maintain this posture causes urine to soak the perineal region and ventrum. Urine may also collect in perineal skin folds in rabbits with excessive folds.
  ◦ Feces (perineal, ventral)—uneaten cecotrophs, chronic diarrhea.
  ◦ Environment—water bowls (dewlap), urine-soaked bedding (perineal, ventral)

RISK FACTORS
• Dental disease—periapical or tooth root abscesses, tooth root impaction, fractured teeth, food lodged between teeth and/or gingival mucosal; malocclusion causing sharp points on crowns, which penetrate oral mucosal; may cause ptyalism or blockage of nasolacrimal duct leading to epiphora; may inhibit grooming
• Chronic upper respiratory tract infection—may cause obstruction of the nasolacrimal duct leading to epiphora
• Obesity—interferes with normal grooming; prevents normal posture while urinating; excessive skin folds retain moisture
• Musculoskeletal disease—arthritis, spondylosis, spinal injury, fractures, and pododermatitis—interferes with normal grooming and/or prevents normal posture while urinating; may prevent ingestion of cecotrophs
• Excessive skin folds—in dewlap or perineal region—trap moisture, debris, and bacteria
• Husbandry—urine- or water-soaked bedding; water bowls may cause chronic soaking of the chin and dewlap in rabbits with large dewlaps
• Parasites—fleas, cheyletiella
• Contact irritants
• Fungal infection—dermatophyte
• Immune incompetency—glucocorticoids; young animals
• Trauma pressure points; scratching; bite wounds; injection site reaction

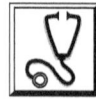 **DIAGNOSIS**

DIFFERENTIAL DIAGNOSIS
• Barbering—hair loss along the flanks, body wall. Close examination reveals broken hairs. Dominant cage mate pulls/chews hairs on submissive rabbit; owners may not observe this behavior. Self-barbering may be due to a craving for fiber seen in rabbits fed diets deficient in hay, or as a nesting behavior in reproductively active females.
• *Cheyletiella* or *Leporacarus gibbus*—lesions are usually located in the intrascapular or tail base region and associated with copious amounts of large white scale. Mites are

readily identified in skin scrapes or acetate tape preparations under low magnification.
• Ear mites—alopecia around ear base, pinna; may extend to face, neck, abdomen, perineal region; intense pruritus; brown, beige crusty exudate in the ear canal and pinna
• Fleas—patchy alopecia; finding flea dirt will help to differentiate; secondary pyoderma sometimes seen
• Injection reactions—alopecia, scabs, scale, erythema, usually in the intrascapular region as this is a common site of subcutaneous injections, most common seen with Penicillin G injections
• Lack of grooming—may cause alopecia and an accumulation of scale in intrascapular or tail base regions
• Dermatophytosis—partial to complete alopecia with scaling; with or without erythema; not always ringlike; may begin as small papules
• *Treponema cuniculi* (rabbit syphilis)— alopecia, crusts at mucocutaneous junctions, especially nose, lips, and genitalia
• Neoplasia—basal cell tumors, cutaneous lymphoma, cutaneous epitheliotropic lymphoma (mycoses fungoides), or mast cell tumors—rare in rabbits; focal or diffuse truncal alopecia; scaling and erythema; may see plaque formation
• Sebaceous adenitis—large amounts of white scale; alopecia; usually begins around the head and neck; may be associated with thymic lymphoma or thymoma. Differentiate by skin biopsy and histologic examination.

CBC/BIOCHEMISTRY/URINALYSIS
• May reflect the underlying cause (e.g., causes of polydipsia/polyuria, diarrhea, and urinary tract infection)
• CBC changes due to pyoderma alone are usually not present.

IMAGING
• Dental or skull radiographs—to identify type and extent of dental disease in rabbits with facial or dewlap pyoderma; perform under general anesthesia
• Radiographs are generally very useful in identifying the underlying cause of perineal pyoderma (e.g., spinal lesions, osteoarthritis, and urinary tract disease)
• Ultrasonography—may be useful in the diagnosis of underlying urinary or gastrointestinal disorders

DIAGNOSTIC PROCEDURES
• Skin scrapings, dermatophyte culture— identify the underlying cause
• Skin biopsy—to rule out neoplasia, if suspected
• Culture—usually positive for *S. aureus*, other organisms may be identified; may be useful to direct antibiotic therapy

PATHOLOGIC FINDINGS
• Folliculitis
• Furunculous
• Inflammatory reaction—suppurative or pyogranulomatous
• Special stains—identify gram-negative bacteria or treponema

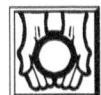

TREATMENT
APPROPRIATE HEALTH CARE
Usually outpatient, unless treatment of underlying cause requires hospitalization
NURSING CARE
• Matted hair must be removed in order for treatment to be effective. Be extremely cautious when clipping hair or pulling on mats since rabbit skin is extremely fragile and will easily tear. Electric clippers are often ineffective in removing thick mats. Curved scissors work best. Work slowly and carefully so as not to damage the skin. Rabbits with large, matted areas will require sedation.
• Bathing should not be performed until all mats are removed. Wet hair mats readily, retains moisture, and may exacerbate pyoderma. After removing matted hair, or on alopecic areas, gentle cleaning with chlorhexidine shampoos will remove surface debris.
• Use extreme caution when dipping or bathing rabbits due to the high risk of skeletal fractures, excessive chilling, and severe stress when performed by inexperienced owners.
• Thoroughly dry the rabbit after bathing.

ACTIVITY
No restriction
DIET
No restrictions
CLIENT EDUCATION
• Inform owner that resolution of dermatitis requires correction of underlying cause. Some conditions, such as chronic dental disease and orthopedic disorders, require a long-term time and financial commitment.
• Stress the importance of good hygiene— clean wet, soiled bedding

SURGICAL CONSIDERATIONS
Fold pyodermas may require surgical correction to prevent recurrence.

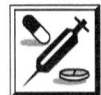

MEDICATIONS
DRUG(S) OF CHOICE
• Treat underlying disease
• Superficial—initially may be treated empirically with broad-spectrum antibiotics

such as enrofloxacin (10–20 mg/kg PO, SC, IM q12–24h), marbofloxacin (5 mg/kg PO q24h), and trimethoprim-sulfa (30 mg/kg PO q12h)
• Recurrent, resistant, or deep—base antibiotic therapy on culture and sensitivity testing
• Superficial, moist dermatitis—apply zinc oxide + menthol powder (Gold Bond, Martin Himmel, Inc.) to clean, clipped skin q24h
• Perineal dermatitis can be extremely painful—administer meloxicam (1 mg/kg PO q24h) or carprofen (2–4 mg/kg PO q12–24h)

CONTRAINDICATIONS
• Oral administration of antibiotics that select against gram-positive bacteria (penicillins, macrolides, lincosamides, and cephalosporins) can cause fatal enteric dysbiosis and enterotoxemia.
• Steroids, topical or systemic—will encourage resistance and recurrence even when used concurrently with antibiotics
• Topical antibiotic creams or ointments— may be ingested by rabbit and lead to enteric dysbiosis

PRECAUTIONS
Use extreme caution when dipping or bathing rabbits due to the high risk of skeletal fractures and excessive chilling when performed by inexperienced owners; sudden death has been reported following bathing.

FOLLOW-UP
PATIENT MONITORING
Administer antibiotics for a minimum of 2 weeks beyond clinical cure.

PREVENTION/AVOIDANCE
• Prevent progressive dental disease by selecting pets without congenital predisposition (when possible), providing high-fiber foods and good-quality hay, discontinuing or limiting the feeding of pellets and soft fruits or vegetables, and periodically trimming overgrown crowns.
• Prevent obesity.
• Provide clean, appropriate surface substrates.

POSSIBLE COMPLICATIONS
• Myiasis
• Pododermatitis
• Bacteremia and septicemia

EXPECTED COURSE AND PROGNOSIS
Likely to be recurrent or nonresponsive if underlying cause is not identified and effectively managed

PYODERMA

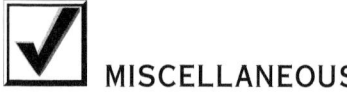

MISCELLANEOUS

ASSOCIATED CONDITIONS
Gastrointestinal hypomotility

SEE ALSO
Cheek teeth maloclussion
Dysuria and hematuria
Hypercalciuria and urolithiasis
Lameness
Obesity
Ptyalism (slobbers)
Ulcerative pododermatitis (sore hocks)

Suggested Reading
Meredith A. Dermatoses. In: Meredith A, Lord B, eds. BSAVA Manual of Rabbit Medicine. Gloucester: British Small Animal Veterinary Association, 2014:255–263.

Palmerio BS, Roberts H. Clinical approach to dermatologic disease in exotic animals. Vet Clin North Am Exot Anim Pract. 2013;16(3):523–577.

Snook TS, White SD, Hawkins MG et al. Skin diseases in pet rabbits: a retrospective study of 334 cases seen at the University of California at Davis, USA (1984–2004). Vet Dermatol 2013;24:613–618.

Varga M. Skin diseases. In: Varga M, ed. Textbook of Rabbit Medicine, 2nd ed. Elsiver, 2014:224–248.

Varga M, Patterson S. Dermatologic diseases of rabbits. In: Quesenberry KE, Carpenter JW, eds. Ferrets, Rabbits and Rodents, 4th Ed). Clinical Medicine and Surgery. 2021 ed. St. Louis: Saunders, 2020:220–222.

Author Barbara Oglesbee, DVM, DABVP (Avian)

RABBITS

PYOMETRA AND NONNEOPLASTIC ENDOMETRIAL DISORDERS

BASICS

OVERVIEW
• Pyometra—develops when bacterial invasion of abnormal endometrium leads to intraluminal accumulation of purulent exudate. Occurs less commonly than other endometrial disorders, including adenocarcinoma.
• Endometrial disorders—common endometrial disorders of rabbits include endometiral hyperplasia (most common), endometrial venous aneurysms, endometriosis, and endometritis. Less common disorders include hydrometra and mucometra.
• Most endometrial disorders can result in significant uterine hemorrhage.
• Frequently see more than one disorder in the same rabbit, especially in rabbits with uterine adenocarcinoma. For instance, many rabbits with uterine neoplasia also have areas of cystic endometrial hyperplasia.
• May be difficult clinically to differentiate nonneoplastic endometrial disorders from uterine adenocarcinoma prior to ovariohysterectomy.
• Normal-cycling rabbits (female rabbit is called a doe)—become reproductively active as early as 4 months of age; induced ovulators with silent estrus; estrous cycles last 7–14 days; most does receptive to males approximately 14 of every 16 days.
• Pseudopregnancy—can occur even in solitary does; lasts 16–17 days (normal gestation 30–33 days); commonly followed by hydrometra, pyometra, or endometrial hyperplasia.
• Bacteria—endometrial secretions provide excellent media for growth; ascend from the vagina through the partially open cervix during proestrus and estrus; may be transmitted from male during copulation; hematogenous spread also reported
• The cause of endometrial venous aneurysm is unknown; often multiple aneurysms are present; rupture results in significant, possibly life-threatening hemorrhage.

SIGNALMENT
• Intact females
• Highest incidence in does >3–4 years old
• All breeds are at risk

SIGNS
Historical Findings
• Hematuria—most common presenting complaint. Not true hematuria since blood originates from the uterus but is released during micturition. Hematuria is often reported as intermittent or cyclic; usually occurs at the end of micturition
• Does with mild or early endometrial disease may have no clinical signs
• Serosanguinous to purulent, blood-tinged vaginal discharge
• Increased aggressiveness
• May have had signs of pseudopregnancy—pulling hair, nest building
• Closed cervix pyometra—signs of systemic illness, may progress to signs of septicemia and shock
• Breeding does—small litter size; increased number of stillborn or resorbed fetuses; infertility; dystocia; abandonment of litters
• Polydipsia and polyuria may be seen with pyometra

Physical Examination Findings
• Uterus—often palpably large; careful palpation may allow determination of size; overly aggressive palpation may induce rupture in rabbits with pyometra, as the uterus can be extremely friable
• Serosanguinous to purulent, blood-tinged vaginal discharge
• Blood-stained perineum
• Enlarged mammary gland—one or multiple, may be firm and multilobulated (mammary tumors), or fluid filled (cystic); septic mastitis may also occur
• Pale mucous membranes, tachycardia in rabbits that have had significant uterine hemorrhage
• Depression, lethargy, anorexia in rabbits with pyometra or uterine hemorrhage

CAUSES AND RISK FACTORS
• Intact sexual status
• Risk increases with age—seen more often in rabbits over 3 years of age
• Risk may increase with sterile mating, or when does mount each other
• Common bacterial pathogens in pyometra—*Pasteurella multocida* and *Staphylococcus aureus* most common; others include *Chlamydia, Listeria monocytogenes, Moraxella bovis, Actinomyces pyogens, Brucella melitensis,* and *Salmonella* spp.

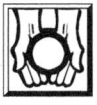

DIAGNOSIS

DIFFERENTIAL DIAGNOSIS
• Pregnancy
• Uterine adenocarcinoma—more common uterine disorder
• Other uterine neoplasia (leiomyoma)

CBC/BIOCHEMISTRY/URINALYSIS
• Often unremarkable
• Neutrophilia—sometimes seen in rabbits with pyometra; most often with relative lymphopenia; TWBC elevations usually not seen
• Regenerative (and occasionally nonregenerative) anemia possible in rabbits with uterine hemorrhage
• Azotemia, increases in ALT, electrolyte disturbances—all can be abnormal in rabbits with pyometra, septicemia, or severe dehydration, depending on clinical course
• Urinalysis—sample collected by ultrasound-guided cystocentesis to differentiate hematuria from uterine bleeding

OTHER LABORATORY TESTS
• Cytologic examination of vaginal discharge—polymorphonuclear cells and bacteria
• Bacterial culture and sensitivity test of uterine contents—obtained during ovariohysterectomy to direct antibiotic therapy; vaginal culture not helpful in confirming diagnosis (bacteria cultured are usually normal vaginal flora)
• Histopathologic examination of uterus following ovariohysterectomy—necessary for definitive diagnosis

IMAGING
Radiography
• Detect a large uterus
• Rule out pregnancy—average gestation lasts 30–33 days, calcification of skeletons occurs in last trimester
• Pyometra—uterus may appear as a distended, tubular structure in the caudal ventral abdomen.

Ultrasonography
• Assess size of uterus and nature of uterine contents.
• Rule out pregnancy.

TREATMENT

APPROPRIATE HEALTH CARE
Inpatient in does with pyometra, or uterine hemorrhage; can be life threatening

NURSING CARE
• Supportive care—immediate intravenous fluid administration and antibiotics in does with pyometra
• Blood transfusion may be required in does with significant uterine hemorrhage.

DIET
• Many affected rabbits are anorectic or have a decreased appetite. It is an absolute requirement that the patient continue to eat during and following treatments. Anorexia may cause or exacerbate gastrointestinal hypomotility and cause derangement of the gastrointestinal microflora and overgrowth of intestinal bacterial pathogens. If the patient refuses these foods, syringe-feed Critical Care for Herbivores (Oxbow Animal Health, Murdock, NE) or Emeraid Herbivore (Lafeber Company, Cornell, IL) diet at approximately 10–15 mL/kg PO q6–8h. Larger volumes and more frequent feedings are often accepted; feed as much as the patient will readily accept. Alternatively, pellets can be

PYOMETRA AND NONNEOPLASTIC ENDOMETRIAL DISORDERS (CONTINUED)

ground and mixed with fresh greens, vegetable baby foods, or water to form a gruel

CLIENT EDUCATION

• Inform client that ovariohysterectomy is indicated with any uterine disorder.
• Medical treatment is not recommended—uterus contains thick exudate that does not drain in does with endometritis or pyometra.
• Most other uterine disorders carry risk of hemorrhage into the uterus; can become life threatening; can progress; all are at risk for developing uterine adenocarcinoma; reproductive performance is reduced in does with endometrial disorders
• Inform client that medical treatment does not cure underlying endometrial disease; progression of disease can be life threatening

SURGICAL CONSIDERATIONS

• Ovariohysterectomy preferred treatment for all uterine disorders
• Proceed cautiously; enlarged uterus may be friable, adhesions, and ovarian abscesses may accompany pyometra
• Ligate caudal to the cervix in the proximal vagina, so that the bicornate cervix (double cervix) is also removed.
• Handle tissues minimally and keep tissues moist intraoperatively to help prevent postoperative adhesion formation.
• Avoid reactive suture materials, use hemoclips or nonreactive suture to prevent postoperative adhesion formation.
• Uterine rupture or leakage of purulent material from the uterine stump—repeated lavage of the peritoneal cavity with sterile saline

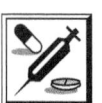

MEDICATIONS

DRUG(S) OF CHOICE

Antibiotics
• Empirical, pending results of bacterial culture and sensitivity test
• All patients with pyometra or endometritis
• Use broad-spectrum antibiotics such as enrofloxacin (10–20 mg/kg PO, SC, IM, IV q12h), marbofloxacin (5 mg/kg PO q24h), trimethoprim-sulfa (15–30 mg/kg PO q12h), or chloramphenicol (50 mg/kg PO q8h).

Acute Pain Management
• Butorphanol (0.1–0.5 mg/kg SQ, IM, IV q4–6h); may cause profound sedation; short acting
• Buprenorphine (0.02–0.05 mg/kg SQ, IM IV q8–12h); less sedating, longer acting than butorphanol
• Hydromorphone (0.1 mg/kg SC IM q2–4h) or oxymorphone (0.05–0.2 mg/kg SC IM q8–12h)
• Meloxicam (1 mg/kg PO, SC, IM q24h)
• Carprofen (2–4 mg/kg PO, SC q12–24h)

Long-Term Pain Management
• Nonsteroidal anti-inflammatories—have been used for short- or long-term therapy to reduce pain and inflammation; meloxicam (1.0 mg/kg PO q24h; carprofen (2 mg/kg PO q12h)
• Tramadol—5–15 mg/kg PO q8–12h
• Gabapentin—5–20 mg/kg PO q8–12h

CONTRAINDICATIONS

• Oral administration of most antibiotics effective against anaerobes will cause a fatal gastrointestinal dysbiosis in rabbits. Do not administer penicillins, macrolides, lincosamides, and cephalosporins orally.
• Corticosteroids—associated with gastrointestinal ulceration and hemorrhage, delayed wound healing, and heightened susceptibility to infection; rabbits are very sensitive to the immunosuppressive effects of both topical and systemic corticosteroids; use may exacerbate subclinical bacterial infection

PRECAUTIONS

• Chloramphenicol—avoid human contact with chloramphenicol due to potential blood dyscrasia. Advise owners of potential risks.
• Meloxicam and other NSAIDs—use with caution in rabbits with compromised renal function
• Oral administration of any antibiotic may potentially cause enteric dysbiosis; discontinue use if diarrhea or anorexia occurs.

ALTERNATIVE DRUGS

Prostaglandins—PGF2a has not been used successfully in rabbits.

FOLLOW-UP

PATIENT MONITORING

• Monitor carefully for signs of pain (reluctance to move, teeth grinding) postoperatively.
• Make certain the doe continues to eat postoperatively.
• If owners elect not to perform surgery, monitor carefully for signs of uterine hemorrhage (blood passed during micturition) or sepsis in rabbits with endometritis or mastitis.

PREVENTION/AVOIDANCE

• Ovariohysterectomy for all nonbreeding rabbits; usually performed between 6 months and 2 years of age
• For breeding rabbits—recommend stop breeding and spay after 4 years of age, as this is when most endometrial disorders (including adenocarcinoma) occur.

POSSIBLE COMPLICATIONS

• Peritonitis, sepsis in does with endometritis or pyometra
• Postoperative intra-abdominal adhesions—may contribute to chronic pain, gastrointestinal motility disorders

• Uterine adenocarcinoma in does over 3 years of age
• Hemorrhage, possible death in rabbits with bleeding uterine disorders

EXPECTED COURSE AND PROGNOSIS

• Good prognosis with timely ovariohysterectomy for most uterine disorders, including adenocarcinoma that has not metastasized
• Guarded prognosis in does with vigorous vaginal hemorrhage; emergency stabilization and hysterectomy are indicated to control hemorrhage.
• Guarded to poor in does with pyometra that is not treated early; sepsis or peritonitis may follow

MISCELLANEOUS

ASSOCIATED CONDITIONS

• Mammary neoplasia
• Mastitis
• Ovarian neoplasia
• Ovarian abscess
• Pyometra of the uterine stump in spayed animals—may develop any time after ovariohysterectomy

AGE-RELATED FACTORS

Risk increases with age

SEE ALSO

Mastitis, cystic and septic
Uterine Adenocarcinoma

ABBREVIATIONS

ALP = alkaline phosphatase
ALT = alanine transferase
GI = gastrointestinal
NSAID = nonsteroidal anti-inflammatory drug
PGF2a = prostaglandin F2a

Suggested Reading
Di Girolamo N, Selleri P. Disorders of the urinary and reproductive system. In: Quesenberry KE, Carpenter JW, eds. Ferrets, Rabbits and Rodents, 4th Ed). Clinical Medicine and Surgery ed. St. Louis: Saunders, 2020:201–220.
Hallman RM, Brandão J. Diagnostic imaging of the renal system in exotic companion mammals. Vet Clin Exot Anim 2020;23:195–214.
Mancinelli E, Lord B. Urogenital and reproductive disease. In: Meredith A, Lord B, eds. BSAVA Manual of Rabbit Medicine. Gloucester: British Small Animal Veterinary Association, 2014:191–204.
Reavill DR, Lennox AM. Disease overview of the urinary tract in exotic companion mammals and tips on clinical management. Vet Clin Exot Anim 2020;23(1):169–193.
Author Barbara Oglesbee, DVM, DABVP (Avian)

RABBIT HEMORRHAGIC DISEASE VIRUS (RHDV)

BASICS

DEFINITION
Rabbit hemorrhagic disease virus (RHDV) is an extremely contagious and fatal viral disease of *Oryctolagus cuniculus* rabbits. RHDV is a calicivirus (lagovirus) that causes severe losses in unvaccinated animals (up to 80% morbidity and 80%–90% mortality rates) and major economic losses in industry rabbits.

PATHOPHYSIOLOGY
• Most commonly spread by direct contact with infected animals via oral, nasal, or conjunctival mucosa. Other routes include an infected carcass or hair and fomites (including contaminated food, bedding, and water). Importation of infected rabbit meat may be the main transmission method of RHDV to a new area. Meat contains high levels of virus-infected blood, which survives freezing well. Flies and other insects are very efficient mechanical vectors; only a few virions are needed to infect a rabbit by the conjunctival route.
• Virus replication does not seem to occur in predators, but predators can excrete RHDV in feces after ingestion of infected rabbits.
• The duration of shedding by rabbits that survive RHD is unknown. Low levels of antibodies are sufficient to protect rabbits. PCR has demonstrated persistence of viral RNA for up to 2 months in recovered or vaccinated rabbits. Liver has the highest concentration of virus, followed by the spleen and serum. Urine, feces, and respiratory secretions can contain virus.
• Virus replication occurs in the liver, lungs, spleen, and intestines, with subsequent viremia and diffuse hemorrhage. Disseminated intravascular coagulation (DIC) likely plays an import role.

SYSTEMS AFFECTED
Multiorgan system involvement, especially hepatic and respiratory

GENETICS
N/A

INCIDENCE/PREVALENCE
• RHDV has become endemic in Europe, Cuba, Australia, and New Zealand. Limited outbreaks have occurred in the Middle East, South America, Mexico, and the United States.

GEOGRAPHIC DISTRIBUTION
• Disease has been recognized in North America, Europe, Cuba, Mexico, South America, Africa, China, North Korea, Australia, and New Zealand.
• While considered a foreign animal disease in the North America, there have been several outbreaks in the United States, often of unknown origin. Classical RHDV and RHDVa (an antigenic variant) are in one serotype but are defined as different subtypes. A recently emerged serotype—RHDV2 was identified in Europe. In February 2018, an outbreak of RHDV2 was reported in British Columbia, Canada, in the United States. There are many strains of RHDV, which can lead to confusion that it is a different/new serotype. Fr example, Czech CAPM 351RHDV was the strain accidentally introduced in Australia in 1995 that led to a temporary crash (10 million dead rabbits in eight weeks) in feral domestic rabbit population. After the population rebounded due to resistance, Australia intentionally introduced strain RHDV1 K5, to continue lethal control of the invasive species. Suspect cases should be immediately reported to state and federal veterinarians.

SIGNALMENT
Species
• RHDV affects wild and domesticated European rabbits (*Oryctolagus cuniculus*).
• Cottontails (*Sylvilagus floridanus*), black-tailed jackrabbits (*Lepus californicus*), and volcano rabbits (*Romerolagus diazzi*) are *not susceptible*. Similarly, all hare species (*Lepus* spp.) are not affected by RHDV, although they are affected by a different calicivirus (European brown hare syndrome). Virus replication has not been reported in other mammals, although seroconversion can occur.

Breed Predilections
All breeds of domestic rabbits are susceptible.

Mean Age and Range
• Disease is seen in rabbits greater than 8 weeks of age; usually subclinical in animals younger than 8 weeks old
• Animals less than four weeks of age are unaffected. This "youth" resistance is still poorly understood. Surviving rabbits develop immunity and become resistant to related strains of RHDV.

Predominant Sex
None

SIGNS
Historical Findings
• The incubation period is 1–3 days, with death 12–36 hours after the onset of fever.
• Suspect an outbreak when there are multiple cases of sudden death following acute lethargy, fever, and characteristic hepatic necrosis or evidence of DIC at necropsy.
• In wild rabbits, can be seasonal, has been associated with breeding season.

Physical Examination Findings
• RHD can be peracute, acute, subacute, or chronic; clinical signs usually seen in the peracute form; the subacute form is characterized by similar but milder signs.
• May be found dead with no premonitory signs
• Anorexia
• Lethargy
• Prostration
• Neurologic signs (convulsion, ataxia, paralysis, opisthotonos, and paddling)
• Groans and cries
• Respiratory signs (dyspnea, frothy and bloody nasal discharge)
• Cyanosis of mucous membranes
• During an outbreak, 5%–10% may show a chronic form with severe and generalized jaundice, loss of weight, and lethargy. These animals often die 1–2 weeks later, due to liver dysfunction.

CAUSES
Exposure to RHDV, a calicivirus

RISK FACTORS
Exposure to infected rabbits, rabbit products, and fomites such as cages, bedding, food, and water. Virus remains viable for months in frozen rabbit meat and decomposing carcasses.

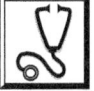

DIAGNOSIS
If RHD is suspected, immediately contact state and federal veterinary regulatory agencies.

DIFFERENTIAL DIAGONSIS
• Septicemic pasteurellosis
• Tularemia
• Poisoning
• Heat stroke
• Atypical myxomatosis
• Other causes of severe septicemia with secondary DIC (*E. coli, Clostridium perfrigens* Type E)

CBC/BIOCHEMISTRY/URINALYSIS
• Often shows a lymphopenia and a gradual decline in the number of thrombocytes
• May see elevated liver enzymes

OTHER LABORATORY TESTS
• In most moribund rabbits, prothrombin and thrombin times are prolonged, and fibrin degradation products can be detected.
• Hemagglutination test, electron microscopy, virus detection ELISA, immunostaining, western blot, RT-PCR, and in situ hybridization are all advanced testing that may be performed at the discretion of the governmental entity involved in the outbreak. In the United States, tissue samples are often submitted to the National Veterinary Services Laboratories (NVSL) Foreign Animal Disease Diagnostic Laboratory (FADDL) at the governmental veterinarian-in-charge's discretion.
• Collect both fresh and formalin-fixed liver, spleen, lung, and kidney, and blood (whole

and EDTA). The liver is the organ of choice for viral identification in patients with peracute and acute disease; the spleen is a better with chronic or subacute disease.
• RT-PCR can detect viral RNA in a many organs, urine, feces, or serum.
• Serum should be collected for serology (hemagglutination inhibition test; indirect or competitive ELISA).

IMAGING
N/A

DIAGNOSTIC PROCEDURES
N/A

PATHOLOGIC FINDINGS
• Due to the rapid course of this disease, deceased animals are usually found in good body condition.
• Gross pathological lesions are variable, may be subtle; usually see diffuse hepatomegaly and hepatic necrosis, splenomegaly, pulmonary hemorrhage, and serosal ecchymoses and petechiation in multiple organs.
• The most severe lesions are in the liver, trachea, and lungs. The liver appears yellowish-brown, brittle, and degenerated, with a marked lobular pattern. The tracheal mucosa is hyperemic, containing abundant frothy fluid, and the lungs are edematous and congested.
• In subacute and chronic disease, an icteric discoloration of the ears, conjunctiva, and subcutis may be noted.

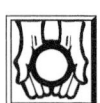

TREATMENT

APPROPRIATE HEALTH CARE
To be determined by governmental veterinarian-in-charge. Quarantine, disinfection of infected premises/establishment(s); once confirmed, likely euthanasia of all affected and exposed animals

NURSING CARE
Generally not advised

ACTIVITY
Confine to quarantine area

DIET
N/A

CLIENT EDUCATION
Follow directives of governmental veterinarian-in-charge.

SURGICAL CONSIDERATIONS
N/A

MEDICATIONS

DRUG(S) OF CHOICE
N/A

CONTRAINDICATIONS
N/A

PRECAUTIONS
N/A

ALTERNATIVE DRUG(S)
N/A

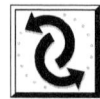

FOLLOW-UP

PATIENT MONITORING
N/A

PREVENTION/AVOIDANCE
• RHDV is very stable. Survives temperatures of 50°C for an hour, as well as freeze–thaw cycles. Stable at pH 4.5–10.5. Survives pH 3.0, but inactivated at pH >12.
• Inactivated with sodium hydroxide (1%) or formalin (1%–2%). The World Organization for Animal Health (OIE) Code recommends formalin (3%) for disinfecting pelts. Other suggested disinfectants include substituted phenolics (e.g., 2% One-stroke Environ) and 0.5% sodium hypochlorite.
• RHDV is very resistant to inactivation, particularly when protected by organic material. Virus may persist in chilled or frozen rabbit meat, as well as in decomposing carcasses in the environment or on fomites for months.
• If wild rabbit populations are not affected, eradication can be accomplished by depopulation, disinfection, surveillance, and quarantines.
• In the United States, the USDA granted Emergency Use Authorization for an inactivated recombinant subunit vaccine against RHDV2 produced by Medgene Labs. This is administered SC as a 2-dose regimen, with the booster given 21 days following the initial dose, with annual boosters.
• Two inactivated vaccines against RHDV2 are a licensed by the European Union.

POSSIBLE COMPLICATIONS
Side effects of the RHDV2 vaccine include swelling at the injection site and lethargy.

EXPECTED COURSE AND PROGNOSIS
Exposed rabbits will likely die, or euthanasia is recommended to prevent spread.

MISCELLANEOUS

ASSOCIATED CONDITIONS
None

AGE-RELATED FACTORS
Very young rabbits (<8 weeks of age) often unaffected

ZOONOTIC POTENTIAL
N/A

PREGNACY/FERTILITY/BREEDING
Vulvar hemorrhages were noted in some pregnant does.

ABBREVIATIONS
DIC = disseminated intravascular coagulopathy
EDTA = ethylenediaminetetraacetic acid
ELISA = enzyme-linked immunosorbent assay
PCR = polymerase chain reaction
RHD = rabbit hemorrhagic disease
RHDV = rabbit hemorrhagic disease virus
RT-PCR = reverse transcriptase polymerase chain reaction

SYNONYMS
Necrotic hepatitis of rabbits
Rabbit calicivirus disease
Rabbit hemorrhagic disease syndrome
X disease

INTERNET RESOURCES
https://cdn.ymaws.com/www.aazv.org/resource/resmgr/IDM/IDM_Rabbit_Hemorrhagic_Disea.pdf. Accessed 21 November 2018.
http://www.cfsph.iastate.edu/Factsheets/pdfs/rabbit_hemorrhagic_disease.pdf. Accessed 21 November 2018.
https://www.oie.int/fileadmin/Home/eng/Animal_Health_in_the_World/docs/pdf/Disease_cards/RHD.pdf. Accessed 21 November 2018.
https://en.wikipedia.org/wiki/Rabbit_haemorrhagic_disease. Accessed 21 November 2018.

Suggested Reading
Hall RN, Mahar JE, Haboury S et al. Emerging rabbit hemorrhagic disease virus 2 (RHDVb), Australia. Emerg Infect Dis 2015;21(12):2276–2278.
Lavazza A, Cavadini P, Barbieri I et al. Field and experimental data indicate that the eastern cottontail (*Sylvilagus floridanus*) is susceptible to infection with European brown hare syndrome (EBHS) virus and not with rabbit haemorrhagic disease (RHD) virus. Vet Res 2015;46:13.
Mahar JE, Read AJ, Gu X et al. Detection and circulation of a novel rabbit hemorrhagic disease virus in Australia. Emerg Infect Dis 2018;24(1):22–31.
Marschang R, Weider K, Erhard H et al. Rabbit hemorrhagic disease viruses detected in pet rabbits in a commercial laboratory in Europe. J Exot Pet Med 2018;27(4):27–30.

Author Eric Klaphake, DVM, Dipl. ABVP, Dipl. ACZM

BASICS

DEFINITION
Hyperemia of the eyelids, conjunctiva, or ocular vasculature or hemorrhage within the eye

PATHOPHYSIOLOGY
• Active dilation of ocular vessels—in response to extraocular or intraocular inflammation or passive congestion
• Hemorrhage from existing or newly formed blood vessels
• Many rabbits with ocular disease have underlying chronic respiratory or dental disease
• Most dental disease is secondary to tooth root elongation

SYSTEMS AFFECTED
• Ophthalmic—eye and/or ocular adnexa
• Oral Cavity—related dental disease
• Respiratory—related respiratory infections and apical (tooth root) invasion of the sinuses

SIGNALMENT
• Middle-aged to older rabbits—acquired cheek tooth elongation causing blockage of nasolacrimal duct or intrusion into the retrobulbar space
• Young animals—congenital tooth malocclusion, congenital eyelid deformities
• Dwarf and lop breeds—congenital tooth malocclusion
• Dwarf and Himalayan breeds—glaucoma more common
• Rex and New Zealand white breeds—entropion and trichiasis more common
• Other ocular diseases—no breed, age, or sex predilection

SIGNS

Historical Findings
• Depend on cause
• History of previous treatment for dental disease
• History of nasal discharge or previous upper respiratory infection
• Facial asymmetry, masses, or exophthalmos in rabbits with tooth root abscesses or facial nerve paralysis
• Unilateral or bilateral alopecia, crusts, matted fur in periocular area, cheeks, and/or nasal rostrum

Physical Examination Findings
• Depend on cause
• Blepharospasm
• Ocular discharge—serous, mucoid, or mucopurulent
• Thick, white exudate accumulation in medial canthus in rabbits with dacryocystitis

• Corneal ulcers associated with dacryocystitis are usually superficial and ventrally located; ulcers secondary to exposure keratitis are usually central and may be superficial or deep.
• Chemosis
• Excessive conjunctival tissue—may partially or completely occlude the cornea
• Facial pyoderma—alopecia, erythema, matted fur, in periocular area, cheeks, and/or nasal rostrum. Due to constant moisture in rabbits with epiphora

Oral Examination
• A thorough examination of the oral cavity is indicated in every rabbit with epiphora. A thorough examination includes the incisors, molars, and buccal and lingual mucosa to rule out dental disease. Use of an otoscope or speculum may be useful in identifying severe abnormalities; however, many problems will be missed by using this method alone. Complete exam requires heavy sedation or general anesthesia and specialized equipment.
• A focused, directed light source and magnification (or a rigid endoscope) will provide optimal visualization.
• Use a rodent mouth gag and cheek dilators (Jorgensen Laboratories, Inc., Loveland, CO) to open the mouth and pull buccal tissues away from teeth surfaces to allow adequate exposure. Use a cotton swab or tongue depressor to retract tongue from lingual surfaces.
• Identify cheek teeth elongation, irregular crown height, spikes, curved teeth, tooth discoloration, tooth mobility, missing teeth, purulent exudate, oral ulceration, or abscesses.
• Significant tooth root abnormalities may be present despite normal-appearing crowns. Skull films are required to identify apical disorders.
• Incisors—may see overgrowth, horizontal ridges or grooves, malformation, discoloration, fractures, increased or decreased curvature

CAUSES
Virtually every case fits into one or more of the following categories:
• Blepharitis—bacterial, *Treponema cuniculi* (rabbit syphilis) or myxomatosis
• Conjunctivitis—primary (rare), secondary to eyelid or lash disorders, foreign bodies, environmental irritants, dacryocystitis, or upper respiratory tract disease
• Aberrant conjunctival overgrowth—unknown cause; conjunctiva grows from the limbus, is nonadherent to the cornea, and may completely cover the cornea; does not appear to be painful or associated with significant inflammation

• Keratitis—traumatic most common; exposure keratitis following anesthesia, facial nerve paralysis; corneal abrasion in rabbits with torticollis; secondary to eyelash or eyelid disorder, trichiasis, or keratoconjunctivitis sicca
• Anterior uveitis—most commonly bacterial or encephalitozoon cuniculi
• Episcleritis or scleritis
• Glaucoma
• Hyphema—trauma, iridal abscess or *Encephalitozoan cuniculi* most common causes
• Orbital disease—usually the orbital abnormality is more prominent
• Dacryocystitis—inflammation of the canaliculi, lacrimal sac, or nasolacrimal ducts. May be sterile and secondary to blockage from dental disease—inflammatory cells, oil, and debris present. Bacterial infection secondary to chronic respiratory infection: *Staphylococcus* spp., *Pseudomonas* spp., *Moraxella* spp., *Pasteurella multocida, Niesseria* spp., *Bordetella* spp. frequently cultured.

RISK FACTORS
• Systemic infectious or inflammatory diseases
• Immunocompromise
• Coagulopathies
• Topical ophthalmic medications—aminoglycosides; pilocarpine; epinephrine
• Neoplasia
• Trauma
• Malocclusion and tooth root elongation

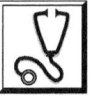

DIAGNOSIS

DIFFERENTIAL DIAGNOSIS
More than one cause may occur simultaneously.

Similar Signs
• Persistent elevation of nictians (third eyelid)—common sign in rabbits with thymoma due to increased mediastinal pressure
• Palpebral conjunctiva—normally redder than bulbar conjunctiva
• One or two large episcleral vessels—may be normal if the eye is otherwise quiet
• Transient mild hyperemia—with excitement, exercise, and straining
• Horner's syndrome—may cause mild conjunctival vascular dilation; differentiated by other signs and pharmacologic testing

Causes
• Superficial (conjunctival) vessels—originate near the fornix; move with the conjunctiva; branch repeatedly; blanch quickly with topical 2.5% phenylephrine or 1:100,000 epinephrine; suggest ocular surface disorders

RED EYE (CONTINUED)

(e.g., conjunctivitis, superficial keratitis, and blepharitis)
• Deep (episcleral) vessels—originate near the limbus; branch infrequently; do not move with the conjunctiva; blanch slowly or incompletely with topical sympathomimetics; suggest episcleritis or intraocular disease (e.g., anterior uveitis or glaucoma)
• Discharge—mucopurulent to purulent: typical of ocular surface disorders and blepharitis; serous or none: typical of intraocular disorders or blockage of the nasolacrimal duct
• Unilateral condition with ocular pain (blepharospasm)—usually indicates a tooth root disorder, keratitis, foreign body. Can be seen with anterior uveitis secondary to *E. cuniculi*, iridal or corneal stromal abscess.
• Chronic, bilateral condition—can indicate a congenital problem or chronic upper respiratory tract infection; bilateral tooth root disorders also seen
• Acute, bilateral condition with severe eyelid edema—consider myxomatosis
• Bilateral blepharitis—rule out *Treponema cuniculi* (rabbit syphilis); most have perineal and perioral dermatitis
• Facial pain, swelling, nasal discharge, or sneezing—seen with tooth root elongation or abscess; may indicate nasal or sinus infection; may indicate obstruction from neoplasm
• White discharge confined to the medial canthus—usually indicates dacryocystitis
• Corneal opacification, neovascularization, or fluorescein stain retention—suggests keratitis
• Aqueous flare or cell (increased protein or cells in the anterior chamber)—confirms diagnosis of anterior uveitis
• Pupil—miotic: common with anterior uveitis; dilated: common with glaucoma; normal: with blepharitis and conjunctivitis
• Abnormally shaped or colored irides—suggests anterior uveitis, iridal abscess, *E. cuniculi*
• Luxated or cataractous lenses—suggests glaucoma or anterior uveitis
• IOP—high: diagnostic for glaucoma; low: suggests anterior uveitis
• Loss of vision—suggests glaucoma, anterior uveitis, or severe keratitis. Vision can be difficult to assess in rabbits; rabbits typically do not menace; pupillary light response may not correlate well with vision; rabbits often refuse to negotiate obstacles, may not respond to objects such as cotton balls tossed near face.
• Glaucoma and anterior uveitis—may complicate hyphema

CBC/BIOCHEMISTRY/URINALYSIS
Usually normal, except with underlying systemic disease

OTHER LABORATORY TESTS
• Serologic testing for *E. cuniculi* in rabbits with cataracts or phacoclastic uveitis—many tests are available, but usefulness is limited since a positive titer indicates only exposure, and does not confirm *E. cuniculi* as the cause of uveitis. *E. cuniculi* can be definitively diagnosed only by finding organisms and resultant lesions on ocular histopathology or by positive DNA probe (PCR) on removed lens material. Antibody titers usually become positive by 2 weeks post-infection but may not continue to rise with active infection or decline with treatment. No correlation exits between antibody titers and shedding of organism, or presence or severity of disease.

IMAGING
• Skull radiographs are needed to identify dental disease, nasal, sinus, or maxillary bone lesions and, if present, to plan treatment strategies and to monitor progression of treatment.
• Perform under general anesthesia or heavy sedation
• Five views are recommended for thorough assessment: ventral-dorsal, lateral, two lateral obliques, and rostral-caudal.
• CT—superior to radiographs to localize obstruction and characterize associated lesions
• Dacryocystorhinography—radiopaque contrast material to help localize nasolacrimal duct obstruction
• Chest radiographs—consider with anterior uveitis or for which intraocular neoplasia is a possibility
• Abdominal radiography or ultrasonography—may help rule out infectious or neoplastic causes
• Ocular ultrasonography—if the ocular media are opaque; may define the extent and nature of intraocular disease or identify an intraocular tumor

DIAGNOSTIC PROCEDURES
• Tonometry—must perform in every patient with an unexplained red eye. Normal intraocular pressure is reported as 10–20 mmHg when measured by applanation tonometry.
• Schirmer tear test—average values are reported as 5 mm/min; however, even lower values can be seen in normal rabbits.
• Cytologic examination of affected tissue—lid; conjunctiva; cornea
• Fluorescein stain—rule out ulcerative keratitis; test for nasolacrimal function and patency, dye flows through the nasolacrimal system and reaches the external nares in approximately 10 seconds in normal rabbits.
• Conjunctival biopsies—with chronic conjunctivitis or with a mass lesion

• Perform a nasolacrimal flush—rule out nasolacrimal disease; may dislodge foreign material. Topical administration of an ophthalmic anesthetic is generally sufficient for this procedure; nervous rabbits may require mild sedation. Rabbits have only a single nasolacrimal punctum located in the ventral eyelid at the medial canthus. A 23-gauge lacrimal cannula or a 24-gauge Teflon intravenous catheter can be used to flush the duct. Irrigation will generally produce a thick, white exudate from the nasal meatus.
• Aerobic bacterial culture and sensitivity—consider with mucopurulent discharge; ideally, specimens taken before anything is placed in the eye (e.g., topical anesthetic, fluorescein, and flush) to prevent inhibition or dilution of bacterial growth; not routinely indicated for KCS and a mucopurulent discharge (secondary bacterial overgrowth almost certain). Often, only normal organisms are isolated (*Bacillus subtilis, Staphylococcus aureus*, and *Bordetella* spp.)

TREATMENT
• Usually outpatient
• Elizabethan collar—considered to prevent self-trauma
• Avoid dirty environments or those that may lead to ocular trauma.
• Because there is a narrow margin for error, consider referral if you cannot attribute the condition to one of the listed causes, if you cannot rule out glaucoma on the initial visit, or if the diagnosis is so uncertain that administration of a topical antibiotic alone or a topical corticosteroid alone would be questionable.
• Underlying tooth root disorders—trimming of cheek teeth (coronal reduction) may correct or control progression of root elongation. If tooth extraction is required or tooth root abscess is diagnosed—may require referral to a veterinarian with special expertise, if feasible. Because rabbits have very long, deeply embedded tooth roots, extraction per os can be extremely time consuming and labor intensive as compared with that in dogs and cats. In rabbits with extensive tooth root abscesses, aggressive debridement is indicated. Maxillary and retrobulbar abscesses can be particularly challenging.
• Aberrant conjunctival overgrowth—surgical excision of the excessive conjunctiva; often only palliative, may reform
• Few causes are fatal; however, a workup may be indicated (especially with anterior

uveitis and hyphema) to rule out potentially fatal systemic diseases.
• Deep corneal ulcers and glaucoma—may be best treated surgically

MEDICATIONS

DRUG(S) OF CHOICE
• Depends on specific cause
• Generally, control ocular pain, inflammation, and infection and IOP
• Topical broad-spectrum antibiotic ophthalmic solutions—keratitis, conjunctivitis, dacryocystitis; while waiting for results of diagnostic tests, may try triple antibiotic solution, ciprofloxacin, ofloxacin, gentocin, or ophthalmic chloramphenicol solution q4–6h
• 1% atropine q12–24h may help reduce ciliary spasm in patients with corneal ulcer or anterior uveitis; however, some rabbits produce atropinase; application may not be effective.
• Dacryocystitis—based on bacterial culture and sensitivity test results; continued for at least 21 days
• Systemic antibiotics—indicated in rabbits with tooth root abscess or upper respiratory tract infection causing dacryocystitis or conjunctivitis
• Topical nonsteroidal anti-inflammatory agents—0.5% ketorolac or 1% diclofenac may help reduce inflammation and irritation associated with flushes.

CONTRAINDICATIONS
• Topical corticosteroids—never use if the cornea retains fluorescein stain.
• Oral administration of most antibiotics effective against anaerobes will cause a fatal gastrointestinal dysbiosis in rabbits. Do not administer penicillins, macrolides, lincosamides, and cephalosporins by oral administration.

PRECAUTIONS
• Topical corticosteroids or antibiotic—corticosteroid combinations—avoid; associated with gastrointestinal ulceration

and hemorrhage, delayed wound healing, and heightened susceptibility to infection; rabbits are very sensitive to the immunosuppressive effects of both topical and systemic corticosteroids; use may exacerbate subclinical bacterial infection
• Topical aminoglycosides—may be irritating; may impede reepithelization if used frequently or at high concentrations
• Topical solutions—may be preferable to ointments if corneal perforation is possible
• Atropine—may exacerbate KCS and glaucoma
• NSAIDs—use with caution in hyphema

POSSIBLE INTERACTIONS
N/A

ALTERNATIVE DRUGS
N/A

FOLLOW-UP

PATIENT MONITORING
• Depends on cause
• Repeat ophthalmic examinations—as required to ensure that IOP, ocular pain, and inflammation are well controlled
• The greater the risk of loss of vision, the more closely the patient needs to be followed; may require daily or more frequent examination

POSSIBLE COMPLICATIONS
• Chronic epiphora
• Loss of the eye or permanent vision loss
• Chronic ocular inflammation and pain

MISCELLANEOUS

ASSOCIATED CONDITIONS
• Dental disease
• GI hypomotility

AGE-RELATED FACTORS
N/A

ZOONOTIC POTENTIAL
N/A

PREGNANCY/FERTILITY/BREEDING
N/A

SEE ALSO
Anterior uveitis
Conjunctivitis
Epiphora

ABBREVIATIONS
CT = computed tomograpy
ELISA = enzyme-linked immunosorbent assay
IFA = immunofluorescence assay
IOP = intraocular pressure
KCS = keratoconjunctivitis sicca
MRI = magnetic resonance imaging
PCR = polymerase chain reaction

Suggested Reading
Bedard KM. Ocular surface disease of rabbits. Vet Clin Exot Anim 2019;922:1–14.
Florin M, Rusanen E, Haessig M et al. Clinical presentation, treatment, and outcome of dacryocystitis in rabbits: a retrospective study of 28 cases (2003–2007). Vet Ophthalmol 2009;12(6):350–356.
Lennox AM, Capello V, Legendre LF. Small mammal dentistry. In: Quesenberry KE, Carpenter JW, eds. Ferrets, Rabbits and Rodents, 4th Ed). Clinical Medicine and Surgery. 2021 ed. St. Louis: Saunders, 2020:514–535.
Van der Woerdt A. Ophthalmologic diseases of small mammals. In: Quesenberry KE, Carpenter JW, eds. Ferrets, Rabbits and Rodents, 4th Ed). Clinical Medicine and Surgery. 2021 ed. St. Louis: Saunders, 2020:583–594.
Williams DL. Laboratory animal ophthalmology. In: Gelatt KN, ed. Veterinary Ophthalmology, 3rd ed. Philadelphia: Lippincott, Williams & Wilkins, 1999:151–181.
Author Georgina Newbold, DVM, Dipl. ACVO

RENAL FAILURE

BASICS

DEFINITION
• Azotemia and an inability to concentrate urine in the absence of dehydration
• Acute renal failure (ARF) is a syndrome characterized by sudden onset of filtration failure by the kidneys, accumulation of uremic toxins, and dysregulation of fluid, electrolyte, and acid–base balance.
• Chronic renal failure (CRF) results from primary renal disease that has persisted for months to years; it is characterized by irreversible renal dysfunction that tends to deteriorate progressively.

PATHOPHYSIOLOGY
• Reduction in functional renal mass results in impaired urine-concentrating ability (leading to polyuria and polydipsia—PU/PD) and retention of nitrogenous waste products of protein catabolism (leading to azotemia).
• Adrenaline release in response to anesthesia, pain, or stress can cause significant reduction in renal plasma flow and glomerular filtration rate, predisposing anesthetized or stressed rabbits to ARF.
• In rabbits, nearly all calcium in the diet is absorbed. Calcium excretion occurs primarily through the kidneys; the fractional urinary excretion is 45%–60% in rabbits, compared to less than 2% in most other mammals. This predisposes rabbits to urinary and renal calculi and may cause renal failure.
• Ascending lower urinary tract infection may cause pyelonephritis and subsequent renal failure.

SYSTEMS AFFECTED
• Renal/Urologic—impaired renal function leading to PU/PD and signs of uremia
• Nervous, gastrointestinal, musculoskeletal, and other body systems—secondarily affected by uremia

GENETICS
N/A

INCIDENCE /PREVALENCE
Not well documented; however, renal failure is a common sequela to many conditions affecting rabbits

SIGNALMENT
Animals of any age can be affected, but prevalence increases with increasing age.

Predominant Sex
None

SIGNS

General Comments
Clinical signs are related to the severity of renal dysfunction and presence or absence of complications.

Historical Findings
• ARF—sudden onset of anorexia, listlessness, diarrhea or lack of stool production (ileus), ataxia, seizures, known toxin exposure, recent medical or surgical conditions, and oliguria/ anuria or polyuria
• CRF—PU/PD, anorexia, diarrhea or lack of stool production (ileus), weight loss, lethargy, and poor hair coat.

Physical Examination Findings
• ARF—depression, dehydration (sometimes overhydration), hypothermia, fever, tachypnea, bradycardia, nonpalpable urinary bladder if oliguric, and kidneys may be painful on palpation
• CRF—small, irregular kidneys sometimes palpable, dehydration, cachexia, mucous membrane pallor; evidence of GI hypomotility (stomach full of desiccated ingesta, gas or fluid in cecum) is common.

CAUSES
• Shock, severe stress, prolonged anesthesia, heat stroke, heart failure, or septicemia can cause ARF.
• ARF or CRF—nephroliths, glomerulonephritis, pyelonephritis, chronic urinary obstruction, drugs (e.g., aminoglycoside, sulfonamides, and nchemotherapeutic agents), heavy metals, lymphoma or other neoplasia, *Encephalitozoon cuniculi*, amyloidosis

RISK FACTORS
• ARF—preexisting renal disease, dehydration, hypovolemia, severe stress, hypotension, advanced age, concurrent disease, prolonged anesthesia or surgery, and administration of nephrotoxic drugs
• CRF—aging, nephroliths, urinary tract infection, and diabetes mellitus

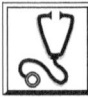

DIAGNOSIS

DIFFERENTIAL DIAGNOSIS
• For polyuria/polydipsia—hypercalciuria/ bladder sludge, pyometra, hepatic failure, diabetes mellitus (rare), postobstructive diuresis, behavioral
• For renomegaly—renal neoplasia (lymphoma), hydronephrosis, renal abscess, cystic kidneys (rare)
• Prerenal azotemia—(decreased renal perfusion) characterized by azotemia with concentrated urine (specific gravity >1.020); correctable with fluid repletion; seen commonly in stressed rabbits
• Postrenal azotemia—characterized by azotemia with obstruction or rupture of the excretory system

CBC/BIOCHEMISTRY/URINALYSIS
• Nonregenerative anemia with CRF, normal or high PCV with ARF
• BUN elevation (normal 9.1–22.7 mg/dL); creatinine elevation (normal 0.5–2.0 mg/dL)
• Normal serum calcium concentration in rabbits is high (12–16 mg/dL) and corresponds directly with dietary calcium intake. In some cases of renal failure, calcium absorption from the intestines continues, while renal elimination is impaired and may result in increases in serum calcium concentration; however, this is not a consistent finding.
• Hyperphosphatemia is seen with decreased GFR, and elevations may be prerenal, renal, or postrenal. Hyperphosphatemia is more commonly observed in rabbits with CRF.
• Hyperkalemia is occasionally seen with ARF or postrenal obstruction.
• Inability to concentrate urine, mild to moderate proteinuria, glucosuria; WBCs, RBCs, and variable bacteriuria may be seen depending on the underlying cause.
• White blood cell casts should prompt consideration of pyelonephritis.
• Urinary sediment evaluation often reveals calcium oxalate or calcium carbonate crystals; however, this is a normal finding in rabbits, and the presence of large amounts of crystals in the urine does not necessarily indicate disease. Disease occurs only when the concentration of crystals is excessive, forming thick, white to brown, sandlike urine and subsequent inflammatory cystitis, partial to complete blockage of the urethra, or nephrolithiaisis.

OTHER LABORATORY TESTS
• Serum lead or zinc concentration
• *Encephalitizooan cuniculi* titers—the usefulness of serum antibody testing is limited in pet rabbits since a positive titer indicates only exposure and does not confirm *E. cuniculi* as the cause of clinical signs. A combination of IgM, IgG, and C-reactive protein appears to be most reliable. *E. cuniculi* is not a common cause of renal failure.

IMAGING
• Abdominal radiographs may reveal calcium oxalate uroliths or calcium "sand" or sludge in the bladder, either as an incidental finding or in association with renal failure.
• Calculi may also form in the renal pelvis and/or ureters. The presence of renal calculi

alone does not imply renal failure; excretory urography is necessary to determine if the affected kidney is patent.
• Abdominal radiographs may demonstrate small kidneys (or large kidneys secondary to hydronephrosis, renal cysts, renal abscess, or neoplasia) in animals with CRF.
• Rabbits with ARF often have normal sized to large kidneys.
• Metastatic calcification of soft tissues, including kidneys and aorta, or hyperostosis is sometimes seen in rabbits with chronic renal failure. Absorption of calcium from the GI tract is not dependent on vitamin D and continues normally in rabbits with renal failure. However, in some cases, renal excretion of calcium is impaired, leading to excessive mineralization of bone and soft tissues.
• Ultrasonography may be useful in identifying pyelonephritis, renal cysts, renal abscess, degeneration, or neoplasia.

DIAGNOSTIC PROCEDURES
• Evaluation of ultrasound-guided fine-needle aspirates of the kidney may be helpful in the diagnosis of renal neoplasia, abscess, or cysts.
• Although not indicated in most rabbits, renal biopsy may be helpful in selected patients to document underlying cause.

PATHOLOGIC FINDINGS
• Gross findings—small kidneys with a lumpy or granular surface may be seen with CRF. Rabbits with previous *E. cuniculi* infections often have focal, irregular areas of pitting on the surface of the kidney. This is usually an incidental finding. Large, irregular kidneys with neoplasia or abscess.
• Histopathologic findings—frequently nonspecific; chronic generalized nephropathy or end-stage kidneys; findings are specific for diseases causing CRF in some patients. Rabbits with previous *E. cuniculi* infectious have focal interstitial fibrosis, usually an incidental finding without clinical significance. Nephrosis or nephritis may be seen in rabbits with ARF.

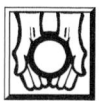

TREATMENT
APPROPRIATE HEALTH CARE
Patients with compensated CRF may be managed as outpatients; patients in ARF or uremic crisis should be managed as inpatients.

NURSING CARE
• Patients in ARF or uremic crisis—correct estimated fluid deficits with normal (0.9%) saline or balanced polyionic solution within 4–6 hours to prevent additional renal injury

from ischemia; once the patient is hydrated, ongoing fluid requirements are provided balanced electrolyte solution (maintenance fluids are estimated at 60 mL/kg/day for larger breeds and 80–100 mL/kg/day for small or dwarf breeds)
• Use caution when hydrating extremely stressed rabbits. Severe stress may cause a decrease in GFR and subsequent overhydration. Be sure that the volume of urine excreted is appropriate to the amount of fluids received.
• Hypervolemia—stop fluid administration and eliminate excess fluid by diuretic administration
• Patients in CRF—subcutaneous fluid therapy (daily or every other day) may benefit patients with moderate to severe CRF.

ACTIVITY
Unrestricted

DIET
• Increase water consumption. Provide multiple sources of fresh water. Flavoring the water with fruit or vegetable juices (with no added sugars) may be helpful. Provide a variety of clean, fresh, leafy vegetables sprayed or soaked with water.
• Many affected rabbits are anorectic or have a decreased appetite. It is an absolute requirement that the patient continue to eat during and following treatments. Anorexia may cause or exacerbate gastrointestinal hypomotility and cause derangement of the gastrointestinal microflora and overgrowth of intestinal bacterial pathogens. If the patient refuses food, syringe-feed Critical Care for Herbivores (Oxbow Animal Health, Murdock, NE) or Emeraid Herbivore (Lafeber Company, Cornell, IL) diet at approximately 10–15 mL/kg PO q6–8h. Larger volumes and more frequent feedings are often accepted; feed as much as the patient will readily accept. Alternatively, pellets can be ground and mixed with fresh greens, vegetable baby foods, water, or sugar-free juice to form a gruel
• High-carbohydrate, high-fat nutritional supplements are contraindicated.
• Further protein restriction is not indicated; the normal recommended diet for rabbits is already protein restricted.
• Following treatment for hypercalciuria/bladder sludge, reduction in the amount of calcium in the diet may help to prevent or delay recurrence. Eliminate feeding of alfalfa pellets, and switch to a high-fiber timothy-based pellet (Oxbow Pet Products, Murdock, NE). Feed timothy and grass hay instead of alfalfa hay and offer large volumes of fresh, green, leafy vegetables.

CLIENT EDUCATION
• CRF—tends to progress over months, possibly to years. Many rabbits with CRF will maintain a good quality of life with periodic SC fluid administration and supportive care for years.
• ARF—inform of the poor prognosis for complete recovery, potential for morbid complications of treatment (e.g., fluid overload, sepsis, and multiple organ failure), expense of prolonged hospitalization

SURGICAL CONSIDERATIONS
Avoid hypotension during anesthesia to prevent additional renal injury.

MEDICATIONS
DRUG(S) OF CHOICE
• Inadequate urine production (anuric or oliguric renal failure)—ensure patient is fluid-volume replete; provide additional isonatric fluid to achieve mild (3%–5%) volume expansion; failure to induce diuresis by fluid replacement indicates severe parenchymal damage or underestimation of fluid deficit.
• If fluid replete, administer furosemide (2 mg/kg IV q8h) to induce diuresis in patients with oliguric renal failure. Urinary flow should increase within 1 hours. If diuresis does not ensue within an hour, increase dosage to 4–6 mg/kg IV. Furosemide may be more effective when administered as a constant rate infusion at 0.1–1.0 mg/kg/hr.
• Reduce stress.
• If these treatments fail to induce diuresis within 4–6 hours, the prognosis is grave.
• Severe chronic anemia—erythropoietin (50–150 IU/kg SC q2–3d until PCV normalizes, then q7d × 4 weeks)

CONTRAINDICATIONS
Avoid nephrotoxic agents (NSAIDs, aminoglycosides).

PRECAUTIONS
Modify dosages of all drugs that require renal metabolism or elimination.

POSSIBLE INTERACTIONS
N/A

ALTERNATIVE DRUGS
N/A

FOLLOW-UP
PATIENT MONITORING
• ARF—monitor urinalysis, PCV, BUN, creatinine, and electrolytes; body weight, urine output, and clinical status—daily
• CRF—monitor at 1–3 month intervals, depending on therapy and severity of disease

RENAL FAILURE (CONTINUED)

PREVENTION/AVOIDANCE

Anticipate the potential for ARF in patients that are hemodynamically unstable, receiving nephrotoxic drugs, have multiple organ failure, or are undergoing prolonged anesthesia and surgery; maintenance of hydration and/or mild saline volume expansion may be preventive.

POSSIBLE COMPLICATIONS

• ARF—seizures, gastrointestinal bleeding, cardiac arrhythmias, congestive heart failure, pulmonary edema, hypovolemic shock, coma, cardiopulmonary arrest, and death
• CRF—gastroenteritis, anemia, and death

EXPECTED COURSE AND PROGNOSIS

• Nonoliguric ARF—milder than oliguric; recovery may occur, but the prognosis remains guarded to unfavorable.
• Oliguric ARF—extensive renal injury, is difficult to manage, and has a poor prognosis for recovery
• Anuric ARF—generally fatal
• CRF—short-term prognosis depends on severity; long-term prognosis guarded because CRF tends to be progressive

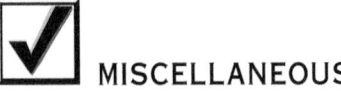

MISCELLANEOUS

ASSOCIATED CONDITIONS

• Hypercalciuria
• Urolithiasis
• Gastrointestinal hypomotility

AGE-RELATED FACTORS

Increased incidence in older animals; normal renal function decreases with aging

ZOONOTIC POTENTIAL

N/A

PREGNANCY/FERTILITY/BREEDING

ARF is a rare complication of pregnancy in animals; promoted by acute metritis, pyometra, and postpartum sepsis or hemorrhage

SYNONYMS

Kidney failure

SEE ALSO

Hypercalciuria and urolithiasis
Polyuria and polydipsia

ABBREVIATIONS

ARF = acute renal failure
BUN = blood urea nitrogen
CRF = chronic renal failure
GI = gastrointestinal
NSAIDs = nonsteroidal anti-inflammatory drugs
PCV = packed cell volume
PU/PD = polyuria/polydipsia

Suggested Reading
Di Girolamo N, Selleri P. Disorders of the urinary and reproductive system. In: Quesenberry KE, Carpenter JW, eds. Ferrets, Rabbits and Rodents, 4th Ed). Clinical Medicine and Surgery ed. St. Louis: Saunders, 2020:201–220.
Hallman RM, Brandão J. Diagnostic imaging of the renal system in exotic companion mammals. Vet Clin Exot Anim 2020;23:195–214.
Mancinelli E, Lord B. Urogenital and reproductive disease. In: Meredith A, Lord B, eds. BSAVA Manual of Rabbit Medicine. Gloucester: British Small Animal Veterinary Association, 2014:191–204.
Reavill DR, Lennox AM. Disease overview of the urinary tract in exotic companion mammals and tips on clinical management. Vet Clin Exot Anim 2020;23(1):169–193.
Author Barbara Oglesbee, DVM

RHINITIS AND SINUSITIS

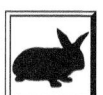

BASICS

DEFINITION
• Rhinitis—inflammation of the mucous membrane of the nose
• Sinusitis—inflammation of the associated paranasal sinuses
• Rabbits are obligate nasal breathers. The rim of the epiglottis is normally situated dorsal to the elongated soft palate to allow air passage from the nose to the trachea during normal respiration. Obstruction of the nasal passages with discharge or mucus can cause severe dyspnea.

PATHOPHYSIOLOGY
• May be acute or chronic, noninfectious, or infectious
• All causes are often complicated by opportunistic secondary microbial invasion.
• In rabbits, the most common cause is bacterial infection. Infection usually begins in the nasal cavity and may spread via the eustachian tubes to the ears, into the sinuses and bones of the face; via the nasolacrimal duct to the eye; and via the trachea to the lower respiratory tract and hematogenously to joints, bones, and other organ systems.
• Recurrent or refractory bacterial infections are common due to foci in inaccessible regions (deep within the sinuses, bone, etc.) and destruction of turbinates.
• Turbinate and facial bone destruction commonly occurs secondary to dental disease and tooth root abscesses.
• Turbinate and facial bone destruction may also develop with neoplastic or fungal disease (less common).

SYSTEMS AFFECTED
• Respiratory—mucosa of the upper respiratory tract, including the nasal cavities, sinuses, and nasopharynx
• Ophthalmic—extension to the eyes via nasolacrimal duct
• Musculoskeletal—extension of infection into bones of the skull
• Neurologic—extension of infection thru eustachian tube causing vestibular signs from otitis interna/media
• Oral cavity—dental disease; tooth root abscess

GENETICS
Unknown

INCIDENCE/PREVALENCE
• Bacterial respiratory infection—one of the most common diseases encountered in clinical practice
• Tooth roots extending into sinuses may contribute
• Nasal tumors and foreign bodies seen occasionally

GEOGRAPHIC DISTRIBUTION
Worldwide

SIGNALMENT
No breed or sex predilection

Mean Age and Range
• Infectious and congenital disease—younger animals
• Tumor, infectious disease, and dental disease—middle-aged to old animals

SIGNS

Historical Findings
• Sneezing, nasal discharge, staining of the front paws, epistaxis
• Ptyalism, anorexia, preference for soft foods with dental disease
• Epiphora, ocular discharge with extension into the eyes via nasolacrimal duct or with nasolacrimal duct obstruction (dried exudates, strictures)
• Head tilt, rolling, nystagmus, and other vestibular signs with extension into the ears via eustachian tubes

Physical Examination Findings
• Nasal discharge—unilateral suggests foreign body, tooth root abscess, or neoplasm, secretions, or dried discharges on the hair around the nose and front limbs, facial alopecia, and pyoderma
• Epistaxis—suggests neoplastic disease; tooth root abscesses, invasive bacterial infection and foreign body erosion may bleed; violent sneezing may cause traumatic epistaxis
• Diminished nasal airflow—unilateral or bilateral
• Ocular discharge—serous or purulent with nasolacrimal obstruction; purulent with extension of bacterial infection to conjunctiva; exophthalmos with retrobulbar abscess.
• Frontal and facial bone deformity—bacterial or neoplastic disease

CAUSES

Infectious
• *Staphylococcus aureus, Bordetella bronchiseptica, Moraxella catarrhalis, Pseudomonas aeruginosa, Mycobacterium* spp., *Pasteurella multocida*, and various anaerobes have been implicated.

Noninfectious
• Dental disease—periapical or tooth root abscesses, elongated maxillary tooth roots penetrating into nasal passages with secondary bacterial infection
• Facial trauma
• Foreign body—mostly inhaled vegetable matter (e.g., grass and seeds)
• Allergic or irritant—inhaled pollen, moldy bedding, dusty hay or litter, or cigarette smoke

• Neoplasia—squamous cell carcinoma, osteosarcoma, chondrosarcoma, and fibrosarcoma

RISK FACTORS
• Immunosuppression—caused by stress, concurrent disease, or corticosteroid use most important risk factor in developing bacterial disease
• Poor husbandry—dirty, molding bedding; ammonia buildup from urine-soaked bedding, dusty cat litter, cleaning agents. Dietary—diets too low in coarse fiber content (long-stemmed hay) predispose to dental disease

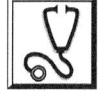

DIAGNOSIS

DIFFERENTIAL DIAGNOSIS
• Epistaxis—coagulopathy or hypertension
• Facial swelling—abscess, neoplasia, primary dental disease
• Epiphora—incisor root impaction, abscess or dried exudate blocking the nasolacrimal duct, primary conjunctivitis, irritation
• Allergic rhinitis—anecdotally reported

CBC/BIOCHEMISTRY/URINALYSIS
• Hemogram—TWBC elevations are usually not seen with bacterial diseases. A relative neutrophilia and/or lymphopenia are more common.

OTHER LABORATORY TESTS
• Serology for *Pasteurella*—ELISA—high IG G results may corelate with active infection. Low positive results may occur due to cross-reaction with other, nonpathogenic bacteria (false positive). False-negative results are common with immunosuppression or early infection. Titers may not correlate well to the presence or absence of disease. Test may be useful to monitor SPF colonies.
• *Pasteurella* PCR assay may also be performed on samples taken from deep nasal swabs. PCR may be more sensitive in detecting the presence of *Pasteurella*; however, it should be combined with anaerobic and aerobic culture to identify other bacterial primary or copathogens.

IMAGING
• Thoracic radiographs are indicated in rabbits with bacterial rhinitis. Subclinical pneumonia is common; often detected only radiographically. Lung abscesses are also common and can be seen radiographically.
• Skull radiographs—must be taken under heavy sedation. Useful to rule out dental disease; may see turbinate atrophy, bone destruction in severe cases
  ◦ Bony lysis or proliferation of the turbinate and facial bones important

radiographic finding, consistent with chronic bacterial or neoplastic invasion
  ○ Assess the apical roots of all teeth.
• CT scans are extremely helpful in detecting the extent of bony changes and to rule out other causes of nasal discharge.

DIAGNOSTIC PROCEDURES
• Cytology—nasal swab or flush rarely yields diagnostic sample; nonspecific inflammation is most commonly found
• Cultures—may be difficult to interpret, since commonly isolated bacteria (e.g., *Bordetella* spp.) often represent only commensal organisms or opportunistic pathogens. A heavy growth of a single organism is usually significant. Deep cultures obtained by inserting a mini-tipped culturette 2–4 cm into each nostril are sometimes reliable. However, samples taken from the nostrils should not be overinterpreted, since the causative agent may be located only deep within the sinuses, and not present at the rostral portion of the nostrils, where samples are readily accessible.
• A lack of growth does not rule out bacterial disease, since the infection may be in an inaccessible, deep area of the nasal cavity or sinuses, and many organisms (especially anaerobes and *Pasteurella* spp.) can be difficult to grow on culture.
• Biopsy of the nasal cavity is indicated in any animal with chronic nasal discharge in which neoplasia is suspected. Specimens may be obtained by direct endoscopic biopsy or rhinotomy. Multiple samples may be necessary to ensure adequate representation of the disease process.
• Rhinoscopy can be extremely valuable to visualize nasal abnormalities, retrieve foreign bodies, or obtain biopsy samples; sometimes the only method of identifying foreign bodies

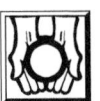

TREATMENT
APPROPRIATE HEALTH CARE
• Severe dyspnea requires hospitalization for supplemental oxygen administration and supportive care; supply O$_2$ enrichment (O$_2$ cage or induction chamber) in a quiet environment.

NURSING CARE
• Provide oxygen supplementation if patient appears to be dyspneic; rabbits are obligate nasal breathers; and nasal discharge can cause severe dyspnea.
• Keep nostrils clear of discharge. Use gentle suction with a bulb syringe or pediatric aspirator to clear nasal discharges
• Symptomatic treatment and nursing care are important in the treatment of rabbits with

nasal discharge. Patient hydration, nutrition, warmth, and hygiene (keeping nostrils clean) are important.
• Humidification of environment often helps mobilize nasal discharge; enhances patient comfort
• Nebulization with normal saline may be useful to humidify airways.
• If epiphora or ocular discharge is present, and the patient is not dyspneic, cannulate, and flush the nasolacrimal duct. Topical administration of an ophthalmic anesthetic is generally sufficient for this procedure.
• Remove environmental allergens/irritants (dusty litters, moldy hay, or betting); provide clean bedding and airspace.

ACTIVITY
No change

DIET
• If the patient refuses food, syringe-feed a gruel such as Critical Care for Herbivores (Oxbow Pet Products) or Emeraid Herbivore (Lafeber Company, Cornell, IL) 10–15 mL/kg PO q6–8h. Alternatively, pellets can be ground and mixed with fresh greens, vegetable baby foods, water, or juice to form a gruel.
• Encourage oral fluid intake by offering fresh water from multiple sources, wetting leafy vegetables.

CLIENT EDUCATION
• If underlying disease (dental disease, severe tissue destruction, chronic bacterial disease) is not correctable, warn client that a cure is unlikely in rabbits. The goal of treatment is to control the more severe clinical signs with medication, and that treatment may be lifelong.

SURGICAL CONSIDERATIONS
Treat associated dental disease—extractions, debride abscesses

MEDICATIONS
DRUG(S) OF CHOICE
Antibiotics
• Relapse common with cessation of treatment
• Systemic therapy—at least 4–6 weeks often indicated to help prevent deep colonization by the resident flora; lifelong treatment may be indicated in some cases
• Base selection on results of nasal culture whenever possible
• Choose broad-spectrum antibiotics such as enrofloxacin (10–20 mg/kg PO, SC, IM, IV q12h), marbofloxacin (5 mg/kg PO q24h), trimethoprim-sulfa (15–30 mg/kg PO q12h), chloramphenicol (50 mg/kg PO q8h), or

penicillin G procaine (40,000–60,000 IU/kg SC q24h).
• Nebulization—used in conjunction with systemic treatment. Nebulize for 15 minutes 1–3 times daily. Choices include: enrofloxacin 100 mg in 10 mL saline; doxycycline 200 mg in 15 mL saline; gentamicin 50 mg I 10 mL saline; and amikacin 50 mg in 10 mL saline
• Topical ophthalmic preparations, such as those containing quinolones, to treat associated conjunctivitis

CONTRAINDICATIONS
• Topical nasal decongestants containing phenylephrine can exacerbate nasal inflammation and cause nasal ulceration and purulent rhinitis.
• Oral administration of antibiotics that select against gram-positive bacteria (penicillins, macrolides, lincosamides, and cephalosporins) can cause fatal enteric dysbiosis and enterotoxemia.
• The use of corticosteroids (systemic or topical in otic preparations) can severely exacerbate bacterial infection.

PRECAUTIONS
• Chloramphenicol—avoid human contact with chloramphenicol due to potential blood dyscrasia. Advise owners of potential risks.
• Nebulization or oral administration of any antibiotic may potentially cause enteric dysbiosis; discontinue use if diarrhea, or anorexia occurs.

POSSIBLE INTERACTIONS
N/A

ALTERNATIVE DRUGS
• Antihistamines have been used rabbits with suspected allergic rhinitis and symptomatically in rabbits with infectious rhinitis. Use is anecdotal and dosages have been extrapolated from feline dosages; hydroxyzine (2 mg/kg PO q8–12h); diphenhydramine (2.0 mg/kg PO, SC q8–12h)

FOLLOW-UP
PATIENT MONITORING
Clinical assessment and monitoring for relapse of clinical signs

PREVENTION/AVOIDANCE
• Avoid stressful conditions, corticosteroid use; provide excellent diet and husbandry
• Prevent dental disease by providing high-fiber foods, especially good-quality hay. Yearly veterinary exams with periodic trimming of overgrown teeth as needed.

POSSIBLE COMPLICATIONS
• Extension of infection into the brain, mouth, eyes, ears, or lungs

- Loss of appetite
- Dyspnea as a result of nasal obstruction

EXPECTED COURSE AND PROGNOSIS
- Prognosis depends on cause and chronicity
- Chronic infection prognosis guarded to poor for complete resolution of clinical signs, depending on invasiveness (e.g., poor with extensive turbinate destruction, CNS signs)
- Neoplasms—prognosis grave to poor

 MISCELLANEOUS

ASSOCIATED CONDITIONS
- Dental disease
- Gastrointestinal hypomotility
- Abscessation
- Pneumonia

AGE-RELATED FACTORS
- Most of the infectious causes are found in young animals.
- Neoplasia or dental disease—more common in old animals

ZOONOTIC POTENTIAL
N/A

PREGNANCY/FERTILITY/BREEDING
N/A

SEE ALSO
Abscessation
Dyspnea and tachypnea
Incisor malocclusion and overgrowth
Pasteurellosis

ABBREVIATIONS
ELISA = enzyme-linked immunosorbent assay
IFA = immunofluorescence assay
PCR = polymerase chain reaction
TWBC = total white blood cell count

Suggested Reading
Capello V, Lennox AM. Diagnostic imaging of the respiratory system in exotic companion mammals. Vet Clin Exot Anim 2011;14:369–389.
DeCubellis J. Common emergencies in rabbits, guinea pigs, and chinchillas. Vet Clin Exot Anim 2016;19:411–429.
Hedley J. Respiratory disease. In: Meredith A, Lord B, eds. BSAVA Manual of Rabbit Medicine. Gloucester: British Small Animal Veterinary Association, 2014:160–167.
Jekl V. Respiratory disorders in rabbits. Vet Clin Exot Anim 2021;24:459–482.
Lennox AM, Mancinelli E. Respiratory diseases. In: Quesenberry KE, Carpenter JW, eds. Ferrets, Rabbits and Rodents, 4th Ed). Clinical Medicine and Surgery ed. St. Louis: Saunders, 2020:188–201.
Varga M. Cardiorespiratory diseases. In: Varga M, ed. Textbook of Rabbit Medicine, 2nd ed. London, UK: Elsevier, 2014:390–405.

Author Barbara Oglesbee, DVM, DABVP-Avian

SEIZURES

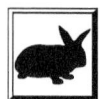

BASICS

DEFINITION
• Clinical manifestation of excessive discharges of hyperexcitable cerebrocortical neurons
• Clinical signs vary depending on the area of the cortex involved.

PATHOPHYSIOLOGY
• Intracranial and extracranial—result in focal or diffuse hyperexcitability of cerebrocortical neurons
• High-frequency and sustained activity may recruit other parts of the brain into the epileptic discharge and cause neuronal damage, leading to more frequent and refractory seizures (in both acute and chronic disorders).

SYSTEMS AFFECTED
Nervous

SIGNALMENT
• White, blue-eyed rabbits may be more likely to have idiopathic epilepsy.
• Dwarf breeds, older, and immunosuppressed rabbits may be more predisposed to infection with *E. cuniculi.*
• Lop-eared rabbits may be predisposed to otitis interna/media with subsequent brain involvement.

SIGNS

General Comments
• Auditory stimulation is more likely to trigger seizures in rabbits.
• Usually sudden onset; short duration (<2 minutes); abrupt termination; often followed by postictal disturbances (e.g., mental confusion, apparent blindness)
• May occur as isolated events, cluster seizures (more than two within 24 hours), or status epilepticus
• Generalized more common than partial

Historical Findings
• Seizure history (e.g., age at first seizure; type; initial and subsequent frequency)—may reveal clues about the underlying cause
• History of upper respiratory infection or otitis externa/interna in rabbits with bacterial encephalitis or brain abscesses
• History of grazing outdoors consistent with parasitic encephalitis (*Baylisascaris, Toxoplasma*)
• History of head trauma

Physical Examination Findings
• Physical abnormalities—may be related to the seizures, indicating multisystemic disease (e.g., infectious, metabolic)
• Head tilt accompanied by other vestibular signs often seen in rabbits with brain abscess or encephalitozoonosis

• In rabbits with otitis, thick, white, creamy exudate may be found in the horizontal and/or vertical canals; however, most rabbits with otitis interna/media have normal-appearing external ear canals, since most infections occur by extension via the nasolacrimal duct.

CAUSES

Extracranial Causes
• Metabolic—severe hypoglycemia and hypocalcemia; advanced hepatic encephalopathy
• Toxicities—heavy metal; many other intoxications in their advanced stages
• Hypoxic—cardiovascular diseases, choke, and pneumonia

Intracranial Causes (Most Common)
• Functional (idiopathic and genetic) epilepsy—poorly documented
• Structural brain lesions—infectious encephalitides (bacterial infections, encephalitozoonosis, toxoplasmosis, and *Baylisascaris*) most common; less frequent: ischemic encephalopathy and brain tumors
• Ischemic—stroke, atherosclerosis

RISK FACTORS
Any brain lesion involving the forebrain

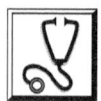

DIAGNOSIS

DIFFERENTIAL DIAGNOSIS

Similar Signs
• Severe vestibular disease—continuous rolling, distress, paddling may mimic seizures or accompany seizures; differentiated by history and physical examination (torticollis, abnormal nystagmus)
• Syncope—rare in rabbits; sudden loss of consciousness and muscle tone resulting in flaccid recumbency and followed by complete recovery within seconds; differentiated by history and physical examination (e.g., episodes induced by stress or exercise, cardiovascular abnormalities such as heart murmur and arrhythmias)

Causes
• Metabolic and hypoxic disorders—other historical, clinical, and laboratory signs
• Toxins—history of exposure to lead: may have intermittent seizures; other toxins: a progression from shaking to trembling and finally to sustained status epilepticus until treatment or death;
• Structural brain lesions—acute onset of high-frequency seizures with no sign of extracranial causes

CBC/BIOCHEMISTRY/URINALYSIS
Usually normal unless multisystemic disease exists

OTHER LABORATORY TESTS
• Serologic testing for *E. cuniculi*—many tests are available, but usefulness is extremely limited since a positive titer only indicates exposure and does not confirm *E. cuniculi* as the cause of neurologic signs. *E. cuniculi* can only be definitively diagnosed by finding organisms and resultant lesions on histopathologic examination in areas that anatomically correlate with observed clinical signs. A combination of IgM, IgG, and C-reactive protein appears to be most reliable.
• Serologic testing for toxoplasmosis—ELISA testing for IgM and IgG is commercially available. The overall seroprevalence is low, and most seropositive rabbits are asymptomatic.

IMAGING
• Skull radiography—may help rule out otitis interna/media; however, normal radiographs do not rule out bulla disease—CT is more accurate
• CT and MRI—extremely valuable for confirming bulla lesions and CNS extension from peripheral locations; document or localize tumor, granuloma, and extent of inflammation

DIAGNOSTIC PROCEDURES
• CSF analysis—sample from the cerebellomedullary cistern; may be valuable for evaluating central disease; detect inflammatory process; sample collection may put the patient at risk for herniation if there is a mass or high intracranial pressure. May see increased protein, lymphocyte, and monocytes with *E. cuniculi* infection. Studies were unable to find organism or evidence of organism utilizing PCR testing on CSF

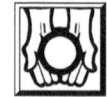

TREATMENT
• Known cause—treat, if possible
• Outpatient—isolated seizures
• Inpatient—cluster seizures; status epilepticus; treat rapidly and aggressively

NURSING CARE
• Constantly supervise hospitalized patient
• Cool down if hyperthermic
• Install IV line for drug and fluid administration

CLIENT EDUCATION
• Emphasize the importance of the diagnostic workup.
• Inform client that antiepileptic treatment is only symptomatic and may not consistently help unless a primary cause can be identified and treated.
• Instruct the client to keep a seizure calendar.

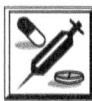

MEDICATIONS

DRUG(S) OF CHOICE

Severe Cluster Seizures and Status Epilepticus
• Diazepam (1–5 mg/kg IV, IM) or midazolam (0.5–2 mg/kg IV, IM) begin with 0.5–1.0 mg/kg IV bolus; may repeat if gross seizure activity has not stopped within 5 minutes; can be administered rectally if IV access cannot be obtained; may diminish or stop the gross motor seizure activity to allow IV catheter placement
• Constant rate infusion protocols used in dogs and cats have been anecdotally used.

Chronically Recurrent Seizures
• Levetiracetam (Keppra)—20 mg/kg PO q8h—anecdotally most effective treatment with fewest side effects
• Phenobarbital—has been anecdotally used at dosages for dogs and cats: 1–2.5 mg/kg PO q12h
For bacterial meningoencephalitis; abscess:
• Antibiotics; choice is ideally based on results of culture and susceptibility testing when possible (otitis, extension from sinuses). Use broad-spectrum antibiotics such as enrofloxacin (10–20 mg/kg PO, SC, IM, IV q12h), marbofloxacin (5 mg/kg PO q24h), trimethoprim-sulfa (15–30 mg/kg PO q12h), or chloramphenicol (50 mg/kg PO q8h)
For encephalitozoonosis:
• Fenbendazole (20 mg/kg q24h × 28 days) is the most common treatment and has been shown to reduce clinical signs and increase survival rates in symptomatic patients. Benzimidazole anthelmintics are effective against E. cuniculi in vitro and have been shown to prevent experimental infection in rabbits. However, efficacy in rabbits with clinical signs is unknown. Long-term treatment has been recommended, as treatment only prevents replication, rather than kills the parasite.
For toxoplasmosis:
• Trimethoprim-sulfa 15–30 mg/kg PO q12h; sulfadiazine in combination with pyrimethamine for 2 weeks has also been recommended

CONTRAINDICATIONS
• Dexamethasone—contraindicated in patients with infectious diseases, but may help decrease brain edema when impending brain herniation or life-threatening edema is suspected
• Oral administration of antibiotics that select against gram-positive bacteria (penicillins, macrolides, lincosamides, and cephalosporins) can cause fatal enteric dysbiosis and enterotoxemia.
• Acepromazine, ketamine, xylazine, bronchodilators (e.g., aminophylline, terbutaline, and theophylline)—do not administer to any patient with documented or potential seizures; lower seizure threshold

PRECAUTIONS
• Intensive parenteral antiepileptic drug therapy—requires constant monitoring and care; hypothermia common; persistent subtle seizure activity difficult to recognize; potential cardiovascular and respiratory depression with overdosage
• Never leave a patient with historical, actual, or potential seizures hospitalized without constant supervision; if monitoring cannot be provided on a 24-hour basis, send the patient home or refer to an emergency clinic.

POSSIBLE INTERACTIONS
Cimetidine, ranitidine, and chloramphenicol—may decrease the metabolism of phenobarbital

ALTERNATIVE DRUGS
Phenobarbital, propofol for status epilepticus; potassium bromide—anecdotally used following canine and feline protocols

FOLLOW-UP

PATIENT MONITORING
• CBC, biochemistry, and urinalysis—evaluate before initiation of maintenance oral antiepileptic drug therapy; then monitor every 6–12 months
• Have owners keep a diary of seizure activity—adjust medications based on clinical response
• Measurement of serum phenobarbital concentration after treatment initiation—optimal concentration unknown in rabbits; anecdotally lower than expected; may not correlate well with clinical control of seizures
• Epilepsy secondary to treated primary disease—slowly and gradually wean patient off the antiepileptic drug after 6 months without seizures; if seizures recur, reinstate the drug

POSSIBLE COMPLICATIONS
• Phenobarbital—hepatotoxicity possible with chronic use; although not reported in rabbits, thrombocytopenia, neutropenia, pruritus, and swelling of the feet may occur in other mammals
• Seizures may continue despite adequate antiepileptic therapy; refractoriness to diazepam may develop.
• Hypoglycemia and hyperthermia with prolonged seizures
• Status epilepticus, leading to death
• Permanent neurologic deficits may follow severe status epilepticus regardless of the cause.
• Progression of disease with deterioration of mental status

EXPECTED COURSE AND ROGNOSIS
• Prognosis—guarded depending on underlying cause; varied response to drug treatment

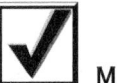

MISCELLANEOUS

ASSOCIATED CONDITIONS
• Upper respiratory infections
• Otitis interna/media
• Gastrointestinal hypomotility

AGE-RELATED FACTORS
Encephalitozoonosis and bacterial disease may be more common in older, especially immunosuppressed animals

ZOONOTIC POTENTIAL
Encephalitozoon cuniculi—unlikely, but possible in immunosuppressed humans. Mode of transmission and susceptibility in humans is unclear
Toxoplasma gondi—zoonosis possible with consumption of infected meat rabbits if undercooked

SEE ALSO
Ataxia
Encephalitis
Encephalitozoonosis
Toxoplasmosis

ABBREVIATIONS
CSF = cerebrospinal fluid
CT = computed tomography
ELISA = enzyme-linked immunosorbent assay
IFA = immunofluorescence assay
MRI = magnetic resonance imaging
PCV = packed cell volume

Suggested Reading
DeCubellis J. Common emergencies in rabbits, guinea pigs, and chinchillas. Vet Clin Exot Anim 2016;19:411–429.
Fisher PG, Künzel F, Rylander H. Neurologic and musculoskeletal disease. In: Quesenberry KE, Carpenter JW, eds. Ferrets, Rabbits and Rodents, 4th Ed). Clinical Medicine and Surgery ed. St. Louis: Saunders, 2020:583–594.
Harkness JE, Turner PV, VandeWoude S, Wheeler CL. Clinical signs and differential

RABBITS

diagnoses: nervous and musculoskeletal conditions. In: Harkness JE, Turner PV, VandeWoude S, Wheeler CL, eds. Biology and Medicine of Rabbits and Rodents, 5th ed. Ames: Wiley-Blackwell, 2010:214–216.

Keeble E. Nervous system and musculoskeletal disorders. In: Meredith A, Lord B, eds. BSAVA Manual of Rabbit Medicine. Gloucester: British Small Animal Veterinary Association, 2014:233–248.

Lennox AM, Gladden JN. Emergency and critical care of small mammals. In: Quesenberry KE, Carpenter JW, eds. Ferrets, Rabbits and Rodents, 4th Ed). Clinical Medicine and Surgery. 2021 ed. St. Louis: Saunders, 2020:595–608.

Varga M. Neurological and locomotive disorders. In: Varga M, ed. Textbook of Rabbit Medicine, 2nd ed. London, UK: Elsevier, 2014:367–389.

Author Barbara Oglesbee, DVM, DABVP (Avian)

SHOPE PAPILLOMA VIRUS

BASICS

OVERVIEW
• A sporadic cutaneous viral disease of pet rabbits caused by a virus in the Papovaviridae family
• Virus is oncogenic; characteristic cutaneous lesions can progress to malignant squamous cell carcinoma; metastasis may occur.
• Seen in domestic and wild rabbits
• Virus is spread via biting arthropods, primarily mosquitos and ticks.
• Clinical signs in pet rabbit consist of characteristic skin lesions.

SIGNALMENT
• Pet rabbits (*Oryctolagus cuniculus*) and wild cottontail rabbits (*Sylviagus* spp.)
• Outdoor rabbits may be at greater risk due to mode of viral transmission.
• Highest incidence rabbits living in California; occurs sporadically over North America

SIGNS
• Raised, red, well-demarcated, rough, usually circular cutaneous lesions; often 1 cm or more in diameter
• Lesions are often friable; bleed readily with trauma
• Cutaneous nodules occur most commonly on the eyelids, nose, ears, and feet in domestic (pet) rabbits
• Nodules occur around the neck and shoulder areas most commonly in wild rabbits.
• Lesions often spontaneously regress

CAUSES AND RISK FACTORS
• Oncogenic, DNA virus in the Papovaviridae family
• Outbreaks may be more likely when mosquitos are numerous (summer, fall)

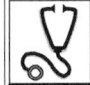

DIAGNOSIS

CBC/BIOCHEMISTRY/URINALYSIS
N/A

OTHER LABORATORY TESTS
Virus isolation

IMAGING
N/A

DIAGNOSTIC PROCEDURES
Histologic examination of excised nodules to confirm diagnosis

PATHOLOGIC FINDINGS
• Cutaneous nodules—raised, round, red, keratinized epithelial nodules
Histopathologic
• Hyperkeratosis; may contain characteristic inclusions bodies

TREATMENT
• Surgical excision of nodules is indicated. Nodules are frequently friable and bleed easily; may transform into malignant squamous cell carcinoma
• Nodules often regress spontaneously—make take weeks to months to resolve

MEDICATIONS

DRUG(S) OF CHOICE
N/A

CONTRAINDICATIONS/POSSIBLE INTERACTIONS
N/A

FOLLOW-UP

PREVENTION/AVOIDANCE
Control of vectors—screening to keep out insects; flea control; keep indoors

MISCELLANEOUS

ZOONOTIC POTENTIAL
None.

Suggested Reading
Meredith A. Dermatoses. In: Meredith A, Lord B, eds. BSAVA Manual of Rabbit Medicine. Gloucester: British Small Animal Veterinary Association, 2014:255–263.
Palmerio BS, Roberts H. Clinical approach to dermatologic disease in exotic animals. Vet Clin North Am Exot Anim Pract 2013;16(3):523–577.
Snook TS, White SD, Hawkins MG et al. Skin diseases in pet rabbits: a retrospective study of 334 cases seen at the University of California at Davis, USA (1984–2004). Vet Dermatol 2013;24:613–618.
Varga M. Skin diseases. In: Varga M, ed. Textbook of Rabbit Medicine, 2nd ed. Elsevier, 2014:224–248.
Varga M, Patterson S. Dermatologic diseases of rabbits. In: Quesenberry KE, Carpenter JW, eds. Ferrets, Rabbits and Rodents, 4th Ed). Clinical Medicine and Surgery. 2021 ed. St. Louis: Saunders, 2020:220–222.
Author Barbara Oglesbee DVM, DABVP (Avian)

RABBITS

SPONDYLOSIS DEFORMANS AND SPINAL ARTHRITIS

BASICS

OVERVIEW
- Degenerative, noninflammatory condition of the vertebral column characterized by the production of osteophytes along the ventral, lateral, and dorsolateral aspects of the vertebral endplates
- Lumbar spine most common
- Spinal root impaction may cause ataxia, weakness, and lameness

SIGNALMENT
- Seen more often in medium to large breeds
- Occurrence increases with age; most often in rabbits over 3 years old

SIGNS

General Comments
- Signs are most often referable to an inability to properly groom or attain a normal stance while urinating due to stiffness or pain. Affected rabbits may be unable to groom the intrascapular, perineal or tail head region, or may be unable to consume cecotrophs from the rectum. If unable to attain a normal stance while urinating, urine may soak the ventrum, resulting in urine scald.
- Gait abnormalities, reluctance to jump reported as second most common clinical sign associated with spinal pain

Physical Examination Findings
- Neurologic deficits referable to the spinal cord or nerve root compression
- Ataxia, rear limb weakness
- Ulcerative pododermatitis
- Perineal dermatitis—matted fur, urine-soaked perineum or ventrum, feces pasted to perineum, alopecia, erythema, ulceration, myiasis
- Alopecia, flaking, cheyletiella mites in intrascapular or tail head region due to inadequate grooming
- Accumulation of wax in ear canals from inadequate grooming
- Hypercalciuria secondary to insufficient voiding
- Obesity

CAUSES AND RISK FACTORS
- Age
- Repeated microtrauma
- Major trauma
- Inherited predisposition possible
- May be related to small cage size, lack of exercise
- Obesity may predispose

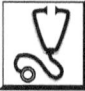

DIAGNOSIS

DIFFERENTIAL DIAGNOSIS
- Pain from nonorthopedic disorders—rabbits may be reluctant to ambulate or groom when painful, regardless of the source of pain.
- Diskospondylitis—differentiated by radiographic evidence of end-plate lysis
- Spinal osteoarthritis—degeneration of the articular facet joints
- Degenerative joint disease
- Intervertebral disc disease

CBC/BIOCHEMISTRY/URINALYSIS
CBC/biochemistry profile usually normal

OTHER LABORATORY TESTS
N/A

IMAGING
- Spinal radiography—initially shows osteophytes as projecting from the edge of the vertebral body; with progression, they appear to bridge the intervertebral space. Signs do not always correlate well with clinical signs.
- Skull radiographs—to rule out dental disease as a cause of pain and reluctance to groom or ambulate
- Whole body radiographs—to rule out other causes of pain and reluctance to groom or ambulate (arthritis, urolithiasis, etc.)
- CT—to rule out intervertebral disc disease or other spinal disorders; in unusual cases of spondylosis, may demonstrate an atypical dorsal osteophyte compressing the spinal cord or nerve roots or encroaching on critical soft tissue structures

TREATMENT

APPROPRIATE HEALTH CARE
- Treat as outpatient with limited exercise and analgesic administration
- Obesity—recommend a weight-reduction program

NURSING CARE
For all rabbits that do not groom or are nonambulatory:
- Keep perineum clean, dry, and free of fecal matter
- Remove matted hair. Be extremely cautious when clipping hair or pulling on mats since rabbit skin is extremely fragile and will easily tear. Sedation may be required.

- Use soft bedding, keep bedding clean and dry to prevent dermatitis or bed sores
- Clean wax from ears as needed

MEDICATIONS

DRUG(S) OF CHOICE
- Nonsteroidal anti-inflammatories—have been used for short- or long-term therapy to reduce pain and inflammation in rabbits with musculoskeletal disease; meloxicam (1.0 mg/kg PO q24h; carprofen (2 mg/kg PO q12h)
- Tramadol—5–15 mg/kg PO q8–12h
- Gabapentin—5–20 mg/kg PO q8–12h
- Dermatitis—initially may be treated empirically with broad-spectrum antibiotics such as enrofloxacin (10–20 mg/kg PO, SC, IM q12–24h), marbofloxacin (5 mg/kg PO q24h), and trimethoprim-sulfa (30 mg/kg PO q12h)
- Superficial, moist dermatitis—apply zinc oxide + menthol powder (Gold Bond, Martin Himmel, Inc) to clean, clipped skin q24h

CONTRAINDICATIONS
- Oral administration of antibiotics that select against gram-positive bacteria (penicillins, macrolides, lincosamides, and cephalosporins) can cause fatal enteric dysbiosis and enterotoxemia.
- Corticosteroids—associated with gastrointestinal ulceration and hemorrhage, delayed wound healing, and heightened susceptibility to infection; rabbits are very sensitive to the immunosuppressive effects of both topical and systemic corticosteroids; use may exacerbate subclinical bacterial infection

PRECAUTIONS
- Meloxicam or other NSAIDs—use with caution in rabbits with compromised renal function

ALTERNATIVE DRUGS
- Chondroitin sulfate (Cosequin, Nutramax) has been used anecdotally using feline dosage protocols; polysulfated glycosaminoglycan (Adequan, Luitpold) 2.2 mg/kg SC, IM q3d × 21–28 days, then q14d
- Acupuncture may be effective for rabbits with chronic pain.

FOLLOW-UP
- Gradually return the animal to normal activity after signs have subsided for several weeks.
- Relapse can occur with strenuous activity.

(CONTINUED) SPONDYLOSIS DEFORMANS AND SPINAL ARTHRITIS

PREVENTION/AVOIDANCE
- Prevent obesity.
- Encourage regular exercise throughout life.

POSSIBLE COMPLICATIONS
- Dermatitis, urine scald, ulcerative pododermatitis (sore hocks), myiasis
- Hypercalciuria

EXPECTED COURSE AND PROGNOSIS
Clinical signs are likely to be progressive with age

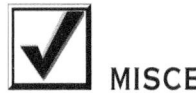 **MISCELLANEOUS**

ABBREVIATIONS
CT = computed tomography
NSAID = nonsteroidal anti-inflammatory drug

Suggested Reading
Bays TB. Geriatric care of rabbits, guinea pigs, and chinchillas. Vet Clin Exot Anim 2020;23:567–593.
Fisher PG, Künzel F, Rylander H. Neurologic and musculoskeletal disease. In: Quesenberry KE, Carpenter JW, eds. Ferrets, Rabbits and Rodents, 4th Ed). Clinical Medicine and Surgery ed. St. Louis: Saunders, 2020:583–594.
Harkness JE, Turner PV, VandeWoude S, Wheeler CL. Clinical signs and differential diagnoses: nervous and musculoskeletal conditions. In: Harkness JE, Turner PV, VandeWoude S, Wheeler CL, eds. Biology and Medicine of Rabbits and Rodents, 5th ed. Ames: Wiley-Blackwell, 2010: 214–216.
Keeble E. Nervous system and musculoskeletal disorders. In: Meredith A, Lord B, eds. BSAVA Manual of Rabbit Medicine. Gloucester: British Small Animal Veterinary Association, 2014:233–248.
Varga M. Neurological and locomotive disorders. In: Varga M, ed. Textbook of Rabbit Medicine, 2nd ed. London, UK: Elsevier, 2014:367–389.

Author Barbara Oglesbee, DVM, DABVP (Avian)

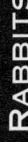

TESTICULAR TUMORS

BASICS

OVERVIEW
• Relatively common tumor of older intact male rabbits. In most cases, owners notice swelling of the affected testicle(s), with no other clinical signs reported.
• Tumors can be functional (hormone secreting)
• Most tumors are benign
• Most common types include seminoma and interstitial (Leydig or granular) cell tumors. Less common are Sertoli cell tumors, adenocarcinoma, teratoma, lymphoma, and mixed cell tumors. More than one tumor types may be present.
• May be more common in rabbits with undescended testicles

SIGNALMENT
• Intact males
• Highest incidence in bucks >6 years old, can occur as early as 3 years of age
• No information on breed risk

SIGNS

Historical Findings
• Often asymptomatic, other than finding scrotal asymmetry
• Bucks with functional Sertoli cell tumors (estrogen-secreting) may develop gynecomastia or behavior changes; those with functional Leydig cell (testosterone secreting) tumors may show increased aggression.
• Occasionally, owners note pain or discomfort if inflammation is present

Physical Examination Findings
• Firm, nodular, usually nonpainful enlargement of one or both testicles.
• If unilateral, the normal testicle may shrink in size
• May be painful or become large enough to interfere with locomotion and become ulcerated
• Metastasis is rare, but can spread to regional lymphodes and/or lungs. May see weight loss, lethargy, GI stasis.

CAUSES AND RISK FACTORS
Intact sexual status
Age
Undescended testicles

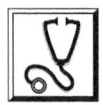

DIAGNOSIS

DIFFERENTIAL DIAGNOSIS
• Abscess
• Hematoma
• Hernia
• Testicular torsion
• Orchitis

CBC/BIOCHEMISTRY/URINALYSIS
• Usually normal

OTHER LABORATORY TESTS
N/A

IMAGING
• Radiographs—to rule out lung metastasis
• Ultrasonography—to distinguish between hernia, hematoma, and abscess

DIAGNOSTIC PROCEDURES
• Histopathologic examination—for definitive diagnosis; submit both testicles and spermatic cord to check for local invasion

TREATMENT
• Castration—treatment of choice; usually curative if metastasis has not occurred.

MEDICATIONS

DRUG(S) OF CHOICE
• Chemotherapy—success in metastatic disease has not been reported in rabbits.
• Pain management is essential during and following surgery, Perioperative choices include butorphanol (0.1–0.5 mg/kg SQ, IM, IV q4–6h, buprenorphine (0.02–0.05 mg/kg SQ, IM IV q8–12h), hydromorphone (0.1 mg/kg SC IM q2–4h), or oxymorphone (0.05–0.2 mg/kg SC IM q8–12h). To manage long-term pain: meloxicam (1.0 mg/kg PO q24h; carprofen (2 mg/kg PO q12h), tramadol (5–15 mg/kg PO q8–12h), and/or gabapentin (5–20 mg/kg PO q8–12h)

FOLLOW-UP

PATIENT MONITORING
Consider thoracic and abdominal radiographs every 3 months for the first 6–12 months post castration. Not all metastases are grossly visible at the time of surgery.

PREVENTION/AVOIDANCE
Routine castration

EXPECTED COURSE AND PROGNOSIS
• Excellent (cure) if castrated prior to metastasis. Metastasis is rare. If owners elect not to castrate, palliative pain management.

MISCELLANEOUS

ASSOCIATED CONDITIONS
• None

AGE-RELATED FACTORS
Risk increases with age. Most commonly seen in rabbits over 6 years of age.

ZOONOTIC POTENTIAL
N/A

PREGNANCY/FERTILITY/BREEDING
Breeding status has no effect on risk of tumor development.

SEE ALSO
Abscesses

Suggested Reading
Di Girolamo N, Selleri P. Disorders of the urinary and reproductive system. In: Quesenberry KE, Carpenter JW, eds. Ferrets, Rabbits and Rodents, 4th Ed). Clinical Medicine and Surgery ed. St. Louis: Saunders, 2020:201–220.
Hallman RM, Brandão J. Diagnostic imaging of the renal system in exotic companion mammals. Vet Clin Exot Anim 2020;23:195–214.
Mancinelli E, Lord B. Urogenital and reproductive disease. In: Meredith A, Lord B, eds. BSAVA Manual of Rabbit Medicine. Gloucester: British Small Animal Veterinary Association, 2014:191–204.
Reavill DR, Lennox AM. Disease overview of the urinary tract in exotic companion mammals and tips on clinical management. Vet Clin Exot Anim 2020;23(1):169–193.
Van Zeeland Y. Rabbit oncology, diseases, diagnostics and treatments. Vet Clin Exot Anim 2017;20:135–182.
Author Barbara Oglesbee, DVM, DABVP (Avian)

RABBITS

THYMOMA AND THYMIC LYMPHOMA

BASICS

OVERVIEW
- Slow growing mediastinal tumor originating from thymic epithelium
- Benign, but ultimately fatal due to space occupying effects with progressive compression of the heart and lungs
- Infiltrated with small, mature lymphocytes and reticular epithelial cells
- Local invasion is possible, metastasis is rare
- Thymic lymphoma has similar appearance, but is less common—tumors consist of lymphoblasts

SIGNALMENT
- Most common cause of mediastinal mass in rabbits
- Seen in middle aged to older rabbits, usually >6 years of age, but has been seen in rabbits as young as 3 years of age.
- Lionhead and dwarf breeds may be predisposed
- No sex predilection

SIGNS

Historical Findings
- Dyspnea—initially may present as exercise intolerance; progresses to increased respiratory effort at rest, often with abdominal effort and nasal flare
- Exophthalmos, third eyelid protrusion—bilateral, due to increased venous pressure from space-occupying effects of the tumor (cranial caval syndrome). This is often the only clinical sign that owners notice. May be intermittent, especially with exertion or stress; often becomes persistent with progression of disease
- Weight loss
- Lethargy, malaise

Physical Examination Findings
- Dyspnea—varies with stage of disease and tumor size from mild increase in effort with stress to severe dyspnea with abdominal effort and nasal flare
- Exophthalmos, third eyelid protrusion—bilateral, nonpainful, globes can be retropulsed
- Heart murmur common due to compression of great vessels
- Often thin body condition
- Swelling of the head, neck, or forelimbs—less common
- Exfoliative dermatitis or sebaceous adenitis—reported as occasionally occurring with thymomas

CAUSES AND RISK FACTORS
N/A

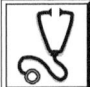

DIAGNOSIS

DIFFERENTIAL DIAGNOSIS
- Normal thymus—the thymus does not completely regress with age in rabbits and is visible radiographically in the mediastinum
- Thyroid carcinoma
- Abscess
- Intrathoracic fat pad
- For bilateral exophthalmos—tooth root abscess, retrobulbar neoplasia—usually painful, eyes cannot be retropulsed; with thymoma, eyes can be retropulsed and no pain is present

CBC/BIOCHEMISTRY/URINALYSIS
- Leukocytosis with WBC >10,000 and lymphocytes comprising >70% of differential count has been reported as a common finding, but not all rabbits will have changes in WBC
- Hemolytic anemia—reported in one case

OTHER LABORATORY TESTS
N/A

IMAGING
- Thoracic radiographs—demonstrates a cranial mediastinal mass. Often see elevated trachea and caudal displacement of the heart shadow. May appear as 2 heart shadows. May see pleural effusion. Important to differentiate from normal thymic remnant, which is visible radiographically but does not elevate the trachea or displaced the heart.
- Thoracic ultrasound—thymomas are often cystic; use to guide aspiration of fluid or needle aspirate for diagnosis
- CT scan—useful to rule out other causes of mediastinal mass

DIAGNOSTIC PROCEDURES
- Fine-needle aspiration of mass—ultrasound guided, under heavy sedation. Useful to drain intralesional cysts, if present, which can have a temporary therapeutic effect. Cytologic examination shows lymphocytes and thymic epithelial cells; difficult to differentiate thymoma vs. thymic lymphoma on aspirate alone
- Thoracocentesis—if pleural effusion is present, both as a diagnostic and therapeutic procedure

TREATMENT

APPROPRIATE HEALTH CARE
- Treatment goal is reduction in size to improve quality of life and temporarily improve symptoms. Although surgical excision has been reported, the survival rate is very low.

- Radiotherapy—conventional radiotherapy (RT), volumetric-modulated arc radiotherapy (VMAT), and intensity-modified radiation treatment (IMRT) have all been successfully used
- Chemotherapy with prednisolone alone—reduction in tumor size and survival times are similar to rabbits treated with radiation treatment
- Aspiration of pleural fluid and/or intralesional cysts when present to temporarily reduce pressure on lungs and heart

NURSING CARE
- Oxygen therapy—for respiratory distress
- General supportive care

ACTIVITY
- Restrict during treatment and in patients that are dyspneic

DIET
- If the patient refuses food, syringe-feed a gruel such as Critical Care for Herbivores (Oxbow Pet Products) or Emeraid Herbivore (Lafeber Company, Cornell, IL) 10–15 mL/kg PO q6–8h. Alternatively, pellets can be ground and mixed with fresh greens, vegetable baby foods, water, or juice to form a gruel
- Encourage oral fluid intake by offering fresh water from multiple sources, wetting leafy vegetable

CLIENT EDUCATION
- The decision as to treatment with radiation therapy vs prednisolone treatment is based on the availability of facilities offering radiation therapy, cost and comorbid, or underlying disorders. Radiation may be cost-prohibitive. Palliative treatment with prednisolone may risk exacerbation or development of clinical signs of potentially life-threatening infectious disorders.
- Advise owners that neither treatment is curative. The goal is to decrease the size of the tumor and improve quality of life for as long as possible. Survival times vary with treatment, but average 200–300 days.

SURGICAL CONSIDERATIONS
- Although complete excision of tumor would potentially be curative, postoperative mortality rates exceed 70%
- If this treatment is elected, referral to a surgeon with experience in rabbit thoracotomy is advised

MEDICATIONS

DRUG(S) OF CHOICE
Prednisolone—
- Prednisolone as a sole agent is an inexpensive and relatively effective palliative

THYMOMA AND THYMIC LYMPHOMA

treatment. However, keep in mind that this may cause significant immunosuppression. Rabbits with subclinical diseases such as *E. cuniculi* or chronic bacterial rhinitis may develop clinical signs, and disease may be exacerbated in symptomatic animals.
• Starting doses range from 0.5 to 2.0 mg/kg PO q12–24h. The dosage and time interval between doses are gradually reduced based on response to treatment, titrating to the lowest effective dose.
• Survival times reported to vary between 2 and 18 months, with a median survival time of 270 days.

CONTRAINDICATIONS/POSSIBLE INTERACTIONS
Immunosuppressive drugs—use with caution and only with definitive diagnosis; immunosuppression may exacerbate subclinical *Encephalitozoon cuniculi* or bacterial infections, the result of which could be fatal.

FOLLOW-UP

PATIENT MONITORING
• Clinical response, with improvement in dyspnea is usually seen within 2–3 following the first RT.
• After completion of RT, monitor with CT (preferable) or radiographs every 2–3 months.
• With prednisone treatment, monitor for emergence of subclinical infection (particularly respiratory)

POSSIBLE COMPLICATIONS
• Death, due to anesthetic complications during RT—occurs most often during first treatment. If first treatment is successful, most patients do well
• Side effects of RT include thrombosis of thoracic vessels, pulmonary fibrosis, pneumonitis, heart failure, and alopecia
• Emergence or exacerbation of underlying infectious disease in rabbits treated with prednisolone
• Exacerbation of heart disease in rabbits treated with prednisolone

EXPECTED COURSE AND PROGNOSIS
• Without treatment—depends on size of tumor at diagnosis; average survival time is 92 days
• With radiation treatment—rabbits surviving the first treatment average a reduction in tumor size by up to 50% after first treatment. Survival times vary, but average 1–2 years.
• With prednisolone alone—also variable depending on the size of tumor at diagnosis; average survival time of 270 days

MISCELLANEOUS

SEE ALSO
Dyspnea and tachypnea
Exophthalmos and orbital diseases

ABBREVIATIONS
RT = radiation therapy
VMAT = volumetric-modulated arc radiotherapy
IMAT = intensity-modified radiation treatment

Suggested Reading
McCready JE, Poirier VJ, Fleck A, Darco J, Beaufrère HH. Adaptive radiation therapy using weekly hypofractionation for thymoma treatment: a retrospective study of 10 rabbits. Vet Comp Oncol 2022;20(3):559–567.
Palmer A, Wu CC, Miwa Y, Turek M, Sladky KK. Outcomes and survival times of client-owned rabbits diagnosed with thymoma and treated with either prednisolone or radiotherapy, or left untreated. J Exot Pet Med 2021;38:35–43.
Quesenberry KA, Pilny AA, St Vincent RS. Lymphoreticular disorders, thymoma and other neoplastic diseases. In: Quesenberry KE, Carpenter JW, eds. Ferrets, Rabbits and Rodents, 4th Ed). Clinical Medicine and Surgery ed. St. Louis: Saunders, 2020:258–269.
Varga M. Cardiorespiratory diseases. In: Varga M, ed. Textbook of Rabbit Medicine, 2nd ed. London, UK: Elsevier, 2014:390–405.

Author Barbara Oglesbee, DVM, DABVP-Avian

TREPONEMATOSIS (RABBIT SYPHILIS)

BASICS

OVERVIEW
• A sexually transmitted bacterial infection caused by the spirochete *Treponema paraluiscuniculi* (formerly *T. cuniculi*)
• Transmission occurs via sexual contact or other direct contact with lesions, or from does to offspring during passage through the vagina at birth.
• Incubation period can be prolonged, as long as 3–12 weeks
• Lesions are confined to mucocutaneous junctions, beginning in the prepuce or vulva, may progress to the anus and perianal region, and spread to the lips, nose, and eyelids during grooming

SIGNALMENT
• Clinical signs are uncommon in pet rabbits; serologic findings suggest approximately 25% of asymptomatic rabbits may have been infected.
• Clinical signs most commonly seen in young rabbits

SIGNS
Historical Findings
• History of recent breeding in adult rabbits or contact with infected animals
• Seen in young rabbits with no breeding history if transmitted from doe
• History of erythema and swelling around the vulva or prepuce, anus, lips, and nose followed by papules and crusts
• Occasionally, a history of abortion or neonatal death in breeding does
• Signs may wax and wane, spontaneously resolve, and reappear following stress

Physical Examination Findings
• Initially erythema, swelling at mucocutaneous junction surrounding the external genitalia, spreading to anus then mouth, nose, and sometimes periocular region with grooming
• Lesions sometimes found on the face only, in the absence of genital lesions (contact by sniffing affected rabbits)
• Lesions progress to papules, vesicles which ulcerate, and form crusts
• Lesions may be painful

CAUSES AND RISK FACTORS
• *Treponema paraluiscuniculi*, a spirochete antigenically similar to *Treponema pallidum*, the causative agent of human syphilis
• Rabbit to human transmission does not occur
• Risk factor—sexual or direct contact with affected rabbits; transmission by asymptomatic animals possible

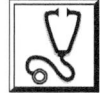

DIAGNOSIS

Although a serologic test is available, false negatives are common. Diagnosis is often presumptive, based on history, characteristic clinical signs, and response to treatment.

DIFFERENTIAL DIAGNOSIS
• Ear mites—although lesions may be seen around the face, neck, abdomen, and perineal region, the majority of lesions are around ear base and pinnae; intense pruritus
• Contact hypersensitivity—may see lesions around face or perineal region, does not progress to papules, ulceration, or crusts
• Pyoderma—moist pyoderma in perineal region or face extremely common, secondary to chronic exposure to moisture; larger area usually affected than with *T. parluiscuniculi*; dry crusts usually not present with pyoderma; underlying cause usually identifiable
• Autoimmune dermatoses—not reported in rabbits

CBC/BIOCHEMISTRY/URINALYSIS
N/A

OTHER LABORATORY TESTS
• Serologic testing—demonstrates exposure to *T. paraluiscuniculi*; titers may take 12 weeks to develop following exposure; lesions may be present before titers become positive; titers eventually decline over several months with treatment but usually remain elevated following spontaneous resolution of clinical signs. False negatives are common, and testing should be repeated several times to verify a true negative response in suspected carrier animals.

IMAGING
N/A

DIAGNOSTIC PROCEDURES
• History, physical examination findings, and response to treatment are usually sufficient for diagnosis
• Skin biopsy and histologic examination—identify organisms with silver staining. Lesions consist of ulcers, and necrotic crusts are surrounded by inflammatory cells. Secondary bacterial infections are common and may confuse the diagnosis.

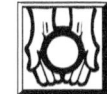

TREATMENT
• Outpatient treatment
• Treat all rabbits in contact with affected rabbit
• Topical treatment, other than keeping the lesions clean and dry, is generally not needed

MEDICATIONS
Penicillin G 42,000–84,000 IU/kg SC, IM q7d × 3wk. Lesions often diminish significantly after only 1 or 2 injections.

CONTRAINDICATIONS/POSSIBLE INTERACTIONS
Do not administer any penicillin by an oral route—can cause fatal dysbiosis

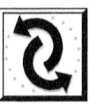

FOLLOW-UP

PATIENT MONITORING
• Treat all in-contact rabbits; monitor for resolution of lesions.
• Monitor for signs of dysbiosis (diarrhea, anorexia) in treated rabbits; dysbiosis is unlikely but possible with high doses of parenteral penicillin.

PREVENTION/AVOIDANCE
Avoid contact with clinically affected or seropositive rabbits.

EXPECTED COURSE AND PROGNOSIS
Prognosis is excellent with treatment; treatment is considered to be curative, and lesions typically resolve in 1–3 weeks; treat all in-contact rabbits to prevent reinfection

MISCELLANEOUS

ZOONOTIC POTENTIAL
T. paraluiscuniculi is not transmissible to humans.

Suggested Reading
Meredith A. Dermatoses. In: Meredith A, Lord B, eds. BSAVA Manual of Rabbit Medicine. Gloucester: British Small Animal Veterinary Association, 2014:255–263.
Palmerio BS, Roberts H. Clinical approach to dermatologic disease in exotic animals. Vet Clin North Am Exot Anim Pract. 2013;16(3):523–577.
Saito K, Hasegawa A. Clinical features of skin lesions in rabbit syphilis: a retrospective study of 63 cases (1999–2003). J Vet Med Sci 2004;66:1247–1249.
Snook TS, White SD, Hawkins MG et al. Skin diseases in pet rabbits: a retrospective study of 334 cases seen at the University of California at Davis, USA (1984–2004). Vet Dermatol 2013;24:613–618.
Varga M. Skin diseases. In: Varga M, ed. Textbook of Rabbit Medicine, 2nd ed. Elsiver, 2014:224–248.
Varga M, Patterson S. Dermatologic diseases of rabbits. In: Quesenberry KE, Carpenter JW, eds. Ferrets, Rabbits and Rodents, 4th Ed). Clinical Medicine and Surgery. 2021 ed. St. Louis: Saunders, 2020:220–222.
Author Barbara Oglesbee DVM, DABVP (Avian)

RABBITS

ULCERATIVE PODODERMATITIS (SORE HOCKS)

BASICS

DEFINITION
• Avascular necrosis, usually followed by abscessation, cellulitis, osteomyelitis, and synovitis, occurring on the plantar or palmar aspect of the feet. Ulcerative pododermatitis occurs more commonly on the rear feet, hence the lay term *sore hocks*; however, the front feet or any portion of the plantar surface can be affected.
• Deep pyoderma/cellulitis secondary to prolonged contact with abrasive, wet, or urine/feces-soaked surfaces, hard or rough surfaces, or excessive weight bearing
• Ulcerative pododermatitis is a painful and often irreversible condition.

PATHOPHYSIOLOGY
• During locomotion, rabbits normally bear weight on the hind digits (digitigrade stance). At rest, weight is born in the area between the hind claws and hock (plantigrade stance). Rabbits do not have foot pads, but instead rely on a covering of thick fur on the plantar aspect of the feet, combined with a compliant surface, to protect the feet. Any condition that disrupts normal digitigrade locomotion or cushioning of the plantar aspect of the feet may lead to the formation of pressure sores on the feet. Increased pressure often occurs due to obesity or decreased weight bearing on other feet.
• Avascular necrosis occurs as a consequence of constant pressure applied to skin and soft tissues pressed between the bones of the feet and a hard surface. Necrosis of these tissues is followed by sloughing, ulceration, and secondary bacterial infection.
• Dermatitis on the plantar aspect of the foot is common in rabbits housed on abrasive surfaces (wire, carpeting, or astroturf) or those that sit in soiled cat litter or corn cob litter or on soiled bedding. Prolonged contact with wire, abrasive or moist surfaces, leads first to hair loss, followed by superficial dermatitis, deep pyoderma, cellulitis, and abscess formation. Untreated, it may progress to osteomyelitis and synovitis.
• Pain associated with necrosis and infection often causes affected rabbits to remain sedentary; continued weight bearing on affected feet in sedentary rabbits extends areas of pressure necrosis, exacerbating the condition. Eventually, some affected rabbits develop osteomyelitis and synovitis with permanent damage to tendons, so that maintenance of a normal stance is no longer possible. In these rabbits, damage is often irreversible.
• Conditions leading to ulcerative pododermatitis may be environmental (e.g., wire cages, hard surfaces, soiled or damp bedding) or an underlying condition (e.g., obesity, urine scald, and spondylosis)

SYSTEMS AFFECTED
• Skin/Exocrine—percutaneous
• Musculoskeletal—osteomyelitis, tendonitis

INCIDENCE/PREVALENCE
Extremely common in commercial rabbits or pet/show rabbits housed in wire cages or hutches. Frequently seen in house rabbits housed on hard floors or carpeting.

SIGNALMENT
• No age or sex predilection
• Rex, Angoras, and large breeds may be more susceptible.

SIGNS

Historical Findings
• Husbandry history—very important in determining underlying cause. Seen in rabbits confined to small wire cages or hutches; rabbits housed on noncompliant surfaces such as bare floors, or carpeting; rabbits kept on soiled feces and urine-soaked bedding
• History of sitting in the litter box—sitting on soiled litter, especially corn cob litter and scoopable litters
• A history of shaving the thick, protective hair on the plantar aspect of the hocks
• History of obesity, musculoskeletal disorder causing sedentary life, decreased weight bearing on the contralateral limb, or urine scalding in the perineal and hind limb region
• History of alopecia on the plantar surface of the hock early in the course of disease; progresses to erythema, ulceration, scab formation, abscess
• Anorexia, depression, lameness, reluctance to move—from pain

Physical Examination Findings
• Early, asymptomatic disease (Grade I)—hair loss on the plantar or plantar aspect of the feet or hocks
• Mild disease (Grade II)—erythema, swelling with overlying skin intact
• Moderate disease (Grade III)—ulceration, scab formation
• Severe disease (Grade IV)—abscess, inflammation of tendons or deeper tissues
• Severe, often irreversible disease (Grade V)—osteomyelitis; synovitis and tendonitis leading to abnormal stance and gait

Other Findings
• Anorexia, depression, lameness, reluctance to move—from pain
• Obesity
• Examine other limbs for musculoskeletal disorders causing a decrease in weight bearing.

CAUSES
• Pressure sores; avascular necrosis caused by entrapment of soft tissues of the hind leg between bone and hard surfaces
• Excoriation, friction, or constant moisture on the skin and soft tissues of the plantar aspect of the hock. Caused by lack of protective fur covering and/or feces, urine, or water coating the feet
• Pyogenic bacteria—secondary infection with *Staphylococcus aureus* most common; *Pseudomonas*; *Escherichia coli*; b-hemolytic *Streptococcus* spp.; *Proteus* spp.; *Bacteroides* spp.; *Pasteurella multocida*

RISK FACTORS
• Environmental—sitting on soiled litter (cat litter, corn cob litter); wire floored cages, hard floor surfaces, abrasive carpeting, and soiled bedding. A lack of footpads requires a soft, compliant surface (grass, dirt in nature; hay or other dry, soft bedding in captivity) for protection of the feet
• Lack of exercise—small cages or housing; abnormal amount of time spent with weight borne on the hocks; this combined with an abrasive/hard surface or soiled litter/bedding will predispose to disease
• Obesity—increased amount of weight supported by hocks; long periods of recumbency
• Musculoskeletal disease or other painful conditions (dental disease, urolithiasis)—reluctance to move increases time spent on hocks; may prevent rabbit from adopting a normal stance while micturating, resulting in urine scalding; may prevent eating of cecotrophs and accumulation of cecotrophs on perineal region and feet; may prevent normal locomotion or weight bearing at rest
• Urinary tract disease or gastrointestinal disease—may cause polyuria or diarrhea leading to urine scald or pasting of feces on feet and perineal region
• Clipping or shaving the protective layer of fur on the plantar or palmar aspect of the hock or feet
• Nervous, stressed rabbits—thump and stamp the rear limbs
• Trauma or puncture wounds to the plantar or palmar aspect of the hock or feet
• Some breeds, especially New Zealand White, normally lose fur on the ventral aspect of the hock with age. This may be a normal finding or may predispose to sore hocks.

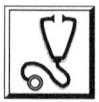

DIAGNOSIS

DIFFERENTIAL DIAGNOSIS
• Abscess secondary to bacteremia or trauma
• Neoplasia

- Granuloma
- Fracture

CBC/BIOCHEMISTRY/URINALYSIS
- CBC—normal or relative neutrophilia and lymphopenia; TWBC elevations not usually seen in rabbits with abscesses
- Urinalysis and serum chemistry profile—depend on underlying cause and system affected

OTHER LABORATORY TESTS
N/A

IMAGING
- Radiography—to determine the extent of bone involvement; essential in guidance of treatment plan and expected prognosis; osteomyelitis carries poorer prognosis, prolonged treatment
- Skull radiographs—to rule out dental disease as a cause of pain and reluctance to groom or ambulate
- Whole-body radiographs—to rule out other causes of pain and reluctance to groom or ambulate (arthritis, urolithiasis, problems with contralateral limb)
- Ultrasonography—may be useful to determine underlying causes; organ system affected; extent of disease

DIAGNOSTIC PROCEDURES
- Aspiration—may reveal a thick, creamy to caseous, white exudate in rabbits with secondary bacterial infection; high nucleated cell count; primarily degenerative neutrophils with lesser numbers of macrophages and lymphocytes
- Biopsy if mass lesion is present—to rule out neoplasia, granuloma, and other causes of masses; sample should contain both normal and abnormal tissue in the same specimen; submit for histopathologic examination and culture
- Culture—sterile, deep sample from affected tissue and/or exudate—aerobic and anaerobic bacteria; bacterial susceptibility testing to direct antibiotic therapy

PATHOLOGIC FINDINGS
- Exudate—large numbers of neutrophils in various stages of degeneration; other inflammatory cells; necrotic tissue
- Surrounding tissue—avascular or suppurative necrosis; ulceration; large number of neutrophils; variable number of lymphocytes; plasma cells; macrophages, fibrous connective tissue
- Osteomyelitis—bone resorption, severe septic arthritis

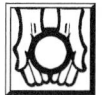

TREATMENT

APPROPRIATE HEALTH CARE
- It is essential to remove/correct the underlying cause for long-term success
- Outpatient—early disease (erythema, alopecia)

- Inpatient—surgical procedures; daily debridement and bandaging

NURSING CARE
- Depends on severity of disease
- Caging on soft, dry bedding alone may be effective in early disease (Grade I or II: erythema, alopecia prior to ulceration or abscess). Clean hay, pine shavings, or shredded paper over a padded surface that can be completely cleaned and dried works well
- More severe disease—requires frequent debridement and flushing of exudate and necrotic tissue (daily in severe cases), frequent bandage changes, long-term antibiotics, and pain control.
- Bandaging—depends on severity of disease. Usually only necessary in rabbits with open wounds or following debridement. Severely affected rabbits may require daily debridement or flushing. This is a painful procedure requiring general anesthesia (isoflurane). Following debridement, application of wet-to-dry bandages may be required initially until a granulation bed is formed; postdebridement application of silver sulfadiazine cream followed by bandaging may also be effective. Once infection is controlled, hydrocolloidial wound dressing can be applied over ulceration. Bandage change interval increases with improvement; wet bandages should be changed immediately.

ACTIVITY
- Restrict until adequate healing of tissues has taken place.
- Long term—encourage activity; prolonged inactivity may cause or exacerbate pododermatitis.

DIET
- It is important that the rabbit continue to eat during and following treatment. This condition is often painful, resulting in anorexia. Anorexia will often cause GI hypomotility, derangement of the gastrointestinal microflora, and overgrowth of intestinal bacterial pathogens.
- Offer a large selection of fresh, moistened greens such as cilantro, romaine lettuce, parsley, carrot tops, dandelion greens, spinach, collard greens, etc., and good-quality grass hay. Many rabbits will begin to eat these foods, even if they were previously anorectic.
- If the patient refuses these foods, syringe-feed a gruel such as Critical Care for Herbivores (Oxbow Pet Products) or Emeraid Herbivore (Lafeber Company, Cornell, IL) 10–15 mL/kg PO q6–8h. Alternatively, pellets can be ground and mixed with fresh greens, vegetable baby foods, water, or juice to form a gruel. If sufficient volumes of food are not accepted in this manner, nasogastric intubation is indicated.
- High-carbohydrate, high-fat nutritional supplements are contraindicated.

- Encourage oral fluid intake by offering fresh water, wetting leafy vegetables, or flavoring water with vegetable juices.
- Dietary modification to correct underlying obesity when present

CLIENT EDUCATION
- Discuss need to correct or prevent risk factors. Correction of underlying disease and husbandry problems is imperative for a successful outcome. Discuss appropriate bedding material; do not house rabbits on wire flooring.
- Severe disease, involving bone and tendon, carries a guarded to poor prognosis for complete resolution. Most will require surgical debridement, sometimes multiple surgeries and multiple follow-up visits. Recurrences are common, especially if the underlying cause cannot be corrected. Clients must be aware of the monetary and time investment.

SURGICAL CONSIDERATIONS
- Debride all visibly necrotic tissue.
- In the majority of cases, no abscess is present. If an abscess is present, simple lancing, flushing, and draining are not adequate. Thick exudates do not drain well, and the abscess will recur. Instead of draining, curette all visible exudates and flush copiously. Repeated, sometimes daily, debridement and flushing are often required.
- Treat as open wound—flush and debride would daily initially, followed by twice weekly to weekly debridement as healing occurs. Irrigate wound with dilute antiseptic solution (chlorhexidine or iodine) daily until healthy granulation bed forms, followed by hydrocolloidal wound dressings or silver sulfadiazine cream until re-epithelialization occurs. Follow debridement with application of soft, padded bandages. Bandages must be changed immediately if they become wet.
- Remove any foreign objects(s) or nidus of infection.
- Place on long-term antibiotic therapy; appropriate pain management
- Severe osteomyelitis may require amputation; mid-femoral amputation of hind limb better tolerated; may be precluded by the presence of bilateral disease.
- Correct underlying cause—provide soft bedding, improve husbandry, and weight loss

MEDICATIONS

DRUG(S) OF CHOICE
Antimicrobial drugs effective against the infectious agent; gain access to site of infection. Choice of antibiotic is ideally based on results of culture and susceptibility testing. Depending on the severity of infection,

ULCERATIVE PODODERMATITIS (SORE HOCKS) (CONTINUED)

long-term antibiotic therapy is required (4–6 weeks minimum). Use broad-spectrum antibiotics such as enrofloxacin (10–20 mg/kg PO, SC, IM, IV q12–24h), marbofloxacin (5 mg/kg PO q24h), trimethoprim-sulfa (30 mg/kg POq12h); if anaerobic infections are suspected use chloramphenicol (25 mg/kg PO q8–12h), metronidazole (20 mg/kg PO q12h), or azithromycin (15–30 mg/kg PO q24h), penicillin G procaine (40,000–60,000 IU/kg SQ q24h). Combine with topical treatment listed above.

Acute Pain Management
• Butorphanol (0.1–0.5 mg/kg SQ, IM, IV q4–6h); may cause profound sedation; short acting
• Buprenorphine (0.02–0.05 mg/kg SQ, IM IV q8–12h); less sedating, longer acting than butorphanol
• Meloxicam (1 mg/kg PO, SC, IM q24h)
• Carprofen (2–4 mg/kg SC q12–24h)
• Gabapentin (10–20 mg/kg PO q8–12h)
• Tramadol (15–30 mg/kg PO, SC q12h)

Long-Term Pain Management
• Nonsteroidal anti-inflammatories (listed above) combined with gabapentin or tramadol—have been used long-term therapy to reduce pain and inflammation in rabbits with spinal cord disease;
• For sedation—light sedation with midazolam (0.5–2 mg/kg IM); for deeper sedation and longer procedures, the author prefers ketamine (10–20 mg/kg IM) plus midazolam (0.5–1.0 mg/kg IM) or dexmedetomidine (0.03–0.05 mg/kg IM) plus hydromorphone (0.1 mg/kg IM) and ketamine (5–15 mg/kg IM); many other sedation protocols exist

CONTRAINDICATIONS
• Oral administration of antibiotics that select against gram-positive bacteria (penicillins, macrolides, lincosamides, and cephalosporins) can cause fatal enteric dysbiosis and enterotoxemia.
• The use of corticosteroids (systemic or topical preparations) can severely exacerbate infection.
• Topical application of antibiotic ointment or creams—the rabbit may ingest these; may cause enteric dysbiosis

PRECAUTIONS
• If amputation of a limb is necessary, the contralateral limb will be at increased risk of developing pododermatitis due to increase in weight bearing.

• Azithromycin—use with caution due to risk of enteric dysbiosis
• Chloramphenicol—avoid human contact with chloramphenicol due to potential blood dyscrasia. Advise owners of potential risks.
• Meloxicam or other NSAIDs—use with caution in rabbits with compromised renal function; monitor renal values
• Oral administration of any antibiotic may potentially cause enteric dysbiosis; discontinue use if diarrhea or anorexia occurs.

POSSIBLE INTERACTIONS
N/A

ALTERNATIVE DRUGS
N/A

 FOLLOW-UP

PATIENT MONITORING
Monitor for progressive decrease in exudate, resolution of inflammation, and improvement of clinical signs.

PREVENTION/AVOIDANCE
• Provide clean, appropriate surface substrates; provide separate litter box and hide box or bed to prevent prolonged sitting on soiled litter; clean soiled substrates daily; avoid wet bedding (rain, spilled water bowlsa or bottles)
• Prevent obesity
• Encourage exercise; provide large spaces to encourage movement

POSSIBLE COMPLICATIONS
• Severe osteomyelitis; irreversible tendon damage
• Sepsis
• Development of pododermatitis on other feet due to increase in weight bearing
• Urine scald from immobility; myiasis

EXPECTED COURSE AND PROGNOSIS
• Depend on the amount of tissue destruction
• Alopecia of weight-bearing foot surfaces—hair often will not regrow—these animals are at risk lifelong; closely control environmental factors and monitor feet
• Superficial disease (erythema, alopecia, swelling without involvement of deeper tissues)—good to fair prognosis; recurrence if husbandry problems are not addressed
• Osteomyelitis, tendon damage, extensive abscesses—prognosis for return to normal

anatomy is grave; prognosis for return to functional weight bearing depends on the severity of bone involvement and extent of abscesses. Amputation or euthanasia may be warranted in animals with intractable pain.

 MISCELLANEOUS

ASSOCIATED CONDITIONS
• Immunosuppression
• Gastrointestinal hypomotility

AGE-RELATED FACTORS
N/A

ZOONOTIC POTENTIAL
N/A

PREGNANCY/FERTILITY/BREEDING
N/A

SYNONYMS
Bumble foot
Sore hocks

SEE ALSO
Abscessation
Obesity

ABBREVIATIONS
GI = gastrointestinal
NSAID = nonsteroidal anti-inflammatory drug

Suggested Reading
Deeb BJ, Carpenter JW. Neurologic and musculoskeletal diseases. In: Quesenberry KE, Carpenter JW, eds. Ferrets, Rabbits, and Rodents: Clinical Medicine and Surgery, 2nd ed. St Louis: WB Saunders, 2004:203–210.
Harcourt-Brown F. Neurological and locomotor diseases. In: Harcourt-Brown F, ed. Textbook of Rabbit Medicine. Oxford, UK: Butterworth-Heinemann, 2002:307–323.
Hess L. Dermatologic diseases. In: Quesenberry KE, Carpenter JW, eds. Ferrets, Rabbits, and Rodents: Clinical Medicine and Surgery, 2nd ed. St Louis: WB Saunders, 2004:194–202.
Kapatkin A. Orthopedics in small mammals. In: Quesenberry KE, Carpenter JW, eds. Ferrets, Rabbits, and Rodents: Clinical Medicine and Surgery, 2nd ed. St Louis: WB Saunders, 2004:383–391.
Author Barbara Oglesbee, DVM, DABVP (Avian)

RABBITS

BASICS

OVERVIEW
• Most common neoplasm in rabbits; incidence of up to 60% in females >3 years old; higher incidence in some breeds
• Arises from the endometrial glandular epithelium
• May be preceded by endometriosis, endometritis, endometrial hyperplasia, or endometrial venous aneurysms.
• Tumors or associated venous aneurysms frequently bleed. Hemorrhage may become life threatening.
• No difference in incidence in breeding vs. nonbreeding does
• Age is the most significant risk factor.
• Relatively slow growing, but will eventually metastasize locally by extension into the myometrium and peritoneum, or will metastasize hematogenously
• Most common site of distant metastasis is the lung; brain, ocular, cutaneous, bone, and hepatic metastasis may also occur
• Average interval between onset of clinical signs and death from metastasis is 12–24 months
• Tumors are usually multicentric; present in both uterine horns
• Tumors may occur simultaneously with endometrial venous aneurysms, pyometra, or pregnancy.
• Mammary neoplasia or cystic mastitis often found in does with uterine neoplasia

SIGNALMENT
• Intact females
• Highest incidence in does >3–4 years old
• All breeds are at risk; highest incidence reported in tan, French silver, Havana, and Dutch breed (up to 80%)

SIGNS
Historical Findings
• Hematuria—most common presenting complaint. Not true hematuria since blood originates from the uterus but is released during micturition. Hematuria is often reported as intermittent or cyclic; usually occurs at the end of micturition, blood clots sometimes seen
• Serosanguinous to purulent, blood-tinged vaginal discharge
• Mastitis (mammary gland cysts)—usually cystic, involving one or more mammary glands; cysts contain clear to cloudy fluid; may be seen in up to 30% of rabbits with uterine adenocarcinoma

• Mammary gland neoplasia
• Increased aggressiveness
• Breeding does—small litter size; increased number of stillborn or resorbed fetuses; infertility; dystocia; abandonment of litters
• Late disease, with metastasis—lethargy, anorexia, pale mucous membranes, dyspnea (pulmonary metastases)

Physical Examination Findings
• Firm, often multiple midcaudal abdominal mass; usually palpable dorsal to the bladder between the bladder and the colon
• Abdominal masses may not be palpable until up to 6 months following the onset of reproductive dysfunction.
• Mammary masses
• Blood-stained perineum

CAUSES AND RISK FACTORS
Intact sexual status

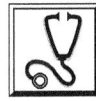

DIAGNOSIS

DIFFERENTIAL DIAGNOSIS
• Pregnancy
• Endometrial venous aneurysms (especially if blood passed with micturition)—may occur simultaneously with adenocarcinoma
• Endometrial hyperplasia, hydrometra, or mucometra—may occur simultaneously with adenocarcinoma
• Pyometra—may occur simultaneously with adenocarcinoma
• Other uterine tumors
• Other mid-caudal abdominal masses

CBC/BIOCHEMISTRY/URINALYSIS
• Anemia with significant uterine hemorrhage
• May see increased liver enzymes with metastasis

OTHER LABORATORY TESTS
N/A

IMAGING
• Abdominal radiographs—may detect a caudal abdominal mass, sometimes fluid-filled, dorsal to the bladder
• Thoracic radiographs—always recommended; assess for metastasis
• Ultrasonography—very useful to delineate uterine mass and to differentiate between uterine bleeding and hematuria if blood is expelled during micturition

DIAGNOSTIC PROCEDURES
• Ultrasound-guided cystocentesis—to differentiate hematuria from uterine blood expelled with urination

• Cytologic evaluation—of associated mammary masses
• Histopathologic examination—necessary for definitive diagnosis

PATHOLOGIC FINDINGS
Gross—usually multicentric; may involve one or both horns; may appear cauliflower-like, papillary- or polyp-like projections into the uterine lumen. Often have necrotic or hemorrhagic center, or may secrete mucus. Tumors may occur simultaneously with endometriosis, endometrial venous aneurysms, pyometra, or pregnancy. May find metastases in local lymph nodes, peritoneum, liver, lung, bone, eyes, or skin.

Histologic—usually well-differentiated adenocarcinoma

TREATMENT
• Ovariohysterectomy—treatment of choice; usually curative if metastasis has not occurred.
• Examine the mesentery and liver to check for metastases.
• Occasionally, local metastasis is not yet grossly visible at time of surgery; advise owner of a guarded prognosis until recheck at 3–6 month intervals.
• Assist feed any rabbit that is anorexic to avoid secondary gastrointestinal disorders.
• Blood transfusion may be indicated in rabbits with significant uterine hemorrhage.
• Excise neoplastic or abscessed mammary glands; cystic mastitis will resolve with ovariohysterectomy alone and does not require excision.

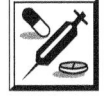

MEDICATIONS

DRUG(S) OF CHOICE
• Chemotherapy—success in metastatic disease has not been reported in rabbits.
• Pain management is essential during and following surgery, Perioperative choices include butorphanol (0.1–0.5 mg/kg SQ, IM, IV q4–6h, buprenorphine (0.02–0.05 mg/kg SQ, IM IV q8–12h), hydromorphone (0.1 mg/kg SC IM q2–4h), or oxymorphone (0.05–0.2 mg/kg SC IM q8–12h). To manage long-term pain: meloxicam (1.0 mg/kg PO q24h; carprofen (2 mg/kg PO q12h), tramadol (5–15 mg/kg PO q8–12h), and/or gabapentin (5–20 mg/kg PO q8–12h)

UTERINE ADENOCARCINOMA (CONTINUED)

FOLLOW-UP

PATIENT MONITORING
Consider thoracic and abdominal radiographs every 3 months for the first 6–12 months post ovariohysterectomy. Not all metastases are grossly visible at the time of surgery.

PREVENTION/AVOIDANCE
Ovariohysterectomy for all nonbreeding rabbits; usually performed between 6 months and 2 years of age. For breeding rabbits—recommend stop breeding and spay before 4 years of age, as this is when most tumors occur.

EXPECTED COURSE AND PROGNOSIS
- Excellent (cure) if ovariohysterectomy prior to metastasis or mammary neoplasia; poor to grave if metastasis has occurred (5 month to 2 years to metastasize); after chemotherapy, unknown
- Without ovariohysterectomy—metastasis, death in 12–24 months
- Associated cystic mastitis will resolve with ovariohysterectomy alone unless secondary infection has developed.

MISCELLANEOUS

ASSOCIATED CONDITIONS
- Mammary neoplasia
- Mastitis
- Pyometra or other nonneoplastic endometrial disorders
- Ovarian neoplasia

AGE-RELATED FACTORS
Rare in rabbits under 2 years of age; risk increases with age; seen in up to 60% of does over 3 years old

ZOONOTIC POTENTIAL
N/A

PREGNANCY/FERTILITY/BREEDING
Uterine neoplasia may be concurrent with pregnancy.

SEE ALSO
Hematuria
Mastitis, cystic, and septic
Pyometra and nonneoplastic endometrial disorders

Suggested Reading
Di Girolamo N, Selleri P. Disorders of the urinary and reproductive system. In: Quesenberry KE, Carpenter JW, eds. Ferrets, Rabbits and Rodents, 4th Ed). Clinical Medicine and Surgery ed. St. Louis: Saunders, 2020:201–220.

Hallman RM, Brandão J. Diagnostic imaging of the renal system in exotic companion mammals. Vet Clin Exot Anim 2020;23:195–214.

Mancinelli E, Lord B. Urogenital and reproductive disease. In: Meredith A, Lord B, eds. BSAVA Manual of Rabbit Medicine. Gloucester: British Small Animal Veterinary Association, 2014:191–204.

Reavill DR, Lennox AM. Disease overview of the urinary tract in exotic companion mammals and tips on clinical management. Vet Clin Exot Anim 2020;23(1):169–193.

Author Barbara Oglesbee, DVM, DABVP (Avian)

VAGINAL DISCHARGE

BASICS

DEFINITION
Any substance emanating from the vulvar labia; in rabbits, fresh blood or serosanguinous discharge is most common

PATHOPHYSIOLOGY
• May originate from several distinct sources, depending in part on the age and reproductive status of the patient; from uterus (most common), urinary tract, vagina, vestibule, or perivulvar skin; except for a small amount of lochia postpartum, vaginal discharge is always abnormal.
• No discharge is seen during estrus in normal does (female rabbit is called a doe). When receptive, the vulva may be slightly swollen, moist, and deep red to purple in color.
• Normal cycling rabbit—become reproductively active as early as 4 months of age; induced ovulators with silent estrus; estrous cycles last 7–14 days
• Serosanguinous discharge or fresh blood is usually mistaken for hematuria since blood is often expelled from the uterus during micturition.

SYSTEMS AFFECTED
• Reproductive
• Renal/Urologic
• Skin/Exocrine

SIGNALMENT
• Intact females
• Highest incidence of uterine disorders seen in does >3–4 years old
• All breeds are at risk
• Postpartum does—normal bloody or greenish discharges common

SIGNS

Historical Findings
• Hematuria—most common presenting complaint. Not true hematuria since blood originates from the uterus but is expelled during micturition. Hematuria is often reported as intermittent or cyclic.
• Discharge from the vulva adhering to perineal fur
• Spotting—usually bloody
• May have had signs of pseudopregnancy—pulling hair, nest building
• Increased aggressiveness
• Recent parturition—with postpartum discharge
• Breeding does—may have history of small litter size; increased number of stillborn or resorbed fetuses; infertility; dystocia; abandonment of litters

Physical Examination Findings
• Blood or serosanguinous discharge—most commonly expelled during urination, but can appear independent of micturition; may see discharge adhered to fur
• Purulent discharge is extremely uncommon.
• Uterus—may be palpably large; careful palpation may allow determination of size; overly aggressive palpation may induce rupture in rabbits with pyometra
• Enlarged mammary gland—one or multiple, may be firm and multilobulated (mammary tumors), or fluid filled (cystic)
• Pale mucous membranes, tachycardia in rabbits that have had significant uterine hemorrhage
• Depression, lethargy, and anorexia in rabbits with pyometra or uterine hemorrhage

CAUSES

Serosanguinous or Frank Blood
• Uterine adenocarcinoma—extremely common cause, other uterine neoplasia possible
• Endometrial disorders—extremely common; endometrial hyperplasia (most common), endometrial venous aneurysms, endometriosis, and endometritis; one or more of these disorders often seen concurrently
• Foreign body—rare
• Vaginal neoplasia or vaginal hematoma—rare
• Vaginal trauma
• Urinary tract infection (unusual)

Greenish/Lochia
• Immediately postpartum
• Dystocia

Purulent Exudate
• Usually not seen with pyometra or vaginitis since exudate is thick and does not drain well
• Exudate from acquired perivulvar dermatitis can be mistaken for vaginal discharge.
• Vaginitis—rare in rabbits
• Fetal death

RISK FACTORS
• Intact sexual status
• Risk for uterine disorders, including neoplasia, increases with age—seen more often in rabbits over 3 years of age
• Risk may increase with sterile mating, or when does mount each other.

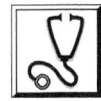

DIAGNOSIS

DIFFERENTIAL DIAGNOSES
• Perivulvar dermatitis—moist dermatitis (urine scald); feces pasted around perineum.
• Serosanguinous or bloody discharge—may be difficult clinically to differentiate nonneoplastic endometrial disorders from uterine adenocarcinoma prior to ovariohysterectomy. Frequently see more than one disorder in the same rabbit, especially in rabbits with uterine adenocarcinoma. For instance, many rabbits with uterine neoplasia also have areas of cystic endometrial hyperplasia.
• Hematuria—use ultrasound-guided cystocentesis to collect urine; differentiates true hematuria from blood expelled from the uterus

CBC/BIOCHEMISTRY/URINALYSIS
• Often unremarkable in rabbits with uterine adenocarcinoma or other uterine disorders
• Neutrophilia—sometimes seen in rabbits with pyometra
• Regenerative anemia possible in rabbits with uterine hemorrhage
• Azotemia, increases in ALT, electrolyte disturbances—all can be abnormal in rabbits with pyometra, septicemia, or severe dehydration, depending on clinical course
• Urinalysis—sample collected by ultrasound-guided cystocentesis to differentiate hematuria from uterine bleeding

OTHER LABORATORY TESTS
Histopathologic examination of uterus following ovariohysterectomy—necessary for definitive diagnosis

IMAGING
• Abdominal radiography—may detect a large uterus (soft tissue or fluid density) in patients with uterine adenocarcinoma, endometrial disorder, or pyometra and later stages of fetal death
• Thoracic radiographs—always recommended; assess for metastasis

Ultrasonography
• With blood filled uterus/vagina, may appear as fluid filled sac cranial to urinary bladder.
• Assess size of uterus and nature of uterine contents
• Rule out pregnancy

DIAGNOSTIC PROCEDURES
• Vaginal cytologic examination—may be helpful in determining if the discharge is purulent or blood; cytology does not establish stage of estrus
• Cystocentesis and bacterial culture—help rule out urinary tract disorders
• Biopsy of vaginal mass—rule out neoplasia

TREATMENT
• Ovariohysterectomy—treatment of choice for uterine adenocarcinoma; usually curative if metastasis has not occurred
• Ovariohysterectomy—treatment of choice for all uterine disorders. All uterine disorders

RABBITS

VAGINAL DISCHARGE   (CONTINUED)

carry risk of hemorrhage into the uterus; can become life threatening; can progress; all are at risk for developing uterine adenocarcinoma; reproductive performance is reduced in does with endometrial disorders.
• In does with neoplasia, local metastases are sometimes not grossly visible at time of surgery; advise owner of a guarded prognosis and recheck at 3–6 month intervals.
• Assist-feed any rabbit that is anorexic to avoid secondary gastrointestinal disorders.
• Blood transfusion may be indicated in rabbits with significant uterine hemorrhage.
• Excise neoplastic or abscessed mammary glands; cystic mastitis will resolve with ovariohysterectomy alone and does not require excision.

MEDICATIONS

DRUG(S) OF CHOICE
• Bacterial vaginitis—antibiotics; empirical pending results of bacterial culture and sensitivity test. Use broad-spectrum antibiotics such as enrofloxacin (10–20 mg/kg PO, SC, IM, IV q12h), marbofloxacin (5 mg/kg PO q24h), trimethoprim-sulfa (15–30 mg/kg PO q12h), or chloramphenicol (50 mg/kg PO q8h).
• Pyometra—medical treatment alone ineffective as exudate does not drain; administer antibiotics perioperatively
• Acute pain management—hydromorphone (0.05–02 mg/kg IV, IM, SC q6–8h), buprenorphine (0.02–0.05 mg/kg SC, IM, IV q8–12h); use preoperatively
• Postoperative/long-term pain management—meloxicam (1 mg/kg PO, SC, IM q24h) or carprofen (2 mg/kg PO q12h)

CONTRAINDICATIONS
• Oral administration of most antibiotics effective against anaerobes will cause a fatal gastrointestinal dysbiosis in rabbits. Do not administer penicillins, macrolides, lincosamides, and cephalosporins by oral administration.
• Corticosteroids—associated with gastrointestinal ulceration and hemorrhage, delayed wound healing, and heightened susceptibility to infection; rabbits are very sensitive to the immunosuppressive effects of both topical and systemic corticosteroids; use may exacerbate subclinical bacterial infection

PRECAUTIONS
• Chloramphenicol—avoid human contact with chloramphenicol due to potential blood dyscrasia. Advise owners of potential risks.

• Meloxicam and other NSAIDs—use with caution in rabbits with compromised renal function.
• Oral administration of any antibiotic may potentially cause enteric dysbiosis; discontinue use if diarrhea or anorexia occurs.

POSSIBLE INTERACTIONS
N/A

ALTERNATIVE DRUGS
Prostaglandins—PGF2a has not been used successfully in rabbits.

FOLLOW-UP

PATIENT MONITORING
• Monitor carefully for signs of pain (reluctance to move, teeth grinding) postoperatively.
• Make certain the doe continues to eat postoperatively.
• If owners elect not to perform surgery— monitor carefully for signs of uterine hemorrhage (blood passed during micturition) or sepsis in rabbits with endometritis or mastitis.

PREVENTION/AVOIDANCE
• Ovariohysterectomy, for all nonbreeding rabbits; usually performed between 6 months and 2 years of age.
• For breeding rabbits—recommend stop breeding and spay after 4 years of age, as this is when most endometrial disorders (including adenocarcinoma) occur.

POSSIBLE COMPLICATIONS
• Peritonitis, sepsis in does with endometritis or pyometra
• Postoperative intra-abdominal adhesions— may contribute to chronic pain, gastrointestinal motility disorders
• Uterine adenocarcinoma, metastasis, and mammary neoplasia in does over 3 years of age
• Hemorrhage, possible death in rabbits with bleeding uterine disorders

EXPECTED COURSE AND PROGNOSIS
• Good prognosis with timely ovariohysterectomy for most uterine disorders, including adenocarcinoma that has not metastasized.
• Guarded prognosis in does presented with vigorous vaginal hemorrhage; emergency stabilization and hysterectomy are indicated to control hemorrhage.
• Guarded to poor in does with pyometra that is not treated early; sepsis or peritonitis may follow

• Excellent (cure) of uterine adenocarcinoma if ovariohysterectomy prior to metastasis or mammary neoplasia; poor to grave if metastasis has occurred (5 months to 2 years to metastasize); after chemotherapy, unknown; without ovariohysterectomy— metastasis, death in 12–24 months.
• Associated cystic mastitis will resolve with ovariohysterectomy alone unless secondary infection has developed.

MISCELLANEOUS

ASSOCIATED CONDITIONS
• Mammary neoplasia
• Mastitis
• Ovarian neoplasia
• Ovarian abscess

AGE-RELATED FACTORS
Uterine neoplasia—rare in rabbits under 2 years of age; risk increases with age; seen in up to 60% of does over 3 years old

ZOONOTIC POTENTIAL
N/A

PREGNANCY/FERTILITY/BREEDING
Many antibiotics and corticosteroids are contraindicated during pregnancy.

SEE ALSO
Mastitis, cystic, and septic
Pyometra and nonneoplastic endometrial disorders
Uterine adenocarcinoma

Suggested Reading
Di Girolamo N, Selleri P. Disorders of the urinary and reproductive system. In: Quesenberry KE, Carpenter JW, eds. Ferrets, Rabbits and Rodents, 4th Ed). Clinical Medicine and Surgery ed. St. Louis: Saunders, 2020:201–220.
Hallman RM, Brandão J. Diagnostic imaging of the renal system in exotic companion mammals. Vet Clin Exot Anim 2020; 23:195–214.
Mancinelli E, Lord B. Urogenital and reproductive disease. In: Meredith A, Lord B, eds. BSAVA Manual of Rabbit Medicine. Gloucester: British Small Animal Veterinary Association, 2014:191–204.
Reavill DR, Lennox AM. Disease overview of the urinary tract in exotic companion mammals and tips on clinical management. Vet Clin Exot Anim 2020;23(1):169–193.
Author Barbara Oglesbee, DVM, DABVP (Avian)

VERTEBRAL FRACTURE OR LUXATION

BASICS

OVERVIEW
• Common cause of acute posterior paresis and paralysis in pet rabbits
• Rabbits have strong muscles in the hindquarters, used for hopping. With improper handling, or when caged rabbits are suddenly startled and jump, the hindquarters twist at the lumbosacral junction, resulting in vertebral fracture or luxation, most commonly at L7.
• Fractures occur more often than dislocations.
• Many affected rabbits are unable to voluntarily express their bladders and may lose anal sphincter tone. Complications secondary to urine retention or urinary/fecal incontinence (uremia, hypercalciuria, moist dermatitis, and fly strike) and decubital ulcer formation are common and often lead to the decision to euthanize.

SIGNALMENT
No specific age, breed, or gender predisposition

SIGNS
General Comments
Acute onset of posterior paresis most common finding

Historical Findings
• Owner may describe an abnormal gait; the rabbit may be unable to hop, may drag the affected limbs, or may be unable get up.
• Sudden onset of paresis/paralysis
• History of improper restraint—inexperienced handlers or owners; restraint for mask induction of anesthesia; very nervous animals escaping from appropriate restraint
• Trauma may not have been witnessed. Rabbits can fracture or luxate vertebrae by suddenly jumping while in their cages. History may include startling event such as a loud thunderstorm, fireworks, or unfamiliar people or pets in the house.

Physical Examination Findings
• Patient usually alert
• Pain or hyperesthesia can usually be elicited at site of spinal cord damage.
• If in pain, patient may resent handling and manipulation during the examination.
• Superficial and deep pain perception may be decreased or absent in the rear limbs.
• Decreased or absent anal tone
• Decreased or absent proprioception in the rear limbs
• Decreased or absent voluntary movement in the rear limbs and/or tail
• Forelimb function is normal; occasionally, Schiff–Sherrington phenomena may cause increased muscle tone in the forelimbs.

• Bladder may also be paralyzed in rabbits with severe spinal cord damage, negating voluntary urination.
• Urine scald in the perineal region; dermatitis or alopecia due to inappropriate grooming or urinary incontinence—sequela to vertebral trauma, days to months following event

CAUSES AND RISK FACTORS
Inappropriate Restraint
• Rabbits often try to jump or twist free of restraint. Injury to L7 is most common result.
• When restraining rabbits, always restrain both front and rear quarters simultaneously. Rabbits can be restrained by using one hand to hold the scruff or hold between the front limbs, and one to hold the hindquarters; also by tucking the head under one arm while holding the hindquarters with the other hand and holding the rabbit against your body.
• On an exam table, always apply pressure to the front and hindquarters simultaneously; use a towel to firmly wrap the body.
• Covering the eyes will calm some rabbits.
• Cradle the rabbit on its back to examine ventral areas; hold nervous rabbits close to the floor as they may jump during examination.
• Use a well-trained assistant for restraint.
• Most rabbits particularly object to examination of the mouth and ears. Be especially cautious with restraint during these procedures.
• When in doubt, administer sedation or anesthesia to perform noxious procedures.

Trauma During Anesthetic Induction
• Many rabbits object to the odor of gas anesthetics. They often appear calm, then suddenly and forcibly jump or kick. Chamber or mask induction without pre-anteisthetic sedation is ill-advised.
• Even with preanesthetic sedation, be prepared for sudden, unexpected jumping or kicking. To prevent injury, be certain that the rabbit is securely restrained.

Trauma in Cage
• Caged rabbits can injure themselves when startled.
• Usually follows an event such as noisy thunderstorms, fireworks, or the appearance unfamiliar people or pets
• Return a hospitalized rabbit to the cage rear end first to prevent jumping.

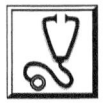

DIAGNOSIS

DIFFERENTIAL DIAGNOSIS
Weak Pelvic Limbs
• Pain or hyperesthesia elicited at site of spinal cord damage usually seen with trauma, Spondylosis/spinal arthritis; IVD disease, discospondylitis, and bone tumors are less common

• Lack of pain along spinal column—consider *E. cuniculi*, CNS lesions, systemic or metabolic disease; vascular disease (rare), degenerative myelopathy, neoplasia
• Acute onset—most common with spinal cord trauma
• Gradual onset or intermittent weakness—usually systemic or metabolic disease; occasionally with spondylosis
• Other clinical signs—lethargy, weight loss, signs referable to a specific system seen in rabbits with weakness due to metabolic disease
• Severe obesity—can cause rear limb weakness
• Spinal reflexes—localize weakness to the thoracolumbar, or lower lumbar cord segments
• Musculoskeletal disorders—typically produce lameness and a reluctance to move; rule out bilateral hind limb fracture or coxofemoral luxation

CBC/BIOCHEMISTRY/URINALYSIS
Usually normal

IMAGING
• Spinal radiographs—lesion localized to the spinal cord; usually reveals fracture or luxation; occasionally spinal column luxates, damaging the cord, then returns to normal-appearing radiographic position; prognosis in these cases can vary widely. Severely displaced, overriding segments or compression fractures generally result in more severe spinal cord injury and poorer prognosis. Use spinal radiographs to rule out other causes, such as spondylosis, intravertebral disc disease, diskospondylitis, bony tumor, congenital vertebral malformation
• Skull films or thoracic radiographs—to rule out other causes of weakness if vertebral abnormalities are not seen
• CT—more accurate evaluation for both spinal and soft tissue abnormalities

TREATMENT

APPROPRIATE HEALTH CARE
Inpatient—with severe weakness/paralysis or until bladder function can be ascertained

NURSING CARE
• Bedding—move paralyzed, paretic, or painful rabbits away from soiled bedding, check and clean frequently to prevent urine scalding and moist pyoderma; use padded bedding to help prevent decubital ulcer formation.
• Keep fur clean and dry.
• Turning—turn recumbent patients from side to side four to eight times daily; prevent hypostatic lung congestion and decubital ulcer formation.
• Manual expression of the bladder if unable to urinate
• Carts available for small breed dogs can sometimes be fitted for larger rabbits and may be tolerated.

VERTEBRAL FRACTURE OR LUXATION (CONTINUED)

ACTIVITY
Restricted to cage rest only in rabbits with spinal trauma

DIET
• It is imperative that the rabbit continue to eat during and following treatment. Painful rabbits may become anorexic. Anorexia will cause GI hypomotility, derangement of the gastrointestinal microflora, and overgrowth of intestinal bacterial pathogens. Hand-feed or bring food to nonambulatory rabbits.
• If the patient refuses food, syringe-feed a gruel such as Critical Care for Herbivores (Oxbow Pet Products) or Emeraid Herbivore (Lafeber Company, Cornell, IL) 10–15 mL/kg PO q6–8h. Alternatively, pellets can be ground and mixed with fresh greens, vegetable baby foods, water, or juice to form a gruel.
• High-carbohydrate, high-fat nutritional supplements are contraindicated.
• Encourage oral fluid intake by offering fresh water and by wetting leafy vegetables. Place water bottles or dishes within reach of recumbent rabbits.

MEDICATIONS

DRUG(S) OF CHOICE

For Spinal Trauma
• Corticosteroids have been used in rabbits with acute spinal cord trauma with some success. Although clinical improvement has been anecdotally reported, rabbits are very sensitive to the immunosuppressive and gastrointestinal side effects of corticosteroids; immunosuppression may exacerbate subclinical bacterial infections or *E. cuniculi*. Methylprednisolone sodium succinate administered IV at doses used in canine/feline patients may be of benefit with acute fracture or luxation. Administer with GI protectant to reduce risk of ulceration—ranitidine (2 mg/kg IV q24h)

Acute Pain Management
• Butorphanol (0.1–0.5 mg/kg SQ, IM, IV q4–6h); may cause profound sedation; short acting
• Buprenorphine (0.02–0.05 mg/kg SQ, IM IV q8–12h); less sedating, longer acting than butorphanol
• Hydromorphone (0.1 mg/kg SC IM q2–4h) or oxymorphone (0.05–0.2 mg/kg SC IM q8–12h)
• Meloxicam (1 mg/kg PO, SC, IM q24h)
• Carprofen (2–4 mg/kg PO, SC q12–24h)

Long-Term Pain Management
• Nonsteroidal anti-inflammatories—have been used for short- or long-term therapy to reduce pain and inflammation in rabbits with musculoskeletal disease; meloxicam (1.0 mg/kg PO q24h; carprofen (2 mg/kg PO q12h)
• Tramadol—5–15 mg/kg PO q8–12h

• Gabapentin—5–20 mg/kg PO q8–12h

Sedation
Light sedation with midazolam (0.5–1.0 mg/kg IM, IV), combined with butorphanol (0.1–0.5 mg/kg IV, IM); many other sedation protocols exist

CONTRAINDICATIONS
• Oral administration of antibiotics that select against gram-positive bacteria (penicillins, macrolides, lincosamides, and cephalosporins) can cause fatal enteric dysbiosis and enterotoxemia.
• Corticosteroids—do not use with NSAIDs because of combined negative effects on the gastrointestinal tract

PRECAUTIONS
Corticosteroids—use with caution, only in acute spinal trauma; associated with gastrointestinal ulceration and hemorrhage, delayed wound healing, and heightened susceptibility to infection; rabbits are very sensitive to the immunosuppressive effects of both topical and systemic corticosteroids; use may exacerbate subclinical bacterial infection

ALTERNATIVE DRUGS
• For acute spinal trauma—prednisolone (0.25 mg/kg PO q12h × 5d); dexamethasone (0.5–2 mg/kg IV, IM); use with caution, if at all
• Chondroprotective agents, nutraceuticals (oral glycosaminoglycans, cosequin)—use not well described in rabbits; have been anecdotally used at feline dosages in addition to analgesics
• Acupuncture may be effective for rabbits with chronic pain.

FOLLOW-UP

PATIENT MONITORING
• Neurologic examinations—daily to monitor status
• Bladder—evacuate (via manual expression or catheterization) three to four times a day to prevent overdistension and subsequent bladder atony; patient can be managed at home if bladder function returns, or owners can be taught to express the bladder. Monitor for bladder enlargement, bladder atony, or uremia secondary to urine retention.

POSSIBLE COMPLICATIONS
• GI stasis
• Urinary tract infection, bladder atony, urine scalding and pyoderma, decubital ulcer formation
• Permanent paralysis warranting euthanasia

EXPECTED COURSE AND PROGNOSIS
• Depends on the severity of spinal cord injury
• Rabbits with rear limb paresis or paralysis due to mild to moderate spinal cord trauma

may regain partial or full function with exercise restriction, supportive care, and long-term administration of NSAIDs.
• Most paralyzed rabbits with severe spinal trauma do not regain mobility; euthanasia may be warranted; rate of complicating conditions (bladder, cutaneous) is very high; quality of life often poor
• Wheeled carts manufactured for small dogs have been used successfully in rabbits.

MISCELLANEOUS

ASSOCIATED CONDITIONS
Gastrointestinal hypomotility

ABBREVIATIONS
CNS = central nervous system
CT = computed tomography
GI = gastrointestinal
IVD = intervertebral disc
NSAID = nonsteroidal anti-inflammatory drug

Suggested Reading
Bays TB. Geriatric care of rabbits, guinea pigs, and chinchillas. Vet Clin Exot Anim 2020;23:567–593.
DeCubellis J. Common emergencies in rabbits, guinea pigs, and chinchillas. Vet Clin Exot Anim 2016;19:411–429.
Fisher PG, Künzel F, Rylander H. Neurologic and musculoskeletal disease. In: Quesenberry KE, Carpenter JW, eds. Ferrets, Rabbits and Rodents, 4th Ed). Clinical Medicine and Surgery ed. St. Louis: Saunders, 2020:583–594.
Harkness JE, Turner PV, VandeWoude S, Wheeler CL. Clinical signs and differential diagnoses: nervous and musculoskeletal conditions. In: Harkness JE, Turner PV, VandeWoude S, Wheeler CL, eds. Biology and Medicine of Rabbits and Rodents, 5th ed. Ames: Wiley-Blackwell, 2010:214–216.
Keeble E. Nervous system and musculoskeletal disorders. In: Meredith A, Lord B, eds. BSAVA Manual of Rabbit Medicine. Gloucester: British Small Animal Veterinary Association, 2014:233–248.
Lennox AM, Gladden JN. Emergency and critical care of small mammals. In: Quesenberry KE, Carpenter JW, eds. Ferrets, Rabbits and Rodents, 4th Ed). Clinical Medicine and Surgery. 2021 ed. St. Louis: Saunders, 2020:595–608.
Varga M. Neurological and locomotive disorders. In: Varga M, ed. Textbook of Rabbit Medicine, 2nd ed. London, UK: Elsevier, 2014:367–389.

Author Barbara Oglesbee, DVM, DABVP (Avian)

BASICS

DEFINITION
• Weight loss is considered clinically important when it exceeds 10% of the normal body weight and is not associated with fluid loss.
• Cachexia is defined as the state of extreme poor health and is associated with anorexia, weight loss, weakness, and mental depression.

PATHOPHYSIOLOGY
• Weight loss can result from many different pathophysiologic mechanisms that share a common feature—insufficient caloric intake or availability to meet metabolic needs.
• Insufficient caloric intake or availability can be caused by (1) a high energy demand (e.g., that characteristic of a hypermetabolic state); (2) inadequate energy intake, including insufficient quantity or quality of food, or inadequate nutrient assimilation (e.g., with anorexia, dysphagia, or malabsorptive disorders); or (3) excessive loss of nutrients or fluid, which can occur in patients with gastrointestinal losses, glucosuria, or proteinuria.
• Caloric requirements reported for rabbits: 2,500 kCal/kg of feed for growing, pregnant, or lactating rabbits; 2,100 kCal/kg of feed for adult maintenance

SYSTEMS AFFECTED
Any can be affected by weight loss, especially if severe or the result of systemic disease.

SIGNALMENT
No age or sex predilections

SIGNS

Historical Findings
• Determine whether the appetite is normal, increased, decreased, or absent.
• Historical information is very important, especially regarding type of diet, environment, signs of dental disease, chronic respiratory disease, abscesses, signs of gastrointestinal disease (including lack of fecal production, scant feces, or diarrhea), or signs of any specific disease.
• Signs of pain, such as teeth grinding, a hunched posture, and reluctance to move, are extremely common in rabbits with oral disease or GI hypomotility.
• Pseudoanorectic patients commonly display excessive drooling, difficulty in prehension and mastication of food, halitosis, dysphagia, bruxism, and odynophagia (painful eating).

Physical Examination Findings
• Most underlying causes of pseudoanorexia can be identified by a thorough examination

of the face, mandible, teeth, neck, oropharynx, and esophagus for dental disease, ulceration, traumatic lesions, masses, foreign bodies, and neuromuscular dysfunction.
• A thorough exam of the oral cavity, including the incisors, cheek teeth, and mucosa, is necessary to rule out dental disease. Use of an otoscope or speculum is required to perform screening examination of the oral cavity. A complete examination requires sedation or anesthesia.
• Examine the face for evidence of chronic upper respiratory disease, such as secretions or dried discharges around the nose and front limbs, ocular discharge, exophthalmos, facial swelling, or pain.
• Abdominal palpation is a valuable tool in the diagnosis of GI stasis. Ingesta is always palpable in the stomach of a normal rabbit. The normal stomach should be easily deformable, feel soft and pliable, and not remain pitted on compression. A firm, noncompliant stomach, or stomach contents that remain pitted on compression, is an abnormal finding.
• Gas distension of the intestines or cecum is common in rabbits with GI tract disease.
• Abdominal palpation may also reveal the presence of organomegaly, masses, or GI foreign bodies.
• Auscultation of the thorax may reveal cardiac murmurs, arrhythmias, or abnormal breath sounds.
• Auscultation of the abdomen reveals decreased borborygmi in most rabbits with GI hypomotility.

CAUSES AND RISK FACTORS

Excessive Use of Calories
• Increased catabolism—fever, inflammation, cancer—common, especially chronic upper respiratory disease, abscesses (subcutaneous, joint, facial, intrathoracic, intra-abdominal)
• Increased physical activity
• Pregnancy or lactation

Pseudoanorexia
• Inability to prehend, or chew food—dental disease is extremely common
• Dysphagia

Maldigestive/Malabsorptive Disorders
• Gastrointestinal hypomotility/stasis—very common
• Cecal disbiosis/chronic intermittent diarrhea—very common
• Cocccidiosis—young or debilitated animals

Metabolic Disorders
• Organ failure—cardiac failure, hepatic failure, and renal failure—very common
• Cancer cachexia—(lymphoma, uterine adenocarcinoma)—common
• Hyperthyroidism—rare, but possible

Dietary Causes
• Insufficient long-stemmed hay and excessive simple carbohydrates—very common, leads to secondary gastrointestinal disorders and dental disease
• Insufficient quantity
• Poor quality

Neuromuscular Disease and Pain
• Dental disease—extremely common
• Otitis interna/media; vestibular disorders—very common
• Degenerative joint disease, spinal arthritis—common
• Urolithiasis/hypercalciuria—very common
• Joint or facial abscesses—very common
• Ulcerative pododermatitis (sore hocks)—common
• CNS disease—brain abscess (and, possibly, *Encephalitozoon cuniculi*)—can be associated with anorexia or pseudoanorexia

Excessive Nutrient Loss
• Protein-losing enteropathy (secondary to infectious or infiltrative diseases)
• Protein-losing nephropathy (rare)

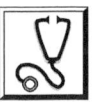

DIAGNOSIS

• If previous weights are not available, subjectively assess the patient for cachexia, emaciation, dehydration, or other clues that would confirm the owner's complaint of weight loss.
• After weight loss is confirmed, seek the underlying cause.

DIFFERENTIAL DIAGNOSIS
• Categorize the weight loss as occurring with a normal, increased, or decreased appetite.
• The list of likely differential diagnoses for a patient with weight loss despite a normal or increased appetite is much different and much shorter than that for patients with decreased appetite or anorexia.
• Determine what the patient's appetite was at the onset of weight loss; any condition can lead to anorexia if it persists long enough for the patient to become debilitated.
• Seek causes of pseudoanorexia—dental disease is one of the most common causes of weight loss in rabbits.
• Some loss of muscle mass may be a normal aging change.

CBC/BIOCHEMISTRY/URINALYSIS
• Help identify infectious, inflammatory, and metabolic diseases, including organ failure
• Especially helpful when the history and physical examination do not provide much useful information

RABBITS

WEIGHT LOSS AND CACHEXIA

OTHER LABORATORY TESTS
• Determined by the clinician's list of most likely differential diagnoses on the basis of the specific findings of the history and physical examination
• Fecal direct examination, fecal flotation to rule out coccidian

IMAGING
• Abdominal radiography and ultrasonography should be utilized to evaluate gastrointestinal disorders; hepatic, renal, and urogenital diseases; or internal abscesses. Secondary hepatic lipidosis is best evaluated through imaging using ultrasonography.
• Skull radiography may help rule out dental disease, but CT provides a broader evaluation of the relationship of the teeth to one another, the nasal cavity, and the bones of the skull.
• Thoracic radiography is used initially to evaluate for cardiac and respiratory diseases. Because of the small thorax, ultrasonography can sometimes be used to localize and guide aspiration of respiratory masses/abscesses. Echocardiography is used to evaluate for specific cardiac diseases.

DIAGNOSTIC PROCEDURES
• Vary depending on initial diagnostic findings and the suspected underlying cause of weight loss
• A thorough examination of the oral cavity is indicated in every rabbit with anorexia or pseudoanorexia. A thorough examination includes the incisors, molars, and buccal and lingual mucosa to rule out dental disease. Use of an otoscope or speculum may be useful in identifying severe abnormalities; however, many problems will be missed by using this method alone. Complete exam requires heavy sedation or general anesthesia and specialized equipment.

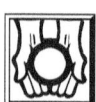

TREATMENT
• The most important treatment principle is to treat the underlying cause of the weight loss.
• Symptomatic therapy includes attention to fluid and electrolyte derangements, reduction in environmental stressors, and modification of the diet to improve palatability.
• Anorexia—it is absolutely imperative that the rabbit begin eating as soon as possible, regardless of the underlying cause. Continued anorexia will exacerbate GI hypomotility and cause further derangement of the gastrointestinal microflora and overgrowth of intestinal bacterial pathogens.

• Offer a large selection of fresh, moistened greens such as cilantro, romaine lettuce, parsley, carrot tops, dandelion greens, spinach, collard greens, etc., and good-quality grass hay. Many rabbits will begin to eat these foods, even if they were previously anorectic. Also offer the rabbit's usual, pelleted diet, as the initial goal is to get the rabbit to eat.
• If the patient refuses these foods, syringe-feed a gruel such as Critical Care for Herbivores (Oxbow Pet Products, Murdock, NE) 10–15 mL/kg PO q6–8h. Larger volumes and more frequent feedings are often accepted; feed as much as the rabbit will readily accept. Alternatively, pellets can be ground and mixed with fresh greens, vegetable baby foods, canned pumpkin, water, or juice to form a gruel. If sufficient volumes of food are not accepted in this manner, nasogastric intubation is indicated.
• High-carbohydrate, high-fat nutritional supplements are contraindicated.

CLIENT EDUCATION
• Virtually any disease in the pet rabbit can cause weight loss and, in a previously obese patient, may lead to hepatic lipidosis, which requires hospitalization, aggressive supportive care, and can still carry a guarded prognosis.
• Evaluate the environment and husbandry and ensure appropriate general care; modify as necessary depending upon the disease process identified.

MEDICATIONS
DRUG(S) OF CHOICE
Depend on the underlying cause of the weight loss; see specific topic for each condition, including anorexia.

CONTRAINDICATIONS
N/A

PRECAUTIONS
N/A

POSSIBLE INTERACTIONS
N/A

ALTERNATIVE DRUGS
N/A

FOLLOW-UP
PATIENT MONITORING
The necessity for frequent patient monitoring and the methods required depend on the underlying cause of the weight loss; however, the patient should be weighed regularly and often.

POSSIBLE COMPLICATIONS
See Causes

MISCELLANEOUS
ASSOCIATED CONDITIONS
See Causes

AGE-RELATED FACTORS
N/A

ZOONOTIC POTENTIAL
N/A

PREGNANCY/FERTILITY/BREEDING
Pregnancy and lactation can be associated with weight loss due to increased calorie expenditure.

SYNONYMS
N/A

SEE ALSO
Abscesses
Anorexia and pseudoanorexia
Gastrointestinal hypomotility and gastrointestinal stasis

ABBREVIATIONS
CNS = central nervous system
CT = computed tomography
GI = gastrointestinal

Suggested Reading
Bays TB. Geriatric care of rabbits, guinea pigs, and chinchillas. Vet Clin Exot Anim 2020;23:567–593.
Harkness JE, Turner PV, VandeWoude S, Wheeler CL. Clinical signs and differential diagnoses: nervous and musculoskeletal conditions. In: Harkness JE, Turner PV, VandeWoude S, Wheeler CL, eds. Biology and Medicine of Rabbits and Rodents, 5th ed. Ames: Wiley-Blackwell, 2010: 214–216.
Lennox AM, Capello V, Legendre LF. Small mammal dentistry. In: Quesenberry KE, Carpenter JW, eds. Ferrets, Rabbits and Rodents, 4th Ed). Clinical Medicine and Surgery. 2021 ed. St. Louis: Saunders, 2020:514–535.
Oglesbee B, Lord B. Gastrointestinal diseases of rabbits. In: Quesenberry KE, Carpenter JW, eds. Ferrets, Rabbits and Rodents, 4th Ed). Clinical Medicine and Surgery. 2021 ed. St. Louis: Saunders, 2020: 174–187.
Varga M. Digestive disorders. In: Varga M, ed. Textbook of Rabbit Medicine, 2nd ed. London, UK: Elsevier, 2014:303–349.
Author Barbara Oglesbee, DVM, DABVP (Avian)

RODENTS

ACUTE RESPIRATORY DISTRESS

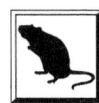

BASICS

DEFINITION
Acute onset of dyspnea or increased respiratory rate and effort. May be accompanied by other evidence of respiratory or cardiac disease

PATHOPHYSIOLOGY
• Multiple etiologies
• While bacterial etiology is most common, other causes of primary respiratory disease include other infectious organisms (viral, parasitic), neoplasia, toxin exposure, or trauma (hemothorax). Also consider cardiac failure as a cause of dyspnea.
• Upper respiratory disease can produce severe respiratory symptoms in rodents, since they are obligate nasal breathers. When dyspneic, rodents often become anxious and increase their respiratory rate and effort. This leads to further nasal congestion and edema, and a vicious circle ensues, leading to acute, severe respiratory distress that may rapidly become life threatening.
• Cardiovascular disease may present as acute respiratory distress.

SYSTEMS AFFECTED
• Respiratory
• Cardiovascular

GENETICS
N/A

INCIDENCE/PREVALENCE
• Common problem in pet rats with history of respiratory tract disorders
• Occasionally seen in mice and hamsters

GEOGRAPHIC DISTRIBUTION
Ubiquitous

SIGNALMENT
• Seen most often in rats
• No specific sex or age predilection for primary respiratory disease
• Cardiovascular disease is more commonly seen in older rodents, in particular, older hamsters.
• Infectious disease may be more common in older, debilitated animals.

SIGNS

Historical Findings
• Rats often have a history of recent or recurrent signs of respiratory tract disease, or a history of exposure to rats with signs of respiratory tract disease.
• Many animals present for acute exacerbation of disease that is currently being treated.

Physical Examination Findings
• May see evidence of respiratory disease such as red tears, naso-ocular discharge,

sneezing, head shaking, and dried discharge on face or front paws
• Increased respiratory rate and effort, often rapidly progressive in severity
• Severe anxiety, distress with progressive dyspnea
• Auscultation findings variable and include increased to decreased or absent airway noise
• May progress to respiratory arrest
• Poor hair coat, weight loss, and dehydration
• Patients may otherwise appear bright and alert to severely depressed.

CAUSES

Infectious
• Chronic upper respiratory disease occurs frequently in rats. This is a multifactorial respiratory infection, generally with more than one pathogen involved. Most are infected with one or more viruses: Sendai virus (parainfluenza), sialodacryoadenitis virus, rat respiratory virus (hantavirus), or pneumonia virus of rats (paramyxovirus), along with *Mycoplasma pulmonis* (murine respiratory mycoplasmosis) and one or more bacteria, including *S. pneumoniae*, *Corynebacterium kutscheri*, or cilia-associated respiratory bacillus.
• A similar respiratory complex, with a combination of Sendai virus, mycoplasma pulmonis, and other bacterial pathogens, exists in mice.
• Sendai and other viral pathogens of mice and rats are nonpathogenic in hamsters. Pneumonia in hamsters is generally bacterial, with *Streptococcus* spp. most common.

Noninfectious
• Trauma (blunt force, falls)
• Environmental and airborne toxins
• Cardiovascular disease occasionally encountered in older rodents and may present as acute respiratory distress
• Respiratory allergens reported anecdotally but not have been documented in pet rodents
• Primary respiratory neoplasia is rare but occasionally encountered
• Pulmonary metastatic neoplasia is rare but has been reported most commonly in mice with mammary and liver neoplasia
• Abdominal distension—organomegaly, neoplasia, ascites

RISK FACTORS
• Presence of respiratory disease
• Poor husbandry, especially overcrowding and poor sanitation
• Other sources of immune suppression may predispose to respiratory disease
• Poor handling techniques increase risk for falls and injuries

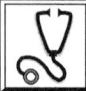

DIAGNOSIS

DIFFERENIAL DIAGNOSIS
• Careful attention to breathing pattern and auscultation may help differentiate between upper and lower respiratory disease
• Trauma/toxin—history and evidence of injury
• Diagnosis of cardiac disease requires thoracic radiography and ultrasound.
• Careful abdominal palpation and radiographs to rule out causes of abdominal distension

CBC/BIOCHEMISTRY/URINALYSIS
• Complete blood count may support but cannot confirm or rule out specific causes of acute respiratory distress.
• Regenerative anemia may support trauma and hemothorax.
• Biochemistry panel is useful to identify underlying disease conditions.

OTHER LABORATORY TESTS
• Culture and susceptibility testing is ideal when indicated but impractical in most cases due to patient size and sample collection difficulty.
• Fluid analysis and culture of thoracocentesis samples

IMAGING
• Radiography and ultrasound are especially useful to help distinguish between pulmonary and cardiovascular disease.
• In cases of suspected *Mycoplasma* sp. pneumonia in rats, imaging may identify abnormalities such as collapsed lungs and pulmonary abscess.
• Ultrasound is essential for confirmation and characterization of cardiovascular disease.

DIAGNOSTIC PROCEDURES
• In larger rodents, ultrasound-guided biopsy of thoracic masses can be attempted.
• Thoracocentesis and fluid analysis as indicated
• Response to antibiotic therapy as a trial
• Response to cardiac drug therapy as a trial when cardiac disease is suspected

TREATMENT

APPROPRIATE HEALTH CARE
Patients with acute respiratory distress should be managed as inpatients.

NURSING CARE
• Administer oxygen therapy—place in an oxygen cage; mask administration may increase anxiety and exacerbate dyspnea. If an

oxygen cage is not available, small patients may be placed directly into an upended large face mask.
• A darkened, quiet area will minimize stress.
• Make sure that the oxygen cage/mask is cool, as dyspneic patients often become hyperthermic, and hyperthermia will exacerbate dyspnea.
• Patients in respiratory distress often benefit from low-dose sedation, which reduces anxiety and respiratory effort.
• Patients with plural space disease benefit from thoracocentesis to remove fluid or air.

ACTIVITY
Strict cage confinement until dyspnea resolves

DIET
Once respiratory distress is relieved, offer high-quality diet.

CLIENT EDUCATION
• Acute respiratory distress carries a guarded prognosis.
• Patients with chronic respiratory disease may be difficult to treat; lifelong treatment may be necessary with recurrent episodes of distress.

SURGICAL CONSIDERATIONS
Thoracotomy for removal of thoracic masses is described in larger exotic companion mammals but is unlikely to be beneficial in smaller patients.

MEDICATIONS
DRUG(S) OF CHOICE
Acute, Severe Respiratory Distress in Rats
• Oxygen should always be administered until the patient is stable.
• Bronchodilators—administer terbutaline (0.01 mg/kg IM—dilute 1:10 with sterile water); if dyspnea persists, deliver 1 puff of albuterol via a feline inhaler
• Low-dose sedation with midazolam (0.5–1.0 mg/kg IM) alone or combined with butorphanol (0.2 mg/kg IM)
• If dyspnea persists, administer furosemide (4 mg/kg IM) to decrease pulmonary edema.

Antibiotic Treatment
• Systemic antibiotics choice is ideally based on results of culture and susceptibility testing, when possible
• In rats, if *Mycoplasma pulmonis* is suspected or confirmed, treat with a combination of enrofloxacin (10 mg/kg PO q12h) and doxycycline (5 mg/kg PO q12h) for a minimum of 2 weeks.
• For other bacterial infections, initially use broad-spectrum antibiotics such as

enrofloxacin (5–10 mg/kg PO, SC, IM q12h), ciprofloxacin (10 mg/kg PO q12h), or trimethoprim-sulfa (15–30 mg/kg PO q12h); if anaerobic infections are suspected use chloramphenicol (30–50 mg/kg PO q8h) or azithromycin (50 mg/kg PO q24h × 14d).

Congestive Heart Failure
The following cardiac drugs have been used in hamsters and may be beneficial in other species as well: digoxin (0.05–0.1 mg/kg PO q12–24h), furosemide (2–10 mg/kg PO, SQ q12h), enalapril (0.5–1.0 mg/kg PO q24h), and verapamil (0.25–0.5 mg SQ q12h).

CONTRAINDICATIONS
Do not administer penicillins, ampicillin, amoxicillin, erythromycin, or lincomycin to hamsters due to the risk of potentially fatal enteric dysbiosis.

PRECAUTIONS
All therapeutic agents, especially drugs used to treat cardiovascular disease, should be used with caution in debilitated, dehydrated patients. Ideally, vascular abnormalities (dehydration, hypotension) are addressed prior to initiating drug therapy.

POSSIBLE INTERACTIONS
N/A

ALTERNATIVE DRUGS
There is some anecdotal evidence that immune boosting drugs/agents have been useful in some cases of infectious respiratory disease.

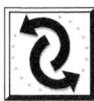

FOLLOW-UP
PATIENT MONITORING
• Patients in acute respiratory distress should be monitored continually until resolution.
• Monitor patient weight.
• Ensure adequate intake of food and water, as patients in respiratory distress are often reluctant to eat or drink.
• Surviving rats are at increased risk for lifelong infection and recurrent episodes of respiratory distress. These episodes can sometimes be managed long term with an orally administered bronchodilator, home nebulization, and albuterol inhalers. It is extremely important to provide excellent husbandry. Provide recycled paper bedding and avoid fragrant woodchip beddings that emit hydrocarbon vapors. House in an open cage to allow adequate ventilation and clean the cage frequently to avoid buildup of ammonia. Avoid using chemicals; avoid dusty environments. Keep on an excellent diet.
• Patients receiving cardiac medications should be monitored carefully for potential untoward effects. There is little information

on the treatment of cardiovascular disease in rodents; precautions used for traditional companion mammals should be observed.

PREVENTION/AVOIDANCE
• Treating respiratory disease in early stages may prevent development of more severe respiratory distress.
• Careful handling helps to avoid trauma.

POSSIBLE COMPLICATIONS
Patients in respiratory distress may progress rapidly to respiratory arrest.

EXPECTED COURSE AND PROGNOSIS
• Mortality is high, even with aggressive treatment.
• Surviving animals are likely to have recurrent episodes.

MISCELLANEOUS
ASSOCIATED CONDITIONS
• Upper respiratory disease or chronic respiratory disease
• Cardiac disease

ZOONOTIC POTENTIAL
Most rodent respiratory pathogens are not zoonotic; however, any animal disease may be of concern to humans with immunocompromise; recent surveys show mycoplasma antibodies in laboratory and veterinary personnel (association with clinical disease unknown).

PREGNANCY/FERTILITY/BREEDING
N/A

SYNONYMS
N/A

SEE ALSO
Congestive heart failure
Mycoplasmosis and chronic respiratory disease
Pneumonia
Rhinitis and sinusitis

Suggested Reading
Capello V, Lennox AM. Diagnostic imaging of the respiratory system in exotic companion mammals. Vet Clin Exot Anim 2011;14:369–389.
Dutton M. Selected veterinary concerns of geriatric rats, mice, hamsters, and gerbils. Vet Clin Exot Anim 2020;23(3): 525–548.
Fitzgerald BC, Dias S, Martorell J. Cardiovascular drugs in avian, small mammal, and reptile medicine. Vet Clin Exot Anim 2018;21:399–442.
Frolich J. Rats and mice. In: Quesenberry KE, Carpenter JW, eds. Ferrets, Rabbits and Rodents, 4th Ed). Clinical Medicine

and Surgery. 2021 ed. St. Louis: Saunders, 2020:345–367.

Jekl V, Knotek Z. Evidence-based advances in rodent medicine. Vet Clin Exot Anim 2017;20:805–816.

Lennox AM, Gladden JN. Emergency and critical care of small mammals. In: Quesenberry KE, Carpenter JW, eds.

Ferrets, Rabbits and Rodents, 4th Ed). Clinical Medicine and Surgery. 2021 ed. St. Louis: Saunders, 2020:595–608.

Mayer J, Mans C. Rodents. In: Carpenter JW, ed. Exotic Animal Formulary, 5th ed. St Louis: Elsevier, 2018:459–493.

Miwa Y, Mayer J. Hamsters and gerbils. In: Quesenberry KE, Carpenter JW, eds.

Ferrets, Rabbits and Rodents, 4th Ed). Clinical Medicine and Surgery. 2021 ed. St. Louis: Saunders, 2020:368–384.

Author Angela M. Lennox, DVM, Dipl ABVP (Avian), ECM; DECZM-Small Mammal

BASICS

DEFINITION
The loss or absence of hair, from focal or patchy to complete hair loss

PATHOPYSIOLOGY
The pathophysiology of alopecia is dependent on the causative factors. Mechanisms of hair loss may include poor development, self-trauma, inflammation, and irritation resulting in damage to the hair follicle and weakening of the hair shaft, tissue necrosis or fibrosis, invasion by ectoparasites, and immune-mediated responses.

SYSTEMS AFFECTED
Skin/Exocrine

GENETICS
There is no known genetic predisposition for many of the underlying causes of alopecia. Genetically hairless rats and mice are not uncommon, but this is not a pathologic process.

INCIDENCE/PREVALENCE
Alopecia resulting from a variety of medical conditions is a very common presenting complaint.

GEOGRAPHIC DISTRIBUTION
N/A

SIGNALMENT
Gender, age, and species predisposition are dependent on the specific condition causing the alopecia.

Breed Predilections
Gerbils
• "Sore nose" or alopecia of the muzzle resulting from rubbing on inappropriate cage materials or excessive humidity
• Barbering by cage mates
• Secondary bacterial dermatitis
• Demodecosis
Mice
• Barbering by cage mates
• Bacterial pyoderma
• Inappropriate caging and sanitation
• Alopecia of ventral thorax and abdomen during nursing and lactation
• Deficiencies of vitamin A, linoleic and arachadonic acid, zinc deficiency
• Genetics
Rats
• Ectoparasites, dermatophytes, bacterial pyoderma, poor housing, mites, barbering by conspecifics, excessive dietary fat, deficiencies of specific amino acids, vitamins, and minerals
Hamsters
• Poor husbandry and sanitation
• *Demodex* mites

• Dermatophytes
• Inadequate protein
• Renal amyloidosis or neoplasia
• Hyperadrenocorticism
• Genetics

SIGNS
Physical Examination Findings
Loss of hair ranging from focal to patchy to generalized. Depending on the causative factor, skin irritation, flaking, erythema, pruritus, discharge, odor, or other symptoms may also be present.

CAUSES
• Genetics (hairless rat, hairless mouse)
• Nutrition
• Infectious
• Stress
• Iatrogenic
• Endocrinopathy
• Secondary to disorders of other systems

RISK FACTORS
The risk factors vary depending on the primary cause of the alopecia. Inadequate husbandry and nutrition, poor sanitation, and overcrowding are common predisposing factors.

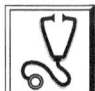

DIAGNOSIS

DIFFERENTIAL DIAGNOSIS
• Environmental/cage rubbing/bite wounds
• Bacterial dermatitis
• Dermatophytosis
• Trauma
• Injection site reaction
• Mites/lice (*Demodex, Cheyletiella*)
• Endocrinopathy (hyperadrenocorticism)
• Nutritional (protein deficiency)
• Immune mediated
• Allergic reaction

CBC/BIOCHEMISTRY/URINALYSIS
For regional or generalized alopecia, the minimum database should include serum biochemistry, complete blood count, and urinalysis where possible, to screen for the presence of underlying metabolic disease processes, infection, and inflammation.

OTHER LABORATORY TESTS
Rarely, endocrine profiles may helpful if commercially available.

IMAGING
In systemically ill patients with generalized alopecia, radiographs may help confirm the presence of organomegaly, dystrophic mineralization, or the presence of masses. Rarely, CT scans could be helpful in diagnosing pituitary tumors or endocrinopathies.

DIAGNOSTIC PROCEDURES
• Skin scrapings and dermatophyte cultures should be included as part of the minimum database.
• Skin biopsies for histopathologic evaluation may be indicated.
• Bacterial culture and susceptibility testing
• Response to therapy as a trial

PATHOLOGIC FINDINGS
Results of diagnostic tests and histopathology will vary depending on the cause of the alopecia.

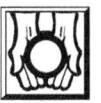

TREATMENT

APPROPRIATE HEALTH CARE
• Treatment will vary depending on the causative factor in each individual case.
• Patients with genetic baldness, such as hairless rats and mice, do not require treatment.

NURSING CARE
Unless systemically ill, almost all cases of alopecia are treated on an outpatient basis. In severe cases, basic supportive care including thermal regulation, fluid administration, and assisted feeding may be needed to stabilize the patient.

ACTIVITY
In most cases, activity restriction is not necessary. If self-mutilation is a concern, restraint with an Elizabethan collar or mild sedation may be indicated.

DIET
Supplementation is appropriate if dietary deficiencies are identified as the cause of alopecia.

CLIENT EDUCATION
• Review of appropriate husbandry for the species in question
• Awareness of zoonotic potential if present

SURGICAL CONSIDERATIONS
• Skin biopsies where indicated
• Repair of traumatic wounds
• Removal of masses if appropriate
• Ovariohysterectomy in cases of cystic ovarian disease

MEDICATIONS

DRUG(S) OF CHOICE
• Varies with the underlying cause of the alopecia
• For bacterial dermatitis, select appropriate antibiotics based on safety and bacterial culture and sensitivity. Antibiotics commonly

used in small rodents include trimethoprim/sulfa (15–30 mg/kg PO, SC q12h), enrofloxacin (5–20 mg/kg PO, SC, IM q12h), chloramphenicol palmitate (30–50 mg/kg PO q8h), azithromycin (10–30 mg/kg PO q24h), and amoxicillin/clavulanic acid (20 mg/kg PO q12 *Do not use in hamsters)

• For dermatophyes—miconazole, topically, q24h for 2–4 weeks for focal or regional lesions; antifungal shampoos that are safe for use in cats may be helpful in treating dermatophytes in small rodents; griseofulvin (15–25 mg/kg PO q24h for up to 60 days). Absorption is enhanced if given with a fatty meal. Gastrointestinal irritation is the most common side effect and can be alleviated by dividing the dose for more frequent administration. Bone marrow suppression is a possible idiosyncratic reaction, or can result from prolonged therapy. Neurologic side effects and teratogenicity in the first two trimesters of pregnancy have been reported. Biweekly monitoring of the CBC is recommended; Lime sulfur dip, 1:40 dilute with water has been used; dip once every 7 days for 4–6 treatments.

• For ectoparasites: ivermectin (0.3–0.5 mg/kg SQ every 7–14 days) for 3 treatments or until infestation is resolved, or 1:100 dilute ivermectin in propylene glycol placed on the head to be spread by normal grooming activity; selamectin (15–30 mg/kg topically every 14–28 days); fipronil (7.5 mg/kg topically every 30–60 days); pyrethrin powder topically every 3–7 days for 3 weeks. May be incorporated into the dust bath for chinchillas and gerbils.

• Postoperative analgesia for surgical patients. Commonly used pain medications include buprenorphine (0.05–0.1 mg/kg SQ, IM q6–8h), meloxicam (1–2 mg/kg PO, SQ, IM q24h), tramadol (1–4 mg/kg PO q8–12h), and midazolam (0.25–1.0 mg/kg IM, IV), which may help reduce postoperative self-mutilation.

CONTRAINDICATIONS

• Application of any topical substance may increase itching and discomfort and draw the patient's attention to the affected area.

• Steroids are not commonly used in small rodents, and their use is contraindicated in patients with dermatophyte infections.

• There is a risk of life-threatening antibiotic-induced enterotoxemia in many rodent species associated with orally administered penicillin, ampicillin, cephalosporins, carbenicillin, lincomycin, clindamycin, streptomycin, gentamycin, neomycin, erythromycin, vancomycin, and tetracycline.

PRECAUTIONS

• The use of griseofulvin should be avoided in pregnant animals and in patients with immune system suppression.

• Tramadol should be used with caution in geriatric or severely debilitated patients, in animals with seizures or those taking other medications that lower the seizure threshold, and in pregnant animals.

• Midazolam may increase the cardiorespiratory effects of other medications. It should be used with caution in debilitated or geriatric patients, in patients with hepatic or renal disease, during the first trimester of pregnancy, and during lactation and nursing.

POSSIBLE INTERACTIONS
N/A

ALTERNATIVE DRUGS

If gastrointestinal distress accompanies antibiotic therapy, concurrent administration of a probiotic may help alleviate the symptoms.

 FOLLOW-UP

PATIENT MONITORING

• Varies with each cause of alopecia
• Patients with ectoparasites should be evaluated 2 weeks and 4 weeks after starting therapy.
• Hair loss in all cases should be evaluated in 6 and again in 12 weeks after the start of treatment.
• All patients should be monitored for potential adverse effects of medications.

PREVENTION/AVOIDANCE

Appropriate husbandry, caging, substrate, sanitation, and population density

POSSIBLE COMPLICATIONS

Possible adverse effects of long-term medication, depending on the cause and treatment of the alopecia

EXPECTED COURSE AND PROGNOSIS

• Most cases of alopecia will resolve with appropriate therapy.
• Some ectoparasite infestations may be difficult to resolve and can require long-term therapy. For persistent cases, evaluation for underlying systemic disease is indicated.
• Environmental decontamination in the case of dermatophyte and some ectoparasite infections is important to prevent spread or reinfection.
• Some endocrinopathies such as hyperadrenocorticism or renal amyloidosis may be fatal.

 MISCELLANEOUS
N/A

ASSOCIATED CONDITIONS
N/A

AGE-RELATED FACTORS
N/A

ZOONOTIC POTENTIAL

• Dermatophytosis
• Some bacterial infections
• Some ectoparasites

PREGNANCY/FERTILITY/BREEDING

Some patients may develop transient hair loss associated with hormonal changes at the time of pregnancy, parturition, and lactation. Some patients may pull fur to line the nest. Evaluate antibiotics and other medications for safety during pregnancy and lactation.

SYNONYMS
Hair loss

SEE ALSO
Dermatophytosis
Ectoparasites
Hyperadrenocorticism
Scent gland disorders
Ulcerative pododermatitis (bumblefoot)

ABBREVIATIONS
N/A

INTERNET RESOURCES
Exotic DVM forum for eDVM readers: www.pets.groups.yahoo.com/group/Exotic DVM
IACUC guidelines, rodent anesthesia, and analgesia formulary: www.upenn.edu/regulatoryaffairs/Documents/GUIDE LINES_RODENT_ANESTHESIA_AND_ ANALGESIA_FORMULARY.pdf
Veterinary Information Network: www.vin.com

Suggested Reading
Dutton M. Selected veterinary concerns of geriatric rats, mice, hamsters, and gerbils. Vet Clin Exot Anim 2020;23(3):525–548.
Frolich J. Rats and mice. In: Quesenberry KE, Carpenter JW, eds. Ferrets, Rabbits and Rodents, 4th Ed). Clinical Medicine and Surgery. 2021 ed. St. Louis: Saunders, 2020:345–367.
Jekl V, Knotek Z. Evidence-based advances in rodent medicine. Vet Clin Exot Anim 2017;20:805–816.
Miwa Y, Mayer J. Hamsters and gerbils. In: Quesenberry KE, Carpenter JW, eds. Ferrets, Rabbits and Rodents, 4th Ed). Clinical Medicine and Surgery. 2021 ed. St. Louis: Saunders, 2020:368–384.

RODENTS

Palmerio BS, Roberts H. Clinical approach to dermatologic disease in exotic animals. Vet Clin North Am Exot Anim Pract. 2013;16(3):523–577.

White SD, Bourdeau PJ, Brément T et al. Companion rats (*Rattus norvegicus*) with cutaneous lesions: a retrospective study of 470 cases at two university veterinary teaching hospitals (1985–2018). Vet Dermatol 2019;30:237–272.

Author Christine Eckermann-Ross, DVM, CVA, CVH

AMYLOIDOSIS

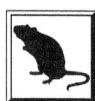

BASICS

DEFINITION
A group of conditions of diverse causes in which extracellular deposition of insoluble fibrillar protein (amyloid) in various organs and tissues compromises their normal function

PATHOPHYSIOLOGY
• Primary amyloidosis is naturally occurring disease in mice, associated with deposition of amyloid proteins consisting primarily of immunoglobulin light chains.
• Secondary amyloidosis is associated with antecedent and often chronic inflammation or neoplasia. It results from a complex cascade reaction involving release of multiple cytokines that stimulate amyloid synthesis in the liver.
• A "hamster female protein" with functional characteristics similar to amyloid protein has been identified in female hamsters and is synthesized under estrogenic influence.
• Amyloidosis is a progressive disease. Kidneys are the organ of predilection for amyloid deposit. Once a glomerulus has been irreversibly damaged by amyloidosis, the entire nephron becomes nonfunctional and is replaced by scar tissue. As more and more nephrons become involved, glomerular filtration decreases, and chronic renal failure ensues.
• Degu develop spontaneous amyloidosis in which the amyloid protein deposit is mostly in the Langherans Islet. This condition leads to a diabetes mellitus.

SYSTEMS AFFECTED
• Renal/Urologic—predilection for amyloid deposition
• Liver, spleen, adrenal glands, pancreas (in degu), and gastrointestinal tract might be affected.

GENETICS
Certain strains of mice seem to me more affected by amyloidosis.

INCIDENCE/PREVALENCE
Renal amyloidosis is a major disease in laboratory mice; it is also common in Syrian hamster (Mesocricetus *auratus*) and described in Mongolian gerbil and degu.

GEOGRAPHIC DISTRIBUTION
Worldwide

SIGNALMENT
Breed Predilections
N/A

Mean Age and Range
• More common in the older mouse

• Common geriatric disease in Syrian hamsters (over 18 month)

Predominant Sex
• Hamster: three times more common in female than male
• None in mouse

SIGNS
General Comments
• Severity of signs depends on the organ affected, the amount of amyloid, and the reaction of the affected organs to amyloid deposit.
• Clinical signs are usually due to renal involvement, occasionally due to hepatic involvement

Historical Findings
• Anorexia
• Weight loss
• Lethargy
• Polyuria/polydipsia
• Diarrhea (uncommon)

Physical Examination Findings
• Related to renal failure—emaciation and dehydration; kidneys usually small, firm, and irregular
• Signs of nephrotic syndrome (e.g., ascites, subcutaneous edema concentrated in the ventral half of the body, hydrothorax)
• May see signs related to the primary inflammatory or neoplastic disease process
• May see signs of hepatic disease (e.g., jaundice, cachexia, and spontaneous hepatic rupture with intraperitoneal bleeding)
• Thromboembolic phenomena (not yet described in rodents)—may occur, signs vary with the location of the thrombus; patient may develop pulmonary thromboembolism (e.g., dyspnea) or iliac or femoral artery throboembolism (e.g., causal paresis)

CAUSES
• Chronic inflammation—inflammatory disease, acariasis, ectoparasitism, chronic bacterial infection (e.g., osteomyelitis, bronchopneumonia, pleuritis, steatitis, pyometra, pyelonephritis, chronic suppurative dermatitis, chronic suppurative arthritis, chronic peritonitis, nocardiosis, and chronic stomatitis), and immune-mediated diseases (e.g., systemic lupus erythematous)
• Neoplasia (e.g., lyphosarcoma, plasmacytoma, multiplemyeloma, mammary tumors, and testicular tumors)
• Stress—crowding, fighting

RISK FACTORS
• Chronic inflammation or neoplasia (mouse)
• Poor husbandry, too many animals in the same cage (overcrowding)
• Familial predisposition

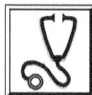

DIAGNOSIS

DIFFERENTIAL DIAGNOSIS
• Glomerulonephritis—proteinuria tends to be more severe in animal with glomerular amyloidosis than those with glomerulonephritis
• Medullary amyloidosis—consider other causes of medullary renal disease (e.g., pyelonephritis, chronic intestinal disease)
• Renal biopsy is necessary for definitive diagnosis

CBC/BIOCHEMISTRY/URINALYSIS
• Nonregenerative anemia is found in some animals with amyloid-induced renal failure.
• May see hypercholesterolemia, elevated triglycerides, hypoalbuminemia, azotemia, hyperphosphatemia, hypocalcemia, and metabolic acidosis
• Proteinuria—with an inactive sediment is suggestive of amyloidosis in rodents

OTHER LABORATORY TESTS
Proteinuria—quantify by 24-hour urinary protein excretion or urinary protein:creatinine ratio.

IMAGING
• Abdominal radiographic findings—kidneys could be small, normal, or enlarged
• Abdominal ultrasonography findings— kidneys are usually hyperechoic

DIAGNOSTIC PROCEDURES
Renal biopsy is needed to differentiate amyloidosis from glomerulonephritis.

PATHOLOGIC FINDINGS
• Gross—small, normal, or large kidneys
• Histopathology—amyloid deposits appear homogenous and eosinophilic when stained by hematoxylin and eosin and viewed by conventional light microscopy. They demonstrate green birefringence after Congo red staining when viewed under polarized light. Evaluation of Congo red–stained section before and after permanganate oxidation permits presumptive diagnosis of AA amyloidosis (versus other type) because AA amyloidosis loses its Congo red affinity after permanganate oxidation.

TREATMENT

APPROPRIATE HEALTH CARE
• Hospitalize patients with chronic renal failure and dehydration for initial medical management.
• Can manage stable patients and those with asymptomatic proteinuria as outpatient

• Change husbandry (e.g., reduce population per cage, identify stressors, and remove them)

NURSING CARE
Correct dehydration with 0.9% NaCl solution or lactated Ringer's solution; patient with severe metabolic acidosis may require bicarbonate supplementation

ACTIVITY
Normal in stable patient with chronic renal failure; restrict if the patient is debilitated due to acute renal failure

DIET
• Patients with chronic renal failure—restrict phosphorus and moderately restrict protein
• Patients with hypertension—restrict sodium

CLIENT EDUCATION
• Discuss progression of the disease
• Discuss familial predisposition
• Discuss potential complication (e.g., hypertension, thromboembolism)

SURGICAL CONSIDERATIONS
N/A

MEDICATIONS
DRUG(S) OF CHOICE
• Identify underlying inflammatory and neoplastic process and treat if possible.
• Manage renal failure according to the principles of conservative medical treatment (see Renal Failure)
• Normalize blood pressure in patient with hypertension
• DMSO—may help patients by solubilizing amyloid fibrils, reducing serum concentration of SAA, and reducing interstitial inflammation and fibrosis in the affected kidneys; may cause lens opacification. Perivascular inflammation and local thrombosis may occur if undiluted DMSO is administered intravenously. Subcutaneous administration of undiluted DMSO may be painful (dilute with saline). Considered to be ineffective in hamster. Has been administered to mice via drinking water.
• Colchicine—impairs release of SAA from hepatocytes; prevents development of amyloidosis and stabilized renal function in patient with nephritic syndrome but without overt renal failure; no evidence of benefit once patient develops renal failure; may cause diarrhea and idiosyncratic neutropenia. A single dose of 0.03 mg IV has been used in laboratory mice.

CONTRAINDICATIONS
Avoid use of nephrotoxic drugs (e.g., aminoglycosides).

PRECAUTIONS
• Dosage of drugs excreted by the kidney needs adjustment in patient with renal failure.
• Use nonsteroidal anti-inflammatory drugs cautiously in patient with medullary amyloidosis; they can decrease renal blood flow in dehydrated patients.

POSSIBLE INTERACTIONS
None

ALTERNATIVE DRUGS
Testosterone administration will inhibit the expression of the female amyloid protein and reduce the incidence of amyloidosis in female hamsters

FOLLOW-UP
PATIENT MONITORING
• Appetite and activity level daily by the owner; body weight weekly
• Serum albumin, creatinine, and BUN concentration every 2–6 months in stable patients
• Can assess the degree of proteinuria serially by urine protein:creatinine ratio

PREVENTION/AVOIDANCE
Do not breed affected animals.

POSSIBLE COMPLICATIONS
• Renal failure
• Nephrotoxic syndrome
• Systemic hypertension
• Hepatic rupture causing intraperitoneal hemorrhage
• Thromboembolic disease

EXPECTED COURSE AND PROGNOSIS
This is a progressive disease that is usually advanced at the time of diagnosis. Disease generally occurs in aged animals; the prognosis is poor.

MISCELLANEOUS
ASSOCIATED CONDITIONS
• Urinary tract infection
• Polyarthritis

AGE-RELATED FACTORS
Older animals are more likely to develop this disease.

ZOONOTIC POTENTIAL
None

PREGNANCY/FERTILITY/BREEDING
High risk in affected animals

SYNONYMS
N/A

SEE ALSO
Renal failure

BBREVIATIONS
AA = amyloid A protein
DMSO = dimethylsulfoxide
SAA = serum amyloid A protein

INTERNET RESOURCES
N/A

Suggested Reading
Dutton M. Selected veterinary concerns of geriatric rats, mice, hamsters, and gerbils. Vet Clin Exot Anim 2020;23(3):525–548.
Frolich J. Rats and mice. In: Quesenberry KE, Carpenter JW, eds. Ferrets, Rabbits and Rodents, 4th Ed). Clinical Medicine and Surgery. 2021 ed. St. Louis: Saunders, 2020:345–367.
Hallman RM, Brandão J. Diagnostic imaging of the renal system in exotic companion mammals. Vet Clin Exot Anim 2020;23: 195–214.
Jekl V, Knotek Z. Evidence-based advances in rodent medicine. Vet Clin Exot Anim 2017;20:805–816.
Lennox AM, Gladden JN. Emergency and critical care of small mammals. In: Quesenberry KE, Carpenter JW, eds. Ferrets, Rabbits and Rodents, 4th Ed). Clinical Medicine and Surgery. 2021 ed. St. Louis: Saunders, 2020:595–608.
Miwa Y, Mayer J. Hamsters and gerbils. In: Quesenberry KE, Carpenter JW, eds. Ferrets, Rabbits and Rodents, 4th Ed). Clinical Medicine and Surgery. 2021 ed. St. Louis: Saunders, 2020:368–384.
Percy DH, Barthold SW. Rat amyloidosis. In: Percy DH, Barthold SW, eds. Pathology of laboratory rodents and rabbits, 3rd ed. Ames: Blackwell, 2007:200–202.
Reavill DR, Lennox AM. Disease overview of the urinary tract in exotic companion mammals and tips on clinical management. Vet Clin Exot Anim 2020;23(1):169–193.
Author Charly Pignon, DVM, Dip ECZM (Small Mammal)

ANOREXIA AND PSEUDOANOREXIA

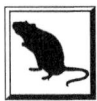

BASICS

DEFINITION
• Lack or loss of appetite for food; in true anorexia, the animal refuses to eat, versus pseudoanorexia whereby there is a mechanical inability or health issue that directly impacts the animal's ability to apprehend or chew food.
• The lack or loss of appetite for food; appetite is psychologic and depends on memory and associations, compared with hunger, which is physiologically aroused by the body's need for food; the existence of appetite in animals is assumed.
• The term *pseudoanorexia* is used to describe animals that have a desire for food but are unable to eat because they cannot prehend, chew, or swallow food.

PATHOPHYSIOLOGY
• Anorexia is most often associated with systemic disease but can be caused by many different mechanisms.
• The control of appetite is a complex interaction between the CNS and the periphery.
• Inflammatory, infectious, metabolic, or neoplastic diseases can cause inappetence, probably as a result of the release of a variety of chemical mediators.

SYSTEMS AFFECTED
Gastrointestinal, any other system could be affected based upon the illness that is causing the lack of appetite.

GENETICS
N/A

INCIDENCE/PREVALENCE
N/A

GEOGRAPHIC DISTRIBUTION
N/A

SIGNALMENT
Animal of any age or breed; depends on the underlying cause

SIGNS

Historical Findings
• No interest in food (anorexia)
• Interest in food with inability to eat (pseudoanorexia)
• Decreased fecal output
• Varying degrees of lethargy, for example, not using exercise wheel
• Other signs vary depending on the underlying cause.

Physical Examination Findings
• Weight loss or gain (as in abdominal masses)

• Decreased activity level
• Poor coat quality
• Incisors may be obviously maloccluded
• In pseudoanorexia, there may be excessive drooling and dysphagia.
• Eyes sunken (especially in hamsters, a very vague sign of illness/disease)
• Findings are variable, depending on cause of anorexia; many other findings possible

CAUSES
Almost any disease process can lead to anorexia in the small rodent. The sick or painful rodent will not eat as much and weight loss is a very common consequence.

Infectious
• Enteritis; salmonellosis (*S. typhimurium* or *S. enteritidis*)
• Sialodacryoadenitis (coronavirus) causing inflammation of salivary glands.
• Chronic respiratory disease complex
• Septicemia
• Pyometra

Metabolic Disorder
• Nutritional (wrong diet offered)
• Renal failure (commonly amyloidosis)
• Hepatic disease (commonly amyloidosis)

Neoplasia
Multiple forms

Other
• Cysts, other abdominal mass
• Trauma
• Arthritis
• Heart disease; congestive heart failure
• Stress
• Anemia

Pseudoanorexia
• Malocclusion of incisors or molars
• Impacted cheek pouch

RISK FACTORS
• Poor husbandry (e.g., wrong bedding, cage type, and poor sanitation)
• Inappropriate diet

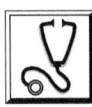

DIAGNOSIS

DIFFERENTIAL DIAGNOSIS
• First differentiate between anorexia and pseudoanorexia.
• If the animal lives with a group of other animals, it may be necessary to separate him from the group to determine if the animal is truly anorexic.
• Since anorexia can be a consequence of any health problem in the small rodent, a large number of differentials exist. Also consider pregnancy, environmental changes, and other stressors.

CBC/BIOCHEMISTRY/URINALYSIS
• Hypoproteinemia and hypoalbuminemia can result from protein loss caused by anorexia/starvation; also may be due to hemorrhage or parasitism.
• Due to the extensive list of causes of anorexia, any abnormalities in standard diagnostic tests are important in determining the cause of anorexia.

OTHER LABORATORY TESTS
• Fecal exam (direct and floatation)
• Bacterial culture and susceptibility testing (e.g., may need to swab oral cavity in hamster pouch impaction or obtain a rectal swab if diarrhea present)
• Cytology of thoracic or abdominal fluid or mass, if present

IMAGING
• Radiographs (full body and/or skull, if oral disease process suspected)—rule out dental disease, organomegaly, respiratory, and cardiac disease
• The need for more extensive imaging depends on findings of physical examination, survey radiographs, and suspected underlying cause of anorexia.

DIAGNOSTIC PROCEDURES
A good oral exam under general anesthesia using cheek dilators and specula made for rodents may be necessary (Jorgenson laboratories Inc., Loveland, CO). A small rigid endoscope can be helpful in performing a complete oral exam. The oral exam will help to identify oral abscess, gingivitis/ stomatitis, ulcers, check pouch impactions (hamsters), and more.

PATHOLOGIC FINDINGS
Variable, depending on the cause of the anorexia

TREATMENT

APPROPRIATE HEALTH CARE
• If anorexia is complete and has been going on for more than 24 hours, inpatient medical care is appropriate. Many anorexic small rodents are present in critical condition and will need to be stabilized before diagnostics can be performed.
• If the anorexia is acute and the cause is determined early, outpatient medical care is acceptable.

NURSING CARE
• Keep the patient warm; if hypothermic an incubator may be required.
• Fluid therapy is used to correct hydration following standard protocols (5%–10% of

(CONTINUED)

body weight administered in SQ boluses). Fluids should be kept warm to prevent hypothermia and can be warmed by placing the prepared syringe in a warm water bath prior to administration. Administration via a 22–25-gauge butterfly needle can reduce stress on the patient by minimizing restraint.
• The critical patient may require fluid therapy via intraosseous (IO) catheter. In addition to crystalloids, the patient may need colloids such as hetastarch at 10 mL/kg IO per day in several small boluses.

ACTIVITY
Based on the cause of anorexia, activity may or may not need to be restricted. Most small rodents that do not feel well will be less active of their own accord. Due to the fact that most live in small cages, cage rest is not required. If activity must be restricted, a smaller cage or removal of an exercise wheel will usually suffice.

DIET
• It is imperative that the animal receive nutritional support if it is not eating. Supplementation with a liquid diet may be required, such as Oxbow Carnivore or Omivore Care (Oxbow Enterprises, Inc., Murdock, NE) or Emeraid Exotic Carnivore or Omnivore (Lafeber's, Cornell, IL). If these commercial formulas are not available, a gruel may be made with rodent block ground into nutritional supplements such as Ensure (Abott Nutrition, Columbus, OH) or human baby food cereals may be used.
• A diet change should never be made abruptly in the anorexic patient. If the diet is inappropriate, wait until the patient is stable and eating again, then convert to an appropriate diet such as one with a rodent block, vegetables/greens, and limited seed content.

CLIENT EDUCATION
Educate small rodent pet owners about proper bedding choices and diet. No matter the cause of anorexia, client consultation should include a thorough discussion of proper husbandry (caging, diet) and the need for regular examinations. The author recommends a wellness examination every 6 months.

SURGICAL CONSIDERATIONS
If surgery is required, or if oral exam, dental procedures, blood, or other sample collection requires general anesthesia, always observe these precautions:
• Fasting is not required prior to general anesthesia, however, always remove all food from the oral cavity using cotton swabs to prevent aspiration.
• It is essential to maintain core body temperature; use of a Bair Hugger (Arizant

Health Care, Eden Prairie, MN), water circulating heating pad, or other warming device is crucial.
• Minimize alcohol used during preparation of any sample site (e.g., for blood collection, needle aspirates), as alcohol can increase loss of body heat.
• Due to the difficulty of intubating small rodents, an appropriate-sized, snug-fitting face mask should be used.
• A Doppler probe can be placed directly over the heart for monitoring anesthesia.

MEDICATIONS
DRUG(S) OF CHOICE
The cause of anorexia should be identified before dispensing any medication.
If the animal is painful:
• Meloxicam (1–3 mg/kg PO, SC, IM q24h)
• Tramadol HCL (10–20 mg/kg PO q8–12h)
• Buprenorphine (0.05–0.1 mg/kg SQ, IM q6–8h)
For bacterial infection:
• Antibiotic-based on culture and sensitivity
• Begin empirical treatment with broad-spectrum antibiotics such as trimethoprim sulfa (15–30 mg/kg PO q12h), enrofloxacin (5–20 mg/kg PO, SC, IM q12h), or ciprofloxacin (10–20 mg/kg PO q12h) for hamsters, gerbils, mice, or rats.
• For rats (do not use in hamsters), amoxicillin/clavulanic acid (20 mg/kg PO q12h) may also be used.
As an appetite stimulant:
    Vitamin B complex (0.02–0.2 mL/kg SQ, IM) may be used.

CONTRAINDICATIONS
• Do not administer penicillins, ampicillin, amoxicillin, erythromycin, or lincomycin to hamsters or gerbils due to the risk of potentially fatal enteric dysbiosis.
• The cause of anorexia should be identified before dispensing any medication.

PRECAUTIONS
• Almost all drugs dispensed to the small rodent are considered off-label and doses have been extrapolated.
• Use caution in dispensing drugs that have been compounded in-house; may achieve better results using a compounding pharmacy or a liquid form of the drug
• Do not use trimethoprim-sulfa if liver or kidney failure is suspected.

POSSIBLE INTERACTIONS
N/A

ALTERNATIVE DRUGS
N/A

FOLLOW-UP
PATIENT MONITORING
• Weigh daily (owner should buy a gram scale if needed).
• Frequent follow-up visits (at least weekly) are required until the patient is no longer anorexic and a normal weight is achieved.

PREVENTION/AVOIDANCE
Depends on the cause of the anorexia

POSSIBLE COMPLICATIONS
• Severe dehydration
• May progress to cachexia

EXPECTED COURSE AND PROGNOSIS
With assisted feeding and rehydration, life can often be prolonged. However, the long-term prognosis will be based largely on identification and correction of the underlying cause. In the older patient (>1 years), prognosis worsens due to age-related complications and the possibility of multiple causes of anorexia.

MISCELLANEOUS
ASSOCIATED CONDITIONS
Many possibilities based on underlying cause

AGE-RELATED FACTORS
N/A

ZOONOTIC POTENTIAL
N/A

PREGNANCY/FERTILITY/BREEDING
The small rodent that is pregnant will need special attention to ensure that caloric needs are met. Reproductive pathology should be considered as a cause for the anorexia.

SYNONYMS
Inappetence

SEE ALSO
Ascites
Congestive heart failure
Dental malocclusion
Diarrhea
Pneumonia
Renal failure

ABBREVIATIONS
N/A

INTERNET RESOURCES
www.vin.com
Suggested Reading
Dutton M. Selected veterinary concerns of geriatric rats, mice, hamsters, and gerbils. Vet Clin Exot Anim 2020;23(3):525–548.

ANOREXIA AND PSEUDOANOREXIA   (CONTINUED)

Frolich J. Rats and mice. In: Quesenberry KE, Carpenter JW, eds. Ferrets, Rabbits and Rodents, 4th Ed). Clinical Medicine and Surgery. 2021 ed. St. Louis: Saunders, 2020:345–367.

Lennox AM, Gladden JN. Emergency and critical care of small mammals. In: Quesenberry KE, Carpenter JW, eds. Ferrets, Rabbits and Rodents, 4th Ed). Clinical Medicine and Surgery. 2021 ed. St. Louis: Saunders, 2020:595–608.

Mayer J, Mans C. Rodents. In: Carpenter JW, ed. Exotic Animal Formulary, 5th ed. St Louis: Elsevier, 2018:459–493.

Miwa Y, Mayer J. Hamsters and gerbils. In: Quesenberry KE, Carpenter JW, eds. Ferrets, Rabbits and Rodents, 4th Ed). Clinical Medicine and Surgery. 2021 ed. St. Louis: Saunders, 2020:368–384.

Authors Renata Schneider, DVM and Barbara Oglesbee, DVM, DABVP (Avian)

ASCITES AND ABDOMINAL DISTENSION

BASICS

DEFINITION
• Ascites: abnormal accumulation of serous (edematous) fluid in the peritoneal cavity characterized by distension of the abdomen, a fluid thrill on percussion, a typical ground glass appearance on radiography, and a positive result on paracentesis
• Abdominal distension can also be caused by space occupying lesions such as organomegaly, abscess or cysts (especially in hamsters)

PATHOPHYSIOLOGY
Abdominal distension can be caused by the following:
• Ascites
• Intraabdominal neoplasia
• Intraabdominal abscesses
• Intraabdominial cysts: ovarian cysts, polycystic diease in hamsters—liver is most commonly affected
• Organomegaly—liver most commonly affected
• Uterine—pyometra, pregnancy
Ascites can be caused by the following:
• CHF and associated interference in venous return
• Neoplastic effusion
• Depletion of plasma proteins, loss, or lack of production. Loss can occur through the gastrointestinal or renal systems
• Liver cirrhosis
• Renal failure (amyloidosis)

SYSTEMS AFFECTED
• Cardiovascular
• Gastrointestinal
• Hemic/Lymphatic/Immune
• Hepatobiliary
• Renal/Urologic

SIGNALMENT
Depends on cause
• Ascites: more common in older animals, especially secondary to organ failure
• Abdominal distension—polycystic disease is common in hamsters; ovarian cysts more common in older rats. Neoplasia in geriatric animals

SIGNS

Historical Findings
• The owner will often complain that the animal has become obese or lethargic.
• Anorexia
• Signs related to organ system affected

Physical Examination Findings
• Abdominal distension
• Abdominal discomfort on palpation
• Dyspnea
• Difficulty ambulating
• Lethargy

CAUSES
See above

RISK FACTORS
N/A

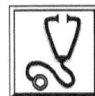

DIAGNOSIS

DIFFERENTIAL DIAGNOSIS
• Obesity
• Gastrointestinal distension/ileus
• Hemoabdomen
• Peritonitis

CBC/BIOCHEMISTRY/URINALYSIS
• Elevated white cell count if infectious
• Low total protein suggests edema and ascites.
• Amyloidosis in aging hamsters is associated with decreased albumin and elevated globulins.
• Liver enzymes may be low to normal if synthesis is impaired or may be elevated if there is inflammation and chronic passive congestion.
• BUN and creatinine may be high in renal failure.

OTHER LABORATORY TESTS
• Protein electrophoresis can be used to characterize hypoproteinemia.
• Culture and sensitivity of exudate/transudate
• Urinalysis—lack of concentration with renal failure

IMAGING
• Radiographs (full-body images are readily obtained given the size of the patient). Used to rule out organomegaly and evaluate heart size. Loss of abdominal detail can make it very difficult to detect the source of the ascites.
• Ultrasonography. Can be used as a guide to drain pockets of fluid in the abdomen and obtain diagnostic samples.
• Echocardiography: useful to evaluate presence of cardiac disease depending on the experience and expertise of the ultrasonographer.

DIAGNOSTIC PROCEDURES
Abdominocentesis/Fine-Needle Aspiration
• Transudate: clear, low specific gravity, low total protein, minimal cells (neutrophils may be present)
• Modified transudate: red or pink, slightly cloudy, moderate proteins, higher specific gravity, moderate cells (neutrophils, mesothelial, erythrocytes, and lymphocytes)
• Exudate (nonseptic): pink or white, cloudy, moderate protein, higher specific gravity, numerous cells (neutrophils, mesothelial, macrophages, erythrocytes, and lymphocytes)
• Exudate (septic): red, white, or yellow, high proteins, higher specific gravity, numerous cells (neutrophils, mesothelial, macrophages, erythrocytes, lymphocytes, and bacteria)
• Hemorrhage: red (spun supernatant clear and sediment red), high proteins, moderate specific gravity, cells consistent with peripheral blood, does not clot
• Urine: clear to pale yellow, moderate proteins, moderate specific gravity, numerous cells (neutrophils, macrophages, erythrocytes, and lymphocytes)

PATHOLOGIC FINDINGS
Depends on the cause. With ascites, degenerative changes and amyloidosis of liver and spleen, neoplasia, and cysts are the most common findings.

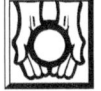

TREATMENT

APPROPRIATE HEALTH CARE
• Outpatient care is appropriate if the animal is otherwise fine and if it is eating and drinking.
• Abdominocentesis can be performed as needed to alleviate clinical signs and provide comfort. If necessary, use isoflurane gas for sedation; however, in the author's experience, this can usually be performed with minimal stress on the awake patient. The author has safely removed up to 50 mL from a teddy bear hamster with ascites using a butterfly needle and 5–10 mL syringes.

NURSING CARE
• It is imperative that the animal receive nutritional support if it is not eating. Supplementation with a liquid diet may be required, such as Oxbow Carnivore Care (Oxbow Enterprises, Inc., Murdock, NE) or Emeraid Exotic Carnivore (Lafeber's, Cornell, IL). If these commercial formulas are not available, a gruel may be made with rodent block ground into Ensure, or baby food may be used.
• Ensure that the patient is kept warm (if hypothermic, an incubator may be required).
• Fluid therapy is used to correct hydration following standard protocols (5%–10% of body weight administered in SQ boluses). Fluids should be kept warm to prevent hypothermia and can be warmed by placing the prepared syringe in hot water for a few minutes prior to administering them. The author finds that using a 22–25 gauge butterfly needle to administer the fluids can reduce stress on the patient by minimizing restraint.

ASCITES AND ABDOMINAL DISTENSION (CONTINUED)

• The critical patient may require fluid therapy via an intraosseous catheter.

ACTIVITY
Based on the cause of ascites, activity may or may not need to be restricted. Most small rodents that do not feel well will be less active of their own accord. Because most live in small cages, cage rest is not required. If activity must be restricted, a smaller cage or removal of an exercise wheel will usually suffice.

DIET
N/A

CLIENT EDUCATION
It is always important, especially in the older patient, to discuss the limited life span of the small rodent pet with ascites of unknown origin. Obtaining a timely diagnosis will help to determine prognosis more easily and allow the client to choose a course of treatment.

SURGICAL CONSIDERATIONS
• Exploratory surgery may be diagnostic and possibly curative (e.g., cysts or neoplasia can be removed). Depending upon findings of abdominal exploratory surgery, euthanasia may be indicated.
• Fasting is not necessary in the small rodent patient prior to surgery.
• It is essential to maintain body temperature; use of a Bair Hugger (Arizant Health Care, Eden, Prairie, MN), water circulating heating pad, or other warming device is crucial.
• Care should be taken in preparation of any surgery site, as alcohol can increase loss of body heat.
• Due to the difficulty of intubation in small rodents, an appropriate size mask should be used.
• A Doppler can be placed on the skin directly overlying the heart for monitoring anesthesia.

MEDICATIONS
DRUG(S) OF CHOICE
• The underlying cause should be determined prior to the use of any medication.
• If septic exudate is present, treat with antibiotic pending culture and sensitivity results. Begin empirical treatment with

broad-spectrum antibiotics such as trimethoprim sulfa (15–30 mg/kg PO q12h), enrofloxacin (5–20 mg/kg PO, SC, IM q12h), ciprofloxacin (10–20 mg/kg PO q12h), or chloramphenicol (30–50 mg/kg q8h).
• Furosemide (2–10 mg/kg PO, SC, IM, IV q12h) may help to alleviate ascites.

CONTRAINDICATIONS
N/A

PRECAUTIONS
• Almost all drugs dispensed to the small rodent are considered off-label, and doses have been extrapolated.
• Be especially careful of compounding drugs in-house; may have better results using a compounding pharmacy or a liquid form of the drug.
• Do not use trimethoprim sulfa if liver or kidney failure is suspected.

POSSIBLE INTERACTIONS
N/A

ALTERNATIVE DRUGS
N/A

FOLLOW-UP
PATIENT MONITORING
• If the fluid in the abdomen is removed, time for recurrence should be monitored. The owner should be given guidelines as to when to return for further fluid removal. After the first visit, the patient should be rechecked within 1 week. If the ascites is controlled, monthly visits may be sufficient.
• If a diagnosis is made, effectiveness of treatment in reducing ascites should be monitored closely. Until the patient is stable, weekly rechecks are highly recommended.

PREVENTION/AVOIDANCE
N/A

POSSIBLE COMPLICATIONS
• Anorexia
• Death

EXPECTED COURSE AND PROGNOSIS
• Fluid will re-accumulate within cysts after drainage
• In the older animal, prognosis is always extremely guarded.

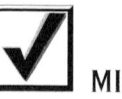

MISCELLANEOUS
ASSOCIATED CONDITIONS
N/A

AGE-RELATED FACTORS
N/A

ZOONOTIC POTENTIAL
N/A

PREGNANCY/FERTILITY/BREEDING
N/A

SYNONYMS
Abdominal effusion

SEE ALSO
Amyloidosis
Congestive heart failure
Hyperadrenocorticism
Lymphoma
Ovarian cysts
Uterine disease

ABBREVIATIONS
BUN = blood urea nitrogen
CHF = congestive heart failure
FNA = fine-needle aspirate

INTERNET RESOURCES
www.vin.com

Suggested Reading
Dutton M. Selected veterinary concerns of geriatric rats, mice, hamsters, and gerbils. Vet Clin Exot Anim 2020;23(3):525–548.
Frolich J. Rats and mice. In: Quesenberry KE, Carpenter JW, eds. Ferrets, Rabbits and Rodents, 4th Ed). Clinical Medicine and Surgery. 2021 ed. St. Louis: Saunders, 2020:345–367.
Lennox AM, Gladden JN. Emergency and critical care of small mammals. In: Quesenberry KE, Carpenter JW, eds. Ferrets, Rabbits and Rodents, 4th Ed). Clinical Medicine and Surgery. 2021 ed. St. Louis: Saunders, 2020:595–608.
Mayer J, Mans C. Rodents. In: Carpenter JW, ed. Exotic Animal Formulary, 5th ed. St Louis: Elsevier, 2018:459–493.
Miwa Y, Mayer J. Hamsters and gerbils. In: Quesenberry KE, Carpenter JW, eds. Ferrets, Rabbits and Rodents, 4th Ed). Clinical Medicine and Surgery. 2021 ed. St. Louis: Saunders, 2020:368–384.

Authors Renata Schneider, DVM and Barbara Oglesbee, DVM, DABVP (Avian)

BASICS

DEFINITION
• A sign of sensory dysfunction that produces incoordination of the limbs, head, and/or trunk
• Three clinical types—sensory (proprioceptive), vestibular, and cerebellar. All produce changes in limb coordination, but vestibular and cerebellar ataxia also produce changes in head and neck movement.

PATHOPHYSIOLOGY
• Cerebellar: characterized by defects in rate, range, force, and direction of movement of limbs; inability to maintain head in proper position so that it oscillates, hypermetria or hypometria, direction cannot be maintained and the animal falls easily, often in an exaggerated way.
• Sensorimotor: caused by moderate spinal cord lesions, manifested by weakness of movement, scuffing of toes, incomplete limb extension, knuckling wobbly gait, easy falling, difficulty rising.
• Vestibular: loss of balance with preservation of strength. If unilateral, the abnormality is asymmetrical, if bilateral, it is symmetrical.

SYSTEMS AFFECTED
• Nervous; spinal cord (and brain stem), cerebellum, vestibular system
• Neuromuscular
• Respiratory—with otitis interna/media

GENETICS
N/A

INCIDENCE/PREVALENCE
N/A

GEOGRAPHIC DISTRIBUTION
N/A

SIGNALMENT
Any age or sex

SIGNS

Historical Findings
Owner may report that the animal is limping, not walking normally, has a head tilt, or is showing nonspecific signs. Investigate the possibility of a cage accident (stuck in bars) or other trauma, such as being dropped.

Physical Examination Findings
• May be difficult to determine type of ataxia due to size and ambulation of small rodent patient, but it is particularly useful to do so
• Abnormal gait; if only one limb affected consider lameness, if rear limbs only are affected may be due to weakness or a spinal cord disorder

• Falling over; all or both ipsilateral limbs affected—cerebellar
• Head tilt—vestibular. Look for discharge or blood from ears.
• Evidence of trauma
• Other signs seen as a consequence of ataxia include anorexia, dehydration, and decreased activity (not using wheel, spending a lot of time in hide box)

CAUSES
• Infectious; otitis, encephalitis, viral infections
• May be a sequela to rhinitis and URI
• Neoplastic; pituitary adenomas in older rats
• Idiopathic (common especially in the case of head tilt)
• Trauma to the brain, ear, or spinal cord (may have been dropped or squeezed)
• Poisoning, including lead (rare)

RISK FACTORS
Inappropriate caging (e.g., cage door does not close properly and animal can get stuck or escape and get injured; small rodents are escape artists)

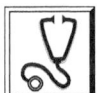

DIAGNOSIS

DIFFERENTIAL DIAGNOSIS
It is important to differentiate ataxia from weakness. Many systemic diseases may cause weakness that resembles ataxia.

CBC/BIOCHEMISTRY/URINALYSIS
Can be normal unless there is an infectious cause or metabolic disorder

OTHER LABORATORY TESTS
Bacterial culture and sensitivity testing from ear swab in rodents with signs of otitis and vestibular disorder

IMAGING
• Skull radiographs to identify or rule out ear pathology
• Full-body radiographs; identify spinal injury, injury that would explain lameness (versus ataxia); identify neoplasia, cardiopulmonary disease, or abdominal masses that may explain difficulty ambulating
• CT—provide better imaging to rule out vestibular disease, but may be cost prohibitive or not accessible to the exotic patient, depending on the area

DIAGNOSTIC PROCEDURES
Culture and sensitivity of ear swab if vestibular syndrome suspected, especially if discharge present

PATHOLOGIC FINDINGS
Depends on cause

TREATMENT

APPROPRIATE HEALTH CARE
As long as the patient is eating and drinking, outpatient care is appropriate; often depends on severity and acuteness of clinical signs

NURSING CARE
• Ensure that the patient is kept warm (if hypothermic an incubator may be required).
• Fluid therapy is used to correct hydration following standard protocols (5%–10% of body weight administered in SQ boluses). Fluids should be kept warm to prevent hypothermia and can be warmed by placing the prepared syringe in hot water for a few minutes prior to administering them. Using a 22–25 gauge butterfly needle to administer the fluids can reduce stress on the patient by minimizing restraint.
• The critical patient may require fluid therapy via an intraosseous catheter.

ACTIVITY
Exercise should be restricted when trauma is suspected, especially spinal. Removal of any ramps, exercise wheels; limit to one level of the cage.

DIET
• It is imperative that the animal receive nutritional support if it is not eating. Supplementation with a liquid diet may be required, such as Oxbow Carnivore Care (Oxbow Enterprises, Inc., Murdock, NE) or Emerald Exotic Carnivore (Lafeber's, Cornell, IL). If these commercial formulas are not available, a gruel may be made with rodent block ground into nutritional supplements such as Ensure (Abott Nutrition, Columbus, OH) or human baby food cereals.
• No change required unless the consultation reveals that the animal has always been on an inappropriate diet, in which case diet counseling is essential.

CLIENT EDUCATION
• Client should be trained to monitor progress of condition (worsening of ataxia to more severe paresis/paralysis).
• Appetite and fecal/urine output should be monitored carefully.

SURGICAL CONSIDERATIONS
N/A

MEDICATIONS

DRUG(S) OF CHOICE
• If convulsions or torticollis present: midazolam (0.5–2 mg/kg IM, IV, IO) or diazepam (0.5–2 mg/kg IM, IV, IO)

ATAXIA

• NSAIDs may be useful in patients with vestibular disorders or spinal trauma; carprofen (5 mg/kg PO, SQ q24h—rats) or meloxicam (1–2 mg/kg PO, SQ, IM q24h)

• For pain: buprenorphine (0.05–0.1 mg/kg SQ, IM q6–8h), meloxicam (1–2 mg/kg PO, SC, IM q24h), or tramadol (1–4 mg/kg q8–12h)

• If an infectious cause is suspected (e.g., otitis interna/externa, encephalitis) choose broad-spectrum antibiotics such as enrofloxacin (5–20 mg/kg PO, SC, IM q12h), ciprofloxacin (10–20 mg/kg PO q12h), and trimethoprim-sulfa (15–30 mg/kg PO q12h); if anaerobic infections are suspected, chloramphenicol (30–50 mg/kg PO q8h), azithromycin (10–30 mg/kg PO q24h), or metronidazole (20 mg/kg PO q12h) can be used in rodent species.

CONTRAINDICATIONS
• Do not administer penicillins, ampicillin, amoxicillin, erythromycin, or lincomycin to hamsters or gerbils due to the risk of potentially fatal enteric dysbiosis.

• All efforts should be made to find the cause of the ataxia prior to dispensing medication.

PRECAUTIONS
• Almost all drugs dispensed to the small rodent are considered off-label, and doses have been extrapolated.

• Do not use trimethoprim-sulfa if liver or kidney failure is suspected.

POSSIBLE INTERACTIONS
N/A

ALTERNATIVE DRUGS
N/A

FOLLOW-UP

PATIENT MONITORING
Patient should be seen at least weekly for follow-up exams until the condition resolves.

PREVENTION/AVOIDANCE
Ensure a safe cage environment. If the rodent is being allowed to run free in the household, monitor closely to avoid exposure to toxins and to avoid injury.

POSSIBLE COMPLICATIONS
Depends on the underlying cause

EXPECTED COURSE AND PROGNOSIS
• Depends on the underlying cause.

• In some cases, mild ataxia or head tilt persists when the animal is eating, drinking, and otherwise doing well. The owner should be informed that so long as quality of life is good, it is acceptable for the pet to live this way.

MISCELLANEOUS

ASSOCIATED CONDITIONS
N/A

AGE-RELATED FACTORS
N/A

ZOONOTIC POTENTIAL
N/A

PREGNANCY/FERTILITY/BREEDING
N/A

SYNONYMS
N/A

SEE ALSO
Head tilt (vestibular disease)

ABBREVIATIONS
CT = computed tomography
MRI = magnetic resonance imaging
NSAID = nonsteroidal anti-inflammatory drug
URI = upper respiratory infection

INTERNET RESOURCES
www.vin.com

Suggested Reading
Dutton M. Selected veterinary concerns of geriatric rats, mice, hamsters, and gerbils. Vet Clin Exot Anim 2020;23(3):525–548.
Frolich J. Rats and mice. In: Quesenberry KE, Carpenter JW, eds. Ferrets, Rabbits and Rodents, 4th Ed). Clinical Medicine and Surgery. 2021 ed. St. Louis: Saunders, 2020:345–367.
Lennox AM, Gladden JN. Emergency and critical care of small mammals. In: Quesenberry KE, Carpenter JW, eds. Ferrets, Rabbits and Rodents, 4th Ed). Clinical Medicine and Surgery. 2021 ed. St. Louis: Saunders, 2020:595–608.
Mayer J, Mans C. Rodents. In: Carpenter JW, ed. Exotic Animal Formulary, 5th ed. St Louis: Elsevier, 2018:459–493.
Miwa Y, Mayer J. Hamsters and gerbils. In: Quesenberry KE, Carpenter JW, eds. Ferrets, Rabbits and Rodents, 4th Ed). Clinical Medicine and Surgery. 2021 ed. St. Louis: Saunders, 2020:368–384.

Authors Renata Schneider, DVM and Barbara Oglesbee, DVM, DABVP (Avian)

CHEEK POUCH DISORDERS (HAMSTERS)

BASICS

DEFINITION
• Hamsters have large, distensible pouches located within the lateral buccal wall which are used to store food and transport bedding materials.
• Cheek pouches may become impacted, develop secondary infections, become everted and distend from the mouth and/or traumatized
• Neoplasia is uncommon, but may occur

PATHOPHYSIOLOGY
• Impaction and infection—overfeeding may cause overdistension, rough foods or bedding causing abrasion and secondary infection; extension from tooth infection
• Eversion—unknown cause when spontaneous. Neoplasia, abscess may cause eversion. Secondary trauma is common.

SIGNALMENT
May occur in any age or gender

SIGNS
• Pawing at the mouth
• Persistent, unilateral swelling (normal swelling from cheek pouches should change as food is removed and consumed)
• Difficulty chewing, anorexia, and weight loss
• Tubular hyperemic mass protruding from the mouth
• Blood on bedding or cage furnishings
• Foul odor with secondary infection or tissue necrosis

CAUSES AND RISK FACTORS
• Over feeding
• Rough foods or bedding
• Tooth infection/gingivitis
• Neoplasia or abscess formation

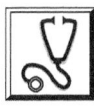

DIAGNOSIS

DIFFERENTIAL DIAGNOSIS
• Neoplasia
• Abscess
• Stomatitis, tooth infection

CBC/BIOCHEMISTRY
• Usually normal
• May reflect underlying cause (e.g., inflammatory leukogram with infection)

OTHER LABORATORY TESTS
• Fine-needle aspirate or biopsy if neoplasia suspected
• Culture should be performed if bacterial infection is suspected

IMAGING
• Skull radiographs or CT to identify bone involvement.

DIAGNOSTIC PROCEDURES
• Sedated oral examination and/or endoscopic oral examination.

PATHOLOGIC FINDINGS
• Vary with cause and severity of diarrheic condition
• Gross pathology may reveal lesions suggestive of etiology.
• Histopathology to obtain a definitive diagnosis for neoplasia—squamous cell carcinoma most commonly reported.

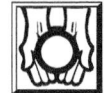

TREATMENT

APPROPRIATE HEALTH CARE
• Must identify and treat underlying cause
• Assisted feeding is typically required for debilitated patients
• Fluid therapy—rehydration and correction of electrolyte imbalances are indicated in most cases, particularly when diarrhea is involved.

CHEEK POUCH EVERSION/PROLAPSE
• Replace under general anesthesia. Debride and close any necrotic tissue. Place 1–2 tacking sutures percutanously extending full thickness into the lumen of the cheek pouch. Suture should be removed in 10–14 days.
• Amputation if the entire pouch is necrotic

CHEEK POUCH IMPACTION
• Careful manual removal of contents under general anesthesia. Flush with saline when emptied.

ABSCESS/NEOPLASIA
• Surgical debridement, excision

MEDICATIONS

DRUG(S) OF CHOICE
• Pain management: meloxicam (0.3–0.5 mg/kg PO q24h)
• Antibiotics for secondary infections, trauma—chloramphenicol (30–50 mg/kg PO q12h), doxycycline (2.5–5 mg/kg PO q12h), enrofloxacin (10–20 mg/kg PO q12h), or trimethoprim-sulfa (15–30 mg/kg PO q12h)

CONTRAINDICATIONS
• Antibiotics that are primarily gram-positive in spectrum will suppress the growth of commensal flora, allowing potentially fatal overgrowth of enteric pathogens. These include lincomycin, clindamycin, erythromycin, ampicillin, amoxicillin, cephalosporins, and penicillins.

PRECAUTIONS
• Antibiotic therapy can predispose small rodents (particularly hamsters) to bacterial dysbiosis and overgrowth of pathogenic bacteria (e.g., *Clostridium difficile*). If signs worsen or do not improve, therapy should be adjusted.
• Chloramphenicol may cause aplastic anemia in susceptible people. Clients and staff should use appropriate precautions when handling this drug.

FOLLOW-UP

PATIENT MONITORING
Remove tacking sutures in 10–14 days

PREVENTION/AVOIDANCE
• Feed small meals
• Avoid rough bedding material and foods

POSSIBLE COMPLICATIONS
• Recurrence

EXPECTED COURSE AND PROGNOSIS
• Good for uncomplicated impaction or eversion
• Good following amputation of damaged/necrotic eversion
• Prognosis is poor in debilitated, aged animals with cheek pouch abscess or neoplasia

MISCELLANEOUS

ASSOCIATED CONDITIONS
Crowding
Poor diet

AGE-RELATED FACTORS
• Older individuals may be more prone to neoplasia or abscesses.

ZOONOTIC POTENTIAL
None

PREGNANCY/FERTILITY/BREEDING
N/A

SYNONYMS
Cheek pouch prolapse

SEE ALSO
N/A

ABBREVIATIONS
N/A

INTERNET RESOURCES
N/A

Suggested Reading
Dutton M. Selected veterinary concerns of geriatric rats, mice, hamsters, and gerbils. Vet Clin Exot Anim 2020;23(3):525–548.
Frolich J. Rats and mice. In: Quesenberry KE, Carpenter JW, eds. Ferrets, Rabbits and Rodents, 4th Ed). Clinical Medicine and Surgery. 2021 ed. St. Louis: Saunders, 2020:345–367.

Lennox AM, Gladden JN. Emergency and critical care of small mammals. In: Quesenberry KE, Carpenter JW, eds. Ferrets, Rabbits and Rodents, 4th Ed). Clinical Medicine and Surgery. 2021 ed. St. Louis: Saunders, 2020:595–608.
Mayer J, Mans C. Rodents. In: Carpenter JW, ed. Exotic Animal Formulary, 5th ed. St Louis: Elsevier, 2018:459–493.

Miwa Y, Mayer J. Hamsters and gerbils. In: Quesenberry KE, Carpenter JW, eds. Ferrets, Rabbits and Rodents, 4th Ed). Clinical Medicine and Surgery. 2021 ed. St. Louis: Saunders, 2020:368–384.
Author Barbara Oglesbee, DVM, Dipl. ABVP (Avian)

BASICS

DEFINITION
• Left-sided congestive heart failure (L-CHF)—failure of the left side of the heart to advance blood at a sufficient rate to meet the metabolic needs of the patient or to prevent blood from pooling within the pulmonary venous circulation
• Right-sided congestive heart failure (R-CHF)—failure of the right side of the heart to advance blood at a sufficient rate to meet the metabolic needs of the patient or to prevent blood from pooling within the systemic venous circulation

PATHOPHYSIOLOGY
• L-CHF: Low cardiac output causes lethargy, exercise intolerance, syncope, and prerenal azotemia. High hydrostatic pressure causes leakage of fluid from pulmonary venous circulation into pulmonary interstitium and alveoli. When fluid leakage exceeds ability of lymphatics to drain the affected areas, pulmonary edema develops.
• R-CHF: High hydrostatic pressure leads to leakage of fluid from venous circulation into the pleural and peritoneal space and interstitium of peripheral tissue. When fluid leakage exceeds ability of lymphatics to drain the affected areas, pleural effusion, ascites, and peripheral edema develop.

SYSTEMS AFFECTED
All organ systems can be affected by either poor delivery of blood or the effects of passive congestion from backup of venous blood.

INCIDENCE/PREVALENCE
• Pet Syrian hamsters have a reported 6% incidence of cardiac disease; this estimate may be low.
• Teddy bear hamsters are derived from a line that had genetic cardiomyopathy. Both hypertrophic and dilated cardiomyopathies are caused by mutation of the same gene (defect in o-sarcoglycan.)
• Although anecdotally reported as common, very little published information on pet rodent heart disease is available.

SIGNALMENT
• Most commonly reported in aging hamsters and, to a lesser extent, gerbils
• Cardiomyopathy is a major cause of death in aged rats but has been reported as early as 3 months of age; males may be more commonly affected than females.
• Older Syrian hamsters (>1.5 years) and female hamsters more likely to develop

cardiomyopathy, as androgens appear to have a protective effect.

SIGNS
General Comments
Signs vary with underlying cause.

Historical Findings
• Weakness, lethargy, exercise intolerance
• Anorexia or inappetence, weight loss
• Dyspnea or tachypnea
• Syncope
• Abdominal distension with ascites

Physical Examination Findings
L-CHF
• Tachypnea
• Inspiratory and expiratory dyspnea when animal has pulmonary edema
• Prolonged capillary refill time
• Possible murmur
• Possible arrhythmia
R-CHF
• Hepatomegaly
• Ascites
• Cold extremities
• Possible murmur
• Rapid, shallow respiration if animal has pleural effusion

CAUSES
• In rats, both dilated and hypertrophic cardiomyopathy are common causes of death in older animals. Rats with chronic lower respiratory tract disease may develop R-CHF. Valvular disease such as endocardiosis or myxomatous thickening has been reported as a cause of CHF.
• In mice, left atrial thrombosis resulting in L-CHF is common. Other causes include amyloidosis, vitamin deficiencies, and septicemia.
• In hamsters, atrial thrombosis and calcifying vasculopathy may result in L-CHF. A number of congenital cardiac abnormalities have been identified in certain lines of laboratory hamsters; sporadic cases of infectious myocarditis have been reported. Hamsters are used as a hypercholesterolemia model for humans; induced by feeding high concentrations of lipids.
• In gerbils, arteriosclerosis and focal myocardial degeneration most commonly reported

RISK FACTORS
• Incidence increases with age for most rodents.
• Increased food intake may predispose rats to cardiomyopathy; the incidence of disease can be reduced by mild caloric restriction.

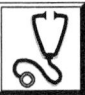

DIAGNOSIS

DIFFERENTIAL DIAGNOSIS
• Pleural effusion—neoplasia, trauma resulting in diaphragmatic hernia, pulmonary hemorrhage, pneumothorax, pneumonia
• Dyspnea—rhinitis or sinusitis (rodents are obligate nasal breathers) and primary pulmonary disease (abscess, pneumonia) most common; neoplasia (heart based tumors, metastatic neoplasia), pleural effusion
• Ascites, abdominal distension—consider hypoproteinemia, severe liver disease, ruptured bladder, peritonitis, abdominal neoplasia, and abdominal hemorrhage
• Diagnosis is based on history and physical examination findings but is aided with diagnostic imaging, including radiographs and ultrasound.

CBC/BIOCHEMISTRY/URINALYSIS
While nonspecific for cardiac disease, may help to rule out other underlying disease conditions

OTHER LABORATORY TESTS
N/A

IMAGING
• Radiography can often identify cardiomegaly and pulmonary effusion and help rule out primary pulmonary disease.
• Ultrasonography may help confirm cardiac disease; however, patient size may complicate evaluation. Reference ultrasonographic measurements have been established for mice, hamsters, and rats.

DIAGNOSTIC PROCEDURES
• Electrocardiography is potentially useful; however, reference ranges may not be readily available for many rodent species; placing alcohol-soaked cotton balls between the patient and clips will aid in obtaining a reading.
• Response to therapy as a trial

PATHOLOGIC FINDINGS
Cardiac findings vary with disease.

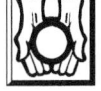

TREATMENT

APPROPRIATE HEALTH CARE
• Inpatient—severely debilitated patients or those in respiratory distress
• Discharge stable patients

NURSING CARE
• Oxygen therapy for patients in respiratory distress

CONGESTIVE HEART FAILURE

- If pleural effusion is present, thoracocentesis has both diagnostic and therapeutic benefits. Sedation can be achieved with midazolam (1–2 mg/kg IM) and butorphanol (0.25–1 mg/kg IM). Supportive care including correction of dehydration and other fluid deficits.
- Ensure that the patient is kept warm (if hypothermic, an incubator may be required).

ACTIVITY
Restrict activity—remove exercise wheels, ramps from cage

DIET
- Provide adequate nutrition; dyspneic animals may be reluctant to eat and may need assisted feeding with a liquid diet such as Oxbow Carnivore Care (Oxbow Enterprises, Inc., Murdock, NE) or Emeraid Exotic Carnivore (Lafeber's, Cornell, IL). If these commercial formulas are not available, a gruel may be made with rodent block ground into nutritional supplements such as Ensure (Abott Nutrition, Columbus, OH) or human baby food cereals.
- If the animal is on an inappropriate diet, for example, seed based, it is important to transition to healthier foods when the appetite returns. Removing the normal diet in the clinically ill patient can cause anorexia and lead to complications.

CLIENT EDUCATION
- CHF is not curable and will progress. Inform client that cardiac disease is difficult to manage, and prognosis for longer term survival is poor; aim of treatment is palliative as long as quality of life can be maintained.

SURGICAL CONSIDERATIONS
N/A

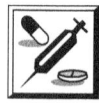

MEDICATIONS
DRUG(S) OF CHOICE
- Drugs for treatment of cardiac disease in dogs and cats have been extrapolated and are used with variable results in pet rodents.
- Furosemide is recommended at the lowest effective dose to eliminate pulmonary edema and pleural effusion. If fulminate cardiac failure is evident, administer furosemide at 1–4 mg/kg q6–12h IM. Initially, furosemide should be administered parenterally. Long-term therapy should be continued orally at 2–10 mg/kg PO q12h.
- Predisposes the patient to dehydration, prerenal azotemia, and electrolyte disturbances.
- Digoxin is used in animals with dilated cardiomyopathy, mitral or tricuspid regurgitation, or to treat supraventricular

arrhythmias in animals with CHF. In hamsters, 0.05–0.1 mg/kg PO q12–24h has been used. Doses for other species have been extrapolated from feline doses.
- Verapamil has been shown to preserve cardiac contractility in some hamsters with cardiomyopathy at a dose of 0.25–0.5 mg SQ q12h.
- Enalapril 0.5–1.0 mg/kg PO q24h has been used in hamsters with cardiomyopathy. It has been anecdotally used in other rodent species; the dose is extrapolated from feline doses.
- Beta-blockers may be beneficial in patients with hypertropic cardiomyopathy; doses are extrapolated from feline doses.
- Pimobenden q12h) (0.2–0.4 mg/kg PO has been used in experimental models of cardiomyopathy in rats and mice and significantly improved cardiac function in these animals.

CONTRAINDICATIONS
- Positive inotropic drugs should be avoided in patients with HCM.

PRECAUTIONS
- Treatment regimens in most rodent species are extrapolated from canine or feline doses and should be used with caution and careful patient monitoring.
- ACE inhibitors and digoxin must be used cautiously in patients with renal disease.
- Overzealous diuretic therapy may cause dehydration and hypokalemia.

POSSIBLE INTERACTIONS
- The use of a calcium channel blocker in combination with a beta blocker should be avoided as clinically significant bradyarrhythmias can develop in other small animals and are likely to also occur in rodents.
- Combination of high-dose diuretics and ACE inhibitor may alter renal perfusion and cause azotemia.

ALTERNATIVE DRUGS
There are numerous reports of herbs and other supplements used in laboratory hamsters to treat cardiovascular-related diseases. These include flax oil at 0.25 mL/kg q24h, coenzyme q10 at 10–30 mg/day, L-carnitine at 25 mg/day, and taurine at 50 mg/day.

FOLLOW-UP
PATIENT MONITORING
- Cardiac disease is likely to be progressive; therefore, frequent recheck evaluation is recommended.
- Monitor response to therapy and adjust drug dosages as indicated.

- Radiographs should be repeated 1 week after treatment is started.
- Monitor patient weight.
- Monitor intake of food and water.

PREVENTION/AVOIDANCE
It is unclear at this time how to prevent development of cardiac disease in rodents; however, decreased fat intake and adequate exercise are beneficial in many species and should be considered for these patients as well.

POSSIBLE COMPLICATIONS
- Disease is likely to be progressive.
- Sudden death due to arrhythmias
- Iatrogenic problems associated with medical management

EXPECTED COURSE AND PROGNOSIS
Cardiomyopathy is progressive, and the owner should be advised that treatments are to increase patient comfort and control clinical signs. Given the short life span of the small rodent pet, prognosis is always guarded.

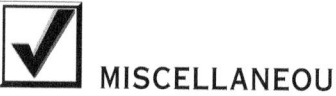

MISCELLANEOUS
ASSOCIATED CONDITIONS
- Lower respiratory disease
- Amyloidosis

ZOONOTIC POTENTIAL
N/A

PREGNANCY/FERTILITY/BREEDING
N/A

SYNONYMS
Heart disease
Heart failure

SEE ALSO
Acute respiratory distress
Pneumonia

ABBREVIATIONS
ACE = angiotensin-converting enzyme
DCM = dilated cardiomyopathy
HCM = hypertrophic cardiomyopathy
L-CHF = left-sided congestive heart failure
R-CHF = right-sided congestive heart failure

Suggested Reading
Carpenter JW. Rodents. In:Exotic Animal Formulary, 5th ed. St Louis: Elsevier-Saunders, 2017:400–494.
Fitzgerald BC, Dias S, Martorell J. Cardiovascular drugs in avian, small mammal, and reptile medicine. Vet Clin Exot Anim 2018;21:399–442.
Goodman G. Rodents: respiratory and cardiovascular system disorders. In: Keeble E, Meredith A, eds. BSAVA Manual of

Rodents and Ferrets. Gloucester, UK: British Small Animal Veterinary Association, 2009.

Heatley JJ. Cardiovascular anatomy, physiology and disease of rodents and small exotic mammals. Vet Clin North Am Exot Anim Pract 2009;12(1):99–113.

Salemi VMC, Bilate A, Ramires FJA et al. Reference values from M-mode Doppler echocardiography for normal Syrian hamsters. Eur J Echocardiogr 2005;6(1):41–46.

Schmidt RE, Reavill DR. Cardiovascular disease in hamsters: review and retrospective study. J Exot Pet Med 2007;16(1):49–51.

Author Angela M. Lennox, DVM, Dipl. ABVP (Avian, ECM); DECZM-Small Mammal

CONSTIPATION (LACK OF FECAL PRODUCTION)

BASICS

DEFINITION
• Constipation—infrequent, incomplete, or difficult defecation with passage of scant, small, hard, or dry fecal pellets
• Intractable constipation and prolonged retention of hard, dry feces leads to obstipation, in which defecation becomes impossible.
• Scant fecal production or lack of fecal production in rodents is often the result of anorexia and/or gastrointestinal hypomotility.

PATHOPHYSIOLOGY
• Constipation can develop with any disease that impairs passage of feces through the colon. Delayed fecal transit allows removal of additional salt and water, producing drier feces.
• Inadequate dietary fiber can decrease gastrointestinal motility; as motility slows, fecal pellets become smaller, less numerous, and drier than normal.
• Diets low in fiber typically contain high simple carbohydrate concentrations, which provide a ready source of fermentable products that can alter the resident microflora, promote the growth of bacterial pathogens, and further suppress gastrointestinal motility.
• Anorexia due to infectious or metabolic disease, pain, stress, or starvation may cause or exacerbate gastrointestinal hypomotility.

SYSTEMS AFFECTED
Gastrointestinal

SIGNALMENT
• Occurs occasionally in mice, rats, hamsters, and gerbils
• No breed or gender predilections reported

SIGNS

Historical Findings
• Scant or no production of fecal pellets
• Small, hard, dry feces
• Infrequent defecation
• Inappetence or anorexia
• Signs of pain, hunched posture, reluctance to move
• Inappropriate diet or abrupt diet change
• Recent illness or stressful event
• Weight loss or other evidence of systemic disease
• Confinement, lack of exercise

Physical Examination Findings
• Small, hard fecal pellets or absence of fecal pellets palpable in the colon
• Firm, dry contents may be palpable within the cecum (cecal impaction)

• Gas, fluid, or firm, doughy, or dry gastrointestinal contents may be palpable depending on the underlying cause.
• Anorectal prolapse, mass, or other lesion
• Abnormal function of hind limbs
• Obesity

CAUSES

Dietary and Environmental Causes
• Lack of dietary fiber—indigestible coarse fiber promotes gastrointestinal motility, adds bulk to the ingesta, and holds water, producing plump, moist fecal pellets.
• Excessive carbohydrate—feeding large amounts of simple carbohydrates can promote the growth of *E. coli* and *Clostridium* spp., which can cause enterotoxemia and ileus. High-carbohydrate, seed-based diets can also promote obesity.
• Obesity—cage confinement, lack of exercise
• Stress—pain, fighting among cage mates, surgery, hospitalization, and new environment
• Dehydration—water bottle malfunction, bad tasting water, and accidental oversight
• Anorexia—malocclusion, excessive fasting, and starvation
• Foreign material—ingestion of/impaction with bedding, fibers, and hair (barbering)

Drugs
• Anesthetic agents, anticholinergics, opioids
• Barium sulfate, kaolin/pectin, sucralfate
• Diuretics

Painful Defecation
• Anorectal disease—rectal prolapse, anal stricture, abscess, and rectal foreign body
• Trauma—fractured pelvis, fractured limb, dislocated hip, perineal bite wound or laceration, and perineal abscess

Mechanical Obstruction
• Extraluminal—healed pelvic fracture with narrowed pelvic canal, intrapelvic neoplasia, intestinal compression secondary to large fetuses
• Intraluminal and intramural—intussusception (*Lawsonia* infection in hamsters, *Syphacia* spp. pinworms), intestinal impaction (*Rodentolepis* tapeworms, bedding, and hair), rectal prolapse, colonic or rectal neoplasia or polyp, rectal stricture, perineal hernia, and congenital defect (atresia ani)

Neuromuscular Disease
• Central nervous system—paraplegia, spinal trauma/disease, intervertebral disk disease, and cerebral trauma/disease
• Peripheral nervous system—sacral nerve trauma/disease

Metabolic and Dental Disease
• Conditions that result in inappetence or anorexia may also promote gastrointestinal

hypomotility. Common causes include incisor malocclusion, metabolic disease (renal disease, liver disease), pain (oral, trauma, and postoperative), neoplasia, and toxins.
• Debility—general muscle weakness, dehydration, and neoplasia

RISK FACTORS
• Gastrointestinal parasitism (oxyurids, cestodes)
• *Lawsonia intracellularis* infection (proliferative ileitis) in hamsters
• *Citrobacter rodentium* infection (transmissible colonic hyperplasia) in mice, gerbils
• Diets with inadequate indigestible coarse fiber content
• Inactivity due to pain, obesity, and cage confinement
• Anesthesia and surgical procedures
• Metabolic disease resulting in dehydration
• Ingestion of bedding substrate, fibers, and fabric
• Barbering, excessive grooming
• Underlying dental, gastrointestinal tract, or metabolic disease
• Spinal, pelvic, or hind-limb trauma

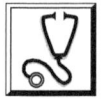

DIAGNOSIS

DIFFERENTIAL DIAGNOSIS
• Dyschezia and tenezmus—may be mistaken for constipation by owners; associated with increased frequency of attempts to defecate and frequent production of small amounts of liquid feces containing blood and/or mucous
• Stranguria—may be mistaken for constipation by owners; can be associated with hematuria and abnormal findings on urinalysis

CBC/BIOCHEMISTRY/URINALYSIS
• Usually normal
• May be used to identify underlying causes of gastrointestinal hypomotility or dehydration
• PCV and TS elevation in dehydrated patients

OTHER LABORATORY TESTS
Fecal direct examination, fecal floatation, and zinc sulfate centrifugation may demonstrate gastrointestinal parasite (cestode) ova.

IMAGING
• Rodents should not be fasted prior to taking radiographs.
• The abdomen of small rodents is much larger than the thorax.
• In small rodents, images of individual organs may be poorly defined.

(CONTINUED) CONSTIPATION (LACK OF FECAL PRODUCTION)

• In cases where there is significant gas in the intestines, radiographic contrast may be poor.
• Contrast radiography may be useful in evaluating gastrointestinal transit time and locating obstructions and displacement of the gastrointestinal tract.
• Abdominal radiography may reveal colonic or rectal foreign body, colonic or rectal mass, spinal fracture, fractured pelvis, or dislocated hip.

PATHOLOGIC FINDINGS
• Vary with cause and severity of constipation
• Gross pathology may reveal lesions suggestive of etiology (e.g., cestodiasis).
• Histopathology is often the best method to obtain a definitive diagnosis for neoplasia, infiltrative or inflammatory conditions, and certain infections (e.g., *Lawsonia intracellularis*).

 TREATMENT

APPROPRIATE HEALTH CARE
• Consider emergency treatment for rodents that have not produced feces or have been anorectic for over 24 hours.
• Outpatient care may be appropriate in some cases, but inpatient hospitalization and support should be considered for the majority.

NURSING CARE
• Remove or ameliorate underlying cause, if possible.
• Discontinue any medications that may cause constipation.
• A warm, quiet environment should be provided.

Fluid Therapy
• Fluid therapy is an essential component of the medical management of all patients with anorexia, gastrointestinal hypomotility, and/or constipation.
• Fluids may be administered by the oral, subcutaneous, intravenous, and/or intraosseous route as indicated by patient condition.
• Mildly affected patients usually respond well to oral and subcutaneous fluids.
• Intravenous or intraosseous fluids are indicated in patients that are severely dehydrated or depressed.
• In most patients, lactated Ringer's solution or Normosol crystalloid fluids are appropriate for parenteral fluid administration.
• Direct oral administration of products such as Gatorade (PepsiCo, Purchase, NY) or Pedialyte (Abbott Nutrition, Lake Forest, IL) are indicated if the patient is not drinking.

• Maintenance fluid requirements are estimated at 100 mL/kg/day.

ACTIVITY
If the patient is not debilitated, exercise should be encouraged as activity promotes gastric motility.

DIET
• Patients should be encouraged to eat during and following treatment. Continued anorexia will exacerbate gastrointestinal hypomotility, promote dysbiosis, and encourage the overgrowth of intestinal pathogens.
• Offer the patient's favorite foods and treats as well as the usual pelleted diet.
• If the patient refuses these foods, syringe-feeding may be indicated: Critical Care for Omnivores (Oxbow Animal Health, Omaha, NE) or Emeraid Omnivore (Lafeber Company, Cornell, IL). If these commercial formulas are not available, a gruel may be made with rodent block ground into nutritional supplements such as Ensure (Abbott Nutrition, Lake Forest, IL), human baby food cereals or blenderized rodent pellets.
• Assisted or forced feeding is contraindicated in cases of intestinal obstruction (e.g., intussusception, rectal prolapse, and cestode impaction)
• Encourage oral fluid intake by offering fresh water, high-moisture-content fruits and vegetables, or by flavoring the water with fruit/vegetable juices.
• Based upon history, diet may need to be permanently modified to include sufficient amounts of indigestible, course fiber and limited simple carbohydrates.

CLIENT EDUCATION
• Discuss the importance of dietary modification, if indicated.
• Advise owners to regularly monitor food consumption and fecal output; seek veterinary attention with a noticeable decrease in either.
• Recommend regular follow-up and monitoring for rodents with incisor malocclusion; owners may also be taught how to do this.

SURGICAL CONSIDERATIONS
• In many cases, constipation and lack of fecal production will resolve with medical treatment alone.
• Surgical manipulation of the intestinal tract, hypothermia, anesthetic agents, and pain all exacerbate gastrointestinal hypomotility. Combined, these factors may worsen the prognosis with surgical treatment.
• Surgery may be indicated for rectal prolapse, intussusception, intestinal foreign body (e.g., bedding, hair), extraluminal

compression of the gastrointestinal tract, intestinal neoplasia, abscesses, and orthopedic problems.

 MEDICATIONS
• Dehydrated patients should be rehydrated with a balanced electrolyte solution.
• Use parenteral medications in animals with severely compromised intestinal motility; oral medications may not be properly absorbed; begin oral medication when intestinal motility begins to return (fecal production, return of appetite, radiographic evidence).

DRUG(S) OF CHOICE
• Antiparasite drugs—praziquantal (6–10 mg/kg PO, SQ, repeat in 10 days) for cestodes; fenbendazole (20 mg/kg PO q24h × 5 days) for oxyurids
• Antibiotics—for *Lawsonia* infection in hamsters: chloramphenicol (30–50 mg/kg PO q12h), tetracycline (10–20 mg/kg PO q12h), enrofloxacin (5–20 mg/kg PO q12h), or trimethoprim sulfa (15–30 mg/kg PO q12h); may also be indicated in patients with bacterial overgrowth that sometimes occurs secondary to gastrointestinal hypomotility; indicated in patients with diarrhea, abnormal fecal cytology, and disruption of the intestinal mucosa (evidenced by blood in the feces). For *Clostridium* spp. overgrowth: metronidazole (20–40 mg/kg PO q12h)
• Analgesics—buprenorphine (0.05–0.1 mg/kg SC, IM q6–8h), carprofen (2–5 mg/kg PO, SC q12–24h), or meloxicam (1–3 mg/kg PO, SC q4h). Intestinal pain, regardless of cause, impairs mobility and decreases appetite and may severely inhibit recovery.
• Laxatives—mineral oil, lactulose as indicated
• Motility modifiers—cisapride (0.1–0.5 mg/kg PO q12h), metoclopramide (0.2–1.0 mg/kg PO, SC, IM q12h); may be indicated in patients with gastrointestinal hypomotility (see Contraindications)

CONTRAINDICATIONS
• Anticholinergics
• Assisted or forced feeding is contraindicated in cases of gastrointestinal tract obstruction or rupture.
• Gastrointestinal motility enhancers in patients with suspected mechanical obstruction (e.g., impaction, intussusception, rectal prolapse, and neoplasia)
• Antibiotics that are primarily Gram-positive in spectrum will suppress the growth of commensal flora, allowing overgrowth of enteric pathogens. These include lincomycin, clindamycin, erythromycin, ampicillin, amoxicillin, cephalosporins, and penicillins.

CONSTIPATION (LACK OF FECAL PRODUCTION) (CONTINUED)

PRECAUTIONS
• Hamsters have antibiotic sensitivities similar to rabbits and other hind-gut fermenters. Do not use oral penicillins, cephalasporins in these species.
• Chloramphenicol may cause aplastic anemia in susceptible people. Clients and staff should use appropriate precautions when handling this drug.
• Metronidazole neurotoxic if overdosed
• Meloxicam—use with caution in cases with suspected renal function

 FOLLOW-UP

PATIENT MONITORING
Monitor appetite and fecal production. Rodents that are successfully treated will regain a normal appetite; fecal volume and consistency will return to normal.

PREVENTION/AVOIDANCE
• Strict feeding of diets containing adequate indigestible coarse fiber and low simple carbohydrate content along with access to fresh water may prevent episodes.
• Obesity prevention; encourage exercise (e.g., provide running wheel) and limit the intake of high-calorie, high-carbohydrate foods, especially seed-based diets.
• Routine fecal examination; internal parasite treatment
• Reduction of stress and prompt treatment of conditions that cause pain
• Be certain that postoperative patients are eating and passing feces prior to release.

POSSIBLE COMPLICATIONS
• Chronic constipation or recurrent obstipation could lead to acquired megacolon, rectal prolapse.

• Death due to gastrointestinal tract rupture, hypovolemic or endotoxic shock
• Postoperative gastrointestinal stasis
• Overgrowth of bacterial pathogens

EXPECTED COURSE AND PROGNOSIS
• Early medical management of constipation and gastrointestinal hypomotility due to dietary causes, obesity, anesthesia/surgery, or anorexia secondary to pain or other stress usually carries a good to excellent prognosis.
• Surgical removal of foreign material, neoplasia, or surgical correction of intussusception or rectal prolapse carries a guarded to poor prognosis.
• Prognosis for *Lawsonia intracellularis* infection in hamsters is guarded.
• The prognosis for other causes varies.

 MISCELLANEOUS

ASSOCIATED CONDITIONS
• Dental disease
• Hepatic lipidosis
• Renal disease

PREGNANCY/FERTILITY/BREEDING
• Pregnancy can produce extraluminal intestinal compression and obstruction.
• With mechanical obstruction due to narrowed pelvic canal, risk of dystocia is increased.

SYNONYMS
Fecal impaction
Gastrointestinal stasis
Ileus

SEE ALSO
Diarrhea
Intestinal parasitism
Rectal prolapse

ABBREVIATIONS
PCV = packed cell volume
TS = total solids

Suggested Reading
Dutton M. Selected veterinary concerns of geriatric rats, mice, hamsters, and gerbils. Vet Clin Exot Anim 2020;23(3):525–548.
Frolich J. Rats and mice. In: Quesenberry KE, Carpenter JW, eds. Ferrets, Rabbits and Rodents, 4th Ed). Clinical Medicine and Surgery. 2021 ed. St. Louis: Saunders, 2020:345–367.
Hrapkiewicz K, Colby L, Denison P, eds. Clinical Laboratory Animal Medicine: An Introduction, 4th ed. Ames: Wiley-Blackwell, 2013:83–92, 128–133, 156–159, 182–187.
Jekl V, Knotek Z. Evidence-based advances in rodent medicine. Vet Clin Exot Anim 2017;20:805–816.
Mayer J, Mans C. Rodents. In: Carpenter JW, ed. Exotic Animal Formulary, 5th ed. St Louis: Elsevier, 2018:459–493.
Mitchell MA, Tully TN, eds. Manual of Exotic Pet Practice. St Louis: Elsevier, 2009:326–344, 406–432.
Miwa Y, Mayer J. Hamsters and gerbils. In: Quesenberry KE, Carpenter JW, eds. Ferrets, Rabbits and Rodents, 4th Ed). Clinical Medicine and Surgery. 2021 ed. St. Louis: Saunders, 2020:368–384.
Author Dan H. Johnson, DVM, Dipl. ABVP (Exotic Companion Mammal)

CUTANEOUS AND SUBCUTANEOUS MASSES

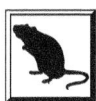

BASICS

DEFINITION
A swelling or mass within or under the skin

PATHOPHYSIOLOGY
• Any process that elicits an inflammatory response resulting in accumulation of inflammatory products and fluid in or under the skin
• Infection and the resultant accumulation of inflammatory or purulent material
• Neoplastic processes and growth of tumors

SYSTEMS AFFECTED
• Skin/Exocrine
• Other systems may be affected, depending on the type of mass present.

GENETICS
N/A

INCIDENCE/PREVALENCE
Subcutaneous and cutaneous masses are common presentations. Incidence will vary with the species being treated.

GEOGRAPHIC DISTRIBUTION
N/A

SIGNALMENT
Breed Predilections
• Gerbils: squamous cell carcinoma, basal cell tumors, melanoma, and tumors of the ventral abdominal gland
• Rats: abscesses, basal cell carcinoma, squamous cell carcinoma, mammary tumors, and papilloma
• Mice: abscesses, mammary adenocarcinoma, fibrosarcoma, squamous cell carcinoma, mouse pox/ectromelia (uncommon in the United States but observed in China, Japan, and Europe)
• Hamsters: benign follicular tumors, epithelioma, keratocanthoma, squamous papilloma, melanoma, SCC, BCC, Harderian gland adenoma, cutaneous lymphoma, and cutaneous hemangiosarcoma

Mean Age and Range
Masses in general are more common in older animals regardless of the species. The incidence of neoplasia in rats over 2 years of age has been reported to be as high as 87%.

Predominant Sex
The incidence of mammary tumors is high in female rats.

SIGNS
Physical Examination Findings
Gerbils:
Squamous cell carcinoma, basal cell tumors, melanoma—particularly on the ears, feet, and base of the tail, tumors of the ventral abdominal gland; lesions may appear raised,

ulcerated, or scabbed with varying degrees of inflammation
Rats:
• Abscesses—swelling that may be fluctuant, possible ulceration, purulent material on aspiration, often accompanied by pruritus
• Mammary tumors—semifirm subcutaneous swelling often located in the inguinal or axillary area. Due to the abundance of mammary tissue in the rat, swellings due to mammary adenoma may occur on the neck, shoulders, or thorax. In some cases, may be accompanied by discharge from an associated teat.
Mice:
• Abscesses—swellings that may be fluctuant, possible ulceration, purulent material on aspiration, often accompanied by pruritus; preputial gland abscesses possible
• Mouse pox/ectromelia—hunched posture, rough fur, facial edema, solitary or generalized rash, papules, swelling, or erosions, particularly on the face and extremities
Hamsters:
Cutaneous lymphoma, cutaneous hemangiosarcoma—patchy alopecia, scabs, and exfoliative erythroderma; may see lethargy, anorexia, and weight loss

CAUSES
Varies with the type of mass; infection, trauma, and neoplasia

RISK FACTORS
Exposure to infectious agents, inadequate husbandry, and overcrowding

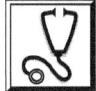

DIAGNOSIS

DIFFERENTIAL DIAGNOSIS
• In many small rodents, normal anatomic structures may be mistaken for masses, such as the flank glands of hamsters, full cheek pouches in hamsters, and the ventral abdominal gland in gerbils. Pet owners will often mistake the testicles of small rodents for masses.
• Abscess
• Benign masses—trichofolliculoma, sebaceous cysts
• Neoplasia—BCC, SCC, mammary tumors, lipoma
• Infectious—papillomatous lesions, pox lesions
• Ectoparasite hypersensitivity
• Myiasis

CBC/BIOCHEMISTRY/URINALYSIS
For systemically ill patients or those that may be treated surgically, the minimum database should include serum biochemistries, complete blood count, and urinalysis.

OTHER LABORATORY TESTS
N/A

IMAGING
Three-view survey radiographs and/or ultrasonographic imaging should be used to screen for potential metastasis if malignant neoplasia is suspected. Radiographs may also be used to evaluate bony structures for osteomyelitis in cases of neoplasia or abscess.

DIAGNOSTIC PROCEDURES
The most useful tools in diagnosing the cause of subcutaneous and cutaneous swellings include fine-needle aspirates and cytology, biopsy and histopathology, and bacterial cultures if indicated for abscesses or secondary infections. Biopsy and histopathology generally provide a more accurate means of diagnosis than fine-needle aspirates, as many swellings and masses do not exfoliate well and only an acellular sample is obtained by aspiration.

PATHOLOGIC FINDINGS
Variable depending on the etiology

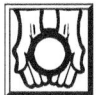

TREATMENT

APPROPRIATE HEALTH CARE
Many cases can be treated on an outpatient basis unless debilitated or requiring postoperative monitoring.

NURSING CARE
Supportive care including thermal regulation, fluid administration, and assisted feeding for stabilization of debilitated patients. Postoperative supportive care for patients treated surgically.

ACTIVITY
Activity restriction usually not necessary except as indicated postoperatively for patients treated surgically.

DIET
N/A

CLIENT EDUCATION
Discuss appropriate husbandry and postoperative care. Educate regarding follow-up care and likelihood of recurrence for specific condition.

SURGICAL CONSIDERATIONS
• Surgical removal of masses or removal/debridement of abscesses are the treatments of choice. Where neoplasia is suspected, every attempt should be made to excise masses completely with wide margins.
• Abscesses are often difficult to resolve, and surgical removal of the abscess including the capsule may be required. Where complete removal is not possible, implantation of AIPMMA beads or treatment of the open

CUTANEOUS AND SUBCUTANEOUS MASSES (CONTINUED)

wound may be needed. Therapeutic lasers may also be employed in the treatment of abscesses.

• Ovariohysterectomy in rats may reduce the incidence of mammary tumors.

MEDICATIONS

DRUG(S) OF CHOICE
• Antibiotics based on culture and sensitivity for abscesses and secondary infections. Antibiotics commonly used in small rodents include trimethoprim/sulfa (15–30 mg/kg PO, SC q12h), enrofloxacin (5–20 mg/kg PO, SC, IM q12h), chloramphenicol (30–50 mg/kg PO q8h), azithromycin (10–30 mg/kg PO q24h), and amoxicillin/clavulanic acid (20 mg/kg PO q12h *Do not use in hamsters)
• Postoperative pain management—buprenorphine (0.05–0.1 mg/kg SQ, IM q6–8h), meloxicam (1–2 mg/kg PO, SQ, IM q24h), tramadol (1–4 mg/kg PO q8–12h)

CONTRAINDICATIONS
Risk of potentially fatal antibiotic-induced enterotoxemia in many species is associated with orally administered penicillin, ampicillin, cephalosporins, carbenicillin, lincomycin, clindamycin, streptomycin, gentamicin, neomycin, erythromycin, vancomycin, and tetracycline.

PRECAUTIONS
Tramadol should be used with caution in geriatric or severely debilitated patients, in animals with seizures or those taking other medications that lower the seizure threshold, and in pregnant animals.

POSSIBLE INTERACTIONS
N/A

ALTERNATIVE DRUGS
• Chemotherapy has been described for conditions such as cutaneous lymphoma in hamsters; however, the prognosis is poor.
• If gastrointestinal distress accompanies antibiotic therapy, concurrent treatment with a probiotic may help resolve symptoms.

FOLLOW-UP

Reevaluate patients within 1–2 weeks for resolution of clinical signs and for surgical follow-up as indicated.

PATIENT MONITORING
Reevaluate at least once every 3–4 months for recurrence of neoplastic conditions.

PREVENTION/AVOIDANCE
Optimize husbandry to avoid injury and exposure to infectious agents.

POSSIBLE COMPLICATIONS
• Metastasis or local recurrence of neoplastic lesions following surgical removal is possible.
• Some infections and abscesses may be resistant to treatment and require long-term therapy.

EXPECTED COURSE AND PROGNOSIS
Variable depending on the species and etiology:
• Cutaneous tumors of gerbils are most often benign and metastasis is uncommon.
• BCCs in rats are locally invasive but do not typically metastasize, while SCCs are locally invasive with the potential for metastasis.
• Mammary adenomas in rats are usually benign, though recurrence is common after surgical excision.
• Fibrosarcoma and SCC in mice are often aggressive and invasive.
• Cutaneous lymphoma in hamsters carries a poor prognosis.

MISCELLANEOUS

ASSOCIATED CONDITIONS
N/A

AGE-RELATED FACTORS
Neoplasias are more common in older animals.

ZOONOTIC POTENTIAL
N/A

PREGNANCY/FERTILITY/BREEDING
It has been suggested that the incidence of mammary tumors in rats may be reduced by ovariohysterectomy.

SYNONYMS
Cancer
Neoplasia

SEE ALSO
N/A

ABBREVIATIONS
AIPMMA = antibiotic-impregnated polymethylmethacrylate
BCC = basal cell carcinoma
SCC = squamous cell carcinoma

INTERNET RESOURCES
Veterinary Information Network: www.vin.com
Exotic DVM forum for eDVM readers: www.pets.groups.yahoo.com/group/ExoticDVM

Suggested Reading
Dutton M. Selected veterinary concerns of geriatric rats, mice, hamsters, and gerbils. Vet Clin Exot Anim 2020;23(3):525–548.
Frolich J. Rats and mice. In: Quesenberry KE, Carpenter JW, eds. Ferrets, Rabbits and Rodents, 4th Ed). Clinical Medicine and Surgery. 2021 ed. St. Louis: Saunders, 2020:345–367.
Jekl V, Knotek Z. Evidence-based advances in rodent medicine. Vet Clin Exot Anim 2017;20:805–816.
Miwa Y, Mayer J. Hamsters and gerbils. In: Quesenberry KE, Carpenter JW, eds. Ferrets, Rabbits and Rodents, 4th Ed). Clinical Medicine and Surgery. 2021 ed. St. Louis: Saunders, 2020:368–384.
Palmerio BS, Roberts H. Clinical approach to dermatologic disease in exotic animals. Vet Clin North Am Exot Anim Pract. 2013;16(3):523–577.
Vergneau-Grosset C, Keel MK, Goldsmith D et al. Description of the prevalence, histologic characteristics, concomitant abnormalities, and outcomes of mammary gland tumors in companion rats (*Rattus norvegicus*): 100 cases (1990–2015). JAVMA 2016;249(10):1170–1179.
White SD, Bourdeau PJ, Brément T et al. Companion rats (*Rattus norvegicus*) with cutaneous lesions: a retrospective study of 470 cases at two university veterinary teaching hospitals (1985–2018). Vet Dermatol 2019;30:237–272.

Author Christine Eckermann-Ross, DVM, CVA, CVH

BASICS

DEFINITION
A cutaneous fungal infection affecting the cornified regions of the nails, hair, and superficial layers of the skin

PATHOPHYSIOLOGY
Exposure to or contact with a dermatophyte may result in active infection with skin inflammation, scaling, and hair loss or may result in a latent infection or prolonged asymptomatic carrier state. Stress, immune compromise, or the use of medications such as corticosteroids may prolong infection. The incubation period for dermatophyte infection is typically 1–4 weeks. Dermatophytes grow in the keratinized layers of the skin, hair, and nails but do not thrive in living tissue.

SYSTEMS AFFECTED
Skin/Exocrine

GENETICS
N/A

INCIDENCE/PREVALENCE
Variable depending on the species and population surveyed

GEOGRAPHIC DISTRIBUTION
Ubiquitous, but may be more commonly diagnosed in regions with a hot, humid climate

SIGNALMENT
Breed Predilections
• Gerbils: infection rarely reported. Dermatophytes most frequently encountered include *Trichophyton mentagrophytes*, followed by *Microsporum* spp.
• Mice: *T. mentagrophytes* and *M. gypsum* most common
• Rats: *T. mentagrophytes* and *Microsporum* spp.
• Hamsters: infection uncommon, *T. mentagrophytes* and *M. canis*

Mean Age and Range
May be more common in older animals debilitated by concurrent disease or immunosupression

Predominant Sex
N/A

SIGNS
Physical Examination Findings
• Clinical signs vary from asymptomatic carrier state to alopecia, which may consist of focal, circular, circumscribed lesions to coalescing or generalized dermatitis. Skin is typically hyperkeratotic and scaling, erythema, brittle hair, hyperpigmentation, and pruritus are variable.

• Gerbils: usually exhibit focal areas of dry, hyperkeratotic, skin with alopecia or brittle hair
• Mice: typically asymptomatic unless debilitated
• Rats: lesions usually present on the neck, tail, back, and appear as slightly raised, alopecic, erythemic areas that may be moist or dry; asymptomatic carriers possible
• Hamsters: asymptomatic or presenting with dry circular lesions on the head, limbs, ears, and body

CAUSES
Trichophyton mentagrophytes and Microsporum species (gypsum, canis, audoiunii) are the most common causes of dermatophytosis in small rodents.

RISK FACTORS
Poor husbandry, overcrowding, poor sanitation, and inappropriate nutrition increase the risk of infection with dermatophytes. Immune-suppressing disease or medications predispose animals to dermatophytosis and increase the potential for more severe and protracted infections.

DIAGNOSIS

DIFFERENTIAL DIAGNOSIS
• Ectoparasites
• Bacterial pyoderma
• Cutaneous neoplasia
• Sebaceous adenitis
• Immune-mediated dermatitis

CBC/BIOCHEMISTRY/URINALYSIS
In systemically ill pets or those with refractory dermatophytosis, serum biochemistries, complete blood count, and urinalysis may help identify underlying problems that are contributing factors in the development of dermatophytosis.

OTHER LABORATORY TESTS
N/A

IMAGING
N/A

DIAGNOSTIC PROCEDURES
• Fungal culture with microscopic identification of microconidia
• Wood's lamp illumination is useful only for identification of *Microsporum*. Both false-positive and false-negative results are possible, so this technique should only be used in conjunction with other screening tools.
• Microscopic evaluation of hair after using a clearing solution such as KOH and toluidine blue
• Response to treatment with antifungal medication

• Skin biopsy may be indicated in refractory cases.

PATHOLOGIC FINDINGS
Folliculitis, perifolliculitis, and/or furunculosis are common. Hyperkeratosis, pyogranulomatous inflammation, and epidermal pustules may also be observed. While some fungal hyphae may be observed with routine H&E staining, special stains are typically needed for better visualization of the fungal organisms.

TREATMENT

APPROPRIATE HEALTH CARE
Treatment with appropriate topical or systemic antifungal medications on an outpatient basis is usually appropriate.

NURSING CARE
Quarantine may be considered in some cases due to the zoonotic potential of dermatophyte infections.

ACTIVITY
Activity restriction is not indicated.

DIET
As long as adequate nutrition is provided, diet changes are not indicated. If griseofulvin is used to treat the infection, consumption of a fatty meal improves absorption of the medication.

CLIENT EDUCATION
• Advise clients of the zoonotic potential of dermatophytes.
• In multipet households, treatment of the environment and all individuals in the collection may be necessary.
• 1:10 dilute bleach has demonstrated efficacy in environmental decontamination.
• Asymptomatic carriers exist, some individuals may have spontaneous resolution of lesions, and some cases of dermatophytosis may be recurrent in nature.

SURGICAL CONSIDERATIONS
N/A

MEDICATIONS

DRUG(S) OF CHOICE
• Focal or regional lesions may be treated with topical agents such as miconazole, once daily for 2–4 weeks.
• Antifungal shampoos that are safe for use in cats may be helpful in treating dermatophytes in small rodents.
• Griseofulvin is the most widely used therapeutic agent (15–25 mg/kg PO q24h for up to 60 days). Absorption is enhanced if

DERMATOPHYTOSIS

given with a fatty meal. Gastrointestinal irritation is the most common side effect and can be alleviated by dividing the dose for more frequent administration. Bone marrow suppression is a possible idiosyncratic reaction or can result from prolonged therapy. Neurologic side effects and teratogenicity in the first two trimesters of pregnancy have been reported. Biweekly monitoring of the CBC is recommended.
• Lime sulfur dip, 1:40 dilute with water has been used; dip once every 7 days for 4–6 treatments.
• Environmental decontamination to prevent spread or reinfection.

CONTRAINDICATIONS
• Application of any topical substance may increase itching and discomfort and draw the patient's attention to the affected area.
• Steroids are not commonly used in small rodents, and their use is contraindicated in patients with dermatophyte infections.

PRECAUTIONS
The use of griseofulvin should be avoided in pregnant animals and in patients with immune system suppression.

POSSIBLE INTERACTIONS
N/A

ALTERNATIVE DRUGS
Itraconzaole (5 mg/kg q24h × 4–10 weeks) has been anecdotally used in rodents.

FOLLOW-UP

PATIENT MONITORING
Repeat fungal cultures are recommended toward the end of treatment as some animals may clinically improve but remain culture positive. Treatment should be continued until a negative culture result is obtained.

PREVENTION/AVOIDANCE
Spread to other animals and reinfection can be reduced by quarantine of infected pets until dermatophyte cultures are negative. Any new animals introduced to the collection

should also undergo a quarantine period to prevent introduction of organisms. Prophylactic treatment of exposed animals with griseofulvin for 10–14 days is advisable.

POSSIBLE COMPLICATIONS
• Both false-positive and false-negative dermatophyte cultures are possible. When dermatophytes are present, the culture medium turns pink in response to protein metabolism, which alters the pH of the medium, causing it to become alkaline. Most dermatophytes cause this color change within a few days, while saprophytes do not effect this change until they have exhausted the carbohydrate in the medium and begin to metabolize the protein. Thus, the culture should be examined daily, and microscopic examination of microconidia should be employed to confirm the presence of pathogenic dermatophytes.
• Wood's lamp illumination is prone to false-positive and false-negative interpretation. Most pathogenic dermatophytes do not fluoresce under Wood's lamp examination. Only *M. canis* infection can be confirmed by this method. The lamp must be allowed to warm up for 5 minutes prior to examination. Keratin from sebum and epidermal scales can produce false-positive fluorescence.

EXPECTED COURSE AND PROGNOSIS
Most animals will respond to treatment and clear dermatophyte infections, and some infections may clear on their own within a few months. Persistent or refractory infections can be a problem in debilitated patients, multipet situations, or in animals with long hair.

MISCELLANEOUS

ASSOCIATED CONDITIONS
N/A

AGE-RELATED FACTORS
N/A

ZOONOTIC POTENTIAL
Dermatophyte infections can be transmitted to humans.

PREGNANCY/FERTILITY/BREEDING
N/A

SYNONYMS
Ringworm

SEE ALSO
Alopecia
Pruritus

ABBREVIATIONS
H&E = hematoxylin and eosin

INTERNET RESOURCES
Exotic DVM forum for eDVM readers: www.pets.groups.yahoo.com/group/ExoticDVM
Veterinary Information Network: www.vin.com

Suggested Reading
Frolich J. Rats and mice. In: Quesenberry KE, Carpenter JW, eds. Ferrets, Rabbits and Rodents, 4th Ed). Clinical Medicine and Surgery. 2021 ed. St. Louis: Saunders, 2020:345–367.
Jekl V, Knotek Z. Evidence-based advances in rodent medicine. Vet Clin Exot Anim 2017;20:805–816.
Miwa Y, Mayer J. Hamsters and gerbils. In: Quesenberry KE, Carpenter JW, eds. Ferrets, Rabbits and Rodents, 4th Ed). Clinical Medicine and Surgery. 2021 ed. St. Louis: Saunders, 2020:368–384.
Palmerio BS, Roberts H. Clinical approach to dermatologic disease in exotic animals. Vet Clin North Am Exot Anim Pract 2013;16(3):523–577.
Pollock C. Fungal diseases of laboratory rodents. Vet Clin North Am 2003;6(2):401–413.
White SD, Bourdeau PJ, Brément T et al. Companion rats (*Rattus norvegicus*) with cutaneous lesions: a retrospective study of 470 cases at two university veterinary teaching hospitals (1985–2018). Vet Dermatol 2019;30:237–272.
Author Christine Eckermann-Ross, DVM, CVA, CVH

BASICS

DEFINITION
Abnormal frequency, liquidity, and volume of feces

PATHOPHYSIOLOGY
• Caused by imbalance in the absorptive, secretory, and motility actions of the intestines
• Can result from a combination of factors: increased membrane permeability, hypersecretion, and malabsorption
• Death occurs from loss of electrolytes and water, acidosis, and from the manifold effects of toxins.
• May or may not be associated with inflammation of the intestinal tract (enteritis)
• A common predisposing cause of diarrhea in small rodents is disruption of enteric commensal flora by antibiotic usage, stress, or poor nutrition. In a process known as bacterial dysbiosis, resident enteric microflora populations are altered by changes in intestinal motility, carbohydrate fermentation, pH, and substrate production. Beneficial bacteria are destroyed while pathogenic bacteria such as *Escherichia coli* and *Clostridium* spp. are promoted. Bacterial dysbiosis can lead to acute diarrhea, enterotoxemia, ileus, chronic intermittent diarrhea, and/or bloating.
• Antibiotic usage can cause severe, acute, often fatal diarrhea due to alteration of normal gut flora. Diarrhea follows the oral administration of antibiotics that are effective against gram-positive bacteria and some gram-negative anaerobes, such as lincomycin, clindamycin, erythromycin, ampicillin, amoxicillin, cephalosporins, and penicillins. These antibiotics should not be orally administered to hamsters.

SYSTEMS AFFECTED
• Gastrointestinal
• Endocrine/Metabolic—fluid, electrolyte, and acid–base imbalances

GENETICS
N/A

INCIDENCE/PREVALENCE
N/A

GEOGRAPHIC DISTRIBUTION
N/A

SIGNALMENT
• No specific age or gender predilection to noninfectious causes
• Younger animals are more commonly affected by infectious causes, particularly during weaning.

• The term "wet tail" is often used in reference to proliferative ileitis, a diarrheic disease of hamsters that may occur at any age, caused by the intracellular bacterium *Lawsonia intracellularis*.
• Enteritis is the most common disease in hamsters.

SIGNS
General Comments
• Diarrhea can occur with or without systemic illness.
• Signs can vary from diarrhea in an apparently healthy patient to severe systemic signs.
• The choice of diagnostic and therapeutic measures depends on the severity of illness.
• Patients that are not systemically ill tend to have normal hydration and minimal systemic signs.
• Signs of more severe illness (e.g., anorexia, weight loss, severe dehydration, depression, and shock) should prompt more aggressive diagnostic and therapeutic measures.

Historical Findings
• Stool production ranging from soft, formed to liquid consistency
• Owner may report fecal accidents, changes in fecal consistency and volume, blood or mucous in the feces, or straining to defecate.
• History of sudden diet change, weaning, overfeeding fresh green foods or fruit, excessive carbohydrates or sugars, or food that is spoiled
• Stress—hospitalization, transportation, environmental changes, and concurrent illness may contribute to alterations in intestinal commensal flora.
• Antibiotic usage—the use of antibiotics that are primarily gram positive in spectrum, suppressing the growth of commensal flora and allowing overgrowth of enteric pathogens

Physical Examination Findings
• Vary with the severity of disease
• Anorexia, lethargy, depression
• Rough hair coat, decreased grooming behavior
• Abdominal pain characterized by hunched posture, reluctance to move, bruxism, and/or pain on abdominal palpation
• Fecal staining of the perineum
• Tenesmus, hematochezia, rectal prolapse
• Dehydration, hypothermia, hypotension, weakness
• Fever
• Abdominal distention—due to thickened or fluid-filled bowel loops, impaction, bloat, masses, or organomegaly
• Fluid or gas may be palpable within the gastrointestinal tract
• Weight loss in chronically infected animals

• Animals may be found dead in the absence of clinical signs.

CAUSES
• Dietary—abrupt change in diet, weaning, excessive fresh green foods or fruit, excessive carbohydrate/sugar, or spoiled food
• Bacterial infection/enterotoxemia—*E. coli*, *Clostridium* spp., *Salmonella* spp., and *Lawsonia intracellularis* (hamsters)
• Obstruction—neoplasia, foreign body, intussusception
• Drugs/toxins—oral administration of lincomycin, clindamycin, erythromycin, ampicillin, amoxicillin, cephalosporins, and penicillins; streptomycin toxic in hamsters; plant toxins; mycotoxins
• Metabolic disorders—liver disease, renal disease
• Intestinal amyloidosis
• Viral infection
• Parasitic causes—protozoans, cestodes, and nematodes
• Systemic illness may also result in diarrhea as a secondary event.
• Neoplasia—primary gastrointestinal tumor, or as a sequela to other organ involvement

RISK FACTORS
• Environmental stressors—improper temperature, poor sanitation, overcrowding, and transportation stress
• Immunosuppressors (radiation, corticosteroids, concurrent disease, thymectomy), heavy parasite load, and poor nutrition are considered to be additional predisposing factors.
• Weaning, dietary changes, and carbohydrate overload
• Improper antibiotic usage
• Intestinal amyloidosis (hamsters)

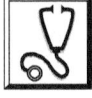

DIAGNOSIS

DIFFERENTIAL DIAGNOSIS
General
• Consider all causes of enteropathy, including diet change, inappropriate antibiotics, enterotoxemia, systemic or metabolic disease, as well as specific intestinal disorders
• Infectious and parasitic causes vary by species.
• True "wet tail" or proliferative ileitis of hamsters is caused by the intracellular bacterium *Lawsonia intracellularis*. Affected animals may have palpably thickened bowel loops and are prone to ileal obstruction, impaction, intussusception, peritonitis, tenesmus, dyschezia, and rectal prolapse.

DIARRHEA

• *Syphacia obvelata* pinworm infestation may be associated with intestinal impaction, intussusception, and rectal prolapse in mice.
• *Salmonella* infection is associated with fresh blood in the feces in some cases.

Mice/Rats
• Viruses—mouse hepatitis virus (coronavirus), epizootic diarrhea of infant mice (rotavirus), reovirus, others; neonates especially susceptible
• Bacteria—*Salmonella* spp., *Helicobacter* spp., *Citrobacter rodentium*, *Clostridium piliforme*, *E. coli*, *Enterococcus* spp., others
• Protozoa—*Entamoeba muris, Trichomonas muris, Spironucleus muris, Giardia muris, Eimeria* spp.
• Cestodes—*Rodentolepis* spp. (formerly *Hymenolepis*)
• Pinworms—*Syphacia* spp., *Aspiculuris tetraptera*

Gerbils
• Bacteria—*Salmonella* spp., *E. coli, Clostridium piliforme, Citrobacter rodentium*
• Cestodes—*Rodentolepis* spp.
• Pinworms—*Dentostomella* spp., *Syphacia* spp.

Hamsters
• Bacteria—*Lawsonia intracellularis, Clostridium piliforme, Clostridium difficile, Campylobacter jejuni, E. coli,* and *Salmonella* spp.
• Protozoa—*Trichomonas* spp., *Spironucleus* spp., and *Giardia*
• Cestodes—*Rodentolepis* spp.
• Pinworms—*Syphacia* spp.

CBC/BIOCHEMISTRY
• Often normal with mild illness
• Moderate to severe illness should prompt a complete evaluation.
• Increased PCV and TS seen with dehydration
• Anemia may be seen with chronic gastrointestinal bleeding.
• TWBC elevation with neutrophilia may be seen with bacterial enteritis.
• Hemogram abnormalities may be consistent with sepsis and/or systemic infection.
• Hypoalbuminemia may be seen with protein loss from the intestinal tract.
• Serum biochemistry abnormalities may suggest renal or hepatic disease.
• Electrolyte abnormalities secondary to anorexia, fluid loss, and dehydration.

OTHER LABORATORY TESTS
Fecal Examination
• Fecal direct examination (with and without Lugol's iodine), fecal floatation, and zinc sulfate centrifugation may demonstrate gastrointestinal parasites or spore-forming bacteria.

• Fecal cytology—may reveal red blood cells or fecal leukocytes, which are associated with inflammation or infection of the intestines
• Fecal Gram stain—may demonstrate large numbers of spore-forming bacteria consistent with *Clostridium* spp. or excessive numbers of Gram-negative bacteria
• Fecal culture should be performed if bacterial infection is suspected; however, interpretation may be difficult since *E. coli* and clostridia may be normal inhabitants in some cases.
• Fecal occult blood testing—to confirm melena when suspected

IMAGING
• Survey abdominal radiography may indicate intestinal obstruction, organomegaly, mass, foreign body, or ascites.
• Contrast radiography may indicate mucosal irregularities, mass, ileus, foreign body, stricture, or thickening of the intestinal wall.
• Abdominal ultrasonography may demonstrate intestinal wall thickening, gastrointestinal mass, foreign body, ileus, or mesenteric lymphadenopathy. Hyperechogenicity may be seen with hepatic lipidosis or fibrosis; hypoechoic nodules are suggestive of hepatic necrosis, abscess, or neoplasia.

PATHOLOGIC FINDINGS
• Vary with cause and severity of diarrheic condition
• Gross pathology may reveal lesions suggestive of etiology
• Histopathology is often the best method to obtain a definitive diagnosis for neoplasia, infiltrative or inflammatory conditions, and certain infections (e.g., *Lawsonia intracellularis, Clostridium piliforme*).

TREATMENT
APPROPRIATE HEALTH CARE
• Treatment must be specific to the underlying cause to be successful.
• Patients with mild diarrhea that are otherwise bright and alert usually respond to outpatient treatment.
• Patients with moderate to severe diarrhea usually require hospitalization and supportive care including parenteral medication, fluid therapy, and thermal support.
• Patients exhibiting signs of lethargy, depression, dehydration, and/or shock should be hospitalized even if diarrhea is mild or absent.
• When infectious disease is suspected, strict isolation of affected and exposed animals is indicated.

NURSING CARE
• Fluid therapy—rehydration and correction of electrolyte imbalances are essential to treatment success in severely ill rodents.
• Severe volume depletion can occur with acute diarrhea, and aggressive shock fluid therapy may be necessary.
• In most patients, crystalloids (e.g., lactated Ringer's solution, Normosol; 20 mL/100 g/24 hours) are appropriate for SQ or IV administration. Crystalloids can also be given PO.
• Oral administration of products such as Gatorade (PepsiCo, Purchase, NY) or Pedialyte (Abbott Nutrition, Lake Forest, IL)
• Maintenance fluid requirements are estimated at 100 mL/kg/day.

DIET3
• It is imperative that rodents continue to eat during treatment and recovery. Prolonged anorexia promotes further derangement of gastrointestinal microflora, encourages overgrowth of intestinal bacterial pathogens, and negatively affects gastrointestinal motility.
• Assisted feeding is typically required until the patient is eating, eliminating, and maintaining body weight.
• A highly digestible, liquefied, elemental diet such as Emeraid Omnivore (Lafeber Company, Cornell, IL) may be indicated in case of suspected enteropathy. If commercial formula is not available, a gruel may be made with rodent block ground into enteral liquid diet such as Ensure (Abbott Nutrition, Lake Forest, IL), blenderized rodent pellets, or human baby food cereals.
• Encourage oral fluid intake: offer fresh water, administer oral fluids via syringe, wet the food, or flavor water with fruit or vegetable juices.
• Direct oral administration of fluids (water, crystalloids, and electrolyte solutions) for patients that are not drinking

MEDICATIONS
DRUG(S) OF CHOICE
Antibiotic Therapy
• Indicated in patients with bacterial inflammatory lesions of the gastrointestinal tract; also indicated in patients with disruption of the intestinal mucosa evidenced by blood in the feces
• Selection should be broad-spectrum antibiotics, based on results of culture and susceptibility testing when possible.
• Some choices for empirical use while waiting for culture results include chloramphenicol (30–50 mg/kg PO q8–12h),

(CONTINUED)

trimethoprim-sulfa (15–30 mg/kg PO q12h), or enrofloxacin (5–20 mg/kg PO, SC, IM q12h)
• Wet tail (*Lawsonia intracellularis*) in hamsters may respond to chloramphenicol (30–50 mg/kg PO q12h), tetracycline (10 mg/kg PO q12h), enrofloxacin (5–10 mg/kg PO q12h), or trimethoprim-sulfa (30 mg/kg PO q12h).
• For *Clostridium* spp. overgrowth: metronidazole (20 mg/kg PO q12h)

Antiparasitic Agents
• Indicated based upon fecal examination for internal parasites, ova, or cysts
• For oxyurid nematodes—fenbendazole (20 mg/kg PO q24h × 5 days), pyrantel pamoate (50 mg/kg PO; dosing interval for small rodents not reported, but dose is repeated in 10 days for most other exotic companion mammals)
• For cestodes—praziquantal (6–10 mg/kg PO or SQ, repeat in 10 days)
• For coccidia—sulfadimethoxine (50 mg/kg PO once, then 25 mg/kg q24h × 10–20 days)
• For *Giardia*—metronidazole (20–40 mg/kg PO q12h; dose cited is anecdotal and lower than that found in many citations; duration of treatment for small rodents not reported, but 5 days is typical for other small mammals), fenbendazole (20 mg/kg PO q24h × 5 days)

Gastrointestinal Agents
• Bismuth subsalicylate (0.3–0.6 mL/kg PO q4–6h PRN; recommended for *Lawsonia intracellularis* in hamsters without a published dose; dose cited is extrapolated from rabbit dose)
• Kaolin/pectin (0.2–0.3 mL/kg PO q6–8h PRN; dose cited is extrapolated from guinea pig dose)
• Loperamide (0.1 mg/kg PO q8h × 3 days, then q24h × 2 days; give in 1 mL water) may be helpful in the treatment of acute diarrhea (see Contraindications).

CONTRAINDICATIONS
• Anticholinergics (loperamide) in patients with suspected intestinal obstruction, glaucoma, intestinal ileus, liver disease, enterotoxin-producing bacteria, and invasive bacterial enteritis.
• Antibiotics that are primarily gram-positive in spectrum will suppress the growth of commensal flora, allowing overgrowth of enteric pathogens. These include lincomycin, clindamycin, erythromycin, ampicillin, amoxicillin, cephalosporins, and penicillins, especially in hamsters.

PRECAUTIONS
• It is important to determine the cause of diarrhea. A general "shotgun" approach with antibiotics may be ineffective or detrimental.

• Antibiotic therapy can predispose small rodents (particularly hamsters) to bacterial dysbiosis and overgrowth pathogenic bacteria (particularly *Clostridium difficile*). If signs worsen or do not improve, therapy should be adjusted.
• Chloramphenicol may cause aplastic anemia in susceptible people. Clients and staff should use appropriate precautions when handling this drug.
• Metronidazole is neurotoxic if overdosed.
• Isolate affected and exposed animals when infectious disease is suspected.

POSSIBLE INTERACTIONS
N/A

ALTERNATIVE DRUGS
N/A

FOLLOW-UP

PATIENT MONITORING
• Fecal volume and character, appetite, attitude, and body weight
• If diarrhea does not resolve, consider reevaluation of the diagnosis.

PREVENTION/AVOIDANCE
• Providing appropriate diet and husbandry
• Reducing stress and providing sanitary conditions
• When infectious disease is suspected, strict isolation of affected and exposed animals is indicated.

POSSIBLE COMPLICATIONS
• Antibiotic therapy can promote bacterial dysbiosis and overgrowth of pathogenic bacteria, especially in hamsters. Use antibiotics with caution, and only use those that are considered safe in the rodent species affected.
• Dehydration due to fluid loss
• Ileal obstruction, intussusception, tenesmus, rectal prolapse, particularly with wet tail (*Lawsonia intracellularis*) in hamsters
• Septicemia due to bacterial invasion of enteric mucosa
• Shock, death from enterotoxicosis

EXPECTED COURSE AND PROGNOSIS
• Depends on cause and severity of disease
• Prognosis for *Lawsonia intracellularis* infection in hamsters is guarded.

MISCELLANEOUS

ASSOCIATED CONDITIONS
• Dehydration
• Malnutrition

• Hypoproteinemia
• Anemia
• Septicemia
• Peritonitis
• Rectal prolapse

AGE-RELATED FACTORS
• All ages susceptible to diarrhea
• Young and recently weaned animals are most severely affected by infectious and parasitic organisms that may cause diarrhea.

ZOONOTIC POTENTIAL
• *Campylobacter jejuni*
• *Salmonella*
• *Rodentolepis*
• *Giardia*

PREGNANCY/FERTILITY/BREEDING
• Severe diarrhea and associated metabolic disturbance may reduce fertility or cause abortion.
• Some infections (e.g., *Salmonella*) can cause abortion.

SYNONYMS
• Diarrhea in hamsters is commonly referred to as "wet tail" regardless of etiology, although in veterinary terminology this term refers exclusively to *Lawsonia intracellularis* infection.
• Wet tail in hamsters caused by *Lawsonia intracellularis* is also known as proliferative ileitis and transmissible ileal hyperplasia.
• Cestodes of the genus *Rodentolepis* are also referred to by the former name *Hymenolepis* in some references.

SEE ALSO
Intestinal parasitism
Rectal prolapse

ABBREVIATIONS
PCV = packed cell volume
TS = total solids
TWBC = total white blood cell count

Suggested Reading
Dutton M. Selected veterinary concerns of geriatric rats, mice, hamsters, and gerbils. Vet Clin Exot Anim 2020;23(3):525–548.
Frolich J. Rats and mice. In: Quesenberry KE, Carpenter JW, eds. Ferrets, Rabbits and Rodents, 4th Ed). Clinical Medicine and Surgery. 2021 ed. St. Louis: Saunders, 2020:345–367.
Hrapkiewicz K, Colby L, Denison P, eds. Clinical Laboratory Animal Medicine: An Introduction, 4th ed. Ames: Wiley-Blackwell, 2013:83–92, 128–133, 156–159, 182–187.
Jekl V, Knotek Z. Evidence-based advances in rodent medicine. Vet Clin Exot Anim 2017;20:805–816.
Lennox AM, Gladden JN. Emergency and critical care of small mammals. In:

RODENTS

Quesenberry KE, Carpenter JW, eds.
Ferrets, Rabbits and Rodents, 4th Ed).
Clinical Medicine and Surgery. 2021 ed.
St. Louis: Saunders, 2020:595–608.
Mayer J, Mans C. Rodents. In: Carpenter
JW, ed. Exotic Animal Formulary, 5th ed.
St Louis: Elsevier, 2018:459–493.

Mitchell MA, Tully TN, eds. Manual of
Exotic Pet Practice. St Louis: Elsevier,
2009:326–344, 406–432.
Miwa Y, Mayer J. Hamsters and gerbils. In:
Quesenberry KE, Carpenter JW, eds.
Ferrets, Rabbits and Rodents, 4th Ed).

Clinical Medicine and Surgery. 2021 ed.
St. Louis: Saunders, 2020:368–384.

Author Dan H. Johnson, DVM, Dipl. ABVP
(Exotic Companion Mammal)

BASICS

DEFINITION
• Dysuria—difficult or painful urination
• Pollakuria—voiding small quantity of urine with increased frequency

PATHOPHYSIOLOGY
The urinary bladder normally serves as a reservoir for storage and periodic release of urine. Inflammatory and noninflammatory disorders of the lower urinary tract may decrease bladder compliance and storage capacity by damaging the structural components of the bladder wall or by stimulating sensory nerve endings located in the bladder or urethra. Sensation of bladder fullness, urgency, and pain stimulate premature micturition and reduce the functional bladder capacity. Dysuria and pollakiuria are caused by lesions of the urinary bladder and/or urethra as well as outflow obstruction and provide evidence of lower urinary tract disease; these clinical signs do not exclude concurrent involvement of the upper urinary tract or disorders of other body system.

SYSTEMS AFFECTED
Renal/Urologic—bladder, urethra

GENETICS
N/A

INCIDENCE/PREVALENCE
Common

GEOGRAPHIC DISTRIBUTION
Worldwide

SIGNALMENT
Breed Predilections
N/A

Mean Age and Range
N/A

Predominant Sex
N/A

SIGNS
Historical Findings
• Hematuria
• Thick white- or tan-appearing urine
• Urine straining in the perineum
• Anorexia, weight loss, lethargy, tooth grinding, tenesmus, and hunched posture in animal with chronic or obstructive lower urinary tract disease

Physical Examination Findings
• May be normal
• Abdominal palpation may induce pain, especially when the bladder is palpate.

• A large urinary bladder may be palpable in patients with partial or complete urethral obstruction.
• Manual expression of the bladder may reveal thick, beige- to brown-colored urine even in animals that have normal-appearing voided urine.

CAUSES
Urinary Bladder
• Urinary tract infection—bacterial
• Urolithiasis, crystals (calcium carbonate, calcium oxalate, and magnesium ammonium phosphate)
• Neoplasia
• Trauma
• Iatrogenic—for example, catheterization, overdistension of the bladder during contrast radiography, and surgery

Urethra
• Urinary tract infection
• Urethrolithiasis
• Urethral plugs—parts of copulatory plug (rat)
• Trauma—especially bite wounds
• Neoplasia

Reproductive
• Endometrial hyperplasia
• Uterine adenoma or adenocarcinoma
• Paraphimosis

RISK FACTORS
• Feeding diet preparations with a low calcium-to-phosphorus ratio may predispose to cystic calculi.
• Obese, sedentary animals
• Intact female likely to develop uterine disease
• Diseases or diagnostic procedures that alter normal host of urinary tract defenses and predispose to infection, formation of uroliths, or damage the urothelium or other tissues of the urinary tract
• Mural or extramural diseases that compress the bladder or urethral lumen

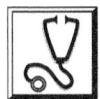

DIAGNOSIS

DIFFERENTIAL DIAGNOSIS
Differential from other abnormal pattern of micturition:
• Rule out polyuria—frequency and volume of urine
• Rule out urethral obstruction—stranguria, anuria, overdistended urinary bladder, and signs of postrenal uremia
Differentiate cause of dysuria and pollakiuria:
• Rule out urinary tract infection—hematuria, bacteriuria; painful, thickened bladder

• Rule out urolithiasis—hematuria, radiopaque bladder
• Rule out neoplasia—hematuria; ultrasound may differentiate
• Rule out neurogenic disorders—flaccid bladder wall; residual urine in bladder lumen after micturition; other neurologic deficits to hind legs, tail perineum, and anal sphincter
• Rule out iatrogenic disorders—history of catheterization, reverse flushing, contrast radiography or surgery
• Rule out uterine disease—females with uterine disease often strain and expel blood when urinating. Blood may mix with urine and be mistaken for hematuria.

CBC/BIOCHEMISTRY/URINALYSIS
• Results may be normal.
• Elevated serum calcium concentration may be present.
• Lower urinary tract disease complicated by urethral obstruction may be associated with azotemia.
• Patients with concurrent pyelonephritis may have impaired urine-concentrating capacity, leukocytosis, and azotemia.
• Disorders of the urinary bladder are best evaluated with a urine specimen collected by cystocentesis.
• Pyuria, hematuria, and proteinuria indicate urinary tract inflammation, but these are nonspecific findings that may result from infectious and noninfectious causes of lower urinary tract disease.
• Identification of bacteria in urine sediment suggests that urinary tract infection is causing or complicating lower urinary tract disease. Identification of neoplastic cells in urine sediment indicates urinary tract neoplasia.
• Crystals in the urine sediment: ammonium magnesium phosphate, mixed carbonate and oxalate, and mixed carbonate, phosphate, magnesium, and calcium may be found

OTHER LABORATORY TESTS
Quantitative urine culture—the most definitive means of identifying and characterizing bacterial urinary tract infection; negative urine culture results suggest a noninfectious cause.

IMAGING
Ultrasonography of the urinary tract and uterus, abdominal radiography, and contrast cystography are important means of identifying and localizing causes of dysuria and pollakiuria.

DIAGNOSTIC PROCEDURES
Cystoscopy—only possible in rats, allow to detect and treat urinary stones (lithotripsy), to visualize the bladder and urethra wall and to collect samples

PATHOLOGIC FINDINGS
Depends on the underlying cause

TREATMENT

APPROPRIATE HEALTH CARE
• Patients with nonobstructive lower urinary tract diseases are typically managed as outpatients; diagnostic evaluation may require brief hospitalization.
• Dysuria and pollakiuria associated with systemic signs of illness (e.g., pyrexia, depression, anorexia, and dehydration) or laboratory findings of azotemia or leukocytosis warrant aggressive diagnostic evaluation and initiation of supportive and symptomatic treatment.
• Treatment depends on the underlying cause and specific sites involved.

MEDICATIONS

DRUG(S) OF CHOICE
• Depend on the underlying cause
• If bacterial cystitis is demonstrated, begin treatment with broad-spectrum antibiotic such as trimethoprim-sulfa (15–30 mg/kg PO q12h), chloramphenicol (30–50 mg/kg PO q12h), or as a second line, enrofloxacin (5–20 mg/kg PO, SC, IM q12h). Modify antibacterial treatment based on result of urine culture and sensibility testing.
• Pain management may aid urination and promote appetite. NSAIDs (meloxicam 1–2 mg/kg PO, SC, IM q24h) reduce pain and may decrease inflammation in the bladder.

CONTRAINDICATIONS
• Glucocorticoids or other immunosuppressive agents
• Potentially nephrotoxic drugs (e.g., aminoglycosides, NSAIDs) in patients that are febrile, dehydrated, or azotemic or that are suspected of having pyelonephritis, septicemia, or preexisting renal disease
• Large amount of fluids if the patient is suffering from obstruction of the urinary tract

PRECAUTIONS
Enrofloxacin SC could cause some skin necrosis, needs to be diluted 1:1 with SC fluids

POSSIBLE INTERACTIONS
N/A

ALTERNATIVE DRUGS
N/A

FOLLOW-UP

PATIENT MONITORING
Response to treatment by clinical signs, serial physical examination, laboratory testing, radiographic, and ultrasonic evaluation appropriate for each specific cause

PREVENTION/AVOIDANCE
• Depends on the underlying cause
• Increase water consumption for the remainder of the animal's life
• Place patient on an appropriate diet
• One successful case report suggested that almitoylethanolamide, glucosamine, and hesperidin supplementation can reduce recurrence of calcium carbonate vesical urolithiasis after surgical treatment in Syrian hamsters.
• Increase exercise
• Provide good hygiene

POSSIBLE COMPLICATIONS
N/A

EXPECTED COURSE AND PROGNOSIS
Good to guarded depending on the underlying cause

MISCELLANEOUS

ASSOCIATED CONDITIONS
• Obesity
• Pyoderma (urine scald)

AGE-RELATED FACTORS
Uroltihs and neoplasia are more common in middle-aged to older animals.

ZOONOTIC POTENTIAL
N/A

PREGNANCY/FERTILITY/BREEDING
N/A

SYNONYMS
N/A

SEE ALSO
Lower urinary tract infection
Renal failure
Uterine disorders

ABBREVIATIONS
NSAID = nonsteroidal anti-inflammatory drug

Suggested Reading
Dutton M. Selected veterinary concerns of geriatric rats, mice, hamsters, and gerbils. Vet Clin Exot Anim 2020;23(3):525–548.
Frolich J. Rats and mice. In: Quesenberry KE, Carpenter JW, eds. Ferrets, Rabbits and Rodents, 4th Ed). Clinical Medicine and Surgery. 2021 ed. St. Louis: Saunders, 2020:345–367.
Hallman RM, Brandão J. Diagnostic imaging of the renal system in exotic companion mammals. Vet Clin Exot Anim 2020;23:195–214.
Jekl V, Knotek Z. Evidence-based advances in rodent medicine. Vet Clin Exot Anim 2017;20:805–816.
Lennox AM, Gladden JN. Emergency and critical care of small mammals. In: Quesenberry KE, Carpenter JW, eds. Ferrets, Rabbits and Rodents, 4th Ed). Clinical Medicine and Surgery. 2021 ed. St. Louis: Saunders, 2020:595–608.
Miwa Y, Mayer J. Hamsters and gerbils. In: Quesenberry KE, Carpenter JW, eds. Ferrets, Rabbits and Rodents, 4th Ed). Clinical Medicine and Surgery. 2021 ed. St. Louis: Saunders, 2020:368–384.
Percy DH, Barthold SW. Rat amyloidosis. In: Percy DH, Barthold SW, eds. Pathology of Laboratory Rodents and Rabbits, 3rd ed. Ames: Blackwell, 2007:200–202.
Petrini D, Di Giuseppe M, Deli G et al. Cystolithiasis in a Syrian hamster: a different outcome. Open Vet J 2016;6(2):135–138.
Reavill DR, Lennox AM. Disease overview of the urinary tract in exotic companion mammals and tips on clinical management. Vet Clin Exot Anim 2020;23(1):169–193.
Author Charly Pignon, DVM, Dip ECZM (Small Mammal)

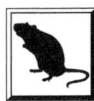

BASICS

DEFINITION
The presence of parasites such as mites, lice, or fleas on the skin, fur, or in the hair follicles

PATHOPHYSIOLOGY
• Varies depending on the parasite
• The presence of large numbers of ectoparasites in the hair follicles exceeds the capacity of the immune system to tolerate the infestation, leading to furunculosis and often to secondary bacterial infection (e.g., *Demodex*).
• Mites that burrow through the stratum corneum cause mechanical irritation and secrete allergenic substances and irritating by-products, which result in intense pruritus (e.g., sarcoptic mites such as *Trixacaris caviae*).
• The bite of some parasites (fleas, some lice, and mites) initiates a hypersensitivity reaction, and the saliva of some ectoparasites (e.g., fleas) contains histamine-like compounds that irritate the skin.

SYSTEMS AFFECTED
Skin, in severe cases psychological/ neurologic

GENETICS
N/A

INCIDENCE/PREVALENCE
Mites and lice are very common presenting complaints in pet rodents.

GEOGRAPHIC DISTRIBUTION
N/A

SIGNALMENT
Breed Predilections
Ectoparasites most commonly diagnosed in small rodents include:
• Hamsters: *Demodex criceti, D. aurati, Notoedres notoedres, N. cati,* and *Liponyssus bacoti*
• Gerbils: *Demodex meroni, D. merioni*
• Mice: *Myobia musculi, Myocoptes musculinus, Radfordia affinis, Liponyssus bacoti,* and *Polyplax senata*
• Rats: *Radfordia ensifera (Myobia ratti), Notoedres muris, Demodex, Polyplax spinuosa, Liponyssus bacoti,* and *fleas*

Mean Age and Range
Ectoparasites are most commonly observed in very young or in aging patients, or in animals with other underlying medical conditions causing generalized debilitation.

Predominant Sex
N/A

SIGNS
Physical Examination Findings
General: patchy to generalized alopecia, scaly skin and/or erythema, pruritus and self-trauma, visualization of lice, nits, fleas, or flea dirt, ill thrift
Hamsters:
• Demodex criceti, *D. aurati*—usually asymptomatic unless the animal is aged, stressed, or debilitated; nonpruritic, dry, scaly patches of alopecia over the hindquarters, back, neck, and abdomen
• *Notoedres, N. cati*—pruritus, crusty lesions on the muzzle, limbs, perineal and genital areas
• *Liponyssus bacoti*—transient infestation, pruritus associated with bites
Gerbils:
Demodex meroni, D. merioni—alopecia, scabs and ulceration, secondary pyoderma
Mice:
• *Myobia musculi*—ruffled, thinning fur; alopecia of the head, back, neck, and shoulders; hypersensitivity and pruritus
• *Myocoptes musculinus*—patchy alopecia and pruritus
• *Radfordia affinis*—pruritus, small scabs to extensive ulceration
• *Liponyssus bacoti*—pruritus associated with bites
• *Polyplax senata*—ill thrift, restlessness, pruritus, and anemia
Rats:
• *Radfordia ensifera (Myobia ratti)*—surface-dwelling fur mite causing alopecia, scaling, pruritus, ill thrift, secondary pyoderma, and allergic hypersensitivity
• *Liponyssus bacoti*—feeds on blood of host, lives in environment. Leads to ill thrift, anemia, and vectors of other diseases
• *Notoedres muris*—burrowing mite typically found in the cornified aural epithelium and other hairless areas
• *Demodex, Polyplax spinuosa, fleas*—also observed but less common

CAUSES
Exposure to infected animals or environments

RISK FACTORS
• Substandard husbandry, inappropriately rough or irritating bedding material, overcrowding, poor sanitation, or other environmental stressors, as well as underlying or concurrent disease states may predispose the patient to ectoparasite infestation and prolong the course of the infection.
• Some ectoparasites serve as vectors for other parasitic or viral disease: *Liponyssus bacoti*—vector for typhus, tularemia, Q fever, plague; *Polyplax senata*—vector for *E. cuniculi, Eperythrozoon coccoides,* and *Haemobartonalla muus*; flea—vector for *Yersinia pestis,* rickettsia, typhus, and intermediate host for *Hymenolepis* tapeworms.

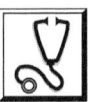

DIAGNOSIS

DIFFERENTIAL DIAGNOSIS
• Bacterial pyoderma
• Dermatophytosis
• Trauma or bite wounds
• Barbering
• Cutaneous manifestation of endocrine disease
• Immune-mediated skin disease
• Cutaneous lymphoma

CBC/BIOCHEMISTRY/URINALYSIS
In debilitated or systemically ill patients, CBC, serum biochemistry, and urinalysis should be included in the minimum database where possible to evaluate for concurrent medical conditions. Leukocytosis, including heterophilia, eosinophilia, monocytosis, and basophilia, may be observed on the CBC. In severe cases, anemia of blood loss may be noted.

OTHER LABORATORY TESTS
N/A

IMAGING
N/A

DIAGNOSTIC PROCEDURES
• Skin scrapings should be performed in all suspected cases to evaluate for the presence of parasites or their ova.
• Skin cytology may reveal inflammatory cells or the presence of bacterial or fungal dermatitis.
• Dermatophyte cultures
• Skin biopsies may be indicated in refractory cases to confirm the diagnosis.

PATHOLOGIC FINDINGS
• Varies depending on the type of ectoparasite present
• Superficial perivascular dermatitis
• Eosinophilic intraepidermal microabscesses
• The presence of eosinophils as a major dermal cellular component
• Furunculosis and the presence of parasites within the hair follicle

TREATMENT

APPROPRIATE HEALTH CARE
• Most cases of ectoparasite infestation will be treated on an outpatient basis.
• Trim toenails to prevent self-trauma if pruritic.

ECTOPARASITES

NURSING CARE
Systemically ill or debilitated animals should be hospitalized for appropriate supportive care, including hand feeding, fluids, and appropriate environmental conditions for the species in question, until stabilized.

ACTIVITY
Activity restriction is typically not necessary. If severe pruritus results in self-mutilation, physical restraint such as a collar or mild sedation may be indicated.

DIET
If nutrition is adequate, no changes are indicated.

CLIENT EDUCATION
Prophylactic treatment of in-contact animals in multipet households is advised.

Environmental decontamination is often necessary, including frequent cage cleaning and bedding changes. Emphasize appropriate nutrition and husbandry for the species in question.

SURGICAL CONSIDERATIONS
N/A

MEDICATIONS

DRUG(S) OF CHOICE
- Ivermectin—0.3–0.5 mg/kg SQ q7–14d for 3 treatments or until infestation is resolved, or 1:100 dilution of ivermectin in propylene glycol placed topically on the head to be spread by normal grooming activity
- Selamectin (15–30 mg/kg topically q14–28d)
- Fipronil (7.5 mg/kg topically q30–60d)
- Pyrethrin powder topically every 3–7 days for 3 weeks. May be incorporated into the dust bath for chinchillas and gerbils.

PRECAUTIONS
- In mice and rats, overdose of ivermectin resulting in neurotoxicity (ataxia, weakness, coma, and death) has been reported.
- Potential side effects of selamectin and imidacloprid include transient local alopecia, lethargy, seizures, vomiting, and diarrhea

POSSIBLE INTERACTIONS
N/A

ALTERNATIVE DRUGS
Animal and surroundings may be treated with pyrethrin or 5% carbaryl powder weekly for several weeks.

FOLLOW-UP

PATIENT MONITORING
Examination of multiple skin scrapings or follow-up skin cytology, as well as clinical resolution of the presenting complaints, is used to monitor progress.

PREVENTION/AVOIDANCE
- Appropriate husbandry and sanitation
- Avoid exposure to carrier animals.

POSSIBLE COMPLICATIONS
N/A

EXPECTED COURSE AND PROGNOSIS
Most ectoparasite infections will improve or resolve within 2 weeks. If there is no improvement, make sure that there is compliance with drug administration, cage disinfection, and other husbandry recommendations and use appropriate diagnostic tests to screen for possible underlying medical conditions.

MISCELLANEOUS

ASSOCIATED CONDITIONS
N/A

AGE-RELATED FACTORS
N/A

ZOONOTIC POTENTIAL
- Some ectoparasite infections, including *Liponyssus bacoti*, *Cheyletiella* spp., have zoonotic potential.
- Ectoparasites can act as vectors of other diseases with zoonotic potential (*Yersinia pestis*, *Hymenolepis* tapeworms).

PREGNANCY/FERTILITY/BREEDING
N/A

SYNONYMS
N/A

SEE ALSO
Alopecia
Pruritus

ABBREVIATIONS
N/A

INTERNET RESOURCES
Exotic DVM forum for eDVM readers: www.pets.groups.yahoo.com/group/ExoticDVM
Veterinary Information Network: www.vin.com

Suggested Reading
Frolich J. Rats and mice. In: Quesenberry KE, Carpenter JW, eds. Ferrets, Rabbits and Rodents, 4th Ed). Clinical Medicine and Surgery. 2021 ed. St. Louis: Saunders, 2020:345–367.
Hoppmann E, Barron HW. Rodent dermatology. J Exot Pet Med 2007;16(4):238–255.
Jekl V, Knotek Z. Evidence-based advances in rodent medicine. Vet Clin Exot Anim 2017;20:805–816.
Meredith A, Redrobe S. BSAVA Manual of Exotic Pets, 4th ed. Gloucester, UK: British Small Animal Veterinary Association, 2002:20–21, 28–30, 39–41, 55–60.
Miwa Y, Mayer J. Hamsters and gerbils. In: Quesenberry KE, Carpenter JW, eds. Ferrets, Rabbits and Rodents, 4th Ed). Clinical Medicine and Surgery. 2021 ed. St. Louis: Saunders, 2020:368–384.
Palmerio BS, Roberts H. Clinical approach to dermatologic disease in exotic animals. Vet Clin North Am Exot Anim Pract 2013;16(3):523–577.
White SD, Bourdeau PJ, Brément T et al. Companion rats (*Rattus norvegicus*) with cutaneous lesions: a retrospective study of 470 cases at two university veterinary teaching hospitals (1985–2018). Vet Dermatol 2019;30:237–272.

Author Christine Eckermann-Ross, DVM, CVA, CVH

EXOPHTHALMOS AND ORBITAL DISEASES

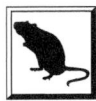

BASICS

DEFINITION
• Abnormal position of the globe
• Exophthalmos—anterior displacement of a normal globe
• Enophthalmos—posterior displacement of a normal globe
• Strabismus—deviation of the globe from a correct position of gaze; not readily corrected by the patient

PATHOPHYSIOLOGY
• Malposition of globe—caused by changes in volume (loss or gain) of the orbital contents or abnormal extraocular muscle function
• Exophthalmos—caused by space-occupying mass lesions posterior to the equator of the globe
• Enophthalmos—caused by reduced volume of orbital contents or by space-occupying mass lesions anterior to the equator of the globe
• Strabismus—caused by either muscular or neurological lesions affecting the tone or function of the extraocular muscles

SYSTEMS AFFECTED
• Ophthalmic
• Respiratory—due to proximity of orbit to nasal cavity, frontal and maxillary sinuses; pneumonia possible with SDA
• Gastrointestinal—proximity of oral cavity to ventral orbit—malocclusion and apical root abscess extension

GENETICS
N/A

INCIDENCE/PREVALENCE
SDA viral infection—common in laboratory commercial colonies

GEOGRAPHIC DISTRIBUTION
N/A

SIGNALMENT

Breed Predilections
• Adenoma of Harderian gland—BALB/c strain of mice
• Microphthalmos—F344 strain of rat

Mean Age and Range
• SDA—weanling and young animals more commonly affected
• Neoplasia—older patients

Predominant Sex
Microphthalmos of the F344 strain of rat more common in females

SIGNS

Historical Findings
• Sudden onset exophthalmos—SDA virus or trauma (e.g., orbital hemorrhage, and proptosis)
• Chronic, progressive exophthalmos—neoplasia
• Chromodacryorrhea (red tears)—see physical exam findings below
• Apparent visual dysfunction—may be seen with microphthalmia and associated ocular anomalies
• Weight loss, difficulty in eating or in prehension, anorexia—dental disease

Physical Examination Findings
Exophthalmos
• SDA virus—sneezing, blepharospasm, photophobia, conjunctivitis, exophthalmos, and epiphora; intermandibular swelling due to lymphadenopathy and inflammation of the submandibular salivary glands
• Chromodacryorrhea—an overflow of red tears—porphyrin pigmented tears are produced in normal amounts by the Harderian gland in several rodent species, particularly in the rat; associated with increase in parasympathetic stimulation of the Harderian gland; can produce characteristic red deposits on the periocular fur, nose, and paws; often a consequence of stress caused by illness, pain, or restraint; often an indication of a chronic underlying condition and warrants full examination
• Additional ocular signs (keratitis, conjunctivitis, and periocular swelling) can be primary or secondary to reduced tear production (KCS) associated with reactive lacrimal gland adenitis and hyperplasia.
• Dental disease—drooling ("slobbers"); bleeding from oral cavity
Enophthalmos
• Ptosis
• Elevation of nictitans
• Extraocular muscle atrophy
• Entropion—with severe disease
Strabismus
• Deviation of globe from normal position—unilateral or bilateral
• May have associated enophthalmos or exophthalmos
Oral examination
• Unlike guinea pigs, rabbits, and chinchillas, the apical roots of the molars of adult mice, rats, gerbils, and hamsters are closed; thus, malocclusion disorders affecting the molars and subsequently the neighboring orbit are less common.
• Specialized equipment is required—rodent dental speculum (Rodent mouth gag, Jorgensen Lab, Loveland, CO) and a set of buccal speculae (Cheek dilator, Jorgensen

Labs); cotton swabs and tongue depressor to retract the tongue and examine lingual surfaces
• Heavy sedation or general anesthesia may be required.
• Tooth root abnormalities may be present in spite of normal-appearing crowns; skull radiographs may be necessary to identify apical root abnormalities if index of suspicion is high for dental involvement

CAUSES

Exophthalmos
• Sialodacryoadenitis—inflammation of the salivary glands and the orbital Harderian gland; caused by highly contagious SDA virus, a common coronavirus; capable of generating epizootic infection, it is generally a self-limiting viral infection, but is a major source of ocular morbidity in affected groups. Acute inflammation of the Harderian gland results in exposure of the globe as well as reduced tear production, predisposing to both exposure keratitis and KCS—severe corneal disease resulting in perforation is possible. Uveitis can be secondary to corneal disease (anterior uveitis) or due to extension of orbital inflammation to the globe (panophthalmitis) in severe cases.
• Orbital hemorrhage—iatrogenic trauma to orbital structures during retrobulbar blood collection—laboratory rats
• Neoplasia of orbital structures—adenocarcinoma, carcinoma, and poorly differentiated sarcomas most commonly reported; benign Harderian gland adenoma—common in mice; optic nerve tumors with orbital extension—meningioma reported in rats
• Prolonged exposure to artificial light—can cause Harderian gland swelling and subsequent necrosis—laboratory rats
• Dental disease—adult mice, rats, gerbils, and hamsters have open incisor roots but molar apical roots are closed; orbital extension of dental disease less common than in rodents with open molar roots (e.g., guinea pigs, chinchillas); abscessation with orbital extension still possible
• Cheek pouch impaction in hamsters—inflammation may extend to periocular region if severe

Enophthalmos
• Ocular pain—retraction of globe
• Horner's syndrome
• Loss of orbital fat or muscle
• Severe weight loss or dehydration
• Neoplasia extending from rostral orbit displacing globe posteriorly

Strabismus
• Abnormal innervation to extraocular muscles

EXOPHTHALMOS AND ORBITAL DISEASES (CONTINUED)

• Posttraumatic restriction of extraocular muscle motility by scar tissue—can occur following orbital blood collection
• Avulsion of extraocular muscle attachment following globe proptosis

RISK FACTORS
• Infection with SDA virus—highly contagious and readily transmitted by direct contact, aerosol, or fomites; the disease varies between different strains and in different environments, which is typical of viral pathogenesis and resultant morbidity
• Orbital blood collection—although previously advocated as a rapid method of blood collection from anesthetized mice and rats, the technique is now generally discouraged
• Head trauma, excessive restraint—proptosis; strabismus
• Dental disease—caries of molars can predispose to tooth root abscesses; can be due to inappropriate physical form and composition of diet (e.g., fruit and grain treats bound together by chocolate, honey, or molasses are readily consumed but should be minimized)

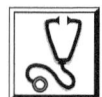

DIAGNOSIS

DIFFERENTIAL DIAGNOSIS

Exophthalmos
• Conformational—prominence of the globe is a normal feature of the small rodent—evaluate bilateral symmetry; observe grossly from position above head of patient
• Buphthalmos—enlargement of the globe due to intraocular disease (i.e., glaucoma)—uncommon in small mammals; in rodents, most often associated with lesions in the anterior uvea that are either congenital or secondary to inflammatory disease; open-angle glaucoma reported in hamsters
• Episcleritis—inflammation of the episcleral tissues can cause focal or diffuse thickening of the fibrous tunic, often mimicking a buphthalmic or exophthalmic globe
• Traumatic proptosis—acute onset related to trauma to head/periocular area—eyelids typically entrapped behind globe; can occur with overzealous restraint in small rodents

Enophthalmos
• Perforated/collapsed globe—acute trauma; perforation of corneal descemetocele
• Phthisis bulbi—acquired shrinkage of the globe, usually secondary to trauma and/or chronic inflammation
• Microphthalmos—congenitally smaller than normal globe, which can include other

anatomical abnormalities—may be blind or vision impaired; occurs with significant frequency in the F344 strain of rat
• Anophthalmos—congenital absence of globe—rare but reported in rats, mice, and hamsters

Strabismus
• Microphthalmos
• Phthisis bulbi

CBC/BIOCHEMISTRY/URINALYSIS
Usually normal; WBC count may be elevated with orbital abscesses

OTHER LABORATORY TESTS
Can consider serologic testing for SDA coronavirus

IMAGING
• Orbital ultrasound—localize and characterize space-occupying mass lesions; guide aspirate or biopsy diagnostic procedures
• Skull radiographs—orbital and dental assessment
• CT—evaluate extent of orbital disease and determine involvement of other cavities (nasal, oral)

DIAGNOSTIC PROCEDURES
• Resistance to globe retropulsion—confirms space-occupying mass
• Tonometry—rule out glaucoma; rebound tonometer best suited to small eyes of rodent and provides accurate assessment of IOP (reported mean 16–18 mmHg in mice and rats)
• Oral examination, skull radiographs, and fine-needle aspiration or biopsy of space-occupying mass lesion in orbit—perform after anesthetizing patient
• Fine-needle aspiration (use 20–22 gauge needle)—if retrobulbar mass is accessible; submit samples for aerobic, anaerobic, and fungal cultures; gram's staining; and cytological evaluation
• Cytology—often diagnostic for abscess and neoplasia; rodent abscesses typically produce thick purulent material
• Biopsy—indicated if needle aspiration is nondiagnostic and mass lesion is accessible
• Forced duction test with strabismus—grasp conjunctiva with a pair of fine forceps following topical anesthesia; differentiates neurological disease (in which the globe moves freely) from restrictive muscle condition (in which the globe cannot be moved manually)

PATHOLOGIC FINDINGS
• SDA—microscopic lesions in Harderian and lacrimal glands include necrosis of secretory and ductal epithelium with both acute and chronic inflammatory cell infiltrates, filling of ducts with inflammatory

exudates, and squamous metaplasia of the ductal epithelium
• Neoplasia—characteristic features of malignancy (anisocytosis, anisokaryosis, increase in mitotic figures)
• Cellulitis, abscess—inflammatory cells, intracellular bacteria

TREATMENT

APPROPRIATE HEALTH CARE
• SDA—supportive—there is no specific treatment for the viral infection; quarantine patient to avoid viral transmission and practice appropriate hygiene with handling; prevent secondary bacterial infections or ocular tissue and respiratory tract
• Orbital neoplasm—consultation with oncologist once diagnosis is made; most are primary and malignant
• Proptosis—temporary tarsorrhaphy indicated to avoid exposure keratitis until retro-orbital swelling subsides; anti-inflammatory therapy
• Retrobulbar abscess—aggressive surgical debridement of orbital abscess and related affected tissues (dentition, maxilla) followed by long-term local and systemic antibiotic treatment; limited (palliative) response to antibiotic treatment alone
• Cheek pouch impaction—hamster—evert pouch to empty and flush; treat abrasions with topical antibiotic; evaluate dentition
• Enophthalmos—depends on cause
• Strabismus—muscle reattachment difficult

NURSING CARE
• Exophthalmos—lubrication of exposed cornea while diagnostics and treatment are carried out
• Supportive care in debilitated or anorectic patients; assisted feeding; subcutaneous or intravenous fluid therapy
• Inflammatory conditions—warm compressing of periocular tissues q6h—encourages blood flow to area—helps decrease swelling and cleans discharges

ACTIVITY
N/A

DIET
Minimize changes in diet during treatment and recovery; may require syringe feeding if anorectic or during perioperative period

CLIENT EDUCATION
SDA—highly infectious; therefore, isolation of patient is necessary; affected patient may continue to shed virus after active symptoms abate—limit new susceptible rodents into the environment

SURGICAL CONSIDERATIONS
- Enucleation/exenteration—the orbital vasculature of rodents varies and is important to consider with surgical technique to avoid significant blood loss in small rodents; orbital venous sinus is present in mice, gerbils, and hamsters; rats have an orbital vascular plexus. The venous sinus can be avoided during enucleation by using a subconjunctival technique to remain close to the sclera during transection of extraocular muscles and the optic nerve.
- Use anticholinergic treatment preoperatively to avoid vagus-induced bradyarrhythmia associated with globe manipulation: atropine 0.1–0.4 mg/kg SC, IM; glycopyrrolate 0.01–0.02 mg/kg SC

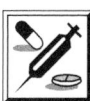

MEDICATIONS
DRUG(S) OF CHOICE
- Exophthalmos (all patients)—lubricate exposed cornea to prevent desiccation and ulceration (e.g., artificial tear ointment or gel)
- Corneal ulceration—topical antibiotic (e.g., neomycin-polymyxin-bacitracin, ciprofloxacin, or ofloxacin q6–8h) and cycloplegic (e.g., atropine 1% q12–24h) to prevent infection and reduce ciliary spasm, respectively
- Antibiotics—broad spectrum pending results of culture and susceptibility testing; enrofloxacin (5–20 mg/kg PO, SC, IM q12h); trimethoprim-sulfa (15–30 mg/kg PO, SC q12h); and chloramphenicol (30–50 mg/kg PO, SC, IM, IV q8h) are safe choices
- Anti-inflammatory therapy—systemic NSAID, e.g., meloxicam (1–2 mg/kg PO, SC, IM q24h)
- Pain management—buprenorphine (0.05–0.1 mg/kg SQ, IM q6–8h); topical nalbuphine 1.2%—corneal ulceration

CONTRAINDICATIONS
- Avoid steroid-containing ophthalmic preparations—in case of corneal ulceration; steroids may cause gastrointestinal stasis
- Hamsters have a marked, often lethal GI tract sensitivity to antibiotic therapy (dysbiosis)—the anaerobic flora is sensitive to antibiotics with a gram-positive spectrum; disturbances of the flora caused by antibiotics may cause an overcolonization of clostridia, particulary *Clostridium difficile*, with resultant fatal toxin elaboration. Penicillins (including ampicillin, amoxicillin), bacitracin, erythromycin, lincomycin, oral gentamicin, clindamycin, cephalosporins, dihydrostreptomycin, streptomycin,

vancomycin, and tylosin at therapeutic doses carry the risk of inducing the syndrome and are contraindicated in hamsters.
- Low-risk antibiotics include chloramphenicol, aminoglycosides, sulphonamides, and the quinolones.
- Avoid systemic fluoroquinolones in young or pregnant rodents—may cause arthropathy; limit SC or IM injections

PRECAUTIONS
- Great care is required when considering the use of antibiotics in hamsters, including topical preparations.
- Trimethoprim-sulfamethoxazole given orally may decrease tear production in the hamster
- Chloramphenicol—avoid human contact due to potential blood dyscrasia. Advise owners of potential risk.

POSSIBLE INTERACTIONS
N/A

ALTERNATIVE DRUGS
N/A

FOLLOW-UP
PATIENT MONITORING
- SDA—monitor for corneal ulceration due to exposure (exophthalmos) and desiccation (KCS); monitor for secondary bacterial infections
- Dental abscess—evaluate entire oral cavity and skull at each recheck and repeat skull radiographs at 3–6 month intervals to monitor for recurrence at the surgical site or other locations

PREVENTION/AVOIDANCE
- SDA—purchase from reputable sources—never purchase an obviously or even suspiciously ill rodent; quarantine or isolation of all newly acquired rodents (~4 weeks) helps to prevent disease among pet rodents. A rat that has been exposed to SDA virus can still shed virus after all symptoms have subsided. Reduce crowding and stress; separate unaffected companions if SDA is identified.
- Orbital hemorrhage—avoid orbital blood collection
- Proptosis—avoid excessive restraint

POSSIBLE COMPLICATIONS
- Permanent lacrimal gland damage with atrophy and KCS
- Keratitis, corneal ulceration, and corneal perforation
- Anterior uveitis, glaucoma, cataracts, and retinal degeneration—less common sequelae of SDA
- Vision loss

- Loss of globe
- Permanent malposition of globe
- Death

EXPECTED COURSE AND PROGNOSIS
- SDA—virus is self-limiting, but morbidity can be high—chronic side effects relate to severity and duration of inflammation—severe disease can result in intraocular inflammation, blindness, and phthisis bulbi
- Orbital neoplasia—fair to poor depending on tumor type, extent of involvement at presentation, and response to therapy
- Retrobulbar tooth root abscess—depends on severity of bone involvement, underlying disease, condition of the cheek teeth, and presence of other abscesses. Fair to guarded with single isolated retrobulbar abscess, adequate surgical debridement, and medical treatment. Abscesses in the nasal passages or with multiple or severe maxillary abscesses have a guarded to poor prognosis—euthanasia may be warranted

MISCELLANEOUS
ASSOCIATED CONDITIONS
N/A

AGE-RELATED FACTORS
Young rats are especially susceptible to SDA, and the infection can occur in the lower respiratory tract, resulting in pneumonia

ZOONOTIC POTENTIAL
N/A

PREGNANCY/FERTILITY/BREEDING
Avoid fluoroquinolones in pregnancy.

SYNONYMS
N/A

SEE ALSO
Red tears (Chromodacryorrhea)
Sialoadacryoadenitis virus

ABBREVIATIONS
CT = computed tomography
GI = gastrointestinal
IOP = intraocular pressure
KCS = keratoconjunctivitis sicca
SDA = sialodacryoadenitis
WBC = white blood cell

Suggested Reading
Beaumont SL. Ocular disorders of pet mice and rats. Vet Clin Exot Anim 2002;5:311–324.
Carpenter JW. Exotic Animal Formulary, 3rd ed. St Louis: Elsevier-Saunders, 2005.
Frolich J. Rats and mice. In: Quesenberry KE, Carpenter JW, eds. Ferrets, Rabbits and Rodents, 4th Ed). Clinical Medicine and Surgery. 2021 ed. St. Louis: Saunders, 2020:345–367.

EXOPHTHALMOS AND ORBITAL DISEASES   (CONTINUED)

Miwa Y, Mayer J. Hamsters and gerbils. In: Quesenberry KE, Carpenter JW, eds. Ferrets, Rabbits and Rodents, 4th Ed). Clinical Medicine and Surgery. 2021 ed. St. Louis: Saunders, 2020:368–384.

Monk C. Ocular surface disease in rodents (guinea pigs, mice, rats, chinchillas). Vet Clin Exot Anim 2019;22:15–26.

Rajaei SM, Ansari Mood M, Selk Ghaffari M et al. Effects of short-term oral administration of trimethoprim-sulfamethoxazole on tear production in clinically normal Syrian hamsters. Vet Ophthalmol 2015;18(1):83–85.

Van der Woerdt A. Ophthalmologic diseases of small mammals. In: Quesenberry KE, Carpenter JW, eds. Ferrets, Rabbits and Rodents, (4th Ed). Clinical Medicine and Surgery. 2021 ed. St. Louis: Saunders, 2020:583–594.

Williams DL. Ocular disease in rats: a review. Vet Ophthalmol 2002;5(3):183–191.

Author Georgina Newbold, DVM, Dipl. ACVO

HEAD TILT (VESTIBULAR DISEASE)

BASICS

DEFINITION
- Tilting of the head away from its normal orientation with the trunk and limbs; associated with disorders of the vestibular system
- Infection/inflammation, neoplasia, trauma, toxicity, or other disease process involving the vestibular apparatus

PATHOPHYSIOLOGY
- Most commonly involves infection/inflammation of the vestibular apparatus
- Often associated with otitis media and interna—inflammation most commonly caused by bacterial infection
- Extension of infection of the external ear through the tympanic membrane or extension from the oral and nasopharyngeal cavities via the eustachian tube
- Interna—may also result from hematogenous spread of a systemic infection
- May be accompanied by evidence of respiratory disease
- Brain stem lesions, including neoplasia, abscess, or trauma, may result in vestibular signs.

SYSTEMS AFFECTED
- CNS—vestibulocochlear receptors in the inner ear and the facial nerve in the middle ear (peripheral) with possible extension of infection intracranially (central)
- Auditory
- Respiratory—infectious disease may be linked to upper respiratory disease via eustachian tube

SIGNALMENT
- Common presentation in rodents, most commonly seen in rats
- No specific sex or age predilection
- Stress, aging, and concurrent disease may predispose

SIGNS
- Vestibular signs, including head tilt, ataxia, rolling, circling, nystagmus
- In cases of otitis, may see discharge from ear canal, accumulation of debris below ear; may be foul smelling; scratching at the ear
- Evidence of respiratory disease
- Other evidence of CNS disease: seizures, depression

CAUSES
- Bacterial otitis in any species
- In mice, opportunistic infections with *Klebsiella oxytoca* primarily result in otitis media.
- *Mycoplasma pulmonis* may cause otitis media in rats.
- Respiratory syncytial virus may play a role in otitis in rodents.
- *Clostridium piliforme* in the hamster or gerbil
- Neoplasia of the nervous system: glioblastoma and astrocytoma in the hamster, aural cholesteatoma, aural papilloma or polyp in the gerbil; pituitary hyperplasia and adenoma in rats and other rodents
- Head trauma in all species
- Ototoxicity, including gentamicin toxicity
- Parasitic encephalitis, including *Baylisascaris procyonis*

RISK FACTORS
- Presence of upper respiratory disease
- Poor husbandry, especially overcrowding and poor sanitation
- Other sources of immune suppression may predispose to infectious disease.
- Exposure to raccoon or other predator feces—contaminated bedding and feed in the case of *Baylisascais procyonis*
- Unsafe handling practices linked to head trauma
- Improper drug dosing linked to rare cases of drug toxicity

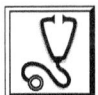

DIAGNOSIS

DIFFERENTIAL DIAGNOSIS
- Central vestibular diseases—pituitary tumors common in rodents; may see lethargy, somnolence, stupor, and other brain stem signs
- Trauma—history and physical evidence of injury
- Diagnosis of otitis media/interna is based on history, physical examination, endoscopic examination of the ear canal (diagnostic otoscopy), and diagnostic imaging of the skull.
- History of recent drug administration, especially gentamicin

CBC/BIOCHEMISTRY/URINALYSIS
Testing is useful to identify other concurrent disease processes but does not provide a specific diagnosis.

OTHER LABORATORY TESTS
If disease includes rupture of the tympanum and otitis externa, cytology and culture and sensitivity of exudate may be useful; note presence of inflammatory cells and bacteria.

IMAGING
Imaging of the skull can be extremely useful but is increasingly difficult as patient size decreases. Some cases of severe otitis interna/media may produce bony abnormalities or filling within the tympanic bulla.

DIAGNOSTIC PROCEDURES
- Response to antibiotic therapy as a trial (parental and/or otic)
- Otoscopic examination or diagnostic otoscopy
- Diagnostic imaging

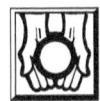

TREATMENT

APPROPRIATE HEALTH CARE
- Inpatient—severe debilitating infection; neurologic signs
- Discharge stable patients, pending further diagnostics and surgery, if indicated.

NURSING CARE
Supportive care, including correction of dehydration, if present, and support feeding; some animals with vestibular disease may be unable to take in adequate nutrition

CLIENT EDUCATION
- Inform client that many causes of vestibular disease will not respond to therapy, and discovery of exact etiology may not be possible antemortem.
- Warn client that some patients may be left with a permanent disability.

SURGICAL CONSIDERATIONS
- Lateral ear canal resection and bulla osteotomy may be possible in larger patients; most commonly described in the chinchilla
- Specific treatment of other underlying disorders

MEDICATIONS

DRUG(S) OF CHOICE
For treatment of suspected otitis:
- Systemic antibiotics—choice is ideally based on results of culture and susceptibility testing, when possible
- Often, exudate in the bullae is thick and limits penetration of systemic antibiotics. Treatment with antibiotics may be effective in preventing extension of infection and may be effective in treating concurrent bacterial respiratory infection.
- In rats, if *Mycoplasma pulmonis* is suspected or confirmed, treat with a combination of enrofloxacin (10 mg/kg PO q12h) and doxycycline (5 mg/kg PO q12h) for a minimum of 2 weeks.
- Initailly, use broad-spectrum antibiotics such as enrofloxacin (5–10 mg/kg PO, SC, IM q12h), ciprofloxacin (10 mg/kg PO q12h), or trimethoprim-sulfa (15–30 mg/kg PO q12h); if anaerobic infections are suspected, use chloramphenicol (30–50 mg/kg

HEAD TILT (VESTIBULAR DISEASE) (CONTINUED)

PO q8h) or azithromycin (10–30 mg/kg PO q24h).

• Consider topical antibiotic therapy in cases involving otitis externa.

• Anti-inflammatory medications may help reduce inflammation in cases of vestibular disease. For pain management or as an anti-inflammatory medication (NSAID)—meloxicam (1–2 mg/kg PO, SC, IM q24h)

• Some animal's refractory to antibiotic therapy (especially those with vestibular signs or pituitary tumors) may respond to temporary steroid therapy; this should be weighed against potential untoward effects of steroids.

• For *Baylisascaris procyonis*: selected nonrodent species with suspected infections responded to albendazole (5 mg/kg q8h × 14d). There are no reports of successful treatment of rodents.

CONTRAINDICATIONS

Do not administer penicillins, ampicillin, amoxicillin, erythromycin, or lincomycin to hamsters due to the risk of potentially fatal enteric dysbiosis.

PRECAUTIONS

• All therapeutic agents should be used with caution in debilitated, dehydrated patients. Ideally, vascular abnormalities (dehydration, hypotension) are addressed prior to initiating antibiotic therapy.

• Steroid therapy should be approached with caution and reserved for cases of vestibular syndrome nonresponsive to antibiotic therapy.

POSSIBLE INTERACTIONS

N/A

ALTERNATIVE DRUGS

There is some anecdotal evidence that immune-boosting drugs/agents have been useful in some cases of infectious respiratory disease.

FOLLOW-UP

PATIENT MONITORING

• Ensure adequate intake of food and water, especially in animals with vestibular disease.

• Monitor patient weight.

PREVENTION/AVOIDANCE

• Treating otitis or upper respiratory infections in early stages may prevent otitis media/interna.

• Careful dosing of potentially ototoxic drug

• Prevent exposure to raccoon/predator feces.

• Practice safe handling of rodents.

POSSIBLE COMPLICATIONS

• Signs associated with vestibular and facial nerve damage may persist.

• Severe infections—may spread to the brain stem

MISCELLANEOUS

ASSOCIATED CONDITIONS

• Upper respiratory infection or chronic respiratory disease

• Aural abscess or neoplasia

• Otitis externa

ZOONOTIC POTENTIAL

Most diseases producing head tilt and ataxia in rodents are not zoonotic; however, all animal diseases may be of concern in immunocompromised humans.

PREGNANCY/FERTILITY/BREEDING

N/A

SYNONYMS

Head tilt
Vestibular syndrome

SEE ALSO

Otitis media and interna
Rhinitis and sinusitis

ABBREVIATIONS

CNS = central nervous system
NSAID = nonsteroidal anti-inflammatory drug

Suggested Reading

Capello V, Lennox AM. Diagnostic imaging of the respiratory system in exotic companion mammals. Vet Clin Exot Anim 2011;14:369–389.

Dutton M. Selected veterinary concerns of geriatric rats, mice, hamsters, and gerbils. Vet Clin Exot Anim 2020;23(3):525–548.

Fitzgerald BC, Dias S, Martorell J. Cardiovascular drugs in avian, small mammal, and reptile medicine. Vet Clin Exot Anim 2018;21:399–442.

Frolich J. Rats and mice. In: Quesenberry KE, Carpenter JW, eds. Ferrets, Rabbits and Rodents, 4th Ed). Clinical Medicine and Surgery. 2021 ed. St. Louis, Saunders, 2020:345–367.

Jekl V, Knotek Z. Evidence-based advances in rodent medicine. Vet Clin Exot Anim 2017;20:805–816.

Lennox AM, Gladden JN. Emergency and critical care of small mammals. In: Quesenberry KE, Carpenter JW, eds. Ferrets, Rabbits and Rodents, 4th Ed). Clinical Medicine and Surgery. 2021 ed. St. Louis: Saunders, 2020:595–608.

Mayer J, Mans C. Rodents. In: Carpenter JW, ed. Exotic Animal Formulary, 5th ed. St Louis: Elsevier, 2018:459–493.

Miwa Y, Mayer J. Hamsters and gerbils. In: Quesenberry KE, Carpenter JW, eds. Ferrets, Rabbits and Rodents, 4th Ed). Clinical Medicine and Surgery. 2021 ed. St. Louis: Saunders, 2020:368–384.

Author Angela M. Lennox, DVM, Dipl. ABVP (Avian), ECM; DECZM-Small Mammal

BASICS

DEFINITION
Presence of blood in the urine. It is important to differentiate true hematuria from blood originating from the reproductive tract in females.

PATHOPHYSIOLOGY
• Secondary to loss of the endothelial integrity in the urinary tract
• Clotting factor deficiency or thrombocytopenia possible but not commonly reported
• Must distinguish from blood originating from the reproductive tract in females. Blood expressed from the uterus or the vaginal vault during micturition is a much more common cause of perceived hematuria than urinary tract bleeding.

SYSTEMS AFFECTED
• Renal/Urologic
• Reproductive

GENETICS
N/A

INCIDENCE/PREVALENCE
True hematuria is not common, but hematuria due to bleeding from the genital tract in female is frequent.

GEOGRAPHIC DISTRIBUTION
World wide

SIGNALMENT

Breed Predilections
Intermittent hematuria has been reported in hybrid Lewis and brown Norway rats, predominantly in males and associated with hydronephrosis.

Mean Age and Range
N/A

Predominant Sex
N/A

SIGNS

Historical Findings
• Red-tinged urine with or without pollakiuria
• Blood expelled during micturition

Physical Examination Findings
• May be normal
• Turgid, sometimes painful bladder on abdominal palpation in animals with urinary stones or cystitis
• With chronic disease, the bladder may markedly increase in size and may even fill most of the abdomen.
• Petechiae or ecchymoses in patients with coagulopathy

CAUSES

Lower Urinary Tract (Most Common)
• Uroliths (calcium carbonate, calcium oxalate, and magnesium ammonium phosphate)
• Infectious—bacterial: *Esherichia coli* and *Pseudomonas* spp. are common causes of bacterial cystitis; parasitic cystitis: *Trichomoide crassicauda* in rat
• Neoplasia
• Trauma

Upper Urinary Tract
• Nephrolithiasis
• Infectious—bacterial
• Inflammatory—glomerulonephritis
• Trauma

Uterine
• Females with uterine disease often expel blood when urinating. Blood may mix with urine and be mistaken for hematuria.
• Most common cause of perceived hematuria in intact females
• Uterine neoplasia, endometrial hyperplasia, or endometrial venous aneuryrism
• Pyometra
• Trauma

Systemic
• Coagulopathy (anticoagulant rodenticides)
• Thrombopenia

RISK FACTORS
• Sedentary, obese animal on diets consisting mainly of mineral unbalanced commercial pellets at high risk of urolithiasis and nephrolithiasis
• Middle-aged to older intact female has risk for uterine neoplasia or pyometra

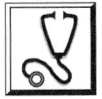

DIAGNOSIS

DIFFERENTIAL DIAGNOSIS
• Rule out blood originating from the uterus in intact females—perform urinalysis with sample collected via ultrasound-guided cystocentesis to differentiate true hematuria from uterine bleeding
• Rule out other cause of discolored urine (myoglobinuria, hemoglobinuria)

CBC/BIOCHEMISTRY/URINALYSIS
• Leukocytosis—may be seen with urinary tract infection
• Azotemia—in some patients with bilateral renal disease or urinary tract obstruction
• Increase in GGT if renal epithelium is damaged
• Thrombocytopenia, anemia—with bleeding disorders
• Crystals in urinary sediment—ammonium magnesium phosphate, mixed carbonate and oxalate, and mixed carbonate, phosphate, magnesium, and calcium may be found
• Pyuria, hematuria, and proteinuria—indicate a urinary tract inflammation, but these are nonspecific findings that may result from infectious and noninfectious cause of lower urinary tract disease
• Bacteria—rarely observed on urinalysis, even in animals with significant lower urinary tract infection
• Neoplastic cells—in urine sediment indicates urinary tract neoplasia

OTHER LABORATORY TESTS
Bacterial culture of urine to identify urinary tract infection

IMAGING
Ultrasonography, radiography, and possibly contrast radiographs may be useful in finding the underlying cause of the hematuria.

DIAGNOSTIC PROCEDURES
Cystoscopy—only possible in rats, allow to detect and treat urinary stones (lithotripsy), to visualize the bladder and urethra wall, and to take samples

PATHOLOGIC FINDINGS
N/A

TREATMENT

APPROPRIATE HEALTH CARE
Depending on the status of the patient and the underlying cause, the patient could be treated as an outpatient or need to be hospitalized.

NURSING CARE
• Fluid therapy for dehydrated patients
• Blood transfusion may be necessary if patient is severely anemic

ACTIVITY
N/A

DIET
• Increase water consumption. Provide multiple sources of fresh water. Flavoring the water with fruit juice (with no added sugar) or artificial sweetener is usually helpful. Provide a variety of clean, fresh, leafy vegetables sprayed or soaked with water.
• Provide a diet with a good calcium-to-phosphorus ratio and an adequate magnesium level.

CLIENT EDUCATION
• Urolith removal does not alter the factors responsible for their formation; eliminating risk factors such as obesity, sedentary life, and poor diet combined with increasing water consumption is necessary to minimize

HEMATURIA (CONTINUED)

recurrence. Even with these changes, however, recurrence is likely.
• Encourage owners to spay females if nonbreeders.

SURGICAL CONSIDERATIONS
Uroliths and uterine disease require surgical intervention.

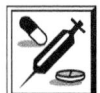

MEDICATIONS

DRUG(S) OF CHOICE
• Pain management may aid urination and promote appetite. NSAIDs (meloxicam 1–2 mg/kg PO, SC, IM q24h) reduce pain and may decrease inflammation in the bladder.
• Antibiotics that concentrate in the urine are most appropriate for bacterial infections. Initial choices include trimethoprim-sulfa (15–30 mg/kg PO q12h) and chloramphenicol (30–50 mg/kg PO q12h). Base choice of the antibiotic on result of bacterial culture of the urine and sensitivity testing. Enrofloxacin (5–20 mg/kg PO, SC, IM q12h) could be used as a second line.
• Antispamodic: diazepam (1–2 mg/kg IM) and midazolam (1 mg/kg IM)
• Ivermectin (0.3–0.5 mg/kg SC repeated 10 days after the first treatment) for rats with bladder threadworm

CONTRAINDICATIONS
N/A

PRECAUTIONS
• Check renal function before using any NSAIDs.
• Enrofloxacin SC could cause some skin necrosis, needs to be diluted 1:1 with fluids

POSSIBLE INTERACTIONS
N/A

ALTERNATIVE DRUGS
N/A

FOLLOW-UP

PATIENT MONITORING
Monitor response to treatment by clinical signs, serial physical examinations, laboratory testing, and radiographic and ultrasonographic evaluation appropriate for each specific cause.

PREVENTION/AVOIDANCE
• Increase water consumption for the remainder of the animal's life.
• Place patient on an appropriate diet.
• One successful case report suggested that almitoylethanolamide, glucosamine, and hesperidin supplementation can reduce recurrence of calcium carbonate vesical urolithiasis after surgical treatment in Syrian hamsters.
• Increase exercise.
• Spay nonbreeding females.

POSSIBLE COMPLICATIONS
• Anemia
• Urinary tract obstruction with urolithiasis
• Renal failure with urolithiasis or hypercalciuria
• Metastasis with uterine neoplasia

EXPECTED COURSE AND PROGNOSIS
Depends on the underlying cause

MISCELLANEOUS

ASSOCIATED CONDITIONS
• Genital infections
• Dermatitis of the inguinal area

AGE-RELATED FACTORS
Neoplasia tends to occur in middle-aged to older animals.

ZOONOTIC POTENTIAL
N/A

PREGNANCY/FERTILITY/BREEDING
Infertile if involvement of the uterus

SEE ALSO
Lower urinary tract infection
Uterine disorders
Vaginal discharge

ABBREVIATIONS
NSAID = nonsteroidal anti-inflammatory drug

Suggested Reading
Dutton M. Selected veterinary concerns of geriatric rats, mice, hamsters, and gerbils. Vet Clin Exot Anim 2020;23(3):525–548.
Frolich J. Rats and mice. In: Quesenberry KE, Carpenter JW, eds. Ferrets, Rabbits and Rodents, 4th Ed). Clinical Medicine and Surgery. 2021 ed. St. Louis: Saunders, 2020:345–367.
Hallman RM, Brandão J. Diagnostic imaging of the renal system in exotic companion mammals. Vet Clin Exot Anim 2020;23:195–214.
Jekl V, Knotek Z. Evidence-based advances in rodent medicine. Vet Clin Exot Anim 2017;20:805–816.
Martorell J. Reproductive disorders in pet rodents. Vet Clin Exot Anim 2017;20:589–608.
Miwa Y, Mayer J. Hamsters and gerbils. In: Quesenberry KE, Carpenter JW, eds. Ferrets, Rabbits and Rodents, 4th Ed). Clinical Medicine and Surgery. 2021 ed. St. Louis: Saunders, 2020:368–384.
Miwa Y, Sladky K. Common surgical procedures of rodents, ferrets, hedgehogs, and sugar gliders. Vet Clin Exot Anim 2016;19:205–244.
Reavill DR, Lennox AM. Disease overview of the urinary tract in exotic companion mammals and tips on clinical management. Vet Clin Exot Anim 2020;23(1):169–193.
Petrini D, Di Giuseppe M, Deli G et al. Cystolithiasis in a Syrian hamster: a different outcome. Open Vet J 2016;6(2):135–138.
Author Charly Pignon, DVM, Dip ECZM (Small Mammal)

HYPERADRENOCORTICISM

BASICS

DEFINITION
Hyperadrenocorticism is a disease resulting from elevated circulating cortisol concentrations and its effect on multiple organ systems.

PATHOPHYSIOLOGY
Disease results from excessive production of cortisol by the adrenal cortex. This can be secondary to pituitary corticotroph tumors or hyperplasia producing increased adrenocorticoptropic hormone (ACTH), which leads to bilateral adrenocortical hyperplasia. Hyperadrenocorticism can also result from functional cortisol-secreting adrenocortical neoplasms. Excessive use of exogenous glucocorticoids can result in iatrogenic hyperadrenocorticism.

SYSTEMS AFFECTED
- Renal/Urologic
- Skin/Exocrine
- Cardiovascular
- Respiratory
- Endocrine/Metabolic
- Renal- and skin-related symptoms are most common; presentation may vary from patient to patient.

GENETICS
While a genetic predisposition has not been clearly elucidated, a report of three related hamsters developing hyperadrenocorticism suggests a possibility of genetic predisposition in this species.

INCIDENCE/PREVALENCE
While hyperadrenocorticism is not widely reported in small rodents, its incidence may be underestimated due to the long list of differential diagnoses and the lack of reliable and readily available diagnostic testing.

GEOGRAPHIC DISTRIBUTION
N/A

SIGNALMENT
Breed Predilections
Hyperadrenocorticism has been reported in hamsters and guinea pigs. Rats with pituitary adenoma may develop hyperadrenocorticism, and hypercortisolism has been demonstrated in fur-chewing chinchillas.

Mean Age and Range
Typically, middle-aged to older animals are affected.

Predominant Sex
N/A

SIGNS
Physical Examination Findings
- Hamsters: generalized, progressive, nonpruritic, bilaterally symmetric alopecia, hyperpigmentation, comedones and ulcerations, polyuria/polydypsia (PU/PD), polyphagia, and abdominal distension
- Rats: usually secondary to pituitary adenoma, symptoms first observed include sudden onset ataxia, inability to pick up food, and torticollis

CAUSES
- Increased production of ACTH by pituitary neoplasms
- Increased secretion of cortisol by adrenal neoplasms or adrenal hyperplasia
- Excessive administration of exogenous glucocorticoids

RISK FACTORS
N/A

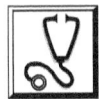

DIAGNOSIS

DIFFERENTIAL DIAGNOSIS
- Ectoparasites
- Hypothyroidism
- Dermatophytosis
- Cutaneous lymphosarcoma
- Fur chewing
- Alopecia of late pregnancy
- Cystic ovarian disease
- Hypovitaminosis C in guinea pigs
- Diabetes mellitus

CBC/BIOCHEMISTRY/URINALYSIS
CBC, serum biochemistry, and urinalysis should be included in the minimum database of all patients with clinical signs suggesting hyperadrenocorticism.

Increased alkaline phosphatase is the most commonly reported biochemical abnormality, and low potassium has been reported in a guinea pig.

High liver enzyme activity, cholesterol, and blood glucose may be noted in some patients.

Eosinopenia, lymphopenia, and leukocytosis are also sometimes observed.

Low urine specific gravity, proteinuria, hematuria, pyuria, and bacteriuria in some patients.

OTHER LABORATORY TESTS
- Measurement of serum cortisol levels
- Urine cortisol/creatinine ratio (low specificity as the ratio can be increased as a result of nonadrenal illness)

IMAGING
- Abdominal radiography to screen for mineralized adrenal tumors, hepatomegaly

- Thoracic radiography to screen for metastasis
- Ultrasound may be used to further evaluate the adrenal glands; CT or MRI could be employed to screen for pituitary adenoma.

DIAGNOSTIC PROCEDURES
- Skin scrape—for ectoparasites and cytologic examintion
- Dermatophyte culture

PATHOLOGIC FINDINGS
- Pituitary chromophobe adenoma—normal to enlarged hypophosis, bilateral adrenocortical enlargement. Microscopically, pituitary adenoma or corticotroph hyperplasia of pars distalis of pars intermedia and adrenocortical hyperplasia
- Adrenal tumor—adrenal mass ± contralateral gland atrophy, metastasis may be present in cases of adrenal carcinoma. Microscopically adrenocortical adenoma or carcinoma.

TREATMENT

APPROPRIATE HEALTH CARE
Will depend on the severity of the presenting signs

NURSING CARE
Hospitalization and supportive care as appropriate depending on the presenting signs

ACTIVITY
N/A

DIET
N/A

CLIENT EDUCATION
Treatment protocols for hyperadrenocorticism are not well established. Lifelong therapy is necessary. Prognosis and potential for adverse reactions to therapy have not been decribed.

SURGICAL CONSIDERATIONS
- Surgical treatment of hyperadrenocorticism is not described in small rodents due to their small size and difficulty and expense of the procedures.
- Hypophysectomy is not recommended due to the difficulty of the procedure and the need for intensive follow-up and lifelong hormone supplementation.

MEDICATIONS

DRUG(S) OF CHOICE
- Very little information is available regarding the efficacy of treatment in rodent

species; medical treatment is anecdotal or limited to individual case reports.
• Trilostane 2–16 mg/kg once daily resulted in good clinical outcome in a guinea pig.

CONTRAINDICATIONS
N/A

PRECAUTIONS
N/A

POSSIBLE INTERACTIONS
N/A

ALTERNATIVE DRUGS
• Ketoconazole (5 mg/kg PO q12h)
• Mitotane (o,p'-DDD) did not result in improvement in a hamster; empirical use of mitotane in guinea pigs has been reported.
• Metyrapone (8 mg PO q24h for 30 days) resulted in hair regrowth in one hamster.

FOLLOW-UP

PATIENT MONITORING
Monitor resolution of clinical symptoms. Where possible, reevaluate serum cortisol and urinalysis in 7 days, 1, 3, and 6 months, and every 6–12 months thereafter.

PREVENTION/AVOIDANCE
N/A

POSSIBLE COMPLICATIONS
N/A

EXPECTED COURSE AND PROGNOSIS
Few reports of treatment of hyperadrenocorticism in small rodents exist. Treatment with metyrapon and trilostane

resulted in improvement of clinical signs for a period of approximately 30 days. The prognosis for this condition in small rodents is poor.

MISCELLANEOUS

ASSOCIATED CONDITIONS
• Neurologic signs in patients with pituitary tumors
• Increased incidence of urinary tract infections and pyoderma

AGE-RELATED FACTORS
N/A

ZOONOTIC POTENTIAL
N/A

PREGNANCY/FERTILITY/ BREEDING
N/A

SYNONYMS
Cushing's disease

SEE ALSO
Alopecia

ABBREVIATIONS
ACTH = adrenocorticotropic hormone
CT = computed tomography
MRI = magnetic resonance imaging
PD = polydypsia
PU = polyuria

INTERNET RESOURCES
Exotic DVM forum for eDVM readers: www. pets.groups.yahoo.com/group/ ExoticDVM Veterinary Information Network: www. vin.com

Suggested Reading
Bauck L, Orr JP, Lawrence KH. Hyperadrenocorticism in three teddy bear hamsters. Can Vet J 1984;25(6):247–250.
Collins BR. Endocrine diseases of rodents. Vet Clin North Am Exot Anim Pract 2008;11(1):153–162.
Frolich J. Rats and mice. In: Quesenberry KE, Carpenter JW, eds. Ferrets, Rabbits and Rodents, 4th Ed). Clinical Medicine and Surgery. 2021 ed. St. Louis: Saunders, 2020:345–367.
Hoppmann E, Barron HW. Rodent dermatology. J Exot Pet Med 2007;16(4):238–255.
Miwa Y, Mayer J. Hamsters and gerbils. In: Quesenberry KE, Carpenter JW, eds. Ferrets, Rabbits and Rodents, 4th Ed). Clinical Medicine and Surgery. 2021 ed. St. Louis: Saunders, 2020:368–384.
Palmerio BS, Roberts H. Clinical approach to dermatologic disease in exotic animals. Vet Clin North Am Exot Anim Pract 2013;16(3):523–577.
Vannevel JY. Clinical presentation of pituitary adenomas in rats. Vet Clin Exot Anim 2006;9(3):673–676.
White SD, Bourdeau PJ, Brément T et al. Companion rats (*Rattus norvegicus*) with cutaneous lesions: a retrospective study of 470 cases at two university veterinary teaching hospitals (1985–2018). Vet Dermatol 2019;30:237–272.

Author Christine Eckermann-Ross, DVM, CVA, CVH

INCISOR MALOCCLUSION AND OVERGROWTH

BASICS

OVERVIEW
This section will review malocclusion in rat-like pet rodents (mouse, hamster, rats, and gerbils). In these species, only the incisors are continuously growing.

Species Differences
• Rodents are grouped into three suborders: the Caviomorph or Hystrycomorph ("guinea pig-like" or "porcupine-like"); the Miomorph ("mouselike" or "ratlike") and the Sciuromorph ("squirrel-like").
• The rat-like group includes the rat (*Rattus* spp.), the mouse (*Mus musculus*), the golden hamster (*Mesocricetus auratus*), the Russian hamster (*Phodopus sungorus, P. campbelli, and P. roborowskii*), the Chinese hamster (*Cricetulus griseus*), the gerbil (*Meriones unguiculatus*), and the duprasi (or "fat-tailed" gerbil, *Pachyuromys duprasi*).
• The squirrel-like group includes many species that can be kept as pets in different countries. Among the most important are the prairie dog (*Cynomis ludovicianus*), the chipmunk (*Tamias striatus*), and the European citellus (*Citellus citellus*).

Anatomy
• All rodent species are Simplicidentata. They have one single row of maxillary incisor teeth.
• All rodent species have one pair of well-developed maxillary and mandibular incisor teeth, representing the best-known anatomical peculiarity of this order.
• While incisor teeth vary slightly in shape, color, and thickness, they are continually growing, open rooted (elodont) in all rodent species.
• All rodents lack canine teeth and have a diastema between the incisor and the first premolar (or molar) tooth.
• Rat-like and squirrel-like rodent species have elodont incisor teeth but anelodont (rooted, not growing throughout life) cheek teeth.
• Rat-like rodents lack premolar teeth; therefore, their dental formula is 2 × 1I 0C 0P 3M = 16
• Dental formula of sciuromorphs is 2 × 1I 0C 1–2/1P 3M = 20–22
• Cheek teeth of rat-like rodents and squirrels have multiple roots

PATHOPHYSIOLOGY
• The primary cause of dental disease in other common pet mammals, such as rabbits, guinea pigs, and chinchillas, is insufficient or improper wearing of cheek teeth due to inappropriate diet, in particular, lack of fiber.

• This syndrome does not occur in rodent species with anelodont cheek teeth. However, these patients can develop dental problems of the cheek teeth due to excessive wearing.
• Primary congenital malocclusion of the incisors in growing rats, hamsters, and squirrels has been reported. This may be difficult to distinguish from malocclusion due to incisor fractures in adult animals, as owners often are not aware that an injury has occurred.
• In these species, acquired malocclusion and severe deviation of incisor teeth occur most often following repeated trauma and fractures.
• Repeated trauma, which interferes with normal tooth eruption, is the most important cause of dysplastic changes (pseudo-odontomas) in prairie dogs. Severe apical deformities act as a space-occupying mass and lead to progressive obstruction of the nasal opening.

SIGNS
Historical Findings
• Rats, hamsters, and other ratlike rodent species are often presented for evident malocclusion of incisor teeth.
• Other historical signs include reduced activity, reduced food intake, emaciation, and ptyalism; diseases of the incisor teeth are often missed by the owner.
• Rat-like rodents generally do not display symptoms related to diseases of the cheek teeth. More common signs include facial swellings related to periapical infection and abscessation, which occasionally affect the ocular and periocular structures.
• Fracture and malocclusion of incisor teeth is common but often missed by the owners. Many owners incorrectly consider frequent incisor fracture and regrowth as normal "shedding" of these teeth.

Physical Examination Findings
• Inspection of the oral cavity while awake is challenging in rodent species; therefore, proper diagnosis of dental disease must be performed under general anesthesia.
• Oral inspection and treatment of dental disease in rodents requires specialized equipment.
• The "tabletop mouth gag and restrainer" is effective on small rodents.
• Inspection by oral endoscopy provides optimal oral visualization for all rodent species. A 14- to 18-cm long, 2.7-mm thick, 30-degree rigid endoscope is commonly used. Other magnification devices are helpful but not always sufficient, and many lesions can be missed without the help of stomatoscopy.
• In rat-like rodents, common findings include slightly elongated or fractured

mandibular incisors and maxillary incisors curved toward the palate.
• Fractures and cavities of the cheek teeth are frequently found in older rodents. The prognosis is poor due to the difficulty of extracting cheek teeth in patients of this size.
• Secondary lesions of the lips, tongue, and palate can be present, including perforation of the hard palate and subsequent oral-nasal fistulas.

CAUSES AND RISK FACTORS
Trauma, such as being dropped, falling, or excessive chewing on hard surfaces such as nuts or cage bars

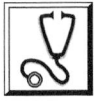

DIAGNOSIS

DIFFERENTIAL DIAGNOSIS
For anorexia—gastrointestinal disease, pain, metabolic disease

CBC/BIOCHEMISTRY/URINALYSIS
Usually normal unless secondary infection or other underlying metabolic disease is present

OTHER LABORATORY TESTS
N/A

IMAGING
• A good to optimal complete radiologic study must include five basic projections (lateral; oblique in two directions; ventrodorsal and rostrocaudal) using very high-definition cassettes and films such as those for mammography.
• Modern CT scans provide excellent detail in small species like rodents.

TREATMENT
The goal of treatment is restoration of dental anatomy to as close to normal as possible.

APPROPRIATE HEALTH CARE
• Unless severely debilitated, coronal reduction is performed on an outpatient basis.
• Provide supportive care, such as fluid therapy and assist feeding, in patients that are not eating.

SURGICAL CONSIDERATIONS
Trimming of Incisors
• A rotating dental unit with a straight handpiece is used, with the addition of smaller metal or silicon burs.
• Trimming should be performed under general anesthesia.
• The mandibular incisors of most rodent species are slightly mobile. Perform trim with

INCISOR MALOCCLUSION AND OVERGROWTH (CONTINUED)

care to avoid separation of the mandible at the symphysis.
• Never perform coronal reduction of cheek teeth in rat-like and squirrel-like rodent species.

Extraction of Incisors
• Extraction of incisor teeth in rats and other smaller rat-like rodents is performed with careful dissection of the periodontal ligament using small (25-gauge) contoured needles.
• The most frequent complications are fracture of the maxillary incisor teeth or separation of the mandibular symphysis during extraction of mandibular incisors.
• Extraction of incisor teeth through an extraoral approach is similar to that described for rabbits. Alternative surgical options are the transpalatal approach, and a dorsal approach via dorsal rhinotomy; lateral approach has been also described.

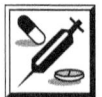

MEDICATIONS

DRUG(S) OF CHOICE
• Antimicrobial drugs are indicated if bacterial infection is evident. Initailly, use broad-spectrum antibiotics such as enrofloxacin (5–20 mg/kg PO, SC, IM q12h), ciprofloxacin (10–20 mg/kg PO q12h), and trimethoprim-sulfa (15–30 mg/kg PO q12h); if anaerobic infections are suspected, use chloramphenicol (30–50 mg/kg PO q8h) or azithromycin (10–30 mg/kg PO q24h).
• Pain management—commonly used pain medications in rats, mice, and hamsters include buprenorphine (0.05–0.1 mg/kg SQ, IM q6–8h), meloxicam (1–2 mg/kg PO, SQ, IM q24h), and tramadol (10–20 mg/kg PO q8–12h).

CONTRAINDICATIONS
Extensive surgery on a debilitated animal

PRECAUTIONS
N/A

FOLLOW-UP

PATIENT MONITORING
• Monitor appetite and the ability to eat following treatment. Some patients may require assist feeding. The duration of assist feeding depends on the severity of disease.
• Reevaluate and trim as needed. Evaluate the entire oral cavity with each recheck.

PREVENTION/AVOIDANCE
N/A

POSSIBLE COMPLICATIONS
Periapical abscesses, recurrence, chronic pain, or inability to chew.

EXPECTED COURSE AND PROGNOSIS
• Dental disease of small rat-like or squirrel-like rodents carries a fair prognosis in cases of uncomplicated malocclusion of incisor teeth.
• Prognosis for diseases related to cheek teeth is guarded to poor due to patient size and the difficulties related to any surgical approach.

MISCELLANEOUS

AGE-RELATED FACTORS
N/A

ZOONOTIC POTENTIAL
N/A

PREGNANCY/FERTILITY/BREEDING
N/A

SYNONYMS
N/A

SEE ALSO
Anorexia and pseudoanorexia

Suggested Reading
Capello V, Gracis M. Lake worth: zoological education network. In: Lennox AM, ed. Rabbit and Rodent Dentistry Handbook, vol. 2007. Ames: Wiley-Blackwell, 2005:276.
Capello V, Lennox AM. Clinical Radiology of Exotic Companion Mammals. Ames: Wiley-Blackwell, 2008.
Dutton M. Selected veterinary concerns of geriatric rats, mice, hamsters, and gerbils. Vet Clin Exot Anim 2020;23(3):525–548.
Frolich J. Rats and mice. In: Quesenberry KE, Carpenter JW, eds. Ferrets, Rabbits and Rodents, 4th Ed). Clinical Medicine and Surgery. 2021 ed. St. Louis: Saunders, 2020:345–367.
Legendre LFJ. Oral disorders of exotic rodents. Vet Clin Exot Anim 2003;6:601–628.
Lennox AM, Capello V, Legendre LF. Small mammal denistry. In: Quesenberry KE, Carpenter JW, eds. Ferrets, Rabbits and Rodents, 4th Ed). Clinical Medicine and Surgery. 2021 ed. St. Louis: Saunders, 2020:514–535.
Mancinelli E, Capello V. Anatomy and disorders of the oral cavity of rat-like and squirrel-like rodents. Vet Clin Exot Anim 2016;19:871–900.
Miwa Y, Mayer J. Hamsters and gerbils. In: Quesenberry KE, Carpenter JW, eds. Ferrets, Rabbits and Rodents, 4th Ed). Clinical Medicine and Surgery. 2021 ed. St. Louis: Saunders, 2020:368–384.
Miwa Y, Sladky K. Common surgical procedures of rodents, ferrets, hedgehogs, and sugar gliders. Vet Clin Exot Anim 2016;19:205–244.

Authors Vittorio Capello, DVM and Barbara Oglesbee, DVM

BASICS

OVERVIEW

• Infection of the gastrointestinal tract by protozoan, cestode, and/or nematode parasites
• Parasites may derive their nutrition from ingesta, microbes within the gut, directly from the host, or a combination of these.
• Concurrent infection by two or more intestinal parasites is possible.
• Some intestinal parasites are copathogens with other enteric infectious agents; may predispose animals to bacterial enteritis, particularly clostridial enterotoxemia and colibacillosis
• The majority of intestinal parasites cause asymptomatic infection in adults and healthy individuals; clinical infection is more likely in young, recently weaned, and immunosuppressed individuals.
• Some parasitic organisms are host specific while others have a broad host range.
• Most parasites affect only a specific part of the digestive tract.
• Clinical signs can be due to competition for nutrients, physical obstruction, malabsorption, blood or protein loss, inflammatory reaction, or tissue destruction.
• Choice of diagnostic and therapeutic measures depends on the severity of illness

SIGNALMENT

• No age, gender, or breed predilection for most parasites.
• Male hosts are generally more heavily parasitized than females.
• Clinical signs tend to be more severe in young and recently weaned animals.

SIGNS

• Vary according to the organ systems and segments of digestive tract affected
• Vary with parasite load and severity of disease
• Range from subclinical to severe; may occur with or without systemic illness
• Anorexia, lethargy, and depression
• Rough hair coat, decreased grooming behavior
• Abdominal pain characterized by hunched posture, reluctance to move, bruxism, and/or pain on abdominal palpation
• Diarrhea, fecal staining of the perineum
• Tenesmus, hematochezia, intestinal obstruction, and rectal prolapse
• Dehydration, hypothermia, hypotension, and weakness
• Abdominal distention—due to thickened or fluid-filled bowel loops, impaction, bloat, masses, or organomegaly

• Fluid or gas may be palpable within the gastrointestinal tract.
• Weight loss in chronically infected animals
• Animals may be found dead in the absence of clinical signs.

CAUSES

Coccidia

• *Eimeria* spp.—protozoan parasites, strictly host specific, affecting mice and rats
• Each species of *Eimeria* typically inhabits a specific segment of the intestine; infection is usually asymptomatic; may cause severe clinical disease in naive, young, or immuno-compromised host
• Multiplication of coccidia in intestinal epithelial cells causes cellular damage and disease; oocysts are shed in the feces; infection occurs by ingestion of oocysts in the environment

Flagellate Protozoans

• *Spironucleus muris*—opportunistic pathogen of mice, rats, and hamsters; inhabits the upper small intestine, feeds on bacteria, invades intervillar crypts, and causes lymphocytic infiltration
• *Giardia* spp.—inhabits the small intestine and cecum and is found in both healthy and symptomatic individuals; organisms attach to surface of enterocytes in small intestine, causing malabsorption. *Giardia* affects mice and hamsters; experimental infection has been reported in gerbils.
• *Giardia* and *Spironucleus* may occur as copathogens, and each organism may act synergistically with other enteric pathogens to cause disease. Primary infections are rare.
• Transmission is by the fecal-oral route; environmentally resistant cysts are ingested from the environment or contaminated water.

Cestodes

• *Rodentolepis* spp. (formerly *Hymenolepis* spp.) tapeworms affect mice, rats, gerbils, and hamsters.
• Tapeworm masses migrate into the anterior two-thirds of the small intestine after the host ingests a meal and then retreat to the posterior two-thirds of the small intestine once the stomach is empty.
• *R. nana* has direct and indirect life cycles. In the former, proglottids are passed in the feces and ova are consumed by another definitive host, or ova can mature in the intestinal lumen and autoinfection can occur. In the latter, an intermediate host (e.g., beetle, cockroach, and flea) consumes the ova before being ingested by another definitive host. In the direct life cycles, tissue migration occurs, causing host reaction. In the indirect life cycle, there is no tissue migration, and minimal host reaction occurs.

• *R. diminuata* only exhibits the indirect life cycle, and minimal host reaction occurs.

Oxyurids

• *Syphacia* spp., *Aspiculuris tetraptera*, and *Dentostomella* spp. pinworms are commensal, mildly or nonpathogenic, ubiquitous, bacteria-feeding nematodes seen in the lower intestinal tract.
• Oxyurids have a direct life cycle. Hosts are infected by ingesting embryonated ova in feces, fecal-contaminated feed, water, or debris, or ova adhered to perianal skin (*Syphacia* spp. only). Oxyurid ova are light and easily aerosolized.
• Male hosts are generally more heavily parasitized than females. Clinical signs are uncommon even with high worm burden, the result of colonic or rectal inflammation. High-fiber diets are reported to reduce worm burdens.
• *Syphacia* spp. infestation may be associated with intestinal impaction, intussusception, and rectal prolapse in mice.
• *Dentostomella* spp. affect gerbils, while *Aspiculuris* spp. affect mice and rats, and *Syphacia* spp. affect mice, rats, gerbils, and hamsters.

RISK FACTORS

• Infected animals in the environment
• Contamination of food or bedding
• Inappropriate husbandry, unsanitary conditions
• Weaning, overcrowding, chilling, stress, and debilitation
• Concurrent illness, presence of copathogens
• Infection may be subclinical until a high parasite load develops.
• Absence of previous exposure predisposes host to more severe effects of infection

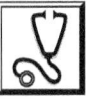

DIAGNOSIS

DIFFERENTIAL DIAGNOSIS

General

• Consider all causes of enteropathy, including diet change, inappropriate antibiotics, enterotoxemia, systemic or metabolic disease, and specific intestinal disorders.
• Infectious causes of enteritis vary by species.

Mice/Rats

• Viruses—mouse hepatitis virus (coronavirus), epizootic diarrhea of infant mice (rotavirus), reovirus, others; neonates especially susceptible
• Bacteria—*Salmonella* spp., *Helicobacter* spp., *Citrobacter rodentium*, *Clostridium piliforme*, *E. coli*, *Enterococcus* spp., others

Gerbils
Bacteria—*Salmonella* spp., *E. coli*, *Clostridium piliforme*, and *Citrobacter rodentium*

Hamsters
Bacteria—*Lawsonia intracellularis*, *Clostridium difficile*, *E. coli*, *Salmonella*, and *Clostridium piliforme*

CBC/BIOCHEMISTRY/URINALYSIS
Usually normal; may be hemoconcentrated if dehydrated

OTHER LABORATORY TESTS
N/A

IMAGING
N/A

DIAGNOSTIC PROCEDURES
• Fecal floatation will reveal nematode and cestode ova, coccidia oocysts, and protozoan cysts; not reliable for tapeworm detection as cestode ova are not shed individually but reach the environment via proglottids shed in the feces
• Fecal direct examination under saline reveals motile protozoans; the addition of Lugol's iodine stops motion, stains intracellular nuclear structures and glycogen masses, and helps to identify protozoan cysts.
• Fecal ELISA for *Giardia*
• Intestinal scraping wet mount or impression smear of necropsy specimens for coccidia detection
• Histopathology or PCR for *Spironucleus*

PATHOLOGIC FINDINGS
• Coccidia—no gross lesions, or dilatation of the small intestine with watery or hemorrhagic content, serosal hyperemia, and edema
• Flagellates—*Spironucleus* anterior small intestinal distention with bubbly froth, possibly with blood; thickened duodenal wall; enlarged mesenteric lymph nodes; ascites. *Giardia* inhabits the small intestine but causes little or no damage; it may disrupt intestinal epithelium during attachment, or less likely by direct invasion
• Cestodes—adult tapeworms are found in the intestinal lumen, and occasionally in the pancreatic and biliary ducts
• Oxyurids—pinworm infection rarely causes gross lesions; intussusception and catarrhal enteritis may be evident; adult worms are visible in the intestinal contents and in close association with the mucosa

TREATMENT
• Usually treated as an outpatient
• Inpatient treatment if debilitated
• Fluid therapy if dehydrated

MEDICATIONS
DRUG(S) OF CHOICE
• Coccidia—toltrazuril (10 mg/kg PO q24h × 3 days, skip 3–5 days, repeat for 3 days); sulfadimethoxine (50 mg/kg PO once, then 25 mg/kg q24h × 10–20 days)
• Flagellates—metronidazole (20 mg/kg PO q12h); dose cited is anecdotal and lower than that found in many citations; duration of treatment for small rodents not reported, but 5 days is typical for other small mammals); also, for *Giardia*—fenbendazole (20 mg/kg PO q24h × 5 days). Reports suggest there may be no effective treatment for *Spironucleus*.
• Cestodes—praziquantal (6–10 mg/kg PO or SQ, repeat in 10 days)
• Oxyurids—fenbendazole (20 mg/kg PO q24h × 5 days), pyrantel pamoate (50 mg/kg PO; dosing interval for small rodents not reported, but dose is repeated in 10 days for most other exotic companion mammals)
• Treat all identified copathogens.

PRECAUTIONS
Metronidazole is neurotoxic if overdosed.

FOLLOW-UP
PATIENT MONITORING
Fecal examination to confirm efficacy of treatment

PREVENTION/AVOIDANCE
• Reducing stress, providing excellent husbandry
• Good sanitation, clean food and bedding
• Screening and quarantine of incoming stock
• Control of vectors and wild animal parasite hosts

MISCELLANEOUS
ZOONOTIC POTENTIAL
• *Rodentolepis* spp. tapeworms
• *Giardia* is the most common intestinal parasite in humans in North America; *Giardia* spp. may not be highly host specific and zoonotic transmission from animals to humans may occur.

SEE ALSO
Diarrhea
Rectal prolapse

ABBREVIATIONS
ELISA = enzyme-linked immunosorbent assay
PCR = polymerase chain reaction

Suggested Reading
Dutton M. Selected veterinary concerns of geriatric rats, mice, hamsters, and gerbils. Vet Clin Exot Anim 2020;23(3):525–548.
Frolich J. Rats and mice. In: Quesenberry KE, Carpenter JW, eds. Ferrets, Rabbits and Rodents, 4th Ed). Clinical Medicine and Surgery. 2021 ed. St. Louis: Saunders, 2020:345–367.
Hrapkiewicz K, Colby L, Denison P, eds. Clinical Laboratory Animal Medicine: An Introduction, 4th ed. Ames: Wiley-Blackwell, 2013:83–92, 128–133, 156–159, 182–187.
Jekl V, Knotek Z. Evidence-based advances in rodent medicine. Vet Clin Exot Anim 2017;20:805–816.
Mayer J, Mans C. Rodents. In: Carpenter JW, ed. Exotic Animal Formulary, 5th ed. St Louis: Elsevier, 2018:459–493.
Mitchell MA, Tully TN, eds. Manual of Exotic Pet Practice. St Louis: Elsevier, 2009:326–344, 406–432.
Miwa Y, Mayer J. Hamsters and gerbils. In: Quesenberry KE, Carpenter JW, eds. Ferrets, Rabbits and Rodents, 4th Ed). Clinical Medicine and Surgery. 2021 ed. St. Louis: Saunders, 2020:368–384.

Author Dan H. Johnson, DVM, Dipl. ABVP (Exotic Companion Mammal)

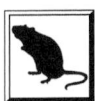

BASICS

DEFINITION
Result of microbial colonization of the urinary bladder and/or the proximal portion of the urethra

PATHOPHYSIOLOGY
• Microbes, usually aerobic bacteria, ascend the urinary tract under conditions that permit them to persist in the urine or adhere to the epithelium and subsequently multiply. Urinary tract colonization requires at least transient impairment of the mechanisms that normally defend against infection. This could be induced by any cause of inflammation in the urinary tract (uroliths, crystals in the urine, neoplasia, and parasites) or by ascending or descending infection (infection of the genital tract or of the kidneys).
• Inflammation of infected tissues results in the clinical signs and laboratory test abnormalities exhibited by patients.

SYSTEMS AFFECTED
Renal/Urologic—lower urinary tract

GENETICS
N/A

INCIDENCE/PREVALENCE
• Urinary tract infection secondary to uroliths are rare in mice and rats; described in hamsters
• Copulatory plug infections are common in rats.

GEOGRAPHIC DISTRIBUTION
Worldwide

SIGNALMENT
Breed Predilections
N/A

Mean Age and Range
More common in older animals

Predominant Sex
N/A

SIGNS
Historical Findings
• None in some patients
• Pollakiuria—frequent voiding of small volume
• Urinating in places that are not customary
• Hematuria
• Urine scald

Physical Examination Findings
• The bladder may be enlarged and painful on palpation
• Automutilation of the penis (mice)
• No abnormalities in some animals

CAUSES
• Bacterial—*Esherichia coli* and *Pseudomonas* spp. are common causes of bacterial cystitis. Urethral obstruction as a result of *S. aureus* in the preputial gland and *P. pneumotropica* bulbourethral infections is described in rats.
• Parasitic—bladder threadworm *Trichomoide crassicauda* in rats
• Uroliths and crystals—bladder stones consisting of struvite; crystals of ammonium magnesium phosphate, mixed carbonate and oxalate, and mixed carbonate, phosphate, magnesium, and calcium in rats
• Mucoid calculi—part of copulatory plugs found in the urethra and bladder of rats

RISK FACTORS
• Conditions that cause urine stasis or incomplete emptying of the bladder—inadequate exercise, cage confinement, or painful conditions (reluctance to move)
• Inadequate water intake—dirty water bowls, unpalatable water, changing water source, and inadequate water provision
• Urine retention—underlying bladder pathology, neuromuscular disease
• Inadequate cleaning of the cage—may cause some animals to avoid urinating for abnormally long periods
• Injury of the penis—as a result of aggressive breeding activity and abrasion on the cage in male mice
• Obesity, lack of exercise
• Diet—high calcium diet or magnesium deficiency, elevated dietary phosphorus, and diet preparations with a low calcium-to-phosphorus ratio

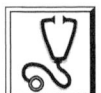

DIAGNOSIS

DIFFERENTIAL DIAGNOSIS
• Females with pyometra, uterine neoplasia, or other uterine disorders may expel blood or a thick, often blood-tinged vaginal discharge when urinating. This discharge may mix with urine and mimic lower urinary tract infection. Obtain urine sample via cystocentesis to differentiate.
• Lower urinary tract neoplasia
• Differentiate from other causes by urinalysis, urine culture, radiography, and ultrasonography.

CBC/BIOCHEMISTRY/URINALYSIS
• Leukocytosis—may be seen, but this finding is rare
• Postrenal azotemia (e.g., high BUN, creatinine, and phosphorus)—if complete urinary outflow obstruction
• Crystals in urinary sediment—ammonium magnesium phosphate, mixed carbonate and oxalate, mixed carbonate, phosphate, magnesium, and calcium
• Pyuria, hematuria, and proteinuria—indicate a urinary tract inflammation, but these are nonspecific findings that may result from infectious and noninfectious causes of lower urinary tract disease; mild proteinuria is often normal in these species
• Bacteria—rarely observed on urinalysis even in animals with significant lower urinary tract infection

OTHER LABORATORY TESTS
• Urine culture and sensitivity testing—necessary for definitive diagnosis. Correct interpretation of the urine culture results requires obtaining the specimen in a manner that minimizes contamination, handling and storing the specimen so that numbers of viable bacteria do not change in vitro, and using a quantitative culture method. Place the specimen in a sealed, sterile container; if the culture is not started right away, the urine can be refrigerated for up to 8 hours without important change in the results.
• Cystocentesis—preferred technique for obtaining urine for culture
• Culture biopsy—sample collected from the bladder wall if cystotomy is performed

IMAGING
• Survey and contrast radiographic studies—could demonstrate a radiopaque stone in the bladder or the urethra
• Ultrasound—detection of urolith, crystalluria, inflammation of the bladder or the urethra (thickening of the wall), mass on the bladder or the urethra. Ultrasound can also assess the uterus to rule out genital disorder.

DIAGNOSTIC PROCEDURES
Cystoscopy—only possible in rats, allow to detect and treat urinary stones (lithotripsy by laser), to visualize the bladder and urethra wall, and to take samples.

PATHOLOGIC FINDINGS
N/A

TREATMENT

APPROPRIATE HEALTH CARE
Treat as outpatient unless another urinary abnormality (e.g., obstruction) requires inpatient treatment.

NURSING CARE
• Fluid therapy—if patient dehydrated, 200 mL/kg/24h (double maintenance fluids); if subcutaneous, give bolus q8h
• Treat associated urine scald with gentle cleaning; keep the area clean and dry; and apply zinc oxide plus menthol powder to clean the skin q24h.

LOWER URINARY TRACT INFECTION (CONTINUED)

ACTIVITY
N/A

DIET
• Increase water consumption. Provide multiple sources of fresh water. Flavoring the water with fruit juice (with no added sugar) or artificial sweetener is usually helpful. Provide a variety of clean, fresh, leafy vegetables sprayed or soaked with water.
• Provide a diet with a good calcium-to-phosphorus ratio and an adequate magnesium level.

CLIENT EDUCATION
• Urolith removal does not alter the factors responsible for their formation; eliminating risk factors such as obesity, sedentary life, and poor diet combined with increasing water consumption is necessary to minimize recurrence. Even with these changes, however, recurrence is likely.
• Frequent cleaning of the cage is essential to prevent recurrence of the infection.

SURGICAL CONSIDERATIONS
Except when a concomitant disorder requires surgical intervention, management does not involve surgery.

Uroliths within the bladder, urethra, or mass obstructing the lower urinary tract must be removed surgically. The procedure is similar to those performed in dogs and cats.

MEDICATIONS
DRUG(S) OF CHOICE
• Base choice of antibiotic on result of sensitivity testing; antibiotics that concentrate in the urine are most appropriate. Initial choices include trimethoprim-sulfa (15–30 mg/kg PO q12h), chloramphenicol (30–50 mg/kg PO q 12h), or as a second line enrofloxacin (5–20 mg/kg PO, SC, IM q12h).
• Pain management may aid urination and promote appetite. NSAIDs (meloxicam 1–2 mg/kg PO, SC, IM q24h) reduce pain and may decrease inflammation in the bladder.
• Antispasmodic: diazepam (1–2 mg/kg IM) and midazolam (1 mg/kg IM)
• Ivermectin (0.3–0.5 mg/kg SC repeated 10 days after the first treatment) for rats with bladder threadworm

CONTRAINDICATIONS
• Large amount of fluids if the patient is suffering from a total obstruction of the urinary tract
• Glucocorticoids or other immunosuppressive agents
• Potentially nephrotoxic drugs (e.g., aminoglycosides, NSAIDs) in patients that are febrile, dehydrated, or azotemic or that

are suspected of having pyelonephritis, septicemia, or preexisting renal disease

PRECAUTIONS
Enrofloxacin SC could cause some skin necrosis, needs to be diluted at least 1:1 with saline

POSSIBLE INTERACTIONS
N/A

ALTERNATIVE DRUGS
N/A

FOLLOW-UP
PATIENT MONITORING
• When antibacterial drug efficacy is in doubt, culture the urine 2–3 days after starting treatment. If the drug is effective, the culture will be negative.
• Rapid recrudescence of signs when treatment is stopped generally indicates either a concurrent urinary tract abnormality or that the infection extends into some deep-seated site (e.g., renal parenchyma)
• Successful cure of an episode of urinary tract infection is best demonstrated by performing a urine culture 7–10 days after completing antimicrobial therapy.

PREVENTION/AVOIDANCE
• Increase water consumption for the remainder of the animal's life.
• Place patient on an appropriate diet.
• Increase exercise.
• Provide good hygiene of the cage.

POSSIBLE COMPLICATIONS
• Urine scald; myasis; pododermatitis
• Failure to detect or to treat effectively may lead to pyelonephritis

EXPECTED COURSE AND PROGNOSIS
• If not treated, expect infection to persist indefinitely.
• Generally, the prognosis for animals with uncomplicated lower urinary tract infection is good to excellent. The prognosis for an animal with complicated infection is determined by the prognosis of the other urinary abnormality.
• The prognosis following the surgical removal of a urolith or urohydropropulsion for the removal of calcium sand is fair to good. Although dietary management may decrease the likelihood of recurrence, many animals will develop clinical disease again within 1–2 years.

MISCELLANEOUS
ASSOCIATED CONDITIONS
• Genital infections

• Dermatitis of the inguinal area
• Obesity

AGE-RELATED FACTORS
Complicated infection is more common in middle-aged to old than young animals.

ZOONOTIC POTENTIAL
Leptospirosis—rat and mouse are capable of carrying leptospirosis without showing any clinical signs; rodents are the prime vector of the disease

PREGNANCY/FERTILITY/BREEDING
N/A

SYNONYMS
Bacterial cystitis

SEE ALSO
Hematuria
Renal failure

ABBREVIATIONS
BUN = blood urea nitrogen
NSAID = nonsteroidal anti-inflammatory drug

Suggested Reading
Dutton M. Selected veterinary concerns of geriatric rats, mice, hamsters, and gerbils. Vet Clin Exot Anim 2020;23(3):525–548.
Frolich J. Rats and mice. In: Quesenberry KE, Carpenter JW, eds. Ferrets, Rabbits and Rodents, 4th Ed). Clinical Medicine and Surgery. 2021 ed. St. Louis: Saunders, 2020:345–367.
Hallman RM, Brandão J. Diagnostic imaging of the renal system in exotic companion mammals. Vet Clin Exot Anim 2020;23:195–214.
Jekl V, Knotek Z. Evidence-based advances in rodent medicine. Vet Clin Exot Anim 2017;20:805–816.
Lennox AM, Gladden JN. Emergency and critical care of small mammals. In: Quesenberry KE, Carpenter JW, eds. Ferrets, Rabbits and Rodents, 4th Ed). Clinical Medicine and Surgery. 2021 ed. St. Louis: Saunders, 2020:595–608.
Miwa Y, Mayer J. Hamsters and gerbils. In: Quesenberry KE, Carpenter JW, eds. Ferrets, Rabbits and Rodents, 4th Ed). Clinical Medicine and Surgery. 2021 ed. St. Louis: Saunders, 2020:368–384.
Percy DH, Barthold SW. Rat amyloidosis. In: Percy DH, Barthold SW, eds. Pathology of Laboratory Rodents and Rabbits, 3rd ed. Ames: Blackwell, 2007:200–202.
Petrini D, Di Giuseppe M, Deli G et al. Cystolithiasis in a Syrian hamster: a different outcome. Open Vet J 2016;6(2):135–138.
Reavill DR, Lennox AM. Disease overview of the urinary tract in exotic companion mammals and tips on clinical management. Vet Clin Exot Anim 2020;23(1):169–193.
Author Charly Pignon, DVM Dip ECZM (Small Mammal)

RODENTS

BASICS

DEFINITION
Malignant and benign tumors involving the mammary gland tissue

PATHOPHYSIOLOGY
• Rats—prolactin favors the multiplication of the tumor cells and inhibits their apoptosis. Because estrus in rats happens every 3–5 days and induces secretion of prolactin, tumors grow rapidly. This growth can be accelerated by autonomous secretion of prolactin by the tumor itself, lactation, or could be accelerated by a pituitary adenoma that secretes prolactin. 90% of rat mammary tumors are benign fibroadenomas but can recur. 10% are malignant adenocarcinomas; however, their potential for local invasion is slow and metastasis occurs late.
• Mice and gerbils—most mammary tumors are malignant (90% in mice), rapidly metastasize, are invasive, and are difficult to remove. In mice, tumor growth can be prolactin, progesterone, or estrogen dependent.
• Hamster—most mammary tumors are benign

SYSTEMS AFFECTED
• Reproductive
• Metastasis sites—lungs, lymph nodes, and other system
• Nervous (in rats with pituitary tumors)

GENETICS
In lab animals, it has been shown that certain strains of rats and mice were predisposed to develop mammary tumor.

INCIDENCE/PREVALENCE
• Mammary tumors are the most common tumor type in female rats and develop in 30%–90% of intact female rats (depending on the strain of rat). The incidence is 0.5%–16% of intact males. They are uncommon in rats younger than 1 year of age.
• Seen in 1%–6% of mice
• Tumors are rare in gerbils and hamsters.

GEOGRAPHIC DISTRIBUTION
Worldwide

SIGNALMENT

Breed Predilections
Certain laboratory rodents have a genetic predisposition.

Predominant Sex
Females are more commonly affected, but males can also develop mammary tumors.

SIGNS

Historical Findings
• Growth can occur rapidly, becoming very large in a period as short as a few weeks and become half or more of the body size of the rat.
• In rats and mice, tumors can be located anywhere from the cervical to the inguinal region ventrally, dorsally over the shoulder regions, and on the flanks.
• In hamsters and gerbils, tumors are generally confined to ventral thorax and abdomen.

Physical Examination Findings
• Single or multiple (less common) large, spherical, firm subcutaneous masses; usually not attached to deeper structures.
• A mass less spherical in shape and with adhesion to underlying musculature suggests a malignant tumor.
• Masses can be very large (up to one-third of the animal body weight) and can become ulcerated.
• Concurrent reproductive tract disorders are common in female rats. May find vaginal discharge, hematuria (due to blood expelled from the uterus during micturition), or palpable uterine enlargement

CAUSES
• In rats, mammary tumors can be secondary to prolactin-secreting pituitary adenomas; genetic predisposition in many strains
• Mouse mammary tumor virus (MMTV-S or Bittner virus) predisposes to the development of mammary adenocarcinoma and is passed transplacentally and through the milk.

RISK FACTORS
• Intact female
• Age—more common in rats >2 years old. Older rats of both sexes develop high levels of prolactin secretion, stimulating tumor growth and formation
• Chronic stress
• Obesity—in rats, more common in obese animals on high-fat diets
• Prolactin-secreting pituitary tumors (rats)

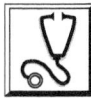

DIAGNOSIS

DIFFERENTIAL DIAGNOSIS
• Subcutaneous abscess—secondary to trauma or bites by cage mate
• Mastitis—common in hamsters after parturition when the young are 7–10 days old. The affected glands are warm and swollen with a hemorrhagic discharge.

• Hyperplasia or cyst of the mammary gland. With continuous stimulation of mammary tissue, can progress to mammary tumor.
• Lipoma
• Mast cell tumor
• Sarcoma
• Squamous cell carcinoma

CBC/BIOCHEMISTRY/ URINALYSIS
Nonspecific findings, usually normal

OTHER LABORATORY TESTS
• Fine-needle aspiration of the mass—may be helpful in differentiating benign, malignant tumor, mastitis
• Fine-needle aspiration of the regional lymph node—to identify metastasis if adenocarcinoma suspected

IMAGING
Thoracic radiography—to detect metastasis if malignant tumor suspected. Rare occurrence in rats, but radiographs are highly recommended in mice as pulmonary metastases are frequent.
   Whole body radiographs or ultrasound to identify concurrent reproductive disease (uterine, ovarian) in female rats.

DIAGNOSTIC PROCEDURES
Excisional biopsy—histologic evaluation for definitive diagnosis

PATHOLOGIC FINDINGS
• Gross—most tumors are well-circumscribed, round or multilobular, and easily separated from surrounding tissues. Malignant tumors sometimes invade into skin and underlying musculature.
• Histopathology—adenoma, fibroadenoma, fibroma, adenolipoma (rare), and adenocarcinoma. In Djungarians hamster, a retrospective pathology study described adenomas, adenocarcinomas, lipid-rich carcinoma, adenoacanthomas, malignant adenomyoepitheliomas, and "balloon cell" carcinosarcomas.

TREATMENT

APPROPRIATE HEALTH CARE
• Even very large masses are generally well tolerated by the animal; however, early surgical removal is recommended.
• Most are treated as outpatients following surgical excision.

NURSING CARE
Assist feeding and fluid therapy if the patient is not able to eat and drink

ACTIVITY
Decrease activity level following surgical removal by confining to cage and removing exercise wheels.

DIET
- Assist feed anorexic patients.
- Provide a high-quality, low-fat diet to prevent obesity

CLIENT EDUCATION
- Advise client to monitor for mammary tumors in all rodents. The prognosis improves with early removal and diagnosis; however, even with benign tumors, recurrence in the same or other locations is common.
- Advice clients of the benefits of ovariohysterectomy in nonbreeding animals.

SURGICAL CONSIDERATIONS
- A nodulectomy is recommended as excision of the entire mammary chain is not possible due to the extensive nature of mammary tissue.
- With benign small masses, removal can be achieved via a simple incision in the overlying skin, shelling out the underlying mass.
- With ulcerated large masses, or suspected malignant masses, remove via an elliptical incision with wide margins.
- With large or malignant tumors, pay particular attention to hemostasis, as large blood vessels are often supplying the tumor.
- The skin is closed with a subcutaneous or intradermal continuous pattern. Tissue glue is used to close the skin. Skin sutures should be avoided because of the risk of the rodent chewing the sutures.
- Local block with lidocaine around the incision in addition to general anesthesia is recommended.
- Radiation therapy could be considered in malignant tumors if the excision margins are not clear.
- Ovariohysterectomy should be performed if concurrent reproductive disorders are identified or suspected.
- Ovariohysterectomy in rats prior to 90 days of age may prevent tumor formation. It is possible that OHE in older rats with or without tumors may prevent future recurrence.

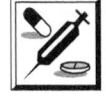

MEDICATIONS

DRUG(S) OF CHOICE

Pain Management
- Buprenorphine (0.05–1.0 mg/kg SC, IV q6–8h)
- Oxymorphone (0.2–0.5 mg/kg SC IM q6–12h)
- Morphine (2–5 mg/kg IM q4h)
- Meloxicam (1–2 mg/kg SC, PO q24)

Antibiotics
Indicated in large masses with ulceration. Use trimethoprim-sulfa (15–30 mg/kg PO q12h).

Chemotherapy
Doxorubicin and toceranib have been used in mice with malignant mammary tumors.

PRECAUTIONS
- Meloxicam—use with caution in animals with compromised renal function
- Doxorubicin—myelotoxicity, compromised myocardial function

POSSIBLE INTERACTIONS
N/A

ALTERNATIVE DRUGS
- Cabergoline (0.6 mg/kg q72h)—antidopaminergic molecule that decreases the secretion of prolactin, thereby inhibiting the stimulation of the mammary tissue by the prolactin. This is particularly useful if a pituitary adenoma is suspected, but also may prevent tumor recurrence in rats without pituitary tumors as it decreased prolactin secretion.
- Deslorelin acetate 4.7 mg implants SC q12 months—anecdotally may be effective in preventing mammary tumors in some rats when given at an early age, but definitive supportive data is lacking.
- Tamoxifen, used in the treatment of mammary tumors in humans, should not be used in rats, as tumors are mediated by prolactin secretion, not estrogens.

FOLLOW-UP

PATIENT MONITORING
- Postoperatively, monitor the suture line. Rodents are extremely likely to chew sutures and open the wound. An Elizabethan collar and/or bandaging may be needed.
- Monitor for signs of pain (reluctance to move, teeth grinding) postoperatively.
- Monitor the appetite.
- Recheck at 1 week to assess the healing of the surgical wound.
- Complete physical examination bimonthly, with emphasis on palpation of the mammary tissue and axillary and inguinal lymph node region for recurrence.

PREVENTION/AVOIDANCE
Ovariohysterecomy or castration may be helpful in preventing tumors or tumor recurrence after mass removal. It has been observed that spaying rats surgically or with a deslorelin acetate implant at 3–6 months of age had a protective effect against the formation of a mammary tumor.

POSSIBLE COMPLICATIONS
- Suture line dehiscence
- Self-mutilation
- Regrowth of the mass if the margins are not clean
- Recurrence of fibroadenoma in rats

EXPECTED COURSE AND PROGNOSIS
The prognosis is fair in rats and hamsters, guarded in gerbils, poor in mice.

MISCELLANEOUS

ASSOCIATED CONDITIONS
Pituitary tumors

AGE-RELATED FACTORS
Older animals are more likely to develop a mammary tumor.

ZOONOTIC POTENTIAL
N/A

PREGNANCY/FERTILITY/BREEDING
Tumors grow more rapidly in pregnant rats due to high levels of prolactin secretion.

SYNONYMS
N/A

SEE ALSO
N/A

ABBREVIATIONS
N/A

INTERNET RESOURCES
N/A

Suggested Reading
Bennett AR. Mammary gland neoplasia. In: Quesenberry KE, Carpenter JW, eds. Ferrets, Rabbits, and Rodents: Clinical Medicine and Surgery, 3rd ed. Elsevier, 2012:282–284.
Greenacre CB. Spontaneous tumors of small mammals. Vet Clin Exot Anim 2004;7:627–652.
Hotchkiss C. Effect of surgical removal of subcutaneous tumors on survival of rats. J Am Vet Med Assoc 1995;206:1575–1579.
Martorell J. Reproductive disorders in pet rodents. Vet Clin Exot Anim 2017;20: 589–608.
Planas-Silva MD, Rutherford TM, Stone MC. Prevention of age-related spontaneous mammary tumors in outbred rats by late ovariectomy. Cancer Detect Prev 2008;32:65–71.

Richardson VCG. Hamster reproductive system. In: VCG R, ed.. Diseases of Small Domestic Rodents. Oxford, UK: Blackwell, 2003a:147–153.

Richardson VCG. Mice reproductive system. In: VCG R, ed.. Diseases of Small Domestic Rodents. Oxford, UK: Blackwell, 2003b:188–193.

Vergneau-Grosset S, Keel MK, Goldsmith D et al. Description of the prevalence, histologic characteristics, concomitant abnormalities, and outcomes of mammary gland tumors in companion rats (*Rattus Norvegicus*). J Am Vet Med Assoc 2016;249(10):1170–1179.

Vergneau-Grosset S, Pena L, Hubbard NE et al. Evaluation of deslorelin implant on mammary fibroadenoma recurrence in rats (*Rattus Norvegicus*). Proc ICARE 2017:107–108.

Yoshimura H, Kimura-Tsukada N, Michishita M et al. Characterization of spontaneous mammary tumors in domestic Djungarian hamsters (*Phodopus sungorus*). Vet Pathol 2015;52(6):1227–1234.

Author Charly Pignon, DVM, Dip ECZM (Small Mammal)

MYCOPLASMOSIS AND CHRONIC RESPIRATORY DISEASE

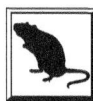

BASICS

DEFINITION
• Chronic respiratory disease (CRD) is a condition defined by persistent infection despite appropriate and aggressive treatment.
• *Mycoplasma* spp. are gram negative, cell wall free, facultative anaerobic bacteria, often implicated in respiratory disease of rats and mice.
• *Mycoplasma pulmonis* is the major pathogen causing CRD in rats. *M. arthritidis* or *M. neurolyticum* (mice) may also play a role.

PATHOPHYSIOLOGY
• Mycoplasma are common inhabitants of the respiratory tract of rats and occasionally mice. Disease depends on the virulence of individual strains of mycoplasma, along with genetic susceptibility and immunocompetence of the host.
• *Mycoplasma* spp. have been isolated in other rodents but rarely associated with clinical disease
• Transmission is primarily aerosol via respiratory secretions; however, intrauterine transmission may also occur.
• Although *M. pulmonis* alone is often the primary pathogen causing respiratory disease in rats and mice, most CRD is caused by a combination of mycoplasma and other agents. Viruses such as Sendai virus (parainfluenza), sialodacryoadenitis virus, rat respiratory virus (hantavirus), or pneumonia virus of rats (paramyxovirus) can act as synergistic agents. Secondary bacterial infections are common, especially with *Streptococcus pneumoniae*, *Corynebacterium kutscheri*, or cilia-associated respiratory bacillus.
• *Mycoplasma* spp. attach to respiratory epithelial cells, causing destruction of cilia, which predisposes to secondary bacterial infections.
• In genetically susceptible rats, virulent strains of *Mycoplasma pulmonis* can cause destruction of mucosa, cartilage, and bone in nasal passages, or bronchioectasis and chronic pneumonia.
• Infection stimulates excessive production and decreased clearance of respiratory mucus. This excessive mucus contributes significantly to symptoms (stertor, dyspnea) and produces a bacterial biofilm that protects bacteria from antibiotic treatment.
• Mycoplasma incite a marked lymphocytic response in susceptible rats, suggestive of an exaggerated immune response.
• Chronic mycoplasmosis often causes irreversible changes in the lungs such as bronchioectasis and consolidation of lung lobes. Eradication from these animals is unlikely, and chronic reccurring respiratory disease is common.
• Mycoplasma organisms may spread to the inner ear via the eustachian tube, causing otitis interna/media.

SYSTEMS AFFECTED
• Respiratory
• Neurologic—with otitis interna/media
• Cardiovascular secondarily affected

GENETICS
N/A

INCIDENCE/PREVALENCE
• Very common disease in both pet populations and research colonies of rats. Intensive efforts to eliminate from laboratory colonies resulted in marked reduction but not elimination.
• A single survey in laboratory rats showed that while prevalence of mycoplasma approached 100%, most animals remained asymptomatic
• Less common in mice
• Surveys of wild rats in the United States demonstrate the presence of antibodies in 72.9%.

GEOGRAPHIC DISTRIBUTION
Ubiquitous

SIGNALMENT
• Common in rats, less so in mice; rare in other rodents
• No specific sex predilection
• More common in older animals (not seen in animals under 3 months of age)
• Stress, aging, and concurrent disease predispose to outbreaks.

SIGNS

Historical Findings
• Exposure to other rodents
• Rats/mice with CRD often have history of past upper respiratory infection
• Often a history of recurrent episodes of respiratory signs, with or without treatment

Physical Examination Findings
• Upper respiratory tract disease—sneezing, nasal and ocular discharge, increased respiratory sounds (stertor, "snoring"), porphyrin discharge (red tears)
• Acute respiratory distress—increased respiratory rate, profound dyspnea; may progress to respiratory arrest
• Otitis interna/media—head tilt, circling, and nystagmus
• Lower respiratory tract disease—poor hair coat, weight loss, emaciation, and dyspnea
• Auscultation findings variable and may be related to upper or lower respiratory tract
• Patients may otherwise appear bright and alert to severely depressed or comatose, with varying degrees of anorexia and dehydration.

CAUSES
• *Mycoplasma pulmonis* most common primary pathogen; *M. arthritidis* or *M. nerolyticum* (in mice) may also play a role.
• Other viruses such as Sendai virus (parainfluenza), sialodacryoadenitis (SDA) virus, rat respiratory virus (RRV; hantavirus), or pneumonia virus of rats (paramyxovirus) act synergetically as copathogens.
• Secondary bacterial infections are common and include *Streptococcus pneumoniae*, *Corynebacterium kutscheri*, and cilia-associated respiratory bacillus.

RISK FACTORS
• Contact with other infected animals, although probability of obtaining a mycoplasma-free rat is unlikely
• Poor husbandry, especially overcrowding; poor sanitation; and poor airflow increase risk for development of clinical disease.
• Other sources of immune suppression may predispose to clinical disease.

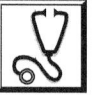

DIAGNOSIS

DIFFERENTIAL DIAGNOSIS
• Upper respiratory disease produced by other conditions such as neoplasia, dental disease, nasal foreign body, facial trauma, allergy, or irritants
• Lower respiratory disease produced by other conditions such as cardiac disease, trauma (pulmonary contusions, hemo- or pneumothorax), and neoplasia
• Cardiac disease may present as increased respiratory rate and effort; differentiate based on physical examination and radiographs
• Young rats (<3 months of age) with upper respiratory tract signs are more likely to have viral disease (SDA virus) alone that is usually self-limiting.
• History and signalment are usually suggestive of CRD

CBC/BIOCHEMISTRY/URINALYSIS
Testing is useful to identify other concurrent disease processes but does not confirm the diagnosis of mycoplasma pneumonia.

OTHER LABORATORY TESTS
• Serologic testing (ELISA) is available for *Mycoplasma* spp., SDA, RRV, and Sendai virus.
• Polymerase chain reaction testing is available for *Mycoplasma* sp. in both mice and rats and is more reliable than isolation on culture.
• Culture—*Mycoplasma* spp. are extremely difficult and time consuming to demonstrate on culture, and it may fail to detect the organism. Culture and susceptibility testing

(CONTINUED) MYCOPLASMOSIS AND CHRONIC RESPIRATORY DISEASE

for other, concurrent bacterial infections is helpful in directing antibiotic therapy.

IMAGING
• Radiography and ultrasonography—may identify abnormalities such as collapsed lungs and pulmonary abscess, which is extremely helpful in formulating prognosis
• Useful in ruling out cardiac disease

DIAGNOSTIC PROCEDURES
• Response to antibiotic therapy as a trial
• Diagnostic procedures such as transtracheal washing and bronchoaveolar lavage are not possible due to small patient size.

PATHOLOGIC FINDINGS
• Serous to catarrhal exudate found in nasal passages, trachea, and major airways
• With CRD—bronchioectasis with mucoid to purulent exudate in lumina; macrophages, neutrophils, and lymphocytic infiltration into respiratory epithelium and alveolar spaces.

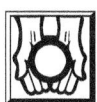

TREATMENT

APPROPRIATE HEALTH CARE
• Inpatient—severely debilitated animals or those in respiratory distress require hospitalization
• Outpatient care for stable animals

NURSING CARE
• Patients in respiratory distress require oxygen therapy.
• Supportive care, including correction of dehydration and hypovolemia, and support feeding
• Specific treatment of other underlying disorders

CLIENT EDUCATION
• Inform clients that *Mycoplasma* spp. in rats is extremely difficult to eliminate; many cases are chronic and recurrence is common. Cases with severe lung lesions will likely not respond.
• Advise owners to correct husbandry deficiencies, in particular, to improve sanitation and remove irritating bedding.

MEDICATIONS

DRUG(S) OF CHOICE
Antibiotics
• In rats, if *Mycoplasma pulmonis* is suspected or confirmed, treat with a combination of enrofloxacin (10 mg/kg PO q12h) and doxycycline (5 mg/kg PO q12h) for a minimum of 2 weeks. With CRD, long-term treatment or lifelong intermittent treatment

may be needed. The combination of these two antibiotics is generally more effective than either used alone. Doxycycline is the treatment of choice for mycoplasmosis in rats since it is effective against most *Mycoplasma* species and is actively secreted into respiratory mucosa. Enrofloxacin is usually effective as an empirical choice for secondary bacterial infections generally associated with CRD.
• Azithromycin (alone or in combination with doxycycline) may be an effective alternative antibiotic treatment for rats no longer responsive to treatment with enrofloxacin and doxycycline. Anecdotally, a dose of 10 mg/kg q24h × 5 days, then twice weekly has controlled infection. Doses as high as 50 mg/kg q12h ×14d may be required.
• Bronchodilators
• Terbutaline—for acute respiratory distress, administer 0.01 mg/kg IM (dilute 1:10 with sterile water); for long term, 5 mg/kg PO q12h has been used. Alternatively, use aminophylline (10 mg/kg PO q12–24h) or theophylline (10–20 mg/kg PO q12h).
• Albuterol can be administered via a metered dose inhaler (MDI)—one puff as needed during episodes of acute respiratory distress, or q12–24h in severely affected rats in a commercial or home-made chamber. Also consider albuterol 0.05 mg/kg PO q8h.

Nebulization
• Various protocols for nebulization exist and anecdotally can be very helpful, although no data on efficacy exists. For chronic use, owners may purchase nebulizers intended for human use and construct a nebulization chamber by drilling holes into large plastic food storage containers, into which the rodent can comfortably fit, or by placing plastic wrap over a small cage.
• Place the rodent into the chamber and nebulize for 10–15 minutes up to three times a day.
• Sterile water or saline alone may be beneficial to moisten airways.
• Hypertonic saline solutions nebulized once to twice daily for 10–15 minutes may be helpful in breaking down mucus in the respiratory tract.
• Other commonly nebulized agents include enrofloxacin (2–10 mg/mL of sterile saline); acetylcysteine, as a mucolytic (50 mg as a 2% solution diluted with saline); or aminophylline (3 mg/mL of sterile saline).

Anti-inflammatory
• Due to inflammatory nature of mycoplasmosis, meloxicam (1–2 mg/kg PO, SC, IM q24h) may be helpful in patients nonresponsive to antibiotic therapy. Other

recommendations include prednisone at 0.5 mg/kg PO q12–24h.

Other Medications
Furosemide: 1–4 mg/kg PO, IM q4–6h when pulmonary congestion or edema is present

CONTRAINDICATIONS
• Do not administer penicillins, ampicillin, amoxicillin, erythromycin, or lincomycin to hamsters due to the risk of potentially fatal enteric dysbiosis.
• Doxycycline should be avoided in very young or pregnant animals.

PRECAUTIONS
All therapeutic agents should be used with caution in debilitated, dehydrated patients. Ideally, vascular abnormalities (dehydration, hypotension) are addressed prior to initiating antibiotic therapy.

POSSIBLE INTERACTIONS
N/A

ALTERNATIVE DRUGS
There is some anecdotal evidence that immune-boosting agents have been useful in some cases of infectious respiratory disease.

FOLLOW-UP

PATIENT MONITORING
• Patients in respiratory distress are often reluctant to eat or drink. Patients should be monitored carefully to ensure adequate intake.
• Monitor patient weight.
• Rats with suspected *Mycoplasma* sp. should be monitored for response to therapy and for recurrence of disease, which is common.

PREVENTION/AVOIDANCE
• Keep in a well-ventilated, clean environment. Clean bedding frequently to prevent the buildup of ammonia fumes.
• Provide a high-quality diet.

POSSIBLE COMPLICATIONS
Chronic mycoplasmosis often results in bronchioectasis, lung lobe consolidation, and abscessation, which significantly lowers prognosis for recovery.

MISCELLANEOUS

ASSOCIATED CONDITIONS
Respiratory disease produced by other bacterial and viral coinfectors

AGE-RELATED FACTORS
Middle-aged to older rats are more likely to have chronic, recurrent disease.

MYCOPLASMOSIS AND CHRONIC RESPIRATORY DISEASE (CONTINUED)

ZOONOTIC POTENTIAL
A 2017 survey demonstrated positive PCR for mycoplasma in oropharyngeal swabs from 24.4 to 76.3% of veterinarians, lab workers, and others; however, association with clinical disease in humans is currently unknown.

PREGNANCY/FERTILITY/BREEDING
N/A

SYNONYMS
Murine respiratory mycoplasmosis

SEE ALSO
Acute respiratory distress
Congestive heart failure
Pneumonia
Rhinitis and sinusitis

ABBREVIATIONS
CRD = chronic respiratory disease
ELISA = enzyme-linked immunosorbent assay
MDI = metered dose inhaler
RRV = rat respiratory virus
SDA = sialodacryoadenitis virus

Suggested Reading
Capello V, Lennox AM. Diagnostic imaging of the respiratory system in exotic companion mammals. Vet Clin Exot Anim 2011;14:369–389.
Dutton M. Selected veterinary concerns of geriatric rats, mice, hamsters, and gerbils. Vet Clin Exot Anim 2020;23(3):525–548.
Ferreira JB, Yamaguti M, Marques LM et al. Detection of mycoplasma pulmonis in laboratory rats and technicians. Zoonoses Public Health 2008;55(5):229–234.
Frolich J. Rats and mice. In: Quesenberry KE, Carpenter JW, eds. Ferrets, Rabbits and Rodents, 4th Ed). Clinical Medicine and Surgery. 2021 ed. St. Louis: Saunders, 2020:345–367.
Graham JE, Schoeb TR. Mycoplasma pulmonis in rats. J Exotic Pet Med 2011;20(4):270–276.
Jekl V, Knotek Z. Evidence-based advances in rodent medicine. Vet Clin Exot Anim 2017;20:805–816.
Mayer J, Mans C. Rodents. In: Carpenter JW, ed. Exotic Animal Formulary, 5th ed. St Louis: Elsevier, 2018:459–493.
Miwa Y, Mayer J. Hamsters and gerbils. In: Quesenberry KE, Carpenter JW, eds. Ferrets, Rabbits and Rodents, 4th Ed). Clinical Medicine and Surgery. 2021 ed. St. Louis: Saunders, 2020:368–384.
Piasecki T, Chrzastek K, Kasprzykowska U et al. Mycoplasma pulmonis of rodents as a possible human pathogen. Vector Borne Zoonotic Dis 2017;17(7):475–477.

Author Angela M. Lennox, DVM, Dipl ABVP (Avian, ECM); Dipl ECZM-Small Mammal

NASAL DISCHARGE AND SNEEZING

BASICS

DEFINITION
Inflammation of the nasal cavity and sinuses

PATHOPHYSIOLOGY
• May be acute or chronic, noninfectious or infectious
• Often complicated by opportunistic secondary microbial invasion.
• Associated mucosal vascular congestion, friability, excessive mucus gland secretion, and dacryocystitis lead to congestion, obstructed airflow, sneezing, epistaxis, nasal discharge, and epiphora
• In genetically susceptible rats, virulent strains of *Mycoplasma pulmonis* can cause destruction of mucosa, cartilage, and bone in nasal passages, predisposing to chronic, recurrent infections.
• Upper respiratory disease can produce severe respiratory symptoms in rodents, as they are obligate nasal breathers.

SYSTEMS AFFECTED
• Respiratory—mucosa of the upper respiratory tract, including the nasal cavities, sinuses, and nasopharynx
• Ophthalmic—extension to the eyes via nasolacrimal duct
• Otic extention of infection via the Eustachian tube to the middle/inner ear
• Musculoskeletal—osteomyelitis involving bones of the skull
• Neurologic—vestibular signs due to otitis media/interna

INCIDENCE/PREVALENCE
Very common in pet rats and mice, less common in hamsters and other rodents

SIGNALMENT
• Young rats (<3 months of age) with upper respiratory tract signs are more likely to have viral disease (SDAV) alone that is usually self-limiting.
• Disease caused by *Mycoplasma* spp. may be more common in aged or stressed animals and/or those with concurrent disease.
• No specific sex or age predilection for other primary respiratory pathogens

SIGNS
• Sneezing, nasal discharge, and epistaxis
• Chromodacryorrhea (porphyrin discharge appearing as red tears), epiphora, and blepharospasm
• Submandibular swelling (salivary glands)
• Increased respiratory sounds (stertor, "snoring")
• Increased respiratory rate and effort; rodents are obligate nasal breathers and may experience severe dyspnea if nasal passages become obstructed.

• Otitis interna/media—head tilt, circling, nystagmus with spread through the eustachian tube
• Auscultation findings variable and include increased to decreased or absent airway noise
• Patients may otherwise appear bright and alert to depressed.

CAUSES
• *Mycoplasma pulmonis* is the most common primary pathogen in rats and mice.
• Other bacterial infections are common and include *Streptococcus pneumoniae*, *Corynebacterium kutscheri*, or cilia-associated respiratory bacillus in rats and mice and *Pasteurella* spp., *Corynebacterium kutscheri*, or *Streptococcus* spp. in hamsters.
• Sialodacryoadenitis virus (SDAV) is a common primary pathogen in young rats.
• Sendai virus (a parainfluenza virus) is a common primary pathogen in mice and can act as a copathogen in rats and hamsters.
• Other viruses such as rat respiratory virus (RRV; a hantavirus) or pneumonia virus of rats (a paramyxovirus) act syngertically as copathogens.
• Head trauma
• Odontogenic abscesses
• Nasal foreign body
• Neoplasia of the sinuses is rare.
• Irritants from dusty or dirty bedding often contribute to disease.
• Respiratory allergens reported anecdotally but not have been documented in pet rodents

RISK FACTORS
• Poor husbandry, especially overcrowding and poor sanitation, increases risk for development of upper respiratory disease
• Other sources of immune suppression may predispose to respiratory disease.

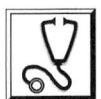

DIAGNOSIS

DIFFERENTIAL DIAGNOSIS
• Trauma—may be history or evidence of an injury
• Careful attention to breathing pattern and auscultation may help differentiate between upper and lower respiratory disease.
• Young rats with serous nasal discharge, chromodacryorrhea, and swollen salivary glands are more likely to have SDAV, which is often self-limiting.

CBC/BIOCHEMISTRY/URINALYSIS
• Complete blood count may support but cannot confirm or rule out respiratory disease.
• Biochemistry panel is useful to identify predisposing underlying disease.

OTHER LABORATORY TESTS
• Serologic testing (ELISA) is available for *Mycoplasma*, SDAV, RRV, and Sendai virus.
• Polymerase chain reaction testing is available for *Mycoplasma* in both mice and rats and is more reliable than isolation on culture.
• Culture—*Mycoplasma* spp. are extremely difficult and time consuming to demonstrate on culture, which may fail to detect the organism.
• Culture and susceptibility testing for other bacterial pathogens is helpful in directing antibiotic therapy. However, patient size may preclude sample collection.

IMAGING
• Radiography of the skull can be helpful, but it is increasingly difficult to obtain diagnostic-quality images as patient size decreases.
• Computed tomography has been reported to be helpful in the diagnosis of larger mammals such as rabbits and guinea pigs; utility is anecdotal in smaller rodents.

DIAGNOSTIC PROCEDURES
• Response to antibiotic therapy as a trial
• Cytologic examination of nasal discharge has limited diagnostic utility.
• Patient size precludes procedures used in larger patients such as endoscopy or nasal mucosal biopsy.

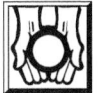

TREATMENT

APPROPRIATE HEALTH CARE
• Inpatient—severe debilitating disease or respiratory distress
• Discharge stable patients pending further diagnostic testing.

NURSING CARE
• Patients in respiratory distress require oxygen therapy.
• Supportive care, including correction of dehydration and hypovolemia, and assisted feeding
• Humidified air may help to moisten and clear nasal secretions.
• Keep the nares clean.

CLIENT EDUCATION
Inform clients that mycoplasma in rats and mice, if present, is extremely difficult to eradicate; many cases are chronic and reoccurrence is common.

SURGICAL CONSIDERATIONS
Rhinotomy for treatment of severe nonresponsive rhinitis has been described in rabbits but not in smaller animals; may be useful in severe disease

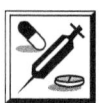

MEDICATIONS

DRUG(S) OF CHOICE

Antibiotics

• In rats and mice, if *Mycoplasma pulmonis* is suspected or confirmed, treat with a combination of enrofloxacin (10 mg/kg PO q12h) and doxycycline (5 mg/kg PO q12h) for a minimum of 2 weeks. With chronic respiratory disease, long-term treatment or lifelong intermittent treatment may be needed. The combination of these two antibiotics is generally more effective than either used alone. Doxycycline is the treatment of choice for mycoplasmosis in rats since it is effective against most *Mycoplasma* spp. and is actively secreted into respiratory mucosa. Enrofloxacin is usually effective as an empirical choice for secondary bacterial infections generally associated with pneumonia.

• Azithromycin (alone or in combination with doxycycline) may be an effective alternative antibiotic treatment for rats no longer responsive to treatment with enrofloxacin and doxycycline. Anecdotally, a dose of 10 mg/kg q24h × 5 days, then twice weekly has controlled infection. Doses as high as 50 mg/kg q12h × 14d may be required.

• For other bacterial pathogens, initially, use broad-spectrum antibiotics such as enrofloxacin (5–10 mg/kg PO, SC, IM q12h), ciprofloxacin (10 mg/kg PO q12h), or trimethoprim-sulfa (15–30 mg/kg PO q12h), pending results of culture and susceptibility testing.

• *Pasteurella pneumotropica*—enrofloxacin (5–10 mg/kg PO q12–24h)

• *Streptococcus pneumoniae*—penicillin (22,000 IU/kg SQ, IM q24h)

• *Corynebacterium kutscheri*—tetracycline (10–20 mg/kg PO q8–12h)

Nebulization

• Various protocols for nebulization exist, but no data on clinical efficacy exists. A 2018 study showed that inhaled fluorescein delivered by nebulization was distributed to the lungs, suggesting this route may be useful in rats.

• For chronic use, owners may purchase nebulizers intended for human use and construct a nebulization chamber by drilling holes into large plastic food storage containers, into which the rodent can comfortably fit, or by placing plastic wrap over a small cage.

• Sterile water or saline alone may be beneficial to moisten airways.

• Hypertonic saline solutions nebulized once to twice daily for 10–15 minutes may be helpful in breaking down mucus in the respiratory tract.

• Other commonly nebulized agents include enrofloxacin (2–10 mg/mL of sterile saline);

acetylcysteine, as a mucolytic (50 mg as a 2% solution diluted with saline), or aminophylline (3 mg/mL of sterile saline)

Anti-inflammatory

Due to inflammatory nature of mycoplasmosis, the addition of anti-inflammatory medication such as meloxicam (1–2 mg/kg PO, SC, IM q24h) may be helpful in patients nonresponsive to antibiotic therapy.

CONTRAINDICATIONS

• Do not administer penicillins, ampicillin, amoxicillin, erythromycin, or lincomycin to hamsters due to the risk of potentially fatal enteric dysbiosis.

• Doxycycline is not recommended for very young or pregnant animals.

PRECAUTIONS

All therapeutic agents should be used with caution in debilitated, dehydrated patients. Ideally, vascular abnormalities (dehydration, hypotension) are addressed prior to initiating therapy.

POSSIBLE INTERACTIONS

N/A

ALTERNATIVE DRUGS

There is some anecdotal evidence that immune-boosting drugs/agents have been useful in some cases of infectious respiratory disease.

FOLLOW-UP

PATIENT MONITORING

Dyspneic patients are often reluctant to eat or drink. Patients should be monitored carefully to ensure adequate intake.

PREVENTION/AVOIDANCE

• Keep in a well-ventilated, clean environment. Clean bedding frequently to prevent the buildup of ammonia fumes.

• Provide a high-quality diet.

• Avoid contact with other rodents exhibiting signs of respiratory tract disease.

POSSIBLE COMPLICATIONS

• Mycoplasma infections frequently cause permanent damage to nasal turbinates and progress to chronic pulmonary disease, which significantly lowers prognosis for recovery.

• Patients with chronic disease may not fully respond to therapy, and recurrence is common.

MISCELLANEOUS

ASSOCIATED CONDITIONS

Acute respiratory distress

ZOONOTIC POTENTIAL

In general, infectious agents producing sinusitis and rhinitis in rodents are nonzoonotic; however, any animal disease is of concern to immunocompromised humans.

PREGNANCY/FERTILITY/BREEDING

Avoid tetracycline in very young or pregnant animals.

SYNONYMS

N/A

SEE ALSO

Mycoplasma and chronic respiratory disease
Pneumonia
Sialodacryoadenitis virus

ABBREVIATIONS

RRV = rat respiratory virus
SDAV = sialodacryoadenitis virus

Suggested Reading

Burn CC, Peters A, Day MJ et al. Long term effects of cage-cleaning frequency and bedding type on laboratory rat health, welfare and handle ability: a cross-laboratory study. Lab Anim 2006;40(4):353–370.

Capello V, Lennox AM. Diagnostic imaging of the respiratory system in exotic companion mammals. Vet Clin Exot Anim 2011;14:369–389.

Dutton M. Selected veterinary concerns of geriatric rats, mice, hamsters, and gerbils. Vet Clin Exot Anim 2020;23(3):525–548.

Ferreira JB, Yamaguti M, Marques LM et al. Detection of mycoplasma pulmonis in laboratory rats and technicians. Zoonoses Public Health 2008;55(5):229–234.

Frolich J. Rats and mice. In: Quesenberry KE, Carpenter JW, eds. Ferrets, Rabbits and Rodents, 4th Ed). Clinical Medicine and Surgery. 2021 ed. St. Louis: Saunders, 2020:345–367.

Graham JE, Schoeb TR. Mycoplasma pulmonis in rats. J Exotic Pet Med 2011;20(4):270–276.

Jekl V, Knotek Z. Evidence-based advances in rodent medicine. Vet Clin Exot Anim 2017;20:805–816.

Mayer J, Mans C. Rodents. In: Carpenter JW, ed. Exotic Animal Formulary, 5th ed. St Louis: Elsevier, 2018:459–493.

Miwa Y, Mayer J. Hamsters and gerbils. In: Quesenberry KE, Carpenter JW, eds. Ferrets, Rabbits and Rodents, 4th Ed). Clinical Medicine and Surgery. 2021 ed. St. Louis: Saunders, 2020:368–384.

Piasecki T, Chrzastek K, Kasprzykowska U et al. Mycoplasma pulmonis of rodents as a possible human pathogen. Vector Borne Zoonotic Dis 2017;17(7):475–477.

Author Angela M. Lennox, DVM, Dipl. ABVP (Avian, ECM); DECZM-Small Mammal

RODENTS

BASICS

DEFINITION
• Inflammation of the middle (otitis media) and inner (otitis interna) ears, most commonly caused by bacterial infection
• May be accompanied by evidence of respiratory disease

PATHOPHYSIOLOGY
• May arise from extension of infection of the external ear through the tympanic membrane or extension from the oral and nasopharyngeal cavities via the eustachian tube
• Interna—may also result from hematogenous spread of a systemic infection
• The chinchilla is a laboratory model for otitis media in humans.

SYSTEMS AFFECTED
• Auditory
• Respiratory—may be linked to upper respiratory disease via eustachian tube
• Nervous—vestibulocochlear receptors in the inner ear and the facial nerve in the middle ear (peripheral) with possible extension of infection intracranially (central)
• Ophthalmic—cornea and conjunctiva; from exposure and/or lack of tear production after nerve damage

INCIDENCE/PREVALENCE
Uncommon disorder in pet rodents

GEOGRAPHIC DISTRIBUTION
N/A

SIGNALMENT
• Most commonly described in the rat
• No specific sex or age predilection
• Stress, aging, and concurrent disease may predispose

SIGNS
• Vestibular signs, including head tilt, nystagmus, ataxia, rolling, or walking in circles
• Discharge from ear canal, accumulation of debris below ear; may be foul smelling
• Scratching at ear
• Holding affected ear down
• Evidence of respiratory disease

CAUSES
• Bacteria—most common primary agents
• In mice, opportunistic infections with *Pasteurella pneumotropica* or *Klebsiella oxytoca* may result in otitis media.
• *Mycoplasma pulmonis* may cause otitis media in rats and mice.
• *Streptococcus pneumoniae* may cause primary otitis interna/media in rats.

• Sendai virus may play a role in otitis in rodents.
• Neoplasia, including Zymbal's gland tumor may present with secondary otitis media/interna

RISK FACTORS
• Presence of upper respiratory disease
• Poor husbandry, especially overcrowding and poor sanitation
• Other sources of immune suppression may predispose to infectious disease.

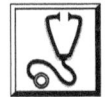

DIAGNOSIS

DIFFERENTIAL DIAGNOSIS
• Central vestibular diseases—pituitary tumors common in rodents; may see lethargy, somnolence, stupor, and other brain stem signs
• Neoplasia—adenoma or adenocarcinoma of Zymbal's glands in rats; usually appears as unilateral swelling at ear base; may develop secondary bacterial infection/abscess resembling refractory otitis; diagnosed by histologic examination and imaging of the head
• Trauma—history and physical evidence of injury
• Diagnosis of otitis media/interna is based on history, physical examination, endoscopic examination of the ear canal (diagnostic otoscopy), and diagnostic imaging of the skull

CBC/BIOCHEMISTRY/URINALYSIS
Testing is useful to identify other concurrent disease processes but does not provide a specific diagnosis.

OTHER LABORATORY TESTS
• If disease includes rupture of the tympanum and otitis externa, cytology of otic exudate may be useful; note presence of inflammatory cells and bacteria
• Bacterial culture and susceptibility testing of otic discharge

IMAGING
Imaging of the skull (radiography/ computed tomography) can be extremely useful but is increasingly difficult as patient size decreases. Some affected animals may develop abnormalities of the tympanic bulla, including evidence of fluid/masses and bony changes.

DIAGNOSTIC PROCEDURES
• Response to antibiotic therapy as a trial (parental and/or otic)
• Otoscopic examination or diagnostic otoscopy

TREATMENT

APPROPRIATE HEALTH CARE
• Inpatient—severe debilitating infection; neurologic signs
• Discharge stable patients

NURSING CARE
Supportive care, including correction of dehydration if present, and assisted feeding; some animals with vestibular disease may be unable to take in adequate nutrition

ACTIVITY
Restrict with substantial vestibular signs to avoid injury; encourage return to activity as soon as safely possible; activity may enhance recovery of vestibular function.

CLIENT EDUCATION
• Inform client that otitis interna/media can be extremely frustrating to treat, especially in chronic cases.
• Warn client that neurologic signs, especially head tilt, may persist. Some patients improve minimally or not at all, even with aggressive therapy.

SURGICAL CONSIDERATIONS
Lateral ear canal resection and bulla osteotomy as described in other species may be possible in larger rodents.

MEDICATIONS

DRUG(S) OF CHOICE
• Systemic antibiotics—choice is ideally based on results of culture and susceptibility testing, when possible.
• Often, exudate in the bullae is thick and limits penetration of systemic antibiotics. Treatment with antibiotics may be effective in preventing extension of infection and may be effective in treating concurrent bacterial respiratory infection.
• In rats, if *Mycoplasma pulmonis* is suspected or confirmed, treat with a combination of enrofloxacin (10 mg/kg PO q12h) and doxycycline (5 mg/kg PO q12h) for a minimum of 2 weeks.
• Initailly, use broad-spectrum antibiotics such as enrofloxacin (5–10 mg/kg PO, SC, IM q12h), ciprofloxacin (10 mg/kg PO q12h), and trimethoprim-sulfa (15–30 mg/kg PO q12h); if anaerobic infections are suspected use chloramphenicol (30–50 mg/kg PO q8h) or azithromycin (10–30 mg/kg PO q24h).
• Consider topical antibiotic therapy in cases involving otitis externa.

• Anti-inflammatory medications may help reduce inflammation in cases of vestibular disease. For pain management or as an anti-inflammatory medication, use meloxicam (1–2 mg/kg PO, SC, IM q24h).

• Some animals refractory to antibiotic therapy (especially those with vestibular signs or pituitary tumors) may respond to temporary steroid therapy; this should be weighed against potential untoward effects of steroids.

CONTRAINDICATIONS

Do not administer penicillins, ampicillin, amoxicillin, erythromycin, or lincomycin to hamsters due to the risk of potentially fatal enteric dysbiosis.

PRECAUTIONS

• All therapeutic agents should be used with caution in debilitated, dehydrated patients. Ideally, vascular abnormalities (dehydration, hypotension) are addressed prior to initiating antibiotic therapy.

• Steroid therapy should be approached with caution and reserved for cases of vestibular syndrome nonresponsive to antibiotic therapy.

POSSIBLE INTERACTIONS

N/A

ALTERNATIVE DRUGS

There is some anecdotal evidence that immune-boosting drugs/agents have been useful in some cases of infectious respiratory disease.

FOLLOW-UP

PATIENT MONITORING

• Ensure adequate intake of food and water, especially in animals with vestibular disease.

• Monitor patient weight.

PREVENTION/AVOIDANCE

• Treating otitis or upper respiratory infections in early stages may prevent otitis media/interna.

POSSIBLE COMPLICATIONS

• Signs associated with vestibular and facial nerve damage may persist.

• Severe infections—may spread to the brain stem

EXPECTED COURSE AND PROGNOSIS

• May require months of systemic antibiotic therapy; most will improve, but some are nonresponsive to medical treatment

• When medical management is ineffective, a surgical evaluation should be explored.

• Residual deficits (especially neurologic) cannot be predicted until after a course of therapy.

MISCELLANEOUS

ASSOCIATED CONDITIONS

• Upper respiratory infection or chronic respiratory disease

• Aural abscess or neoplasia

• Otitis externa

ZOONOTIC POTENTIAL

Most diseases producing otitis in rodents are not zoonotic; however, all animal diseases may be of concern in immunocompromised humans.

PREGNANCY/FERTILITY/BREEDING

N/A

SYNONYMS

Middle and inner ear infection

SEE ALSO

Head tilt (vestibular disease)
Mycoplasmosis and chronic respiratory disease
Rhinitis and sinusitis

ABBREVIATIONS

N/A

Suggested Reading

Capello V, Lennox AM. Diagnostic imaging of the respiratory system in exotic companion mammals. Vet Clin Exot Anim 2011;14:369–389.

Dutton M. Selected veterinary concerns of geriatric rats, mice, hamsters, and gerbils. Vet Clin Exot Anim 2020;23(3):525–548.

Frolich J. Rats and mice. In: Quesenberry KE, Carpenter JW, eds. Ferrets, Rabbits and Rodents, 4th Ed). Clinical Medicine and Surgery. 2021 ed. St. Louis: Saunders, 2020:345–367.

Jekl V, Knotek Z. Evidence-based advances in rodent medicine. Vet Clin Exot Anim 2017;20:805–816.

Mayer J, Mans C. Rodents. In: Carpenter JW, ed. Exotic Animal Formulary, 5th ed. St Louis: Elsevier, 2018:459–493.

Meredith AL, Richardson J. Neurologic disease of rabbits and rodents. J Exot Pet Med 2015;24:21–33.

Miwa Y, Mayer J. Hamsters and gerbils. In: Quesenberry KE, Carpenter JW, eds. Ferrets, Rabbits and Rodents, 4th Ed). Clinical Medicine and Surgery. 2021 ed. St. Louis: Saunders, 2020:368–384.

Author Angela M. Lennox, DVM, Dipl. ABVP (Avian, ECM); DECZM-Small Mammal

BASICS

DEFINITION
An ovarian cyst is any collection of fluid, surrounded by a very thin wall, within an ovary.

PATHOPHYSIOLOGY
• Cysts can develop spontaneously and increase in size with the age of the animal.
• One or both ovaries can be involved.
• Although ovulation usually continues, litter sizes often become reduced, and some animals will become infertile.

SYSTEMS AFFECTED
• Reproductive
• Endocrine
• Behavioral
• Urologic
• Skin

INCIDENCE/PREVALENCE
• Seen in 50% of gerbils over 400 days old
• Reported in 2% of Russian dwarf hamsters
• Paraovarian cysts are frequent in mice because mouse ovaries are enclosed within membranous pouches.
• Uncommon in rats

SIGNALMENT
Predominant Sex
Female only

SIGNS
Historical Findings
• May see vague signs such as anorexia, lethargy, and depression
• Hair loss
• Bloody urine
• Infertility
• Behavior changes (aggressiveness, nesting behavior)

Physical Examination Findings
• Abdominal distension; mass may be palpable in the midabdomen
• Symmetrical flank alopecia
• Hematuria
• Dyspnea with abdominal distension due to very large cysts

CAUSES
• Continuous light has been reported to cause persistent estrus and ovarian cyst in rats.
• Testosterone production in females is suspected to stimulate ovarian epithelial cell growth.

RISK FACTORS
• Intact female
• Continuous light exposure (rats)

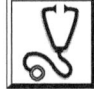

DIAGNOSIS

DIFFERENTIAL DIAGNOSIS
• Neoplasia of abdominal organs
• Renal cysts
• Ectoparasite for the alopecia

CBC/BIOCHEMISTRY/URINALYSIS
• Nonspecific findings, usually normal
• Hematuria sometimes present

OTHER LABORATORY TESTS
Fine-needle aspiration of the cyst will reveal a serous to hemorrhagic fluid.

IMAGING
• Abdominal ultrasound—mass or multiple masses with anechoic content in the ovaries area (caudal to the kidneys)
• Abdominal radiography—mass in the midabdominal region

DIAGNOSTIC PROCEDURES
Excisional biopsy—definitive diagnosis

PATHOLOGIC FINDINGS
• Gross—uni- or multilobulated cyst with a thin membrane surrounding transparent fluid
• Histopathology—theca interna is usually luteinized, and the granulosa may be sparse or absent.

TREATMENT

APPROPRIATE HEALTH CARE
Inpatient if severely depressed, anorexic
Outpatient if stable

NURSING CARE
• If cysts are very large, drain the contents via percutaneous fine-needle aspiration to decompress the abdominal cavity and to facilitate surgery. If cystic contents are spilled into the abdomen during the aspiration or if the cyst ruptures, no systemic problems will usually arise from this event. This is only a stabilization treatment as cysts often refill with fluid after drainage
• Stabilization of the patient (fluid therapy, oxygen therapy, and warming)

ACTIVITY
Restrict postoperatively by confining to cage and removing exercise wheels

DIET
Consider assist feeding the patient if anorectic

CLIENT EDUCATION
Advise clients of the potential benefit of an early ovariohysterectomy in nonbreeding females.

SURGICAL CONSIDERATIONS
Ovariohysterctomy to prevent recurrence of ovarian cyst and to prevent infection of the uterus; perform via paramedian incision in gerbils and Hungarian hamster (*Phodopus sungorus*) to avoid the ventral skin gland

MEDICATIONS

DRUG(S) OF CHOICE
Pain Management
• Buprenorphine (0.05–1.0 mg/kg SC, IV q6–8h)
• Oxymorphone (0.2–0.5 mg/kg SC IM q6–12h)
• Morphine (2–5 mg/kg IM q4h)
• Meloxicam (1–2 mg/kg SC, PO q24)

Antibiotics
Indicated postoperatively only in case of complication. Use trimethoprim-sulfa (15–30 mg/kg PO q12h).

PRECAUTIONS
Meloxicam—use with caution in animals with compromised renal function

FOLLOW-UP

PATIENT MONITORING
• Monitor postoperatively that the animal does not chew his sutures and open his wound.
• Monitor carefully for signs of pain (reluctance to move, teeth grinding) postoperatively.
• Monitor the appetite.
• Recheck at 1 week to assess the healing of the surgical wound.

PREVENTION/AVOIDANCE
Consider ovariohysterectomy

POSSIBLE COMPLICATIONS
Wound dehiscence

EXPECTED COURSE AND PROGNOSIS
The prognosis is good if the patient recovers well from the surgery.

MISCELLANEOUS

ASSOCIATED CONDITIONS
Leiomyoma, cystic endometrial hyperplasia, endometritis

AGE-RELATED FACTORS
The risk increases with the age

PREGNANCY/FERTILITY/BREEDING

Animals with ovarian cyst are often infertile

Suggested Reading

Dutton M. Selected veterinary concerns of geriatric rats, mice, hamsters, and gerbils. Vet Clin Exot Anim 2020;23(3):525–548.

Frolich J. Rats and mice. In: Quesenberry KE, Carpenter JW, eds. Ferrets, Rabbits and Rodents, 4th Ed). Clinical Medicine and Surgery. 2021 ed. St. Louis: Saunders, 2020:345–367.

Lewis W. Cystic ovaries in gerbils. Exot DVM 2003;5(1):12.

Martorell J. Reproductive disorders in pet rodents. Vet Clin Exot Anim 2017;20:589–608.

Miwa Y, Mayer J. Hamsters and gerbils. In: Quesenberry KE, Carpenter JW, eds. Ferrets, Rabbits and Rodents, 4th Ed). Clinical Medicine and Surgery. 2021 ed. St. Louis: Saunders, 2020:368–384.

Miwa Y, Sladky K. Common surgical procedures of rodents, ferrets, hedgehogs, and sugar gliders. Vet Clin Exot Anim 2016;19:205–244.

Norris ML, Adams CE. Incidence of cystic ovaries and reproductive performance in the Mongolian gerbil, Meriones unguiculatus. Lab Anim 1972;6:337–342.

Peluso JJ, England-Charlesworth C. Formation of ovarian cysts in irregularly cycling rats. Biol Reprod 1981;24:1183–1190.

Author Charly Pignon, DVM, Dip ECZM (Small Mammal)

BASICS

DEFINITION
Respiratory disease characterized by the fully developed inflammatory response to virulent bacteria, viruses, deep mycoses, or inhaled foreign material in the lung parenchyma.

PATHOPHYSIOLOGY
• Infectious agents enter the lower respiratory tract primarily by inhalation, aspiration, or hematogenous routes.
• Spread of organisms often occurs via upper respiratory tract.
• Development and severity of infection depends on the virulence of organism and host immunity.
• Viral infection allows bacterial attachment and colonization of respiratory epithelium; reduces mucociliary clearance
• Some pathogenic bacteria, particularly *Mycoplasma* spp. infection in mice and rats, attach to respiratory epithelial cells, causing destruction of cilia, which predisposes to secondary bacterial infections.
• Mycoplasma incite a marked lymphocytic response in susceptible rats, suggestive of an exaggerated immune response. Infection stimulates excessive production and decreased clearance of respiratory mucus. This excessive mucus contributes significantly to symptoms (stertor, dyspnea) and produces a bacterial biofilm that protects bacteria from antibiotic treatment.
• Chronic mycoplasmosis often causes irreversible changes in the lungs such as bronchioectasis and consolidation of lung lobes. Eradication from these animals is unlikely, and chronic reoccurring respiratory disease is common.

SYSTEMS AFFECTED
Respiratory—primary or secondary infections

GENETICS
N/A

INCIDENCE/PREVALENCE
Common in pet rats and mice; relatively rare in hamsters and other small rodents

GEOGRAPHIC DISTRIBUTION
Ubiquitous

SIGNALMENT
• No specific sex predilection
• More common in older animals
• Stress, aging, poor husbandry, and concurrent disease may predispose.

SIGNS
• Upper respiratory signs such as sneezing, nasal and ocular discharge, or porphyrin discharge resembling red tears

(chromodacryorrhea) may precede or accompany lower respiratory tract signs.
• Increased respiratory rate and effort (often expiratory) to profound dyspnea
• May progress to respiratory arrest
• Weight loss, emaciation
• Poor hair coat
• Auscultation findings variable and may be related to upper or lower respiratory tract
• Patients may otherwise appear bright and alert to severely depressed or comatose, with varying degrees of anorexia and dehydration.

CAUSES
• Bacterial agents, especially *Mycoplasma*, cilia-associated respiratory bacillus, *Corynebacterium kutscheri*, *Pasteurella pneumotropica*, and *Streptococcus pneumoniae* in rats and mice
• Although *M. pulmonis* alone is often the primary pathogen causing respiratory disease in rats and mice, most pneumonia is caused by a combination of mycoplasma and other bacterial and/or viral copathogens.
• Viral agents including sialodacryoadenitis virus (SDAV), Sendai virus (a parainfluenza virus), rat respiratory virus (RRV; a hantavirus), or pneumonia virus of rats (a paramyxovirus) may be primary pathogens or act synergetically as copathogens in rats
• *Mycoplamsa pulmonis, Pasteurella pneumotrpica*, Sendai virus in mice
• *Pasteruella pneumotropica, Streptococcus* spp., and pneumonia virus of rat (paramyxovirus) in hamsters
• Other bacteria and viruses may be implicated, especially in debilitated rodents
• Environmental irritants, including aromatic beddings and airborne toxins, may predispose to bacterial or viral pneumonia.
• Aspiration pneumonia is rare, since rodents cannot vomit; may occur when force-fed oral medications or food
• Mycotic pneumonia is extremely rare in rodents; *Aspergillus* spp. and *Pneumocystis* spp. have been reported in immunocompromised rats.

RISK FACTORS
• Presence of upper respiratory disease
• Poor husbandry, especially overcrowding and poor sanitation
• Aging
• Other sources of immune suppression may predispose to infectious disease.

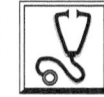 **DIAGNOSIS**

DIFFERENTIAL DIAGNOSIS
• Upper respiratory tract disorder—severe upper respiratory tract disease may resemble pneumonia. Rodents are obligate nasal

breathers, and severe or chronic infection can lead to significant dyspnea and debility. Differentiate based on history, clinical signs, auscultation, and radiography.
• Lower respiratory disease produced by other conditions—cardiac disease, trauma (pulmonary contusions, hemo- or pneumothorax), neoplasia
• Pulmonary metastatic neoplasia is rare but has been reported most commonly in mice with mammary and liver neoplasia.
• Cardiac disease may present as increased respiratory rate and effort; differentiate based on physical examination and radiographs.
• Parasitic pneumonia is uncommon.

CBC/BIOCHEMISTRY/URINALYSIS
Testing is useful to identify other concurrent disease processes but does not confirm the diagnosis of pneumonia.

OTHER LABORATORY TESTS
• Serologic testing (ELISA) is available for *Mycoplasma* spp., SDA, RRV, and Sendai virus.
• Polymerase chain reaction testing is available for *Mycoplasma* spp. in both mice and rats and is more reliable than isolation on culture.
• Culture—*Mycoplasma* spp. are extremely difficult and time consuming to demonstrate on culture, which may fail to detect the organism. Culture and susceptibility testing for other, concurrent bacterial infections is helpful in directing antibiotic therapy.

IMAGING
Radiography and ultrasound are extremely useful, especially to differentiate from cardiac disease and identify pulmonary lesions.

DIAGNOSTIC PROCEDURES
• Response to antibiotic therapy as a trial
• Diagnostic procedures such as transtracheal washing and bronchoalveolar lavage are challenging due to small patient size.

 TREATMENT

APPROPRIATE HEALTH CARE
• Inpatient—severely debilitated animals or those in respiratory distress require hospitalization.
• Outpatient care for stable animals

NURSING CARE
• Patients in respiratory distress require oxygen therapy.
• Supportive care, including correction of dehydration and hypovolemia; maintenance of normal hydration is important to aid mucociliary clearance
• Some animals with dyspnea are reluctant to eat; assist feeding may be necessary.

CLIENT EDUCATION
• Inform clients that pneumonia, especially if chronic or due to mycoplasmosis in rats, is extremely difficult to eliminate; many cases are chronic and recurrence is common. Patients with severe lung lesions will likely not respond.
• Advise owners to correct husbandry deficiencies, in particular, to improve sanitation and remove irritating bedding.

SURGICAL CONSIDERATIONS
While lung lobectomy has been described in larger exotic companion mammals, it is unlikely to benefit smaller mammals.

MEDICATIONS
DRUG(S) OF CHOICE
Antibiotics
• In rats and mice, if *Mycoplasma pulmonis* is suspected or confirmed, treat with a combination of enrofloxacin (10 mg/kg PO q12h) and doxycycline (5 mg/kg PO q12h) for a minimum of 2 weeks. With chronic respiratory disease, long-term treatment or lifelong intermittent treatment may be needed. The combination of these two antibiotics is generally more effective than either used alone. Doxycycline is the treatment of choice for mycoplasmosis in rats since it is effective against most *Mycoplasma* spp. and is actively secreted into respiratory mucosa. Enrofloxacin is usually effective as an empirical choice for secondary bacterial infections generally associated with pneumonia.
• Azithromycin (alone or in combination with doxycycline) may be an effective alternative antibiotic treatment for rats no longer responsive to treatment with enrofloxacin and doxycycline. Anecdotally, a dose of 10 mg/kg q24h × 5 days, then twice weekly has controlled infection. Doses as high as 50 mg/kg q12h x 14d may be required.
• For other bacterial pathogens, initially, use broad-spectrum antibiotics such as enrofloxacin (5–10 mg/kg PO, SC, IM q12h), ciprofloxacin (10 mg/kg PO q12h), or trimethoprim-sulfa (15–30 mg/kg PO q12h), pending results of culture and susceptibility testing.
• *Pasteurella pneumotropica*—enrofloxacin (5–10 mg/kg PO q12–24h)
• *Streptococcus pneumoniae*—penicillin (22,000 IU/kg SQ, IM q24h)
• *Corynebacterium kutscheri*—tetracycline (10–20 mg/kg PO q8–12h)

Bronchodilators
• Terbutaline—for acute respiratory distress, administer 0.01 mg/kg IM (dilute 1:10 with sterile water); for long term 0.3–0.4 mg/kg PO q12h has been used. Alternatively, use aminophylline (10 mg/kg PO q12–24h) or theophylline (10 mg/kg PO q12h).
• Albuterol can be administered to rats via a metered dose inhaler (MDI)—one puff as needed during episodes of acute respiratory distress, or q12–24h in severely or chronically affected rats. Although veterinary brand feline MDIs have been used, the face mask is not form fitting to rats, and stressed rats resist the use of a face mask. Alternatively, inhaled bronchodilators can be administered with a homemade chamber. The bottom is cut from a 2-liter soda bottle, and the rat trained (with a treat) to go to the narrow end, where the puff is delivered.

Nebulization
• Various protocols for nebulization exist, but no data on clinical efficacy exists. A 2018 study showed that inhaled fluorescein delivered by nebulization was distributed to the lungs, suggesting this route may be useful in rats.
• For chronic use, owners may purchase nebulizers intended for human use and construct a nebulization chamber by drilling holes into large plastic food storage containers, into which the rodent can comfortably fit, or by placing plastic wrap over a small cage.
• Sterile water or saline alone may be beneficial to moisten airways.
• Hypertonic saline solutions nebulized once to twice daily for 10–15 minutes may be helpful in breaking down mucus in the respiratory tract.
• Other commonly nebulized agents include enrofloxacin (2–10 mg/mL of sterile saline); acetylcysteine, as a mucolytic (50 mg as a 2% solution diluted with saline), or aminophylline (3 mg/mL of sterile saline)

Anti-inflammatory
• Due to inflammatory nature of mycoplasmosis, the addition of anti-inflammatory medication such as meloxicam (1–2 mg/kg PO, SC, IM q24h) may be helpful in patients nonresponsive to antibiotic therapy.

Other Medications
• Furosemide: 1–4 mg/kg PO, IM q4–6h when pulmonary congestion or edema is present.

CONTRAINDICATIONS
• Do not administer penicillins, ampicillin, amoxicillin, erythromycin, or lincomycin to hamsters due to the risk of potentially fatal enteric dysbiosis.
• Doxycycline is not recommended for very young or pregnant animals.

PRECAUTIONS
All therapeutic agents should be used with caution in debilitated, dehydrated patients. Ideally, vascular abnormalities (dehydration, hypotension) are addressed prior to initiating therapy.

POSSIBLE INTERACTIONS
N/A

ALTERNATIVE DRUGS
There is some anecdotal evidence that immune-boosting drugs/agents have been useful in some cases of infectious respiratory disease.

FOLLOW-UP
PATIENT MONITORING
• Patients in respiratory distress are often reluctant to eat or drink. Patients should be monitored carefully to ensure adequate intake.
• Monitor patient weight.

PREVENTION/AVOIDANCE
• Keep in a well-ventilated, clean environment. Clean bedding frequently to prevent the buildup of ammonia fumes.
• Provide a high-quality diet.
• Early treatment may prevent formation of pulmonary abscess or lung consolidation in cases of bacterial pneumonia.

POSSIBLE COMPLICATIONS
• Bacterial infections frequently produce pulmonary lung lobe collapse, consolidation, and abscessation, which significantly lowers prognosis for recovery.
• Patients with chronic disease may not fully respond to therapy, and recurrence is common.

MISCELLANEOUS
ASSOCIATED CONDITIONS
Pneumonia may develop secondary to underlying metabolic disease, especially in older animals.

AGE-RELATED FACTORS
Middle-aged to older rats are more likely to have chronic, recurrent disease.

ZOONOTIC POTENTIAL
Most respiratory pathogens in rodents are not considered to be zoonotic; however, any animal pathogen may be of significance to immunocompromised humans.

PREGNANCY/FERTILITY/BREEDING
N/A

SYNONYMS
Murine respiratory mycoplasmosis

SEE ALSO
Acute respiratory distress
Congestive heart failure
Mycoplasmosis and chronic respiratory disease
Rhinitis and sinusitis

ABBREVIATIONS
ELISA = enzyme-linked immunosorbent assay
MDI = metered dose inhaler
RRV = rat respiratory virus
SDA = sialodacryoadenitis virus

Suggested Reading
Capello V, Lennox AM. Diagnostic imaging of the respiratory system in exotic companion mammals. Vet Clin Exot Anim 2011;14:369–389.
Dutton M. Selected veterinary concerns of geriatric rats, mice, hamsters, and gerbils. Vet Clin Exot Anim 2020;23(3):525–548.
Ferreira JB, Yamaguti M, Marques LM et al. Detection of mycoplasma pulmonis in laboratory rats and technicians. Zoonoses Public Health 2008;55(5):229–234.
Frolich J. Rats and mice. In: Quesenberry KE, Carpenter JW, eds. Ferrets, Rabbits and Rodents, 4th Ed). Clinical Medicine and Surgery. 2021 ed. St. Louis: Saunders, 2020:345–367.
Graham JE, Schoeb TR. Mycoplasma pulmonis in rats. J Exotic Pet Med 2011;20(4):270–276.
Jekl V, Knotek Z. Evidence-based advances in rodent medicine. Vet Clin Exot Anim 2017;20:805–816.
Mayer J, Mans C. Rodents. In: Carpenter JW, ed. Exotic Animal Formulary, 5th ed. St Louis: Elsevier, 2018:459–493.
Miwa Y, Mayer J. Hamsters and gerbils. In: Quesenberry KE, Carpenter JW, eds. Ferrets, Rabbits and Rodents, 4th Ed). Clinical Medicine and Surgery. 2021 ed. St. Louis: Saunders, 2020:368–384.
Piasecki T, Chrzastek K, Kasprzykowska U et al. Mycoplasma pulmonis of rodents as a possible human pathogen. Vector Borne Zoonotic Dis 2017;17(7):475–477.

Author Angela M. Lennox, DVM, Dipl. ABVP (Avian, ECM); DECZM-Small Mammal

POLYURIA AND POLYDIPSIA

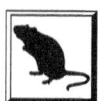 **BASICS**

DEFINITION
• Polyuria is defined as greater than normal urine production, and polydipsia as greater than normal water consumption.
• Average water intake (per 100 g body weight/day)—gerbil 4–7 mL, hamster 8–10 mL, mouse 15 mL, rat >10–12 mL
• Urine production—gerbil 2–4 drops/24 hr, hamster 5.1–8.4 mL/24 hr, mouse 0.5–2.5 mL/24 hr, rat 13–23 mL/24 hr

PATHOPHYSIOLOGY
• Urine production and water consumption (thirst) are controlled by interaction between the kidney, the pituitary gland, and the hypothalamus.
• Usually polydipsia occurs as a compensatory response to polyuria to maintain hydration. The patient's plasma becomes relatively hypertonic and activates the thirst mechanism. Occasionally, polydipsia may be the primary process and polyuria is the compensatory response; the patient's plasma becomes relatively hypotonic because of excessive water intake and ADH secretion is reduced, resulting in polyuria.

SYSTEMS AFFECTED
• Renal/Urologic—kidney
• Endocrine/Metabolic

GENETICS
Certain strains of laboratory rodents could be predisposed.

INCIDENCE/PREVALENCE
• Very common in rats
• Common in mouse and gerbil

GEOGRAPHIC DISTRIBUTION
Worldwide

SIGNALMENT

Mean Age and Range
More likely to be seen in middle-aged to older animals

Predominant Sex
No sex predilection

SIGNS

Historical Findings
• Increased water consumption
• Owner often has difficulty assessing urine production.

Physical Examination Findings
• Nonspecific, or related to the underlying disease process
• If the animal is hospitalized, urine production can be assessed.

CAUSES
• Primary polyuria due to impaired renal response to ADH—renal failure, pyelonephritis, pyometra, hepatic failure, hypokalemia, drugs, hyperadrenocorticism (hamster)
• Primary polyuria caused by osmotic diuresis—diabetes mellitus (rat, mouse, degu, and gerbil), postobstructive diuresis, some diuretics (e.g., mannitol and furosemide), ingestion or administration of large quantities of solute (e.g., sodium chloride or glucose)
• Primary polyuria due to ADH deficiency (rats; very rare)—traumatic, neoplastic; some drugs (e.g., alcohol and phenytoin)
• Primary polydipsia—behavioral problems (especially boredom), pyrexia, or pain; organic disease of anterior hypothalamic thirst center of neoplastic, traumatic, or inflammatory origin

RISK FACTORS
• Renal or hepatic disease
• Selected electrolyte disorders
• Administration of diuretics and anticonvulsivants

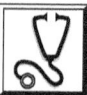 **DIAGNOSIS**

DIFFERENTIAL DIAGNOSIS

Differentiating Similar Signs
Differentiate polyuria from an abnormal increase in the frequency of urination (pollakiuria). Pollakiuria is often associated with dysuria, stranguria, or hematuria. Patients with polyuria void large quantities of urine; patients with pollakiuria typically void small quantities of urine. Measuring urinary specific gravity may provide evidence of adequate urine concentrating ability.

Differentiating Causes
• If associated with progressive weight loss—consider renal failure, hepatic failure, pyometra, neoplasia, pyelonephritis, and possibly diabetes mellitus
• If associated with hypercalciuria—consider renal failure and nephrolithiasis
• If associated with polyphagia—consider diabetes mellitus
• If associated with recent estrus in an intact female—consider pyometra
• If associated with abdominal distension—consider hepatic failure and neoplasia

CBC/BIOCHEMISTRY/URINALYSIS
• Relative hypernatremia or high serum osmolality suggests primary polyuria.
• Hyponatremia or low serum osmolality suggests primary polydipsia.

• BUN elevation; creatinine elevation is consistent with renal cause for PU/PD but may also indicate dehydration resulting from inadequate compensatory polydipsia
• High hepatic enzyme activities are consistent with hepatic disease.
• Hypercalcemia—can be a potential cause of renal failure, rather than the result of a renal failure
• Hypoalbuminemia supports renal or hepatic cause of PU/PD.
• Neutrophilia may suggest infectious or inflammatory disease.
• White blood cell casts and/or bacteriuria should prompt consideration of pyelonephritis.
• Urinary sediment evaluation often reveals struvite in rats, which could induce subsequent inflammatory cystitis or partial to complete blockage of the urethra.
• Pyuria, hematuria, and proteinuria indicate urinary tract inflammation, but these are nonspecific findings that may result from infectious and noninfectious causes of lower urinary tract disease.

OTHER LABORATORY TESTS
Urine culture—chronic pyelonephritis cannot be conclusively ruled out by absence of pyuria or bacteriuria

IMAGING
Abnormal survey radiography and ultrasonography may provide additional evidence of renal (e.g., primary renal disease), hepatic (e.g., microhepatica, hepatic infiltrate), or uterine (e.g., pyometra) disorder that can contribute to PU/PD.

DIAGNOSTIC PROCEDURES
N/A

PATHOLOGIC FINDINGS
Depends on the cause of the PU/PD and the organ involved

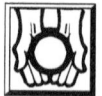 **TREATMENT**

APPROPRIATE HEALTH CARE
Serious medical consequences for the patient are rare if the patient has free access to water and is willing and able to drink. Until the mechanism of polyuria is understood, discourage owners from limiting access to water.

NURSING CARE
• Provide polyuric patients with free access to water. Also provide fluids parenterally when other conditions limit oral intake or dehydration persists despite polydipsia.

(CONTINUED)

• Base fluid selection on knowledge of the underlying cause for fluid loss. In most patients, lactated Ringer's solution is an acceptable replacement fluid. Maintenance fluids are estimated at 100 mL/kg/day. Fluids may be administered via an SC or IO (intraosseous) route in small patients, as IV route is limited by small patient size.

ACTIVITY
N/A

DIET
• Assist-feed if anorexic; adapt the diet to the underlying disease
• Provide multiple sources of fresh water. Flavoring the water with fruit or vegetable juice (with no added sugars) may be helpful. Provide a variety of clean, fresh, leafy vegetables sprayed or soaked with water; baby food; or pellets soaked in water.

CLIENT EDUCATION
• Discuss the importance of access to fresh water for the patient.
• Make sure owner understands natural history of the pet; gerbils often do not need to drink at all if fed an adequate diet. PD/PU can be caused by owner who forces the animal to drink via syringe.

SURGICAL CONSIDERATIONS
N/A

MEDICATIONS

DRUG(S) OF CHOICE
Vary with underlying cause

CONTRAINDICATIONS
N/A

PRECAUTIONS
Until renal and hepatic failure have been excluded as potential causes for PU/PD, use caution in administration of any drug eliminated via these pathways.

POSSIBLE INTERACTIONS
N/A

ALTERNATIVE DRUGS
N/A

FOLLOW-UP

PATIENT MONITORING
• Hydration status by clinical assessment of hydration and serial evaluation of body weight
• Fluid intake and urine output—provide a useful baseline for assessing adequacy of hydration therapy

PREVENTION/AVOIDANCE
Avoid overfeeding the animal; use appropriate diet to prevent diabetes mellitus

POSSIBLE COMPLICATIONS
• Dehydration
• Urine scald, pododermatitis, and myiasis secondary to polyuria

EXPECTED COURSE AND PROGNOSIS
Depends on the underlying cause

MISCELLANEOUS

ASSOCIATED CONDITIONS
Bacterial urinary tract infection

AGE-RELATED FACTORS
The prevalence of most underlying diseases increases with the age of the patient.

ZOONOTIC POTENTIAL
None

PREGNANCY/FERTILITY/BREEDING
N/A

SYNONYMS
N/A

SEE ALSO
Amyloidosis
Hematuria
Lower urinary tract infection
Renal failure

ABBREVIATIONS
ADH = antidiuretic hormone (or vasopressin)
PU/PD = polyuria/polydipsia

INTERNET RESOURCES
N/A

Suggested Reading
Dutton M. Selected veterinary concerns of geriatric rats, mice, hamsters, and gerbils. Vet Clin Exot Anim 2020;23(3):525–548.
Fisher PG. Exotic mammal renal disease: causes and clinical presentation. Vet Clin Exot Anim 2006;9:33–67.
Frolich J. Rats and mice. In: Quesenberry KE, Carpenter JW, eds. Ferrets, Rabbits and Rodents, 4th Ed). Clinical Medicine and Surgery. 2021 ed. St. Louis: Saunders, 2020:345–367.
Hallman RM, Brandão J. Diagnostic imaging of the renal system in exotic companion mammals. Vet Clin Exot Anim 2020;23:195–214.
Jekl V, Knotek Z. Evidence-based advances in rodent medicine. Vet Clin Exot Anim 2017;20:805–816.
Miwa Y, Mayer J. Hamsters and gerbils. In: Quesenberry KE, Carpenter JW, eds. Ferrets, Rabbits and Rodents, 4th Ed). Clinical Medicine and Surgery. 2021 ed. St. Louis: Saunders, 2020:368–384.
Reavill DR, Lennox AM. Disease overview of the urinary tract in exotic companion mammals and tips on clinical management. Vet Clin Exot Anim 2020;23(1):169–193.
Richardson VCG. Gerbil urinary system. In: Richardson VCG, ed. Diseases of Small Domestic Rodents. Oxford, UK: Blackwell, 2003a:106,226–227.
Richardson VCG. Hamster urinary system. In: VCG R, ed. Diseases of Small Domestic Rodents. Oxford, UK: Blackwell, 2003b:153.

Author Charly Pignon, DVM, Dip ECZM (Small Mammal)

PRURITUS

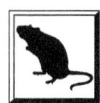

BASICS

DEFINITION
A sensation leading to the desire to scratch, rub, chew, or lick the affected area of inflamed skin.

PATHOPHYSIOLOGY
Though the causative factors of pruritus are many and varied, the sensation of itching is carried to the dorsal root of the spinal cord by A, delta, and C fibers in the peripheral nervous system. These axons ascend the lateral spinothalamic tract to synapse in the thalamus and sensory cortex. At this level, a variety of factors may modify the perception of pruritus.

SYSTEMS AFFECTED
Skin, in some cases mental status, may be affected

GENETICS
N/A

INCIDENCE/PREVALENCE
Pruritus is a very common presenting complaint across all small rodent species.

GEOGRAPHIC DISTRIBUTION
N/A

SIGNALMENT
Highly variable depending on the underlying cause of the pruritus

Breed Predilections
- Gerbils: bacterial dermatitis
- Mice: S. aureus pyoderma, ectoparasites, otitis media, idiopathic ulcerative dermatitis
- Rats: S. aureus pyoderma, ectoparasites
- Hamsters: ectoparasites

Mean Age and Range
N/A

Predominant Sex
N/A

SIGNS

Physical Examination Findings
Observation of the act of chewing, scratching, licking, or rubbing; or in some cases, evidence of inflamed skin, alopecia, and excoriations indicating self-trauma

CAUSES
- Ectoparasites
- Bacterial pyoderma
- Dermatophytosis (most often mild or nonpruritic)
- Poor nutrition, abnormal fatty acid metabolism (mice)
- Vasculitis, immune complex deposition (mice)
- Allergy—parasite hypersensitivity, atopy, food allergy, contact allergy, and drug allergy
- Psychogenic/stress

RISK FACTORS
Inappropriate husbandry, inappropriate humidity level, poor sanitation, poor diet

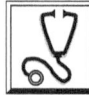

DIAGNOSIS

DIFFERENTIAL DIAGNOSIS
- Ectoparasites
- Bacterial pyoderma
- Dermatophytosis (most often mild or nonpruritic)
- Poor nutrition, dysregulated fatty acid metabolism (mice)
- Vasculitis, immune complex deposition (mice)

CBC/BIOCHEMISTRY/URINALYSIS
In systemically ill animals, serum biochemistry, complete blood count, and urinalysis should be included in the minimum database when possible.

OTHER LABORATORY TESTS
N/A

IMAGING
N/A

DIAGNOSTIC PROCEDURES
- Skin scrapings, epidermal cytology, dermatophyte culture and microscopic identification, and bacterial culture and sensitivity should be used to help identify concurrent or underlying parasitic, fungal, or bacterial disease.
- Skin biopsy and histopathologic evaluation for unusual cases with unclear etiology, expected immune-mediated disease, or poor response to therapy
- Trial therapy such as antiparasitic treatment, change of bedding materials, or hypoallergenic diet trials and monitoring response to treatment. Some parasitic infections, particularly sarcoptic infestations, may be difficult to identify on skin scrapings.

PATHOLOGIC FINDINGS
Variable depending on the etiology of the pruritus

TREATMENT

APPROPRIATE HEALTH CARE
Appropriate care will vary depending on the underlying cause of the itching, and multiple disease processes may be present. In some cases, restraint with a collar or light sedation may be helpful to prevent self-trauma, but mechanical restraint is not an appropriate long-term solution and can be difficult to achieve in small rodent species.

NURSING CARE
Most cases of pruritus will be treated on an outpatient basis.

ACTIVITY
If pruritus is severe and self-mutilation is a concern, activity may be limited by use of a restraining collar or light sedation. In most cases, activity should remain normal.

DIET
- Supplementation is appropriate if dietary deficiencies are identified as the cause of alopecia. Supplementation of essential fatty acids can help relieve dermal dryness and itching.
- If employing hypoallergenic diet trials, the novel diet should be continued for 8–10 weeks or until the animal improves. If the pet improves, the original diet should be reintroduced, and the pet monitored for the return of symptoms within 7–14 days.

CLIENT EDUCATION
- Review of appropriate husbandry for the species in question
- Awareness of zoonotic potential if present

SURGICAL CONSIDERATIONS
N/A

MEDICATIONS

DRUG(S) OF CHOICE
Topical therapy for mild or focal pruritus (antihistamines, antifungals, antibiotics, and aloe vera)

Antibiotics—for primary or secondary bacterial infections. Common antibiotics used in the treatment of small rodents include:
- Trimethoprim-sulfa (15–30 mg/kg PO, SC q12h)
- Enrofloxacin (5–20 mg/kg PO, SC, IM q12h)
- Chloramphenicol (30–50 mg/kg PO q8h)
- Azithromycin (10–30 mg/kg PO q24)
- Amoxicillin/Clavulanic acid (20 mg/kg PO q12h *Do not use in hamsters)

Antiparasitic medications commonly used include:
- Ivermectin—0.3–0.5 mg/kg SQ every 7–14 days for 3 treatments or until infestation is resolved, or 1:100 dilute ivermectin in propylene glycol placed on the head to be spread by normal grooming activity
- Selamectin—15–30 mg/kg topically every 14–28 days
- Fipronil—7.5 mg/kg topically every 30–60 days
- Pyrethrin powder topically every 3–7 days for 3 weeks. May be incorporated into the dust bath for chinchillas and gerbils.

Commonly used antifungals include:
• Topical miconazole, once daily for 2–4 weeks
• Antifungal shampoos that are safe for use in cats
• Griseofulvin 15–25 mg/kg orally once daily for up to 60 days. Absorption is enhanced if given with a fatty meal. Gastrointestinal irritation is the most common side effect and can be alleviated by dividing the dose for more frequent administration. Bone marrow suppression is a possible idiosyncratic reaction or can result from prolonged therapy. Neurologic side effects and teratogenicity in the first two trimesters of pregnancy have been reported. Biweekly monitoring of the CBC is recommended.
• Lime sulfur dip, 1:40 dilute with water has been used; dip once every 7 days for 4–6 treatments.
If pruritus is severe, light sedation may be needed
• Midazolam (0.25–1.0 mg/kg IM, IV)

CONTRAINDICATIONS
• Application of any topical substance may increase itching and discomfort and draw the patient's attention to the affected area.
• Antihistamines and psychoactive medications may cause sedation and have no proven efficacy in treatment of pruritic conditions in small rodents.
• Risk of potentially fatal antibiotic-induced enterotoxemia in Hamsters is associated with orally administered penicillin, ampicillin, cephalosporins, carbenicillin, lincomycin, clindamycin, streptomycin, gentamycin, neomycin, erythromycin, vancomycin, and tetracycline.
• Midazolam may increase the cardiorespiratory effects of other medications. It should be used with caution in debilitated or geriatric patients, in patients with hepatic or renal disease, during the first trimester of pregnancy, and during lactation and nursing.

PRECAUTIONS
Steroid medications are infrequently used in small rodents due to the potential for serious side effects. Topical products should be applied with caution as most of the small mammals groom prodigiously and may ingest excessive amounts of medication.

POSSIBLE INTERACTIONS
N/A

ALTERNATIVE DRUGS
N/A

FOLLOW-UP

PATIENT MONITORING
Patient monitoring and client communication are very important as many causes of pruritus have similar symptoms and concurrent disease processes are common. Resolution of one etiologic agent does not mean that other disease processes are not present. Many of these conditions are chronic in nature or may vary by season, requiring excellent client communication to elucidate treatment success/failure. Any patient on long-term medical therapy should be evaluated every 3–4 months for potential side effects of therapy.

PREVENTION/AVOIDANCE
• Review of appropriate husbandry for the species in question
• Awareness of zoonotic potential, if present

POSSIBLE COMPLICATIONS
• Client frustration is common in many of the chronic cases of pruritus in which diagnostic testing and treatment may appear unrewarding, and prolonged therapy may be necessary.
• Complications are a possibility with any long-term medication.

EXPECTED COURSE AND PROGNOSIS
Prognosis is variable depending on the etiology of the pruritus. Some mite infestations and dermatophyte or bacterial dermatoses resolve quickly and completely with appropriate medications. Other conditions such as allergy, food intolerance, or conditions complicated by underlying medical problems may have a more protracted course and carry a more conservative prognosis.

MISCELLANEOUS

ASSOCIATED CONDITIONS
Pets affected by underlying medical conditions, immune system compromise or stress, or poor husbandry may be predisposed to developing conditions associated with pruritus.

AGE-RELATED FACTORS
Young animals, particularly those just acquired, and animals of advanced age may be more disposed to developing conditions associated with pruritus.

ZOONOTIC POTENTIAL
• Dermatophytes
• Some ectoparasites

PREGNANCY/FERTILITY/BREEDING
N/A

SYNONYMS
Itching

SEE ALSO
Alopecia
Dermatophytosis
Ectoparasites

ABBREVIATIONS
N/A

INTERNET RESOURCES
Exotic DVM forum for eDVM readers:
www.pets.groups.yahoo.com/
group/ExoticDVM
    Veterinary Information Network:
www.vin.com

Suggested Reading
Frolich J. Rats and mice. In: Quesenberry KE, Carpenter JW, eds. Ferrets, Rabbits and Rodents, 4th Ed). Clinical Medicine and Surgery. 2021 ed. St. Louis: Saunders, 2020:345–367.
Hoppmann E, Barron HW. Rodent dermatology. J Exot Pet Med 2007;16(4):238–255.
Jekl V, Knotek Z. Evidence-based advances in rodent medicine. Vet Clin Exot Anim 2017;20:805–816.
Meredith A, Redrobe S. BSAVA Manual of Exotic Pets, 4th ed. Gloucester, UK: British Small Animal Veterinary Association, 2002:20–21, 28–30, 39–41, 55–60.
Miwa Y, Mayer J. Hamsters and gerbils. In: Quesenberry KE, Carpenter JW, eds. Ferrets, Rabbits and Rodents, 4th Ed). Clinical Medicine and Surgery. 2021 ed. St. Louis: Saunders, 2020:368–384.
Palmerio BS, Roberts H. Clinical approach to dermatologic disease in exotic animals. Vet Clin North Am Exot Anim Pract 2013;16(3):523–577.
White SD, Bourdeau PJ, Brément T et al. Companion rats (*Rattus norvegicus*) with cutaneous lesions: a retrospective study of 470 cases at two university veterinary teaching hospitals (1985–2018). Vet Dermatol 2019;30:237–272.
Author Christine Eckermann-Ross, DVM, CVA, CVH

RECTAL PROLAPSE

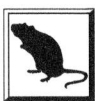

BASICS

DEFINITION
- A protrusion of rectal mucosa through the external anal orifice is an anal prolapse (partial prolapse).
- A double layer of the rectum that protrudes through the anal canal is a rectal prolapse (complete prolapse).
- A prolapse of the colon or small intestine through the rectum and anus is a bowel prolapse.
- The term *rectal prolapse* is commonly applied to all of the above.

PATHOPHYSIOLOGY
Excessive straining promotes intussusception of rectum and/or large intestine with protrusion through the anal opening.

SIGNALMENT
- May occur in any age or gender
- Young and recently weaned animals are predisposed to diarrhea and internal parasites, common predisposing factors for rectal prolapsed.
- Male hosts are generally more heavily parasitized by pinworms—a risk factor for rectal prolapse—than are females.
- The rectum of mice is weakly anchored by the mesocolon and prone to prolapse with straining.

SIGNS
- Persistent tenesmus
- Vocalization when defecating
- Tubular hyperemic mass protruding from the anus
- Blood on bedding or cage furnishings

CAUSES AND RISK FACTORS
- Diarrhea—due to bacterial, parasitic, or viral infection; infiltrative or neoplastic intestinal disease; secondary to systemic illness; improper antibiotic usage; carbohydrate overload
- Constipation—straining to defecate, excessively dry or hard feces due to inappropriate diet, dehydration, and some drugs (anticholinergics, opioids, barium, kaolin/pectin, sucralfate)
- Gastrointestinal obstruction—neoplasia, foreign body, intussusception
- Tenesmus—colonic or rectal disease, pinworm infestation, dyschezia, urogenital discomfort, stranguria, dystocia, pelvic fracture, intrapelvic mass
- Estrogenic stimulation—phytoestrogens, fungal estrogens (mice)

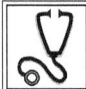

DIAGNOSIS

DIFFERENTIAL DIAGNOSIS

General
- Consider all causes of enteropathy and diarrhea, including diet change, inappropriate antibiotics, enterotoxemia, systemic or metabolic disease, and specific intestinal disorders.
- Infectious and parasitic causes vary by species, as listed below.

Mice/Rats
- Most common cause is pinworm (*Syphacia obvelata, Aspiculuris tetraptera*) infestation, which can be associated with intestinal impaction, intussusception, peritonitis, and rectal prolapse in mice
- *Citrobacter rodentium* infection ("transmissible murine colonic hyperplasia") occasionally causes rectal prolapse in mice.
- Other potential causes—viruses (especially common in neonates; mouse hepatitis virus [coronavirus], epizootic diarrhea of infant mice [rotavirus], reovirus, others); bacteria (*Helicobacter* spp., *Salmonella* spp., *Clostridium piliforme, E. coli, Enterococcus* spp., others); protozoa (*Spironucleus muris, Giardia muris, Eimeria,* others); cestodes (*Rodentolepis* spp., formerly *Hymenolepis*)

Gerbils
Potential causes—bacteria (*Citrobacter rodentium, Salmonella* spp., *E. coli,* and *Clostridium piliforme*); cestodes (*Rodentolepis* spp.); pinworms (*Dentostomella* spp., *Syphacia* spp.)

Hamsters
- Most common cause is "wet tail" or proliferative ileitis of hamsters, caused by the intracellular bacterium *Lawsonia intracellularis.* Affected animals may have palpably thickened bowel loops and are prone to ileal obstruction, impaction, intussusception, peritonitis, tenesmus, dyschezia, and rectal prolapse.
- Other potential causes—bacteria (*Clostridium difficile, E. coli, Salmonella,* and *Clostridium piliforme*); protozoa (*Spironucleus* spp., *Giardia,* others); cestodes (*Rodentolepis* spp.); pinworms (*Syphacia* spp.)

CBC/BIOCHEMISTRY
- Usually normal
- May reflect underlying cause (e.g., inflammatory leukogram with infectious disease)

OTHER LABORATORY TESTS
- Fecal direct examination, fecal floatation, and zinc sulfate centrifugation—may demonstrate gastrointestinal parasites or spore-forming bacteria
- Fecal cytology/gram's stain—detection of inflammation, spore-forming, or gram-negative bacteria

- Fecal culture should be performed if bacterial infection is suspected.
- Cellophane tape impressions of the perineal area—detects *Syphacia* spp. pinworm infection

IMAGING
- Survey abdominal radiography may indicate intestinal obstruction, organomegaly, mass, foreign body, ascites, pregnancy, or urolithiasis.
- Contrast radiography may indicate mucosal irregularities, mass, ileus, foreign body, stricture, or thickening of the intestinal wall.
- Abdominal ultrasonography may demonstrate intestinal wall thickening, gastrointestinal mass, foreign body, ileus, mesenteric lymphadenopathy, or intussusception.

DIAGNOSTIC PROCEDURES
- Determine what has prolapsed by carefully examining the tissue: if the tissue is solid, it may be a rectal mass or polyp that has extruded on a stalk; if there is an orifice at the end of the tissue, it is a section of bowel.
- It the prolapse is bowel, then a small, blunt probe is gently passed along each side of the prolapsed tissue: if the probe easily passes 1 cm or less along the side of the tissue, it is an anal or rectal prolapse; if the probe easily passes greater than 1 cm along the side of the tissue, it is an intestinal or colonic prolapse.
- Exploratory laparotomy and surgical biopsy are indicated if there is evidence of obstruction or intestinal mass and/or for definitive diagnosis of gastrointestinal inflammatory or infiltrative disease.
- Viability of the prolapsed tissue may be assessed by surface appearance and tissue temperature—vital tissue appears swollen and hyperemic, and red blood exudes from the cut surface; devitalized tissue appears dark purple or back, and dark cyanotic blood exudes from the cut surface. Ulcerations of the prolapsed tissue may be present.

PATHOLOGIC FINDINGS
- Vary with cause and severity of diarrheic condition
- Gross pathology may reveal lesions suggestive of etiology.
- Histopathology is often the best method to obtain a definitive diagnosis for neoplasia, infiltrative or inflammatory conditions, and intracellular infections (e.g., *Lawsonia intracellularis, Clostridium piliforme*).

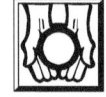

TREATMENT

APPROPRIATE HEALTH CARE
- Must identify and treat underlying cause
- Assisted feeding is typically required for debilitated patients until they are eating, eliminating, and maintaining body weight.

• Fluid therapy—rehydration and correction of electrolyte imbalances are indicated in most cases, particularly when diarrhea is involved.
• If prolapse is mild or intermittent and does not cause straining, treating the underlying cause without replacing the mucosa may be sufficient; keep tissues moist by use of lubricant until underlying problem resolves.
• Conservative medical management—gently replace viable prolapsed tissue through the anus with the use of lubricants; osmotic agents may help if severe swelling exists.
• Placement of an anal purse-string suture may aid in retention and prevent recurrence after reduction; suture placement must allow room for defecation. The purse-string suture is generally removed in 5–7 days.
• Necrotic rectal/bowel prolapses can be amputated using a full-thickness incision through the prolapse at its healthy junction with remaining normal rectum or intestine. Anastomosis is performed 360 degrees around the incision, joining healthy rectum to healthy anus, or healthy bowel to healthy bowel.
• Extensive bowel prolapse may be treated through a ventral midline abdominal approach. Identify and gently reduce the intussuscepted segment. Resect the necrotic portion of the intussusception and perform an end-to-end anastomosis. Colopexy may be indicated to prevent recurrence.

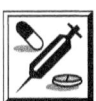

MEDICATIONS
DRUG(S) OF CHOICE
• Appropriate anesthetics/analgesics as needed
• Topical agents to aid in reduction—50% dextrose solution and sterile lubricant jelly
• Specific treatment for the underlying cause
• Mice with pinworm (*Syphacia* spp., *Aspiculuris tetraptera*) infestation—ivermectin (2 mg/kg PO, repeat in 10 days; dose cited is 10× higher than normally used in other species and is reported to be safe and effective in mice), fenbendazole (20 mg/kg PO q24h × 5 days), pyrantel pamoate (50 mg/kg PO; dosing interval for small rodents not reported, but dose is repeated in 10 days for most other exotic companion mammals)
• Hamsters with *Lawsonia intracellularis* infection (wet tail or proliferative ileitis)—chloramphenicol (30–50 mg/kg PO q12h), tetracycline (10–20 mg/kg PO q12h), enrofloxacin (5–10 mg/kg PO q12h), or trimethoprim-sulfa (15–30 mg/kg PO q12h)
• For *Clostridium* spp. overgrowth—metronidazole (20 mg/kg PO q12h)

• Empirical treatment of other suspected bacterial infections, broad-spectrum antibiotics based upon culture/sensitivity where possible: chloramphenicol (30–50 mg/kg PO q8h), trimethoprim-sulfa (15–30 mg/kg PO q12h), or enrofloxacin (5–10 mg/kg PO, SC, IM q12h)

CONTRAINDICATIONS
• Anticholinergics (e.g., loperamide) in patients with suspected intestinal obstruction, glaucoma, intestinal ileus, liver disease, enterotoxin-producing bacteria, and invasive bacterial enteritis
• Antibiotics that are primarily gram-positive in spectrum will suppress the growth of commensal flora, allowing overgrowth of enteric pathogens. These include lincomycin, clindamycin, erythromycin, ampicillin, amoxicillin, cephalosporins, and penicillins.

PRECAUTIONS
• Antibiotic therapy can predispose small rodents (particularly hamsters) to bacterial dysbiosis and overgrowth of pathogenic bacteria (e.g., *Clostridium difficile*). If signs worsen or do not improve, therapy should be adjusted.
• Chloramphenicol may cause aplastic anemia in susceptible people. Clients and staff should use appropriate precautions when handling this drug.
• Metronidazole is neurotoxic if overdosed.
• Meloxicam—use with caution in cases with suspected renal compromise

FOLLOW-UP
PATIENT MONITORING
Purse-string removal in 5–7 days

PREVENTION/AVOIDANCE
• Providing appropriate diet and husbandry
• Reducing stress and providing sanitary conditions
• When infectious disease is suspected, strict isolation of affected and exposed animals is indicated.

POSSIBLE COMPLICATIONS
• Recurrence—especially if uncontrolled underlying problem exists
• Complete elimination of oxyurid pinworms in mice is difficult to achieve.

EXPECTED COURSE AND PROGNOSIS
• Depends on cause and severity of disease
• Rodents with intussuscepted, prolapsed bowel have a poor prognosis for survival because they usually present in a debilitated condition secondary to primary disease that caused the straining and the prolapse.

• Prognosis for *Lawsonia intracellularis* infection in hamsters is guarded
• Pinworm infestations are difficult to eliminate due to the environmental resistance and ease of transmission of oxyurid ova. Anthelmintic treatment alone usually results in only a transient elimination of the intestinal nematodes.

MISCELLANEOUS
ASSOCIATED CONDITIONS
See Causes and Risk Factors

AGE-RELATED FACTORS
• Young and recently weaned animals and those with decreased resistance to infection are most susceptible to infectious and parasitic risk factors for rectal prolapse.
• Adults and older individuals may be more prone to neoplastic intestinal disease, intrapelvic masses, or degenerative systemic disease leading to rectal prolapse.

ZOONOTIC POTENTIAL
Syphacia spp. pinworm infection has been reported in humans, which are a dead-end host for the parasite.

PREGNANCY/FERTILITY/BREEDING
Pinworm infestation may be associated with reproductive depression in small rodents.

SYNONYMS
• The term *rectal prolapse* is commonly applied to any anal prolapse regardless of tissue origin (i.e., anus, rectum, and colon).
• Wet tail in hamsters caused by *Lawsonia intracellularis* infection is also known as proliferative ileitis and transmissible ileal hyperplasia.
• *Citrobacter rodentium* infection is also referred to as transmissible (murine) colonic hyperplasia.
• Cestodes of the genus *Rodentolepis* are referred to by the former name *Hymenolepis* in many references.
• Pinworm infestation is also referred to as oxyuriasis.

SEE ALSO
Diarrhea
Intestinal parasitism

ABBREVIATIONS
N/A

INTERNET RESOURCES
N/A

Suggested Reading
Dutton M. Selected veterinary concerns of geriatric rats, mice, hamsters, and gerbils. Vet Clin Exot Anim 2020;23(3): 525–548.

RECTAL PROLAPSE

Frolich J. Rats and mice. In: Quesenberry KE, Carpenter JW, eds. Ferrets, Rabbits and Rodents, 4th Ed). Clinical Medicine and Surgery. 2021 ed. St. Louis: Saunders, 2020:345–367.

Hrapkiewicz K, Colby L, Denison P, eds. Clinical Laboratory Animal Medicine: An Introduction, 4th ed. Ames: Wiley-Blackwell, 2013:83–92, 128–133, 156–159, 182–187.

Jekl V, Knotek Z. Evidence-based advances in rodent medicine. Vet Clin Exot Anim 2017;20:805–816.

Lennox AM, Gladden JN. Emergency and critical care of small mammals. In: Quesenberry KE, Carpenter JW, eds. Ferrets, Rabbits and Rodents, 4th Ed). Clinical Medicine and Surgery. 2021 ed. St. Louis: Saunders, 2020:595–608.

Mayer J, Mans C. Rodents. In: Carpenter JW, ed. Exotic Animal Formulary, 5th ed. St Louis: Elsevier, 2018:459–493.

Mitchell MA, Tully TN, eds. Manual of Exotic Pet Practice. St Louis: Elsevier, 2009:326–344, 406–432.

Miwa Y, Mayer J. Hamsters and gerbils. In: Quesenberry KE, Carpenter JW, eds. Ferrets, Rabbits and Rodents, 4th Ed). Clinical Medicine and Surgery. 2021 ed. St. Louis: Saunders, 2020:368–384.

Author Dan H. Johnson, DVM, Dipl. ABVP (Exotic Companion Mammal)

RED TEARS (CHROMODACRYORRHEA)

BASICS

DEFINITION
• Accumulation of porphyrin pigment in ocular and respiratory secretions
• Not a primary disease process

PATHOPHYSIOLOGY
• Porphyrin, or porphyrin precursors, are produced in the Harderian glands (lacrimal glands) of rats.
• The exact mechanism for excessive production is uncertain, but it can be caused by obstruction of the lacrimal ducts due to rhinitis or inflammation of the Harderian glands.
• Significant production also occurs with stress (physiologic and psychologic) or pain.

SYSTEMS AFFECTED
• Ocular—primary production of pigmented tears
• Respiratory—pigmented tears traveling through the nasolacrimal duct
• Urinary—also may see porphyrin pigments in the urine

SIGNALMENT
• No specific sex or age predilection
• Associated with stress and concurrent disease, so incidence may increase with age

SIGNS
• Pink- to red-colored nasal and ocular discharge
• Pink- to red-colored urine may also be seen.
• Other signs are related to the presence of underlying disease conditions.

CAUSES
• Has been associated with a number of underlying disease conditions
• In rats is commonly seen with respiratory disease, including both bacterial and viral agents, in particular sialodacryoadenitis (SDAV) virus; in cases of SDAV virus is generally self-limiting
• May also be associated with environmental stress (handling, aggression from cagemates, and overcrowding)
• Environmental and airborne irritants, including aromatic beddings

RISK FACTORS
Any condition producing physiologic or psychologic stress

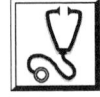

DIAGNOSIS

DIFFERENTIAL DIAGNOSIS
• Hemorrhage from eyes or nose secondary to trauma or inflammation

• Hematuria or blood from vaginal orifice secondary to urinary tract or reproductive disease

CBC/BIOCHEMISTRY/URINALYSIS
Testing is useful to identify other concurrent disease processes.

OTHER LABORATORY TESTS
• Ultraviolet light, Wood's lamp—porphyrin pigments emit a characteristic pink florescence under an ultraviolet light source
• Cytologic preparation of nasal/ocular exudate to rule out the presence of erythrocytes
• Urinalysis/urine cytology will to rule out the presence of erythrocytes in porphyrin-pigmented urine.

IMAGING
• Useful for identification of other underlying disease conditions
• Useful for identification of urolithiasis, which may produce hematuria

DIAGNOSTIC PROCEDURES
• Treatment of underlying disease conditions as a trial
• Thorough diagnostic evaluation to identify underlying disease conditions

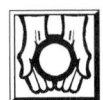

TREATMENT

APPROPRIATE HEALTH CARE
Outpatient—unless severe debilitating disease

NURSING CARE
• Supportive care
• Keep discharge cleaned from face

CLIENT EDUCATION
• Inform client porphyrin discharge is often secondary to an underlying medical condition.
• Ensure ideal husbandry, including reduction of overcrowding and stress.
• Identify and correct stress-producing handling techniques.

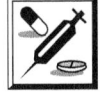

MEDICATIONS

DRUG(S) OF CHOICE
• No specific treatment for chromodacryorrhea
• Treat underlying disease

CONTRAINDICATIONS
• Do not administer penicillins, ampicillin, amoxicillin, erythromycin, or lincomycin to hamsters due to the risk of potentially fatal enteric dysbiosis.
• Doxycycline should be avoided in very young or pregnant animals.

• Do not use corticosteroid-containing topical ophthalmic preparations.

PRECAUTIONS
All therapeutic agents should be used with caution in debilitated, dehydrated patients. Ideally, vascular abnormalities (dehydration, hypotension) are addressed prior to initiating antibiotic therapy.

ALTERNATIVE DRUGS
There is some anecdotal evidence that immune-boosting drugs/agents have been useful in some cases of infectious disease.

FOLLOW-UP

PATIENT MONITORING
• Ensure adequate intake of food and water.
• Monitor response to therapy of underlying disease condition.
• When underlying conditions are corrected, presence of porphyrin discharge should decrease.

MISCELLANEOUS

SYNONYMS
Chromodacryorrhea
Porphyrin staining

SEE ALSO
Rhinitis and sinusitis
Sialodacryoadenitis virus

ABBREVIATIONS
N/A

Suggested Reading
Capello V, Lennox AM. Diagnostic imaging of the respiratory system in exotic companion mammals. Vet Clin Exot Anim 2011;14:369–389.

Dutton M. Selected veterinary concerns of geriatric rats, mice, hamsters, and gerbils. Vet Clin Exot Anim 2020;23(3):525–548.

Ferreira JB, Yamaguti M, Marques LM et al. Detection of mycoplasma pulmonis in laboratory rats and technicians. Zoonoses Public Health 2008;55(5):229–234.

Frolich J. Rats and mice. In: Quesenberry KE, Carpenter JW, eds. Ferrets, Rabbits and Rodents, 4th Ed). Clinical Medicine and Surgery. 2021 ed. St. Louis: Saunders, 2020:345–367.

Graham JE, Schoeb TR. Mycoplasma pulmonis in rats. J Exotic Pet Med 2011;20(4):270–276.

Jekl V, Knotek Z. Evidence-based advances in rodent medicine. Vet Clin Exot Anim 2017;20:805–816.

RODENTS

RED TEARS (CHROMODACRYORRHEA)

Mayer J, Mans C. Rodents. In: Carpenter JW, ed. Exotic Animal Formulary, 5th ed. St Louis: Elsevier, 2018:459–493.

Miwa Y, Mayer J. Hamsters and gerbils. In: Quesenberry KE, Carpenter JW, eds. Ferrets, Rabbits and Rodents, 4th Ed). Clinical Medicine and Surgery. 2021 ed. St. Louis: Saunders, 2020:368–384.

Piasecki T, Chrzastek K, Kasprzykowska U et al. Mycoplasma pulmonis of rodents as a possible human pathogen. Vector Borne Zoonotic Dis 2017;17(7):475–477.

Author Angela M. Lennox, DVM, Dipl. ABVP (Avian, ECM) DECZM-Small Mammal

BASICS

DEFINITION
• Azotemia (higher than normal blood concentration of urea or other nitrogen-containing compounds in the blood) and inability to concentrate urine, or azotemia in the absence of dehydration
• Acute renal failure (ARF) is a syndrome characterized by a sudden onset of filtration failure by the kidneys, accumulation of uremic toxins, and dysfunction of fluid, electrolyte, and acid–base balance.
• Chronic renal failure (CRF) results from primary renal disease that has persisted for a month to years; characterized by irreversible renal dysfunction that tends to deteriorate progressively.

PATHOPHYSIOLOGY
• Reduction in functional renal mass results in impaired urine-concentrating ability (leading to polyuria/polydipsia) and retention of nitrogenous waste products of protein catabolism (leading to azotemia).
• Adrenaline release in response to stress can cause significant reduction in renal plasma flow and glomerular filtration rate, predisposing stressed animal to ARF.
• Renal calculi—rat
• Nephrocalcinosis—rat and gerbil: dietary factors, including magnesium deficiency, elevated dietary phosphorus or calcium, and diet preparations with a low calcium-to-phosphorus ratio
• Chronic progressive nephrosis (CPN)—rats—high-protein diets may promote disease
• Ascending lower urinary tract infection—bacterial, parasitic (in rat: bladder thread-worm *Trichosomoides crassicauda*) may cause pyelonephritis and subsequent renal failure
• With chronicity, decrease of erythropoietin and calcitriol production by the kidneys can result in nonregenerative anemia.
• Anesthesia (with any type of protocol) can cause significant reduction in renal plasma flow and glomerular filtration rate, predisposing animal to ARF.
• Because of their gnawing behavior, their urine-concentrating ability, and their more efficient nephron, gerbils are prone to accumulations of systemic lead and subsequent toxicity.

SYSTEMS AFFECTED
• Renal/Urologic—impaired renal function leading to PU/PD and signs of uremia
• Nervous, gastrointestinal, musculoskeletal, and other body system, secondary to affected by uremia
• Hemic/Lymphatic/Immune—anemia

GENETICS
Certain strains of laboratory rats are more affected (e.g., CPN)

INCIDENCE/PREVALENCE
• CPN—common in rat
• Pyelonephritis/nephritis—common in mice
• Arteriolar nephrosclerosis—common in old female hamsters
• Chronic interstitial nephritis—common in old gerbils
• Chronic nephropathies as a result of aging are common in rodents older than 1 year (especially in rats)

GEOGRAPHIC DISTRIBUTION
Worldwide

SIGNALMENT

Breed Predilections
Sprague-Dawley rat (CPN)

Mean Age and Range
• CPN is a common life-limiting disease in the older rat.
• Animals of all ages can be affected, but prevalence increases with increasing age.
• Pyelonephritis/nepritis—old rats

Predominant Sex
• CPN in male rats is more severe and an earlier disease than in females.
• Nephrocalcinosis is more common in female rats.

SIGNS

General Comments
Clinical signs are related to the severity of renal dysfunction and presence or absence of complications.

Historical Findings
Acute renal failure:
• Sudden onset of anorexia, listlessness
• Diarrhea or lack of stool production (ileus)
• Ataxia or seizures
• Known toxin exposure
• Recent medical or surgical conditions
• Oliguria, anuria, or polyuria
Chronic renal failure:
• PU/PD
• Anorexia
• Diarrhea or lack of stool production (ileus)
• Weight loss, lethargy, or poor hair coat
• Ataxia, seizure, or coma seen in late stages
• Asymptomatic animals with CRF may decompensate, resulting in a uremic crisis.

Physical Examination Findings
Acute renal failure:
• Depression
• Dehydration (sometimes overhydration)
• Hypothermia
• Fever
• Tachypnea
• Bradycardia

• Nonpalpable urinary bladder if oliguric
• Kidneys may be painful on palpation.
Chronic renal failure:
• Small, irregular kidneys sometime palpable
• Dehydration
• Cachexia
• Mucous membrane pallor
• Rats often have unkempt appearance and are reluctant to move.

CAUSES

Acute Renal Failure
• Shock
• Severe stress
• Prolonged anesthesia
• Heatstroke
• Septicemia (e.g., pyometra)

Acute or Chronic Renal Failure
• Nephroliths
• Glomerulonephritis
• Chronic urinary obstruction (proteinaceous plugs or calculi in mice and rats)
• Drugs (e.g., aminoglycosides, sulfanamides, and chemotherapeutic agents)
• Heavy metals
• Lymphoma or other neoplasia
• Amyloidosis

RISK FACTORS

Acute Renal Failure
• Preexisting renal disease
• Pyelonephritis
• Dehydration
• Hypovolemia
• Severe stress
• Hypotension
• Advanced age
• Concurrent disease
• Prolonged anesthesia
• Administration of nephrotoxic agents

Chronic Renal Failure
• Aging
• Nephroliths
• Urinary tract infection
• Diabetes mellitus
• CPN: high-protein diets
• Nephrocalcinosis
• Diet with magnesium deficiency
• Elevated phosphorus or calcium and low calcium-to-phosphorus ratio

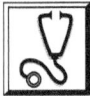

DIAGNOSIS

DIFFERENTIAL DIAGNOSIS
• For PU/PD—hypercalciuria, pyometra, hepatic failure, diabetes mellitus, post-obstructive diuresis, and behavioral disorder
• For renomegaly—renal neoplasia (cortical epithelial carcinoma, adenoma, and adenocarcinoma in rat, lymphoma in

hamster), hydronephrosis (rat, gerbil), renal abscess, polycystic kidneys (rat, hamster)
• Prerenal azotemia (decreased renal perfusion)—characterized by azotemia with concentrated urine, decreased renal perfusion (dehydration, shock, or cardiac disease), or as a result of a high-protein diet or intestinal hemorrhage
• Postrenal azotemia—characterized by azotemia with obstruction or rupture of the excretory system

CBC/BIOCHEMISTRY/ URINALYSIS
• Pyelonephritis may result in a leukocytosis characterized by a left shift or mature neutrophilia.
• Nonregenerative anemia with CRF; normal or high PCV with ARF
• BUN elevation, creatinine elevation
• Significant proteinuria (CPN)—healthy adult mouse, rat, gerbil, and hamster normally have mild proteinuria
• May see hyper- or hypocalcemia
• Hyperphosphatemia
• Hyper- or hypokalemia
• Hypoproteinemia, hypercholesterolemia common
• Inability to concentrate the urine
• Increased WBC in case of pyelonephritis
• Urinary sediment—struvite in rats

OTHER LABORATORY TESTS
Serum lead or zinc to rule out heavy metal intoxication as a cause

IMAGING
• Abdominal ultrasonography may be helpful to assess the size of the kidney, identify pyelonephritis, renal cyst, renal abscess, hydronephrosis, degeneration or neoplasia
• Renal ultrasonography plays a role in discerning tissue architecture, allowing for differentiation between focal and diffuse disease. Ultrasonography can help with the diagnosis of pyelonephritis, hydronephrosis and hydroureter, renal cysts, and abscesses. On ultrasound, the normal length of the left kidney is 19.47 ± 2.3 mm and for the right kidney 19.45 ± 2.18 mm.
• Abdominal radiography may reveal urinary sludge or uroliths, renal calculi (struvite rat). It could also be useful to assess the size of the kidneys. Radiographic measures of the kidneys were evaluated and expressed as a ration to the body length of the second lumbar vertebra. The left kidney ratio length is 2.39–3.85, and the right kidney ratio length is 2.13–3.98.
• Contrast urography—useful in assessing renal anomalies, especially in small species
• Animals with ARF often have normal-sized to large kidneys.

• Animals with CRF often have small kidneys. But enlarged kidneys could be found secondary to hydronephrosis, renal cysts, renal abscess, or neoplasia.

DIAGNOSTIC PROCEDURES
Evaluation of ultrasound-guided fine-needle aspirate of the kidney may be helpful in the diagnosis of renal neoplasia, abscesses, or cysts.

PATHOLOGIC FINDINGS
• Gross findings—small kidneys with a lumpy or granular surface may be seen with CRF. Large, irregular kidneys with neoplasia or abscess are commonly found. CPN: enlarged and pale kidneys, with pitted and irregular renal cortices that often contain pinpoint cysts
• Histologic findings—chronic generalized nephropathy or end-stage kidneys; findings are specific for disease causing CRF; CPN: severe glomerulosclerosis with deposition of protein-rich material in proximal tubules; nephrocalcinosis: deposition of calcium phosphates in the interstitium of the corticomedullary junction, with intratubular aggregations; nephrosis or nephritis may be seen in patients with ARF

TREATMENT
APPROPRIATE HEALTH CARE
• Patients with compensated CRF may be managed as outpatients.
• Patients in ARF or uremic crisis should be managed as inpatients.

NURSING CARE
• Patients in ARF or uremic crisis—correct estimated fluids deficits with normal (0.9%) saline or balanced polyionic solution within 4–6 hours to prevent additional renal injury from the ischemia; once the patient is hydrated, ongoing fluid requirements are provided as a balanced electrolyte solution. Use caution when hydrating stressed animal. Severe stress may cause a decrease in GFR and subsequent overhydration. Be sure that the volume of urine excreted is appropriate to the amount of fluids received. Survey respiratory rate and respiratory effort. Fluids may be administered by IO (intraosseous) or SC routes; IV route is limited by small patient size. Maintenance fluid rate is estimated at 100 mL/kg/day or 3–4 mL/kg/day.
• Hypervolemia—stop fluid administration and eliminate excess fluid by diuretic administration.
• Patient in CRF—subcutaneous fluid therapy (daily or every other day) may benefit patients with moderate to severe CRF.

ACTIVITY
N/A

DIET
• Increase the water consumption. Provide multiple sources of fresh water. Flavoring the water with fruit or vegetable juice (with no added sugars) may be helpful. Provide a variety of clean, fresh, leafy vegetables sprayed or soaked with water; baby food; and pellets soaked in water.
• Provide a diet with correct calcium-to-phosphorous ratio and protein.
• Consider assist feeding the animal if anorexic.
• High-carbohydrate, high-fat nutritional supplements are contraindicated.

CLIENT EDUCATION
• CRF—tends to progress over months, possibly years
• ARF—inform owner of the poor prognosis for complete recovery, potential for morbid complication of treatment (e.g., fluid overload, sepsis, and multiple organ failure), and expense of prolonged hospitalization.
• In any patient with renal failure, quality of life issues and euthanasia should be discussed with the owner.

SURGICAL CONSIDERATIONS
• Avoid hypotension during anesthesia to prevent additional renal injuries.
• Nephrotomy to remove a nephrolith
• Nephrectomy—after assessing that the other kidney is functional

MEDICATIONS
DRUG(S) OF CHOICE
• Inadequate urine production (anuric or oliguric renal failure)—ensure patient is fluid volume replete; provide additional isonatric fluid to achieve mild (3%–5%) volume expansion; failure to induce diuresis by fluid replacement indicates severe parenchymal damage or underestimation of fluid deficit; if fluid replete, administration of diuretic (furosemide [1–4 mg/kg IV] or mannitol [0.5–1 g/kg IV over 20 minutes]) to induce diuresis may be successful; reduce stress. If these treatments fail to induce diuresis within 4–6 hours, the prognosis is grave.
• Hyperphosphatemia—aluminum hydroxide 30–90 mg/kg/day, divided
• Anorexia, inappetence—reduce gastric acid production: famotidine (0.t5–10 PO, SC, q24h) or ranitidine (1–2 mg/kg IV q24h or 2.5 mg/kg PO q12h)
• Severe chronic anemia—erythropoietin (50–150 IU/kg SC q2–3d until PCV normalizes, then q7d × 4 weeks)

• Antibiotics—in pyelonephritis/nephritis based on results of bacterial culture and antimicrobial sensitivity 4–6 weeks
• Treat anemia with vitamin/iron supplementation or human recombinant erythropoietin.

CONTRAINDICATIONS
Avoid nephrotoxic agents (NSAIDS, aminoglycosides)

PRECAUTIONS
Modify dosage of all drugs that require renal metabolism or elimination.

POSSIBLE INTERACTIONS
N/A

ALTERNATIVE DRUGS
• Studies have shown that omega-3 fatty acids have a number of beneficial effects on rat renal disease, including mitigating some of the detrimental effects of a high-fat diet and hyperlipidemia on glomerular function; attenuating the decline in glomerular filtration rate, the rise in blood pressure, and the proteinuria associated with renal disease; and in maintaining significantly lower serum creatinine levels.
• Anabolic steroids and B complex vitamins to stimulate appetite and encourage red blood cell production
• Phosphorus binders, such as aluminum hydroxide, to limit dietary phosphorus absorption and control hyperphosphatemia and secondary renal hyperparathyroidism, and decreased salt intake to help diminish fluid loss and control high blood pressure

 FOLLOW-UP

PATIENT MONITORING
• ARF—monitor urinalysis, PCV, BUN, creatinine and electrolytes, body weight, urine output, and clinical status twice daily.
• CRF—monitor at 1–3 month intervals, depending on the therapy and severity of disease.

PREVENTION/AVOIDANCE
Anticipate the potential for ARF in patients that are hemodynamically unstable, receiving nephrotoxic drugs, have multiple organ failure, or are undergoing prolonged anesthesia and surgery; maintenance of hydration and/or mild saline volume expansion may be preventive.

POSSIBLE COMPLICATIONS
ARF—seizures, gastrointestinal bleeding, cardiac arrhythmia, congestive heart failure, pulmonary edema, hypovolemic shock, coma, cardiopulmonary arrest, and death
  CRF—gastroenteritis, anemia, and death

EXPECTED COURSE AND PROGNOSIS
• Nonoliguric ARF—milder than oliguric; recovery may occur, but the prognosis remains guarded to unfavorable
• Oliguric ARF—extensive renal injury is difficult to manage and has a poor prognosis for recovery
• Anuric ARF—generally fatal
• CRF—short-term prognosis depends on severity; long-term prognosis guarded to poor, since CRF tends to be progressive

 MISCELLANEOUS

ASSOCIATED CONDITIONS
• Hypercalciuria
• Urolithiasis
• Ileus

AGE-RELATED FACTORS
Increased incidence in older animals; normal renal function decreases with aging

ZOONOTIC POTENTIAL
Leptospirosis—rat and mouse can carry leptospirosis, usually without showing any clinical signs

PREGNANCY/FERTILITY/ BREEDING
ARF is a rare complication of pregnancy in animal; promoted by acute metritis, pyometra, and postpartum sepsis or hemorrhage

SYNONYMS
Kidney failure

SEE ALSO
Amyloidosis
Polyuria and polydipsia

ABBREVIATIONS
ARF = acute renal failure
BUN = blood urea nitrogen
CPN = chronic progressive nephrosis
CRF = chronic renal failure
GFR = glomerular filtration rate
NSAID = nonsteroidal anti-inflammatory drug
PCV = packed cell volume
PU/PD = polyuria/polydipsia
WBC = white blood cell count

Suggested Reading
Bezato T, Bellini L, Contiero B et al. Abdominal anatomic features and reference values determined by use of ultrasonography in healthy common rats (*Rattus norvegicus*). AJVR 2014;75(1):67–76.
Dorotea AB, Banzato T, Bellini L et al. Kidney measure in the domestic rat: a radiographic study and a comparison to ultrasonographic reference values. JEPM 2016;25:157–162.
Dutton M. Selected veterinary concerns of geriatric rats, mice, hamsters, and gerbils. Vet Clin Exot Anim 2020;23(3):525–548.
Fisher PG. Exotic mammal renal disease: causes and clinical presentation. Vet Clin Exot Anim 2006;9:33–67.
Frolich J. Rats and mice. In: Quesenberry KE, Carpenter JW, eds. Ferrets, Rabbits and Rodents, 4th Ed). Clinical Medicine and Surgery. 2021 ed. St. Louis: Saunders, 2020:345–367.
Hallman RM, Brandão J. Diagnostic imaging of the renal system in exotic companion mammals. Vet Clin Exot Anim 2020;23:195–214.
Miwa Y, Mayer J. Hamsters and gerbils. In: Quesenberry KE, Carpenter JW, eds. Ferrets, Rabbits and Rodents, 4th Ed). Clinical Medicine and Surgery. 2021 ed. St. Louis: Saunders, 2020:368–384.
Reavill DR, Lennox AM. Disease overview of the urinary tract in exotic companion mammals and tips on clinical management. Vet Clin Exot Anim 2020;23(1): 169–193.
Richardson VCG. Gerbil urinary system. In: VCG R, ed. Diseases of Small Domestic Rodents, vol. 106. Oxford, UK: Blackwell, 2003a:226–227.
Richardson VCG. Hamster urinary system. In: VCG R, ed. Diseases of Small Domestic Rodents. Oxford, UK: Blackwell, 2003, 2003b:153.
Yabuki A, Yoneshige S, Tanaka S et al. Age-related histological changes in kidneys of Brown Norway rat. J Vet Med Sci 2014;76(2):277–280.

Author Charly Pignon, DVM, Dip ECZM (Small Mammal)

SCENT GLAND DISORDERS

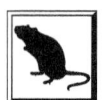

BASICS

DEFINITON
Inflammation, infection, or neoplastic change involving the scent glands

PATHOPHYSIOLOGY
Accumulation of secretions may lead to gland impaction and secondary infection. Infection may also occur secondary to trauma, or may be associated with poor husbandry and sanitation. Neoplasia affecting the scent glands may be a primary problem or may occur secondary to chronic inflammation and infection.

SYSTEMS AFFECTED
Skin/Exocrine

INCIDENCE/PREVALENCE
A common presentation in gerbils

SIGNALMENT

Breed Predilections
• In gerbils, the ventral scent gland is the third most common site of neoplasia (adenocarcinoma).
• Hamsters may develop inflammation of the pigmented flank glands, and melanoma of the scent gland in hamsters is reported.
• Preputial gland abscesses are reported in mice and rats.

Predominant Sex
Medical conditions involving the scent glands are more common in males.

SIGNS

Physical Examination Findings
• Swelling, erythema, discharge, or ulceration in the area of the scent gland
• Self-trauma from pruritus or discomfort
• Purulent exudate or other evidence of primary or secondary bacterial infection

CAUSES
• Introduction of pathogenic bacteria by trauma or self-mutilation.
• Accumulation of glandular secretions associated with poor grooming, general debilitation, and underlying medical conditions, poor sanitation
• Overproduction of glandular secretions resulting from hormonal stimulation, particularly in males
• Idiopathic

RISK FACTORS
Poor sanitation and overcrowding may predispose animals to the development of scent gland abnormalities.

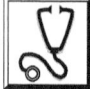

DIAGNOSIS

DIFFERENTIAL DIAGNOSIS
• Neoplasia
• Trauma
• Abscess
• Normal scent gland

DIAGNOSTIC PROCEDURES
• Skin cytology, fine-needle aspiration, or excisional biopsy
• Bacterial culture and sensitivity where appropriate for bacterial infection

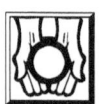

TREATMENT

APPROPRIATE HEALTH CARE
For inflammation of the scent glands, clip and clean the area around the gland and apply topical antibiotics.

NURSING CARE
Most cases may be treated on an outpatient basis. Postoperative supportive care as indicated for patients treated surgically. Supportive care as indicated for debilitated patients.

CLIENT EDUCATION
• Discuss appropriate husbandry for the species presented.
• Neoplasia of the scent gland in gerbils carries a poor prognosis
• Monitor patients for self-trauma during treatment and after surgery.

SURGICAL CONSIDERATIONS
• Castration may reduce secretory activity and help prevent inflammation of the scent glands.
• Surgical removal of suspected neoplasms
• Surgical debridement of abscesses

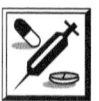

MEDICATIONS

DRUG(S) OF CHOICE
Systemic antibiotics based on bacterial culture and sensitivity where indicated. Antibiotics commonly used in small rodents include trimethoprim-sulfa (15–30 mg/kg PO, SC q12h), enrofloxacin (5–20 mg/kg PO, SC, IM q12h), chloramphenicol (30–50 mg/kg PO q8h), azithromycin (10–30 mg/kg PO q24h), and amoxicillin/clavulanic acid (20 mg/kg PO q12h *Do not use in Hamsters)

CONTRAINDICATIONS
Risk of potentially fatal antibiotic-induced enterotoxemia in Hamsters is associated with orally administered penicillin, ampicillin, cephalosporins, carbenicillin, lincomycin, clindamycin, streptomycin, gentamycin, neomycin, erythromycin, vancomycin, and tetracycline.

ALTERNATIVE DRUGS
If gastrointestinal distress accompanies antibiotic therapy, concurrent administration of a probiotic may help alleviate the symptoms.

FOLLOW-UP

PATIENT MONITORING
Monitor for resolution of the presenting signs. During treatment and after surgery, patients should be monitored for self-mutilation.

PREVENTION/AVOIDANCE
Castration may reduce secretory activity and help prevent inflammation of the scent glands.

POSSIBLE COMPLICATIONS
• Self-trauma following surgical procedures is common.
• Recurrence of neoplastic conditions after surgery

EXPECTED COURSE AND PROGNOSIS
Many neoplasms are locally aggressive, and recurrence is common. Some infections may require long-term antibiotic therapy for complete resolution.

MISCELLANEOUS

SEE ALSO
Cutaneous and subcutaneous masses

ABBREVIATIONS
N/A

INTERNET RESOURCES
Exotic DVM forum for eDVM readers: www.pets.groups.yahoo.com/group/ExoticDVM Veterinary Information Network: www.vin.com

Suggested Reading
Frolich J. Rats and mice. In: Quesenberry KE, Carpenter JW, eds. Ferrets, Rabbits and Rodents, 4th Ed). Clinical Medicine and Surgery. 2021 ed. St. Louis: Saunders, 2020:345–367.

Hoppmann E, Barron HW. Rodent dermatology. J Exot Pet Med 2007;16(4):238–255.

Jekl V, Knotek Z. Evidence-based advances in rodent medicine. Vet Clin Exot Anim 2017;20:805–816.

Meredith A, Redrobe S. BSAVA Manual of Exotic Pets, 4th ed. Gloucester, UK: British Small Animal Veterinary Association, 2002:20–21, 28–30, 39–41, 55–60.

Miwa Y, Mayer J. Hamsters and gerbils. In: Quesenberry KE, Carpenter JW, eds. Ferrets, Rabbits and Rodents, 4th Ed). Clinical Medicine and Surgery. 2021 ed. St. Louis: Saunders, 2020:368–384.

Palmerio BS, Roberts H. Clinical approach to dermatologic disease in exotic animals. Vet Clin North Am Exot Anim Pract. 2013;16(3):523–577.

White SD, Bourdeau PJ, Brément T et al. Companion rats (*Rattus norvegicus*) with cutaneous lesions: a retrospective study of 470 cases at two university veterinary teaching hospitals (1985–2018). Vet Dermatol 2019;30:237–272.

Author Christine Eckermann-Ross, DVM, CVA, CVH

SIALODACRYOADENITIS VIRUS

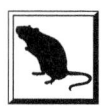

BASICS

DEFINITION
A common, highly contagious coronaviral infection of rats and mice

PATHOPHYSIOLOGY
• Transmitted through direct contact, bedding, and aerosol
• Clinical disease is seen most often in young animals; adults are often asymptomatic. Uncomplicated viral infection is usually self-limiting.
• Often implicated as significant copathogen in rats with chronic respiratory disease (CRD)
• Viral affinity for Harderian, lacrimal, and salivary glands causes inflammation and swelling. Infection in the respiratory and olfactory epithelium results in necrotizing rhinitis. In the lower respiratory tract, infection can result in tracheitis and focal bronchiolitis.
• SDAV-free laboratory colonies are established through screening and culling.

SYSTEMS AFFECTED
• Respiratory
• Ocular
• Lymphatic

SIGNALMENT
• Serious primary disease of young animals only (<3 months of age)
• Infection in adult animals is usually subclinical, unless complicated by *Mycoplasma* sp. or other secondary bacterial infection.
• Actual incidence in pet rats and mice is unknown

SIGNS
• Harderian/lacrimal gland infection: porphyrin discharge (red tears), conjunctivitis, corneal lesions, blepharospasm, and exophthalmia
• Sneezing, nasal discharge
• Cervical swelling with salivary gland infection
• Stunted growth

CAUSES
Sialodacryoadenitis virus is a naturally occurring rat coronavirus.

RISK FACTORS
• Concurrent disease, especially other respiratory pathogens
• Stress, poor husbandry

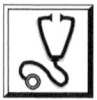

DIAGNOSIS

DIFFERENTIAL DIAGNOSIS
• Other respiratory pathogens, especially *Mycoplasa* sp. and ciliary-associated respiratory bacillus, or viruses such as Sendai virus, rat respiratory virus, or pneumonia virus of rats, can cause clinical signs or act synergistically as copathogens. Disease is usually seen in adult mice and rats.
• Mild respiratory signs in young mice and rats are often due to infection with SDAV alone and may be self-limiting.
• Cervical swelling caused by other organisms or neoplasia

CBC/BIOCHEMISTRY/URINALYSIS
Does not confirm or rule out disease but can be useful to diagnose other underlying disease conditions

OTHER LABORATORY TESTS
• Serologic testing (IFA or ELISA) is available but not often utilized in clinical practice.
• Culture and susceptibility—testing for other, concurrent bacterial infections is helpful in directing antibiotic therapy. *Mycoplasma* spp. are extremely difficult and time consuming to demonstrate on culture; may fail to detect the organism.

IMAGING
Not useful for diagnosis of this virus, but can help identify concurrent disease of the respiratory tract

DIAGNOSTIC PROCEDURES
N/A

TREATMENT

APPROPRIATE HEALTH CARE
• Inpatient—severe debilitating disease, dehydration, and respiratory distress
• Outpatient—stable patients

NURSING CARE
• Supportive care, including correction of dehydration
• Some animals with severe respiratory disease may be reluctant to eat or drink and may require assisted feeding.
• Provide oxygen to dyspneic patients.

CLIENT EDUCATION
Inform clients that virus is likely a copathogen with other organisms and may be part of chronic respiratory disease that is difficult to eradicate.

SURGICAL CONSIDERATIONS
Cervical abscesses may require debridement and flushing.

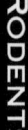

MEDICATIONS

DRUG(S) OF CHOICE
• No specific antiviral treatment
• Treat bacterial copathogens, especially *Mycoplasma*, pending results of culture and susceptibility testing. If mycoplasmosis is suspected as a copathogen, begin treatment with a combination of enrofloxacin (10 mg/kg PO q12h) and doxycycline (5 mg/kg PO q12h) for a minimum of 2 weeks.
• Antibiotic eye ointments—to treat or prevent secondary bacterial infections and to keep the eye lubricated while lacrimal glands heal

CONTRAINDICATIONS
• Do not administer penicillins, ampicillin, amoxicillin, erythromycin, or lincomycin to hamsters due to the risk of potentially fatal enteric dysbiosis.
• Doxycycline should be avoided in very young or pregnant animals.
• Do not use corticosteroid-containing topical ophthalmic preparations.

PRECAUTIONS
All therapeutic agents should be used with caution in debilitated, dehydrated patients. Ideally, vascular abnormalities (dehydration, hypotension) are addressed prior to initiating antibiotic therapy.

POSSIBLE INTERACTIONS
N/A

ALTERNATIVE DRUGS

There is some anecdotal evidence that immune-boosting drugs/agents have been useful in some cases of infectious respiratory disease.

FOLLOW-UP

PATIENT MONITORING

• Patients in respiratory disease are often reluctant to eat or drink. Patients should be monitored carefully to ensure adequate intake.
• Monitor patient weight.

PREVENTION/AVOIDANCE

• Since the incidence of this virus in pet population is unknown and adult animals may be asymptomatic, avoidance is difficult.
• Optimal husbandry and prevention of stress/overcrowding important

POSSIBLE COMPLICATIONS

• SDAV infection alone is often self-limiting
• When SDAV is a component of CRD in rodents, complete elimination of respiratory disease is unlikely and remission is common.
• With significant infection of the lacrimal glands, tear production may be reduced, causing permanent damage to the cornea.

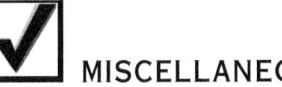

MISCELLANEOUS

ASSOCIATED CONDITIONS

• *Mycoplasma* spp.
• Secondary bacterial infections
• Other viral infections

ZOONOTIC POTENTIAL

Not considered zoonotic

PREGNANCY/FERTILITY/BREEDING

Neonatal mortality and changes in estrous cycle can occur with SDAV.

SYNONYMS

Parker's rat coronavirus

SEE ALSO

Mycoplasmosis and chronic respiratory disease
Pneumonia
Red tears (chromodacryorrhea)
Rhinitis and sinusitis

ABBREVIATIONS

CRD = chronic respiratory disease
ELISA = enzyme-linked immunosorbent assay
IFA = immunofluorescence assay
SDAV = sialodacryoadenitis virus

Suggested Reading

Capello V, Lennox AM. Diagnostic imaging of the respiratory system in exotic companion mammals. Vet Clin Exot Anim 2011;14:369–389.

Dutton M. Selected veterinary concerns of geriatric rats, mice, hamsters, and gerbils. Vet Clin Exot Anim 2020;23(3):525–548.
Ferreira JB, Yamaguti M, Marques LM et al. Detection of mycoplasma pulmonis in laboratory rats and technicians. Zoonoses Public Health 2008;55(5):229–234.
Frolich J. Rats and mice. In: Quesenberry KE, Carpenter JW, eds. Ferrets, Rabbits and Rodents, 4th Ed). Clinical Medicine and Surgery. 2021 ed. St. Louis: Saunders, 2020:345–367.
Graham JE, Schoeb TR. Mycoplasma pulmonis in rats. J Exotic Pet Med 2011;20(4):270–276.
Jekl V, Knotek Z. Evidence-based advances in rodent medicine. Vet Clin Exot Anim 2017;20:805–816.
Mayer J, Mans C. Rodents. In: Carpenter JW, ed. Exotic Animal Formulary, 5th ed. St Louis: Elsevier, 2018:459–493.
Miwa Y, Mayer J. Hamsters and gerbils. In: Quesenberry KE, Carpenter JW, eds. Ferrets, Rabbits and Rodents, 4th Ed). Clinical Medicine and Surgery. 2021 ed. St. Louis: Saunders, 2020:368–384.
Piasecki T, Chrzastek K, Kasprzykowska U et al. Mycoplasma pulmonis of rodents as a possible human pathogen. Vector Borne Zoonotic Dis 2017;17(7):475–477.

Author Angela M. Lennox, DVM, Dipl. ABVP (Avian, ECM); DECZM-Small Mammal

TYZZER'S DISEASE

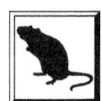

BASICS

OVERVIEW
- Infection of the intestinal tract caused by *Clostridium piliforme* (formerly *Bacillus piliformis*)
- *C. piliforme* is a spore-forming, motile, pleomorphic, filamentous, rod-shaped, Gram-negative, PAS-positive, nonacid-fast, obligate intracellular bacterium.
- Broad host range includes mice, rats, gerbils, hamsters, guinea pigs, rabbits, cats, dogs, horses, cattle, rhesus monkeys, marmosets, and other species; has not been reported in humans.
- Gerbils are particularly susceptible, with high morbidity and mortality in colony outbreaks. Rat, mouse, and hamster colonies may have inapparent infection.
- *C. piliforme* is a common benign intestinal inhabitant that persists for years in spore form outside the host.
- Transmission is thought to be by the fecal-oral route. Infectious spores survive for years in bedding, soil, or contaminated feed.
- Tyzzer's disease occurs more frequently and is usually more severe in recently weaned animals, immunosuppressed animals, and those housed in unfavorable conditions.
- Acute, highly fatal form of disease is seen most often in weanling animals, but adults may be affected also.
- Chronically infected animals in which hepatic lesions may be more pronounced exhibit weight loss, tough hair coat, and eventually death.

SIGNALMENT
- The most common infectious disease in gerbils; also affects hamsters, mice, rats, guinea pigs, and rabbits
- Clinical disease is most common in younger animals, recently weaned individuals, and those that are stressed due to inappropriate environment, poor nutrition, or concurrent illness.

SIGNS

General Comments
Subclinical infection in a colony is probably the most common form of Tyzzer's disease, with sporadic outbreaks of clinical disease occurring when spores in the environment are ingested.

Historical Findings
- In weanling or stressed animals, Tyzzer's is a peracute to acute enzootic disease causing hunched posture, rough hair coat, lethargy, and death within 48–72 hours.
- Watery diarrhea and perineal staining may or may not occur.
- Septicemia may lead to encephalitis and myocardial lesions with additional clinical signs of torticollis, rolling, and sudden death.

Physical Examination Findings
- Vary with the severity of disease
- Anorexia, lethargy, and depression
- Rough haircoat, decreased grooming behavior
- Abdominal pain characterized by hunched posture, reluctance to move, bruxism, and/or pain on abdominal palpation
- Diarrhea, fecal staining of the perineum
- Dehydration, hypothermia, hypotension, and weakness
- Abdominal distention
- Torticolis, rolling
- Weight loss in chronically infected animals
- Animals may be found dead in the absence of clinical signs.

CAUSES AND RISK FACTORS
- Tyzzer's disease may be precipitated by high environmental temperature, poor sanitation, overcrowding, and stress of shipping.
- Immunosuppressors (radiation, corticosteroids, concurrent disease, and thymectomy), heavy parasite load, and poor diet are considered to be additional predisposing factors.

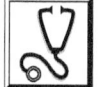

DIAGNOSIS

DIFFERENTIAL DIAGNOSIS

General
- Consider all causes of enteropathy, including diet change, inappropriate antibiotics, enterotoxemia, systemic or metabolic disease, as well as specific intestinal disorders.
- Infectious and parasitic causes vary by species.
- True "wet tail" or proliferative ileitis of hamsters is caused by the intracellular bacterium *Lawsonia intracellularis*. Affected animals may have palpably thickened bowel loops and are prone to ileal obstruction, impaction, intussusception, peritonitis, tenesmus, dyschezia, and rectal prolapse.
- *Syphacia obelata* pinworm infestation may be associated with intestinal impaction, intussusception, and rectal prolapse in mice.
- *Salmonella* infection is associated with fresh blood in the feces in some species.

Mice/Rats
- Viruses—mouse hepatitis virus (coronavirus), epizootic diarrhea of infant mice (rotavirus), reovirus, others; neonates especially susceptible
- Bacteria—*Salmonella* spp., *Helicobacter* spp., *Citrobacter rodentium*, *E. coli*, *Enterococcus* spp., and others
- Protozoa—*Spironucleus muris, Giardia muris, Eimeria* spp., and others
- Cestodes—*Rodentolepis* spp. (formerly *Hymenolepis*)
- Pinworms—*Syphacia* spp., *Aspiculuris tetraptera*

Gerbils
- Bacteria—*Salmonella* spp., *E. coli*, and *Citrobacter rodentium*
- Cestodes—*Rodentolepis* spp.
- Pinworms—*Dentostomella* spp., *Syphacia* spp.

Hamsters
- Bacteria—*Lawsonia intracellularis, Clostridium difficile, E. coli*, and *Salmonella*
- Protozoa—*Spironucleus* spp., *Giardia*, and others
- Cestodes—*Rodentolepis* spp.
- Nematodes—*Syphacia* spp.

CBC/BIOCHEMISTRY/URINALYSIS
- Hemogram abnormalities may be consistent with sepsis and/or systemic infection.
- Blood chemistries are likely to indicate liver disease, dehydration, and/or electrolyte abnormalities.

OTHER LABORATORY TESTS
- Fecal examination (floatation, wet-mount, and cytology) will assist in differentiating *C. piliforme* infection from internal parasite infection.
- Fecal culture may help to rule out other enteric bacterial infection.
- Inoculation of feces from suspected animals into known *C. piliforme*-free weanling gerbils (which are highly susceptible) can detect the presence of Tyzzer's disease in a suspect colony.

IMAGING
N/A

DIAGNOSTIC PROCEDURES
- *C. piliforme* is an intracellular bacterium that will not grow on routine culture media; thus, antemortem diagnosis is difficult.
- Diagnosis is based on signs and demonstration of the intracellular organisms with Giemsa or silver stains in histologic sections of the intestine, liver, or heart.
- *C. piliforme* infection can also be diagnosed by PCR.
- Serologic detection by ELISA is variable.

PATHOLOGIC FINDINGS
- Liver, intestine, and/or heart may be involved.
- Classical lesion is enlarged liver with variable number of gray, white, or yellow, 1–2 mm foci. Absence of liver lesions does not rule out Tyzzer's disease.
- In more acute cases, there may be edema, congestion, hemorrhage, and focal ulceration of the intestine, particularly around the ileocecal-colonic junction. Gut is often atonic and filled with yellowish fluid.
- Mesenteric lymph nodes may be enlarged.
- Abdomen and small intestine may be distended.
- Affected guinea pigs and gerbils may exhibit proteinaceous peritoneal effusion.

(CONTINUED)

• Heart may exhibit pale myocardial foci (rabbits, rats, mice, and hamsters).
• Spleen is usually normal.
• Histopathology of hepatic, intestinal, and myocardial foci are characterized by areas of necrosis surrounded by a scant mixed-inflammatory cell population. Foci are thought to arise by embolic shower of organisms from a primary infection in the intestine. Filamentous organisms in a "pile of sticks" arrangement may be seen within the cytoplasm of cells adjacent to necrotic areas.

TREATMENT
• May be unrewarding
• Supportive care such as fluid therapy, assisted feeding, and thermal support
• Antibiotic therapy
• Isolate affected and exposed animals to limit spread of disease.
• Because the bacteria form spores, the housing environment should be thoroughly sanitized and disinfected.

MEDICATIONS
DRUG(S) OF CHOICE
• Tetracycline (10–20 mg/kg PO q8–12h)
• Oxytetracycline (10–20 mg/kg PO q8h)
• Chloramphenicol (30–50 mg/kg PO q8h)
• Metronidazole (20 mg/kg PO q12h)

CONTRAINDICATIONS
Antibiotics that are primarily gram-positive in spectrum will suppress the growth of commensal flora, allowing overgrowth of enteric pathogens. These include lincomycin, clindamycin, erythromycin, ampicillin, amoxicillin, cephalosporins, and penicillins.

PRECAUTIONS
• It is important to determine the cause of diarrhea. Using a "shotgun" approach with antibiotics may be ineffective or detrimental.
• Antibiotic therapy can predispose small rodents (particularly hamsters) to bacterial dysbiosis and overgrowth of pathogenic bacteria (e.g., *Clostridium difficile*). If signs worsen or do not improve, therapy should be adjusted.
• Chloramphenicol may cause aplastic anemia in susceptible people. Clients and staff should use appropriate precautions when handling this drug.
• Metronidazole is neurotoxic if overdosed.

POSSIBLE INTERACTIONS
N/A

ALTERNATIVE DRUGS
N/A

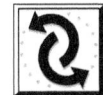

FOLLOW-UP
PATIENT MONITORING
• Fecal volume and character, appetite, attitude, and body weight
• If diarrhea does not resolve, consider reevaluation of the diagnosis.

PREVENTION/AVOIDANCE
• Purchase of stock from reputable vendors who use cesarean derivations, barrier rearing techniques, and good husbandry practices is the best preventive measure.
• Reducing stress and providing sanitary conditions
• Providing appropriate diet and husbandry

POSSIBLE COMPLICATIONS
• Antibiotic therapy can promote bacterial dysbiosis and overgrowth of pathogenic bacteria, especially in hamsters.
• Use antibiotics with caution, and only use those that are considered safe in the rodent species affected.
• Septicemia due to bacterial invasion of enteric mucosa
• Dehydration due to fluid loss
• Shock, death from clostridial enterotoxicosis

EXPECTED COURSE AND PROGNOSIS
• Treatment of Tyzzer's disease is often unrewarding.
• The course of disease may be too rapid for treatment to be effective in some individuals, particularly in gerbils, which are especially susceptible.
• Recovered animals may continue to shed *C. piliforme*. If Tyzzer's disease becomes enzootic in a rodent colony, then intermittent outbreaks of disease are likely to occur in the future, particularly in young or immunosuppressed individuals.

MISCELLANEOUS
ASSOCIATED CONDITIONS
Although not typical of Tyzzer's disease, diarrhea and tenesmus in small rodents may lead to rectal prolapse.

AGE-RELATED FACTORS
Young and recently weaned animals are most often affected.

ZOONOTIC POTENTIAL
Clostridium piliforme infection is not reported in humans.

PREGNANCY/FERTILITY/BREEDING
N/A

SYNONYMS
• *Bacillus piliformis*
• Diarrhea in hamsters is commonly referred to as "wet tail" regardless of etiology, although in veterinary terminology this term refers exclusively to *Lawsonia intracellularis* infection.
• Cestodes of the genus *Rodentolepis* are referred to by the former name *Hymenolepis* in many references.

SEE ALSO
Diarrhea
Intestinal parasitism

ABBREVIATIONS
ELISA = enzyme-linked immunosorbent assay
PAS = periodic acid-Shiff
PCR = polymerase chain reaction

INTERNET RESOURCES
N/A

Suggested Reading
Dutton M. Selected veterinary concerns of geriatric rats, mice, hamsters, and gerbils. Vet Clin Exot Anim 2020;23(3):525–548.
Frolich J. Rats and mice. In: Quesenberry KE, Carpenter JW, eds. Ferrets, Rabbits and Rodents, 4th Ed). Clinical Medicine and Surgery. 2021 ed. St. Louis: Saunders, 2020:345–367.
Hrapkiewicz K, Colby L, Denison P, eds. Clinical Laboratory Animal Medicine: An Introduction, 4th ed. Ames: Wiley-Blackwell, 2013:83–92, 128–133, 156–159, 182–187.
Jekl V, Knotek Z. Evidence-based advances in rodent medicine. Vet Clin Exot Anim 2017;20:805–816.
Mayer J, Mans C. Rodents. In: Carpenter JW, ed. Exotic Animal Formulary, 5th ed. St Louis: Elsevier, 2018:459–493.
Mitchell MA, Tully TN, eds. Manual of exotic pet practice. St Louis: Elsevier, 2009:326–344, 406–432.
Miwa Y, Mayer J. Hamsters and gerbils. In: Quesenberry KE, Carpenter JW, eds. Ferrets, Rabbits and Rodents, 4th Ed). Clinical Medicine and Surgery. 2021 ed. St. Louis: Saunders, 2020:368–384.

Author Dan H. Johnson, DVM, Dipl. ABVP (Exotic Companion Mammal)

RODENTS

ULCERATIVE PODODERMATITIS (BUMBLEFOOT)

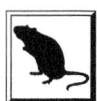

BASICS

DEFINITION
Chronic granulomatous, ulcerative dermatitis on the plantar surface of the foot. In severe cases, secondary bacterial infection and osteomyelitis may be observed.

PATHOPHYSIOLOGY
• Decreased mobility initially leads to the development of calluses on the plantar surfaces of the feet. Common causes of decreased mobility include obesity, arthritis, or other medical conditions. Sitting for long periods on rough bedding materials or wire cage flooring can exacerbate or initiate disease. With long-term pressure on affected feet, pressure necrosis develops, accompanied by ulceration, secondary bacterial infection and, in severe cases, osteomyelitis.
• In rats, chronic inflammation may lead to amyloidosis of the kidney, liver, spleen, adrenal glands, and/or pancreas.

SYSTEMS AFFECTED
• Skin/Exocrine
• Musculoskeletal
• Other organ systems with chronic disease and secondary amyloidosis

GENETICS
N/A

INCIDENCE/PREVALENCE
A very common condition, most prevalent in obese animals and older pets with limited mobility due to osteoarthritis

GEOGRAPHIC DISTRIBUTION
N/A

SIGNALMENT
• Most commonly observed in hamsters, mice, and rats
• No age or gender predilection

SIGNS

Physical Examination Findings
Mice:
• Lesion on the plantar aspect of the foot
• Generally begins with alopecia and erythema
• May be swollen, ulcerated, covered by scabs, or have evidence of secondary infection (erythema, exudate)
• May see altered locomotion
Rat:
• Lesion on the plantar aspect of the foot
• Generally begins with alopecia and erythema
• May be swollen, ulcerated, covered by scabs, or have evidence of secondary infection (erythema, exudate)
• If severe, see limited mobility due to osteomyelitis, osteoarthritis, or tendonitis
• Lethargy, anorexia due to pain

CAUSES AND RISK FACTORS
• Abrasive bedding, wire flooring, poor sanitation, or trauma
• Limited mobility due to obesity, arthritis, or underlying disease conditions
• Poor husbandry or sanitation—sitting in soiled or wet bedding
• Secondary infection caused by *Staphylococcus aureus* or other, opportunistic bacteria

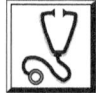

DIAGNOSIS

DIFFERENTIAL DIAGNOSIS
• Trauma
• Abscess
• Neoplasia (fibrosarcoma)

CBC/BIOCHEMISTRY/URINALYSIS
• Results of routine laboratory tests are often normal.
• Leukocytosis may be observed if infection is present.
• In debilitated patients, changes may reflect underlying medical conditions or sequelae of chronic inflammation.

OTHER LABORATORY TESTS
N/A

IMAGING
Radiographic imaging of the feet is indicated if osteomyelitis is suspected.

DIAGNOSTIC PROCEDURES
• Bacterial culture and susceptibility testing if secondary bacterial infection suspected
• Cytology of exudates—may reveal pyogranulomatous exudate or bacteria
• Fine-needle aspiration or biopsy to rule out neoplasia
• Bacterial culture and sensitivity should be performed if infection is present.

PATHOLOGIC FINDINGS
Diagnosis is usually made on the basis of the medical history, clinical signs, and visualization of plantar lesions.

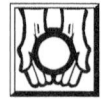

TREATMENT

APPROPRIATE HEALTH CARE
• Most patients with pododermatitis are treated on an outpatient basis.
• Correction of underlying husbandry and nutritional deficiencies is essential to successful treatment.

NURSING CARE
• Supportive care as indicated for debilitated patients
• The degree and duration of wound care depend on the severity of lesions. Early disease may respond to husbandry changes, daily warm soaks in saline or chlorhexidine solution, and application of topical silver sulfadiazine cream, along with pain control and antibiotic treatment if secondary infection is present.
• Chronic, deep infections usually require topical application of hydrocolloidal wound dressings followed by soft, padded bandages to promote epithelialization. The frequency of bandage changes depends on the severity of the lesion. Severe infections may initially require daily bandage changes.
• Analgesia is important to restore mobility.

ACTIVITY
Mobility is often limited early, but activity should be gradually increased to help relieve pressure on the feet and reduce the incidence of obesity.

DIET
Correct any underlying deficiencies. Dietary restriction for weight loss is indicated in obese patients.

CLIENT EDUCATION
• Good husbandry practices are essential for treatment of pododermatitis. Soft bedding materials, bedding that does not contain aromatic oils or other contact irritants, soft, solid flooring versus wire mesh flooring
• Adequate cleaning and sanitation
• Appropriate nutrition for the species being treated

SURGICAL CONSIDERATIONS
Surgical debridement of pododermatitis lesions is rarely effective in their resolution.

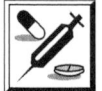

MEDICATIONS

DRUG(S) OF CHOICE

Antibiotic Treatment
• Antibiotics based on culture and sensitivity in patients with secondary bacterial infections. Most chronic lesions are secondarily infected. Treatment often requires a 2–6 month course of antibiotics.
• Antibiotics commonly used in small rodents include trimethoprim-sulfa (15–30 mg/kg PO, SC q12h), enrofloxacin (5–00 mg/kg PO, SC, IM q12h), chloramphenicol (30–50 mg/kg PO q8h), azithromycin (10–30 mg/kg PO q24h), and amoxicillin/clavulanic acid (20 mg/kg PO q24h *Do not use in hamsters)

Pain Management
Long-term pain control is essential for treatment. Painful rodents are sedentary, exacerbating lesions. Commonly used pain medications include buprenorphine (0.05–0.1 mg/kg SQ, IM q6–8h), meloxicam (1–2 mg/kg PO, SQ, IM q24h), and tramadol (10–20 mg/kg PO q8–12h).

CONTRAINDICATIONS

There is a risk of life-threatening antibiotic-induced enterotoxemia in hamsteres associated with orally administered penicillin, ampicillin, cephalosporins, carbenicillin, lincomycin, clindamycin, streptomycin, gentamycin, neomycin, erythromycin, vancomycin, and tetracycline.

PRECAUTIONS

Frequent bandage changes should be performed to monitor the progress of the condition and to prevent complications associated with inappropriately applied bandage materials.

POSSIBLE INTERACTIONS

N/A

ALTERNATIVE DRUGS

If gastrointestinal distress accompanies antibiotic therapy, concurrent treatment with a probiotic may help alleviate symptoms.

FOLLOW-UP

PATIENT MONITORING

Frequent monitoring and bandage changes are required, at least once weekly in advanced cases.

PREVENTION/AVOIDANCE

• Avoid abrasive or irritating bedding and provide appropriate diet and sanitation.
• Avoid obesity.

POSSIBLE COMPLICATIONS

• Secondary infection
• Osteomyelitis

• Osteoarthritis
• Tendonitis
• Sequelae of chronic inflammation such as amyloidosis

EXPECTED COURSE AND PROGNOSIS

The course of treatment may be prolonged and lesions often do not completely resolve. Recurrence is common.

MISCELLANEOUS

ASSOCIATED CONDITIONS

• Obesity
• Osteoarthritis
• Osteomyelitis

AGE-RELATED FACTORS

Older animals with limited mobility due to osteoarthritis may be at greater risk for development of pododermatitis.

ZOONOTIC POTENTIAL

N/A

PREGNANCY/FERTILITY/BREEDING

N/A

SYNONYMS

Bumblefoot

SEE ALSO

N/A

ABBREVIATIONS

N/A

INTERNET RESOURCES

Exotic DVM forum for eDVM readers: www.pets.groups.yahoo.com/group/ExoticDVM
Veterinary Information Network: www.vin.com

Suggested Reading

Frolich J. Rats and mice. In: Quesenberry KE, Carpenter JW, eds. Ferrets, Rabbits and Rodents, 4th Ed). Clinical Medicine and Surgery. 2021 ed. St. Louis: Saunders, 2020:345–367.

Jekl V, Knotek Z. Evidence-based advances in rodent medicine. Vet Clin Exot Anim 2017;20:805–816.

Miwa Y, Mayer J. Hamsters and gerbils. In: Quesenberry KE, Carpenter JW, eds. Ferrets, Rabbits and Rodents, 4th Ed). Clinical Medicine and Surgery. 2021 ed. St. Louis: Saunders, 2020:368–384.

Miwa Y, Sladky K. Common surgical procedures of rodents, ferrets, hedgehogs, and sugar gliders. Vet Clin Exot Anim 2016;19:205–244.

Palmerio BS, Roberts H. Clinical approach to dermatologic disease in exotic animals. Vet Clin North Am Exot Anim Pract 2013;16(3):523–577.

White SD, Bourdeau PJ, Brément T et al. Companion rats (*Rattus norvegicus*) with cutaneous lesions: a retrospective study of 470 cases at two university veterinary teaching hospitals (1985–2018). Vet Dermatol 2019;30:237–272.

Author Christine Eckermann-Ross, DVM, CVA, CVH

UTERINE DISORDERS

BASICS

DEFINITION
Any diseases that involve the uterus

PATHOPHYSIOLOGY
- Pyometra—develops when bacterial invasion of abnormal endometrium leads to intraluminal accumulation of purulent exudate
- Endometrial disorder—hyperplasia, aneurism, and endometritis—can lead into significant uterine hemorrhage; the pathophysiology remains unclear. Hydrometra is a common disease in mice.
- Dystocia—in primary inertia, the uterus fails to respond to fetal signals and is unable to initiate labor; could be caused by small litter size, an inherited predisposition, nutritional imbalances, fatty infiltration of the myometrium, or deficiencies of neuroendocrine regulation. Secondary uterine inertia implies that some fetuses have been delivered, and the remainder are in utero due to exhaustion of the uterine myometrium.

SYSTEMS AFFECTED
- Endocrine
- Reproductive

GENETICS
N/A

INCIDENCE/PREVALENCE
- Cystic endometrial hyperplasia of endometrial glands is a frequent finding in aged female mice.
- Pyometra is rare in pet hamsters; it is often overdiagnosed due to the appearance of a normal, creamy discharge after ovulation.
- Hydrometra common in mice with a genetic predisposition (BALB/c, B6, and DBA strains)

GEOGRAPHIC DISTRIBUTION
Worldwide

SIGNALMENT
- Intact female
- Highest incidence of uterine disorders are seen in females >1 year

SIGNS

Historical Findings
- Hematuria—most common presenting complaint. Not true hematuria, since the blood originates from the uterus but is expelled during micturition. Hematuria is often reported as intermittent or cyclic; it usually occurs at the end of micturition.
- Discharge from the vulva adhering to the perineal fur
- Spotting, usually bloody
- May have signs of pseudopregnancy—pulling hair, nest building (gerbils, hamster)
- Increased aggressiveness
- Recent parturition—with persistent postpartum discharge
- Breeding female—may have history of small litter size, increased number of stillborn or resorbed fetuses, infertility, dystocia, and abandonment of litters

Physical Examination Findings
- Physical examination is sometimes normal.
- Blood or serosanguinous vaginal discharge—most commonly expelled during urination, but can appear independent of micturition; may see discharge adherent to fur
- Purulent vaginal discharge
- Uterus may be enlarged, causing abdominal distension, or may see uterine prolapse
- Pale mucous membrane and tachycardia in animals that have significant uterine hemorrhage
- Depression, lethargy, and anorexia in animals with pyometra or uterine hemorrhage

CAUSES

Neoplasia
- Adenocarcinoma, histiocytic sarcomas, hemangiomas, leiomyosarcoma (hamster) and hemangiosarcomas (mouse)
- Adrenal tumor-secreting estrogens

Infection
Pyometra (*Mycoplasma pulmonis*, *Esherichia coli*, and *Prevotella bivia*), ascending urinary tract infection

Dystocia
Uterine inertia, obstruction of the birth canal (uterine torsion or rupture, congenital malformation)

Postparturient Conditions
- Hemorrhage
- Retained placenta and fetuses
- Acute metritis
- Uterine rupture
- Uterine prolapse

Endometrial Disorders
Endometrial hyperplasia, endometrial venous aneurysms, endometriosis, endometritis, polyps, cystic endometrial hyperplasia of endometrial glands (mice)

RISK FACTORS
- Intact sexual status
- Risk for uterine disorders, including neoplasia, increases with age; seen more often in animals >1 year

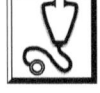

DIAGNOSIS

DIFFERENTIAL DIAGNOSIS
- Hematuria—use ultrasound-guided cystocentesis to collect urine; differentiates true hematuria from blood expelled from the uterus
- Pregnancy
- Other abdominal mass
- Physiologic discharges from the vulva (creamy white after ovulation in hamster, bloody discharge prior to parturition in hamster, degu, rat, and mouse; slight bloody discharge after parturition)

CBC/BIOCHEMISTRY/ URINALYSIS
- Regenerative anemia in animal with uterine hemorrhage
- Increased BUN and creatinine, electrolyte disturbances in animals with pyometra, septicemia, or severe dehydration secondary to the severity of disease
- Urinalysis—sample collected by ultrasound-guided cystocentesis to differentiate hematuria from uterine bleeding

OTHER LABORATORY TESTS
- Vaginal cytology examination—may be helpful in determining if the discharge is purulent or bloody
- Cystocentesis and bacterial culture—help to rule out urinary tract infection
- Uterine bacterial culture—via culture swab; perform after the ovariohysterectomy and opening of the uterus, may be helpful in adjusting the antibiotic therapy
- Urine dipstick to confirm presence of blood.

IMAGING
- Abdominal ultrasound—may detect an enlarged uterus with thickened walls (endometrial disorder) or an abnormal content (pyometra). Irregularity of the uterine wall and adhesion to surrounding tissues could be sign of neoplasia.
- Abdominal radiography—may detect a large uterus in patients with uterine adenocarcinoma, endometrial disorder, or pyometra and later stage of fetal death
- Thoracic radiographs—recommended if suspicion of neoplasia

DIAGNOSTIC PROCEDURES
Histopathologic examination of the uterus following ovariohysterectomy is necessary for definitive diagnosis.

PATHOLOGIC FINDINGS
Gross—neoplasia could involve one or both horns or the body of the uterus; appear cauliflower-like, cystic-like, or with polyp-like projection into the uterine lumen; often have necrotic or hemorrhagic center

TREATMENT

APPROPRIATE HEALTH CARE
- Debilitated patients need to be stabilized, and blood transfusion may be indicated in animals with significant uterine hemorrhage.

• A true vaginal hemorrhage is considered a surgical emergency, as the patient could die rapidly from blood loss. Dystocia is considered an emergency with cesarean section generally necessary for survival of the offspring.

NURSING CARE
Fluid therapy—if the patient is dehydrated, hypovolemic, or in case of suspected pyometra to support kidney function

ACTIVITY
N/A

DIET
Assist feed any animal that is anorexic or inappetant to avoid any secondary hypoglycemia and gastrointestinal disorders.

CLIENT EDUCATION
Advise client of the potential benefits of an early ovariohysterectomy in nonbreeding animals.

SURGICAL CONSIDERATIONS
• Ovariohysterectomy—treatment of choice for uterine neoplasia (usually curative if metastasis has not occurred) and for most uterine disorders because all carry risk of hemorrhage into the uterus
• Cesarean—treatment of choice for dystocia if medical management fails

MEDICATIONS
DRUG(S) OF CHOICE
Antibiotics
Recommended in bacterial vaginitis, pyometra, or endometritis; broad-spectrum antibiotics pending results of bacterial culture and sensitivity test. Trimethoprim-sulfa (15–30 mg/kg PO q12h), chloramphenicol (30–50 mg/kg PO q12h), metronidazole in closed pyometra (20 mg/kg PO q12h), or as a second line enrofloxacin (5–10 mg/kg PO, SC, IM q12h).

Pain Management
• Buprenorphine (0.05–1.0 mg/kg SC, IV q6–8h)
• Oxymorphone (0.2–0.5 mg/kg SC IM q6–12h)
• Morphine (2–5 mg/kg IM q4h)
• Meloxicam (1–2 mg/kg SC, PO q24h)
• Prostaglandin F2 alpha—0.5 mg/animal IM will generally result in delivery within 3 hours
• Calcium gluconate—100 mg/kg IM
• Oxytocin—0.2–0.3 IU/kg SC, IM; if babies are not delivered within 8 hours, perform a cesarean

CONTRAINDICATIONS
Oxytocin—if obstructive dystocia
Do not administer penicillins, ampicillin, amoxicillin, erythromycin, or lincomycin to hamsters due to the risk of potentially fatal enteric dysbiosis.

PRECAUTIONS
• Enrofloxacin—SC could cause some skin necrosis, needs to be diluted 1:1 with fluids
• Meloxicam—use with caution in animal with compromised renal function

POSSIBLE INTERACTIONS
N/A

ALTERNATIVE DRUGS
N/A

FOLLOW-UP
PATIENT MONITORING
• Monitor postoperatively that the animal does not chew her sutures and open the wound.
• Monitor carefully signs of pain (reluctance to move, teeth grinding) postoperatively.
• Monitor the appetite.
• If the owners elect not to perform surgery to treat endometrial disorders, monitor carefully for signs of hemorrhage or sepsis.

PREVENTION/AVOIDANCE
Ovariohysterectomy for all nonbreeding females

POSSIBLE COMPLICATIONS
• Peritonitis, sepsis in animal with endometritis, pyometra, uterine rupture
• Postoperative intra-abdominal adhesions may contribute to chronic pain.
• Metastasis
• Hemorrhage, possible death in animal with bleeding uterine disorders
• Death of the offspring with dystocia

EXPECTED COURSE AND PROGNOSIS
• Good prognosis with timely ovariohysterectomy for most uterine disorders, including neoplasia that has not metastasized
• Poor prognosis in animals presented with vigorous vaginal hemorrhage; emergency stabilization and ovariohysterectomy indicated to control hemorrhage
• Poor in animals with pyometra that is not treated early; sepsis or peritonitis may follow
• Associated mastitis will resolve with ovariohysterectomy alone, unless secondary infection has developed.

MISCELLANEOUS
ASSOCIATED CONDITIONS
• Hamster—pyometra could be a sequel of respiratory infection with *Streptococcus* sp. and *Pasteurella pneumotropica*.
• Mouse—lymphocytic choriomeningitis virus can cause pyometra and infertility.
• Rats—*Mycoplasma pulmonis*, primary pulmonary infection can spread into the genital system and cause infection of the fallopian tubes and uterus
• Mammary neoplasia or mastitis
• Ovarian neoplasia or abscess
• Poor husbandry, poor diet, and obesity

AGE-RELATED FACTORS
Risk of uterine disorders increases with the age of the animal.

ZOONOTIC POTENTIAL
N/A

PREGNANCY/FERTILITY/ BREEDING
• Animals with uterine disorders have decreased fertility or are sterile.
• The treatment of choice remains ovariohysterectomy. Hemostasis during this procedure could be more difficult if the animal is pregnant due to increased uterine blood supply.

SYNONYMS
N/A

SEE ALSO
N/A

ABBREVIATIONS
BUN = blood urea nitrogen

Suggested Reading
Dutton M. Selected veterinary concerns of geriatric rats, mice, hamsters, and gerbils. Vet Clin Exot Anim 2020;23(3):525–548.
Frolich J. Rats and mice. In: Quesenberry KE, Carpenter JW, eds. Ferrets, Rabbits and Rodents, 4th Ed). Clinical Medicine and Surgery. 2021 ed. St. Louis: Saunders, 2020:345–367.
Lewis W. Cystic ovaries in gerbils. Exot DVM 2003;5(1):12.
Martorell J. Reproductive disorders in pet rodents. Vet Clin Exot Anim 2017;20:589–608.
Miwa Y, Mayer J. Hamsters and gerbils. In: Quesenberry KE, Carpenter JW, eds. Ferrets, Rabbits and Rodents, 4th Ed). Clinical Medicine and Surgery. 2021 ed. St. Louis: Saunders, 2020:368–384.
Miwa Y, Sladky K. Common surgical procedures of rodents, ferrets, hedgehogs, and sugar gliders. Vet Clin Exot Anim 2016;19:205–244.
Nagaoka T, Onodera H, Matsushima Y et al. Spontaneous uterine adenocarcninomas in aged rats and their relation to endocrine imbalance. J Cancer Res Clin Oncol 1990;116:623–628.
Richardson VCG. Hamster reproductive system. In: VCG R, ed. Diseases of Small Domestic Rodents. Oxford, UK: Blackwell, 2003a:147–153.
Richardson VCG. Mice reproductive system. In: VCG R, ed. Diseases of Small Domestic Rodents. Oxford, UK: Blackwell, 2003b:188–193.

Author Charly Pignon, DVM, Dip ECZM (Small Mammal)

VAGINAL DISCHARGE

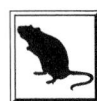

BASICS

DEFINITION
Any substance emanating from the vulvar labia

PATHOPHYSIOLOGY
• Discharge may originate from several distinct sources, depending in part on the age and reproductive status of the patient; from the uterus (most common), urinary tract, vagina, vestibule, or perivulvar skin
• Serosanguineous discharge or fresh blood is usually mistaken for hematuria, since blood is often expelled from the uterus during micturition. This is not seen in hamsters, where the urinary and the genital orifice are separated.
• After ovulation in hamsters, a creamy white, stringy discharge is normal.
• Prior to parturition—in hamsters, degus, rats, and mice, a bloody discharge is normally present.
• Postpartum—a slight bloody discharge is normal in rats and mice.

SYSTEMS AFFECTED
• Endocrine
• Renal/Urologic
• Skin/Exocrine

GENETICS
N/A

INCIDENCE/PREVALENCE
• Cystic endometrial hyperplasia of endometrial glands is a frequent finding in aged female mice.
• Pyometra rare in pet hamster, but often misdiagnosed due to the presence of a normal, white postovulatory discharge
• A discharge is always present physiologically a few hours prior to parturition in hamsters, degus, rats, and mice; often confused with an abnormal discharge

GEOGRAPHIC DISTRIBUTION
N/A

SIGNALMENT
• Intact female
• Highest incidence of uterine disorders is seen in females >1 year

SIGNS

Historical Findings
• Hematuria—most common presenting complaint. Not true hematuria, since the blood originates from the uterus but is expelled during micturition. Hematuria is often reported as intermittent or cyclic; it usually occurs at the end of micturition.
• Discharge from the vulva adhering to the perineal fur. This discharge is usually foul smelling.
• Spotting, usually bloody

• May have signs of pseudopregnancy—pulling hair, nest building (gerbils, hamster)
• Increased aggressiveness
• Recent parturition—with persistent postpartum discharge
• Breeding female—may have history of small litter size, increased number of stillborn or resorbed fetuses, infertility, dystocia, or abandonment of litters

Physical Examination Findings
• Blood or serosanguineous discharge—most commonly expelled during urination, but can appear independent of micturition; may see discharge adherent to fur
• Purulent vaginal discharge
• Uterus may be enlarged, causing abdominal distension
• Pale mucous membranes and tachycardia in animals that have significant uterine hemorrhage
• Depression, lethargy, and anorexia in animals with pyometra or uterine hemorrhage

CAUSES

Serosanguineous or Frank Blood
• Uterine neoplasia—adenocarcinoma, histocytic sarcomas, hemangiomas, and hemangiosarcomas (mouse)
• Endometrial disorders—endometrial hyperplasia, endometrial venous aneurysms, endometriosis, endometritis, and cystic endometrial hyperplasia of endometrial glands (mouse)
• Urinary tract infection
• Vaginal trauma
• Foreign body
• Normal parturition
• Dystocia

Colored Discharge
• Prepartum (few hours before)
• Postpartum
• Dystocia
• Purulent exudate usually not seen with pyometra or vaginitis since the exudate is thick in rodents and does not drain well
• Vaginitis
• Fetal death

RISK FACTORS
• Intact sexual status
• Risk for uterine disorders, including neoplasia, increases with age; seen more often in animals >1 year old

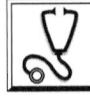

DIAGNOSIS

DIFFERENTIAL DIAGNOSIS
• After copulation—hamsters, rats, and mice form copulatory plugs: opaque, waxy, thick white plugs on the urogenital orifice; formed

by accessory sex glands of the male. Remain in place for 18–24 hours in the mouse, 4 hours in the rat
• Perivulvar dermatitis—moist dermatitis (urine scald); feces pasted around perineum
• Serosanguineous or bloody discharge—may be difficult to clinically differentiate nonneoplastic uterine disorders from neoplasia prior to ovariohysterectomy and histopathologic diagnosis
• Hematuria—use ultrasound-guided cystocentesis to collect urine; differentiates true hematuria from blood expelled from the uterus

CBC/BIOCHEMISTRY/ URINALYSIS
• Neutrophilia possible with pyometra
• Regenerative anemia in animals with uterine hemorrhage
• Increase BUN and creatinine, electrolyte disturbances in animals with pyometra, septicemia, or severe dehydration secondary to severe disease
• Urinalysis—sample collected by ultrasound-guided cystocentesis to differentiate hematuria from uterine bleeding

OTHER LABORATORY TESTS
• Vaginal cytology—may be helpful in determining if the discharge is purulent or bloody
• Cystocentesis and bacterial culture—help to rule out urinary tract infection
• Uterine bacterial culture—via culture swab; perform after the ovariohysterectomy and opening of the uterus, may be helpful in adjusting the antibiotic therapy
• Urine dipstick to confirm blood

IMAGING
• Abdominal ultrasound—may detect an enlarged uterus with thickened walls (endometrial disorder) or an abnormal content (pyometra). Irregular uterine walls and adhesion to surrounding tissues could be sign of neoplasia.
• Abdominal radiography—may detect a large uterus in patients with uterine adenocarcinoma, endometrial disorder, or pyometra or the later stages of fetal death
• Thoracic radiographs—recommended if suspicion of a neoplasia

DIAGNOSTIC PROCEDURES
• A case report described the use of a 2.7 mm rigid endoscope with a 3 mm examination sheath to explore a vaginal hemorrhage in a rat. The hemorrhage originated from a polyp and the vaginoscopy allowed to perform a biopsy.
• Histopathologic examination of the uterus following ovariohysterectomy is necessary for definitive diagnosis.

PATHOLOGIC FINDINGS
N/A

(CONTINUED)

VAGINAL DISCHARGE

TREATMENT

APPROPRIATE HEALTH CARE
• Debilitated patients need to be stabilized and blood transfusion may be indicated in animal with significant uterine hemorrhage.
• A true vaginal hemorrhage is considered a surgical emergency, as the patient could die rapidly from blood loss.

NURSING CARE
Fluid therapy—if the patient is dehydrated, hypovolemic; or in cases of suspected pyometra to support kidney function

ACTIVITY
N/A

DIET
Assist-feed any animal that is anorexic or inappetant to avoid any secondary hypoglycemia and gastrointestinal disorders.

CLIENT EDUCATION
Advise client of the potential benefits of an early ovariohysterectomy in nonbreeding animals.

SURGICAL CONSIDERATIONS
• Ovariohysterectomy—treatment of choice for uterine adenocarcinoma; usually curative if metastasis has not occurred
• Ovariohysterectomy is also the treatment of choice for most other uterine disorders. All uterine disorders carry risk of hemorrhage into the uterus; can become life threatening and can progress; all are at risk for developing uterine adenocarcinoma; reproductive performance is reduced in females with endometrial disorders.

MEDICATIONS

DRUG(S) OF CHOICE

Antibiotics
Recommended in bacterial vaginitis, pyometra, or endometritis; broad-spectrum antibiotics pending results of bacterial culture and sensitivity test. Trimethoprim-sulfa (15–30 mg/kg PO q12h), chloramphenicol (30–50 mg/kg PO q12h), metronidazole in closed pyometra (20 mg/kg PO q12h), or as a second-line enrofloxacin (5–20 mg/kg PO, SC, IM q12h).

Pain Management
• Buprenorphine (0.05–1.0 mg/kg SC, IV q6–8h)

• Oxymorphone (0.2–0.5 mg/kg SC IM q6–12h)
• Morphine (2–5 mg/kg IM q4h)
• Meloxicam (1–3 mg/kg SC, PO q24h)

CONTRAINDICATIONS
Do not administer penicillins, ampicillin, amoxicillin, erythromycin, or lincomycin to hamsters due to the risk of potentially fatal enteric dysbiosis.

PRECAUTIONS
• Enrofloxacin—SC could cause some skin necrosis, needs to be diluted 1:1 with fluids
• Meloxicam—use with caution in animal with compromised renal function

POSSIBLE INTERACTIONS
N/A

ALTERNATIVE DRUGS
N/A

FOLLOW-UP

PATIENT MONITORING
• Monitor postoperatively that the animal does not chew her sutures and open the wound.
• Monitor carefully signs of pain (reluctance to move, teeth grinding) postoperatively.
• Monitor the appetite.
• If the owners elect not to perform surgery to treat endometrial disorders, monitor carefully for signs of hemorrhage or sepsis.

PREVENTION/AVOIDANCE
Ovariohysterectomy for all nonbreeding females

POSSIBLE COMPLICATIONS
• Peritonitis, sepsis in animal with endometritis, pyometra, and uterine rupture
• Postoperative intra-abdominal adhesions may contribute to chronic pain.
• Metastasis
• Hemorrhage, possible death in animal with bleeding uterine disorders

EXPECTED COURSE AND PROGNOSIS
• Good prognosis with timely ovariohysterectomy for most uterine disorders, including neoplasia that has not metastasized
• Poor prognosis in animals presented with vigorous vaginal hemorrhage; emergency stabilization and ovariohysterectomy indicated to control hemorrhage
• Poor in animals with pyometra that is not treated early; sepsis or peritonitis may follow
• Associated mastitis will resolve with ovariohysterectomy alone, unless secondary infection has developed.

✓

MISCELLANEOUS

ASSOCIATED CONDITIONS
• Hamster—pyometra could be a sequel of respiratory infection with *Streptococcus* spp. and *Pasteurella pneumotropica*.
• Mouse—lymphocytic choriomeningitis virus can cause pyometra and infertility.
• Rats—*Mycoplasma pulmonis*, primary pulmonary infection can spread into the genital system and cause infection of the fallopian tubes and uterus
• Mammary neoplasia or mastitis
• Ovarian neoplasia or abscess
• Poor husbandry, poor diet, and obesity
• Ovarian neoplasia
• Ovarian abscess

AGE-RELATED FACTORS
Risk of uterine disorders increases with the age of the animal.

ZOONOTIC POTENTIAL
N/A

PREGNANCY/FERTILITY/ BREEDING
• Animals with uterine disorders have decreased fertility or are sterile.
• The treatment of choice remains ovariohysterectomy. Hemostasis during this procedure could be more difficult if the animal is pregnant due to increased uterine blood supply.

SYNONYMS
N/A

SEE ALSO
N/A

ABBREVIATIONS
BUN = blood urea nitrogen

Suggested Reading
Dutton M. Selected veterinary concerns of geriatric rats, mice, hamsters, and gerbils. Vet Clin Exot Anim 2020;23(3): 525–548.
Frolich J. Rats and mice. In: Quesenberry KE, Carpenter JW, eds. Ferrets, Rabbits and Rodents, 4th Ed). Clinical Medicine and Surgery. 2021 ed. St. Louis: Saunders, 2020:345–367.
Lewis W. Cystic ovaries in gerbils. Exot DVM 2003;5(1):12.
Martorell J. Reproductive disorders in pet rodents. Vet Clin Exot Anim 2017;20:589–608.
Miwa Y, Mayer J. Hamsters and gerbils. In: Quesenberry KE, Carpenter JW, eds. Ferrets, Rabbits and Rodents, 4th Ed).

RODENTS

VAGINAL DISCHARGE

Clinical Medicine and Surgery. 2021 ed. St. Louis: Saunders, 2020:368–384.

Miwa Y, Sladky K. Common surgical procedures of rodents, ferrets, hedgehogs, and sugar gliders. Vet Clin Exot Anim 2016;19:205–244.

Nagaoka T, Onodera H, Matsushima Y et al. Spontaneous uterine adenocarcninomas in aged rats and their relation to endocrine imbalance. J Cancer Res Clin Oncol 1990;116:623–628.

Richardson VCG. Gerbils reproductive system. In:Diseases of Small Domestic Rodents. Oxford, UK: Blackwell, 2003a:103–106.

Richardson VCG. Hamster reproductive system. In:Diseases of Small Domestic Rodents. Oxford, UK: Blackwell, 2003b:147–153.

Richardson VCG. Mice reproductive system. In: VCG R, ed. Diseases of Small Domestic Rodents. Oxford, UK: Blackwell, 2003c:188–193.

Richardson VCG. Rats reproductive system. In: VCG R, ed. Diseases of Small Domestic Rodents. Oxford, UK: Blackwell, 2003d:221–226.

Author Charly Pignon, DVM, Dip ECZM (Small Mammal)

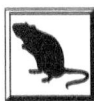

BASICS

DEFINITION
• Weight loss is clinically significant when it exceeds 10% of the normal body weight and is not associated with fluid loss.
• Cachexia indicates an animal in poor condition; it is weight loss that has led to weakness and an altered physiological state due to a chronic disease condition.

PATHOPHYSIOLOGY
• Weight loss and cachexia stem from reduced caloric intake, hypermetabolism, and altered metabolism of glucose and protein synthesis.
• There are many mechanisms that can cause the patient to consume an insufficient caloric intake and thus create an altered metabolic state. The three main mechanisms are (1) increased demand, (2) inadequate intake based on quantity or quality, and (3) excessive loss of nutrients.

SYSTEMS AFFECTED
Depending on the underlying cause, any system can be affected. The consequences of cachexia can also impact many different systems:
• Endocrine/Metabolic
• Gastrointestinal
• Musculoskeletal
• Behavioral (altered mental state)

GENETICS
N/A

INCIDENCE/PREVALENCE
N/A

GEOGRAPHIC DISTRIBUTION
N/A

SIGNALMENT
Any age, breed, or sex

SIGNS

Historical Findings
• Animal may or may not be eating.
• Weight loss may be significant and noticeable to owner, or owner may not have noticed weight loss.
• Owner may only report lethargy.
• Obtaining a time line will help in narrowing the differential diagnoses.

Physical Examination Findings
• Weight loss (if previous weights are available)
• Any other changes can be observed on physical exam and will help in narrowing down the cause of the weight loss/cachexia.
• A thorough exam of the oral cavity will be useful and may require sedation in the rodent patient.

CAUSES

Infectious
• Enteritis; salmonellosis (*S. typhimurium* or *S. enteritidis*), *Clostridium piliformes*, proliferative ileitis (wet tail)
• Parasitism
• Sialodacryoadenitis (coronavirus) causing inflammation of salivary glands
• Chronic respiratory disease complex
• Septicemia
• Pyometra

Metabolic Disorder
• Nutritional (wrong diet offered, poor-quality diet)
• Renal failure (commonly amyloidosis)
• Hepatic disease (commonly amyloidosis), hepatic cirrhosis
• Hyperadrenocorticism (rare)

Neoplasia
Multiple forms

Other
• Heart disease and failure
• Cysts, other abdominal mass
• Arteriosclerosis
• Arthritis
• Stress/environmental factors
• Anemia
• Foreign bodies (rare)

Inability to Eat
• Malocclusion of incisors or molars
• Impacted pouch

RISK FACTORS
N/A

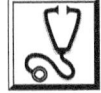

DIAGNOSIS

DIFFERENTIAL DIAGNOSIS
Weight loss and cachexia are objective, not subjective. As such, the condition is more of a clinical manifestation of all of the above causes.

CBC/BIOCHEMISTRY/URINALYSIS
• These basic diagnostic tests are usually helpful in identifying the underlying cause.
• Hypoproteinemia and hypoalbuminemia can result from protein loss caused by hemorrhage, parasitism, or starvation.
• Blood collection may require anesthesia; if the patient is cachexic the risks should be discussed with the owner, and blood collection may have to wait until the patient is more stable.

OTHER LABORATORY TESTS
• Fecal direct and float
• If diarrhea is present, a fecal culture and sensitivity may help to direct therapy.
• Plasma protein electrophoresis

IMAGING
Full-body radiographs of the small rodent patient can help to identify masses (chest or abdominal), dental disease, heart disease, and many other abnormalities that may aid in diagnosis.

DIAGNOSTIC PROCEDURES
• Vary depending on initial diagnostic findings and the suspected underlying cause.
• A good oral exam under general anesthesia, using cheek dilators and specula made for rodents, may be necessary (Jorgenson laboratories Inc., Loveland, CO). A small rigid endoscope can be helpful in performing a complete oral exam. The oral exam will help to identify any oral abscess, tooth root elongation/malalignment, ulcers, pouch impactions, and more.

PATHOLOGIC FINDINGS
Vary depending on cause

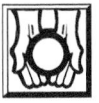

TREATMENT

APPROPRIATE HEALTH CARE
• If the cause is found on physical exam and can be resolved (e.g., malocclusion), outpatient care may be acceptable.
• If the patient is weak and unstable, it may be best to hospitalize and proceed slowly with diagnostics.
• In some cases, home care with assist feeding for a period of time can help the patient to gain weight. If the patient is stable, this can be attempted before performing diagnostic procedures that may put the patient at risk.

NURSING CARE
• It is imperative that the animal receive nutritional support if it is not eating. Supplementation with a liquid diet may be required, such as Oxbow Carnivore Care (Oxbow Enterprises, Inc., Murdock, NE) or Emeraid Exotic Carnivore (Lafeber's, Cornell, IL). If these commercial formulas are not available, a gruel may be made with rodent block ground into Ensure, or human baby foods may be used.
• Ensure that the patient is kept warm (if hypothermic, an incubator may be required).
• Fluid therapy is used to correct hydration following standard protocols (5%–10% of body weight administered in SQ boluses). Fluids should be kept warm to prevent hypothermia and can be warmed by placing the prepared syringe in hot water for a few minutes prior to administering them. Using a 22–25 gauge butterfly needle to administer the fluids can reduce stress on the patient by minimizing restraint.
• The critical patient may require an intraosseous catheter. If hypoproteinemic, administer hetastarch at 10 mL/kg per day in addition to maintenance fluids.

WEIGHT LOSS AND CACHEXIA

ACTIVITY
Based on the cause of weight loss, activity may or may not need to be restricted. Most small rodents that do not feel well will be less active of their own accord. Due to the fact that most live in small cages, cage rest is not required. If activity must be restricted, a smaller cage or removal of an exercise wheel will usually suffice.

DIET
A diet change should never be made abruptly in the anorexic patient. When the patient is stable, changing to an appropriate diet such as rodent block, limited seed, or vegetables/greens should be recommended.

CLIENT EDUCATION
• The small rodent pet owner often needs to be educated regarding bedding choices and diet.
• No matter what the cause of the weight loss, any consultation should include a discussion of caging, diet, and need for regular examinations.
• The author recommends a wellness examination every 6 months.

SURGICAL CONSIDERATIONS
In the event that exploratory surgery or surgical biopsies are required to make a diagnosis, there are several measures that must be taken to increase the prognosis of survival in the small rodent patient.
• Maintenance of body temperature is essential and accomplished through use of a Bair Hugger (Arizant Health Care, Eden, Prairie, MN), water-circulating heating pad, or other warming device.
• Use alcohol sparingly, as this can increase loss of body heat.
• Due to the difficulty of intubating small rodents, an appropriate-sized, snug-fitting face mask should be used.
• A Doppler can be placed directly on the body wall overlying the heart for monitoring anesthesia.
• If general anesthesia is required for blood collection, oral exam, dental work, or other sample collection, the same precautions should be observed.

MEDICATIONS
DRUG(S) OF CHOICE
Choice is based upon the identification of an underlying cause.

If the Animal is Painful
• Meloxicam (1–3 mg/kg PO, SC, IM q24h)
• Tramadol HCL (10–20 mg/kg PO q8–12h)
• Buprenorphine (0.05–0.1 mg/kg SQ, IM q6–8h)

For Bacterial Infection
• Antibiotic-based on culture and sensitivity
• Begin empirical treatment with broad-spectrum antibiotics such as trimethoprim sulfa (15–30 mg/kg PO q12h), enrofloxacin (5–20 mg/kg PO, SC, IM q12h), or ciprofloxacin (10–20 mg/kg PO q12h) for hamsters, gerbils, mice, or rats.
• For rats (do not use in hamsters), amoxicillin/clavulanic acid (20 mg/kg PO q12h) may also be used.

As an Appetite Stimulant
Vitamin B complex 0.02–0.2 mL/kg SQ, IM may be used.

CONTRAINDICATIONS
• Amoxicillin, ampicillin, penicillin, and amoxicillin/clavulanic acid should never be used in hamsters and gerbils.
• The cause of the weight loss should be identified before dispensing any medication.

PRECAUTIONS
• Almost all drugs dispensed to the small rodent are considered off-label, and doses have been extrapolated.
• Be especially careful of compounding drugs in-house; may achieve more favorable results using a compounding pharmacy or a liquid form of the drug.
• Do not use trimethoprim-sulfa if liver or kidney failure is suspected.

POSSIBLE INTERACTIONS
N/A

ALTERNATIVE DRUGS
Booster dietary supplement (Harrison's Products) is a natural, whole-food vitamin supplement with antimicrobial activity for all sick, weak, or immune-compromised animals.

FOLLOW-UP
PATIENT MONITORING
• The owner should purchase a gram scale to monitor the pet's weight at home.
• Rechecks should be frequent (at least weekly) until the patient's weight is normalized.

PREVENTION/AVOIDANCE
N/A

POSSIBLE COMPLICATIONS
• Severe dehydration
• Organ failure and death

EXPECTED COURSE AND PROGNOSIS
The prognosis is based largely on identifying the cause of the weight loss/cachexia; however, a guarded prognosis is generally warranted for cachexia in the older patient.

MISCELLANEOUS
ASSOCIATED CONDITIONS
See Causes

AGE-RELATED FACTORS
N/A

ZOONOTIC POTENTIAL
N/A

PREGNANCY/FERTILITY/BREEDING
Pregnancy and lactation can be associated with weight loss due to increased caloric expenditure.

SYNONYMS
N/A

SEE ALSO
Anorexia and pseudoanorexia
Ascites
Congestive heart failure
Dental malocclusion
Intestinal parasitism
Lymphoma
Pneumonia
Renal failure
Rhinitis and sinusitus

ABBREVIATIONS
N/A

INTERNET RESOURCES
www.vin.com (membership required)

Suggested Reading
Dutton M. Selected veterinary concerns of geriatric rats, mice, hamsters, and gerbils. Vet Clin Exot Anim 2020;23(3):525–548.
Frolich J. Rats and mice. In: Quesenberry KE, Carpenter JW, eds. Ferrets, Rabbits and Rodents, 4th Ed). Clinical Medicine and Surgery. 2021 ed. St. Louis: Saunders, 2020:345–367.
Lennox AM, Gladden JN. Emergency and critical care of small mammals. In: Quesenberry KE, Carpenter JW, eds. Ferrets, Rabbits and Rodents, 4th Ed). Clinical Medicine and Surgery. 2021 ed. St. Louis: Saunders, 2020:595–608.
Mayer J, Mans C. Rodents. In: Carpenter JW, ed. Exotic Animal Formulary, 5th ed. St Louis: Elsevier, 2018:459–493.
Miwa Y, Mayer J. Hamsters and gerbils. In: Quesenberry KE, Carpenter JW, eds. Ferrets, Rabbits and Rodents, 4th Ed). Clinical Medicine and Surgery. 2021 ed. St. Louis: Saunders, 2020:368–384.

Authors Renata Schneider, DVM and Barbara Oglesbee, DVM, DABVP (Avian)

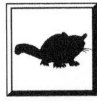

SUGAR GLIDERS

ALOPECIA

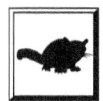

BASICS

DEFINITION
- The loss or absence of hair, from focal or patchy to complete hair loss
- In adult males, focal alopecia on the forehead and chest overlying scent glands is a normal finding.

PATHOPYSIOLOGY
The pathophysiology of alopecia is dependent on the causative factors. Mechanisms of hair loss may include poor development, self-trauma, inflammation, and irritation resulting in damage to the hair follicle and weakening of the hair shaft, tissue necrosis or fibrosis, invasion by ectoparasites, endocrinopathy, and immune-mediated responses.

SYSTEMS AFFECTED
Skin/Exocrine

GENETICS
There is no known genetic predisposition for many of the underlying causes of alopecia.

INCIDENCE/PREVALENCE
Alopecia resulting from a variety of medical conditions is an uncommon presenting complaint in sugar gliders.

GEOGRAPHIC DISTRIBUTION
N/A

SIGNALMENT
Gender and age predisposition are dependent on the specific condition causing the alopecia.

SIGNS

Physical Examination Findings
- Loss of hair ranging from focal to patchy to generalized. Depending on the causative factor, skin irritation, flaking, erythema, pruritus, discharge, odor, or other symptoms may also be present.

CAUSES
- Normal focal alopecia on the forehead and chest in adult males
- Nutrition
- Infectious
- Parasitic
- Stress
- Iatrogenic
- Endocrinopathy
- Secondary to disorders of other systems

RISK FACTORS
The risk factors vary depending on the primary cause of the alopecia. Inadequate husbandry and nutrition, overcrowding, and poor sanitation are common predisposing factors.

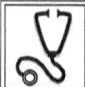

DIAGNOSIS

DIFFERENTIAL DIAGNOSIS
- Environmental/cage rubbing/bite wounds
- Self-mutilation
- Bacterial dermatitis
- Dermatophytosis
- Trauma
- Injection site reaction
- Mites/lice (*Guntheria kowanyam*, *Petauralges rackae*) and fleas
- Endocrinopathy
- Nutritional
- Immune mediated

CBC/BIOCHEMISTRY/URINALYSIS
For regional or generalized alopecia, the minimum database should include serum biochemistry, complete blood count, and urinalysis where possible, to screen for the presence of underlying metabolic disease processes, infection, and inflammation.

OTHER LABORATORY TESTS
Dermatophyte testing, either PCR or fungal culture. Fungal culture results are often delayed due to the long growth time required. Unless lesions are progressive and concerns for zoonosis are present, treatment is typically delayed until a positive test result returns.

Tape preparations or skin scrapes for suspected ectoparasites.

Rarely, endocrine profiles may be helpful, if commercially available.

IMAGING
In systemically ill patients with generalized alopecia, radiographs may help confirm the presence of organomegaly, dystrophic mineralization, or the presence of masses. Rarely, CT scans could be helpful in diagnosing pituitary tumors or endocrinopathies.

DIAGNOSTIC PROCEDURES
- Skin scrapings and dermatophyte cultures should be included as part of the minimum database.
- Skin biopsies for histopathologic evaluation may be indicated.
- Bacterial culture and susceptibility testing
- Response to therapy as a trial

PATHOLOGIC FINDINGS
Results of diagnostic tests and histopathology will vary depending on the cause of the alopecia.

TREATMENT

APPROPRIATE HEALTH CARE
- Treatment will vary depending on the causative factor in each individual case.

NURSING CARE
Unless systemically ill, almost all cases of alopecia are treated on an outpatient basis. In severe cases, basic supportive care including thermal regulation, fluid administration, and assisted feeding may be needed to stabilize the patient.

ACTIVITY
In most cases, activity restriction is not necessary. If self-mutilation is a concern, restraint with an Elizabethan collar or mild sedation may be indicated.

DIET
Supplementation is appropriate if dietary deficiencies are identified as the cause of alopecia.

CLIENT EDUCATION
- Review of appropriate husbandry for the species in question
- Awareness of zoonotic potential if present

SURGICAL CONSIDERATIONS
- Skin biopsies where indicated
- Repair of traumatic wounds
- Removal of masses if appropriate
- Ovariohysterectomy in cases of reproductive pathology

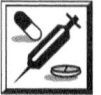

MEDICATIONS

DRUG(S) OF CHOICE
- Varies with the underlying cause of the alopecia
- For bacterial dermatitis, select appropriate antibiotics based on safety and bacterial culture and sensitivity. Antibiotics commonly used in sugar gliders include trimethoprim/sulfa (10–20 mg/kg PO q12h), enrofloxacin (2.5–5 mg/kg PO, SC, IM q12h), chloramphenicol palmitate (50 mg/kg PO q12h), and amoxicillin/clavulanic acid (12.5 mg/kg PO q12h)
- For dermatophytes—miconazole, topically, q24h for 2–4 weeks for focal or regional lesions; antifungal shampoos that are safe for use in cats may be helpful in treating dermatophytes; griseofulvin (20 mg/kg PO q24h for up to 60 days). Absorption is enhanced if given with a fatty meal. Gastrointestinal irritation is the most

common side effect and can be alleviated by dividing the dose for more frequent administration. Bone marrow suppression is a possible idiosyncratic reaction, or can result from prolonged therapy. Neurologic side effects and teratogenicity in the first two trimesters of pregnancy have been reported. Biweekly monitoring of the CBC is recommended; itraconazole (5–10 mg/kg PO q12h × 4 weeks)
• For ectoparasites: ivermectin (0.2–0.4 mg/kg PO, SC repeat on days 14 and 28) for 3 treatments or until infestation is resolved; selamectin (6–18 mg/kg topically repeat in 30 days).
• Postoperative analgesia for surgical patients. Commonly used pain medications include buprenorphine (0.01–0.03 mg/kg PO, SC, IM q8–12h), meloxicam (0.1–0.2 mg/kg PO, SQ q24h).
• For sedation: Light sedation: Midazolam (0.2–0.5 mg/kg SC, IM, IV intranasal) ± butorphanol (0.5 mg/kg SC) or buprenorphine (0.01 mg/kg SC). Heavier sedation/mild anesthesia: ketamine (10–20 mg/kg IM, IV) + midazolam (0.3–0.5 mg/kg SC, IM, IV); other protocols exist.

CONTRAINDICATIONS
• Application of any topical substance may increase itching and discomfort and draw the patient's attention to the affected area.
• Steroids may be used as an anti-inflammatory agent although nonsteroidal anti-inflammatories are preferred. The use of steroids is contraindicated in patients with dermatophyte infections.

PRECAUTIONS
• The use of griseofulvin should be avoided in pregnant animals and in patients with immune system suppression.

POSSIBLE INTERACTIONS
N/A

ALTERNATIVE DRUGS
If gastrointestinal distress accompanies antibiotic therapy, concurrent administration of a probiotic may help alleviate the symptoms.

FOLLOW-UP
PATIENT MONITORING
• Varies with each cause of alopecia
• Patients with ectoparasites should be evaluated 2 weeks and 4 weeks after starting therapy.
• Hair loss in all cases should be evaluated in 6 and again in 12 weeks after the start of treatment.
• All patients should be monitored for potential adverse effects of medications.

PREVENTION/AVOIDANCE
Appropriate husbandry, caging, substrate, sanitation, and population density

POSSIBLE COMPLICATIONS
Possible adverse effects of long-term medication, depending on the cause and treatment of the alopecia

EXPECTED COURSE AND PROGNOSIS
• Most cases of alopecia will resolve with appropriate therapy.
• Some ectoparasite infestations may be difficult to resolve and can require long-term therapy. For persistent cases, evaluation for underlying systemic disease is indicated.
• Environmental decontamination in the case of dermatophyte and some ectoparasite infections is important to prevent spread or reinfection.
• Some endocrinopathies such as hyperadrenocorticism or renal amyloidosis may be fatal.

MISCELLANEOUS
Male sugar gliders have two regions of normal alopecia associated with a scent gland. One is present on the dorsal aspect of the head and a second in the gular region (the ventral neck/cranial thoracic region).

ASSOCIATED CONDITIONS
N/A

AGE-RELATED FACTORS
Some older female gliders may develop bilateral symmetrical alopecia. This is a similar condition to that caused by prolactin-secreting pituitary adenomas in older female short-tailed opossums (*Monodelphis domestica*). The cause of this condition in sugar gliders has not been determined.

ZOONOTIC POTENTIAL
• Dermatophytosis
• Some bacterial infections
• Some ectoparasites

PREGNANCY/FERTILITY/BREEDING
Some patients may develop transient hair loss associated with hormonal changes at the time of pregnancy, parturition, and lactation. Evaluate antibiotics and other medications for safety during pregnancy and lactation.

SYNONYMS
Hair loss

SEE ALSO
Dermatophytosis
Ectoparasites
Nutritional osteodystrophy
Pericloacal gland disorders
Self-mutilation

ABBREVIATIONS
N/A

INTERNET RESOURCES
Exotic DVM forum for eDVM readers: www. pets.groups.yahoo.com/group/ExoticDVM
Veterinary Information Network: www. vin.com

Suggested Reading
Johnson-Delaney C. Sugar gliders. In: Quesenberry KE, Carpenter JW, eds. Ferrets, Rabbits and Rodents, 4th Ed). Clinical Medicine and Surgery. 2021 ed. St. Louis: Saunders, 2020:385–400.
Palmerio BS, Roberts H. Clinical approach to dermatologic disease in exotic animals. Vet Clin North Am Exot Anim Pract 2013;16(3):523–577.
Author Nicholas Jew, DVM

ANOREXIA AND PSEUDOANOREXIA

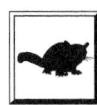

BASICS

DEFINITION
• Lack or loss of appetite for food; in true anorexia the animal refuses to eat, versus pseudoanorexia whereby there is a mechanical inability or health issue that directly impacts the animal's ability to apprehend or chew food.

PATHOPHYSIOLOGY
• Anorexia is most often associated with systemic disease but can be caused by many different mechanisms.
• Inflammatory, infectious, metabolic, or neoplastic diseases can cause inappetence, probably as a result of the release of a variety of chemical mediators.

SYSTEMS AFFECTED
Gastrointestinal, any other system could be affected based upon the illness that is causing the lack of appetite.

GENETICS
N/A

INCIDENCE/PREVALENCE
N/A

GEOGRAPHIC DISTRIBUTION
N/A

SIGNALMENT
Animal of any age or breed; depends on the underlying cause

SIGNS
Historical Findings
• No interest in food (anorexia)
• Interest in food with inability to eat (pseudoanorexia)
• Decreased fecal output
• Varying degrees of lethargy, for example, not using exercise wheel
• Other signs vary depending on the underlying cause.

Physical Examination Findings
• Weight loss or gain (as in abdominal masses)
• Decreased activity level
• Poor coat quality
• Incisors may be fractured or otherwise altered
• In pseudoanorexia, there may be excessive drooling and dysphagia.
• Eyes sunken (a very vague sign of illness/disease)
• Findings are variable, depending on cause of anorexia; many other findings possible

CAUSES
Almost any disease process can lead to anorexia in sugar gliders. The sick or painful sugar glider will not eat as much and weight loss is a very common consequence.

Infectious
• Enteritis (*E. coli*, *Clostridium* species, other bacteria, and rotavirus)
• Parasitic diseases (trematodes, nematodes, Giardiasis, and cryptosporidiosis)
• *Simplicimonas* (Tritrichomonadae)
• Oral abscesses (*Proteus* and *Enterobacter* species)
• Septicemia
• Pyometra

Metabolic Disorder
• Nutritional (wrong diet offered)
• Renal failure
• Hepatic disease

Neoplasia
Multiple forms

Other
• Cysts, other abdominal mass
• Trauma
• Arthritis
• Heart disease; congestive heart failure
• Stress
• Anemia

Pseudoanorexia
• Incisor trauma and infection
• Periodontal disease, caries, tarter accumulation

RISK FACTORS
• Poor husbandry (e.g., cage type, poor sanitation)
• Inappropriate diet

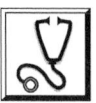

DIAGNOSIS

DIFFERENTIAL DIAGNOSIS
• First differentiate between anorexia and pseudoanorexia.
• If the animal lives with a group of other animals, it may be necessary to separate from the group to determine if truly anorexic.
• Since anorexia can be a consequence of any health problem, a large number of differentials exist. Also consider pregnancy, environmental changes, and other stressors.

CBC/BIOCHEMISTRY/URINALYSIS
• Hypoproteinemia and hypoalbuminemia can result from protein loss caused by anorexia/starvation; also may be due to hemorrhage or parasitism.
• Due to the extensive list of causes of anorexia, any abnormalities in standard diagnostic tests are important in determining the cause of anorexia.

OTHER LABORATORY TESTS
• Fecal exam (direct and floatation)
• Bacterial culture and susceptibility testing (e.g., may need to swab oral cavity or obtain a rectal swab if diarrhea present)
• Cytology of thoracic or abdominal fluid or mass, if present

IMAGING
• Radiographs (full body and/or skull, if oral disease process suspected)—rule out dental disease, organomegaly, respiratory, and cardiac disease
• The need for more extensive imaging depends on findings of physical examination, survey radiographs, and suspected underlying cause of anorexia.

DIAGNOSTIC PROCEDURES
A good oral exam under general anesthesia using cheek dilators and specula made for rodents may be necessary (Jorgenson laboratories inc., Loveland, CO). A small rigid endoscope can be helpful in performing a complete oral exam. The oral exam will help to identify oral abscess, gingivitis/stomatitis, ulcers, dental disorders, or masses.

PATHOLOGIC FINDINGS
Variable, depending on the cause of the anorexia

TREATMENT

APPROPRIATE HEALTH CARE
• If anorexia is complete and lasting greater than 24 hours, inpatient medical care is appropriate. Many anorexic sugar gliders present in critical condition and will need to be stabilized before diagnostics can be performed.
• If the anorexia is acute and the cause is determined early, outpatient medical care is acceptable.

NURSING CARE
• Keep the patient warm; if hypothermic an incubator may be required.
• Fluid therapy is used to correct hydration following standard protocols (5%–10% of body weight administered in SQ boluses). Fluids should be kept warm to prevent hypothermia and can be warmed by placing the prepared syringe in a warm water bath prior to administration. Administration via a 22–25-gauge butterfly needle can reduce stress on the patient by minimizing restraint.
• For critical patients, administer fluid therapy via IV or intraosseous (IO) catheter. In addition to crystalloids, the patient may need colloids such as hetastarch at 10 mL/kg IO per day in several small boluses.

ACTIVITY
Based on the cause of anorexia, activity may or may not need to be restricted. Most small mammals that do not feel well will be less active of their own accord. Cage rest may be required. Due to the larger nature of cages

and the ability to glide, limited vertical mobility may be necessary.

DIET
• It is imperative that the animal receive nutritional support if it is not eating. Supplementation with a liquid diet may be required, such as Oxbow Omnivore Care (Oxbow Enterprises, Inc., Murdock, NE) or Emeraid Omnivore (Lafeber's, Cornell, IL). If these commercial formulas are not available, a gruel may be made with moistened sugar glider pellets into nutritional supplements such as Ensure (Abott Nutrition, Columbus, OH).
• A diet change should never be made abruptly in the anorexic patient. If the diet is inappropriate, wait until the patient is stable and eating again, then convert to an appropriate diet.

CLIENT EDUCATION
Educate sugar glider owners about proper caging choices and diet. No matter the cause of anorexia, client consultation should include a thorough discussion of proper husbandry (caging, diet) and the need for regular examinations. The author recommends a wellness examination every 6 months.

SURGICAL CONSIDERATIONS
If surgery is required, or if oral exam, dental procedures, blood, or other sample collection requires general anesthesia, always observe these precautions:
• A 4-hour fast prior to surgery is recommended. A longer fasting period may be indicated for gastrointestinal surgery.
• It is essential to maintain core body temperature; use of a Bair Hugger (Arizant Health Care, Eden Prairie, MN), water circulating heating pad, or other warming device is crucial.
• Minimize alcohol used during preparation of any sample site (e.g., for blood collection, needle aspirates), as alcohol can increase loss of body heat.
• Due to the difficulty of intubating sugar gliders, an appropriate-sized, snug-fitting face mask should be used. Alternatively, a 1-mm Cook endotracheal tube (Global Veterinary Products, New Buffalo, MI) can be used.
• A Doppler probe can be placed directly over the heart for monitoring anesthesia.

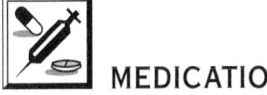

MEDICATIONS
DRUG(S) OF CHOICE
The cause of anorexia should be identified before dispensing any medication.

If the Animal is Painful
• Meloxicam (0.1–0.2 mg/kg PO, SC q24h)
• Buprenorphine (0.02–0.05 mg/kg SQ, IM q12h)

For Bacterial Infection
• Antibiotic-based on culture and sensitivity
• Begin empirical treatment with broad-spectrum antibiotics such as amoxicillin (30 mg/kg PO, IM q24h) and enrofloxacin (2.5–5 mg/kg PO, IM q12h).
• Metronidazole (15 mg/kg PO q24h).

As an Appetite Stimulant
• Vitamin B complex (0.01–0.02 mL/kg SQ, IM) may be used. Stings on injection.
• Capromorelin (1–3 mg/kg PO q24h), anecdotally effective, no published data regarding dose or efficacy.

For Sedation
• Light sedation: Midazolam (0.2–0.5 mg/kg SC, IM, IV intranasal) ± butorphanol (0.5 mg/kg SC) or buprenorphine (0.01 mg/kg SC). Heavier sedation/mild anesthesia: Ketamine (10–20 mg/kg IM, IV) + midazolam (0.3–0.5 mg/kg SC, IM, IV); other protocols exist.

CONTRAINDICATIONS
• The cause of anorexia should be identified before dispensing any medication.

PRECAUTIONS
• Almost all drugs dispensed to sugar gliders are considered off-label and doses have been extrapolated.
• Use caution in dispensing drugs that have been compounded in-house; may achieve better results using a compounding pharmacy or a liquid form of the drug
• Do not use trimethoprim-sulfa if liver or kidney failure is suspected.

POSSIBLE INTERACTIONS
N/A

ALTERNATIVE DRUGS
N/A

FOLLOW-UP
PATIENT MONITORING
• Weigh daily (owner should buy a gram scale if needed).
• Frequent follow-up visits (at least weekly) are required until the patient is no longer anorexic and a normal weight is achieved.

PREVENTION/AVOIDANCE
Depends on the cause of the anorexia

POSSIBLE COMPLICATIONS
• Severe dehydration
• May progress to cachexia

EXPECTED COURSE AND PROGNOSIS
With assisted feeding and rehydration, life can often be prolonged. However, the long-term prognosis will be based largely on identification and correction of the underlying cause. In the older patient, prognosis worsens due to age-related complications and the possibility of multiple causes of anorexia.

MISCELLANEOUS
ASSOCIATED CONDITIONS
Many possibilities based on underlying cause

AGE-RELATED FACTORS
N/A

ZOONOTIC POTENTIAL
N/A

PREGNANCY/FERTILITY/BREEDING
The sugar glider that is pregnant will need special attention to ensure that caloric needs are met. Reproductive pathology should be considered as a cause for the anorexia.

SYNONYMS
Inappetence

SEE ALSO
Dental disease
Diarrhea
Dysuria and hematuria
Nutritional osteodystrophy
Reproductive disease

ABBREVIATIONS
N/A

INTERNET RESOURCES
www.vin.com

Suggested Reading
Brust D, Mans C. Sugar gliders. In: Carpenter JW, ed.. Exotic Animal Formulary, 5th ed. St Louis: Elsevier, 2018:432–442.
Johnson-Delaney C. Sugar gliders. In: Quesenberry KE, Carpenter JW, eds. Ferrets, Rabbits and Rodents, 4th Ed). Clinical Medicine and Surgery. 2021 ed. St. Louis: Saunders, 2020:385–400.
Lennox AM, Gladden JN. Emergency and critical care of small mammals. In: Quesenberry KE, Carpenter JW, eds. Ferrets, Rabbits and Rodents, 4th Ed). Clinical Medicine and Surgery. 2021 ed. St. Louis: Saunders, 2020:595–608.
Author Nicholas Jew, DVM

CONJUNCTIVITIS

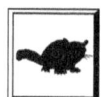 **BASICS**

DEFINITION
Inflammation of the conjunctiva, the vascularized mucosal membrane lining the eyelids, and the nictitating membrane (palpebral conjunctiva) and is continuous with the bulbar conjunctiva which overlies the anterior portion of the globe (bulbar conjunctiva).

PATHOPHYSIOLOGY
• Primary—infectious, environmental irritation
• Secondary to an underlying ocular or systemic disease

SYSTEMS AFFECTED
• Ophthalmic—may include cornea (keratoconjunctivitis), eyelids/periocular skin (e.g., blepharoconjunctivitis), lens (cataracts), and nasolacrimal system (dacryocystitis)
• Respiratory—upper respiratory infections and tooth root invasion of sinuses
• Oral cavity—related dental disease with extension to nasolacrimal system and orbital and nasal cavities

GENETICS
N/A

INCIDENCE/PREVALENCE
Common

GEOGRAPHIC DISTRIBUTION
N/A

SIGNALMENT
Breed Predilections
N/A

Mean Age and Range
N/A

Predominant Sex
Males may be more prone to traumatic injury and retrobulbar abscess due to bite wounds from competing males.

SIGNS
Historical Findings
• History of nasal discharges or sneezing
• History of previous treatment for dental disease
• History of ocular injury or cataract(s).

Physical Examination Findings
• Conjunctival hyperemia
• Chemosis
• Ocular discharge—may be serous (epiphora), mucoid, or mucopurulent
• Conjunctival follicle formation
• Blepharospasm
• Periocular alopecia or matted fur, crusting of discharges on cheeks, and/or nasal rostrum

• Upper respiratory infection—sneezing, nasal discharge
• Oral cavity signs—incisor trauma, swelling, odor, and discharge.
• Signs of pain—depression, lethargy, hiding, and hunched posture
• Symptoms of nutritional osteodystrophy—hind limb paresis, paralysis, and poor body condition
• Cataracts

CAUSES
Bacterial
• The three most commonly isolated bacteria from conjunctival sampling are *Staphylococcus* spp., *Coryneform* spp., and unidentified Gram-positive cocci.
• May be more likely with the introduction of new conspecifics or poor sanitation.

Secondary to Trauma or Environmental Causes
• Conjunctival foreign body—especially if unilateral
• Exposure to environmental irritants (airborne or contact)—may be related to poor hygiene of the local environment
• Irritation from trauma—sexually mature males will often inflict bite wounds on the head and near the eye.

Secondary to Adnexal Disease
• Entropion or aberrant hair (trichiasis) causing mechanical irritation to cornea, conjunctiva, or both
• Nasolacrimal duct obstruction and dacryocystitis—inflammation of the canaliculi, lacrimal sac, or nasolacrimal ducts; may be associated with dental disease
• Orbital disease—orbital abnormality is usually more prominent (e.g., exophthalmos)

Secondary to Other Ocular Diseases
• Ulcerative keratitis
• Anterior uveitis—lens-induced uveitis may accompany cataracts, bilateral uveitis unrelated to cataract may be indicative of systemic disease
• Glaucoma—primary (rare) or related to other intraocular disease

Ectoparasites
Associated periocular dermatitis and alopecia, dermal lichenification—conjunctivitis is due to either direct irritation or secondary to pruritus-induced periocular self-trauma

Neoplastic/Other
• Tumors involving conjunctiva (e.g., lymphosarcoma)—rare

RISK FACTORS
• Recent introduction of new glider(s)—may carry infectious agents

• Poor diet—vitamin A deficiency; diet contains too many soft foods, increasing risk of dental disease
• Dental disease—extension of disease from oral cavity to orbit or nasolacrimal system
• Stress—especially in young gliders
• Environmental stressors—crowding with associated aggression (ocular trauma from fighting); unhygienic housing

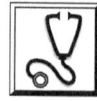 **DIAGNOSIS**

DIFFERENTIAL DIAGNOSIS
Must differentiate primary cause from secondary with a full assessment of eye—more than one cause can occur simultaneously
• Superficial vessels (conjunctival)—originate near fornix; move with the conjunctiva; branch repeatedly; blanch quickly with topical sympathomimetic (e.g., 1:100,000 epinephrine); suggests ocular surface disease (e.g., conjunctivitis, superficial keratitis, and blepharitis)
• Deep vessels (episcleral)—originate near limbus; branch infrequently; do not move with the conjunctiva; blanch slowly or incompletely with topical sympathomimetic; suggests episcleritis or intraocular disease (e.g., anterior uveitis, glaucoma)
• Discharge—mucopurulent or purulent: typical of ocular surface disorders, dacryocystitis, or blepharitis; serous or none: typical of nasolacrimal obstruction or intraocular disease
• Unilateral condition with ocular pain (blepharospasm)—typical of trauma, foreign body or aberrant hair, anterior uveitis, ipsilateral dental disease
• Bilateral chronic condition—congenital problem, chronic upper respiratory tract infection, bilateral tooth root disorders
• Corneal opacification, neovascularization, or fluorescein retention—keratitis
• Pupil—compare to unaffected contralateral eye—miotic pupil may accompany uveitis or corneal ulceration; dilated pupil more common in glaucoma; normal pupil size with blepharitis and conjunctivitis; dyscoria (abnormal shape of pupil) or discoloration of iris: anterior uveitis or iris neoplasia
• Aqueous flare or hyphema—anterior uveitis
• Luxated or cataractous lens—anterior uveitis or glaucoma
• IOP—high: diagnostic for glaucoma; low: suggests uveitis
• Vision loss—severe keratitis or uveitis, cataract, hyphema, or glaucoma; inconsistent menace response, making assessment of vision difficult

- Differentiate from conjunctival masses and infiltrative disease

CBC/BIOCHEMISTRY/URINALYSIS
N/A if primary

OTHER LABORATORY TESTS
- Bacterial C&S—swab conjunctival sac with microtip culturette, taking care to avoid touching periocular fur

IMAGING
- Skull radiographs—to identify dental, nasal sinus, or maxillary bone lesions
- CT—superior to radiographs to localize obstruction and characterize associated lesions; may define extent and nature of intraocular disease
- Ocular ultrasonography—if the ocular media are opaque
- Dacryocystorhinography—radiopaque contrast material to help localize nasolacrimal duct obstruction

DIAGNOSTIC PROCEDURES
- Complete ophthalmic examination—examine intraocular structures for signs of uveitis (miosis, aqueous flare) and adnexa for foreign body, or eyelid abnormalities (aberrant cilia, entropion); ideally use magnification
- Tear production—rule out keratoconjunctivitis sicca—Schirmer tear test may be more informative than phenol red thread (PRT) test due to low values obtained with PRT in normal patients (0.0 ± 0.0 mm/15 s); mean values for STT reported: 2.2 ± 6.7 mm/min
- Aerobic bacterial C&S—acquire sample ideally before any solutions are used (topical anesthetic, fluorescein stain, and flush) to prevent inhibition and dilution of bacterial growth
- Conjunctival cytology—may see degenerate neutrophils and intracellular bacteria with bacterial infection
- Fluorescein stain—rule out corneal ulceration
- Intraocular pressure—rule out glaucoma; mean of 12 ± 2.6 mmHg reported for rebound tonometry
- Conjunctival biopsy may be appropriate in chronic, unresponsive cases

PATHOLOGIC FINDINGS
- Cause of chronic conjunctivitis—inflammatory cell population may suggest cause—neutrophils (bacterial); eosinophils (allergic, parasitic); granulomatous inflammation
- Characteristic features of malignancy (anisocytosis, anisokaryosis, and increase in mitotic figures)

TREATMENT

APPROPRIATE HEALTH CARE
- Primary conjunctivitis—outpatient
- Remove cause of ocular irritation—extract corneal or conjunctival foreign body; keratectomy; surgical correction of entropion; treatment of other primary ocular disease (e.g., ulcerative conjunctivitis, uveitis)
- Secondary to systemic disease—hospitalize only if critical—sugar gliders do not tolerate hospitalization well
- Appropriate dental treatment in cases of related dental disease—if tooth extraction is required or tooth root abscess is diagnosed, it may require referral to a veterinarian with special expertise, if feasible. In patients with extensive tooth root abscesses, aggressive debridement is indicated. Maxillary and retrobulbar abscesses can be particularly challenging.
- General husbandry should be assessed in all ill sugar gliders—avoid crowding and provide multiple locations of security; ensure housing hygiene; adequate diet

NURSING CARE
- Supportive—rinse any mucoid or mucopurulent debris from eye as produced—and always before treating with topical drugs to improve absorption; minimize crusty or moist build-up on periocular fur to reduce risk of secondary dermatitis
- May require change in housing if stressful or if suspect environmental irritant
- Provide hiding box of towel for burrowing for security if hospitalized

ACTIVITY
- Primary—typically no restriction; segregate if infectious cause suspected/confirmed
- Secondary—reduce exposure to at-risk environment or contact with potential irritant

DIET
- Be certain the patient continues to eat
- If vitamin A deficient ensure adequate supplementation
- Provide coarser, harder appropriate dietary items to prevent tarter formation.

CLIENT EDUCATION
- Clean discharge from conjunctival surfaces/cul-de-sacs before treatment
- If multiple topical medications required, use drops followed by ointments or lubricants and allow 5 minutes between different preparations

- If related to dental disease, long-term management may be required to reduce chronic recurrent disease

SURGICAL CONSIDERATIONS
If mass or localized lesion, excisional biopsy recommended

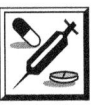

MEDICATIONS

DRUG(S) OF CHOICE
Topical antibiotics preferred over systemic if adequate to avoid GI upset

Primary Bacterial
- Ideally based on culture and sensitivity results
- Initial treatment—based on cytology and gram's stain, or empirical with broad-spectrum agent such as topical oxytetracycline or fluoroquinolone pending C&S results
- Common systemic antibiotics used in sugar gliders include amoxicillin (30 mg/kg PO q24h), amoxicillin/clavulanic acid (12.5 mg/kg PO q12h), enrofloxacin 2.5–5 mg/kg PO q12h), and chloramphenicol (50 mg/kg PO q12h).

Anti-Inflammatory Therapy
- Topical NSAID (e.g., flurbiprofen 0.03% BID-QID or ketorolac 0.5% BID-QID or diclofenac 1% BID-QID) to reduce inflammation if marked
- Systemic NSAID (e.g., meloxicam 0.1–0.2 mg/kg PO, SC q24h)

Analgesics/Sedation
- Buprenorphine 0.01–0.03 mg/kg PO, SC, IM q8–12h
- For sedation: Light sedation: Midazolam (0.2–0.5 mg/kg SC, IM, IV intranasal) ± butorphanol (0.5 mg/kg SC) or buprenorphine (0.01 mg/kg SC). Heavier sedation/mild anesthesia: Ketamine (10–20 mg/kg IM, IV) + midazolam (0.3–0.5 mg/kg SC, IM, IV); other protocols exist.

CONTRAINDICATIONS
- Avoid steroid containing ophthalmic preparations in cases of ulcerative keratitis; steroids may exacerbate infectious disease.

PRECAUTIONS
- Chloramphenicol—avoid human contact due to potential blood dyscrasia. Advise owners of potential risk.

POSSIBLE INTERACTIONS
N/A

ALTERNATIVE DRUGS
N/A

SUGAR GLIDERS

CONJUNCTIVITIS (CONTINUED)

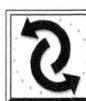

FOLLOW-UP

PATIENT MONITORING

Reevaluate short-term after initiating therapy (i.e., 5–7 days); treat until condition resolved then recheck again 5–7 days after therapy is discontinued—stain cornea with fluorescein at each recheck

PREVENTION/AVOIDANCE

• Therapy for underlying conditions
• Appropriate diet—often a combination of live insects, home-cooked foods, and prepared pellets
• Correct husbandry/clean environment
• Quarantine new arrivals and thoroughly clean environment to prevent infectious disease.

POSSIBLE COMPLICATIONS

• Keratitis—from reduced aqueous tear production, entropion, trichiasis, or foreign body mechanical irritation
• Stenosis of nasolacrimal punctate—from chronic conjunctival inflammation
• Periocular dermatitis from persistent ocular discharges

EXPECTED COURSE AND PROGNOSIS

• Primary/Infectious—usually resolves with appropriate antibiotics or other specific treatment
• Secondary—depends on course of predisposing condition

MISCELLANEOUS

ASSOCIATED CONDITIONS

Cataracts
Nutritional osteodystrophy
Hypovitaminosis A

AGE-RELATED FACTORS

N/A

ZOONOTIC POTENTIAL

N/A

PREGNANCY/FERTILITY/BREEDING

• Use of systemic antibiotics should be used with caution in pregnant females.
• Carriers of chronic infection may not be suitable for breeding.

SYNONYMS

Pink eye

SEE ALSO

Nutritional osteodystrophy
Dental disease
Exophthalmos and orbital diseases

ABBREVIATIONS

C&S = culture and sensitivity results
CT = computed tomography
GI = gastrointestinal
IOP = intraocular pressure
KCS = keratoconjunctivitis sicca
NSAID = nonsteroidal anti-inflammatory drug
PCR = polymerase chain reaction
PRT = phenol red thread test
STT = Schirmer tear test

Suggested Reading
Brust D, Mans C. Sugar gliders. In: Carpenter JW, ed.. Exotic Animal Formulary, 5th ed. St Louis: Elsevier, 2018:432–442.
Fraess GA, Sadar MJ, Daniels JB, Sharkey L, Henriksen MDL. Clinical ophthalmological diagnostic description of 10 healthy sugar gliders (*Petaurus breviceps*) and prevalence of ocular-related presentations in a larger hospital population. Vet Ophthalmol 2021;24:80–92.
Johnson-Delaney C. Sugar gliders. In: Quesenberry KE, Carpenter JW, eds. Ferrets, Rabbits and Rodents, 4th Ed). Clinical Medicine and Surgery. 2021 ed. St. Louis: Saunders, 2020:385–400.

Author Nicholas Jew, DVM

CONSTIPATION (LACK OF FECAL PRODUCTION)

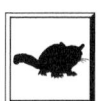

BASICS

DEFINITION
• Constipation—infrequent, incomplete, or difficult defecation with passage of scant, small, hard, or dry fecal pellets
• Intractable constipation and prolonged retention of hard, dry feces leads to obstipation, in which defecation becomes impossible.
• Scant fecal production or lack of fecal production in sugar gliders may result from anorexia, ileus, mechanical obstruction of outflow, and/or disease of the cloaca.

PATHOPHYSIOLOGY
• Constipation can develop with any disease that impairs the passage of feces through the colon. Delayed fecal transit results in the removal of excessive salt and water, producing drier feces.
• Anorexia due to infectious or metabolic disease, pain, stress, or starvation may cause or exacerbate gastrointestinal hypomotility.

SYSTEMS AFFECTED
Gastrointestinal

SIGNALMENT
• Older, overweight sugar gliders may be overrepresented.

SIGNS

Historical Findings
• Scant or no production of fecal pellets
• Small, hard, dry feces
• Infrequent defecation
• Inappetence or anorexia
• Signs of pain, hunched posture, and reluctance to move
• Inappropriate diet or abrupt diet change
• Recent illness or stressful event
• Weight loss or other evidence of systemic disease
• Confinement, lack of exercise

Physical Examination Findings
• Small, hard fecal pellets or absence of fecal pellets palpable in the colon
• Gas, fluid, firm, doughy, or dry gastrointestinal contents may be palpable depending on the underlying cause.
• Enlarged paracloacal glands (common cause)
• Cloacal prolapse, mass
• Abnormal function of hind limbs
• Obesity

CAUSES

Mechanical Obstruction
• Enlarged paracloacal glands—most common cause
• Extraluminal—healed pelvic fracture with narrowed pelvic canal, intrapelvic neoplasia

• Intraluminal and intramural—intussusception, intestinal impaction, cloacal prolapse, colonic or cloacal neoplasia or polyp, stricture, and congenital defect

Dietary and Environmental Causes
• Excessive carbohydrate—feeding large amounts of simple carbohydrates can promote the growth of *E. coli* and *Clostridium* spp., which can cause enterotoxemia and ileus. High-carbohydrate diets can also promote obesity.
• Obesity—cage confinement, lack of exercise
• Stress—pain, fighting among cage mates, surgery, hospitalization, new environment
• Dehydration—lack of access, inappropriate diet
• Anorexia—dental disease, starvation, and secondary to other illness
• Foreign material—ingestion of/impaction with bedding, fibers, and hair (barbering)

Drugs
Anesthetic agents, anticholinergics, and opioids

Painful Defecation
• Cloacal disease—paracloacal gland enlargement, prolapse, and neoplasia
• Trauma—orthopedic abnormalities, poorly aligned healed fractures of the pelvis

Neuromuscular Disease
• Central nervous system—paraplegia, spinal trauma/disease, and cerebral trauma/disease
• Peripheral nervous system—sacral nerve trauma/disease

Metabolic and Dental Disease
• Oral pain from dental disease, metabolic disease (renal disease, liver disease, and nutritional osteodystrophy), pain (oral, trauma, and postoperative), neoplasia, and toxins.
• Debility—general muscle weakness, dehydration, and neoplasia

RISK FACTORS
• Inappropriate diet
• Inactivity due to pain, obesity, and cage confinement
• Anesthesia and surgical procedures
• Metabolic disease resulting in dehydration
• Ingestion of bedding substrate, fibers, and fabric
• Underlying dental, gastrointestinal tract, or metabolic disease
• Spinal, pelvic, or hind-limb trauma

DIAGNOSIS

DIFFERENTIAL DIAGNOSIS
• Dyschezia and tenezmus—may be mistaken for constipation by owners; associated with increased frequency of attempts to defecate and frequent production

of small amounts of liquid feces containing blood and/or mucous
• Stranguria—may be mistaken for constipation by owners; can be associated with hematuria and abnormal findings on urinalysis

CBC/BIOCHEMISTRY/URINALYSIS
• May be used to identify underlying causes of gastrointestinal hypomotility or dehydration
• PCV and TS elevation in dehydrated patients

OTHER LABORATORY TESTS
Fecal direct examination, fecal floatation, and zinc sulfate centrifugation may demonstrate gastrointestinal parasite (cestode) ova.

IMAGING
• In sugar gliders, radiographic detail of individual abdominal organs is often poor.
• Contrast radiography may be useful in evaluating gastrointestinal transit time and locating obstructions and displacement of the gastrointestinal tract.
• Abdominal radiography may reveal a colonic or rectal foreign body, colonic or cloacal mass, spinal fracture, or fractured or dislocated pelvis.
• Computed tomography may provide improved resolution of the abdominal organs and underlying pathology.
• Abdominal ultrasonography may aid in the identification of extra- and intraluminal masses causing compression of the gastrointestinal tract.

PATHOLOGIC FINDINGS
• Vary with cause and severity of constipation

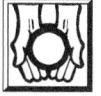

TREATMENT

APPROPRIATE HEALTH CARE
• Consider emergency treatment for sugar gliders that have not produced feces or have been anorectic for over 24 hours.
• Outpatient care may be appropriate in some cases, but inpatient hospitalization and support should be considered for the majority.

NURSING CARE
• Remove or ameliorate underlying cause, if possible.
• If paracloacal glands are enlarged: Gentle expression of contents from impaction. Sedation is required due to pain with expression. Often, thick yellow to ivory color discharge is expressible from the paracloacal glands. This may require significant pressure in more severe cases.
• Discontinue any medications that may cause constipation.
• A warm, quiet environment should be provided.

CONSTIPATION (LACK OF FECAL PRODUCTION)   (CONTINUED)

Fluid Therapy
• Fluid therapy is an essential component of the medical management of all patients with anorexia, gastrointestinal hypomotility, and/or constipation.
• Fluids may be administered by the oral, subcutaneous, intravenous, and/or intraosseous route
• Mildly affected patients usually respond well to oral and subcutaneous fluids.
• Intravenous or intraosseous fluids are indicated in patients that are severely dehydrated or depressed.
• In most patients, lactated Ringer's solution or Normosol crystalloid fluids are appropriate for parenteral fluid administration.
• Maintenance fluid requirements are estimated at 100 mL/kg/day.

ACTIVITY
If the patient is not debilitated, exercise should be encouraged as activity promotes gastric motility.

DIET
• Assisted or forced feeding is contraindicated in cases of intestinal obstruction (e.g., intussusception, rectal prolapse, and cestode impaction)
• If the patient refuses these foods, syringe feeding may be indicated: Critical Care for Omnivores (Oxbow Animal Health, Omaha, NE) or Emeraid Omnivore (Lafeber Company, Cornell, IL). If these commercial formulas are not available, a gruel may be made with blenderized omnivore/sugar glider pellets.
• Encourage oral fluid intake by offering fresh water, high-moisture-content fruits and vegetables, or by flavoring the water with fruit/vegetable juices.

CLIENT EDUCATION
• Discuss the importance of dietary modification, if indicated.
• Advise owners to regularly monitor food consumption and fecal output; seek veterinary attention with a noticeable decrease in either.
• Recommend regular follow-up and monitoring for sugar gliders with constipation.

SURGICAL CONSIDERATIONS
• In most cases, constipation and lack of fecal production will resolve with medical treatment alone.
• Surgery may be indicated for cloacal prolapse, intussusception, intestinal foreign body, extraluminal compression of the gastrointestinal tract, intestinal neoplasia, abscesses, and orthopedic problems.

 ## MEDICATIONS
• Dehydrated patients should be rehydrated with a balanced electrolyte solution.

• Use parenteral medications in animals with severe ileus; oral medications may not be properly absorbed; begin oral medication when intestinal motility begins to return (fecal production, return of appetite, and radiographic evidence).

DRUG(S) OF CHOICE
• Antiparasite drugs—praziquantel (5–10 mg/kg PO, SQ, repeat in 10–14 days) for cestodes and trematodes; fenbendazole (20 mg/kg PO q24h × 3 days) for roundworms, hookworms, whipworms, and cestodes
• Antibiotics—amoxicillin (30 mg/kg PO q12h), amoxicillin/clavulanic acid (12.5 mg/kg PO, SQ q12h), enrofloxacin (2.5–5 mg/kg PO q12h), trimethoprim/sulfamethoxazole (10–20 mg/kg PO q12h), chloramphenicol (50 mg/kg PO q12h); may also be indicated in patients with bacterial overgrowth that sometimes occurs secondary to ileus; indicated in patients with diarrhea, abnormal fecal cytology, and disruption of the intestinal mucosa (evidenced by blood in the feces). For *Clostridium* spp. overgrowth and giardiasis: metronidazole (25 mg/kg PO q12h)
• Analgesics—buprenorphine (0.01–0.03 mg/kg PO, SQ, IM q8–12h), carprofen (2 mg/kg PO, SC q12h), or meloxicam (0.1–0.2 mg/kg PO, SQ q24h). Intestinal pain, regardless of cause, impairs mobility, and decreases appetite and may inhibit recovery.
• Laxatives—mineral oil, lactulose as indicated
• Motility modifiers—cisapride (0.1–0.2 mg/kg PO q8h), metoclopramide (0.5 mg/kg PO, SC q12h); may be indicated in patients with ileus (see Contraindications)
• For sedation: Light sedation: Midazolam (0.2–0.5 mg/kg SC, IM, IV intranasal) ± butorphanol (0.5 mg/kg SC) or buprenorphine (0.01 mg/kg SC). Heavier sedation/mild anesthesia: Ketamine (10–20 mg/kg IM, IV) + midazolam (0.3–0.5 mg/kg SC, IM, IV); other protocols exist.

CONTRAINDICATIONS
• Anticholinergics
• Assisted or forced feeding is contraindicated in cases of gastrointestinal tract obstruction or rupture.
• Gastrointestinal motility enhancers in patients with suspected mechanical obstruction (e.g., impaction, intussusception, rectal prolapse, and neoplasia)

PRECAUTIONS
• Chloramphenicol may cause aplastic anemia in susceptible people. Clients and staff should use appropriate precautions when handling this drug.

• Metronidazole neurotoxic if overdosed
• Meloxicam—use with caution in cases with suspected renal function

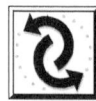 ## FOLLOW-UP
PATIENT MONITORING
Monitor appetite and fecal production. Sugar gliders that are successfully treated will regain a normal appetite; fecal volume and consistency will return to normal.

PREVENTION/AVOIDANCE
• Obesity prevention; encourage exercise (e.g., provide running wheel) and limit the intake of high-calorie, high-carbohydrate foods, especially seed-based diets.
• Routine fecal examination; internal parasite treatment
• Reduction of stress and prompt treatment of conditions that cause pain
• Be certain that postoperative patients are eating and passing feces prior to release.

POSSIBLE COMPLICATIONS
• Chronic constipation or recurrent obstipation could lead to acquired megacolon, cloacal prolapse.
• Death due to gastrointestinal tract rupture, hypovolemic, or endotoxic shock
• Postoperative ileus
• Overgrowth of bacterial pathogens

EXPECTED COURSE AND PROGNOSIS
• Early medical management of constipation or ileus due to dietary causes, obesity, anesthesia/surgery, or anorexia secondary to pain or other stress usually carries a good to excellent prognosis.
• Surgical removal of foreign material, neoplasia, or surgical correction of intussusception or cloacal prolapse carries a guarded to poor prognosis.
• The prognosis for other causes varies.

 ## MISCELLANEOUS
ASSOCIATED CONDITIONS
• Paracloacal gland abscess/infection
• Dental disease
• Hepatic lipidosis
• Renal disease
• Diarrhea
• Nutritional osteodystrophy

PREGNANCY/FERTILITY/BREEDING
• N/A

SYNONYMS
Fecal impaction
Ileus

(CONTINUED)

CONSTIPATION (LACK OF FECAL PRODUCTION)

SEE ALSO
Diarrhea
Dental disease
Nutritional osteodystrophy
Paracloacal gland disorders
Reproductive disease

ABBREVIATIONS
PCV = packed cell volume
TS = total solids

Suggested Reading
Brust DM. Gastrointestinal diseases of marsupials. J Exot Pet Med 2013;22(2):132–140. doi: 10.1053/j.jepm.2013.05.005.
Brust D, Mans C. Sugar gliders. In: Carpenter JW, ed.. Exotic Animal Formulary, 5th ed. St Louis: Elsevier, 2018:432–442.
Johnson-Delaney C. Sugar gliders. In: Quesenberry KE, Carpenter JW, eds. Ferrets, Rabbits and Rodents, 4th Ed). Clinical Medicine and Surgery. 2021 ed. St. Louis: Saunders, 2020:385–400.
Reavill D. Pathology of the exotic companion mammal gastrointestinal system. Vet Clin North Am Exot Anim Pract 2014;17(2):145–164 10.1016/j.cvex.2014.01.002.

Author Nicholas Jew, DVM

DENTAL DISEASE

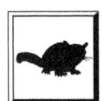

BASICS

OVERVIEW

Anatomy
• Sugar gliders are diprotodonts meaning they have two lower incisors.
• Well-developed first mandibular incisor teeth that are longer than their maxillary counterparts. These teeth are designed for peeling bark.
• All teeth are anelodont and do not grow continuously.
• The mandibular arcades lack canine teeth.
• Dental formula is 2(I 3/2, C 1/0, P 3/3, M 4/4) = 40

PATHOPHYSIOLOGY
• Dental disease in sugar gliders is primarily associated with inappropriate diets that are too soft and carbohydrate rich. These diets often lead to the development of periodontal disease, caries, and tartar accumulation.
• Gingival and oral mucosal abscesses may be present in young gliders. Commonly bacteria from the GI tract are cultured from these (*Proteus* and *Enterobacter* species). It is suspected that this is introduced to the oral cavity following grooming of the vent.
• Primary malocclusion is uncommon compared to other exotic companion mammals.
• Trauma to the teeth may result in pulp exposure and infection.

SIGNS

Historical Findings
• Historical signs often include hyporexia or anorexia, weight loss, discharge or moisture around the mouth, and changes in the dietary items preferred (trending toward softer items).
• Altered feeding and chewing behavior may be observed by owners that should be evaluated further for evidence of dental disease and pain.
• Swellings or mass lesions around the cheeks and eyes may be noted initially by caregivers.
• Fracture and malocclusion of incisor teeth are often missed by the owners.

Physical Examination Findings
• Inspection of the oral cavity while awake is challenging in sugar gliders; therefore, proper diagnosis of dental disease must be performed under deep sedation or general anesthesia.
• Oral inspection and treatment of dental disease in sugar gliders require specialized equipment.
• Inspection by oral endoscopy provides optimal oral visualization. A 14- to 18-cm

long, 2.7-mm thick, 30-degree rigid endoscope is commonly used. Other magnification devices are helpful but not always sufficient, and many lesions can be missed without the help of stomatoscopy.
• Common findings include gingivitis, dental discoloration, tartar and calculus, periodontitis, and mass lesions. Many gliders with dental disease will also be underweight.
• Dental caries and root exposure are commonly identified with thorough oral evaluation. The prognosis is poor due to the difficulty of extracting teeth in patients of this size.

CAUSES AND RISK FACTORS
Diets that lack hard or abrasive elements (chitinous exoskeletons), contain only soft items and are rich in carbohydrates.

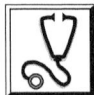

DIAGNOSIS

DIFFERENTIAL DIAGNOSIS
For anorexia—gastrointestinal disease, pain, and metabolic disease

CBC/BIOCHEMISTRY/URINALYSIS
Usually normal unless secondary infection or other underlying metabolic disease is present

OTHER LABORATORY TESTS
N/A

IMAGING
• A complete radiologic study of the skull must include five basic projections (lateral; oblique in two directions; ventrodorsal and rostrocaudal) using high-definition digital radiology equipment or a dental radiology unit.
• Modern CT scans provide excellent detail in small species like sugar gliders.

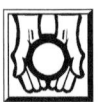

TREATMENT
The goal of treatment is the resolution of bacterial infection, removal of tartar and calculus, and removal of diseased, damaged, or painful dentition.

APPROPRIATE HEALTH CARE
• Thorough dental evaluation, dental scaling, and dental surgery should be completed under general anesthesia with appropriate analgesia.
• Provide supportive care, such as fluid therapy and assist feeding, in patients that are not eating.
• Use of antimicrobials should, ideally, be based on the result of culture and sensitivity testing.

SURGICAL CONSIDERATIONS

Dental Scaling
• General anesthesia is required for dental scaling.
• Hand scalers are preferred over piezoelectric or ultrasonic due to the teeth size and gingiva sensitivity.
• Polishing should be performed after scaling.

Dental Extractions
• Teeth are extracted with careful dissection of the periodontal ligament using small (25-gauge) contoured needles or appropriately sized dental elevators.
• The most frequent complications are fractures of the teeth or root and fractures of the maxilla or mandible especially when osteomyelitis and/or nutritional osteodystrophy are present.
• Dental disease requiring extraction of teeth typically carries a poor prognosis due to the difficulty and complications associated with extraction.

MEDICATIONS

DRUG(S) OF CHOICE
• Antimicrobial drugs are indicated if bacterial infection is evident. Initially, use broad-spectrum antibiotics such as enrofloxacin (5 mg/kg PO, SC, IM q12h), ciprofloxacin (10 mg/kg PO q12h), and amoxicillin/clavulanic acid (12.5 mg/kg PO, SQ q12h); if anaerobic infections are suspected, use chloramphenicol (50 mg/kg PO q12h) or metronidazole (25 mg/kg PO q12h).
• Pain management—commonly used pain medications include buprenorphine (0.02–0.05 mg/kg SQ, IM q12h) and meloxicam (0.1–0.2 mg/kg PO, SQ q12h).

CONTRAINDICATIONS
Extensive surgery on a debilitated animal

PRECAUTIONS
• Chloramphenicol may cause aplastic anemia in susceptible people. Clients and staff should use appropriate precautions when handling this drug.
• Metronidazole is neurotoxic if overdosed.

FOLLOW-UP

PATIENT MONITORING
• Monitor appetite and the ability to eat following treatment. Some patients may require assist feeding. The duration of assist feeding depends on the severity of disease.

• Reevaluate and perform dental prophylaxis regularly. Evaluate the entire oral cavity with each recheck.

PREVENTION/AVOIDANCE

Provision of an appropriate diet with a variety of textures and items of differing hardnesses.
• Sugar gliders are omnivores, and the ideal diet for a captive sugar glider is unknown. Many dietary variations may be adequate.
• Example diet 1
  ○ 75% commercial sugar glider pellets, 25% variety of fruits and vegetables, calcium supplement, small quantities of treat items (<5% of daily diet, this includes live insects)
• Example diet 2
  ○ 50% fruit sugars in the form of sap or nectar, 50% lean protein (insectivore diet, supplemental live insects)

POSSIBLE COMPLICATIONS

Iatrogenic maxilla/mandibular fracture, recurrence, chronic pain, or inability to chew.

EXPECTED COURSE AND PROGNOSIS

• Oral abscesses typically carry a fair prognosis if they respond to medical therapy.
• The prognosis for diseases related to premolar and molar teeth is guarded to poor due to patient size and the difficulties related to any surgical approach.

 MISCELLANEOUS

AGE-RELATED FACTORS

Young gliders have a higher incidence of oral abscess development.

ZOONOTIC POTENTIAL

N/A

PREGNANCY/FERTILITY/BREEDING

N/A

SYNONYMS

N/A

SEE ALSO

Anorexia, nutritional osteodystrophy, and weight loss and cachexia.

Suggested Reading
Brust D, Mans C. Sugar gliders. In: Carpenter JW, ed.. Exotic Animal Formulary, 5th ed. St Louis: Elsevier, 2018:432–442.
Johnson-Delaney C. Sugar gliders. In: Quesenberry KE, Carpenter JW, eds. Ferrets, Rabbits and Rodents, 4th Ed). Clinical Medicine and Surgery. 2021 ed. St. Louis: Saunders, 2020:385–400.
Lennox AM, Miwa Y. Anatomy and disorders of the oral cavity of miscellaneous exotic companion mammals. Vet Clin North Am Exot Anim Pract 2016;19(3):929–945.
Author Nicholas Jew, DVM

DIARRHEA

SUGAR GLIDERS

BASICS

DEFINITION
Abnormal frequency, liquidity, and volume of feces

PATHOPHYSIOLOGY
• Caused by imbalance in the absorptive, secretory, and motility actions of the intestines
• Can result from a combination of factors: increased membrane permeability, hypersecretion, and malabsorption
• Death occurs from loss of electrolytes and water, acidosis, and from the manifold effects of toxins.
• May or may not be associated with inflammation of the intestinal tract (enteritis)

SYSTEMS AFFECTED
• Gastrointestinal
• Endocrine/Metabolic—fluid, electrolyte, and acid–base imbalances

GENETICS
N/A

INCIDENCE/PREVALENCE
N/A

GEOGRAPHIC DISTRIBUTION
N/A

SIGNALMENT
• No specific age or gender predilection to noninfectious causes
• Younger animals are more commonly affected by infectious causes.
• Diet changes can precipitate diarrhea, particularly in joeys.
• Young, stressed, or breeding gliders may have Giardia associated intermittent diarrhea.

SIGNS

General Comments
• Diarrhea can occur with or without systemic illness.
• Signs can vary from diarrhea in an apparently healthy patient to severe systemic signs.
• The choice of diagnostic and therapeutic measures depends on the severity of illness.
• Patients that are not systemically ill tend to have normal hydration and minimal systemic signs.
• Signs of more severe illness (e.g., anorexia, weight loss, severe dehydration, depression, and shock) should prompt more aggressive diagnostic and therapeutic measures.

Historical Findings
• Stool production ranging from soft, formed to liquid consistency

• Owner may report fecal accidents, changes in fecal consistency and volume, blood or mucous in the feces, or straining to defecate.
• History of sudden diet change, weaning, overfeeding fruit, excessive carbohydrates or sugars, or food that is spoiled
• Stress—hospitalization, transportation, environmental changes, and concurrent illness may contribute to alterations in intestinal commensal flora.
• Antibiotic usage—the use of antibiotics may alter the microbiome of the GI tract and subsequent diarrhea.

Physical Examination Findings
• Vary with the severity of disease
• Anorexia, lethargy, and depression
• Poor haircoat; decreased grooming behavior
• Abdominal pain characterized by hunched posture, reluctance to move, bruxism, and/or pain on abdominal palpation
• Fecal staining of the perineum
• Tenesmus, hematochezia, and cloacal prolapse
• Dehydration, hypothermia, hypotension, and weakness
• Fever
• Abdominal distention—due to thickened or fluid-filled bowel loops, impaction, bloat, masses, or organomegaly
• Fluid or gas may be palpable within the gastrointestinal tract
• Weight loss in chronically infected animals
• Animals may be found dead in the absence of clinical signs.

CAUSES
• Dietary—abrupt change in diet, weaning, excessive fresh green foods or fruit, excessive carbohydrate/sugar, or spoiled food
• Bacterial infection/enterotoxemia—*E. coli*, *Clostridium* spp., and *Salmonella* spp.
• Obstruction—neoplasia, foreign body, intussusception
• Drugs/toxins—oral administration of antibiotics; plant toxins; mycotoxins
• Viral—murine rotavirus A
• Metabolic disorders—liver disease, renal disease
• Parasitic causes—protozoans, cestodes, and nematodes
• Systemic illness may also result in diarrhea as a secondary event.
• Neoplasia—primary gastrointestinal tumor, or as a sequela to other organ involvement

RISK FACTORS
• Environmental stressors—improper temperature, poor sanitation, overcrowding, and transportation stress
• Immunosuppressors (radiation, corticosteroids, and concurrent disease),

heavy parasite load, and poor nutrition are considered to be additional predisposing factors.
• Weaning, dietary changes, and carbohydrate overload
• Antibiotic usage

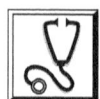

DIAGNOSIS

DIFFERENTIAL DIAGNOSIS

General
• Consider all causes of enteropathy, including diet change, inappropriate antibiotics, enterotoxemia, systemic or metabolic disease, as well as specific intestinal disorders
• Infectious and parasitic causes may be primary or secondary.
• Viral—murine rotavirus A
• Bacteria—*Salmonella* spp., *Clostridium* spp., *E. coli*, and others
• Protozoa—*Simplicomonas and Simplicimonas* spp., *Giardia* spp., cryptosporidiosis
• Nematodes—*Parastrongyloides*, *Paraustrostrongylus, and Paraustroxyuris* spp.

CBC/BIOCHEMISTRY
• Often normal with mild illness
• Moderate to severe illness should prompt a complete evaluation.
• Increased PCV and TS seen with dehydration
• Anemia may be seen with chronic gastrointestinal bleeding.
• TWBC elevation with neutrophilia may be seen with bacterial enteritis.
• Hemogram abnormalities may be consistent with sepsis and/or systemic infection.
• Hypoalbuminemia may be seen with protein loss from the intestinal tract.
• Serum biochemistry abnormalities may suggest renal or hepatic disease.
• Electrolyte abnormalities secondary to anorexia, fluid loss, and dehydration.

OTHER LABORATORY TESTS

Fecal Examination
• Fecal direct examination, fecal floatation, and zinc sulfate centrifugation may demonstrate gastrointestinal parasites or spore-forming bacteria.
• Fecal cytology—may reveal red blood cells or fecal leukocytes, which are associated with inflammation or infection of the intestines
• Fecal gram stain—may demonstrate large numbers of spore-forming bacteria consistent with *Clostridium* spp. or excessive numbers of gram-negative bacteria

• Fecal culture should be performed if a bacterial infection is suspected; however, interpretation may be difficult since *E. coli* and clostridia may be normal inhabitants in some cases.
• Fecal occult blood testing—to confirm melena when suspected

IMAGING
• Survey abdominal radiography may indicate intestinal obstruction, organomegaly, mass, foreign body, or ascites.
• Contrast radiography may indicate mucosal irregularities, mass, ileus, foreign body, stricture, or thickening of the intestinal wall.
• Abdominal ultrasonography may demonstrate intestinal wall thickening, gastrointestinal mass, foreign body, ileus, or mesenteric lymphadenopathy. Hyperechogenicity may be seen with hepatic lipidosis or fibrosis; hypoechoic nodules are suggestive of hepatic necrosis, abscess, or neoplasia.

PATHOLOGIC FINDINGS
• Vary with cause and severity of diarrheic condition
• Gross pathology may reveal lesions suggestive of etiology
• Histopathology is often the best method to obtain a definitive diagnosis for neoplasia, infiltrative or inflammatory conditions, and certain infections.

TREATMENT

APPROPRIATE HEALTH CARE
• Treatment must be specific to the underlying cause to be successful.
• Patients with mild diarrhea that are otherwise bright and alert usually respond to outpatient treatment.
• Patients with moderate to severe diarrhea usually require hospitalization and supportive care including parenteral medication, fluid therapy, and thermal support.
• Patients exhibiting signs of lethargy, depression, dehydration, and/or shock should be hospitalized even if diarrhea is mild or absent.
• When infectious disease is suspected, strict isolation of affected and exposed animals is indicated.

NURSING CARE
• Fluid therapy—rehydration and correction of electrolyte imbalances are essential to treatment success in severely ill sugar gliders.
• Severe volume depletion can occur with acute diarrhea, and aggressive shock fluid therapy may be necessary.
• In most patients, crystalloids (e.g., lactated Ringer's solution, Normosol; 50–100 mL/kg/day) are appropriate for SQ or IV

administration. Crystalloids can also be given PO.
• Maintenance fluid requirements are estimated at 100 mL/kg/day.

DIET
• It is imperative that sugar gliders continue to eat during treatment and recovery. Prolonged anorexia promotes further derangement of gastrointestinal microflora, encourages overgrowth of intestinal bacterial pathogens, and negatively affects gastrointestinal motility.
• Assisted feeding is typically required until the patient is eating, eliminating, and maintaining body weight.
• A highly digestible, liquefied, elemental diet such as Emeraid Omnivore (Lafeber Company, Cornell, IL) may be indicated in case of suspected enteropathy.
• If commercial assist feeding diets are not available, then a liquefied blend can be made of commercial pellets, fresh fruits and vegetables, insectivore diets, and live insects.
• Encourage oral fluid intake: offer fresh water, administer oral fluids via syringe, wet the food, or flavor water with fruit or vegetable juices.
• Direct oral administration of fluids (water, crystalloids, and electrolyte solutions) for patients that are not drinking

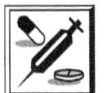

MEDICATIONS

DRUG(S) OF CHOICE
Antibiotic Therapy
• Indicated in patients with bacterial inflammatory disorders of the gastrointestinal tract; also indicated in patients with disruption of the intestinal mucosa evidenced by blood in the feces
• Selection should be broad-spectrum antibiotics, based on the results of culture and susceptibility testing when possible.
• Some choices for empirical use while waiting for culture results include chloramphenicol (50 mg/kg PO q12h) or enrofloxacin (5 mg/kg PO, SC, IM q12h)
• For *Clostridium* spp. overgrowth and *Simplicomonas* and *Simplicomonas* spp.: metronidazole (25 mg/kg PO q24h × 14 days)

Antiparasitic Agents
• Indicated based upon fecal examination for internal parasites, ova, or cysts
• For nematodes—fenbendazole (20–50 mg/kg PO q24h × 3 days, repeat in 14 days)
• For cestodes—praziquantel (5–10 mg/kg PO or SQ, repeat in 10 days)
• For coccidia—sulfadimethoxine (50 mg/kg PO once, then 25 mg/kg q24h × 10–20 days);

dose is anecdotal and extrapolated from other exotic companion mammals
• For *Giardia*—metronidazole (25 mg/kg PO q12h; dose cited is anecdotal; duration of treatment for sugar gliders is not reported, but 5 days is typical for other exotic companion mammals), fenbendazole (20–50 mg/kg PO q24h × 5 days)

CONTRAINDICATIONS
• Antibiotics that are primarily gram-positive in spectrum may suppress the growth of commensal flora, allowing overgrowth of enteric pathogens.

PRECAUTIONS
• It is important to determine the cause of diarrhea. A general "shotgun" approach with antibiotics may be ineffective or detrimental.
• Antibiotic therapy can predispose sugar gliders to bacterial dysbiosis and overgrowth pathogenic bacteria (particularly *Clostridium difficile*). If signs worsen or do not improve, therapy should be adjusted.
• Chloramphenicol may cause aplastic anemia in susceptible people. Clients and staff should use appropriate precautions when handling this drug.
• Metronidazole is neurotoxic if overdosed.
• Isolate affected and exposed animals when infectious disease is suspected.

POSSIBLE INTERACTIONS
N/A

ALTERNATIVE DRUGS
N/A

FOLLOW-UP

PATIENT MONITORING
• Fecal volume and character, appetite, attitude, and body weight
• If diarrhea does not resolve, consider reevaluation of the diagnosis.

PREVENTION/AVOIDANCE
• Providing appropriate diet and husbandry
• Reducing stress and providing sanitary conditions
• When infectious disease is suspected, strict isolation of affected and exposed animals is indicated.

POSSIBLE COMPLICATIONS
• Antibiotic therapy can promote bacterial dysbiosis and overgrowth of pathogenic bacteria.
• Dehydration due to fluid loss
• Ileal obstruction, intussusception, tenesmus, and cloacal prolapse.
• Septicemia due to bacterial invasion of enteric mucosa
• Shock, death from enterotoxicosis

SUGAR GLIDERS

DIARRHEA

EXPECTED COURSE AND PROGNOSIS
- Depends on cause and severity of disease

MISCELLANEOUS

ASSOCIATED CONDITIONS
- Dehydration
- Malnutrition
- Hypoproteinemia
- Anemia
- Septicemia
- Peritonitis
- Cloacal prolapse

AGE-RELATED FACTORS
- All ages susceptible to diarrhea
- Young and recently weaned animals are most severely affected by infectious and parasitic organisms that may cause diarrhea.

ZOONOTIC POTENTIAL
- *Salmonella*
- *Giardia*

PREGNANCY/FERTILITY/BREEDING
- Severe diarrhea and associated metabolic disturbance may reduce fertility or cause abortion.
- Some infections (e.g., *Salmonella*) can cause abortion.

SYNONYMS
- "Sticky Joey Syndrome"—clinical signs include diarrhea, dehydration, anorexia, and death. Adults may be asymptomatic while joeys typically have wet and "sticky" fur that appears poorly groomed. This disease syndrome is described colloquially as "ick." Evaluation of the joey's stool typically reveals a trichmonad that has been identified as *Simplicomonas and Simplicimonas*. Joeys and adults in the environment should be treated concurrently.

SEE ALSO
Anorexia
Nutritional osteodystrophy
Paracloacal gland disorders
Reproductive diseases

ABBREVIATIONS
PCV = packed cell volume
TS = total solids
TWBC = total white blood cell count

Suggested Reading
Brust D, Mans C. Sugar gliders. In: Carpenter JW, ed.. Exotic Animal Formulary, 5th ed. St Louis: Elsevier, 2018:432–442.
Johnson-Delaney C. Sugar gliders. In: Quesenberry KE, Carpenter JW, eds. Ferrets, Rabbits and Rodents, 4th Ed). Clinical Medicine and Surgery. 2021 ed. St. Louis: Saunders, 2020:385–400.
Lennox AM, Gladden JN. Emergency and critical care of small mammals. In: Quesenberry KE, Carpenter JW, eds. Ferrets, Rabbits and Rodents, 4th Ed). Clinical Medicine and Surgery. 2021 ed. St. Louis: Saunders, 2020:595–608.
Pignon C, Mayer J. Zoonoses of ferrets, hedgehogs, and sugar gliders. Vet Clin North Am Exot Anim Pract 2011;14(3):533–549.
Author Nicholas Jew, DVM

DYSURIA AND HEMATURIA

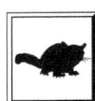

BASICS

DEFINITION
- Dysuria—difficult or painful urination
- Pollakiuria—voiding small quantity of urine with increased frequency
- Hematuria—the presence of blood in urine. It is important to differentiate true hematuria from blood originating from the reproductive tract in females.

PATHOPHYSIOLOGY
- Dysuria and pollakiuria are caused by lesions of the urinary bladder and/or urethra as well as outflow obstruction and provide evidence of lower urinary tract disease; these clinical signs do not exclude concurrent involvement of the upper urinary tract or disorders of other body system.
- Hematuria occurs secondary to loss of the endothelial integrity in the urinary tract. Clotting factor deficiency or thrombocytopenia possible but not commonly reported. Must distinguish from blood originating from the reproductive tract in females.

SYSTEMS AFFECTED
Renal/Urologic—bladder, urethra

GENETICS
N/A

INCIDENCE/PREVALENCE
Common

GEOGRAPHIC DISTRIBUTION
World wide

SIGNALMENT
Breed Predilections
N/A

Mean Age and Range
N/A

Predominant Sex
N/A

SIGNS
Historical Findings
- Hematuria
- Thick white- or tan-appearing urine
- Urine staining in the perineum
- Anorexia, weight loss, lethargy, tooth grinding, tenesmus, and hunched posture in animal with chronic or obstructive lower urinary tract disease

Physical Examination Findings
- May be normal
- Abdominal palpation may induce pain, especially when the bladder is palpated.
- A large urinary bladder may be palpable in patients with partial or complete urethral obstruction.

- Manual expression of the bladder may reveal thick, beige- to brown-colored urine even in animals that have normal-appearing voided urine.

CAUSES
Urinary Bladder
- Urinary tract infection—bacterial
- Urolithiasis, crystals (calcium carbonate, calcium oxalate, and magnesium ammonium phosphate)
- Neoplasia
- Trauma

Urethra
- Cloacal and paracloacal gland disease—most common cause
- Urinary tract infection
- Urethrolithiasis
- Trauma—especially bite wounds
- Neoplasia

RISK FACTORS
- Mural or extramural diseases that compress the bladder or urethral lumen. The most common cause is compression of the urethra by enlargement of the paracloaca glands
- Feeding diet preparations with a low calcium-to-phosphorus ratio may predispose to cystic calculi.
- Obese, sedentary animals
- Diseases or diagnostic procedures that alter normal host of urinary tract defenses and predispose to infection, formation of uroliths, or damage the urothelium or other tissues of the urinary tract

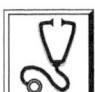

DIAGNOSIS

DIFFERENTIAL DIAGNOSIS
Differentiate from other abnormal patterns of micturition:
- Rule out polyuria—frequency and volume of urine
- Rule out urethral obstruction—stranguria, anuria, overdistended urinary bladder, and signs of postrenal uremia
  Differentiate cause of dysuria and hematuria:
- Rule out paracloacal gland enlargement—careful palpation of the peri-cloacal region will demonstrate firm, round nodules on one of both lateral aspect of the cloaca
- Rule out urinary tract infection—hematuria, bacteriuria; painful, thickened bladder
- Rule out urolithiasis—hematuria, radiopaque bladder, nonproductive straining
- Rule out neoplasia—hematuria; ultrasound may differentiate
- Rule out neurogenic disorders—flaccid bladder wall; residual urine in bladder lumen after micturition; other neurologic

deficits to hind legs, tail perineum, and anal sphincter
- Rule out iatrogenic disorders—history of catheterization, reverse flushing, contrast radiography, or surgery
- Rule out uterine disease—females with uterine disease often strain and expel blood when urinating. Blood may mix with urine and be mistaken for hematuria.

CBC/BIOCHEMISTRY/URINALYSIS
- Results may be normal.
- Leukocytosis—may be seen with urinary tract infection
- Lower urinary tract disease complicated by urethral obstruction may be associated with azotemia.
- Patients with concurrent pyelonephritis may have impaired urine-concentrating capacity, leukocytosis, and azotemia.
- Disorders of the urinary bladder are best evaluated with a urine specimen collected by cystocentesis.
- Pyuria, hematuria, and proteinuria indicate urinary tract inflammation, but these are nonspecific findings that may result from infectious and noninfectious causes of lower urinary tract disease.
- Identification of bacteria in urine sediment suggests that urinary tract infection is causing or complicating lower urinary tract disease. Identification of neoplastic cells in urine sediment indicates urinary tract neoplasia.
- Crystals in the urine sediment: ammonium magnesium phosphate, mixed carbonate and oxalate, and mixed carbonate, phosphate, magnesium, and calcium may be found

OTHER LABORATORY TESTS
Quantitative urine culture—the most definitive means of identifying and characterizing bacterial urinary tract infection; negative urine culture results suggest a noninfectious cause. Administration of antibiotics prior to urine culture may confound the meaning of a negative urine culture.

IMAGING
Ultrasonography of the urinary tract and uterus, abdominal radiography, and contrast cystography are important means of identifying and localizing causes of dysuria and pollakiuria. With increasing access to computed tomography and magnetic resonance imaging, these modalities may play an increasing role in the diagnosis of lower urinary tract disease.

DIAGNOSTIC PROCEDURES
Cloacal endoscopy—due to the nonlinear anatomy and small luminal diameter of the urethra, cystoscopy is not an effective means of evaluating the bladder.

DYSURIA AND HEMATURIA   (CONTINUED)

PATHOLOGIC FINDINGS
Depends on the underlying cause

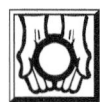

TREATMENT

APPROPRIATE HEALTH CARE
• Patients with nonobstructive lower urinary tract diseases are typically managed as outpatients; diagnostic evaluation may require brief hospitalization.
• Dysuria and pollakiuria associated with systemic signs of illness (e.g., pyrexia, depression, anorexia, and dehydration) or laboratory findings of azotemia or leukocytosis warrant aggressive diagnostic evaluation and initiation of supportive and symptomatic treatment.
• Treatment depends on the underlying cause and specific sites involved.

MEDICATIONS

DRUG(S) OF CHOICE
• Depend on the underlying cause
• If bacterial cystitis is demonstrated, begin treatment with broad-spectrum antibiotic such as trimethoprim-sulfa (10–20 mg/kg PO q12h), amoxicillin (30 mg/kg PO q12h), amoxicillin/clavulanic acid (12.5 mg/kg PO, SC divided q12h), or as a second line, enrofloxacin (2.5–5 mg/kg PO, SC, IM q12h), and chloramphenicol (50 mg/kg PO q12h). Modify antibacterial treatment based on result of urine culture and sensibility testing.
• Pain management may aid urination and promote appetite. NSAIDs (meloxicam 0.1–0.2 mg/kg PO, SC q24h) reduce pain and may decrease inflammation in the bladder.
• For sedation: Light sedation: Midazolam (0.2–0.5 mg/kg SC, IM, IV intranasal) ± butorphanol (0.5 mg/kg SC) or buprenorphine (0.01 mg/kg SC). Heavier sedation/mild anesthesia: Ketamine (10–20 mg/kg IM, IV) + midazolam (0.3–0.5 mg/kg SC, IM, IV); other protocols exist.

CONTRAINDICATIONS
• Glucocorticoids or other immunosuppressive agents
• Potentially nephrotoxic drugs (e.g., aminoglycosides, NSAIDs) in patients that are febrile, dehydrated, or azotemic or that

are suspected of having pyelonephritis, septicemia, or preexisting renal disease

NURSING CARE
For Paracloacal gland impaction:
• Gentle expression of contents from impaction. Sedation is required due to pain with expression. Often, thick yellow to ivory color discharge is expressible. This may require significant pressure in more severe cases.
• Gentle aseptic cleansing of the paracloacal region, particularly if any wounds are present.

CLIENT EDUCATION
• Regular monitoring of urinary and fecal eliminations is critical to avoid potential life-threatening complication of obstructive paracloacal gland disease.

SURGICAL CONSIDERATIONS
• If abscess or impaction of paracloacal glands recurs, consider surgical excision of paracloacal glands.
• If a paracloacal mass is present, surgery may be indicated to alleviate clinical signs and to obtain a definitive diagnosis which is imperative to determine prognosis.

PRECAUTIONS
• Enrofloxacin SC could cause skin necrosis, needs to be diluted 1:1 with SC fluids
• Cautious fluid therapy until patency of the urethra is established
• Urethra catheterization is not possibly anatomically due to the bend in the urethra prior to entering the urinary bladder. Attempts to advance beyond the urethra into the bladder may lead to iatrogenic trauma.

POSSIBLE INTERACTIONS
N/A

ALTERNATIVE DRUGS
N/A

FOLLOW-UP

PATIENT MONITORING
Response to treatment by clinical signs, serial physical examination, laboratory testing, and radiographic and ultrasonic evaluation appropriate for each specific cause

PREVENTION/AVOIDANCE
• Depends on the underlying cause
• Increase water consumption for the remainder of the animal's life
• Place patient on an appropriate diet
• Increase exercise
• Provide good hygiene

POSSIBLE COMPLICATIONS
N/A

EXPECTED COURSE AND PROGNOSIS
Good to guarded depending on the underlying cause

MISCELLANEOUS

ASSOCIATED CONDITIONS
• Paracloacal gland disorders
• Obesity
• Pyoderma (urine scald)

AGE-RELATED FACTORS
Uroliths, paracloacal gland disorders, and neoplasia are more common in middle-aged to older animals.

ZOONOTIC POTENTIAL
N/A

PREGNANCY/FERTILITY/BREEDING
N/A

SYNONYMS
N/A

SEE ALSO
Self-mutilation
Reproductive disorders

ABBREVIATIONS
NSAID = nonsteroidal anti-inflammatory drug

Suggested Reading
Brust D, Mans C. Sugar gliders. In: Carpenter JW, ed. Exotic Animal Formulary, 5th ed. St Louis: Elsevier, 2018:432–442.
Johnson-Delaney C. Sugar gliders. In: Quesenberry KE, Carpenter JW, eds. Ferrets, Rabbits and Rodents, 4th Ed). Clinical Medicine and Surgery. 2021 ed. St. Louis: Saunders, 2020:385–400.
Reavill D, Lennox A. Disease overview of the urinary tract in exotic companion mammals and tips on clinical management. Vet Clin North Am Exot Anim Pract. 2020;23(1):169–193.
Author Nicholas Jew, DVM

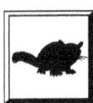

BASICS

DEFINITION
• Abnormal position of the globe
• Exophthalmos—anterior displacement of a normal globe
• Enophthalmos—posterior displacement of a normal globe
• Strabismus—deviation of the globe from a correct position of gaze; not readily corrected by the patient

PATHOPHYSIOLOGY
• Malposition of globe—caused by changes in volume (loss or gain) of the orbital contents or abnormal extraocular muscle function
• Exophthalmos—caused by space-occupying mass lesions posterior to the equator of the globe
• Enophthalmos—caused by reduced volume of orbital contents or by space-occupying mass lesions anterior to the equator of the globe
• Strabismus—caused by either muscular or neurological lesions affecting the tone or function of the extraocular muscles

SYSTEMS AFFECTED
• Ophthalmic
• Respiratory—due to proximity of orbit to nasal cavity, frontal and maxillary sinuses
• Gastrointestinal—proximity of oral cavity to ventral orbit—malocclusion and apical root abscess extension
• Auditory-proximity of inner and middle ear to caudal and medial aspects of orbit-otitis media/interna, aural abscess

GENETICS
N/A

INCIDENCE/PREVALENCE
Trauma occurs frequently due to protruding globes.
Exophthalmos or periorbital swelling are common secondary to dental disease.

GEOGRAPHIC DISTRIBUTION
N/A

SIGNALMENT

Predominant Sex
Males are more likely than females to experience conspecific trauma that can predispose to retrobulbar abscesses.

SIGNS

Historical Findings
• Sudden onset exophthalmos—trauma (e.g., orbital hemorrhage, proptosis)
• Chronic, progressive exophthalmos—neoplasia or tooth root abscess
• Apparent visual dysfunction—may be seen with microphthalmia and associated ocular anomalies
• Weight loss, difficulty in eating or in prehension, anorexia—dental disease

Physical Examination Findings

Exophthalmos
• Additional ocular signs (keratitis, conjunctivitis, and periocular swelling) can be primary or secondary to reduced tear production (KCS) associated with reactive lacrimal gland adenitis and hyperplasia.
• Dental disease—hypersalivation; bleeding from oral cavity; periocular swelling
• Facial abscess-periocular swelling may be present in the retrobulbar space, associated with auditory structures, or oral/dental disease.

Enophthalmos
• Ptosis
• Elevation of nictitans
• Extraocular muscle atrophy
• Entropion—with severe disease

Strabismus
• Deviation of globe from normal position—unilateral or bilateral
• May have associated enophthalmos or exophthalmos

Oral examination
• Specialized equipment is required—rodent dental speculum (Rodent mouth gag, Jorgensen Lab, Loveland, CO) and a set of buccal speculae (Cheek dilator, Jorgensen Labs); cotton swabs and tongue depressor to retract the tongue and examine lingual surfaces
• Heavy sedation or general anesthesia may be required.
• Tooth root abnormalities may be present in spite of normal-appearing crowns; skull radiographs may be necessary to identify apical root abnormalities if index of suspicion is high for dental involvement.

CAUSES

Exophthalmos
• Orbital hemorrhage—trauma to orbital structures
• Neoplasia of orbital structures
• Dental disease—orbital extension of dental disease
• Trauma-bite-induced retrobulbar abscess

Enophthalmos
• Ocular pain—retraction of globe
• Horner's syndrome
• Loss of orbital fat or muscle
• Severe weight loss or dehydration
• Neoplasia extending from rostral orbit displacing globe posteriorly

Strabismus
• Posttraumatic restriction of extraocular muscle motility by scar tissue
• Avulsion of extraocular muscle attachment following globe proptosis

RISK FACTORS
• Head trauma, excessive restraint—proptosis; strabismus
• Dental disease—caries of molars can predispose to tooth root abscesses; can be due to inappropriate physical form and composition of diet (e.g., fruit and grain treats bound together by chocolate, honey, or molasses are readily consumed but should be minimized)
• Inappropriate social groups-competition between males may lead to facial wounds, predominantly bite wounds and less often excoriation

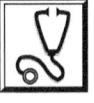

DIAGNOSIS

DIFFERENTIAL DIAGNOSIS

Exophthalmos
• Conformational—prominence of the globe is a normal feature—evaluate bilateral symmetry; observe grossly from a position above the head of the patient
• Buphthalmos—enlargement of the globe due to intraocular disease (i.e., glaucoma)—uncommon in small mammals; most often associated with lesions in the anterior uvea that are either congenital or secondary to inflammatory disease
• Traumatic proptosis—acute onset related to trauma to head/periocular area—eyelids typically entrapped behind globe; can occur with overzealous restraint

Enophthalmos
• Perforated/collapsed globe—acute trauma, perforation of corneal descemetocele
• Phthisis bulbi—acquired shrinkage of the globe, usually secondary to trauma and/or chronic inflammation
• Microphthalmos—congenitally smaller than normal globe, which can include other anatomical abnormalities—may be blind or vision impaired
• Anophthalmos—congenital absence of globe—rare, reported in other small mammals

Strabismus
• Microphthalmos
• Phthisis bulbi

CBC/BIOCHEMISTRY/URINALYSIS
Usually normal; WBC count may be elevated with orbital abscesses

OTHER LABORATRY TESTS
N/A

SUGAR GLIDERS

IMAGING
• Orbital ultrasound—localize and characterize space-occupying mass lesions; guide aspirate or biopsy diagnostic procedures
• Skull radiographs—orbital and dental assessment
• CT—evaluate extent of orbital disease and determine involvement of other cavities (nasal, oral)

DIAGNOSTIC PROCEDURES
• Resistance to globe retropulsion—confirms space-occupying mass
• Tonometry—rule out glaucoma; rebound tonometer best suited to small eyes of rodent and provides accurate assessment of IOP (reported mean 10–15 mmHg)
• Oral examination, skull radiographs, and fine-needle aspiration or biopsy of space-occupying mass lesion in orbit—perform after anesthetizing patient
• Fine-needle aspiration (use 20–22 gauge needle)—if retrobulbar mass is accessible; submit samples for aerobic, anaerobic, and fungal cultures; gram's staining; and cytological evaluation
• Cytology—often diagnostic for abscess and neoplasia
• Biopsy—indicated if needle aspiration is nondiagnostic and mass lesion is accessible
• Forced duction test with strabismus—grasp conjunctiva with a pair of fine forceps following topical anesthesia; differentiates neurological disease (in which the globe moves freely) from restrictive muscle condition (in which the globe cannot be moved manually)

PATHOLOGIC FINDINGS
• Neoplasia—characteristic features of malignancy (anisocytosis, anisokaryosis, and increase in mitotic figures)
• Cellulitis, abscess—inflammatory cells, intracellular bacteria

TREATMENT
APPROPRIATE HEALTH CARE
• Orbital neoplasm—consultation with an oncologist once a diagnosis is made; most are primary and malignant
• Proptosis—temporary tarsorrhaphy indicated to avoid exposure keratitis until retro-orbital swelling subsides, and anti-inflammatory therapy. Enucleation may be indicated if the globe no longer viable or presentation for treatment was delayed.
• Retrobulbar abscess—aggressive surgical debridement of orbital abscess and related affected tissues (dentition, maxilla) followed by long-term local and systemic antibiotic

treatment; limited (palliative) response to antibiotic treatment alone
• Enophthalmos—depends on cause
• Strabismus—muscle reattachment difficult

NURSING CARE
• Exophthalmos—lubrication of exposed cornea while diagnostics and treatment are carried out
• Supportive care in debilitated or anorectic patients; assisted feeding; subcutaneous or intravenous fluid therapy
• Inflammatory conditions—warm compressing of periocular tissues q6h—encourages blood flow to area—helps decrease swelling and cleans discharges

ACTIVITY
N/A

DIET
Minimize changes in diet during treatment and recovery; may require syringe feeding if anorectic or during the perioperative period

CLIENT EDUCATION
Education on an appropriate diet to avoid recurrent dental disease.

SURGICAL CONSIDERATIONS
• Enucleation/exenteration—careful dissection and evaluation during surgery is paramount to avoid excessive hemorrhage.
• Use anticholinergic treatment preoperatively to avoid vagus-induced bradyarrhythmia associated with globe manipulation: atropine 0.01–0.02 mg/kg SC, IM; glycopyrrolate 0.01–0.02 mg/kg SC, IM

MEDICATIONS
DRUG(S) OF CHOICE
• Exophthalmos—lubricate exposed cornea to prevent desiccation and ulceration (e.g., artificial tear ointment or gel)
• Corneal ulceration—topical antibiotic (e.g., neomycin-polymyxin-bacitracin, ciprofloxacin, or ofloxacin q6–8h) and cycloplegic (e.g., atropine 1% q12–24h) to prevent infection and reduce ciliary spasm, respectively
• Antibiotics—broad-spectrum pending results of culture and susceptibility testing; enrofloxacin (2.5–5 mg/kg PO, SC, IM q12h); trimethoprim-sulfa (10–20 mg/kg PO, SC q12h); amoxicillin/clavulanic acid (12.5 mg/kg PO, SC divided q12h) are safe choices
• Anti-inflammatory therapy—systemic NSAID, e.g., meloxicam (0.1–0.2 mg/kg PO, SC, IM q24h)
• Pain management—buprenorphine (0.01–0.03 mg/kg PO, SQ, IM q8–12h)

• For sedation: Light sedation: Midazolam (0.2–0.5 mg/kg SC, IM, IV intranasal) ± butorphanol (0.5 mg/kg SC) or buprenorphine (0.01 mg/kg SC). Heavier sedation/mild anesthesia: Ketamine (10–20 mg/kg IM, IV) + midazolam (0.3–0.5 mg/kg SC, IM, IV); other protocols exist.

CONTRAINDICATIONS
• Avoid steroid-containing ophthalmic preparations—in case of corneal ulceration

PRECAUTIONS
N/A

POSSIBLE INTERACTIONS
N/A

ALTERNATIVE DRUGS
N/A

FOLLOW-UP
PATIENT MONITORING
Dental abscess—evaluate the entire oral cavity and skull at each recheck and repeat skull radiographs at 3–6-month intervals to monitor for recurrence at the surgical site or other locations

PREVENTION/AVOIDANCE
• Close monitoring of social dynamics when introducing new members or juveniles reach sexual maturity. This is particularly important when multiple males are present.
• Proptosis—avoid excessive restraint

POSSIBLE COMPLICATIONS
• Permanent lacrimal gland damage with atrophy and KCS
• Keratitis, corneal ulceration, and corneal perforation
• Vision loss
• Loss of globe
• Permanent malposition of globe
• Death

EXPECTED COURSE AND PROGNOSIS
• Orbital neoplasia—fair to poor depending on tumor type, extent of involvement at presentation, and response to therapy
• Retrobulbar tooth root abscess—depends on severity of bone involvement, underlying disease, condition of the teeth, and presence of other abscesses. Fair to guarded with single isolated retrobulbar abscess, adequate surgical debridement, and medical treatment. Abscesses in the nasal passages or with multiple or severe maxillary abscesses have a guarded to poor prognosis—euthanasia may be warranted

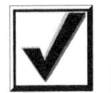 **MISCELLANEOUS**

ASSOCIATED CONDITIONS
N/A

AGE-RELATED FACTORS
N/A

ZOONOTIC POTENTIAL
N/A

PREGNANCY/FERTILITY/BREEDING
Avoid fluroquinolones in pregnancy.

SYNONYMS
N/A

SEE ALSO
Conjunctivitis
Dental disease

ABBREVIATIONS
CT = computed tomography
GI = gastrointestinal
IOP = intraocular pressure
KCS = keratoconjunctivitis sicca
WBC = white blood cell

Suggested Reading
Brust D, Mans C. Sugar gliders. In: Carpenter JW, ed. Exotic Animal Formulary, 5th ed. St Louis: Elsevier, 2018:432–442.
Fraess GA, Sadar MJ, Daniels JB, Sharkey L, Henriksen MDL. Clinical ophthalmological diagnostic description of 10 healthy sugar gliders (*Petaurus breviceps*) and prevalence of ocular-related presentations in a larger hospital population. Vet Ophthalmol. 2021;24:80–92.
Johnson-Delaney C. Sugar gliders. In: Quesenberry KE, Carpenter JW, eds. Ferrets, Rabbits and Rodents, 4th Ed). Clinical Medicine and Surgery. 2021 ed. St. Louis: Saunders, 2020:385–400.
Author Nicholas Jew, DVM

FEMALE REPRODUCTIVE DISORDERS

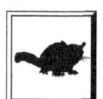

BASICS

DEFINITION
• Origins may include infectious, inflammatory, traumatic, and neoplastic
• The female reproductive tract is smaller than that of placental mammals. There are paired uterine bodies that form two lateral and a central vaginal canal. Unlike other marsupials, sugar gliders lack marsupial bones.

PATHOPHYSIOLOGY
• Disorders of the endometrium can result in mild vaginal discharge to uterine hemorrhage.
• The secretions of the endometrium provide an excellent media for bacterial growth.
• The anatomy of the cloaca provides additional route of ascending infection from the urinary and digestive systems.
• The location of the mammary glands within the pouch provides an opportunity for pouch infection to be primary as well as secondary to mastitis.
• Infertility in females may arise as a result of obesity, inappropriate social situation, and underlying medical conditions. There may be a genetic link to infertility, predominantly in males, in mosaic color mutations.

SYSTEMS AFFECTED
Reproductive

GENETICS
Mosaic color mutations may be more likely to suffer from infertility.

INCIDENCE/PREVALENCE
N/A

GEOGRAPHIC DISTRIBUTION
Worldwide

SIGNALMENT
Predominant Sex
Infertility associated with mosaic color mutations is more commonly reported in male sugar gliders.

SIGNS
Historical Findings
• Lethargy
• Anorexia
• Hematuria
• Cloacal discharge
• Lack of successful breeding
• Masses, subcutaneous, or abdominal
• Self-mutilation
• Premature eviction of joey from pouch
• Death or failure to thrive of joey

Physical Examination Findings
• May be normal
• Abdominal palpation may be painful and/or reveal the presence of a mass. Mammary masses

are located within the pouch and are commonly found concurrently with a uterine mass
• Careful evaluation of the cloaca and pouch may allow for visualization of discharge either directly as a liquid or as crusting around the opening.
• Joeys that have been evicted may have an exudate on their fur, and commonly they are dehydrated.

CAUSES
Pouch
• Bacterial infection—*Pseudomonas aeruginosa*
• Yeast infection
• Neoplasia

Mammary
• Infectious (mastitis)
• Neoplasia—adenocarcinoma and carcinoma reported. Primary mammary neoplasia is often found concurrently with uterine neoplasia (anecdotal per the author)

Vaginal
• Bacterial infection, often ascending from the cloaca—*Staphylococcus aureus, Streptococcus* sp., *Escherichia coli*, and *Proteus* sp., have all been reported.
• Trauma—secondary to breeding or self-mutilation
• Neoplasia—squamous cell carcinoma reported.

Uterine
• Bacterial infection, often ascending from the cloaca—*Staphylococcus aureus, Streptococcus* sp., *Escherichia coli*, and *Proteus* sp., have all been reported.
• Neoplasia

Misc
• Failure-to-thrive—pouch trauma, infection, mastitis, and dislodgement from the nipple.
• Pouch eviction—etiology varies from accidental expulsion during grooming to infectious or neoplastic conditions. The presence of joeys of differing ages may increase the likelihood of eviction of the younger by the older. Underlying pouch pathology should be thoroughly evaluated.
• Genetic—mosaic color mutations may have an increased risk of infertility.
• "Sticky Joey Syndrome"—*Simplicomonas and Simplicimonas.*

RISK FACTORS
• Obese, sedentary animals
• Reduced grooming ability secondary to other disease.
• Diarrhea and/or urinary tract infection.
• Older sugar gliders at increased risk for neoplastic conditions affecting the reproductive system.
• Inappropriate social grouping may lead to infertility.

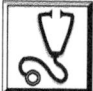

DIAGNOSIS

DIFFERENTIAL DIAGNOSIS
Pouch
• Bacterial infection—*Pseudomonas aeruginosa*
• Yeast infection
• Neoplasia

Mammary
• Infectious (mastitis)
• Neoplasia—adenocarcinoma and carcinoma reported. Primary mammary neoplasia is often found concurrently with uterine neoplasia (anecdotal per the author)

Uterine/Vaginal
• Bacterial infection, often ascending from the cloaca—*Staphylococcus aureus, Streptococcus* sp., *Escherichia coli*, and *Proteus* sp., have all been reported.
• Trauma—secondary to breeding or self-mutilation
• Neoplasia—squamous cell carcinoma report

Infertility
• Genetic—mosaic color mutations may have an increased risk of infertility.
• Obesity
• Inappropriate social groupings
• Physical alterations leading to difficulty with breeding, particularly from self-mutilation.

CBC/BIOCHEMISTRY/URINALYSIS
• Results may be normal.
• Leukocytosis—may be seen with infectious or neoplastic causes
• Anemia, regenerative, or nonregenerative, may be present in the case of uterine hemorrhage.
• Azotemia may be present with dehydration.
• Sepsis may result in elevated BUN, ALT, and GGT.
• Metabolic acidosis may be present with hyperkalemia, hyponatremia, and hypochloremia.
• Urinalysis collected via cystocentesis lacking hematuria indicates that hemorrhage is more likely to be from reproductive tract.

OTHER LABORATORY TESTS
• Cytologic evaluation of discharge from the pouch and vaginal discharge maybe indicative of an infectious or neoplastic etiology. Cytologic findings consistent with infectious etiologies does not rule out neoplasia.
• Culture of fluid or discharge from reproductive tract or pouch should be used to direct antimicrobial therapy.
• Histopathology of any reproductive tissue excised to provide definitive diagnosis, particularly in the case of neoplasia.

IMAGING
• Abdominal radiography may reveal a mass effect in the caudal abdomen. Abdominal effusion may also be present in both infectious and neoplastic causes. Pouch masses may be differentiated from an in-pouch joey via direct visualization or radiographic evaluation.
• Thoracic radiography is always recommended to evaluate for potential metastatic disease where neoplasia is suspected.
• Ultrasonography is often better able to differentiate changes in the reproductive and urinary tract. Obtaining diagnostic images likely requires sedation unless the sugar glider is significantly lethargic.
• Advanced imaging (CT and MRI)—as the access to these imaging modalities become more widely available, CT and MRI are likely to provide a significant improvement in the antemortem and presurgical detection of reproductive tract disease. Sedation or anesthesia is often required for advanced imaging studies.

DIAGNOSTIC PROCEDURES
• Ultrasound guided aspiration—differentiation of uterine hemorrhage from hematuria (cystocentesis), sample collection from prostate
• Fine-needle aspirate—evaluation of mammary and pouch masses

PATHOLOGIC FINDINGS
Depends on the underlying cause

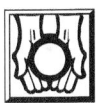

TREATMENT

APPROPRIATE HEALTH CARE
• Diagnostic evaluation may require sedation or general anesthesia.
• Systemic signs of illness (e.g., pyrexia, depression, anorexia, and dehydration) or laboratory findings of anemia, azotemia, or leukocytosis warrant aggressive diagnostic evaluation and initiation of supportive and symptomatic treatment.
• Treatment depends on the underlying cause and specific sites involved.
• For reproductive tract neoplasia or infection, surgical excision may be warranted. In some cases, exploratory surgery acts as both diagnostic evaluation and the initial treatment.

NURSING CARE
• Fluid therapy—rehydration and correction of electrolyte imbalances are essential to treatment success in severely ill sugar gliders.
• Blood transfusion may be required for female sugar gliders with significant uterine hemorrhage.

• Appropriate fluid resuscitation and supplemental nutrition for those sugar gliders that are failing to thrive or have been evicted from the pouch.
• Attempt to replace evicted and displaced joeys under direct supervision.

CLIENT EDUCATION
• Uterine disorders often require ovariohysterectomy.
• Medical treatment for pyometra is not recommended even in cases where discharge is draining from the cloaca.
• Infertility can be challenging to diagnose definitively. Often, infertility is diagnosed based on historical reports of failed breeding.
• In cases of mammary neoplasia, thorough evaluation for uterine neoplasia should always be performed as they commonly occur concurrently.
• Ensuring appropriate husbandry and social grouping are critical to the treatment of failure-to-thrive joeys.

SURGICAL CONSIDERATIONS
• Ovariohysterectomy or ovario-vaginal-hysterectomy is the preferred treatment for all uterine disorders. During surgery, identification of the ureters may be difficult, particularly in obese sugar gliders. If the ureters cannot be isolated, the central and lateral vaginal canals are not removed to avoid inadvertent ureteral trauma during surgery.
• A ventral midline laparotomy incision is made through the inner wall of the pouch.
• Enlarged uterus may be friable and easily rupture. Adhesions may be present. Should uterine rupture or leakage occur, repeated lavage of peritoneal cavity with sterile saline is indicated.
• Thorough evaluation of the abdominal organs when uterine neoplasia is identified should be performed to identify metastatic lesions.

MEDICATIONS

DRUG(S) OF CHOICE
• Depend on the underlying cause
• Postoperative analgesia—meloxicam (0.1–0.2 mg/kg PO, SC q24h, avoid if azotemia present) and buprenorphine (0.02–0.05 mg/kg PO, SC, IM q12h).
• Antimicrobial therapy—indicated in sugar gliders with infectious etiologies. Selection of antimicrobial therapy should d be broad-spectrum and based on the result of culture and sensitivity when possible
• Amoxicillin/Clavulanic acid (12.5 mg/kg PO, SC q12h), ciprofloxacin (10 mg/kg PO q12h), enrofloxacin (2.5–5 mg/kg PO, IM

q12–24h), and chloramphenicol (50 mg/kg PO q12h)
• For sedation: Light sedation: Midazolam (0.2–0.5 mg/kg SC, IM, IV intranasal) ± butorphanol (0.5 mg/kg SC) or buprenorphine (0.01 mg/kg SC). Heavier sedation/mild anesthesia: ketamine (10–20 mg/kg IM, IV) + midazolam (0.3–0.5 mg/kg SC, IM, IV); other protocols exist.

CONTRAINDICATIONS
• Glucocorticoids or other immunosuppressive agents
• Potentially nephrotoxic drugs (e.g., aminoglycosides, NSAIDs) in patients that are febrile, dehydrated, or azotemic or that are suspected of having pyelonephritis, septicemia, or preexisting renal disease.

PRECAUTIONS
• Enrofloxacin SC could cause skin necrosis, needs to be diluted 1:1 with SC fluids
• Antibiotic therapy can predispose sugar gliders to bacterial dysbiosis and overgrowth pathogenic bacteria (particularly *Clostridium difficile*). If signs worsen or do not improve, therapy should be adjusted.
• Chloramphenicol may cause aplastic anemia in susceptible people. Clients and staff should use appropriate precautions when handling this drug.

POSSIBLE INTERACTIONS
N/A

ALTERNATIVE DRUGS
N/A

FOLLOW-UP

PATIENT MONITORING
Response to treatment by clinical signs, serial physical examination, laboratory testing, radiographic, and ultrasonic evaluation appropriate for each specific cause

PREVENTION/AVOIDANCE
• Depends on the underlying cause
• Prophylactic ovariohysterectomy or ovario-vaginal-hysterectomy are not commonly performed in sugar gliders.
• Prophylactic castration to both prevent unwanted pregnancy and prostatitis is recommended.

POSSIBLE COMPLICATIONS
Sepsis
Metastatic neoplasia
Paraneoplastic syndrome
Postoperative hemorrhage

EXPECTED COURSE AND PROGNOSIS
Poor to guarded depending on the underlying cause

SUGAR GLIDERS

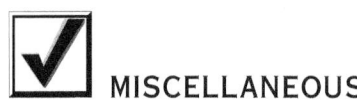

MISCELLANEOUS

ASSOCIATED CONDITIONS
- Obesity
- Diarrhea

AGE-RELATED FACTORS
Neoplasia is more common in older sugar gliders.

ZOONOTIC POTENTIAL
N/A

PREGNANCY/FERTILITY/BREEDING
N/A

SYNONYMS
"Sticky Joey Syndrome"—clinical signs include diarrhea, dehydration, anorexia, and death. Adults may be asymptomatic while joeys typically have wet and "sticky" fur that appears poorly groomed. This disease syndrome is described colloquially as "ick."

Evaluation of the joey's stool typically reveals a trichmonad that has been identified as *Simplicomonas and Simplicimonas*. Joeys and adults in the environment should be treated concurrently.

SEE ALSO
Anorexia
Diarrhea
Dysuria and hematuria
Self-mutilation

ABBREVIATIONS
ALT = alanine transaminase
BUN = blood urea nitrogen
CT = computed tomography
GGT = gamma-glutamyl transferase
MRI = magnetic resonance imaging
NSAID = nonsteroidal anti-inflammatory drug

Suggested Reading
Brust D, Mans C. Sugar gliders. In: Carpenter JW, ed. Exotic Animal Formulary, 5th ed. St Louis: Elsevier, 2018:432–442.
Johnson-Delaney CA. Reproductive medicine of companion marsupials. Vet Clin North Am Exot Anim Pract 2002;5(3):537–553, vi.
Johnson-Delaney C. Sugar gliders. In: Quesenberry KE, Carpenter JW, eds. Ferrets, Rabbits and Rodents, 4th Ed). Clinical Medicine and Surgery. 2021 ed. St. Louis: Saunders, 2020:385–400.
Johnson-Delaney CA, Lennox AM. Reproductive disorders of marsupials. Vet Clin North Am Exot Anim Pract 2017;20(2):539–553.
Miwa Y, Sladky KK. Small mammals: common surgical procedures of rodents, ferrets, hedgehogs, and sugar gliders. Vet Clin North Am Exot Anim Pract 2016;19(1):205–244.
Author Nicholas Jew, DVM

NASAL DISCHARGE AND SNEEZING

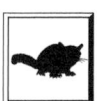

BASICS

DEFINITION
Inflammation of the nasal cavity and sinuses

PATHOPHYSIOLOGY
• May be acute or chronic, noninfectious, or infectious
• Often complicated by opportunistic secondary microbial invasion
• Associated mucosal vascular congestion, friability, and excessive mucus gland secretion lead to congestion, obstructed airflow, sneezing, epistaxis, nasal discharge, and epiphora

SYSTEMS AFFECTED
• Respiratory—mucosa of the upper respiratory tract, including the nasal cavities, sinuses, and nasopharynx
• Ophthalmic—extension to the eyes via the nasolacrimal duct
• Otic—extension of infection via the Eustachian tube to the middle/inner ear
• Musculoskeletal—osteomyelitis involving bones of the skull
• Neurologic—vestibular signs due to otitis media/interna

INCIDENCE/PREVALENCE
Common

SIGNALMENT
• Recently acquired sugar gliders may be overrepresented with upper respiratory signs.
• No specific sex or age predilection.

SIGNS
• Sneezing, nasal discharge, and epistaxis
• Epiphora, blepharospasm
• Increased respiratory sounds (stertor, "snoring")
• Increased respiratory rate and effort
• Otitis interna/media—head tilt, circling, and nystagmus with spread through the eustachian tube
• Auscultation findings variable and include increased to decreased or absent airway noise
• Patients may otherwise appear bright and alert to depressed.

CAUSES
• Primary infectious pathogens causing upper respiratory tract signs are rarely reported on in sugar gliders.
• Bacterial *Pasturella multocida, Streptococcus pneumoniae,* and *Klebsiella* spp.
• Parasitic—*Rilleyella petauri*
• Head trauma
• Odontogenic abscesses
• Nasal foreign body
• Neoplasia of the sinuses is rare.
• Irritants from dusty or dirty bedding often contribute to disease.

• Respiratory allergens reported anecdotally but not have been documented in sugar gliders

RISK FACTORS
• Poor husbandry, especially overcrowding and poor sanitation, increase risk for development of upper respiratory disease.
• Other sources of immune suppression may predispose to respiratory disease.

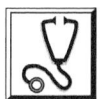

DIAGNOSIS

DIFFERENTIAL DIAGNOSIS
• Trauma—may be history or evidence of an injury
• Careful attention to breathing pattern and auscultation may help differentiate between upper and lower respiratory disease.

CBC/BIOCHEMISTRY/URINALYSIS
• Complete blood count may support but cannot confirm or rule out respiratory disease.
• Biochemistry panel is useful to identify predisposing underlying disease.

OTHER LABORATORY TESTS
• Culture and susceptibility testing for other bacterial pathogens is helpful in directing antibiotic therapy. However, patient size may preclude sample collection.
• DNA sequencing may aid in the identification of infectious pathogens (MiDOG All-in-One Microbial Test).

IMAGING
• Radiography of the skull can be helpful, but it is difficult to obtain diagnostic-quality images as patient size decreases.
• Computed tomography provides better resolution and diagnostic image quality compared to traditional radiographs.

DIAGNOSTIC PROCEDURES
• Response to antibiotic therapy as a trial
• Cytologic examination of nasal discharge has limited diagnostic utility.
• Patient size precludes procedures used in larger patients such as endoscopy or nasal mucosal biopsy.

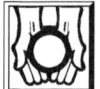

TREATMENT

APPROPRIATE HEALTH CARE
• Inpatient—severe debilitating disease or respiratory distress
• Discharge stable patients pending further diagnostic testing.

NURSING CARE
• Patients in respiratory distress require oxygen therapy.

• Supportive care, including correction of dehydration and hypovolemia, and assisted feeding
• Humidified air may help to moisten and clear nasal secretions.
• Keep the nares clean.

CLIENT EDUCATION
Quarantine from unaffected gliders should be discussed and monitoring for other gliders in the colony to display similar clinical signs.

SURGICAL CONSIDERATIONS
Surgical exploration and removal/debridement of any masses or abscesses may be indicated. Due to the size of patients, caution should be taken not to exacerbate upper airway occlusion further following surgical manipulation.

MEDICATIONS

DRUG(S) OF CHOICE

Antibiotics
• Antibiotic choice should be based on culture and sensitivity whenever possible.
• For other bacterial pathogens, initially, use broad-spectrum antibiotics such as enrofloxacin (2.5–5 mg/kg PO, SQ q12h, dilute for SQ injection), ciprofloxacin (10 mg/kg PO q12h), or trimethoprim-sulfa (10–20 mg/kg PO q12h), pending results of culture and susceptibility testing.

Nebulization
• Various protocols for nebulization exist but no data on clinical efficacy exists. A 2018 study showed that inhaled fluorescein delivered by nebulization was distributed to the lungs, suggesting this route may be useful in sugar gliders.
• For chronic use, owners may purchase nebulizers intended for human use and construct a nebulization chamber by drilling holes into small plastic storage containers, into which the glider can comfortably fit. A commercially manufactured nebulization chamber can also be purchased intended for dogs and cats.
• Sterile saline alone may be beneficial to moisten airways.
• Hypertonic saline solutions nebulized once to twice daily for 10–15 minutes may be helpful in breaking down mucus in the respiratory tract.
• Other commonly nebulized agents include amikacin (0.1–0.5 mL diluted in 5 mL of sterile saline); acetylcysteine, as a mucolytic (50 mg as a 2% solution diluted with saline), or aminophylline (3 mg/mL of sterile saline)

NASAL DISCHARGE AND SNEEZING

Anti-Inflammatory
• The addition of anti-inflammatory medication such as meloxicam (0.1–0.2 mg/kg PO, SC, IM q24h) may be helpful in patients nonresponsive to antibiotic therapy.
• In cases where inflammation does not respond to NSAIDs, a steroid may be considered—dexamethasone (0.1–0.6 mg/kg SC, IM q12–24h) and prednisolone (0.1–0.2 mg/kg PO, SQ q24h)

Sedation
• For sedation: Light sedation: Midazolam (0.2–0.5 mg/kg SC, IM, IV intranasal) ± butorphanol (0.5 mg/kg SC) or buprenorphine (0.01 mg/kg SC). Heavier sedation/mild anesthesia: ketamine (10–20 mg/kg IM, IV) + midazolam (0.3–0.5 mg/kg SC, IM, IV); other protocols exist.

CONTRAINDICATIONS
• Doxycycline is not recommended for very young or pregnant animals.
• Avoid the use of corticosteroids in conjunction with meloxicam or other NSAIDs.

PRECAUTIONS
• All therapeutic agents should be used with caution in debilitated, dehydrated patients. Ideally, vascular abnormalities (dehydration, hypotension) are addressed prior to initiating therapy.
• Do not use steroids in conjunction with NSAIDs.

POSSIBLE INTERACTIONS
N/A

ALTERNATIVE DRUGS
Maropitant (0.2 mg/kg PO, SQ q24h) may help to reduce upper airway inflammation (anecdotal evidence)

FOLLOW-UP
PATIENT MONITORING
Dyspneic patients are often reluctant to eat or drink. Patients should be monitored carefully to ensure adequate intake.

PREVENTION/AVOIDANCE
• Keep in a well-ventilated, clean environment. Clean bedding frequently to prevent the buildup of ammonia fumes.
• Provide a high-quality diet.
• Avoid contact with other sugar gliders exhibiting signs of respiratory tract disease.

POSSIBLE COMPLICATIONS
• Chronic inflammation may cause permanent damage to nasal turbinates and progress to chronic pulmonary disease, which significantly lowers prognosis for recovery.
• Patients with chronic disease may not fully respond to therapy, and recurrence is common.

MISCELLANEOUS
ASSOCIATED CONDITIONS
Acute respiratory distress
Dental disease
Pneumonia

ZOONOTIC POTENTIAL
N/A

PREGNANCY/FERTILITY/BREEDING
Avoid tetracycline in very young or pregnant animals.

SYNONYMS
N/A

SEE ALSO
Conjunctivitis
Dental disease
Exophthalmos and orbital diseases

ABBREVIATIONS
NSAID = non-steroidal anti-inflammatory

Suggested Reading
Fraess GA, Sadar MJ, Daniels JB, Sharkey LC, Henriksen MD. Clinical ophthalmological diagnostic description of 10 healthy sugar gliders (*Petaurus breviceps*) and prevalence of ocular-related presentations in a larger hospital population. Vet Ophthalmol 2021;24(1):80–92.
Johnson DH. Hedgehogs and sugar gliders: respiratory anatomy, physiology, and disease. Vet Clin Exot Anim Pract 2011;14(2):267–285.
Johnson-Delaney C. Sugar gliders. In: Quesenberry KE, Carpenter JW, eds. Ferrets, Rabbits and Rodents, 4th Ed). Clinical Medicine and Surgery. 2021 ed. St. Louis: Saunders, 2020:385–400.
McLaughlin A, Strunk A. Common emergencies in small rodents, hedgehogs, and sugar gliders. Vet Clin Exot Anim Pract 2016;19(2):465–499.
Spratt DM. Rileyella petauri gen. nov., sp. nov. (*Pentastomida: Cephalobaenida*) from the lungs and nasal sinus of Petaurus breviceps (*Marsupialia: Petauridae*) in Australia. Parasite 2003;10(3):235–241. doi: 10.1051/parasite/2003103235.
Author Nicholas Jew, DVM

NUTRITIONAL OSTEODYSTROPHY

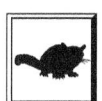

BASICS

DEFINITION
• Also known as nutritional secondary hyperparathyroidism or metabolic bone disease.
• Chronic calcium deficiency leading to overproduction of parathyroid hormone which stimulates osteoclastic activity, weakens bone, and ultimately death if untreated.

PATHOPHYSIOLOGY
• Inappropriate diet will lead to imbalance of calcium, vitamin D, and phosphorous.
• Hypocalcemia may lead to osteoporosis, pathologic fractures, seizures, and paresis/paralysis.
• Sugar gliders are omnivores with seasonal dietary variations. To date, there are no commercially manufactured diets that are comparable to the diet consumed in the wild. During the spring and summer, more animal protein is typically consumed in the form of invertebrates. The remainder of their natural diet consists of sap, gum, nectar, manna, and honeydew.
• Diets high in fat and protein may lead to obesity.
• Soft diets high in carbohydrates increase the risk for periodontal disease and dental calculus.

SYSTEMS AFFECTED
The consequences of nutritional osteodystrophy affect many systems:
• Cardiac
• Gastrointestinal
• Musculoskeletal
• Neurologic
• Renal
• Hepatic

GENETICS
N/A

INCIDENCE/PREVALENCE
N/A

GEOGRAPHIC DISTRIBUTION
N/A

SIGNALMENT
Any age or sex

SIGNS

Historical Findings
• Weakness, lethargy
• Acute collapse
• Seizures
• Hind limb paresis/paralysis

Physical Examination Findings
• Physical examination findings vary widely depending on the severity of disease.

• Weight alteration (if previously measured and recorded)
• Obesity or thin body condition
• Weakness and lethargy
• Seizures
• Hind limb paresis or paralysis
• Dehydration
• Pale mucous membranes
• Long bone fractures
• Periodontal disease
• Corneal opacities or cataracts

CAUSES

Dietary
Chronic use of nutritionally inappropriate diets.

RISK FACTORS
• Excess lean meat, insects, and fruit.
• Lack of appropriate dietary supplementation.
• Diets high in fat.
• Feeding inappropriate dietary items such as processed human foods.

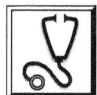

DIAGNOSIS

DIFFERENTIAL DIAGNOSIS
• Pathologic fractures—trauma
• Hind limb paresis/paralysis—hind limb or pelvic fracture, spinal cord disease (degenerative, neoplastic, vascular, and inflammatory)
• Seizures
  ◦ Cranial trauma
  ◦ Parasitic CNS disease—toxoplasmosis, *Baylisascaris*
  ◦ Fungal disease
  ◦ Bacterial meningitis
  ◦ Intoxication—lead
  ◦ Neoplasia
• Corneal opacities
  ◦ Ulceration and edema
  ◦ Scar from prior trauma
• Cataracts
  ◦ Hypovitaminosis A
  ◦ Maternal pouch infection

CBC/BIOCHEMISTRY/URINALYSIS
• Anemia may result from inadequate protein intake and anorexia.
• Biochemical profile and ionized calcium are often helpful in obtaining a definitive diagnosis—hypoproteinemia, hypocalcemia, and hypoglycemia.
• Blood collection may require anesthesia; if the patient is cachexic the risks should be discussed with the owner, and blood collection may have to wait until the patient is more stable.

OTHER LABORATORY TESTS
• Fecal direct and float
• If diarrhea is present, a fecal evaluation may help to direct therapy.

IMAGING
• Full-body radiographs of the sugar glider patient can help to identify masses (chest or abdominal), dental disease, heart disease, and skeletal disease that may aid in diagnosis. Radiographs often reveal thickened bones, long bone fractures, and abnormal cortical bone calcification.
• Advanced imaging (e.g., CT and MRI) may be useful for evaluation of neurologic signs. General anesthesia or heavy sedation may be required. Increasing access to these imaging modalities and improved image resolution for small patients may make CT of greater diagnostic value compared to traditional radiographs.

DIAGNOSTIC PROCEDURES
• Vary depending on initial diagnostic findings.
• A good oral exam under general anesthesia is often necessary for identifying periodontal disease, dental caries, and dental calculus.

PATHOLOGIC FINDINGS
N/A

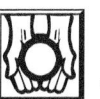

TREATMENT

APPROPRIATE HEALTH CARE
• In weak and debilitated patients, hospitalization and placement of an IV or IO catheter are often indicated; sedation or anesthesia may be necessary for placement
• Correct hypoglycemia and hypocalcemia if present.

NURSING CARE
• It is imperative that the animal receive nutritional support if it is not eating. Supplementation with a liquid diet may be required, such as Oxbow Omnivore Care (Oxbow Enterprises, Inc., Murdock, NE) or Emeraid Intensive Care Omnivore (Lafeber's, Cornell, IL). If these commercial formulas are not available, a gruel may be made with 75% pellet (sugar glider, insectivore, or carnivore) with 25% fresh fruits and vegetables, vitamin, and calcium supplement.
• Ensure that the patient is kept warm (if hypothermic, an incubator may be required).
• Fluid therapy is used to correct hydration following standard protocols (5%–10% of body weight administered in SQ boluses). Fluids should be kept warm to prevent hypothermia and can be warmed by placing

SUGAR GLIDERS

the prepared syringe in hot water for a few minutes prior to administering them. Using a 22–25-gauge butterfly needle to administer the fluids can reduce stress on the patient by minimizing restraint.
• The critical patient may require an intraosseous catheter. If hypoproteinemic, administer hetastarch at 10 mL/kg per day in addition to maintenance fluids.

ACTIVITY
In the presence of debilitation, weakness, and orthopedic compromise, exercise restriction is recommended to avoid additional trauma. Limit access to single-level enclosures without tall cage furniture.

DIET
A diet change should never be made abruptly in the anorexic patient. When the patient is stable, changing to an appropriate diet should be recommended.
  Example diet 1
• 75% commercial sugar glider pelleted diet
• 25% fresh fruits and vegetables
• Vitamin and calcium supplement
• Shall quantities of live insects
  Example diet 2
• 50% commercial insectivore or carnivore diet
• 50% Leadbeater's mixture—150 mL water, 150 mL honey, 1 shelled hard-boiled egg, 25 g high-protein baby cereal, 1 teaspoon vitamin, and mineral powder
• <5% gut-loaded insects

CLIENT EDUCATION
• Education on appropriate diet is essential to treatment and prevention.
• The author recommends a wellness examination every 6 months.

SURGICAL CONSIDERATIONS
• Healing of pathologic fractures may be complicated and delayed due to inappropriate calcium metabolism early in the course of disease.
• Placement of implants for orthopedic surgery may have an increased risk of iatrogenic trauma due to poor bone quality and abnormal cortical mineralization.

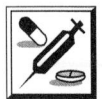

MEDICATIONS
DRUG(S) OF CHOICE
Analgesia/Sedation
• Meloxicam (0.1–0.2 mg/kg PO, SC q24h)
• Buprenorphine (0.02–0.05 mg/kg PO, SC, IM q8–12h)
• For sedation: Light sedation: Midazolam (0.2–0.5 mg/kg SC, IM, IV intranasal) ± butorphanol (0.5 mg/kg SC) or buprenorphine (0.01 mg/kg SC). Heavier sedation/mild anesthesia: Ketamine (10–

20 mg/kg IM, IV) + midazolam (0.3–0.5 mg/kg SC, IM, IV); other protocols exist.

Correction of Hypocalcemia:
• Calcium glubionate (150 mg/kg PO q24h)—this formulation may no longer be available commercially
• Calcium gluconate (100 mg/kg SC q12h, dilute in saline to 10 mg/mL), initial doses may be given IV or IO in the face of seizures and/or severe debilitation—administer slowly and monitor for bradycardia
• Calcitonin (50–100 IU/kg SC) is recommended for severely affected animals when blood calcium levels are within the normal range and with concurrent oral calcium supplementation to decrease resorption of calcium from bone.

Control of Seizures
• Midazolam 0.5–1 mg/kg IN, SC, IM

As an Appetite Stimulant
• Vitamin B complex 0.01–0.02 mL/kg SQ, dilution reduces pain associated with injection.

For Secondary Bacterial Infection
• Enrofloxacin 5 mg/kg PO, SC diluted in fluid pocket q12h
• Ciprofloxacin 10 mg/kg PO q12h
• Amoxicillin/clavulanic acid 12.5 mg/kg PO, SC divided q12h

CONTRAINDICATIONS
N/A

PRECAUTIONS
• Almost all drugs dispensed to the sugar gliders are considered off-label, and doses have been extrapolated.
• Be especially careful of compounding drugs in-house; may achieve more favorable results using a compounding pharmacy or a liquid form of the drug.
• Avoid excess vitamin D_3 supplementation.
• The calcium to phosphorous ratio should be 2:1 or greater.

POSSIBLE INTERACTIONS
N/A

ALTERNATIVE DRUGS
The use of commercially available vitamin and mineral supplements intended for sugar gliders may aid in the prevention of nutritional osteopathy. Do not supplement with extra vitamins, particularly vitamin D_3, to avoid oversupplementation which may worsen nutritional osteopathy.

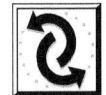

FOLLOW-UP
PATIENT MONITORING
• The owner should purchase a gram scale to monitor the pet's weight at home.

• Repeat biochemical profile and radiograph monitoring to track healing of fractures and bone density and metabolic derangements.
• Rechecks should be frequent to monitor condition. At a minimum, re-evaluation every 1–2 weeks.

PREVENTION/AVOIDANCE
Providing an appropriate diet with 1% calcium, 0.5% phosphorous, and 1500 IU/kg vitamin D_3 on a dry weight basis. If invertebrates are used as a food source, gut load with a calcium-containing diet prior to offering.

POSSIBLE COMPLICATIONS
• Severe dehydration
• Organ failure and death
• Permanent skeletal deformity

EXPECTED COURSE AND PROGNOSIS
• In more debilitated patients, the prognosis may be poor due to concurrent organ dysfunction and long-term orthopedic and/or neurologic deficits that reduce the quality of life long term.
• For those sugar gliders that are not severely debilitated, the prognosis is fair to good with appropriate treatment and improving diet.

MISCELLANEOUS
ASSOCIATED CONDITIONS
Cardiac, hepatic, and pancreatic disease
Renal and hepatic dysfunction
Anemia, hypoproteinemia
Obesity

AGE-RELATED FACTORS
N/A

ZOONOTIC POTENTIAL
N/A

PREGNANCY/FERTILITY/BREEDING
Pregnancy and lactation can be associated with weight loss due to increased caloric expenditure.

SYNONYMS
Nutritional secondary hyperparathyroidism
Metabolic bone disease

SEE ALSO
Anorexia
Dental Disease
Diarrhea
Seizures and Tremors

ABBREVIATIONS
CT = computed tomography
MRI = magnetic resonance imaging

INTERNET RESOURCES
www.vin.com (membership required)

Suggested Reading
Brust D, Mans C. Sugar gliders. In: Carpenter JW, ed. Exotic Animal Formulary, 5th ed. St Louis: Elsevier, 2018:432–442.
Dierenfeld ES. Feeding behavior and nutrition of the sugar glider (*Petaurus breviceps*). Vet Clin North Am Exot Anim Pract 2009;12(2):209–215, xiii–viii.
Dierenfeld ES, Thomas D, Ives R. Comparison of commonly used diets on intake, digestion, growth, and health in captive sugar gliders (*Petaurus breviceps*). J Exot Pet Med 2006;15:218–224.
Johnson-Delaney C. Sugar gliders. In: Quesenberry KE, Carpenter JW, eds. Ferrets, Rabbits and Rodents, 4th Ed). Clinical Medicine and Surgery. 2021 ed. St. Louis: Saunders, 2020:385–400.
Author Nicholas Jew, DVM

SUGAR GLIDERS

OBESITY

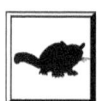

BASICS

DEFINITION
• The presence of body fat in sufficient excess to compromise normal physiologic function or predispose to metabolic, surgical, and/or mechanical problems. Obesity has become an extremely common, and often debilitating, problem in pet sugar gliders.

PATHOPHYSIOLOGY
• Increase caloric intake and/or decreased activity. Most sugar gliders are housed in groups with limited ability to exercise similarly to their wild counterparts.
• Sugar gliders have a particular affinity to high fat, sweet-tasting treats. Many glider owners have difficulty denying their sugar glider treats.
• Meeting the nutritional requirements of sugar gliders in captivity is particularly challenging, and to-date, no commercially formulated diets have been identified as nutritionally complete.

SYSTEMS AFFECTED
• Musculoskeletal—articular and locomotor problems
• Hepatobiliary—hepatic lipidosis
• Cardiovascular

GENETICS
N/A

INCIDENCE/PREVALENCE
N/A

GEOGRAPHIC DISTRIBUTION
N/A

SIGNALMENT
No age or sex predisposition

SIGNS
Historical Findings
• Free choice feeding of pellets, insects, and sugary treats.
• Weight gain may be significant but not noticeable to owner
• Owner may report that they have no current concerns.
• Owners may report lethargy, impaired mobility, and/or difficulty grooming.

Physical Examination Findings
• Excess amounts of body fat for body size; can measure as body condition score >4 on a 1–5 scale in which 1 = cachectic (>20% underweight), 2 = lean (10%–20% underweight), 3 = moderate, 4 = stout (20%–40% overweight), 5 = obese (>40% overweight).
• Sites of adipose tissue to evaluate during physical examination include intraabdominal, inguinal and axillary regions, and in the patagium.

CAUSES
• Most commonly, excessive access to highly palatable food, often combined with insufficient activity; owners usually leave food out continuously and supplement by feeding sugary treats and other palatable foods as part of a social interaction.

RISK FACTORS
Owner lifestyle
Diet palatability and energy density
Inappropriate diet composition
Activity level

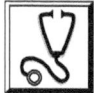

DIAGNOSIS

DIFFERENTIAL DIAGNOSIS
• Joey inhabiting the pouch.
• Ascites
• Intraabdominal neoplasia or organomegaly
• Pouch mass
• Nutritional osteodystrophy (often concurrent)

CBC/BIOCHEMISTRY/URINALYSIS
• Often normal although triglycerides and cholesterol may be elevated.
• In instances of hepatic lipidosis, liver isoenzymes may be normal or elevated.
• If concurrent nutritional osteodystrophy, disturbances in calcium phosphorous may be present. Often relatively or absolute hypocalcemia.
• Blood collection may require sedation or anesthesia.

OTHER LABORATORY TESTS
• N/A

IMAGING
Demonstrates excess body fat.

PATHOLOGIC FINDINGS
May vary depending on the presence of concurrent illnesses.

TREATMENT
• Successful treatment is lifelong amelioration of the problem.
• Gradual reduction in caloric intake and activity level.

ACTIVITY
It is important to provide access to a gradual increase in activity level and exercise.

DIET
A diet change should never be made abruptly. In ill patients, wait until the patient is stable before changing to an appropriate diet.
Example diet 1
• 75% commercial sugar glider pelleted diet
• 25% fresh fruits and vegetables

• Vitamin and calcium supplement
• Small quantities of live insects
Example diet 2
• 50% commercial insectivore or carnivore diet
• 50% Leadbeater's mixture—150 mL water, 150 mL honey, 1 shelled hard-boiled egg, 25 g high-protein baby cereal, 1 teaspoon vitamin, and mineral powder
• <5% gut-loaded insects

CLIENT EDUCATION
• Education on appropriate diet is essential to treatment and prevention.
• The author recommends a wellness examination every 6 months.

CONTRAINDICATIONS
• Abrupt reduction in caloric intake.

PRECAUTIONS
• Avoid excess vitamin D_3 supplementation.
• The calcium to phosphorous ratio should be 2:1 or greater.

FOLLOW-UP

PATIENT MONITORING
• Regular weight checks and documentation of gradual weight loss.

PREVENTION/AVOIDANCE
Avoid oversupplementation with highly palatable, sugary treats.
Provide appropriate access to a large enough enclosure to allow for normal activity.

POSSIBLE COMPLICATIONS
• Severe dehydration
• Organ failure and death

EXPECTED COURSE AND PROGNOSIS
The prognosis is based on the presence of concurrent illness and the owner's ability to achieve weight loss.

MISCELLANEOUS

ASSOCIATED CONDITIONS
Nutritional osteodystrophy

AGE-RELATED FACTORS
N/A

ZOONOTIC POTENTIAL
N/A

PREGNANCY/FERTILITY/BREEDING
Reproductive failure may be more common in obese sugar gliders.

SYNONYMS
N/A

SEE ALSO
Nutritional osteodystrophy

ABBREVIATIONS
N/A

INTERNET RESOURCES
Association of Sugar Glider Veterinarians - http://www.asgv.org/index.php (membership required)

Suggested Reading
Brust D, Mans C. Sugar gliders. In: Carpenter JW, ed. Exotic Animal Formulary, 5th ed. St Louis: Elsevier, 2018:432–442.
Dierenfeld ES. Feeding behavior and nutrition of the sugar glider (*Petaurus breviceps*). Vet Clin North Am Exot Anim Pract 2009;12(2):209–215. doi: 10.1016/j.cvex.2009.01.014.
Dierenfeld ES, Thomas D, Ives R. Comparison of commonly used diets on intake, digestion, growth, and health in captive sugar gliders (*Petaurus breviceps*). J Exot Pet Med 2006;*15*(3). doi: 10.1053/j.jepm.2006.06.008.
Johnson-Delaney CA. Captive marsupial nutrition. Vet Clin North Am Exot Anim Pract 2014;17(3):415–447. doi: 10.1016/j.cvex.2014.05.006.
Johnson-Delaney C. Sugar gliders. In: Quesenberry KE, Carpenter JW, eds. Ferrets, Rabbits and Rodents, 4th Ed). Clinical Medicine and Surgery. 2021 ed. St. Louis: Saunders, 2020:385–400.

Author Nicholas Jew, DVM

PARACLOACAL GLAND DISORDERS

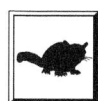

BASICS

DEFINITION
• The paracloacal scent glands are similar to anal glands in placental mammals. These glands are found laterally adjacent to the cloacal opening.
• Both males and females have paracloacal glands.
• Male sugar gliders have two pairs of Cowper's glands.

PATHOPHYSIOLOGY
• During scent marking, secretions are deposited around the perineal region surface.
• Although the underlying etiology is unknown, it is thought to be due to poor nutrition.

SYSTEMS AFFECTED
• Skin/Exocrine
• Gastrointestinal
• Urinary

GENETICS
N/A

INCIDENCE/PREVALENCE
• Older sugar gliders and those that have been de-sexed are more commonly affected. It is believed that reduced sexual activity and scent marking occur in these population leading to decreased expression. Impaction and infection are more common in these populations.

GEOGRAPHIC DISTRIBUTION
N/A

SIGNS
Historical Findings
• Straining to defecate and/or urinate
• Anorexia
• Irritability
• Weight loss
• Constipation
• Lethargy, inappetence
• Pain, relentlessness, and vocalization
• Diarrhea

Physical Examination Findings
• Pain on palpation of the cloacal and paracloacal regions
• Swelling adjacent to and involving the cloaca
• Irritation, excoriation, or wounds of the paracloacal region

CAUSES
• Paracloacal gland impaction
• Infection or abscessation—bacterial
• Cystic mass
• Neoplasia
• Trauma (may be secondary and/or concurrent with other pathology)

RISK FACTORS
• Obese, sedentary gliders
• Spayed and neutered gliders
• Chronic or recurrent diarrhea may predispose to infectious causes or impaction
• Self-trauma

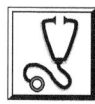

DIAGNOSIS

DIFFERENTIAL DIAGNOSIS
• Primary cloacal pathology
• Herniation of the bladder
• Cystolithiasis, cystitis
• Lower urinary tract infection

CBC/BIOCHEMISTRY/URINALYSIS
• CBC—normal or leukocytosis with a neutrophilia
• Serum chemistry profile—may be normal. In cases of secondary urinary tract obstruction, azotemia may be present. Certain neoplasms may lead to hypercalcemia.
• Assess overall health

OTHER LABORATORY TESTS
N/A

IMAGING
Radiographs—useful for ruling out abdominal organ herniation, cystolithiasis, and for evaluation of the GI tract.

DIAGNOSTIC PROCEDURES
History and Palpation
Visualization of swelling or mass effect in the region of the cloaca and paracloacal gland(s).

Cytologic Examination
• FNA of firm masses within or around the peracloacal gland to rule out neoplasia
• Examination of fluid contents of the glands to look for signs of inflammation, infection, and neoplasia
• Normal cytology—small amount of neutrophil and bacteria; however, if severe neutrophilia or a large number of bacteria are seen, inflammation and infection should be suspected

Culture and Sensitivity
Aerobic and anaerobic bacterial culture of fluid contents of glands—sterile, deep sample from affected tissue or exudate; susceptibility testing to direct antibiotic therapy

PATHOLOGIC FINDINGS
Depends on the underlying cause. Paracloacal gland carcinoma and a cystic mass of the cloacal wall have been reported.

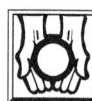

TREATMENT

APPROPRIATE HEALTH CARE
• Patients with nonobstructive lower urinary/gastrointestinal tract diseases are typically managed as outpatients; diagnostic evaluation may require brief hospitalization.
• Systemic signs of illness (e.g., pyrexia, depression, anorexia, and dehydration) or laboratory findings of azotemia or leukocytosis warrant aggressive diagnostic evaluation and initiation of supportive and symptomatic treatment.
• Treatment depends on the underlying cause and specific sites involved.

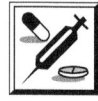

MEDICATIONS

DRUG(S) OF CHOICE
• Depend on the underlying cause
• If abscessed or bacterial infection is suspected, begin treatment with broad-spectrum antibiotic such as trimethoprim-sulfa (10–20 mg/kg PO q12h), amoxicillin (30 mg/kg PO q12h), amoxicillin/clavulanic acid (12.5 mg/kg PO, SC divided q12h), or as a second line, enrofloxacin (2.5–5 mg/kg PO, SC, IM q12h) and chloramphenicol (50 mg/kg PO q12h). Modify antibacterial treatment based on the results of culture and sensibility testing.
• Pain management may aid urination and promote appetite. NSAIDs (meloxicam 0.1–0.2 mg/kg PO, SC q24h) reduce pain and may decrease inflammation.
   ○ For sedation: Light sedation: Midazolam (0.2–0.5 mg/kg SC, IM, IV intranasal) ± butorphanol (0.5 mg/kg SC) or buprenorphine (0.01 mg/kg SC). Heavier sedation/mild anesthesia: ketamine (10–20 mg/kg IM, IV) + midazolam (0.3–0.5 mg/kg SC, IM, IV); other protocols exist.

CONTRAINDICATIONS
• Glucocorticoids or other immunosuppressive agents
• Potentially nephrotoxic drugs (e.g., aminoglycosides, NSAIDs) in patients that are febrile, dehydrated, or azotemic or that are suspected of having pyelonephritis, septicemia, or preexisting renal disease

NURSING CARE
• Gentle expression of contents from impaction. Sedation is required due to pain with expression. Often, thick yellow to ivory color discharge is expressible from the

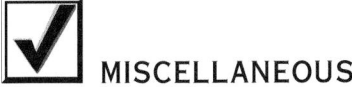

(CONTINUED) PARACLOACAL GLAND DISORDERS

paracloacal glands. This may require significant pressure in more severe cases.
• Gentle aseptic cleansing of the paracloacal region, particularly if any wounds are present.

CLIENT EDUCATION
• Regular monitoring of urinary and fecal eliminations is critical to avoid potential life-threatening complication of obstructive paracloacal gland disease.

SURGICAL CONSIDERATIONS
• If abscess or impaction recurs, consider surgical excision of the affected gland(s)
• If a paracloacal mass is present, surgery may be indicated to alleviate clinical signs and to obtain a definitive diagnosis which is imperative to determine prognosis.

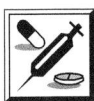

MEDICATIONS

DRUG(S) OF CHOICE

Antimicrobial Therapy
• Topical antibiotics—triple antibiotic (neomycin, polymyxin B sulfates, and bacitracin zinc) without hydrocortisone
• Topical antiseptics—dilute betadine solution
• Broad-spectrum antibiotics can be used if there is a severe infection.
• Therapy should be based on culture and sensitivity, if possible.
  ◦ Commonly used antibiotics include trimethoprim-sulfa (10–20 mg/kg PO q12h), amoxicillin (30 mg/kg PO q12h), amoxicillin/clavulanic acid (12.5 mg/kg PO, SC divided q12h) or as a second line, enrofloxacin (2.5–5 mg/kg PO, SC, IM q12h) and chloramphenicol (50 mg/kg PO q12h).

Analgesic Therapy
• Meloxicam (0.1–0.2 mg/kg PO, SC q24h)
• Buprenorphine (0.02–0.05 mg/kg PO, SC, IM q8–12h)

CONTRAINDICATIONS
N/A

PRECAUTIONS
Painful sugar gliders are more likely to bite, and expression or palpation of painful paracloacal swellings should be performed with appropriate analgesia and sedation. Chloramphenicol may cause aplastic anemia in susceptible people. Clients and staff should use appropriate precautions when handling this drug.

POSSIBLE INTERACTIONS
N/A

ALTERNATIVE DRUGS
N/A

FOLLOW-UP

PATIENT MONITORING
Monitor for resolution of clinical signs with serial examination.

PREVENTION/AVOIDANCE
• Routine examination of the paracloacal area
• Provide proper nutrition
• Place patient on an appropriate diet
• Increase exercise
• Provide good hygiene

POSSIBLE COMPLICATIONS
Paracloacal gland impactions can cause complete blockage of the urethra and colon

EXPECTED COURSE AND PROGNOSIS
Paracloacal gland impaction and infection carry a fair to good prognosis if treated early prior to more systemic illness and debilitation. Prognosis with neoplastic causes may vary based on the biologic behavior of the diagnosed neoplasm.

✓ MISCELLANEOUS

ASSOCIATED CONDITIONS
N/A

AGE-RELATED FACTORS
More prevalent in older sugar gliders.

ZOONOTIC POTENTIAL
N/A

PREGNANCY/FERTILITY/BREEDING
N/A

SYNONYMS
Scent gland impaction

SEE ALSO
Anorexia
Diarrhea
Dysuria and hematuria

ABBREVIATIONS
CBC = complete blood count

Suggested Reading
Chen L, Yu P, Liu C-H, Chi C-h. Paracloacal gland carcinoma in sugar glider (*Petaurus breviceps*). J Exot Pet Med 2017;27:36–40. doi: 10.1053/j.jepm.2017.10.019.
Johnson-Delaney C. Sugar gliders. In: Quesenberry KE, Carpenter JW, eds. Ferrets, Rabbits and Rodents, 4th Ed). Clinical Medicine and Surgery. 2021 ed. St. Louis: Saunders, 2020:385–400.
Johnson-Delaney CA, Lennox AM. Reproductive disorders of marsupials. Vet Clin North Am Exot Anim Pract 2017;20(2):539–553.
Thomas M, Parkinson L, Shaw G, Mans C. Paracloacal cyst in a sugar glider (*Petaurus Breviceps*). J Exot Pet Med 2018;29:40–44. doi: 10.1053/j.jepm.2018.02.046.

Author Nicholas Jew, DVM

SUGAR GLIDERS

PARESIS AND PARALYSIS

BASICS

DEFINITION
• Paresis—partial paralysis; loss of power of voluntary movement
• Paralysis (plegia)—loss of voluntary motor function
• Mono (paresis or plegia)—one limb affected
• Hemi—both limbs on the same side of the body
• Para—both pelvic limbs affected
• Quadri- or tetra-—all four limbs affected

PATHOPHYSIOLOGY
• May be caused by lesions of the central or peripheral nervous system
• Muscle wasting will occur from disuse in as little as 5–7 days.

SYSTEMS AFFECTED
• Nervous
• Musculoskeletal—atrophy or contracture of musculature is a secondary complication.

GENETICS
None

INCIDENCE/PREVALENCE
Common

GEOGRAPHIC DISTRIBUTION
None

SIGNALMENT
No age or gender predispostion

SIGNS
General Comments
• It is important to differentiate paresis or paralysis from generalized weakness; patients with generalized weakness will not exhibit any deficits on neurologic exam. However, this can be difficult to interpret in the debilitated sugar glider.
• Clinical signs may be acute or chronic and may be progressive or static. Onset and progression may be indicative of etiology.
• Acute or peracute onset of signs without progression or with gradual improvement is usually consistent with trauma or vascular events.
• Gradual or subacute onset with gradual improvement in response to treatment usually indicates infection.
• Slow onset and continued progression of clinical signs usually indicates a neoplastic or degenerative process.
• Static clinical signs (or signs present at birth) indicate an anomalous cause.

Historical Findings
• Owner may notice an abnormal gait, leaning to one side, falling, or inability to stand, walk, climb, or glide.

• There may be a known traumatic event such as being dropped or stepped on, or there may be a history of children playing with the pet.
• Inability to right itself from lying down, or an inability to get up without assistance
• Dragging of a limb
• Urine staining around the perineum and/or on limbs (may be unilateral or bilateral)
• Swelling, redness, or pododermatitis of unaffected or less affected limbs may be the first sign identified and is often the result of excessive weight bearing on these limbs.
• Alopecia of the affected limbs may be present from rubbing, excessive grooming, or dragging.
• Owners may report witnessing seizures or tremors.

Physical Examination Findings
• Mentation may be normal.
• Pain on spinal palpation may be present in cases of trauma or injury.
• Muscle wasting may be present in patients with more gradual onset or prolonged disease.
• Patient may be tachypneic in response to pain.
• Urine staining may be present around perineum and/or on limbs (may be unilateral or bilateral).
• Swelling, redness, or pododermatitis of unaffected or less affected limbs may be identified and is often the result of excessive weight bearing on these limbs.
• Alopecia of the affected limbs may be present.
• Gastric dilation (usually mild) may occur as a result of aerophagia; anorexia or diarrhea may be present due to inappetence from pain or an inability to access food or water.

NEUROLOGIC EXAMINATION
Findings
• Pain may be present on spinal palpation in cases of trauma.
• Prioprioceptive deficits may be present in the affected limbs
• Deep pain is assessed by using a toe-pinch (superficial pain) or pinching of the pad/bone (deep pain); withdrawal of the limb is a reflex that alone does not indicate intact pain sensation; conscious response to the pinch is required to indicate spinal cord integrity.
• Neurolocalization is important.
• Cervical (C1–C6)—proprioceptive or motor deficits of all four limbs. Pain may be found on cervical palpation.
• Cervicothoracic (C6–T2)—lower-motor neuron signs to the forelimb, including poor motor function and weak withdrawal with loss of reflexes
• Thoracolumbar (T3–L3)—weakness and proprioceptive abnormalities in the rear limbs

with normal motor function and proprioception in the front limbs. Spinal reflexes are normal. Pain may be found on spinal palpation.
• Lumbosacral (L4–S3)—lower motor neuron signs to the rear limbs, including proprioceptive abnormalities, weakness, poor withdrawal reflexes, and loss of segmental spinal reflexes. Urinary and fecal incontinence may be present.
• Tremors may be present.
• Seizures are often not witnessed during the exam even when reported at home by owners.

CAUSES
• Trauma/injury is the most common cause of paresis or paralysis in pet sugar gliders; an incident may have been directly observed, or there may be a history of contact with children or other pets.
• Meningitis/encephalitis—bacterial (consider spread of otitis media/interna or upper respiratory infection); viral, disseminated infection
• Neoplasia (brain or spinal cord)
• CNS abscess (effects and diagnostics may mimic neoplasia)
• Cerebrovascular accident
• Toxoplasmosis
• Nutritional osteodystrophy with secondary hypocalcemia and hypoglycemia
• Toxicity—heavy metals, lead, and polyvinyl chloride are among toxins that can cause CNS or PNS signs and should be suspected if there is a possibility of ingestion or exposure

RISK FACTORS
• Obesity
• Inappropriate diet
• Fractures, luxations often the result of trauma from improper handling or housing, children, or other pets
• Spondylosis/arthritis

DIAGNOSIS

DIFFERENTIAL DIAGNOSIS
• Weakness (metabolic) may lead to similar clinical presentation.
• Osteoarthritis
• Pododermatitis
• Neoplasia

CBC/BIOCHEMISTRY/URINALYSIS
Usually normal unless infection is present; leukocytosis may be present in cases of infection; elevations in CK are likely in cases of trauma; alterations in calcium, phosphorous, and electrolytes may be present in cases of nutritional osteodystrophy and dehydration.

(CONTINUED)

OTHER LABORATORY TESTS
• Blood lead or heavy metal levels if ingestion is suspected

IMAGING
• Radiography—may reveal spinal fracture or luxation, osteomyelitis, osteoarthritis, discospondylitis, or bone neoplasia. Skull radiographs may reveal bulla disease. Reduced bone density and poorly mineralized cortices may be suspected.
• CT or MRI—more sensitive for evaluation of brain infiltrate, spinal cord compression, or bony lesions

DIAGNOSTIC PROCEDURES
• CSF analysis can be performed via the cisterna magna; indicated if infection or neoplasia is suspected; do not attempt to aspirate but instead collect sample via capillary tube; only a few drops will be obtained

TREATMENT

APPROPRIATE HEALTH CARE
• Inpatient—neurologic signs; severe infections; anorexic patients; nonambulatory patients
• Outpatient—stable patients that are able to eat and drink with little or no assistance

NURSING CARE
• Fluid therapy to maintain hydration—subcutaneous generally adequate unless severe infection/sepsis
• Assisted feeding of anorexic animals
• Maintain clean, soft bedding with padding if necessary.
• Lubricate eyes if blink response is absent or diminished.
• In severe cases, turn patient every 4 hours or as needed to prevent formation of decubitus ulcers.
• Express bladder if patient is unable to void without assistance.
• Keep fur clean and dry.

ACTIVITY
Restrict activity, particularly in cases of trauma. Confine to a very small space initially to prevent falls or further injury.

DIET
• It is essential to maintain food intake during treatment; patients may become anorexic due to pain or neurologic signs; secondary derangements of intestinal microbial populations may occur.
• Offer the normal diet provided at home.
• If anorexic, it is essential to provide adequate nutritional support. Syringe-feed a formulated diet such as Critical Care for Omnivores

(Oxbow Pet Products, Murdock, NE) or Emeraid Omnivore (Lafeber Company, Cornell, IL). If these commercial formulas are not available, a gruel may be made with blenderized omnivore/sugar glider pellets.
• Avoid high-carbohydrate foods, treats, or grains.
• Use caution when syringe feeding, as aspiration pneumonia may occur in patients with central nervous system signs.

CLIENT EDUCATION
Owners should be informed that in cases of spinal trauma or paralysis, motor function may improve gradually or may not improve at all.

SURGICAL CONSIDERATIONS
Surgical repair of fractures should only be undertaken by an experienced surgeon and may be of limited value. Many cases of partial paresis or paralysis will improve without surgery.

MEDICATIONS

DRUG(S) OF CHOICE
• Corticosteroids are recommended in mammals with spinal trauma, care should be taken to monitor for signs of immunosuppression when used in sugar gliders.
• If administered, a short-acting steroid such as methylprednisolone sodium succinate (10–30 mg/kg IV or IM is the canine dose—sugar glider dose not reported) may be preferable to minimize any long-term immunosuppression.
• Anti-inflammatory doses of glucocorticoids may be needed for either short-term use or chronically—prednisolone (0.1–0.2 mg/kg PO, SQ, IM q24h).
• Analgesics should be administered in cases of confirmed or suspected trauma; systemic meloxicam (0.1–0.2 mg/kg PO, SC q24h) for its anti-inflammatory effects alone or in combination with an opioid (avoid if corticosteroids have been administered); buprenorphine (0.01–0.03 mg/kg PO, SC, IM, IV q8–12h), butorphanol (0.1–0.5 mg/kg SC, IM q6–8h), or tramadol (5–10 mg/kg PO q12h) for additional analgesia.
• For suspected or confirmed CNS infections, use systemic antibiotics. Choose broad-spectrum antibiotics that penetrate the CNS, such as enrofloxacin (2.5–5 mg/kg PO, SC, IM q12h), ciprofloxacin (10 mg/kg PO q12h), or trimethoprim-sulfa (10–20 mg/kg PO q12h); for anaerobic infections consider chloramphenicol (50 mg/kg PO q12h) or metronidazole (25 mg/kg PO q12h).

• For sedation: Light sedation: Midazolam (0.2–0.5 mg/kg SC, IM, IV intranasal) ± butorphanol (0.5 mg/kg SC) or buprenorphine (0.01 mg/kg SC). Heavier sedation/mild anesthesia: Ketamine (10–20 mg/kg IM, IV) + midazolam (0.3–0.5 mg/kg SC, IM, IV); other protocols exist.

CONTRAINDICATIONS
• Avoid the use of corticosteroids in conjunction with meloxicam or other NSAIDs.
• Avoid the use of drugs that are potentially toxic to the central nervous system (metronidazole at high doses; aminoglycosides).

PRECAUTIONS
Do not use steroids in conjunction with NSAIDs.
Use caution in choosing antimicrobials.

POSSIBLE INTERACTIONS
Do not use steroids in conjunction with NSAIDs.

FOLLOW-UP

PATIENT MONITORING
Serial neurologic examinations should be performed daily or more frequently initially to monitor for progression of clinical signs.

PREVENTION/AVOIDANCE
Avoid free roaming or unsupervised activity or interactions with children or other pets.

POSSIBLE COMPLICATIONS
• Urine retention, urine scald, urinary tract infection, and ascending renal infection
• Pododermatitis and osteomyelitis from excessive weight bearing of unaffected or lesser affected limbs
• Permanent paralysis
• Pathologic fractures if nutritional osteodystrophy is present

EXPECTED COURSE AND PROGNOSIS
• Depends on etiology
• Without improved husbandry and diet, nutritional osteodystrophy carries a poor prognosis.
• The loss of deep pain perception carries a poor prognosis for recovery.

MISCELLANEOUS

ASSOCIATED CONDITIONS
• Nutritional deficiencies
• Otitis media/interna or upper respiratory infection may serve as a source for CNS infections.

PARESIS AND PARALYSIS

AGE-RELATED FACTORS
None

ZOONOTIC POTENTIAL
N/A

PREGNANCY/FERTILITY/BREEDING
Sugar gliders with paresis or paralysis should not breed; pregnancy and parturition would put excessive strain on any injury.

SYNONYMS
None

SEE ALSO
Nutritional osteodystrophy
Seizures and tremors

ABBREVIATIONS
CK = creatine kinase
CNS = central nervous system
CSF = cerebral spinal fluid
CT = computed tomography
EMG = electromyelogram
MRI = magnetic resonance imaging
NCV = nerve conduction velocity
NSAID = nonsteroidal anti-inflammatory drug
PCR = polymerase chain reaction

Suggested Reading
Johnson DH. Sugar gliders. Exot Anim Emerg Crit Care Med 2021;15:408–430.
Johnson-Delaney C. Sugar gliders. In: Quesenberry KE, Carpenter JW, eds. Ferrets, Rabbits and Rodents, 4th Ed). Clinical Medicine and Surgery. 2021 ed. St. Louis: Saunders, 2020:385–400.
Johnson-Delaney CA. Captive marsupial nutrition. Vet Clin Exot Anim Pract 2014;17(3):415–447.
McLaughlin A, Strunk A. Common emergencies in small rodents, hedgehogs, and sugar gliders. Vet Clin Exot Anim Pract 2016;19(2):465–499.

Author Nicholas Jew, DVM

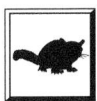

BASICS

DEFINITION
Inability of the glans penis to be retracted partially or fully into the prepuce.

PATHOPHYSIOLOGY
• Trauma—induced by another glider in the colony. Typically, as part of a normal social interaction or interrupted/failed breeding attempt.
• Self-mutilation—inappropriately socialized young, male gliders or as the result of stress and inappropriate husbandry

SYSTEMS AFFECTED
• Reproductive—breeding failure, self-mutilation, and trauma
• Systemic—sepsis with infection; anorexia and weight loss with pain
• Urologic—urinary tract infection, urethral obstruction

INCIDENCE/PREVALENCE
Penile mutilation and necrosis are common conditions in sugar gliders.

SIGNALMENT
Usually breeding age males. Young, inappropriately socialized young males may be overrepresented.

SIGNS

Historical Findings
• May be asymptomatic in early stages.
• Owners may report visualization of penis more frequently. Along with this may come reports of color change or bleeding from penis.
• Excessive grooming around penis
• Breeding failure
• Dysuria, stranguria
• Hyporexia, anorexia, and depression with pain or secondary infection

Physical Examination Findings
• Failure to appropriately retract penis into prepuce.
• Penis may appear desiccated, avascular, discolored, and/or flaccid.
• Typically, the bifid portion of the penis fails to retract although full penile prolapse may also occur.
• Trauma, inflammation, and infection at the base of the bifid portion of the penis may contribute to alteration of the external urethral orifice.
• If infection becomes generalized or urinary outflow is constricted- anorexia, lethargy, fever, dehydration

CAUSES

Trauma
• Failed breeding—first time breeders are overrepresented. Interrupted breeding and hyperextension of penis.

• Bite wounds from other male or unreceptive female gliders.
• Human intervention during unwanted copulation may be a contributing factor.

Self-Mutilation
• Inappropriate socialization of young, male gliders as sexual maturity is approached.
• Stress—changes in husbandry, inappropriate diet, lack of appropriate environmental enrichment, inappropriate husbandry practices.

RISK FACTORS
• Inappropriate husbandry and diet
• Lack of appropriate socialization and social groups

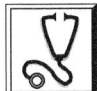

DIAGNOSIS

DIFFERENTIAL DIAGNOSIS
For stranguira, dysuria:
• Paracloacal gland enlargement—impaction, cysts, or neoplasia
• Cystitis—bacteriuria; painful, thickened bladder
• Urolithiasis—palpable uroliths in the bladder, radio-opacities within the bladder
• For flaccid penile prolapse:
• Neurogenic: trauma, neuropathy, myelopathy, and CNS lesions

CBC/BIOCHEMISTRY/URINALYSIS
• CBC—usually normal unless infection is severe or becomes systemic
• Biochemistry panel—if urethral obstruction occurs—may see azotemia, changes in electrolytes such as hyperkalemia, hypochloremia, and hyponatremia
• Urinalysis—to rule out bacterial cystitis

OTHER LABORATORY TESTS
• Cytology of purulent discharge—Diff-Quick and gram's stain to direct therapy
• Bacterial culture and sensitivity testing of exudate

IMAGING
Radiographs to rule out orthopedic causes and urolithiasis

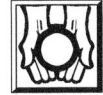

TREATMENT

APPROPRIATE HEALTH CARE
• Patients with nonobstructive penile disorders may be managed as outpatients following reduction of prolapse although amputation may be necessary for those not responding to medical treatment.
• Secondary urinary obstructions should be hospitalized, and emergency supportive and

symptomatic therapy should be provided until the obstruction is resolved.

NURSING CARE
• Frequent lubrication and hydration of the penis to avoid desiccation and necrosis if not already present.
• Clean all accumulation smegma and preputial discharge with dilute (0.125%) chlorohexidine solution
• Applications of hypertonic topical agents (e.g., moistened sugar, dextrose) to reduce swelling and facilitate reduction
• If severely swollen or edematous, forceful reduction should be avoided to prevent further trauma. Application of hydrocolloid gel topically multiple times daily may help to resolve swelling.
• An E-collar, properly fitted, is necessary to prevent further trauma. While wearing an E-collar, hand feeding or assisted feeding may be necessary.

ACTIVITY
• While wearing an E-collar, it may be best to limit opportunities for climbing and gliding to avoid accidental trauma from falling.
• Quarantine from the colony/conspecifics to ensure access to resources and avoid bullying while impaired.

DIET
• If anorectic or have a decreased appetite assist feed Critical Care for Omnivores (Oxbow Animal Health, Omaha, NE) or Emeraid Omnivore (Lafeber Company, Cornell, IL). Alternatively, a blenderized gruel of an insectivore or omnivore pellet may be used.

CLIENT EDUCATION
• Instruct and encourage clients to aid in grooming while the sugar glider is wearing an E-collar to avoid secondary infection of the compromised penis/prepuce.

SURGICAL CONSIDERATIONS
• When reduction fails or necrosis of the penis is present, amputation of the bifid portion of the penis is an appropriate surgical option. The urethral opening is present at the base of the bifurcation of the distal penis, and amputation of the bifid portion does not interfere with the normal outflow of urine.
• Should amputation be necessary below the level of the external urethral orifice, and a urethrostomy may need to be considered. Stricture and secondary obstruction from postoperative inflammation may be concerns.
• Abscesses may require surgical drainage.
• Castration and scrotal ablation are often indicated to aid in resolution when breeding is not intended.

PENILE PROLAPSE

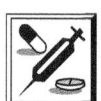

MEDICATIONS

DRUG(S) OF CHOICE
• Antibiotics if bacterial infection is present—ideally based on culture and sensitivity testing. Broad-spectrum antibiotics commonly used include enrofloxacin (2.5–5 mg/kg PO, SQ q12h, dilute for SQ injection), ciprofloxacin (10 mg/kg PO q12h), amoxicillin/clavulanic acid (12.5 mg/kg PO q12h), or trimethoprim-sulfa (10–20 mg/kg PO q12h), pending results of culture and susceptibility testing.
• Analgesics—meloxicam (0.1–0.2 mg/kg PO, SQ q24h), buprenorphine (0.01–0.03 mg/kg PO, SQ, IM q8–12h), gabapentin (3–5 mg/kg PO q8–12h), and and methadone (0.15–0.4 mg/kg SQ q4–6h) in cases of severe pain.
• For sedation: Light sedation: Midazolam (0.2–0.5 mg/kg SC, IM, IV intranasal) ± butorphanol (0.5 mg/kg SC) or buprenorphine (0.01 mg/kg SC). Heavier sedation/mild anesthesia: Ketamine (10–20 mg/kg IM, IV) + midazolam (0.3–0.5 mg/kg SC, IM, IV); other protocols exist.

CONTRAINDICATIONS
If the exposed glans penis is severely edematous, do not force it back into the prepuce

PRECAUTIONS
Monitor for weight loss while wearing E-collar and the ability to eat normally has been impaired.
When concurrent castration is not performed, recurrence of prolapse is common.

POSSIBLE INTERACTIONS
N/A

ALTERNATIVE DRUGS
N/A

FOLLOW-UP

PATIENT MONITORING
• Monitor weight while wearing an E-collar to ensure appropriate intake of food.

PREVENTION/AVOIDANCE
• Regular inspection of the glans penis and prepuce
• Clean environment
• Appropriate socialization, husbandry, and enrichment.

POSSIBLE COMPLICATIONS
• Urinary outflow obstruction and subsequent uremia in more severe cases involving the proximal penis.
• Extension of infection, formation of abscesses, or bacterial sepsis
• Necrosis of the exposed glans penis with chronicity
• Self-mutilation

EXPECTED COURSE AND PROGNOSIS
When castration is not performed, recurrence of prolapse is common.
Amputation of the bifid portion of the penis is well tolerated if the external urethral orifice is not involved.
Trauma to the external urethral orifice/proximal penis carries a more guarded prognosis due to the increased risk of stricture and obstruction of urine outflow.

MISCELLANEOUS

ASSOCIATED CONDITIONS
Self-mutilation

AGE-RELATED FACTORS
Young, males reaching sexual maturity.

ZOONOTIC POTENTIAL
N/A

PREGNANCY/FERTILITY/BREEDING
Can prevent successful breeding.
Following amputation, breeding impaired.

SYNONYMS
N/A

SEE ALSO
Dysuria and hematuria
Nutritional osteodystrophy
Self-mutilation

ABBREVIATIONS
N/A

INTERNET RESOURCES
N/A

Suggested Reading
Johnson-Delaney C. Sugar gliders. In: Quesenberry KE, Carpenter JW, eds. Ferrets, Rabbits and Rodents, 4th Ed). Clinical Medicine and Surgery. 2021 ed. St. Louis: Saunders, 2020:385–400.
Johnson-Delaney CA, Lennox AM. Reproductive disorders of marsupials. Vet Clin North Am Exot Anim Pract 2017;20(2):539–553.
Malbrue RA, Arsuaga CB, Collins TA, Allen JL, Diggs TJ, Langohr IM. Scrotal stalk ablation and orchiectomy using electrosurgery in the male sugar glider (*Petaurus breviceps*) and histologic anatomy of the testes and associated scrotal structures. J Exot Pet Med 2018;27(2):90–94.
Miwa Y, Sladky KK. Small mammals: common surgical procedures of rodents, ferrets, hedgehogs, and sugar gliders. Vet Clin North Am Exot Anim Pract 2016;19(1):205–244.
Pye G. Surgery of sugar gliders. In: Bennett RA, Pye G, eds. Surgery of Exotics Animals. Wiley Blackwell, 2022:332–337.
Reavill DR, Lennox AM. Disease overview of the urinary tract in exotic companion mammals and tips on clinical management. Vet Clin Exot Anim Pract 2020;23(1):169–193.
Tuğba KU, Atespare ZD, Cerkez EE. A case of penile prolapse and treatment in a sugar glider (*Petaurus breviceps*). Turk Vet J 2020;2(2):80–83.
Author Nicholas Jew, DVM

SEIZURES AND TREMORS

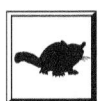

BASICS

DEFINITION
• Seizure—sudden, uncontrolled electrical disturbance in the brain that can cause changes in behavior, movement, and levels of consciousness.
• Tremor—an involuntary, rhythmic muscle contraction causing a shaking movement of one or more parts of the body.

PATHOPHYSIOLOGY
• Common causes of seizures include hypocalcemia, hypoglycemia, toxicosis, neoplasia, and infectious disease.
• Hypoglycemia may result from prolonged anorexia of a variety of causes.
• Hypocalcemia often results from inappropriate diet and lack of supplementation. There are currently no commercially available diets that adequately compare to the diet of wild sugar gliders.
• Toxicosis—reported neurotoxic agents in sugar gliders include polyvinyl chloride (PVC) and heavy metals
• Infectious—reported are *Toxoplasmosis*, *Baylisascaris*, *Listeriosis*, as well as other bacterial and fungal organisms.

SYSTEMS AFFECTED
Neurologic
Musculoskeletal

GENETICS
N/A

INCIDENCE/PREVALENCE
Common

GEOGRAPHIC DISTRIBUTION
Worldwide

SIGNALMENT
Breed Predilections
N/A

Mean Age and Range
Younger sugar gliders may be more affected by toxicities.

Predominant Sex
N/A

SIGNS
Historical Findings
• Anorexia
• Abrupt or recent diet change may be reported. Historical use of a nutritionally inappropriate or incomplete diet.
• Weight loss
• Enclosures with PVC coating
• Introduction of new sugar gliders into a colony
• Recently purchased a new cage or cage furniture

Physical Examination Findings
• May be normal.
• Altered cranial nerve evaluation, mentation, and postural reactions may be present.
• Body condition may vary between emaciated and obese.
• Muscle fasciculations and tremors may be exacerbated by stressful events and handling.
• In some cases, the stress of handling may induce seizure or seizure-like activity.
• Partial or generalized paresis or paralysis may be present.

CAUSES
Infectious
• Toxoplasmosis
• Listeriosis
• Baylisascaris
• Other fungal and bacterial pathogens

Toxicosis
• Polyvinyl chloride (PVC)
• Heavy metals, especially zinc
• Environmental exposure to household chemicals

Nutritional
• Hypocalcemia—often the result of nutritional osteodystrophy
• Hypoglycemia

Other
• Primary CNS neoplasia
• Congenital and structural brain disease
• Head trauma

RISK FACTORS
• Chronic use of an inappropriate diet with a low calcium-to-phosphorus ratio.
• Wild caught or recently introduced sugar gliders into a colony.
• Use of cage material that contains toxins (e.g., PVC and zinc)

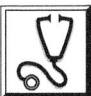

DIAGNOSIS

DIFFERENTIAL DIAGNOSIS
Differentiate from Pruritus
• Rule out ectoparasites that may cause extreme pruritus that can often be mistaken for tremors or seizure activity.

Differentiate from Vestibular Disease
• Rule out otitis media/interna that may induce peripheral vestibular signs such as a head tilt, torticollis, and a horizontal nystagmus.

Differentiate Causes of Tremors and Seizures
• Most commonly, a thorough history and husbandry review will provide relevant information to differential potential nutritional causes and toxicoses.

• Rule out accidental exposure to prescription medications and environmental toxins with a thorough history. Many owners may need to be questioned specifically regarding medications and/or lotions and cremes that may have been accidentally ingested during handling.

CBC/BIOCHEMISTRY/URINALYSIS
• Results may be normal.
• Leukocytosis—may be seen with infectious causes
• Decreased serum calcium concentration may be present.
• Elevated serum phosphorus concentration may be present.
• In the face of normal calcium and phosphorus levels, an inverted calcium-to-phosphorus ratio may be calculated.

OTHER LABORATORY TESTS
• Serologic testing against Toxoplasmosis may be indicated. Care should be taken in the interpretation of single IgM or IgG titers as the interval of expression is not well documented in sugar gliders. Extrapolation from domestic animals may prove useful, and if so, elevated IgM titers (>1:256) may indicate recent infection. IgM antibodies may only persist for 3 months after infection. Conversely, IgG titers may be elevated for years with subclinical infection. Paired IgG titers 3–4 weeks apart with at least a fourfold increase may indicate active infection.
• Histologic samples (collected ante- or post-mortem) may provide the most definitive means of identifying Toxoplasmosis. This may prove particularly useful in a colony of sugar gliders where multiple individuals are ill or acute mortalities are identified. Necropsy may be the most useful diagnostic tool in these situations.
• Heavy metal testing may prove useful for obtaining a definitive diagnosis where this toxicity is of concern. Often the turnaround time on these results will lag behind the need for empirical treatment.
• Cytology and culture (fungal and bacterial) may provide a definitive diagnosis for infectious causes of seizures. Often empirical treatment will have been initiated prior to the return of culture and sensitivity, and treatment plans should be adjusted accordingly. The ability to safely collect sufficient volume of CSF may make these tests less practical.

IMAGING
• Traditional radiography may provide information regarding the skeletal health of affected sugar gliders. Care should be taken in interpretation of bone density on traditional radiography. Differences in

technique and the small size of sugar gliders may hinder the identification of skeletal pathology.

• Advanced imaging (CT and MRI) may be the most appropriate means of imaging the central nervous system. Sedation or anesthesia may be necessary for these imaging modalities. The increasing availability of these imaging modalities may provide the practitioner with the ability to provide an antemortem diagnosis with structural CNS disease.

DIAGNOSTIC PROCEDURES
Contrast-enhanced CT or MRI may aid in the identification of enhancing primary CNS lesions. Placement of an intravenous or intraosseous catheter is required.

PATHOLOGIC FINDINGS
Depends on the underlying cause

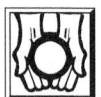

TREATMENT
APPROPRIATE HEALTH CARE
• Treatment depends on the underlying cause and specific sites involved.
• In an emergent situation, anticonvulsants and supportive care are critical.
• In weak and debilitated patients, the best outcome may be achieved through hospitalization and placement of an intravenous intraosseous catheter. Sedation or anesthesia may be necessary.
• Correct hypoglycemia and hypocalcemia if present.
• Antibiotics and antifungals should ideally be chosen based on the result of culture and sensitivity testing.

MEDICATIONS
DRUG(S) OF CHOICE
Anticonvulsants
• Midazolam (0.1–0.5 mg/kg SC, IM, IV, IO, intranasal)
• Diazepam (0.5–2 mg/kg PO, SC, IM, avoid parenteral injection if possible)

Antibiotics/Antifungals
• Amoxicillin/clavulanic acid (12.5 mg/kg PO, SC divided q12)
• Clindamycin (5.5–10 mg/kg PO q12), higher doses may be needed for Toxoplasmosis (12.5 mg/kg PO q12 × 4 weeks)
• Chloramphenicol (50 mg/kg PO q12)
• Enrofloxacin (5 mg/kg PO, SC q12)
• Itraconazole (5–10 mg/kg PO q24)

Anti-Inflammatory
• Meloxicam (0.1–0.2 mg/kg PO, SC q24h)

Sedation
• Light sedation: Midazolam (0.2–0.5 mg/kg SC, IM, IV intranasal) ± butorphanol (0.5 mg/kg SC) or buprenorphine (0.01 mg/kg SC). Heavier sedation/mild anesthesia: Ketamine (10–20 mg/kg IM, IV) + midazolam (0.3–0.5 mg/kg SC, IM, IV); other protocols exist.

Miscellaneous
• Calcium gluconate (100 mg/kg SC q12 × 3–5 days, dilute to 10 mg/mL in saline)
• Vitamin B complex (0.02 mL/kg SC, IM)
• Activated charcoal (1–3 g/kg PO)

CONTRAINDICATIONS
• Glucocorticoids or other immunosuppressive agents
• Potentially nephrotoxic drugs (e.g., aminoglycosides, NSAIDs) in patients that are febrile, dehydrated, or azotemic.

PRECAUTIONS
• Enrofloxacin SC could cause skin necrosis, needs to be diluted 1:1 with SC fluids
• Sample collection and IV or IO access may require sedation or brief anesthesia.
• Chloramphenicol may cause aplastic anemia in susceptible people. Clients and staff should use appropriate precautions when handling this drug.

POSSIBLE INTERACTIONS
N/A

ALTERNATIVE DRUGS
N/A

FOLLOW-UP
PATIENT MONITORING
Response to treatment by clinical signs, serial physical examination, laboratory testing, and imaging evaluation appropriate for each specific cause.

PREVENTION/AVOIDANCE
• Depends on the underlying cause
• Place patient on an appropriate diet
• Provide good hygiene
• Appropriate quarantine practices for any new sugar gliders entering a home or colony. This should include screening for infectious and parasitic disease.

POSSIBLE COMPLICATIONS
N/A

EXPECTED COURSE AND PROGNOSIS
Guarded to poor depending on the underlying cause

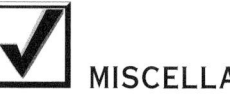

MISCELLANEOUS
ASSOCIATED CONDITIONS
• Nutritional osteodystrophy

AGE-RELATED FACTORS
Younger sugar gliders may have clinical signs of PVC toxicity quicker than adults.

ZOONOTIC POTENTIAL
Toxoplasmosis is a potentially zoonotic disease. Appropriate hygiene should be practiced at all times, and any immunocompromised individuals living with a sugar glider suspected of having Toxoplasmosis should limit their interactions with the animal as much as possible.

PREGNANCY/FERTILITY/BREEDING
N/A

SYNONYMS
N/A

SEE ALSO
Nutritional osteodystrophy

ABBREVIATIONS
NSAID = nonsteroidal anti-inflammatory drug
IgG = immunoglobulin G
IgM = immunoglobulin M
CSF = cerebral spinal fluid
CT = computed tomography
MRI = magnetic resonance imaging
CNS = central nervous system

Suggested Reading
Barrows M. Toxoplasmosis in a colony of sugar gliders (*Petaurus breviceps*). Vet Clin North Am Exot Anim Pract 2006;9(3): 617–623.
Brust D, Mans C. Sugar gliders. In: Carpenter JW, ed. Exotic Animal Formulary, 5th ed. St Louis: Elsevier, 2018:432–442.
Evans EE, Souza MJ. Advanced diagnostic approaches and current management of internal disorders of select species (rodents, sugar gliders, hedgehogs). Vet Clin North Am Exot Anim Pract 2010;13(3):453–469.
Johnson-Delaney C. Sugar gliders. In: Quesenberry KE, Carpenter JW, eds. Ferrets, Rabbits and Rodents, 4th Ed). Clinical Medicine and Surgery. 2021 ed. St. Louis: Saunders, 2020:385–400.
Lennox AM. Emergency and critical care procedures in sugar gliders (*Petaurus breviceps*), African hedgehogs (*Atelerix albiventris*), and prairie dogs (*Cynomys* spp). Vet Clin North Am Exot Anim Pract 2007;10(2):533–555.
Author Nicholas Jew, DVM

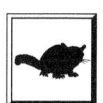

BASICS

DEFINITION
Self-induced trauma, typically from chewing and/or excoriation. In sugar gliders, commonly this behavior is orientated toward the penis and scrotum, tail base, and inguinal region.

PATHOPHYSIOLOGY
• Causes of self-mutilation in sugar gliders may include pain, stress, and boredom.
• Inappropriate social grouping with multiple sexually mature or pubescent male sugar gliders may lead to stress and self-mutilation.
• Paracloacal and perineal-cloacal mutilation has been reported secondary to infection, impaction, and neoplasia.

SYSTEMS AFFECTED
• Genitourinary
• Dermatologic
• Neurologic

GENETICS
N/A

INCIDENCE/PREVALENCE
N/A

GEOGRAPHIC DISTRIBUTION
N/A

SIGNALMENT
• Intact male sugar gliders that have recently reached sexual maturity are overrepresented (12–14 months of age).
• Sugar gliders of either sex that are housed alone with limited social interaction and lack of enrichment.

SIGNS

General Comments
• Clinical signs aside from self-mutilation may vary based on underlying disease/cause of pain.
• The choice of diagnostic and therapeutic measures depends on the cause and severity of mutilation.
• Signs of more severe illness (e.g., anorexia, weight loss, severe dehydration, depression, and shock) should prompt more aggressive diagnostic and therapeutic measures.

Historical Findings
• Owner may report recent loss of another sugar glider from the same social group.
• Owner may report seeing excessive grooming behavior or finding blood on bedding or cage materials.
• Stress—hospitalization, transportation, environmental changes, and concurrent illness may contribute to self-mutilation.

• Lack of environmental enrichment and adequate resources in groups may predispose to self-mutilation.
• Prior injury or trauma may be reported to have occurred immediately or shortly prior to the onset of self-mutilation.

Physical Examination Findings
• Vary with the severity of disease
• Excessive grooming behavior
• Alterations in the fur and skin may be noted. Severity could vary from thinning coat or alopecia in earlier evaluation to superficial abrasions or full thickness wounds at the site of self-mutilation. In severe cases, bleeding may result due to involvement of large vessels.
• Chronic cases may exhibit dehydrated and/or devitalized tissue. An odor may be present as well as purulent discharge.

CAUSES
• Pain—any source of pain may lead to self-mutilation. Infection or impaction of glands, orthopedic and/or soft tissue trauma, lower urinary tract disease, reproductive disease, and neoplasia.
• Stress—environmental and medical stressors may include loss of a conspecific, alteration to enclosure space, lack of appropriate enrichment, inadequate resources for the number of sugar gliders in the social group, inappropriate grouping or housing density, and unwanted or excessive handling.

RISK FACTORS
• Environmental stressors—multiple sexually mature males in a single group.

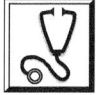

DIAGNOSIS

DIFFERENTIAL DIAGNOSIS

General
• Primary—typically considered to be secondary to environmental or social stressors.
• Secondary to pain—reported causes of pain include but are not limited to trauma, neoplasia, and paracloacal disease.

CBC/BIOCHEMISTRY
• May be normal
• Increased PCV and TS seen with dehydration
• Anemia may be seen with chronic cases and recurrent or ongoing blood loss.
• TWBC elevation with neutrophilia may be seen with bacterial.
• Hemogram abnormalities may be consistent with sepsis and/or systemic infection in severe and chronic cases.
• Electrolyte abnormalities secondary to anorexia, fluid loss, and dehydration.

OTHER LABORATORY TESTS

Imaging
• Survey abdominal radiography may indicate orthopedic trauma, organomegaly, or mass lesion(s).

Pathologic Findings
• Vary with cause and severity of condition
• Gross pathology may reveal lesions suggestive of etiology
• Histopathology is often the best method to obtain a definitive diagnosis for neoplasia, infiltrative or inflammatory conditions, and certain infections.

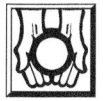

TREATMENT

APPROPRIATE HEALTH CARE
• Treatment must be specific to the underlying cause to be successful.
• Patients with mild clinical signs that are otherwise bright and alert may respond to outpatient treatment.
• Patients with moderate to severe clinical signs usually require hospitalization and supportive care including parenteral medication, fluid therapy, and thermal support. Surgical intervention may be need for devitalized or necrotic tissue.
• When infectious disease is suspected, strict isolation of affected and exposed animals is indicated.

NURSING CARE
• Fluid therapy—rehydration and correction of electrolyte imbalances are essential to treatment success in severely ill sugar gliders.
• Severe volume depletion can occur with acute hemorrhage, and aggressive shock fluid therapy may be necessary.
• In most patients, crystalloids (e.g., lactated Ringer's solution, normosol; 50–100 mL/kg/day) are appropriate for SC or IV administration. Crystalloids can also be given PO.
• Maintenance fluid requirements are estimated at 100 mL/kg/day.

DIET
• It is imperative that sugar gliders continue to eat during treatment and recovery.
• Assisted feeding is typically required until the patient is eating, eliminating, and maintaining body weight.
• A highly digestible, liquefied, elemental diet such as Emeraid Omnivore (Lafeber Company, Cornell, IL) may be indicated in case of suspected enteropathy.
• If commercial assist feeding diets are not available, then a liquified blend can be made of commercial pellets, fresh fruits and vegetables, insectivore diets, and live insects.

• Encourage oral fluid intake: offer fresh water, administer oral fluids via syringe, wet the food, or flavor water with fruit or vegetable juices.
• Direct oral administration of fluids (water, crystalloids, and electrolyte solutions) for patients that are not drinking

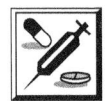

MEDICATIONS

DRUG(S) OF CHOICE

Antibiotic Therapy
• Indicated in patients with bacterial inflammatory lesions of the gastrointestinal tract; also indicated in patients with disruption of the intestinal mucosa evidenced by blood in the feces
• Selection should be broad-spectrum antibiotics, based on results of culture and susceptibility testing when possible.
• Some choices for empirical use while waiting for culture results include amoxicillin (30 mg/kg PO, SC q24h), amoxicillin/clavulanic acid (12.5 mg/kg PO, SC divided q12h), ciprofloxacin (10 mg/kg PO q12h), or enrofloxacin (2.5–5 mg/kg PO, SC, IM q12h)

Analgesia/Anti-Inflammatory
• Meloxicam (0.1–0.2 mg/kg PO, SC q24h)
• Buprenorphine (0.02–0.05 mg/kg PO, SC, IM q12h), gastrointestinal and transmucosal absorption has not been adequately evaluated and use is anecdotal, higher doses may cause sedation

Sedation
• For sedation: Light sedation: Midazolam (0.2–0.5 mg/kg SC, IM, IV intranasal) ± butorphanol (0.5 mg/kg SC) or buprenorphine (0.01 mg/kg SC). Heavier sedation/mild anesthesia: Ketamine (10–20 mg/kg IM, IV) + midazolam (0.3–0.5 mg/kg SC, IM, IV); other protocols exist.

Psychotropic
• Fluoxetine (0.5–1 mg/kg PO q24h), this dose has been reported but no data exists regarding efficacy for self-mutilation

SURGICAL INTERVENTION

Amputation/Debridement
• Devitalized or necrotic tissue of the distal limbs, digits, or penis likely requires surgical amputation or debridement to avoid ongoing infection, sepsis, pain, and reduce the likelihood of ongoing self-mutilation.
• Commonly, male sugar gliders will mutilate their penis to the point of devitalization and necrosis requiring amputation. Amputation does not interfere with the ability to urinate as the urethral opening is located at the base

of the penis. Monitor urethral opening patency closely after surgery as secondary swelling may lead to occlusion and inability to urinate.
• Castration is recommended for any male sugar glider with penile or scrotal self-mutilation.
• Aggressive pain management following surgery may be needed to avoid ongoing self-mutilation at the surgical site.
• Elizabethan collars and restrictive bandages may be required to prevent mutilation of the surgical site.

CONTRAINDICATIONS
• Avoid the use of nonsteroidal anti-inflammatory medication in dehydrated sugar gliders or those with known or suspected renal disease.

PRECAUTIONS
• It is important to determine the cause of self-mutilation. A general "shotgun" approach with antibiotics and pain medication may only be temporarily effective or ineffective.
• Antibiotic therapy can predispose sugar gliders to bacterial dysbiosis and overgrowth pathogenic bacteria (particularly *Clostridium difficile*).
• Isolate affected and exposed animals when infectious disease is suspected.
• Safety data regarding the use of fluoxetine or other psychotropic medications is not available for sugar gliders. Extrapolating from other mammalian species, higher doses or accidental overdose may lead to serotonin syndrome.

POSSIBLE INTERACTIONS
Prior to starting any psychotropic medication, a thorough history regarding over-the-counter supplements or other at home remedies should be taken to avoid potential interaction or additive effect leading to serotonin syndrome.

ALTERNATIVE DRUGS
N/A

FOLLOW-UP

PATIENT MONITORING
Frequent and regular follow-up should be recommended to monitor the healing of any wounds and ensure that self-mutilation does not continue.

PREVENTION/AVOIDANCE
• Providing appropriate diet and husbandry
• Reducing stress and providing sanitary conditions
• When infectious disease is suspected, strict isolation of affected and exposed animals is indicated.

POSSIBLE COMPLICATIONS
• Antibiotic therapy can promote bacterial dysbiosis and overgrowth of pathogenic bacteria.
• Dehydration due to fluid loss
• Serotonin syndrome

EXPECTED COURSE AND PROGNOSIS
• Depends on cause and severity of disease

MISCELLANEOUS

ASSOCIATED CONDITIONS
• Dehydration
• Malnutrition
• Hypoproteinemia
• Anemia
• Septicemia
• Cloacal prolapse

AGE-RELATED FACTORS
• Males that have recently reached sexual maturity more often noted to self-mutilate.

ZOONOTIC POTENTIAL
• N/A

PREGNANCY/FERTILITY/BREEDING
• N/A

SYNONYMS
• N/A

SEE ALSO
Alopecia
Paracloacal gland disorders
Reproductive diseases

ABBREVIATIONS
PCV = packed cell volume
TS = total solids
TWBC = total white blood cell count

Suggested Reading
Brust D, Mans C. Sugar gliders. In: Carpenter JW, ed. Exotic Animal Formulary, 5th ed. St Louis: Elsevier, 2018:432–442.
Hernandez-Divers SM. Principles of wound management of small mammals: hedgehogs, prairie dogs, and sugar gliders. Vet Clin North Am Exot Anim Pract 2004;7(1):1–18, v. doi: 10.1016/j.cvex.2003.09.002. PMID: 14768377.
Johnson-Delaney C. Sugar gliders. In: Quesenberry KE, Carpenter JW, eds. Ferrets, Rabbits and Rodents, 4th Ed). Clinical Medicine and Surgery. 2021 ed. St. Louis: Saunders, 2020:385–400.
Lennox AM. Emergency and critical care procedures in sugar gliders (*Petaurus breviceps*), African hedgehogs (*Atelerix albiventris*), and prairie dogs (*Cynomys* spp). Vet Clin North Am Exot Anim Pract 2007 May;10(2):533–555.

McLaughlin A, Strunk A. Common emergencies in small rodents, hedgehogs, and sugar gliders. Vet Clin North Am Exot Anim Pract 2016 May;19(2):465–499.

Morges MA, Grant KR, MacPhail CM, Johnston MS. A novel technique for orchiectomy and scrotal ablation in the sugar glider (*Petaurus breviceps*). J Zoo Wildl Med 2009;40(1):204–206. doi: 10.1638/2007-0169.1 PMID: 19368264.

Tynes VV. Behavioral dermatopathies in small mammals. Vet Clin North Am Exot Anim Pract 2013;16(3):801–820. doi: 10.1016/j.cvex.2013.05.004. Epub 2013 Jul 19. PMID: 24018038.

Vergneau-Grosset C, Ruel H. Abnormal repetitive behaviors and self-mutilations in small mammals. Vet Clin North Am Exot Anim Pract 2021;24(1):87–102. doi: 10.1016/j.cvex.2020.09.003 PMID: 33189258.

Author Nicholas Jew, DVM

COMMON DOSAGES FOR CHINCHILLAS

Drug	Dosage
Albendazole	25 mg/kg PO q12h × 2 days
Azithromycin	30 mg/kg PO q24h
Buprenorphine	0.1–0.2 mg/kg SC, IV q8–12h
Butorphanol	0.2–2.0 mg/kg SC, IM, IV q4h
Carprofen	2–5 mg/kg PO q12h
Chloramphenicol	30–50 mg/kg PO, SC, IM, IV q12h
Ciprofloxacin	5–25 mg/kg po q12–24h
Cisapride	0.5–1.0 mg/kg PO q8–12h
Enrofloxacin	5–15 mg/kg PO, SC, IM q12h
Fenbendazole	20 mg/kg PO q24h × 5 days
Fluconazole	16 mg/kg q24h
Griseofulvin	25 mg/kg PO q24h × 4–6 weeks
Imidacloprid 10%/moxidectin 1%	0.1 mL/animal
Itraconazole	5–10 mg/kg PO q24h × 4–6 weeks
Ivermectin	0.4 mg/kg SC q10–14d × 3–4 doses
Meclizine	2–12 mg/kg PO q24h
Meloxicam	0.5–1 mg/kg PO, SC q24h
Metoclopramide	0.2–1.0 mg/kg PO, SC, IM q12h
Metronidazole	10–20 mg/kg PO q12h
Oxytocin	0.2–3.0 IU/kg IM or SC
Penicillin G benzathine	40,000–60,000 IU/kg SC q2–7d
Praziquantal	5–10 mg/kg PO or SQ, repeat in 10 days
Selamectin	15–30 mg/kg applied topically q21–28d
Simethicone	20 mg/kg PO q8–12h
Sulfadimethoxine	25–50 mg/kg PO q24h × 10 days
Terbinifine	20–40 mg/kg PO q24h × 4–6 weeks
Trimethoprim-sulfa	15–30 mg/kg PO q12h

NORMAL VALUES FOR CHINCHILLAS

Table 1

Reference Physiologic Values for Chinchillas	
Body weight	450–800 g
Respiratory rate	40–80/min
Heart rate	200–240/min
Erythrocytes	$5.2–10.7 \times 10^6/mm^3$ ($5.2–10.7 \times 10^{12}/L$)
Hematocrit	27%–54% (0.27–0.54 g/L)
Hemoglobin	8–15.4 g/dL (80–154 g/L)
Leukocytes	$4–11.5 \times 10^3/mm^3$ ($4–11.5 \times 10^9/L$)
Neutrophils	9%–45%
Lymphocytes	19%–98%
Eosinophils	0%–9.0%
Monocytes	0%–6%
Basophils	0%–1.0%
Platelets	$254–740 \times 10^3/mm^3$ ($254–740 \times 10^9/L$)
Serum protein	5.0–6.0 g/dL (50–60 g/L)
Albumin	2.4–4.2 g/dL (24–42 g/L)
Sodium	130–155 mEq/L (130–155 mmol/L)
Potassium	5–6.5 mEq/L (5–6.5 mmol/L)
Chloride	105–115 mEq/L (105–115 mmol/L)
Serum calcium	5.6–12.1 mg/dL (1.40–3.02 mmol/L)
Serum phosphate	4–8 mg/dL (1.29–2.58 mmol/L)
Serum glucose	60–120 mg/dL (3.3–6.7 mmol/L)
Blood urea nitrogen	10–25 mg/dL (3.6–8.9 mmol/L)
Total bilirubin	0.4 mg/dL (7 μmol/L)
Cholesterol	40–100 mg/dL 1.03–2.59 mmol/L)
Aspartate aminotransferase (AST)	96 IU/L
Alanine aminotransferase (ALT)	10–35 IU/L
Alkaline phosphatase (ALP)	3–47 IU/L

Note: SI units are in parentheses, where appropriate.
Adapted from Harkness JE, Turner PV, VandeWoude S, et al.

Harkness and Wagner's Biology and Medicine of Rabbits and Rodents, 5th ed. Ames: Wiley-Blackwell, 2010.

NORMAL VALUES FOR CHINCHILLAS

Table 2

Biodata: Chinchillas	
Adult Body Weight	
Male	400–500 g
Female	400–600 g
Birth weight	40–60 g
Body temperature	37–38°C (98.6–100.4°F)
Pulse	200–240 bpm
Respirations	45–80/min
Diploid number	64
Life span	9–18 years
Food consumption	30–40 g/day; 5.5 g/100 g/day
Water consumption	10–20 mL/day; 8–9 mL/100 g/day
GI transit time	12–15 hours
Breeding Onset	
Male	7–9 months
Female	4–5 months
Cycle length	30–50 days
Gestation period	105–120 days; average 112
Postpartum estrus	Fertile
Litter size	2–6
Weaning age (lactation duration)	3–8 weeks
Breeding duration	3 years
Milk composition	7.2% protein, 12.3% fat; 1.7% lactose

Adapted from Harkness JE, Turner PV, VandeWoude S, et al. Harkness and Wagner's Biology and Medicine of Rabbits and Rodents, 5th ed. Ames: Wiley-Blackwell, 2010.

COMMON DOSAGES FOR FERRETS

Drug	Dosage	Indication
Acepromazine	0.01–0.25 SC, IM mg/kg	Light sedation
Acetylsalicylic acid (aspirin)	10–20 mg/kg PO q8–12h	Analgesia, anti-inflammatory, anticoagulant
Amikacin	8–16 mg/kg SC, IM, IV total per day, divided q8–24h	General antibiotic therapy; potentially nephrotoxic
Aminophylline	4–6.5 mg/kg PO, IM q12h	Bronchodilation
Amlodipine	02–.04 mg/kg PO q12h	Calcium agonist, afterload reduction with heart disease
Amoxicillin	20 mg/kg q12h; PO, SC For helicobacter amoxicillin—30 mg/kg PO q8h, plus Metronidazole (20 mg/kg PO q12h) and bismuth subsalicylate (17.5 mg/kg PO q8–12h)	General antibiotic therapy Treatment of *Helicobacter pylori* gastritis can be combined with H_2-receptor blockers; treat for at least 2 weeks
Amoxicillin + clavulanic acid	13–25 mg/kg PO q12h	General antibiotic therapy (dose of combined drugs)
Amphotericin B	0.4–0.8 mg/kg once weekly to a total cumulative	Systemic antifungal therapy
Amprolium	19 mg/kg PO q24h	Coccidiostat
Ampicillin	5–30 mg/kg SC, IM, IV q8–12h	General antibiotic therapy
Apomorphine	5 mg/kg SC single dose	To stimulate emesis
Atenolol	3.125–6.25 mg/kg PO q24h	β-Adrenergic receptor blocker used in treatment of cardiomyopathy
Atipamezole	0.4–1 mg/kg IM 5 times dose of medetomidine on a milligram-to-milligram basis	Reversal agent for medetomidine
Atropine	0.02–0.05 mg/kg SC, IM, IV	Parasympatholytic, treatment of bradycardia
Azathioprine	0.9 mg/kg q24, 48, or 72h (for severe, moderate, or mild gastroenteritis, respectively); PO	For the treatment of inflammatory bowel disease
Barium sulfate	10–15 mL/kg PO	Gastrointestinal contrast radiography (dilute as per product directions for varying opacity)
Benazepril	0.25–0.5 mg/kg PO q24h	ACE inhibitor, vasodilator
Bismuth subsalicylate	0.25–1 mL/kg of regular strength formula q8–12h; PO 17.5 mg/kg q12h (Pepto-Bismol original formula) + amoxicillin (30 mg/kg q8–12h) + metronidazole (20–30 mg/kg q8–12h) PO	Gastric protectant treatment of *H. pylori* gastritis, can be combined with H_2-receptor blockers; treat for at least 2 weeks
Buprenorphine	0.01–0.05 mg/kg oral transmucosal, SC, IM, IV q6–12h	Analgesic
Butorphanol	0.1–0.5 mg/kg SC, IM, IV q8–12h	Analgesic; sedation at high end of dose
Carbaryl (0.5% w/v shampoo, 5.0% w/w powder)	Treat once weekly for 3–6 weeks	Ectoparasite control
Carprofen (Rimadyl, Zoetis)	1–5 mg/kg PO q12–24h; 4 mg/kg SC	Anti-inflammatory, pain control
Captopril	1/8 of a 12.5 mg tablet PO q48h	Vasodilator as part of therapy for congestive heart failure
Cefadroxil	15–20 mg/kg PO q12h	General antibiotic therapy
Cephalexin	15–30 mg/kg PO q12h	General antibiotic therapy
Chloramphenicol	25–50 mg/kg PO, SC, IM, IV q12h	General antibiotic therapy; treatment of choice for proliferative bowel disease with minimum treatment period of 14 days proliferative bowel disease

COMMON DOSAGES FOR FERRETS (CONTINUED)

Drug	Dosage	Indication
Chlorpheniramine	1–2 mg/kg PO q8–12h	Antihistamine
Chorionic gonadotropin	100 IU IM once after second week of estrus, repeat in 2 weeks if neede	To terminate estrus
Cimetidine	5–10 mg/kg PO, SC, IM, IV q6–8h	H_2-receptor blocking agent for gastric ulcer therapy
Ciprofloxacin	10–30 mg/kg PO q12h	General antibiotic therapy
Cisapride	0.5 mg/kg PO q8–12h	Gastrointestinal motility stimulant
Clarithromycin	12.5 mg/kg PO q8–12h plus ranitidine bismuth citrate; or 50 mg/kg PO q24h or divided q12h with omeprazole and metronidazole	Treatment of *H. pylori* gastric infection
Clindamycin	5.5–10 mg/kg PO q12h	General antibiotic therapy
Deslorelin acetate	4.7 mg slow-release deslorelin implants every 8–20 months	Treatment of Adrenal Disease
Desoxycorticosterone pivalate (DOCP)	2 mg/kg IM q21d	Mineralocorticoid for treatment of Addison's disease after bilateral adrenal surgery
Dexamethasone	0.5–2.0 mg/kg IM, IV once	Therapy for shock, anti-inflammatory, after bilateral adrenalectomy
Dexamethasone sodium phosphate	4–8 mg/kg IM, IV, once	As above, also prior to blood transfusion
Dextrose	0.5–2 mL of 50% in slow IV bolus to effect. Continuous IV infusion of 5% dextrose in crystalloid fluids	Hypoglycemia caused by insulinoma
Diazepam	0.2–1 mg/kg IV as needed	For sedation
	0.25–1 mg/kg IV as needed	For seizure control
Diazoxide	5–30 mg/kg PO divided q8–12 has necessary	For treatment of insulinoma
Digoxin elixir	0.005–0.01 mg/kg PO q12–24h	Management of congestive heart failure and cardiomyopathy
Diltiazem	3175–7.5 mg/kg PO q12h	Management of congestive heart failure and cardiomyopathy
Diphenhydramine	0.5–2 mg/kg PO, IM q8–12	Antihistamine
Dobutamine	5–10 mcg/kg/min IV	Hypotension
Doxapram	2–5 mg/kg IV	Respiratory stimulant
Doxycycline	10 mg/kg PO q12h	Respiratory infections
Enalapril	0.25–0.5 mg/kg PO q48h initially, increase to q24h clinically appropriate	Management of congestive heart failure and cardiomyopathy
Enilconazole	Apply topically as required	Antifungal
Enrofloxacin	5–10 mg/kg PO, SC, IM q12h	General antibiotic therapy
Epoetin alpha	50–150 IU/kg 3 times per week until packed cell volume is stable, then 1–2 times per week	Stimulates erythropoiesis
Erythromycin	10 mg/kg PO q6h	General antibiotic therapy
Famotidine	0.25–0.5 mg/kg PO, SC, IV q24h	H_2-receptor blocking agent for gastric ulcer therapy
Fenbendazole	20 mg/kg PO q24h for 5 days	Endoparasites
Fentanyl citrate	Loading dose of 5–10 mcg/kg IV followed by 10–30 mcg/kg/h IV as constant rate infusion	Postoperative analgesia
Ferretonin™	5.4 mg implants, Melatek, LLC) every 4 months	Treatment of adrenal disease
Fipronil (Frontline, Boehringer Ingelheim)	0.2–0.4 mL/animal topically q30d	Flea adulticide
Fluconazole	50 mg/kg PO q12h	Antifungal

Common Dosages for Ferrets (continued)

Drug	Dosage	Indication
Fludrocortisone	0.05–0.1 mg/kg PO q24h or divided q12h. Adjust according to patient's response	Mineralocorticoid; support for Addison's disease after bilateral adrenalectomy
Flutamide	10 mg/kg PO q12–24h	Inhibits androgens; treatment of prostatomegaly in adrenal disease
Furosemide	1–4 mg/kg PO, SC, IM, IV q8–12h	Diuretic, initial management of congestive heart failure
	1–2 mg/kg PO q8–12h	Long-term maintenance therapy of congestive heart failure
Gabapentin	3–5 mg/kg PO q8–12h	Neurotropic pain
Glycopyrrolate	0.01–0.02 mg/kg SC, IM, IV	Anticholinergic preanesthetic
GnRH	0.02 mg/kg SC, IM once after second week of estrus, repeat in 2 weeks if needed	To terminate estrus
Griseofulvin	25 mg/kg PO q24h for 3–6 weeks	Systemic antifungal therapy
Hydrocortisone sodium succinate	25–40 mg/kg IV single dos	Treatment of shock, adrenal insufficiency
Hydromorphone	0.1–0.2 mg/kg SC, IM, IV q6–8h	Pain control
Hydroxyzine hydrochloride	2 mg/kg PO q8–12h	Antihistamine
Imidacloprid	10 mg/kg topically	Flea control
Imidacloprid and moxidectin (Advantage Mutli for Cats, Bayer)	1.9–3.3 mcg/kg topically q30d	External parasites, heartworm prevention
Insulin, NPH	0.1–5 U/kg SC, IM q12h; start with low dose and increase according to patient's response	For treatment of diabetes mellitus; monitor blood/urine glucose
Iron dextran	10 mg/kg IM once	For iron deficiency anemia
Isoproterenol	40–50 mcg/kg PO q12h or 20–25 mcg/kg SC, IM q4–6h	
Isoflurane	3–5% for induction, 0.5–2.5% or as required for maintenance	Inhalant anesthetic of choice
Itraconazole	10–20 mg/kg PO q24h	Antifungal
Ivermectin	0.2–0.5 mg/kg SC q14d × 3 treatments	sarcoptic mange
	0.4 mg/kg PO, SC q14d	Control of ear mites, ticks
	0.05 mg/kg PO q30d	Heartworm microfilaricide, use with prednisolone 1 mg/kg po q24h
	0.02 mg/kg PO q30d	Heartworm prevention
Kaolin-pectin products	1–2 mL/kg of regular strength product; PO q2–6h as needed	Gastrointestinal protectant
Ketamine + acepromazine	10–35 mg/kg + 0.05–0.35 mg/kg; IM, SC	Anesthesia
Ketamine + diazepam	10–20 mg/kg + 1–2 mg/kg; IM	Anesthesia
	5–10 mg/kg + 0.5–1 mg/kg; IV	Anesthesia
Ketamine + dexmedetomidine	5–8 mg/kg + 0.03 mg/kg; IM	Anesthesia
Ketamine + medetomidine	5 mg/kg + 80 µg/kg + 0.1 mg/kg; IM	Anesthesia (use separate syringe for butorphanol)
Ketamine + midazolam	5–10 mg/kg + 0.25–0.5 mg/kg; IV	Anesthetic induction
Ketoconazole	10–50 mg/kg q12–24h	Systemic antifungal therapy

COMMON DOSAGES FOR FERRETS (CONTINUED)

Drug	Dosage	Indication
Lactulose (syrup—15 mg/10 mL)	0.1–0.75 mL/kg PO q12h	In hepatic disease to decrease blood ammonia levels; laxative
Leuprolide acetate (Lupron) 30-day depot	100–250 µg/ferret once monthly; IM; may decrease to q6–8w	Ferret adrenal disease (1-month depot formulation)
Lime sulfur	Dilute 1:40 in water, wash once weekly for 6 weeks	Ectoparasite control (especially mites)
Maropitant citrate (Cerenia)	1 mg/kg PO, SC q24h	Anti-emetic
Medetomidine	See ketamine + medetomidine 0.08–0.2 mg/kg; SC, IM	Dose dependent sedation and immobilization
Melarsomine dihydrochloride	2.5 mg/kg IM once; repeat 1 month later with 2 injections 24 hours apart	Heartworm adulticide treatment; deep IM injection
Melatonin	0.5–1.0 mg/ferret q24h; PO 7–9 hours after sunrise	Symptomatic treatment of ferret adrenal disease
Meloxicam	0.1–0.3 mg/kg PO, SC, IM, IV q24h	Analgesic and anti-inflammatory
Metaproterenol	0.25–1.0 mg/kg PO q12h	Sympathomimetic for treatment of 3rd degree AV block
Metoclopramide	0.2–1 mg/kg PO, SC, IV q6–8h	Gastric motility disorders, vomiting and nausea associated with gastritis
Metronidazole	15–20 mg/kg PO, IV q12h	Antibacterial agent with good anaerobic spectrum
	20 mg/kg q12h + amoxicillin (30 mg/kg PO q8h) + bismuth subsalicylate (17.5 mg/kg q12h, Pepto-Bismol original formula) for at least 2 weeks	Treatment of *H. pylori* gastritis, can be combined with H$_2$-receptor blockers
Midazolam	0.3–1.0 mg/kg; SC, IM	Sedation
Milbemycin oxime	1.15–2.33 mg/kg PO q30d	Broad spectrum antiparasitic; heartworm preventative
Naloxone	0.01–0.03 mg/kg or to effect; SC, IM, IV	Opioid reversal by titration
Nitroglycerine	1/8-in. length of 2% ointment applied topically; once daily to q12h	Management of congestive heart failure
Omeprazole	0.7 mg/kg PO q24h	Proton pump inhibitor; for gastric ulcer therapy
Oxymorphone	0.05–0.2 mg/kg SC, IM, IV q8–12h as needed	Analgesia
Oxytetracycline	20 mg/kg PO q8h	General antibiotic therapy
Oxytocin	0.2–3 IU/kg SC, IM	To stimulate uterine motility or milk letdown
Phenobarbital elixir	1–2 mg/kg PO q8–12h for seizure control, titrate dose for maintenanc	Control and prevention of seizures
Pimobendan	0.5–1.25 mg/kg PO q12h	Phosphodiesterase inhibitor, increase cardiac contractility
Prednisone, Prednisolone	0.5–1.0 mg/kg PO q12h, reduce dose and frequency for long-term therapy	Antiinflammatory
	0.5–2.5 mg/kg PO q12h; start at low dose, increase as necessary	Treatment of hypoglycemia due to insulinoma; reduce dosage if combined with diazoxide therapy
	1.25–2.5 mg/kg PO q24h taper dose to 0.5–1.25 every other day or lowest dose possible	Inflammatory bowel disease
	1 mg/kg PO q24h or divided q12h, for 3 months; taper dose to wean animal at completion of therapy	In conjunction with adulticide treatment for heartworm disease
	1–2 mg/kg PO q24h	Chemotherapy for lymphoma; palliative alone or used with other protocols

COMMON DOSAGES FOR FERRETS (CONTINUED)

Drug	Dosage	Indication
Prednisolone sodium succinate	22 mg/kg; slow IV	Therapy for shock
Propranolol	0.2–1 mg/kg PO, SC q8–12h	Beta-blocker for management of heart failure
Prostaglandin F2α	0.5–1.0 mg/ferret IM as needed	Treatment of dystocia or metritis
Pyrantel pamoate	4.4 mg/kg PO once, repeat in 2 week	Treatment of gastrointestinal nematodes
Pyrethrin products	Use topically as directed; treat once weekly as needed	Treatment of ectoparasites, especially fleas
Ranitidine bismuth citrate	24 mg/kg PO q8–12h	Combine with clarithromycin for treatment of *Helicobacter pylori* gastritis
Ranitidine HCl	3.5 mg/kg PO q12h	H_2-receptor blocking agent for gastric ulcer therapy
Selamectin	15 mg/kg topically q30d	Treatment of ectoparasites, heartworm prevention
Spironolactone	1–2 mg/kg PO q12h	Diuretic
Sucralfate	25 mg/kg PO q6–12h	Treatment of gastric ulceration and gastritis
Sulfadimethoxine	50 mg/kg PO once, then 25 mg/kg daily for 9 days	Treatment of gastrointestinal coccidiosis
Terbutaline	0.01 mg/kg SC, IM	Bronchodilation
Tetracycline	25 mg/kg PO q8–12h	General antibiotic therapy
Theophylline	4.25–10 mg/kg PO q8–12h	Bronchodilation
Tramadol	5–10 mg/kg PO q12–24h	Analgesia
Trimethoprim sulfonamide combinations	15–30 mg/kg PO, SC q12h	General antibiotic therapy
	30 mg/kg PO q24h for 2 weeks	Treatment of gastrointestinal coccidiosis
Ursodiol	15–20 mg/kg PO q12–24h	Treatment of cholangiolar and gallbladder disorders
Vitamin B complex	Dose to thiamine content at 1–2 mg/kg IM as needed	Vitamin B supplementation
Vitamin C	50–100 mg/kg PO q12h	Supportive therapy, as an antioxidant

APPENDICES

Normal Values for Ferrets

Table 3

Parameter	Albino Ferrets	Fitch Ferets
Sodium (mmol/L)	137–162	146–160
Potassium (mmol/L)	4.5–7.7	4.3–5.3
Chloride (mmol/L)	106–125	102–121
Calcium (mg/dL)	8.0–11.8	8.6–10.5
Phosphorus (mg/dL)	4.0–9.1	5.6–8.7
Glucose (mg/dL)	94–207	62.5–134
BUN (mg/dL)	10–45	12–3
Creatinine (mg/dL)	0.4–0.9	0.2–0.6
Total protein (g/dL)	5.1–7.4	5.3–7.2
Albumin (g/dL)	2.6–3.8	3.3–4.1
Globulin (g/dL)	—	2.0–2.0
Total bilirubin (mg/dL)	<1.0	<1.0
Cholesterol	64–296	119–201
Alkaline phosphatase (SAP) (IU/L)	9–84	30–120
Alanine aminotransferase (ALT) (IU/L)	—	82–289
Aspartate aminotransferase (AST) (IU/L)	28–120	74–248

Adapted from Fox, JG. Normal clinical and biologic parameters. In: Fox JG, ed. Biology and Disease of the Ferret. 2nd Ed. Baltimore: Williams and Wilkins, 1998.

Table 4

Parameter	Male Albino	Male Fitch
PCV%	44–61	48–59
Hemoglobin (g/dL)	16.3–18.2	15.4–18.5
RBC ($\times 10^6$/mm³)	7.3–12.18	10.1–13.2
MCV	—	42.6–51
MCH	—	13.7–16
MCHC	—	30.3–34.9
Reticulocytes (%)	1–12	—
Platelets (10^3/mm³)	297–730	—
WBC ($\times 10^3$/mm³)	4.4–19.1	1.7–11.9
Differential (%)		
Bands	—	0–1
Neutrophils	11–82	24–72
Lymphocytes	12–54	26–73
Monocytes	0–9	1–4
Eosinophils	0–7	0–3
Basophils	0–2	0–2.7

Adapted from Fox, JG. Normal clinical and biologic parameters. In: Fox JG, ed. Biology and Disease of the Ferret. 2nd Ed. Baltimore: Williams and Wilkins, 1998.

Normal Values for Ferrets (continued)

Table 5

Adult weight	
Male	1–2 kg
Female	600–950 g
Life span (average)	5–11 years
Body temperature	37.8–0°C (100–104°F)
Dental formula	2 (I 3/3, C 1/1, P4/3, M 1/2)
Vertebral formula	$C_7T_{15}L_5S_3Cd_{14}$
Age of sexual maturity	6–12 months
Length of breeding life	2–5 years
Gestation	42 ± 2 days
Litter size	Average 8 (range 1–18)
Birth weight	6–12 g
Eyes open	34 days
Onset of hearing	32 days
Weaning	6–8 weeks
Food consumption	140–190 g/24 hr
Water intake	75–100 mL/24 hr
Arterial blood pressure:	
Mean systolic	Female 133; male 161 mm Hg (conscious)
Mean diastolic	110–125 mm Hg (anesthetized)
Heart rate	200–400 bpm
Cardiac output	139 mL/min
Blood volume	Male 60 mL, female 40 mL (approximate)
Respiration	33–36 breaths/min

Adapted from Fox, JG. Normal clinical and biologic parameters. In: Fox JG, ed. Biology and Disease of the Ferret. 2nd Ed. Baltimore: Williams and Wilkins, 1998.

COMMON DOSAGES FOR GUINEA PIGS

Drug	Dosage
Aminophylline	50 mg/kg PO q12h
Azithromycin	15–30 mg/kg PO q24h
Buprenorphine	0.05–0.2 mg/kg SC, IM, IV q8–12h or 0.2 mg/kg oral transmucosal q5h
Butorphanol	0.4–2.0 mg/kg SC, IM q4–12h
Carprofen	4 mg/kg SC q24h or 1–2 mg/kg PO q12h
Chloramphenicol	30–50 mg/kg PO, SC, IM, IV q8–12h
Cimetidine	5–10 mg/kg PO, SC, IM, IV q6–12h
Ciprofloxacin	5–25 mg/kg PO q12h
Cisapride	0.5–1 mg/kg PO q8–12h
Doxycycline	2.5–5 mg/kg PO q12h
Enrofloxacin	5–20 mg/kg PO q12–24h
Famotidine	0.5 mg/kg PO, SC, IM, IV q24h
Fenbendazole	20 mg/kg PO q24h
Florfenicol	20–25 mg/kg PO, IM, IV q12h
Fluconazole	16–20 mg/kg PO q24h
Furosemide	2–5 mg/kg SC, IM, IV q4–6h; 1–4 mg/kg PO q12h
Gonadotropin-releasing hormone (GnRH)	25 µg/treatment IM every 2 weeks for 2 injections
Griseofluvin	15–25 mg/kg PO q24h
Human chorionic gonadotropin (hCG)	1000 USP IM repeated in 7–10 days for 3 treatments
Hydromorphone	0.1 mg/kg SC, IV q6–12h
Imidacloprid/moxidectin (Advantage Multi)	0.1 mL/kg topically q30d
Itraconazole	5–10 mg/kg PO q24h
Ivermectin	0.4 mg/kg PO, SC q7–10d
Ketoconazole	10–40 mg/kg PO q24h
Leuprolide acetate	100 µg/kg SC once every 3 weeks
Marbofloxacin	4 mg/kg PO 24h
Maropitant	1–2 mg/kg SC, slow IV q24h
Meclizine	2–12 mg/kg PO q12h
Meloxicam	0.5–1.0 mg/kg PO, SC, IM q24h
Metoclopramide	0.2–1.0 mg/kg PO, SC, IV q12h
Metronidazole	10–20 mg/kg PO, IV q12h
Midazolam	0.4–2.0 mg/kg IM
Oxymorphone	0.2–0.5 mg/kg SC, IM q4–12h
Oxytocin	0.2–3.0 IU/kg SC, IM
Penicillin G	40,000–60,000 IU/kg SC q2–7d
Pradofloxacin	5 mg/kg PO q12h
Praziquantel	5–10 mg/kg PO, SC, IM q10–14d
Pimobendan	0.25 mg/kg PO q12h
Ranitidine	2 mg/kg IV or 2–5 mg/kg PO q24h
Selamectin	15–30 mg/kg topically q21–28d
Sucralfate	25 mg/kg PO q6h
Sulfadimethoxine	25–50 mg/kg PO q24h
Terbinafine	10–40 mg/kg PO q24h
Theophylline	4–10 mg/kg PO q8–12h
Tramadol	5–10 mg/kg PO q12h
Trimethoprim-sulfa	15–30 mg/kg PO q12h
Vitamin C	30–50 mg/kg PO daily or 50–100 mg/kg SC q24h

NORMAL VALUES FOR GUINEA PIGS

Table 6

Reference Physiologic Values for Guinea Pigs	
Body weight	700–1200 g
Respiratory rate	42–104/min
Tidal volume	2.3–5.3 mL/kg
Heart rate	230–380/min
Blood volume	65–85 mL/kg
Blood pressure	80–94/55–58 mmHg
Erythrocytes	$4.5–7.0 \times 10^6/mm^3$ ($4.5–7.0 \times 10^{12}/L$)
Hematocrit	37%–48% (0.37–0.48 L/L)
Hemoglobin	11–15 g/dL (110–150 g/L)
Leukocytes	$7–18 \times 10^3/mm^3$ ($7–18 \times 10^9/L$)
Neutrophils	28%–44%
Lymphocytes	39%–72%
Eosinophils	1%–5%
Monocytes	3%–12%
Basophils	0%–3%
Platelets	$250–850 \times 10^3/mm^3$ ($250–850 \times 10^9/L$)
Serum protein	4.6–6.2 g/dL (46–62 g/L)
Albumin	2.1–3.9 g/dL (21–39 g/L)
Globulin	1.7–2.6 g/dL (17–26 g/L)
Sodium	132–156 mEq/L (132–156 mmol/L)
Potassium	4.5–8.9 mEq/L (4.5–8.9 mmol/L)
Chloride	98–115 mEq/L (98–115 mmol/L)
Serum calcium	5.3–12 mg/dL (1.32–3.00 mmol/L)
Serum phosphate	3.0–12 mg/dL (0.97–3.87 mmol/L
Serum glucose	60–125 mg/dL (3.3–6.9 mmol/L)
Blood urea nitrogen	9.0–31.5 mg/dL (3.2–11.2 mmol/L)
Creatinine	0.6–2.2 mg/dL (53–194 µmol/L)
Total bilirubin	0.3–0.9 mg/dL (5–15 µmol/L)
Serum lipids	95–240 mg/dL (1.0–2.4 g/L)
Phospholipids	25–75 mg/dL (0.3–0.8 g/L)
Triglycerides	0–145 mg/dL (0–1.4 g/L)
Cholesterol	20–43 mg/dL (0.52–1.11 mmol/L)
Alanine aminotransferase (ALT)	10–25 IU/L
Alkaline phosphatase (ALP)	18–28 IU/L

Note: SI units are in parentheses, where appropriate.
Adapted from Harkness JE, Turner PV, VandeWoude S, et al. Harkness and Wagner's Biology and Medicine of Rabbits and Rodents, 5th ed. Ames: Wiley-Blackwell, 2010.

APPENDICES

Normal Values for Guinea Pigs (continued)

Table 7

Biodata: Guinea Pigs	
Adult Body Weight	
Male	900–1200 g
Female	700–900 g
Birth weight	70–100 g
Body surface area (cm^2)	
700–830 g	$9.2 \times$ (weight in grams)$^{2/3}$
200–680 g	$10.1 \times$ (weight in grams)$^{2/3}$
Body temperature	37.2°–39.5°C
Diploid number	64
Life span	5–7 years
Food consumption	6 g/100 g/day
Water consumption	10 mL/100 g/day
GI transit time	13–30 hours
Breeding Onset	
Male	600–700 g (3–4 months)
Female	350–450 g (2–3 months)
Cycle length	15–17 days
Gestation period	59–72 days
Postpartum estrus	Fertile, 60%–80% pregnancy
Litter size	1–6
Weaning age (lactation duration)	150–200 g, 14–21 days
Breeding duration	18 months (4–5 L) to 4 years
Young production (index per female)	0.7–1.4/mo
Milk composition	3.9% fat, 8.1% protein, 3.0% lactose

Adapted from Harkness JE, Turner PV, VandeWoude S, et al. Harkness and Wagner's Biology and Medicine of Rabbits and Rodents, 5th ed. Ames: Wiley-Blackwell, 2010.

APPENDIX IV

COMMON DOSAGES FOR HEDGEHOGS

Afoxolaner (A) + milbemycin oxime (MO) (NexGard Spectra, Merial)	(A) 2.5 mg/kg + (MO) 40 mg/kg PO once
Amikacin sulfate	2.5–5 mg/kg SC, IM q8–12h Nebulization: 5 mg/1 mL sterile saline × 15 min q12–24h
Amoxicillin	15 mg/kg PO, SC, IM q12h
Amoxicillin/Clavulanic acid	12.5–25 mg/kg PO, SC q8–12h
Atropine	0.01–0.05 mg/kg SC, IM, IV
Buprenorphine	0.02–0.05 mg/kg PO, SC, IM q6–8h
Butorphanol	0.2–0.4 mg/kg PO, SC, IM q6–12 prn
Calcium glubionate	150 mg/kg PO q24h
Calcium gluconate (10%)	50–100 mg/kg SC q12h × 3–5 days
Carprofen	1 mg/kg PO, SC q12–24h
Cefovecin (Convenia, Zoetis)	8 mg/kg SC q5–6d
Ceftiofur sodium	20 mg/kg SC q12–24h
Cephalexin	25 mg/kg PO q8h
Chloramphenicol	30–50 mg/kg PO, SC, IM, IV q12h
Ciprofloxacin	5–20 mg/kg PO q12h
Cisapride	0.25 mg/kg PO, SC q8–24h
Clindamycin	10 mg/kg PO q12h
Dexamethasone	0.1–1.5 mg/kg SC, IM, IV
Doxycycline	2.5–10 mg/kg PO, SC, IM q12h
Epinephrine	0.003 mg/kg IV
Enrofloxacin	5–10 mg/kg PO, SC, IM, IV q12h
Enalapril	0.5–1 mg/kg PO q24h
Famotidine	1 mg/kg SC q24h
Fenbendazole	10–30 mg/kg PO q24h × 5 days; or 25 mg/kg PO q14d × 3 treatments
Fipronil spray (Frontline, Merial)	Apply 1 light spray over spiny dorsum ("mantle") repeat in 10–14 days for 1–3 treatments
Fluralaner (Bravecto, Merck)	15 mg/kg PO once
Fluoxetine	0.5–5 mg/kg PO q12–24h
Furosemide	2.5–5 mg/kg PO, SC, IM, IV q6–8h
Glycopyrrolate	0.01–0.02 mg/kg SC, IM, IV
Hydromorphone	0.1 mg/kg SC q4–6h
Itraconazole	5–10 mg/kg PO q12–24h
Imidacloprid	½ puppy/kitten dose topical q30d
Imidacloprid 10% + moxidectin 1% (Advantage Multi for cats)	0.1 mL/kg topical once
Ivermectin	0.2–0.4 mg/kg PO, SC, q7–14d × 3–5 treatments
Ketoconazole	10 mg/kg PO q24h × 6–8 weeks
Lactulose	0.3 mL/kg PO q8–12h
Levamisole (1%)	10 mg/kg SC, repeat q48h; repeat prn q14d
Lufenuron	½ puppy/kitten dose PO q30d
Maropitant	1–2 mg/kg PO, SC q24h
Meloxicam	0.2 mg/kg PO, SC q24h

Common Dosages for Hedgehogs (continued)

Midazolam	0.1–0.5 mg/kg SC, IM, IV
Metoclopramide	0.2–0.5 mg/kg PO, SC q8–12h
Metronidazole	20–25 mg/kg PO q12h
Moxidectin (Cydectin, Bayer)	0.3 mg/kg SC q10d
Nystatin	30,000 IU/kg PO q8–24h
Omeprazole	0.5–1 mg/kg SQ, PO q24**h**
Orbifloxacin	10–20 mg/kg PO q12–24h
Penicillin G procaine	40,000 IU/kg SC, IM q24h
Pimobendan	0.3 mg/kg PO q12h
Piperacillin	10 mg/kg SC q8–12h
Prednisolone	0.5–2 mg/kg PO q12–24h
Praziquantel	7 mg/kg PO, SC, repeat in14 days
Sarolaner (Simparica, Zoetis)	2 mg/kg PO once
Selamectin	20–30 mg/kg topically q21–28d
Sucralfate	10 mg/kg PO q8–12h
Sulfadimethoxine	2–20 mg per day PO, SC, IM treat for 2–5 days, off for 5 days, then repeat
Terbinafine	100 mg/kg PO q12h
Toltrazuril	10 mg/kg PO q24h × 2 treatments then repeated q7d × 3 weeks
Trimethoprim-sulfa	30 mg/kg PO q12h
Tramadol	2–5 mg/kg PO q8–12h
Theophylline	10 mg/kg PO, IM q12h

HEDGEHOGS APPENDIX II

Table 8

Biodata: Hedgehogs	
Body temperature	95.7–98.6°F
Pulse	180–280 bpm
Respiration	25–50 bpm
Body weight	Adult male—400–600 g; adult female—250–400 g
Mean life span	3–5 years, up to 10 years recorded
Sexual maturity	Male 2–6 months, female 6–8 months; females sexually mature at 2 months but should not be bred before 6 months of age
Gestation	34–37 days
Litter size	1–9 pups (average 3–4)
Birth weight	10–18 g
Eyes open	14–18 days
Weaning age	4–6 weeks, begin eating solids at 3 weeks

NORMAL HEMATOLOGIC VALUES FOR HEDGHOGS

PCV (%)	33.50–47.00
HbC (g/dL)	10.71–14.86
RBC (10^6/μL)	4.29–5.96
MCV(fl)	76.34–99.78
MCH (pg)	22.47–31.44
MCHC (g/dL)	27.69–35.19
Total WBC count (10^3/μL)	11.50–21.65
Differential WBC Count (%)	
Neutrophils	52.00–76.00
Lymphocyte	22.00–47.00
Monocyte	0.0–4.00
Eosinophils	0.00–2.00
Basophils	0.00–1.00
Absolute WBC Count (10^3/μL)	
Neutrophils	6.13–14.63
Lymphocyte	3.28–8.88
Monocyte	0.00–0.78
Eosinophils	0.00–0.30
Basophils	0.00–0.20

Normal Biochemistry Values for Hedgehogs

ALT (IU/L)	15.23–28.79
AST (IU/L)	19.00–65.59
ALP (IU/L)	18.18–25.45
Total proteins (g/dL)	4.58–6.86
Albumin (g/dL)	2.67–3.89
Globulin (g/dL)	1.86–3.60
Fasting blood glucose (mg/dL)	60.00–125.00
Cholesterol (mg/dL)	100–150
Triglycerides (mg/dL)	30.77–46.15
Calcium (mg/dL)	8.57–11.43
Urea nitrogen (mg/dL)	34.33–57.33
Creatinine (mg/dL)	0.50–1.00

COMMON DOSAGES FOR RABBITS

Drug	Dosage	Indication
Acepromazine	0.25–1 mg/kg; SC, IM	Light sedation
Activated charcoal	1 g/kg PO q4–6h as needed; dilute 1 g charcoal/5 mL water	To decrease toxin absorption
Alfaxalone (Alfaxan, Jurox)	1–2 mg/kg IV give slowly over 1 min to effect 0.5–1 mg/kg IM when combined with midazolam, opioids, and ketamine 4–6 mg/kg IM	Anesthetic induction Sedation
Azithromycin	15–30 mg/kg; PO q24h	Treatment of anaerobic infections
Benazepril	0.25–0.5 mg/kg PO q24h	Vasodilators
Buprenorphine	0.02–0.05 mg/kg SC, IM, IV q4–6h	Analgesia
Buprenorphine SR	0.12 mg/kg SC	Analgesia
Butorphanol	0.1–0.5 mg/kg SC, IM, IV q4–6h	Analgesia, can cause sedation
Calcium EDTA	27 mg/kg SC q6–12h for 5 days; dilute with saline. Repeat if necessary	Chelation, lead toxicosis
Carbaryl 5% powder	Dust lightly once weekly	Ectoparasites
Carprofen	2–4 mg/kg PO, SC q12–24h	Analgesia
Chloramphenicol	25 mg/kg PO q8–12h 30–50 mg/kg SC, IM, IV q8–12h	General antibiotic therapy
Chlorpheniramine maleate	0.2–0.4mg/kg PO q12h	Antihistamine
Cholestyramine (Questran, Squibb)	2 g/animal PO q24h	Enterotoxaemia treatment
Chondroitin sulfate (Cosequin, Nutramax)	Use feline dose	Arthritis, nutrceutical
Ciprofloxacin	10–20 mg/kg PO q12h	General antibiotic therapy
Cisapride	0.5 mg/kg PO q8–12h	Gastrointestinal promotility agent
Dexmedetomidine	0.03–0.05 IM mg/kg	Sedation
Diazepam	0.5–2 IM, IV mg/kg	Sedation, seizures
Digoxin	0.005–0.01 PO mg/kg q12–24h	Management of congestive heart failure and cardiomyopathy
Diphenhydramine	2 mg/kg PO, SC q8–12h	Antihistamine
Doxapram	2–5 mg/kg SC, IV q15min prn	Respiratory stimulant
Enalapril	0.25–0.5 mg/kg PO q24h	Management of congestive heart failure and cardiomyopathy
Enrofloxacin	10–20 mg/kg PO, SC, IM, IV q12–24h	General antibiotic treatment
Epinephrine	0.2–0.4 mg/kg IM, IV, IT	Cardiac arrest
Famotidine	0.5–1 mg/kg PO, SC, IV q12–24h	Antacid
Fenbendazole	20 mg/kg once daily for 5–28 days; PO.	Intestinal parasites, *E. cuniculi*
Fluconazole	5 mg/kg PO q24h	Systemic antifungal therapy
Flumazenil	0.01–0.1 mg/kg IM, IV	Reversal for benzodiazepines
Furosemide	1–4 mg/kg SC, IM IV q4–6h 2–5 mg/kg PO q12h	Diuretic
Gabapentin	5–20 mg/kg PO q8–12h	Neuropathic pain
Glycopyrrolate	0.01–0.1 mg/kg; SC	Anticholinergic preanesthetic
Griseofulvin	12.5–25 mg/kg PO q24h or divided q12h	Systemic antifungal therapy; may cause bone marrow suppression at high doses

COMMON DOSAGES FOR RABBITS (CONTINUED)

Drug	Dosage	Indication
Hetastarch	5–20 mL/kg IV	Volume expansion
Hydromorphone	0.05–0.2 mg/kg SC, IM, IV q6–8h	Analgesia, can cause sedation
Hydroxyzine	2 mg/kg q12h to q8h; PO	Antihistamine
Imidacloprid (Advantage, Bayer)	10–16 mg/kg topically	Topical flea treatment
Imidacloprid/monidectin (Advantage Multi for Cats, Bayer)	10 mg/kg (i) + 1 mg/kg (m) topically q30d	Topical flea and mite treatment
Iron dextran	4–6 mg/kg once; IM	Iron-deficient anemia
Itraconazole	5–10 mg/kg PO q24h × 30 days	Systemic antifungal therapy
Ivermectin	0.2–0.4 mg/kg SC q8–14d	Ectoparasites
Ketamine	10–20 mg/kg IM	Anesthesia
Ketoconazole	10–40 mg/kg PO q24h × 14 days	Systemic antifungal therapy
Levetiracetam (Keppra, UCB)	20 mg/kg PO q8h	Anticonvulsant
Lidocaine (2% injectable)	1–3 mg/kg	Local anesthetic
	2 mg/kg IV loading dose then 50–100 mcg/kg/min	CRI for analgesia
Lime sulfur 2.5% solution	Apply once weekly for 4–6 weeks	Ectoparasites
Marbofloxacin	5 mg/kg PO q24h 2 mg/kg SC, IM, IV q24h	Antibiotic
Maropitant	2 mg/kg SC, PO q24h	Visceral pain
Meclizine	2–12 mg/kg PO q8–12h	Vestibular disorders
Meloxicam	1 mg/kg PO, SC, IM q24h	Analgesia
Metoclopramide	0.5–1.0 mg/kg PO, SC, IM q12h or 1–2 mg/kg/day IV as a constant rate infusion	Gastrointestinal promotility agent
Metronidazole	20 mg/kg PO q12h 5–20 mg/kg IV slowly q12h	For anaerobic infections
Miconazole (cream or 2% shampoo)	Apply topically as required	Topical antifungal
Midazolam	0.5–2 mg/kg; IM, IV	Sedation
Morphine	0.5–2 mg/kg SC, IM q2–4h	Analgesia
Naloxone	0.01–0.1 mg/kg IM, IV to effect	Opioid reversal by titration
Oxytocin	0.1–3 U/kg SC, IM	To stimulate uterine motility or milk letdown
Penicillin G, procaine	40,000–60,000 IU/kg SC q24h	General antibiotic and treatment of *Treponema cuniculi*. Do not administer orally
Pimobendan	0.1–0.3 mg/kg PO q12h–24h	Increases cardiac contractility
Piperazine citrate	100 mg/kg PO q24h for 2 days	Antiparasitic
Polysulfate glycosaminoglycan (Adequan, Luitpold)	2.2 mg/kg SC q3d for 21–28 days, then q14d;	Nutraceutical treatment for joint inflammation
Ponazuril	20–50 mg/kg PO q24h × 30 days	For treatment of *E. cuniculi*
Potassium Citrate	33 mg/kg PO q8h	Prevention of hypercalciuria
Praziquantel	5–10 mg/kg PO, SC, IM, repeat in 10 days	Cestodes, trematodes
Prednisone	0.5–2 PO mg/kg	Few indications in rabbits; use with caution
Pyrethrin products (0.05% shampoo) or use as directed for cats	Once weekly for 4 weeks	Treatment of ectoparasites, especially fleas
Ranitidine	2–5 mg/kg PO q12h or 2 mg/kg SC, IV q24h	H_2-receptor blocking agent for gastric ulceration

COMMON DOSAGES FOR RABBITS (CONTINUED)

Drug	Dosage	Indication
Selamectin (Revolution, Pfizer)	12 mg/kg applied topically every 30 days	Treatment of ectoparasites
Sevoflurane	Inhalant anesthetic used to effect	Anesthesia
Simethicone	65–130 mg/animal PO q1h as needed	Alleviation of gastrointestinal gas
Sulfadimethoxine	50 mg/kg PO once, then 25 mg/kg q24h × 10–20 days	Coccidiosis
Terbinafine	10 mg/kg PO q24h	Systemic antifungal therapy
Tramadol	5–15 mg/kg PO q8–12h	Analgesia
Trimethoprim/sulfa	15–30 mg/kg PO, SC q12h	General antibiotic therapy; may cause tissue necrosis SC
Vitamin B complex	0.02–0.4 mL/rabbit SC, IM q24h	Thiamine deficiency, possible appetite stimulant
Vitamin K_1	1–10 mg/kg IM prn	Treatment of anticoagulant rodenticide toxicosis; use with caution; anaphylaxis reported

Normal Values for Rabbits

Table 9

Reference Ranges for Serum Biochemistry Values: Rabbits	
Serum protein	2.8–10.0 g/dL^
Albumin	2.7–4.6 g/dL^
Globulin	1.5–2.8 g/dL^
Fibrinogen	0.2–0.4 g/dL^
Serum glucose	75–150 mg/dL^
Blood urea nitrogen	15.0–23.5 mg/dL^
Creatinine	0.5–2.5 mg/dL*
Total bilirubin	0.25–0.74 mg/dL^
Serum lipids	280–350 mg/dL^
Phospholipids	75–113 mg/dL^
Triglycerides	124–156 mg/dL^
Cholesterol	18–35 mg/dL^
Calcium	5.6–12.5 mg/dL*
Phosphorus	4.0–6.9 mg/dL*
Alanine aminotransferase (ALT)	48–80 U/L*
Aspartate aminotransferase (AST)	14–113 U/L*
Alkaline phosphatase (AP)	4–16 U/L*

^ Harkness JE, Wagner JE. The Biology and Medicine of Rabbits and Rodents. 4th Ed. Baltimore: Williams and Wilkins, 1995
* Okerman L. Diseases of Domestic Rabbits. 2nd Ed. Oxford: Blackwell Scientific Publications, 1994

Table 10

Hematologic Values: Rabbit	
Erythrocytes	$4–7.2 \times 10^6/mm^3$
Hematocrit	36–48%
Hemoglobin	10.0–15.5 mg/dL
Leukocytes	$7.5–13.5 \times 10^3/mm^3$
Neutrophils	20–35%
Lymphocytes	55–80%
Monocytes	1–4%
Basophils	2–10%
Platelets	$200–1000 \times 10^3/mm^3$

Adapted from Harkness JE, Wagner JE. The Biology and Medicine of Rabbits and Rodents. 4th Ed. Baltimore: Williams and Wilkins, 1995.

APPENDICES

Normal Values for Rabbits (continued)

Table 11

Physiologic Values: Rabbits	
Body weight	2–6 kg
Respiratory rate	30–60 breaths/min
Tidal volume	4–6 mL/kg
Oxygen use	0.4–0.85 mL/g/hr
Heart rate	103–325 beats/min
Blood volume	57–78 mL/kg
Blood pressure	90–130/60–90 mm Hg
Rectal temperature	38.5–40.0°C (101–104°F)
Life span	5–6 years or more
Water consumption	5–10 mL/100 g/day
Gastrointestinal transit time	4–5 hours
Breeding onset: Male	6–10 months
Breeding onset: Female	4–9 months
Cycle length	Induced ovulator
Gestation period	29–35 days
Postpartum estrus	None
Litter size	4–10
Weaning age	4–6 weeks
Breeding duration	1–3 years
Milk composition	12.2% fat, 10.4% protein, 1.8% lactose

Adapted from Harkness JE, Wagner JE. The Biology and Medicine of Rabbits and Rodents. 4th Ed. Baltimore: Williams and Wilkins, 1995.

COMMON DOSAGES FOR SELECTED RODENT SPECIES

Aminophylline	10 mg/kg PO q12–24h
Amoxicillin/Clavulanic acid	20 mg/kg PO q12h *Do not use in hamsters
Azithromycin	15–30 mg/kg PO q24h
Buprenorphine	0.05–0.1 mg/kg SC, IM q6–8h
Butorphanol	1–2 mg/kg SC q4h
Carprofen	2–5 mg/kg PO, SC q24h
Chloramphenicol	30–50 mg/kg PO q8h
Ciprofloxacin	10–20 mg/kg PO q12h
Cisapride	0.1–0.5 mg/kg PO q12h
Doxycycline	2.5–5 mg/kg PO q12h
Digoxin	0.05–0.1 mg/kg PO q12–24h hamsters
Enalapril	0.5–1 mg/kg PO q24h
Enrofloxacin	5–20 mg/kg PO, SC q12h
Famotidine	0.5 mg/kg PO, SC, IV q24h
Fenbendazole	20 mg/kg PO q24h × 5 days
Fipronil	7.5 mg/kg topically every 30–60 days
Furosemide	1–5 mg/kg PO, SC, IM q12h
Gabapentin	30 mg/kg PO q8h
Griseofulvin	15–25 mg/kg PO q24h
Ivermectin	0.3–0.5 mg/kg SQ q7–14d
Loperamide HCl	0.1 mg/kg PO q8h
Meloxicam	1–3 mg/kg PO, SQ, IM q24h
Metoclopramide	0.2–1.0 mg/kg PO, SC, IM q12h
Metronidazole	20–40 mg/kg PO q12h
Morphine	2–5 mg/kg IM q4h
Oxymorphone	0.2–0.5 mg/kg SC IM q6–12h
Penicillin G	22,000 IU/kg SC, IM q24h
Pimobendan	0.2–0.4 mg/kg PO q12h
Praziquantal	6–10 mg/kg PO, SQ, repeat in 10 days
Selamectin	15–30 mg/kg topically q14–28d
Sulfadimethoxine	50 mg/kg PO once, then 25 mg/kg q24h × 10–20 days
Terbutaline	0.01 mg/kg IM or 0.3–0.4 mg/kg PO q12h
Tetracycline	10–20 mg/kg PO q12h
Theophylline	10 mg/kg PO q12h
Tramadol	10–20 mg/kg PO q8–12h
Trimethoprim-sulfa	15–30 mg/kg PO q12h
Verapamil	0.25–0.5 mg SC q12h hamsters

APPENDICES

Normal Values for Selected Rodent Species

Table 12

Reference Physiologic Values for Hamsters	
Body weight	85–150 g
Respiratory rate	35–135/min
Tidal volume	0.6–1.4 mL
Oxygen use	0.6–1.4 mL/g/hr
Heart rate	250–500/min
Blood volume	65–80 mL/kg
Blood pressure	150/100 mmHg
Erythrocytes	$6–10 \times 10^6/mm^3$ ($6–10 \times 10^{12}/L$)
Hematocrit	36%–55% (0.36–0.55 L/L)
Hemoglobin	10–16 g/dL (100–160 g/L)
Leukocytes	$3–11 \times 10^3/mm^3$ ($3–11 \times 10^9/L$)
Neutrophils	10%–42%
Lymphocytes	50%–94%
Eosinophils	0%–4.5%
Monocytes	0%–3%
Basophils	0%–1%
Platelets	$200–500 \times 10^3/mm^3$ ($200–500 \times 10^9/L$)
Serum protein	4.5–7.5 g/dL (45–75 g/L)
Albumin	2.6–4.1 g/dL (26–41 g/L)
Globulin	2.7–4.2 g/dL (27–42 g/L)
Sodium	128–144 mEq/L (128–144 mmol/L)
Potassium	3.9–5.5 mEq/L (3.9–5.5 mmol/L)
Serum calcium	5–12 mg/dL (1.25–3.00 mmol/L)
Serum phosphate	3.4–8.2 mg/dL (1.10–2.65 mmol/L)
Serum glucose	60–150 mg/dL (3.3–8.3 mmol/L)
Blood urea nitrogen	12–25 mg/dL (4.3–8.9 mmol/L)
Creatinine	0.91–0.99 mg/dL (80–88 µmol/L)
Total bilirubin	0.25–0.60 mg/dL (4–10 µmol/L)
Cholesterol	25–135 mg/dL (0.66–3.49 mmol/L)
Aspartate aminotransferase (AST)	28–122 IU/L
Alanine aminotransferase (ALT)	22–128 IU/L
Alkaline phosphatase (ALP)	45–187 IU/L

Note: SI units are in parentheses, where appropriate.
Adapted from Harkness JE, Turner PV, VandeWoude S, et al. Harkness and Wagner's Biology and Medicine of Rabbits and Rodents, 5th ed. Ames: Wiley-Blackwell, 2010.

Normal Values for Selected Rodent Species (continued)

Table 13

Biodata: Hamsters	
Adult Body Weight	
Male	85–130 g
Female	95–150 g
Birth weight	2 g
Body surface area (cm²)	$11.8 \times$ (wt. in grams)$^{2/3}$
Body temperature	37°–38°C
Diploid number	44
Life span	18–24 months
Food consumption	8–12 g/100 g/day
Water consumption	8–10 mL/100 g/day
Breeding Onset	
Male	10–14 weeks
Female	6–10 weeks
Cycle length	4 days
Gestation period	15–16 days
Postpartum estrus	Infertile, nonovulatory (Golden hamster); fertile (Siberian hamster)
Litter size	5–9
Weaning age (lactation duration)	20–25 days
Breeding duration	10–12 months
Commercial	5–7 L
Young production (index per female)	3/mo
Milk composition	12.0% fat, 9.0% protein, 3.4% lactose

Adapted from Harkness JE, Turner PV, VandeWoude S, et al. Harkness and Wagner's Biology and Medicine of Rabbits and Rodents, 5th ed. Ames: Wiley-Blackwell, 2010.

NORMAL VALUES FOR SELECTED RODENT SPECIES (CONTINUED)

Table 14

Reference Physiologic Values for Gerbils	
Body weight	55–100 g
Respiratory rate	90/min
Oxygen use	1.4 mL/g/hr
Heart rate	360/min
Blood volume	65–80 mL/kg
Erythrocytes	$8–9 \times 10^6/mm^3$ ($8–9 \times 10^{12}/L$)
Reticulocytes	21–54/1000 RBC
Stippled RBC	2–16/1000 RBC
Polychromatophilic RBC	5–30/1000 RBC
Hematocrit	43%–49% (0.43–0.49 L/L)
Hemoglobin	12.6–16.2 g/dL (126–162 g/L)
Leukocytes	$7–15 \times 10^3/mm^3$ ($7–15 \times 10^9/L$)
Neutrophils	5%–34%
Lymphocytes	60%–95%
Eosinophils	0%–4%
Monocytes	0%–3%
Basophils	0%–1%
Platelets	$400–600 \times 10^3/mm^3$ ($400–600 \times 10^9/L$)
Serum protein	4.3–12.5 g/dL (43–125 g/L)
Albumin	1.8–5.5 g/dL (18–55 g/L)
Globulin	1.2–6.0 g/dL (12–60 g/L)
Sodium	144–158 mEq/L (144–158 mmol/L)
Potassium	3.8–5.2 mEq/L (3.8–5.2 mmol/L)
Serum calcium	3.7–6.2 mg/dL (0.92–1.55 mmol/L)
Serum phosphate	3.7–7.0 mg/dL (1.19–2.26 mmol/L
Serum glucose	50–135 mg/dL (2.8–7.5 mmol/L)
Blood urea nitrogen	17–27 mg/dL (6.1–9.6 mmol/L)
Creatinine	0.6–1.4 mg/dL (53–124 µmol/L)
Total bilirubin	0.2–0.6 mg/dL (3–10 µmol/L)
Cholesterol	90–150 mg/dL (2.38–3.88 mmol/L)

Note: SI units are in parentheses, where appropriate.
Adapted from Harkness JE, Turner PV, VandeWoude S, et al. Harkness and Wagner's Biology and Medicine of Rabbits and Rodents, 5th ed. Ames: Wiley-Blackwell, 2010.

Normal Values for Selected Rodent Species (continued)

Table 15

Biodata: Gerbils	
Adult Body Weight	
Male	65–100 g
Female	55–85 g
Birth weight (depends on litter size)	2.5–3.0 g
Blood volume	7.7 mL/100 g
Body surface area (cm^2)	$10.5 \times$ (wt. in grams)$^{2/3}$
Body temperature	37.0°–38.5°C
Diploid number	44
Life span	3–4 years
Food consumption	5–8 g/100 g/day
Water consumption	4–7 mL/100 g/day
Vaginal opening	41 days or 28 g
Breeding Onset	
Male	70–85 days
Female	65–85 days
Estrous cycle length	4–6 days
Gestation period	
Nonlactating	24–26 days
Concurrent lactation	27–48 days
Postpartum estrus	Fertile
Litter size	3–7; 5 average
Weaning age	20–26 days
Breeding duration	12–17 months
Commercial	4–10 L
Litters per year	7 avg
Young production	1/wk per breeding pair

Adapted from Harkness JE, Turner PV, VandeWoude S, et al. Harkness and Wagner's Biology and Medicine of Rabbits and Rodents, 5th ed. Ames: Wiley-Blackwell, 2010.

NORMAL VALUES FOR SELECTED RODENT SPECIES (CONTINUED)

Table 16

Reference Physiologic Values for Mice	
Body weight	20–40 g
Respiratory rate	60–220/min
Tidal volume	0.09–0.23 mL
Oxygen use	1.63–2.17 mL/g/hr
Heart rate	325–780/min
Blood volume	70–80 mL/kg
Erythrocytes	$7.0–12.5 \times 10^6$/mm³ ($7.0–12.5 \times 10^{12}$/L)
Hematocrit	39%–49% (0.39–0.49 L/L)
Hemoglobin	10.2–16.6 g/dL (102–166 g/L)
Leukocytes	$6–15 \times 10^3$/mm³ ($6–15 \times 10^9$/L)
Neutrophils	10%–40%
Lymphocytes	55%–95%
Eosinophils	0%–4%
Monocytes	0.1%–3.5%
Basophils	0%–0.3%
Platelets	$800–1100 \times 10^3$/mm³ ($800–1100 \times 10^9$/L)
Serum protein	3.5–7.2 g/dL (35–72 g/L)
Albumin	2.5–4.8 g/dL (25–48 g/L)
Globulin	0.6 g/dL (6 g/L)
Sodium	112–193 mEq/L (112–193 mmol/L)
Potassium	5.1–10.4 mEq/L (5.1–10.4 mmol/L)
Chloride	82–114 mEq/L (82–114 mmol/L)
Serum calcium	3.2–8.5 mg/dL (0.80–2.12 mmol/L)
Serum phosphate	2.3–9.2 mg/dL (0.74–2.97 mmol/L)
Serum glucose	62–175 mg/dL (33.4–9.7 mmol/L)
Blood urea nitrogen	12–28 mg/dL (4.3–1.0 mmol/L)
Creatinine	0.3–1.0 mg/dL (27–88 µmol/L)
Total bilirubin	0.1–0.9 mg/dL (2.0–15 µmol/L)
Cholesterol	26–82 mg/dL (0.67–2.12 mmol/L)
Aspartate aminotransferase (AST)	54–269 IU/L
Alanine aminotransferase (ALT)	26–77 IU/L
Alkaline phosphatase (ALP)	45–222 IU/L

Note: SI units are in parentheses, where appropriate.
Adapted from Harkness JE, Turner PV, VandeWoude S, et al. Harkness and Wagner's Biology and Medicine of Rabbits and Rodents, 5th ed. Ames: Wiley-Blackwell, 2010.

Normal Values for Selected Rodent Species (continued)

Table 17

Biodata: Mice	
Adult Body Weight	
Male	20–40 g
Female	25–40 g
Birth weight	0.75–2.0 g
Body surface area (cm^2)	$10.5 \times$ (wt. in grams)$^{2/3}$
Rectal temperature	36.5°–38.0°C
Diploid number	40
Life span	1.5–3 years
Food consumption	12–18 g/100 g/day
Water consumption	15 mL/100g/day
GI transit time	8–14 hours
Breeding Onset	
Male	50 days
Female	50–60 days
Cycle length	4–5 days
Gestation period	19–21 days
Postpartum estrus	fertile
Litter size	10–12
Weaning age	21–28 days
Breeding duration	7–9 months
Commercial	6–10 L
Young production	8/mo
Milk composition	12.1% fat, 9.0% protein, 3.2% lactose

Adapted from Harkness JE, Turner PV, VandeWoude S, et al. Harkness and Wagner's Biology and Medicine of Rabbits and Rodents, 5th ed. Ames: Wiley-Blackwell, 2010.

APPENDICES

Normal Values for Selected Rodent Species (continued)

Table 18

Reference Physiologic Values for Rats	
Body weight	250–520 g
Respiratory rate	70–115/min
Tidal volume	0.6–2.0 mL
Oxygen use	0.68–1.10 mL/g/hr
Heart rate	250–450/min
Blood volume	50–70 mL/kg
Blood pressure	84–134/60 mmHg
Erythrocytes	$7–10 \times 10^6$/mm^3 ($7–10 \times 10^{12}$/L)
Hematocrit	36%–48% (0.36–0.48 L/L)
Hemoglobin	11–18 g/dL (110–180 g/L)
Leukocytes	$6–17 \times 10^3$/mm^3 ($6–17 \times 10^9$/L)
Neutrophils	9%–34%
Lymphocytes	65%–85%
Eosinophils	0%–6%
Monocytes	0%–5%
Basophils	0%–1.5%
Platelets	$500–1300 \times 10^3$/mm^3 ($500–1300 \times 10^9$/L)
Serum protein	5.6–7.6 g/dL (56–76 g/L)
Albumin	3.8–4.8 g/dL (38–48 g/L)
Globulin	1.8–3.0 g/dL (18–30 g/L)
Sodium	135–155 mEq/L (135–155 mmol/L)
Potassium	4–8 mEq/L (4–8 mmol/L)
Serum calcium	5.3–13.0 mg/dL (1.32–3.24 mmol/L)
Serum phosphate	5.3–8.3 mg/dL (1.71–2.68 mmol/L)
Serum glucose	50–135 mg/dL (2.8–7.5 mmol/L)
Blood urea nitrogen	15–21 mg/dL (5.4–7.5 mmol/L)
Creatinine	0.2–0.8 mg/dL (18–18 μmol/L)
Total bilirubin	0.20–0.55 mg/dL (3–9 μmol/L)
Serum lipids	70–415 mg/dL (0.7–4.2 g/L)
Phospholipids	36–130 mg/dL (0.4–1.3 g/L)
Triglycerides	26–145 mg/dL (0.3–1.4 g/L)
Cholesterol	34–130 mg/dL (0.88–3.36 mmol/L)
Alanine aminotransferase (ALT)	16–89 IU/L
Alkaline phosphatase (ALP)	16–125 IU/L

Note: SI units are in parentheses, where appropriate.
Adapted from Harkness JE, Turner PV, VandeWoude S, et al. Harkness and Wagner's Biology and Medicine of Rabbits and Rodents, 5th ed. Ames: Wiley-Blackwell, 2010.

Normal Values for Selected Rodent Species (continued)

Table 19

Biodata: Rats	
Adult Body Weight	
Male	450–520 g
Female	250–300 g
Birth weight	5–6 g
Body surface area (cm^2)	$10.5 \times$ (wt. in grams)$^{2/3}$
Rectal temperature	35.9°–37.5°C
Diploid number	42
Life span	2.5–3.5 years
Food consumption	5–6 g/100 g/day
Water consumption	10–12 mL/100 g/day or more
GI transit time	12–24 hours
Breeding Onset	
Male	65–110 days
Female	65–110 days
Cycle length	4–5 days
Gestation period	21–23 days
Postpartum estrus	Fertile
Litter size	6–12
Weaning age	21 days
Breeding duration	350–440 days
Commercial	7–10 L
Young production	4–5/mo
Milk composition	13.0% fat, 9.7% protein, 3.2% lactose

Adapted from Harkness JE, Turner PV, VandeWoude S, et al. Harkness and Wagner's Biology and Medicine of Rabbits and Rodents, 5th ed. Ames: Wiley-Blackwell, 2010.

APPENDICES

COMMON DOSAGES FOR SUGAR GLIDERS

Amikacin sulfate	10 mg/kg SC, IM q12h × 5 days
Amoxicillin	30 mg/kg PO, SC q24h
Amoxicillin/Clavulanic acid	12.5 mg/kg PO, SC q12h
Atropine	0.02–0.04 mg/kg SC, IM, IV
Buprenorphine	0.02–0.05 mg/kg PO, SC, IM q12h
Butorphanol	0.1–0.5 mg/kg SQ, IM q6h
Calcium EDTA	25 mg/kg SC q12h × 5 days
Calcium glubionate	150 mg/kg PO q24h
Calcium gluconate	100 mg/kg SC q12h × 3–5 days
Carprofen	2 mg/kg PO q12h
Chloramphenicol	50 mg/kg PO q12h
Ciprofloxacin	10 mg/kg PO q12h
Cisapride	0.25 mg/kg PO, SC q8–24h
Clindamycin	5.5–10 mg/kg PO q12h
Dexamethasone	0.1–0.6 mg/kg SC, IM, IV
Doxapram	2 mg/kg SC, IM, IV
Epinephrine	0.003 mg/kg IV
Enrofloxacin	2.5–5 mg/kg PO, IM q12–24h
Fenbendazole	20–50 mg/kg PO q24h × 3 days, repeat in 2 weeks
Fluoxetine	0.5–5 mg/kg PO q12–24h
Furosemide	1–4 mg/kg SC, IM, IV q6–8h
Gabapentin	3–5 mg/kg PO q8–12h
Glycopyrrolate	0.01–0.02 mg/kg SC, IM, IV
Griseofulvin	20 mg/kg PO q24h × 30–60 days
Itraconazole	5–10 mg/kg PO q12–24h
Ivermectin	0.2–0.4 mg/kg PO, SC, repeat in 14 and 28 days
Marbofloxacin	2–5 mg/kg PO, SQ, IM q24h
Maropitant	1 mg/kg PO, SC q24h
Meloxicam	0.1–0.2 mg/kg PO, SC q24h
Methadone	0.15–0.4 mg/kg SQ q4–6h for 24–48 hours only
Midazolam	0.1–0.5 mg/kg IM, SC, intranasal
Metronidazole	25 mg/kg PO q12–24h × 7–10 days
Prednisolone	0.1–0.2 mg/kg PO, SC, IM q24h
Praziquantel	5–10 mg/kg PO, SC, repeat in 10–14 days
Selamectin	6–18 mg/kg topically, repeat in 30 days
Tramadol	5–10 mg/kg PO q12h
Vitamin B complex	0.01–0.02 mL/kg SC (dilute to avoid stinging)
Trimethoprim-sulfa	10–20 mg/kg PO q12–24h

SUGAR GLIDERS

Adapted from: Booth, R.J. (2020). Marsupials. In Exotic Animal Laboratory Diagnosis (eds J.J. Heatley and K.E. Russell) John E. Wiley & Sons, Inc.

Table 20

Biodata: Sugar Gliders
Adult weight: 80–160 g; females smaller than males
Adult body length: about 12.7 cm (5 in)
Total length, including tail: about 28 cm (11 in)
Longevity: 12–14 years in captivity
Body temp: average 32°C (89.6°F)
Heart rate: 200–300 beats/min
Respiratory rate: 16–40 breaths/min
Sexual maturity: female at 8–12 months; male 12–14 months; capable of reproducing until over 10 years old
Estrous cycle: 29 days (seasonally polyestrous); they can breed all year in captivity
Mating: usually occurs in the evening
Gestation: 16 days, fetus then migrated to pouch
Litter size: one (19%) or two (89%)
L/yr: 1–2 in the wild; up to 4 L/yr in captivity

Table 21

Sugar Glider Urinalysis	
Specific gravity	1.02–1.04
pH	6.00–6.32
Protein (mg/dL)	9.45–14.58

Table 22

Hematologic Reference Values for Sugar Gliders	
Total erythrocytes (RBC)	8312–8830 cells/μL
Mean corpuscular volume (MCV)	60.2–68.1 fl
Mean corpuscular hemoglobin (MCH)	18.8–19.4 Pg
Mean corpuscular hemoglobin concentration (MCHC)	30.6–31.0 g/dL
Packed cell volume (PCV)	51%–54%
Hemoglobin (Hb)	(15.8–16.9 g/dL
Total leukocytes (WBC)	5500–9300/μL
Neutrophils	1460–2200 C/μL
Lymphocytes	3690–7160 C/μL
Monocytes	110–170/μL
Eosinophils	90–280/μL
Basophils	30–60/μL
Platelets	180–400/μL

SUGAR GLIDERS (CONTINUED)

Table 23

Biochemical Reference Ranges for Sugar Gliders	
Alkaline phosphatase (ALP)	89–115 IU/L
Alanine (ALT) aminotransferase	97–137 IU/L
Aspartate aminotransferase (AST)	54–99 IU/L
Bilirubin (total)	0.1–0.7 mg/dL
Urea nitrogen (BUN)	15.1–18.1 mg/dL
Calcium	8.5–8.9 mg/dL
Chloride	106–109 mEq/L
Cholesterol	112–124 mg/dL
Creatine kinase (CK)	1081–1627 IU/L
Creatinine	0.5–0.6 mg/dL
Glucose	153–171 mg/dL
Phosphorus	4.4–6.1 mg/dL
Potassium	4.6–5.5 mEq/L
Protein—total	6.7–7.0 g/dL
Albumin	3.1–4.6 g/dL
Sodium	139–143 mEq/L

INDEX